The Legacy of Harvey Cushing
Profiles of Patient Care

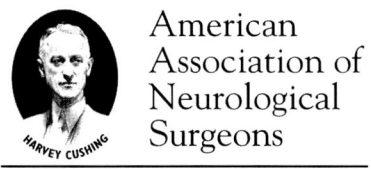

and the American Association of Neurosurgeons

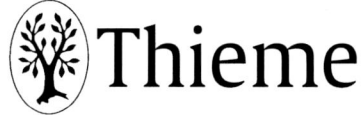

The Legacy of Harvey Cushing
Profiles of Patient Care

Edited by

Aaron A. Cohen-Gadol, M.D., M.Sc.
Indianapolis Neurosurgical Group
Skull base/Cerebrovascular and Epilepsy Surgery Programs
Clarian Health Care System (Methodist Hospital, Indiana
   University Hospital, and Riley Hospital for Children)
Indianapolis, Indiana

Dennis D. Spencer, M.D.
Harvey and Kate Cushing Professor and Chairman
Department of Neurosurgery
Yale University School of Medicine
New Haven, Connecticut

Thieme
New York • Stuttgart

American Association of Neurosurgeons
Rolling Meadows, Illinois

Thieme Medical Publishers, Inc.
333 Seventh Ave.
New York, NY 10001

American Association of Neurosurgeons (AANS)*
5550 Meadowbrook Drive
Rolling Meadows, Illinois, 60008-3852

Editor: Birgitta Brandenburg
Assistant Editor: Ivy Ip
Vice President, Production and Electronic Publishing: Anne T. Vinnicombe
Production Editor: Rebecca Dille
Sales Director: Ross Lumpkin
Associate Marketing Director: Verena Diem
Chief Financial Officer: Peter van Woerden
President: Brian D. Scanlan
Designer: Russell Shaddox
Photo retouching: Terry Dagradi
Printer: Everbest

Library of Congress Cataloging-in-Publication Data

Cohen-Gadol, Aaron A.
　The Legacy of Harvey Cushing : profiles of patient care / Aaron A.
Cohen-Gadol, Dennis D. Spencer.
　　p. ; cm.
　Includes bibliographical references and index.
ISBN 978-1-58890-389-1 (TPN, the Americas : alk. paper) – ISBN
Cushing, Harvey, 1869–1939. 2. Nervous system – Surgery – Case studies.
3. Nervous system – Surgery – History – Sources. I. Spencer, Dennis D.
II. Title.
　[DNLM: 1. Cushing, Harvey, 1869-1939. 2. Yale University. 3.
Central Nervous System Neoplasms – surgery – Connecticut – Case Reports. 4.
Neurosurgical Procedures – history – Connecticut – Case Reports. 5. Brain
Diseases – surgery – Connecticut – Case Reports. WL 11 AC8 C678L 2007]
　RD593.C592 2007
　617.4'8 – dc22
　　　　　　　　　　2006103399

Copyright © 2007 by the Yale University Department of Neurosurgery. This book, including all parts thereof, is legally protected by copyright. Any use, exploitation, or commercialization outside the narrow limits set by copyright legislation without the publisher's consent is illegal and liable to prosecution. This applies in particular to photostat reproduction, copying, mimeographing or duplication of any kind, translating, preparation of microfilms, and electronic data processing and storage.

Important note: Medical knowledge is ever-changing. As new research and clinical experience broaden our knowledge, changes in treatment and drug therapy may be required. The authors and editors of the material herein have consulted sources believed to be reliable in their efforts to provide information that is complete and in accord with the standards accepted at the time of publication. However, in view of the possibility of human error by the authors, editors, or publisher of the work herein or changes in medical knowledge, neither the authors, editors, or publisher, nor any other party who has been involved in the preparation of this work, warrants that the information contained herein is in every respect accurate or complete, and they are not responsible for any errors or omissions or for the results obtained from use of such information. Readers are encouraged to confirm the information contained herein with other sources. For example, readers are advised to check the product information sheet included in the package of each drug they plan to administer to be certain that the information contained in this publication is accurate and that changes have not been made in the recommended dose or in the contraindications for administration. This recommendation is of particular importance in connection with new or infrequently used drugs.

Some of the product names, patents, and registered designs referred to in this book are in fact registered trademarks or proprietary names even though specific reference to this fact is not always made in the text. Therefore, the appearance of a name without designation as proprietary is not to be construed as a representation by the publisher that it is in the public domain.

The material presented in this publication by the AANS is for educational purposes only. The material is not intended to represent the only, nor necessarily the best, method or procedure appropriate for the medical or socioeconomic situations discussed, but rather it is intended to present an approach, view, statement, or opinion of the faculty, which may be helpful to others who face similar situations.

Neither the content, the use of a specific product in conjunction herewith, nor the exhibition of any materials by any parties coincident with this publication, should be construed as indicating endorsement or approval of the views presented, the products used, or the materials exhibited by the AANS, or its Committees, Commissions, or Affiliates.

Printed in China

ISBN 978-1-58890-389-1　(The Americas)

Dedication

This book is dedicated to:

My mother, Hemda, and my father, Soleiman: They have been the exemplary parents, and have taught me the value of hard work, integrity, and perseverance.

My wife, Isabelle: She is the light of my life. She has taught me every day how to become a better person.

My mentors, Drs. M. Gazi Yaşargil, David G. Piepgras, Fredric B. Meyer, Dennis D. Spencer, and Ossama Al-Mefty: All of whom have taught me the importance of commitment to the quest for neurosurgical perfection. They represent the best of Harvey Cushing.

Most importantly, my patients: They have made the practice of neurosurgery all worth it.

Aaron A. Cohen-Gadol, M.D., M.Sc.

My family and the family of Neurosurgery.

Dennis D. Spencer, M.D.

Contents

Contents	iii
Preface	v
Introduction	vii
Cushing Brain Tumor Registry: A Diary of Neurological Surgery During Its Conception	ix
Contributors	xxiii

Chapter 1   Pituitary tumors and other parasellar region masses — 1

- 1.1 Pituitary adenoma
- 1.2 Pituitary adenoma
- 1.3 Glioma of optic chiasm
- 1.4 Suprasellar lesion
- 1.5 Craniopharyngioma
- 1.6 Suprasellar epidermoid
- 1.7 Pituitary adenoma
- 1.8 Glioma of optic chiasm
- 1.9 Craniopharyngioma
- 1.10 Pituitary adenoma
- 1.11 Glioma of optic chiasm
- 1.12 Pituitary adenoma
- 1.13 Pituitary adenoma

Chapter 2   Gliomas and other "malignant" tumors — 93

- 2.1 Parietal neuroblastoma
- 2.2 Pineal region tumor
- 2.3 Glioma of lateral ventricle
- 2.4 Frontal glioma
- 2.5 Adenocarcinoma of skull base
- 2.6 Pineal region tumor
- 2.7 Osteosarcoma of skull
- 2.8 Temporal glioma
- 2.9 Thalamic glioma
- 2.10 Temporal fibrosarcoma
- 2.11 Pineal region tumor
- 2.12 Fronto-temporal medulloblastoma
- 2.13 Myeloma of the frontal bone
- 2.14 Occipital glioma

Chapter 3   Meningiomas — 189

- 3.1 Cerebellar meningioma
- 3.2 Convexity meningioma
- 3.3 Parasagittal meningioma
- 3.4 Olfactory groove meningioma
- 3.5 Sphenoid wing meningioma
- 3.6 Parasagittal meningioma
- 3.7 Parasagittal meningioma
- 3.8 Frontal meningioma
- 3.9 Large parasagittal meningioma
- 3.10 Occipital meningioma
- 3.11 Parasagittal meningioma
- 3.12 Parasagittal meningioma
- 3.13 Meningioma of the sylvian fissure

Chapter 4   Cerebral aneurysms and arteriovenous malformations — 291

- 4.1 Aneurysm of the internal carotid artery
- 4.2 Aneurysm of the internal carotid artery
- 4.3 Congenital aneurysm of the right temporal lobe
- 4.4 Anterior cerebral artery aneurysm
- 4.5 Arteriovenous malformation

Chapter 5   Spinal tumors   317

- 5.1 Spinal meningioma
- 5.2 Metastatic carcinoma of the spine
- 5.3 Cauda equina fibrosarcoma
- 5.4 Spinal cord ganglioneuroma
- 5.5 Spinal meningioma
- 5.6 Spinal meningioma
- 5.7 Spinal meningoma
- 5.8 Spina bifida – Intraspinal lipoma
- 5.9 Spinal cord ependymoma
- 5.10 Spinal neurinoma

Chapter 6   Posterior fossa tumors and other pathologies   375

- 6.1 Trigeminal neuralgia
- 6.2 Myelomeningocele
- 6.3 Porencephalic cyst
- 6.4 Acoustic neuroma
- 6.5 Epidermoid of the fourth ventricle
- 6.6 Brachial plexus tumor
- 6.7 Cervical meningocele
- 6.8 Hemifacial spasm
- 6.9 Craniosynostosis
- 6.10 Hydrocephalus
- 6.11 Progeria
- 6.12 Left rotational torticollis
- 6.13 Acoustic neuroma
- 6.14 Left rotational torticollis
- 6.15 Craniosynostosis
- 6.16 Fungus cerebri
- 6.17 Ulnar nerve decompression
- 6.18 Petroclival epidermoid
- 6.19 Cerebellar hemangioblastoma
- 6.20 Carotid body tumor

Chapter 7   Special illustrations, additional operative sketches, teaching slides, and operating room photographs   471

Index   549

Preface

Neurological surgery is founded in large part on the work of early surgeons such as Horsley and Cushing. Cushing arrived in history just when anesthetic, aseptic, and technical advances had reached the point at which exploration in the human cranium was possible but not necessarily safe or efficient. Cushing's Halstedian conservative personality embedded in his ritual of meticulous handling of tissues was the substance which not only allowed establishment of our discipline but also allowed its further progress in the face of critics.

For Cushing to achieve the dream of establishing and spreading his specialty through his disciples, he needed to first prove the safety of his methods. His patients therefore became the center of his career and their stories, which he carefully recorded, became the diary of neurological surgery in its infancy.

Cushing stored his patient stories in his Tumor Registry. During my fellowship training in epilepsy surgery at the Yale University Department of Neurosurgery, with the generous assistance of Dr. Dennis D. Spencer, I had the privilege of working on the Cushing Brain Tumor Registry. I immediately recognized the value of publishing some of this collection of patient histories. But this was not possible until the Yale Legal Counsel confirmed that publishing these images would not violate patients' confidentiality rights, as the privacy of the patients was of utmost importance.

In the following chapters, the patients' images (originally stored on glass therefore preserving their quality) have been correlated to their hospital history and presented in the chronological order of the date of patient admission or surgery. The reason for the selection of this group of patients was twofold: (1) their images were available in the Tumor Registry and (2) their images carried a special message about their disease. The patients' records have been retyped based on the original patients' charts on microfilm. In the opening paragraph for each patient record under the title "History," we have summarized the presenting symptoms and signs. Similarly, we have inserted short paragraphs in the middle and end of the record to facilitate understanding of the flow of events in the hospital course and during follow-up. The statements of greatest interest are in boldface. In Chapter 3, Meningiomas, Dr. Barker has further discussed the organization of Cushing's patient records in his thorough introduction. For further information, consult Dr. Peter McL. Black and colleagues' *The Surgical Art of Harvey Cushing*, where the precise format of the patient charts is discussed. In addition, Dr. Wahl has discussed the salient features of the Yale Cushing Brain Tumor Registry in his introduction to this book (page xi).

Cushing often dictated his "special note" before the operative note. He dictated these operative notes usually immediately after surgery, when he knew about the results of his intervention. These notes provide us with a reasonable window on Cushing's decision-making processes and are important features of the present offering.

The current generation of neurological surgeons may understand that the roots of their discipline are found in the stories of these patients. **This book is a recognition of the Cushing patients for their gift to neurosurgery. The emotional expression on their faces more than any words convey their suffering and sense of uncertainty. In this book, we witness their suffering and we renew our oath to care for our patients with passion and to honor their trust in our hands.**

Aaron A. Cohen-Gadol, M.D., M.Sc.
Indianapolis, IN

Introduction

Harvey Williams Cushing, destined to become the founder of and most important figure in the history of neurosurgery, was born in Cleveland, Ohio, on April 8, 1869. He was of Puritan descent on both sides of his family, and his father, grandfather, and great-grandfather had been physicians. He received a liberal education at Yale, graduating in 1891, after which he studied medicine at Harvard (MD, 1895), followed by a year's internship at the Massachusetts General Hospital in Boston. He then began a surgical residency at Johns Hopkins Hospital under W.S. Halsted.

Cushing always intended to be a surgeon – there appears to be no truth in the story that he first hoped to train in medicine under Osler at Hopkins – but he drifted into neurosurgery more or less accidentally over a several-year period. His route to the brain evolved out of an early interest in problems of anaesthesia in general surgery, which led him to work with cocaine as a local anaesthetic, which led to an interest in nerve-blocking, which led to an interest in problems of facial pain, and in 1900 resulted in his first important publication, a new surgical approach to trigeminal neuralgia, involving a new route to the juncture of the trigeminal nerve and the brain, where he severed the gasserian ganglion.

Cushing did this innovative work before he went to Europe in 1900–01 on a long-delayed wanderjahr to observe old world surgeons. His European diaries show that he found no masters there, no one who could teach him more than he had learned in the United States. On the beautifully symbolic day of July 4, 1900, Harvey Cushing in London watched the world's then-most acclaimed brain surgeon, Victor Horsley, enter a cranium by rongeuring away big chunks of bone. He concluded that Horsley was disappointing, a better researcher than an operator, and abandoned any plans for more work with Horsley. Later that year he found congenial research opportunities under the great Theodor Kocher in Berne, Switzerland; these took him in a direction he was already going.

It was back at Johns Hopkins, between 1901 and 1910, that Cushing developed the techniques that made him the parent of successful neurosurgery. Unsuccessful neurosurgery had many fathers, including Horsley.

Cushing's work at Hopkins was tolerated by his chief, Halsted, who was barely functional in these years because of his ongoing morphine addiction. Cushing's real spiritual inspiration was Hopkins' chief physician, William Osler, an already surgeon-friendly physician, who commented in 1901 that Cushing was opening the book of surgery at a new page.

Like his predecessors, Cushing approached the central nervous system without the aid of imaging, navigation aids, or antibiotics. He succeeded where others failed because he brought to the previously crude and bloody field of craniotomies and craniectomies Halsted's obsession with hemostasis and caution, his own dexterity, patience, and obsessive attention to detail in every aspect of the surgical experience, and a particularly sophisticated understanding of problems of intracranial and vascular tension that he had developed during his European research.

By 1905 Cushing had overcome the bedevilling problem of herniation leading to the development of fungus cerebri. He relied heavily on a

---

This essay was originally presented to the Congress of Neurological Surgeons as the inaugural John Thompson History of Medicine Lecture at the 2006 annual meeting. It relies upon and summarizes the research underlying the author's fully-documented 2005 biography, *Harvey Cushing: A Life in Surgery*, published by Oxford University Press.

subtemporal decompression procedure that relieved intracranial pressure without causing herniation, gave important palliative relief to victims of tumor, and made possible further exploratory procedures aimed at locating tumors.

By 1908, working only from signs and symptoms in the absence of effective imaging technology, Cushing was beginning to be able to locate and remove benign subdural tumors in human patients – in one case removing a tumor while talking with the patient. He had a particularly dramatic triumph in 1910 when he excised a huge meningioma from the head of Leonard Wood, former governor of Cuba and ranking general in the US army.

Also by 1908, Cushing and his students were developing routes to the pituitary, first in animals, then in humans. He soon began surgical and clinical treatment of pituitary conditions, and he began making pioneering contributions to the understanding of the gland's physiology, as outlined in his 1912 monograph, The Pituitary Body and Its Disorders. Cushing was the first to conceptualize the pituitary's role in secreting hormones that influenced growth, and, as a pituitary man, automatically became a pioneer in the murky field of endocrinology.

By 1910 Cushing at Hopkins had created neurosurgery as a new subspecialty, with an effective population of one. His operative results so far exceeded all others', including Horsley's, as to be non-comparable. In 1913 Cushing relocated to Boston, to become Moseley Professor at Harvard and surgeon-in-chief of the new Peter Bent Brigham hospital. Cushing's early work in Boston was twice interrupted by service in World War I, but in 1917 he published a second major monograph, Tumors of the Nervus Acusticus, which was the first detailed study of acoustic tumors and the possibility of their excision.

In France in 1915, then in 1917–18, he did very extensive battlefield surgery, including being involved in a futile attempt to save the life of William Osler's son, Revere, in August 1917. Under pressure to process head wounds quickly, he developed state-of-the-art techniques of wound debridement. In the final months of the war he fell victim to the Spanish flu and a consequent polyneuritis, which was probably Guillan-Barré syndrome possibly superimposed on a form of Buerger's disease (the latter probably influenced by his heavy smoking).

Trying to rebuild his practice in Boston after the war, Cushing was hindered by what he felt was his duty to acquiesce in Grace Osler's request that he write a biography of her husband, who had died in 1919. Cushing's two-volume Life of Sir William Osler was published to great acclaim in 1925 and won that year's Pulitzer Prize for biography. Cushing was a brilliant, prolific writer of both technical and literary works, at least Osler's equal as an essayist and stylist.

During the 1920s Cushing operated on several hundred patients a year, almost exclusively tumor cases, with continually impressive results. By 1930 Cushing had driven his case mortality below ten percent in an era when most other neurosurgeons still reported mortality in the range of 30-45 percent. His histological work on tumors with Percival Bailey in the 1920s led to a series of articles and monographs that established today's basic classification of brain tumors. In 1926 Cushing's interest in an electric scalpel developed by W.T. Bovie resulted in the first applications of electricity to neurosurgery. Cushing's team continued their study of pituitary conditions, attempted vainly to isolate growth and other pituitary hormones, and often operated on dwarfs, acromegalics, and others suffering from pituitary tumors.

By 1931 Cushing and his surgical team had operated more than two thousand times for brain tumors. Cushing stood to neurosurgery as Henry Ford did to the automobile, Sigmund Freud to psychoanalysis, the Wrights or Lindbergh to aviation, Ty Cobb or Babe Ruth to baseball, Louis Armstrong to jazz. The surgical world had flocked to Cushing's operating room to study how he worked on the brain, and he almost single-handedly trained the first generation of effective neurosurgeons who then fanned out across North America and Europe to begin a new specialty. He was also a founder and inspirer of professional organizations that exist to this day, including the then-named Harvey Cushing Society (currently the American Association of Neurological Surgeons).

In a spectacular last hurrah before retirement, Cushing in 1932 brilliantly synthesized clinical observation and theorizing in his paper, "The Basophil Adenomas of the Pituitary Body and Their Clinical Manifestations (Pituitary Basophilism)" in which he outlined what almost immediately became known as Cushing's syndrome and Cushing's disease. Cushing spent his final years at his alma mater, Yale, bequeathing to it his great personal library and the magnificent Harvey Cushing Brain Tumor Registry. He died in 1939.

Although Cushing became a legend during his surgical lifetime, some younger neurosurgeons began to see him as an establishment figure, cautious and conservative to a fault. In 1918 one of his former students, Walter Dandy, who had remained at Johns Hopkins, published his discovery of ventriculography, the first imaging technique useful in locating tumors. Dandy also began claiming great success in aggressively attacking acoustic and other deep-seated tumors, growths that Cushing often backed away from.

The Cushing-Dandy relationship has not been well understood. It was both personal and highly generational – that of a surgical father-figure trying to temper the enthusiasms of a brilliant but rough-hewn surgical offspring. Dandy seems to have had history on his side, as it were, for ventriculography eventually became very important. On the other hand, in the early years the technique was extremely hazardous and Cushing's and others' conservatism and their scepticism about Dandy's poorly documented series of cases was well justified. More generally, the surgical dispute was between Cushing's conservative approach to tumor issues and Dandy's and other young Turks' willingness to go faster, deeper, and sacrifice healthy tissue. It was a conflict between radical and conservative approaches that resonates to the present.

One of my central interpretations of the life and values of Harvey Cushing is that his personal conservatism, very much in the tradition of his physician father and grandfather, and perhaps of their Puritan forebears, was in large part responsible for the radical breakthroughs he achieved as a surgeon. To do intracranial surgery in Cushing's day required a temperament specially tuned to caution, attention to detail, deliberation, small achievements, and great patience, combined with a willingness to break from convention and journey into unknown surgical territory. The danger with many of Cushing's successors, notably Dandy, was that they might err on the side of impatience in their urge to develop new territory and become, in effect, throwbacks to the aggressive cutters of pre-Cushing, pre-Halsted days.

In everyday life Cushing was a driven workaholic, who achieved so much in substantial part because he worked so hard. He worked 14-16 hour days, six or seven days a week – about a 98 hour week – seldom took holidays, and expected his staff to match the intensity of his own commitment. His residents and other assistants, for whom he set the template of neurosurgical training as an endurance course, found working with him utterly exhausting. He was intensely critical of both human and surgical weakness, and often came across as aloof, unkind, and egotistical, a mean hombre, whom Osler several times at Johns Hopkins had to warn not to be so open in criticizing people he had to work with.

Cushing's egotism was a combination of pride in his achievements and determination that they be recognized in medical history. It was the kind of egotism we see in great athletes or perhaps great adventurers or explorers. It was also tied up with the Cushing family's intense sense of professionalism. Cushing's most severe critics always acknowledge his extraordinary bedside manner, and his total devotion to his patients -- these were some of the values he had in common with his less-driven, more-balanced mentor, Osler.

The cost of Cushing's success was paid not just by the occasional patients he lost – which included Leonard Wood on re-operation in 1927 – and by the people who worked with him, but perhaps above all by his family, whose story is in itself an American saga. In 1902 Harvey Cushing married his high school sweetheart from Cleveland, Kate Crowell, and they had five beautiful and smart children, and enjoyed the best of everything. As the wife of a workaholic brain surgeon, Kate Cushing found herself raising the children practically by herself. As the children entered adulthood, they found it difficult to relate to their distant, Victorian father, who may have achieved tremendous progress in medicine in the "Roaring Twenties" but who disapproved of practically everything else that was happening in that decade. Cushing disliked jazz music, radio, the movies, women wearing make-up, women (but not men) smoking, and anything that smacked of waste or frivolity.

Cushing pushed his sons hard. His eldest son, Bill, managed to get to Yale in the middle of the 1920s, where he was starting to blossom and probably would have chosen medicine. On June 11, 1926, at the height of the age of jazz, flappers, illicit booze, and fast cars, Bill Cushing decided to celebrate the end of his third year at Yale. He and a friend borrowed a roadster, picked up a couple of New Haven floozies, and danced and drank the night away out of town at a Connecticut roadhouse. On the way home the roadster hit a tree, all four of the young people were killed, all of their bodies reeked of alcohol. It is a true story that Cushing received the news of his son's death early that morning just as he was going into the operating room. He carried out the operation, which was a success, then told his team about the family tragedy, then left for Connecticut to claim his son's body. (This, by the way, was a Saturday in the life of a neurosurgeon that in drama and tragedy far surpasses the events of the Saturday imagined by the skilled novelist, Ian McEwan.)

The second son, Henry, eventually dropped out of Yale, distanced himself from his father, and made a quietly successful career in insurance. The three Cushing girls – the fabulous Cushing sisters – had anything but quiet lives, becoming the toast of American society in the 1930s and 1940s. While daughter Betsey linked the Cushings to the presidency of the United States through her marriage to Jimmie Roosevelt (son of Franklin D. Roosevelt), the closest likeness to Harvey seems to me to have been daughter Barbara – eventually Babe Paley – who seemed to replicate her father's driven temperament even as she helped make the lean, nicotine-dependent physical type a model of feminine beauty. In today's world Barbara Cushing would probably have gone into medicine, perhaps surgery. In that era the conservative Cushings, both Harvey and Kate, did not encourage their girls to even attend university, let alone study medicine. It is not true, however, that the Cushing girls were fortune-hunters, if only because the family had always been independently wealthy, and their fortunes quickly recovered from Depression losses.

Indeed Harvey Cushing's personal achievement founding neurosurgery rested partly on American wealth – his own family's wealth and that of the merchant Johns Hopkins' which underlay the Baltimorean's magnificent endowment of a hospital and university mandated to achieve international excellence. The educational roots of Cushing's achievement lay in the residency system that Halsted and Osler established at Hopkins, in their explicit relocation of Old World training standards to the New. They brought the best of Europe to America, and Cushing was the first American fully to profit from it.

He and many of his disciples were also shaped by the high standards of medical care and service that American patients expected from their physicians and Americans' willingness to support advanced research. With figures like Cushing, the United States began assuming global medical leadership. Within a few years of his having found on that July 4, 1900, that the best of Europe had nothing to teach him, Harvey Cushing began teaching his techniques to visiting Europeans. Thus Theodore Kocher of Berne, Switzerland, sent his son to observe Harvey Cushing in Baltimore, Maryland, in 1907, writing "the United States are the place where we have to go and learn more than we are able to show to the many men coming over to see us. Our turn now to admire others."

Harvey Cushing's career is an example of American medical achievement as a product of American puritanism, American wealth, and American democratic egalitarianism. It was also a product of the idealism that often motivates those who choose the medical calling, regardless of nationality. Whatever his blind spots and personal failings, Harvey Cushing was driven by values very similar to those of his friend and mentor Osler. Both men were utterly committed to advancing medicine so as to better treat patients and serve humanity.

Like Osler, Cushing sometimes talked of medicine in almost religious terms. In a 1926 address, "Consecratio Medici," he talked of "the practical religion of the physician," which was "not the promising of bliss in the future but the giving of health and happiness on earth." He concluded with a quote from an earlier physician [Stephen Paget]: "If a doctor's life may not be a divine vocation, then no life is a vocation, and nothing is divine."

Michael Bliss, Ph.D.
Professor Emeritus
University of Toronto
Toronto, Canada

Cushing Brain Tumor Registry
A Diary of Neurological Surgery during its Conception

"I would like to see the day when somebody would be appointed surgeon somewhere who had no hands, for the operative part is the least part of the work."

*Letter from Harvey Cushing
to Henry Christian (1911)*

Harvey Cushing's Brain Tumor Registry is a document that chronicles the foundation of the discipline of neurological surgery. It is an immense collection comprised of more than 2,200 patient case studies: human whole brain specimens, tumor specimens, microscopic slides, notes, journal excerpts, and more than 15,000 compelling photographic negatives – materials dating from as early as 1887. The photographic material illustrates the patients' clinical findings and has inherent artistic value. The registry reveals Cushing's surgical odyssey through the human cranium in the early twentieth century.

Harvey Cushing's Brain Tumor Registry is a collection which characterizes the pinnacle of the Homeric observational method in the early part of the twentieth century. The meticulous acquisition of clinical data by Drs. Cushing, Eisenhardt, and Bailey inductively led to the refinement of neurological surgery as a valid surgical specialty. The archive survives in its relative entirety, providing the opportunity for historical re-evaluation of Cushing's work and embodies a remarkably complete diary of neurological medicine from its conception. Because the history of Cushing's Brain Tumor Registry has never been fully documented in one place, a good portion of this offering will attempt to formally record the conception, organization, storage, and revitalization of the archive.

Even a perfunctory examination of the photographs, specimens, and records that comprise the Cushing Brain Tumor Registry acquaint one with the character of its creator. The registry represents an embodiment of Cushing's passion for meticulously recording, ordering, re-ordering, and interpreting information. The registry is rivaled only by Cushing's personal diaries, for he made daily entries for a great number of years. Indeed, the late Dr. John Fulton, Harvey Cushing's devoted biographer, faced an inordinate challenge to limit his biography to a mere 754 pages; from Cushing's earliest days, a continual theme in his life was his obsession with observation, innovation, and tireless documentation, principles which permeated all of his endeavors. Recently Michael Bliss has further expanded our understanding of Cushing's personality.[1] The evolution of the Brain Tumor Registry is intimately tied to Cushing's life experience.

The Genesis of the Cushing Brain Tumor Registry at Johns Hopkins Hospital

Dr. Cushing returned to Johns Hopkins Hospital in September eager to take his position alongside William S. Halsted and specialize in cases involving neurological surgery. Halsted first suggested to Cushing that he might fare better in orthopædic surgery. Cushing, while a chief resident, had already helped to establish William S. Baer as the director of an orthopaedic clinic at Hopkins; and Baer, in his turn, traveled across Europe to work with the outstanding orthopedic surgeons of his day.

Harvey Cushing seemed to be up against insurmountable odds. Even with the rapid advancement of medicine, surgery on the brain remained largely the same as it had been 400 years earlier in the time of Ambroise Pare. Cushing researched the Johns Hopkins Hospital experience with surgery on the brain and found that over the previous decade, 36,000 patients had been seen at the hospital, of those only 32 received a diagnosis of brain tumor, and of those, 13 had been referred to surgery.[2] However, only two patients ever made it to the operating room, and both died before leaving the hospital. Regardless, Cushing was set on his goal to organize a section of surgery for neurological disorders. He was eventually offered a position as an Associate in Surgery, given the opportunity to direct and teach in Halsted's Hunterian Surgical Laboratory, and expected to help manage Halsted's busy surgical clinic. In return, Harvey Cushing earned his dubious distinction; he would be referred any patient requiring surgical treatment of the nervous system.

In 1902, a golf ball-sized piece of brain tissue, or more to the point, the conspicuous absence of a golf ball-sized piece of tissue, provided the definitive catalyst to a series of events ultimately leading to the conception of the Cushing Brain Tumor Registry. Cushing's opportunities at intracranial tumor surgery were few and far between, and successes were rare. Still, he regularly examined all tissues removed during surgical cases, a habit he learned from both Halsted and Kocher. Following the removal of a "pituitary cyst" from a Ms. M.D., the Johns Hopkins Pathology Department "misplaced" Cushing's tissue specimen. The young surgeon, prone to fits of anger, which occasionally drew admonition from Dr. Osler, failed to contain his fury. He insisted that from that day on, he would be allowed to personally retain all specimens removed during his operative cases or autopsy. Welch and MacCallum agreed, and, at least in theory, the Cushing Brain Tumor Registry was born.

In fact, the stage had been set for the registry's creation, and even if Johns Hopkins Hospital authorities had never misplaced the tissue, it was likely that Cushing would still have demanded to keep his specimens. The event represents a certain psychological investment that Cushing made in his art; he would build a library toward his school of thought.

Within ten years of his return from Europe, Harvey Cushing had introduced and refined many of the surgical techniques he would use for the rest of his career. Utilizing his obscure collection of tumor specimens, microscopic slides, and photographs, he reviewed his labors up to 1910. The results were presented in Cleveland as "The Special Field of Neurological Surgery." His clinic admitted a total of 180 patients referred to him with some type of neurological tumor. Of the most recent 100 in whom an operation was performed, Cushing's mortality rate was 11%. Only three of the postoperative deaths occurred in the last 50 patients. Cushing understood, as Elizabeth Thomson wrote, "This was partly due to the fact that patients were beginning to present themselves before the outlook was completely hopeless, since early signs of tumor were being recognized more readily. Patients less frequently arrived at the clinic already blind, because ophthalmologists had become aware of what conditions indicated pressure on the optic nerves …"[3] Indeed, the surgeon began to amass and publish data on his series at an increasing rate. As he saw patients who were not yet at death's door, his success with tumors increased, and in turn, patients were more likely to agree to an operation. When the outcomes were unfortunate, autopsies were conducted in approximately 90% of intra-hospital deaths. Some of his specimens were seized under "inauspicious circumstances."

Harvard, with the generous support of Peter Bent Brigham, set to establish a benchmark hospital; one which promised to serve the underserved populations of Boston and the United States, and pledged to compare favorably in quality of care with any existing institution. The trustees offered to let Cushing aid in the design of the hospital and its policies, establish an autonomous section of neurological surgery, and to serve as the surgeon-in-chief and the Moseley Professor of Surgery. The chance fortune to fashion a department in his own image stood as a once-in-a-lifetime opportunity, and Harvey Cushing departed from Baltimore in October 1912 to establish his surgical laboratory and registry in Boston.

Maturation of the Cushing Brain Tumor Registry in Boston

Cushing's transition to Boston was relatively smooth. He seized the time available, while work continued on the hospital, to integrate himself into the scientific community. When the wards finally opened, he immediately set to work. The task was undoubtedly simplified by Cushing's decision to bring with him to Boston his entourage of residents and research scientists. Indeed, he also brought surgical notes, sketches, and specimens. By 1915, things were flowing effortlessly, and Cushing again made public his statistics concerning the mortality rates for intracranial operations for tumors. This time, he astonished his colleagues, submitting to the *Journal of the American Medical Association* an overall surgical mortality of only 8.4%. In contrast to the death rates of other leading neurological surgeons of the time – Kuttner, Krause, Eiselberg, and Horsley – whose figures ranged from 38% to 50%, Cushing's results seemed baffling.[4] However, he satisfied his skeptics by offering an explanation for the discrepancy: infection and sepsis played heavily into the disappointing percentages shared by each of the other surgeons; for Cushing, only a handful of patients succumbed to infective complications. He attributed the remarkable lack of postoperative infection to his stringently sterile procedures, and to the careful closing of anatomical layers, particularly the galea.

Despite the tensions and difficult atmosphere created by the First World War, Cushing began a period of intense, prolific writing activity, utilizing his unofficial registry, and especially the numerous pen-and-ink sketches outlining the critical steps of each case. He compiled and recompiled his results, publishing liberally in journal reports, and set to work on another major monograph – *Tumors of the Nervous Acousticus*. To this end, he hired a young, enthusiastic editorial assistant, Louise Eisenhardt, to work with him full-time.

Upon Cushing's return home from World War I, he immediately set to work on matters of intracranial tumors. Louise Eisenhardt remained as his assistant and, in addition, he was approached by a young graduate from the Northwestern Medical School named Percival Bailey. Bailey had the opportunity to witness a craniotomy as an intern, and came to Cushing curious about the possibilities of brain surgery. The pair met for the first time while Cushing operated, Bailey reporting to have won approval by identifying for the chief a "Ballenger swivel knife," invented by a professor of rhinology at the University of Illinois.[5]

Percival Bailey's principal interest lay in the staining, identification, and classifications of pathological tissue – a significant portion of the Tumor Registry consists of the pathological slides. Bailey harbored a temperament perhaps too similar to "the chief," for while Bailey and Cushing set common eyes on scientific problems, they only occasionally saw common solutions. Their relationship was at times volatile (Bailey having left Cushing's service on two occasions after fierce differences of opinion.) The neurosurgical caseload and clinic, boiling with activity on the heels of Cushing's growing reputation, stole away from the surgeon's time to pursue scientific research. In short, the duo developed a somewhat dysfunctional, oftentimes tenuous, but "fruitful co-dependence." Bailey also attempted, with little supervision, to decipher Cushing's diagnostic techniques of visual perimetry, and to work at classifying both his operative cases and materials from previous years.

After their initial meeting, Bailey never received an official appointment. Within a year, he left again for the University of Chicago to further study tissue staining. On one occasion, Bailey made some preparations from removed tissues in which Cushing could find no tumor. Dr. Cushing had been so impressed with the slides that he invited Bailey to return to the Brigham as the Arthur Tracy Cabot Fellow, for 1920-21.[5] At the same time, Louise Eisenhardt, spurred by her own interest in Cushing's work and the laboratory, and perhaps out of necessity created by Cushing and Bailey's fiery relationship, matriculated at the Tufts Medical School in Boston. Bailey again left Cushing in 1921, presumably with the hope of finding smoother waters. He later wrote of his relationship with Dr. Cushing, "We disagreed often, sometimes vigorously. When the tension became too great, I went away for a while. But I always came back. My debt to him was incalculable."[3] With Bailey in and out of the laboratory, Eisenhardt, his assistant, often away at school, and the passing in 1919 of this long-time mentor, Sir William Osler, it must have been a tumultuous time for Cushing. With the dutiful help of a number of particularly outstanding residents, Gilbert Horrax among them, Cushing pressed ahead with his surgeries, and passed much of his spare time preparing the manuscript for his biography of Osler (which had been specifically commissioned to him by Lady Osler).

With 1922 came the *tout ensemble* of Harvey Cushing's surgical and scientific pursuits in the registry. Bailey again returned to Boston and started with some degree of autonomy the program for the histological study of neurological tumors. Louise Eisenhardt, who never officially left Cushing's service, began keeping her obsessively detailed records on Cushing's operations and follow-up, somewhat as a liaison between the surgeon and neuropathologist. Cushing, with the help of his passionate resident staff, operated daily, reserving early mornings and evenings to write. In addition, Cushing brought onboard Mildred Codding, a medical artist who studied with Max Brodel, the German-born illustrator employed at Johns Hopkins.

The protracted study on the registry was financed primarily by the Phillip H. Gray Fund. It had been established in 1923 by Ms. Gray, in memory of her husband, who had succumbed to a malignant glioma. The fund appropriated $10,000 per year for ten years to be utilized toward the study of tumors of the glioma type. In addition, another grant, donated by Mr. Chester C. Bolton of Cleveland (in gratitude to Cushing for the care of Bolton's son Charles after a diving accident), supplemented the Gray Fund some years later. Overall, the project cost an estimated $30,000 per annum – the sum required to purchase materials and pay salaries for the research at the Tumor Registry. Additional funding became available occasionally through wealthier patients who agreed to pay exaggerated fees for Cushing's service. The balance was provided by Dr. Cushing himself, who paid from his own pocket detracting from the $5000 per year salary he maintained throughout his entire 20 years at the Peter Bent Brigham Hospital.[3] The Cushing Brain Tumor Registry evolved as an integrated research tool and matured since its early days at Johns Hopkins and Cushing's misplaced tumor.

Bailey and Eisenhardt took it upon themselves to organize and reclassify the tumors which Cushing had collected over the years. Many of these were ill-defined, the collection was in some degree of disarray, and the vast diversity of the tissues were not readily suited for classification. Eisenhardt contacted each patient on a regular basis (usually the anniversary of their surgery), to establish statistics on the natural behavior of the tumor types.

Later in his career, Cushing's operative mortality percentages continued to plummet. However, Eisenhardt, the savvy young neuropathologist (incidentally, the first female neuropathologist) knew of Harvey Cushing's somewhat competitive, obstinate nature. Rather than facing the skepticism of critics who might question Dr. Cushing's absurdly low mortalities, Dr. Eisenhardt kept the surgical "score" in what came to be known as "the little black book." The book's existence was well established at the Brigham, its contents subject to curiosity, and its whereabouts a complete mystery. Even Dr. Cushing had never been granted access to the document. Yet, its contents eventually divulged the case results, diagnoses, and mortality percentages for all tumor types operated upon at the Peter Bent Brigham Hospital from 1922 until the end of Cushing's career. The book forecasted the event of his 2000th verified tumor operation, an event of some celebration at the Brigham. As an aside, it was not until the occasion of Dr. Cushing's 70th birthday party, long retired from the operating room and teaching at Yale, that Cushing burst into Eisenhardt's office and demanded the document from her secretary. He presented the book to his colleagues at the party with the following playful statement:

"Had it not been for this confounded little book which [Dr. Eisenhardt] was prone to consult at awkward moments, the operative and case mortality percentages for the meningiomas would have been found much lower and the end results much better. For had I been left to myself, the temptation to exclude a case here and there to improve the figures would have been irresistible …"[6]

By 1924, the histological laboratory ran smoothly. A paper on the medulloblastomas was well received both in Philadelphia and at a meeting of the Harvard Medical Society.[2] Bailey worked furiously with the tissues from the operating room and the preparations belonging to the collection. Eventually, he surmised that each of the many varied tumors might have a common cellular origin. In December 1924, he called Dr. Cushing into the laboratory, believing that he had come to a solution of this "glioma problem." Utilizing the tissues and natural histories (as determined by the black book), Percival Bailey arranged these various glial tumors into an evolutionary tree, making careful correlations between their histological appearance and their clinical behavior. Clearly, his occasional sabbaticals from Cushing's laboratory had been valuable to the research; one had taken him to Madrid to study the cellular staining and study methods of Ramon y Cajal and del Rio Hortega, the other off to France for a Guggenheim Fellowship in pathology. Bailey hoped to spend more time defining his categorization of the gliomas, but Dr. Cushing, eager to present some results during the Cameron Lectures in

Edinburgh, insisted they press ahead to publication. Bailey once again became annoyed with Cushing and left Boston. Cushing personally wrote the final chapter on the monograph, and saw the book through to publication in 1926. *A Classification of the Tumors of the Glioma Group on a Histogenetic Basis with a Correlated Study of Prognosis* won instantaneous worldwide acclaim.

In the operating room, Harvey Cushing continued to work much as he had since 1910. He had made several contributions along the years – the ether charts, the blood pressure cuff, the neurodiagnostic utility of the X-ray, a novel approach to the gasserian ganglion, and the silver hemostatic clip to name a few. However, the most radical advance in neurosurgical instrumentation came in 1926, with the introduction of electrosurgical methods to the neurosurgical operating theatre. William T. Bovie, employed by the Harvard Cancer Commission, developed an apparatus specifically designed to help with the removal of tumors. The year of cultivating "the Bovie" for use on the brain was clearly an arduous one, which Hugh Cairns (Cushing's resident that year) would later compare to the Battle of the Marne. However, once suited to its purpose, the instrument allowed Cushing to re-operate on many tumors previously abandoned secondary to their vascularity, and it gave Cushing the confidence to bring to the operating theatre many cases which, without the hemostatic precision of Bovie's tool, could never have been attempted. This seems to be confirmed by a glance at Eisenhardt's little black book, which shows a multitude of re-operations, and a slight rise in overall operative mortality for the years of 1927 and 1928.

By 1930, Cushing knew well that in two years he would be expected to relinquish his position as the Moseley Professor of Surgery at Harvard. He himself and Henry Christian, physician-in-chief at the Brigham, set the retirement age at 63. He again received overtures from Yale and Johns Hopkins to continue his work away from Harvard. These overtures both included provisions for the aging Dr. Cushing to hold a position as a Professor of the History of Medicine – Cushing's private collection of books was already known. But Cushing politely declined, preferring instead to see what provisions might eventually be made available in Boston. In April 1931, Louise Eisenhardt approached Dr. Cushing with some interesting news. Her black book indicated that he was approaching his 2000th verified tumor operation. He had completed 189 verified tumor operations at Johns Hopkins, and completed the remainder at the Brigham. Somewhat to the consternation of the surly surgeon, the event was held with some degree of pomp and theatrics, filmed for posterity before a considerable audience. Dr. Cushing refused to fully cooperate with the filming, but the resulting footage remains adequate. The Brigham staff gave to Dr. Cushing a silver cigarette box as a momento of the occasion.

Louise Eisenhardt helped Cushing compile results of his 2000 verified cases for the meeting of the International Neurological Congress in Berne, Switzerland. Indeed, the paper "Intracranial Tumors. Notes Upon a Series of Two Thousand Verified Cases with Surgical-Mortality Percentages Pertaining Thereto" heralded a certain culmination of Cushing's life work. This would be Cushing's final presentation of his operative mortality statistics – still riveting to his colleagues – and it was only fitting that it occurred on the occasion of his pilgrimage back to Berne, where 28 years before, working with the likes of Kocher and Kronecker, Cushing somehow decided to embark upon his surgical odyssey into the human cranium. William H. Welch, during the particularly enthusiastic ovation that Dr. Cushing received after presenting the results, leaned to his neighbor in the audience to make a bold, but in all likelihood true statement, "Cushing is undoubtedly the outstanding medical figure of the world today."[7]

Emotionally prepared as he might have been, Cushing became the disapprobatory victim of the policy which he helped to author. When 1932 came around (bringing Cushing's 63rd birthday with it) he was already in quite poor health. His vasculopathy, partially a result of the polyneuritis he contracted during the war, no doubt aggravated by his incessant cigarette smoking, prohibited his walking any distance without rest on the wards, and he could no longer stand through long operations. Evidently though, Cushing had a realistic appreciation of his handicaps; he reluctantly but wisely passed an offer to continue as chief of neurosurgery at Case Western Reserve, the position his successor at Harvard, Elliot Cutler, had just vacated.

Dr. Cushing summered again in Europe and, to his chagrin, returned to a quite different Peter

Bent Brigham Hospital. Elliot Cutler considerably reorganized the surgical clinic in Cushing's absence. Knowing Cushing's dictatorial tendencies, Cutler stood hard and made it clear to his predecessor that the senior's clinical role at Harvard would be minimal. Cushing's longtime assistant, Dr. Gilbert Horrax, had already departed to the Lahey Clinic, and Cushing's entourage had been replaced by an unfamiliar junior staff. To add insult to injury, Cushing was given only a small suite in place of his previous offices. Despite his somewhat humiliating surroundings, Cushing and Eisenhardt began work on the Tumor Registry, reviewing tissues, specimens, photographs, and records pertaining to another type of tumor, the meningiomas. He had completed monographs on many of the tumor types, specifically on the glandular and glial varieties. This final monograph would serve to complete the scientific study Cushing intended to conduct on his surgical series of 2,209 verified brain tumor operations. Numerous institutions once again courted Cushing. Richard Light described his predicament:

"He lived in this tomb-like isolation for a year, unable to make up his mind which to choose of the offers made to him by Western Reserve, Johns Hopkins, and Yale. He hated to move and waited expectantly for Harvard to come up with something worthwhile, but Harvard slumbered on, and in the end he returned to his alma mater. As one wag put it, "Harvard fumbled the ball, and Yale fell on it." [8]

Cushing's return to Yale became a viable option for two reasons. First, John Fulton's biography, and private correspondence indicate that the Boston investment firm with whom Cushing entrusted his finances went bankrupt, losing great sums of money for many in the Harvard faculty. Cushing wrote to Mr. J. R. Angell, President of Yale at the time, "I now learn that the people who had my affairs in hand have so manhandled them that I may have to start in afresh as a wage earner, which is not easy at my time of life ..." [2] Secondly, when Cushing respectfully declined the offer to succeed William Welch as the Professor of the History of Medicine at Johns Hopkins in 1931, he suggested the position be offered to Professor Henry Sigerist, Director of the Institute of Medical History at Leipzig. Hopkins acted upon this recommendation and, therefore, in the interval before Cushing's formal retirement from Harvard and Cutler's subsequent abuse, the position had been filled.

Still, Harvey Cushing maintained strong ties to his alma mater throughout his career, and with John Fulton successfully fueling the flames at Yale, in 1933, Cushing agreed to come on staff as the Sterling Professor of Medicine in Neurology, continue his research pursuits, and spend the twilight of his career with Yale's History of Medicine Department, sharing his impressive collection of books and manuscripts. The Tumor Registry was subsequently relocated to Yale since Brigham authorities failed to show any significant interest in preserving the collection in Boston.

Relocation of the Tumor Registry from Boston to New Haven

With his decisive yet apologetic letter of June 27, 1934, James B. Conant, then the President of Harvard University, effectively closed the chapter on Harvey Cushing's official relationship with the Harvard Medical School. The sixty-three-year-old Dr. Cushing had retired from his thirteen-year tenure as Moseley Professor of Surgery in 1932, and returned somewhat disparaged to his alma mater, Yale. At the urging of Dr. S. Burt Wolbach, Chief of the Department of Pathology at Boston's Peter Bent Brigham Hospital, Cushing had left his Brain Tumor Registry to Harvard's Warren Museum.

The registry was an immense document comprised of over 2,200 case studies: human whole brain specimens, tumor specimens, microscopic slides, notes, journal excerpts, and more than 15,000 compelling photographic negatives – materials dating from as early as 1887. It was the embodiment of Cushing's scientific odyssey that chronicled the emergence of neurological surgery as a modern medical specialty, an icon for the relentless pursuit of knowledge, and quite literally, a portrait of human misery, bravery, suffering, and triumph. However, by 1934, Dr. Wolbach was having difficulty promoting the project to keep the Cushing Brain Tumor Registry. His Department of Pathology had little space to spare, and the Warren Museum lacked the funds to make the necessary alterations to house the archive. The correspondence merely confirmed Cushing's suspicions; his aspirations for the registry as a permanent scientific and historic archive would never be realized in Boston.

While Welch and McCallum, the pathologists at Johns Hopkins Hospital, maintained enthusiasm about Cushing's "private" collection, Wolbach had not always been so appreciative. John Fulton suggests that the establishment of the autonomous neuropathological laboratory headed by Percival Bailey contributed to ill-feelings. Certainly the publication of the glioma monograph from the Department of Surgery, with a minor mention of the Harvard's Department of Pathology made matters worse.[2] During Cushing's career at Brigham, Cushing's lab sectioned specimens for study, providing tissues first and foremost to the Department of Pathology. Cushing himself sectioned the gross tissues, and dictated the findings to pathology. Separate microscopic dictations and diagnoses were made by each of the laboratories, and in difficult or obscure cases, the departments conferred on findings. In each case, Cushing provided the Department of Pathology with photographs of patients, gross specimens, and photomicrographs when they were available.[2]

Harvey Cushing labored for a year to see his registry come to fruition. The Warren Museum, which was a possible location to house the registry, was in need of structural modification to accommodate the archive at an estimated cost of $4000. James B. Conant continued working with Cushing on the issue, but several meetings and memos made it clear to Dr. Cushing that the momentum was draining from the project. The arduous struggle to see the Tumor Registry through to its final preservation, made impossible by Cushing's absentee status (he had already moved to New Haven by November 1933) led him to the conclusion that he should move the entire collection to New Haven.

Following the June 27, 1934 letter from President Conant at Harvard, Dr. Cushing urged Dr. Eisenhardt to accompany the Tumor Registry to Yale, which she did in September 1934. Owing to the generous endowment by the Bolton Fund and the Childs Fund, Cushing had photographed onto microfilm the entire set of patient records from his brain tumor surgical series at the Peter Bent Brigham Hospital, and several hundred other records brought for "special purposes."

The registry was comfortably arranged in the Brady Museum at the Yale School of Medicine, and Dr. Eisenhardt, appointed director of the collection, was given ample laboratory space in Yale's Lauder Hall. Cushing and Eisenhardt drafted a bulletin that ran in scientific journals under the heading "Concerning a Registry of Brain Tumors." The bulletin extended invitation to anyone interested in the subject of brain tumors to contribute to or, "… utilize the material for … a general study of tumor types or for the preparation of papers they may have in hand …," it makes reference to, "… an immense number of problems relating to tumor classification and expectancy of life after tumor removal that are as yet unsolved …"

In 1935, Cushing and Eisenhardt completed the photography of patient's clinical records onto microfilm and immediately set to work on the final monograph in Cushing's trilogy on intracranial tumor growths, *The Meningiomas*. Work on the monograph proceeded slowly, as scholars and visitors flocked to the archive almost immediately. Hugh Cairns, the British assistant resident who worked with Cushing during the year that electrocautery was introduced to the specialty, came to New Haven in October 1935 with the idea of publishing on the series of patients whom he treated with Cushing between September 1926 and September 1927. The results of his follow-up appeared in the *Yale Journal of Biology and Medicine* in 1936 under the title "The Ultimate Results of Operations for Intracranial Tumors." Cairns found that during this period, 369 patients had been admitted to the Brigham with symptoms suggestive of a brain tumor. Of those, 157 patients were found to have a verified brain tumor at autopsy or operation. Cushing and Cairns lost 22 patients to postoperative complications, and of the remaining 135 who were discharged alive, 63 were still living 10 years later at the time of the report – 37 of whom were still wage earners.[9]

Despite his declining health, Dr. Cushing managed to labor diligently on the meningioma monograph, which was eventually published in 1938. Beginning with his first paper in 1898 at Johns Hopkins to *The Meningiomas,* Harvey Cushing published 14 books and monographs, over 300 journal articles, and had been awarded the Pulitzer Prize.

Cushing maintained very specific plans for his library at Yale. He insisted that a special building be constructed that could be readily accessible to students and faculty from almost anywhere in the medical school or hospital. Eventually, Dean Winternitz and President Angell agreed to allow Grosvenor Atterbury, an undergraduate classmate and close friend of Cushing to begin drawing up plans for the structure. Four years of revision went into the plans. However, it soon became obvious that a totally separate structure would be prohibitively expensive. By 1938, there emerged another set of plans, which described the Y-shaped building now incorporated into the medical school's Sterling Hall of Medicine.

Still, with plans seemingly secure, Cushing set back to work on his *Bio-bibliography of Andreas Vesalius,* a project that would ultimately contribute to his end. On October 3, 1939, Cushing received word that the Sterling trustees appropriated adequate funds, the Yale Corporation accepted the plans, and work was to begin on the library. Four days later, Dr. Cushing suffered a fatal myocardial infarction precipitated by the lifting of one of the great Vesalian folios to be used in the biography.[5]

Cushing Brain Tumor Registry at Yale

Ironically, the Brain Tumor Registry stayed at Yale in part because of Cushing's death. Prior to Cushing's retirement from the Brigham, Percival Bailey left for the University of Illinois to assume a position in neurology with Dr. Eric Oldberg. After the completion of the meningioma monograph in April 1938, Cushing was fully absorbed in his historical scholarship and had no intentions of proceeding with the scientific classifications. Cushing, Eisenhardt, Oldberg, and Bailey were in accord on the theory that the entire registry should be moved again, this time to Chicago, where Bailey and Eisenhardt could continue the work on problems not yet addressed. However, upon Harvey Cushing's death, Howard M. Hannah of Cleveland (who's only son succumbed to a neurological tumor) endowed the Brain Tumor Registry with a grant to Yale. The gift lifted Cushing's collection to the status he felt it deserved. Louise Eisenhardt and the registry would stay in New Haven.

For two decades, Yale's Brain Tumor Registry, with Louise Eisenhardt at the helm, remained a site of pilgrimage for young neurosurgeons and neuropathologists to study intracranial pathologies. Dr. Elias Manuelidis became Eisenhardt's successor in the Section of Neuropathology and, therefore, curator of the enormous archive. The registry had been enormously popular from 1935, probably reaching its apogee a decade later. Throughout the 1940s and '50s, many young scholars, particularly neurosurgeons and neuropathologists studying for their certification boards, came to utilize the collection. However, incrementally the gross specimens and photographic negatives came to be used little for research purposes. By 1968, the year after Eisenhardt's death, Manuelides faced a tremendous problem; the Section of Neuropathology prepared to secede from Pathology. With the split, laboratory space would be scarce, and the vast bookshelves, stacked floor to ceiling with gallon vesicles containing gross brain specimens and stacks of photographic negatives, played little role in the developing atmosphere of bench scientific research.

The 40-year-old specimens stood in a void – too old to be of scientific value and, ironically, too young to be of historical interest. Coincidentally, the unwieldy archive reeked of formaldehyde. The Edward S. Harkness Medical School Dormitory at Yale, built in 1955, retained rooms in the sub-basement for storage, adjacent to a fallout shelter. Many of the storage cages contained provisions, including large barrel tins of meal, drinking water, and sanitary supplies; others were utilized for the cold storage of building supplies, file cabinets, and discarded medical equipment. Manuelidis acquired permission to stow the entire collection – photographic negatives, gross specimens, laboratory materials and dyes, even an old gurney – into a locked room near the shelter. He employed the help of faculty and students, and moved everything save the microscopic slides (which are still in use today) below the dormitory. The collection remains in this sub-basement today (Figure 1A).

The Importance of Patients' Photographs and Records in the Registry

Unexpectedly, the most revealing source of information related to Cushing's work lay in the 15,000 photographic negatives. Cushing's negatives portray patients pre- and postoperatively, gross specimens, tumor specimens, photomicrographs, journal excerpts, letters, and any other number of images relating to the founding of tumor surgery on the brain. A small number of these patient photographs were published with Cushing's original reports and monographs, others can be found inserted into the Peter Bent Brigham Hospital

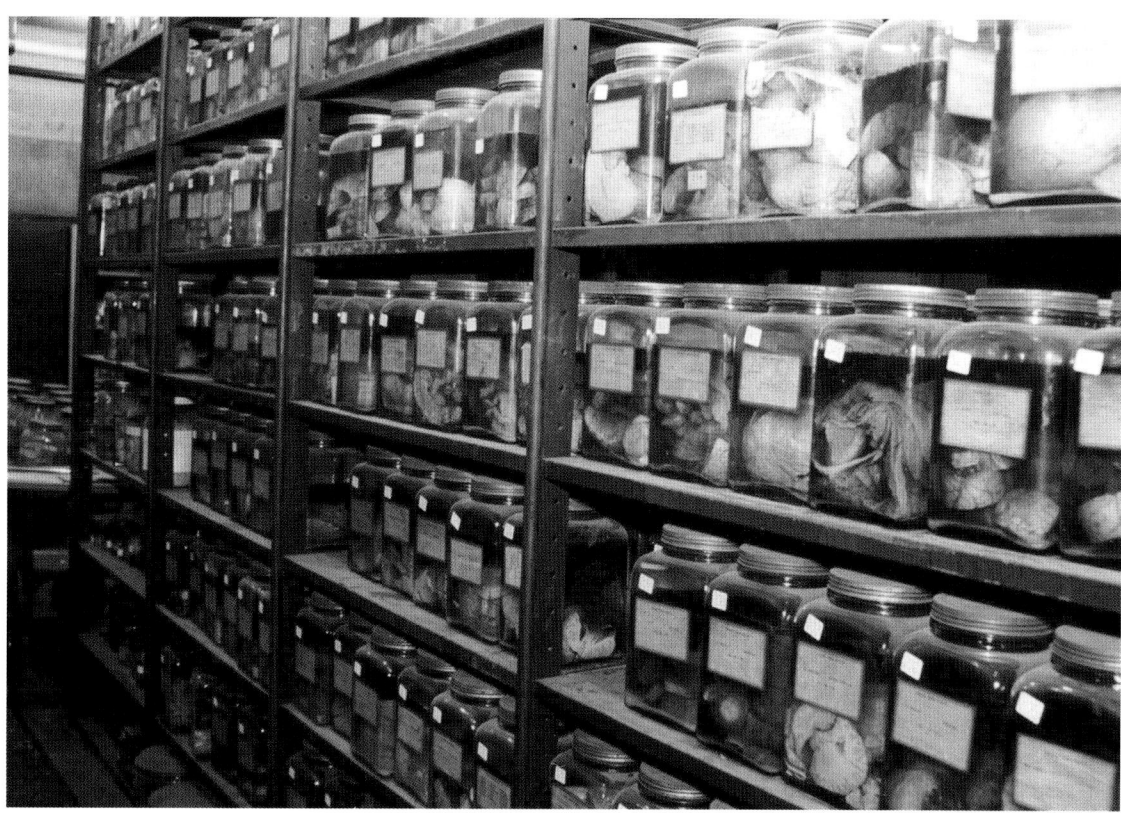

FIG. 1A (ABOVE) AND 1B (BELOW). THE CUSHING TUMOR REGISTRY IN THE SUB-BASEMENT OF THE EDWARD S. HARKNESS MEDICAL SCHOOL DORMITORY AT YALE. THE REGISTRY IS AN IMMENSE DOCUMENT COMPRISED OF OVER 2,200 CASE STUDIES — HUMAN WHOLE BRAIN SPECIMENS, TUMOR SPECIMENS, MICROSCOPIC SLIDES, NOTES, JOURNAL EXCERPTS, AND OVER 15,000 COMPELLING PHOTOGRAPHIC NEGATIVES — MATERIALS DATING FROM AS EARLY AS 1887. SEE COLOR PHOTO SECTION.

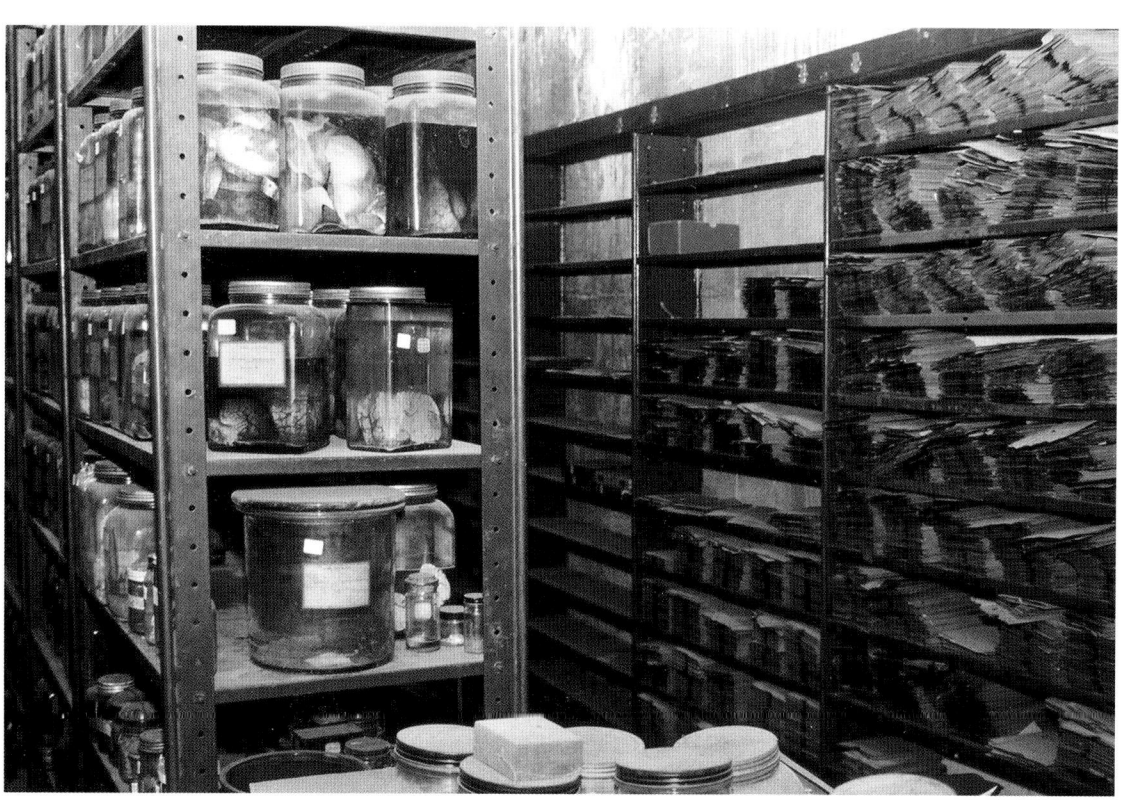

records. A great percentage, however, have never been published (if they were ever even printed.) The photographs often portray obsolete surgical practices, tumors that have grown to proportions rarely seen today outside the third world, and allude to the symptomatology, signs, and diagnostic techniques employed, which led Drs. Cushing, Eisenhardt, and Bailey to the foundations of modern neurosurgery and neuropathology. Approximately 80% of the negatives are etched into the emulsion of 5" x 7" glass plates, the remainder (in poorer condition) appear on 5" x 7" celluloid film (Figure 1B). Owing to the negative's large format, the prints are striking for their clarity in detail.

Because the photographic negatives are in a chronological order, which correlates with the hospital records, Cushing preserved for history a remarkable photographic diary. In the photographic negatives, one can follow the clinical presentation of disease to Dr. Cushing. One sees the sudden emergence of changing surgical approaches, documented in the records and complemented by novel intraoperative drawings and photographs of patients with craniotomy scars indicative of a changing technique. In these images, radiographs evidence the emergence of the silver hemostatic clip, portraits exhibit similarities in morphology leading to Cushing's elucidation of pituitary basophilism, and histological photomicrographs highlight the utilization of staining techniques brought to the Brigham by Percival Bailey.

The hospital records on microfilm, which accompany the photographs, indicate that Dr. Cushing cultivated in his residents the same meticulous attention to factual detail for which he is known. Past medical histories, family histories, complaints, progress notes, laboratory and perimetry results, neurological and physical examinations, operative notes, postmortem reports, telegrams, correspondence, and Cushing's ubiquitous operative sketches make the records so comprehensive that scientific studies of the cases, including the applications of pre-morbidity scales, is possible. The photographic negatives and patient records tell the historian much about Cushing, indeed much about the state of clinical medicine and surgery at the Peter Bent Brigham Hospital in the early part of the twentieth century. Ironically, and perhaps owing to the participation of Eisenhardt, Bailey, and various other residents, the archive seems to boast a special level of objectivity and integrity.

The photographs in the registry are the earliest photographs taken of neurological and neurosurgical problems. Cushing used these photographs as we use modern imaging to record the diagnostic moment in time, to document the results of intervention, and to provide history with chronology of the patient's course.

The Faces of Neurologic Disease and Cushing's Photographic Legacy

To further understand the possible contributing factors behind Cushing's interest in photographing his patients, one needs to review a brief history of photography itself. On August 19, 1839, Louis Jacques Mandé Daguerre presented to the world his technique for developing a photograph based on mercury vapor and silver iodide fixed by hot common salt. The process was made freely available to the world in a unique bargain with the French government that he and his deceased partner's family would receive a moderate annuity. Although fragile, the daguerreotype photo was extremely popular in America between 1839 and 1860, about 3 million being produced each year at a peak in the early 1850s. The medical journals began to photograph patients pre- and post-operatively, primarily for head and neck cancers and plastic procedures.

Following the daguerreotype, collodion, a mixture of gun cotton in alcohol and ether, was used as a wet plate process to make the first photographs on glass. This process was suggested by Dr. J. Milton Sanders to Ezekiel Hawkins and John Locke of Yale. The ambrotype perfected the collodion process in 1854 but was soon replaced by the tintype invented by Hamilton Smith in 1856. By 1900, cheap cellulose film and cameras were available to the public. These dates are important since even though newer flexible cellulose films were available, either Cushing or the unknown photographer at Brigham chose to continue using the dry glass plate technique from the earliest photo available in 1903 to the latest one in 1930. Several later photos were taken with the newer cellulose roll film and they have not withstood the aging process. On the other hand, the glass plates are perfectly preserved and are of incredible quality. Cushing may have understood the importance of preservation of these photographs as his important historical legacy.

Cushing's early 20th century portraits were grounded on the late 19th century tradition of scientific facial photography. Although X-ray was to emerge, as the next visual extension, peeling off one more layer between the viewer and the living brain, Cushing used photographs routinely as an extension of his diagnostic power and a catalogue of his historical sense.

In the Cushing Brain Tumor Registry for 75 years had lain the portraits of every patient Cushing touched, almost always photographed before and after an operation, but many times serially during the hospital stay particularly if the patient was deteriorating, and when there was nothing more Cushing could do – he documented the unrelenting course and death. And, for the majority of his patients that survived, he often chronicled their clinic visits sending the patient down for a "routine photo" as we would repeat an MRI scan today. This process apparently was so second nature to his patient care, like his operative sketches, that he never wrote about it. Unfortunately, we have no clue as to who took these pictures, whether it was the same person or a series of photographers. The quality, however, speaks for a professional who understood how these diseases were to be represented for Cushing and that the quality and permanence of the glass was superior to the more acceptable and common practice of using cellulose films.

Cushing never wrote about his patient portraits or their faces as an emotional response to their disease. Instead, he described disease, often for the first time, through the camera's lens. Cushing's groundbreaking work in identifying and classifying tumors of pituitary and parapituitary origin may have stimulated the first photographs. The phenotypic expression of pituitary tumors such as acromegaly could be identified in pictures, documented for publication, and repeated to look for progression or remission after surgery. However, he did not only photograph those patients with obvious phenotypic expression of their disorders, he photographed essentially every patient. Although it is not clear how most of these images contributed to patient care, education, or research at the time, the possible unintended consequences for art and history are incredibly powerful.

These patients' photographs are most likely the first and the most complete catalogue of neurological disease at the beginning of the twentieth century. What makes them even more powerful is Cushing's compulsive cross-reference process that ties each picture to the available hospital record on microfilm. Therefore, the records can be a glimpse into the person behind each photograph.

Time has helped create a form of art that is far beyond a mere hundred-year-old snapshot. Sometimes the art is the composition, sometimes it is the shading and background, but primarily it is the poignancy of a moment in time that tells a story. Each patient is of historical significance now because our discipline of neurological surgery evolved through his or her care. Cushing also captured in the patients' faces what we do not image today – loneliness, fear, pain, trust, despair, and often just stoicism.

Aside from historical merit, the photographic archive and hospital records give the observer a unique glimpse into the world of Dr. Cushing's patients. While nearly a century old, the photographs afford one the opportunity to witness a timeless emotional undercurrent. By any measure, Harvey Cushing's written and photographic diary of neurosurgery in the early part of the twentieth century steps beyond semantic issues. The technique and large format of the photographic negatives capture a raw emotional energy and oftentimes macabre subject matter that bring the viewer into empathetic participation with Dr. Cushing's patients. This relationship becomes much more sublime when one stops to consider the age of the photographs and senses that while neurosurgery changed so much over this past century, the experience of being a patient has not. In 1969, the year Harvey Cushing would have been a centenarian, Wilder Penfield qualified him as, "an artist, a Leonardo da Vinci devoting his talent to surgery." The passing of time and the re-evaluation of the materials belonging to the Harvey Cushing Brain Tumor Registry buttress the veracity of Penfield's statement.

Christopher J. Wahl, M.D.
Seattle, Washington

Dennis D. Spencer, M.D.
New Haven, CT

Aaron A. Cohen-Gadol, M.D., M.Sc.
Indianapolis, IN

Terry Dagradi
New Haven, CT

References

1. Bliss M: *Harvey Cushing: A Life in Surgery*. Oxford: University Press, 2005
2. Fulton J: *Harvey Cushing: A Biography.* New York: The Classics of Medicine Library, 1974
3. Thomson EH: *Harvey Cushing: Surgeon, Author, Artist*. New York: Neale Watson Academic Publications, Inc, 1981
4. Cushing H: Concerning the results of operations for brain tumors. *JAMA* 64:189-195, 1915
5. Bailey P: Pepper Pot., in Bucy P (ed): *Neurosurgical Giants: Feet of Clay and Iron.* New York: Elsevier, 1985
6. Davey L: Louise Eisenhardt, MD: First editor of the journal of neurosurgery. *J Neurosurg* 80:342-346, 1994
7. Light RU: The contributions of Harvey Cushing to the techniques of neurosurgery. *Surg Neurol* 35:69-73, 1991
8. Light RU: Cushing's handwriting and remembering Harvey Cushing: the closing years. *Surg Neurol* 37:147-157, 1992
9. Cairns H: The ultimate results of operations for intracranial tumors. *Yale J Biol & Med* 8:421-492, 1936

Contributors

Fred G. Barker II, M.D.
Associate Professor of Neurosurgery
Harvard Medical School
Attending Neurosurgeon
Massachusetts General Hospital
Boston, Massachusetts

Stephen B. Tatter, M.D., Ph.D.
Liang Yee and Dixie Soo Professor in Neurosurgery
Attending Neurosurgeon
Wake Forest University School of Medicine
Winston-Salem, North Carolina

Edward R. Laws, M.D.
Professor of Neurosurgery
Clinical Internal Medicine and Pediatrics
Department of Neurological Surgery
University of Virginia Health System
Charlottesville, Virginia

William T. Couldwell, M.D., Ph.D.
Professor and Chairman
Department of Neurosurgery
University of Utah
Salt Lake City, Utah

Martin H. Weiss, M.D.
Professor
Department of Neurological Surgery
University of Southern California
Los Angeles, California

Mitchel S. Berger, M.D.
Professor and Chairman
Department of Neurological Surgery
Kathleen M. Plant Distinguished Professor
University of California, San Francisco
San Francisco, California

Michael Bliss, Ph.D.
Professor Emeritus
University of Toronto
Toronto, Canada

Robert J. Maciunas, M.D., M.P.H., F.A.C.S.
Vice Chairman of University Neurosurgeons
Professor of Neurological Surgery
and Radiation Oncology
CASE School of Medicine
Director
Center for Image-Guided Neurological Surgery
and the Gamma Knife Surgery Center
University Hospitals of Cleveland
Cleveland, Ohio

Joseph M. Piepmeier, M.D.
Nixdorff-German Professor and Vice-Chairman
Department of Neurosurgery
Yale University
New Haven, Connecticut

Fredric B. Meyer, M.D.
Professor and Chairman
Department of Neurologic Surgery
Mayo Clinic College of Medicine
Rochester, Minnesota

William E. Krauss, M.D.
Associate Professor
Department of Neurologic Surgery
Mayo Clinic
Rochester, Minnesota

Paul C. McCormick, M.D., M.P.H., F.A.C.S.
Professor of Neurosurgery
Columbia University
College of Physicians & Surgeons
New York, New York

Amandip S. Gill, B.S.
Medical Student
Department of Neurological Surgery
University of California, Irvine
Irvine, California

Devin Binder, M.D., Ph.D.
Assistant Professor
Department of Neurological Surgery
University of California, Irvine
Irvine, California

Acknowledgments

Many individuals have selflessly devoted their time and effort to the preparation of this book. Some of these individuals have been mentioned below.

Terry Dagradi has been in charge of the Cushing Brain Tumor Registry at Yale University Department of Neurosurgery since 1995. She has had a passion for maintenance, organization, and revival of the Registry. Her altruistic interest in further recognition of these archives has been the most important tool in making this book possible. She completed the digitization, organization, and refinement of the photographs to be presented in the final format in this offering. *Toby Appel* has been instrumental in providing Cushing's special operative sketches (Chapter 7.)

Svetlana Pravdenkova assisted in organization of the patient hospital records. Her sincere work ethic and attention to detail has made the portion of the book related to patient histories a complete diary.

Christopher J. Wahl, Mark P. Piedra, Brian V. Nahed, Michael L. DiLuna and *Jennifer R. Voorhees* have dedicated a large amount of their time to study the Registry and assist with the preparation of the presented material. They also put together the database which allows the correlation of photographs to the appropriate patient records. In addition, *Peter Steiner* refined Cushing's hand-drawn operative sketches in the clear format that is available to you.

Russell Shaddox's special efforts in organizing the book in its final format have greatly facilitated our demonstration of patients' diaries.

Kathy Redelman has refined this offering by her outstanding editorial skills and her selfless time commitment allowed this book to be ready on time for the celebration of the 75th anniversary of the American Association of Neurological Surgeons meeting.

The sincere efforts of the above individuals are immensely appreciated. This book would have not been possible without their support.

Chapter 1

Pituitary tumors and other parasellar lesions

Introduction

"Surgeons have assailed it from below through the nasal cavities, and from above through the skull by elevating the frontal lobe either from in front or the side. It is certain that no method is applicable for all conditions of pituitary tumor and that for some no satisfactory procedure has been devised. Speaking for myself, I find that I am conducting proportionately fewer rather than more transphenoidal operations, though in favorable cases with a large ballooned sella I believe the latter to be the simplest and easiest method, the one most free from risk and most certain to lead to a rapid restoration of vision. However, in increasing numbers, both in children and adults, suprasellar tumors giving secondary hypophyseal symptoms are being recognized, and if the sella is not enlarged an approach from above is necessitated (1921)." [4]

Harvey Cushing

Cushing's surgical approach to parasellar lesions evolved from palliative subtemporal decompression to transsphenoidal partial lesionectomy to subfrontal radical adenomectomy.[14] Early attempts at resection of these lesions were associated with significant risks. Sir Victor Horsley [11] attempted the first recorded intracranial approach to a pituitary adenoma in 1889, albeit unsuccessfully, due to forceful retraction of the frontal lobe. Caton and Paul [2] attempted resection of a pituitary tumor in 1893 based on a subtemporal approach recommended by Horsley; the tumor was never exposed and the patient died three months later. Schloffler [17] in 1906 was the first to embark on resection of a pituitary growth through extensive resection of ethmoid and sphenoid sinuses through a lateral rhinotomy approach. This technique was simplified and improved by Kanavel in 1909,[12] Halstead,[6] Kocher,[13] and Hirsch[8] in 1910.

Prior to December 1910, the contemporary literature, including Osler's textbook of medicine, recognized only two disorders of the pituitary gland: acromegaly, also called hyperpituitarism or Marie's disease resulting from gland hypertrophy; and hypopituitarism, or underdevelopment of the gland. Beginning as early as 1909, Cushing introduced a third term, "dyspituitarism," to describe syndromes in which patients displayed other signs of pituitary malfunction. To Cushing, however, the study of this gland and its disorders became a passion. John Fulton writes:

"Cushing was always fascinated by the circus, particularly by the sideshows where he obtained histories of the giants, fat women, and midgets, and any other freak that might happen to be on display. In this way, he made friends with many circus personalities and over the years managed to keep in touch with several well-known giants and midgets. Sir Arthur Keith, the distinguished curator of the Hunterian Museum, consented some years ago, on Cushing's insistence, to removing the top of the skull of the famous Irish giant whose skeleton had long been on display in the Museum, in order to ascertain the condition of the sella turcica where the pituitary body would have been. Sure enough, the sella was grossly enlarged and there was evidence that there had been a sizeable intracranial extension of the pituitary tumor." [5]

Cushing presented the results of his first 20 pituitary tumor patients to the New York Academy of Medicine as part of the Harvey Lecture series in 1910. The lecture was a resounding success, and Cushing labored over the next two years with another 27 cases. He published the entire series of 47 cases in 1912 under the title, *The Pituitary Body and Its Disorders. Clinical States Produced by Disorders of the Hypophysis Cerebri*. The book drew largely from Cushing's collection of photos, specimens, and histories saved in the registry. He separated the individual case studies into those resembling hyperpituitarism, hypopituitarism, and dyspituitarism. Unlike any work which could be published today, *The Pituitary Body* presented little in the way of physiology, pathology, or chemistry; it is predominantly a book of observations with an end comment on incidence, symptomatology, and therapy. However, the work put the diagnosis of pituitary disorders into the hands of physicians everywhere. Where previously there had been only giants, dwarfs, and bearded women; headaches, blindness, adiposity, and polyuria, suddenly there existed an explanation: malfunction of the hypophysis. Physician Leonard P. Mark illustrated the epiphany when describing his own experience: "For some 15 or 20 years, each day when I looked into the glass to brush my hair or to shave, there was a typical acromegalic literally staring me in the face. Yet I never recognized the fact."[1] The pituitary became the primary focus of much of Dr. Cushing's scientific and clinical career; in 1927, he once again reflected on acromegaly, "Nature in her ugliest mood conceived such a malady."[3] With the 1912 publication, Cushing firmly consolidated his reputation as the foremost authority of surgery on the human brain—particularly in the extirpation of tumors.

Of the 1870 patients listed in the Cushing Tumor Registry database today, 336 (18%) underwent surgery for a pathologically proven pituitary adenoma through a transsphenoidal or transfrontal approach. Based on this database, 89 patients underwent at least one operation for resection of a pituitary tumor between 1926 and 1929. Henderson[7] conducted a comprehensive review of Cushing's pituitary practice in 1939. He reported 91 patients who were operated on in this four-year interval; 2 of these were not found in the current registry database. During World War I, Cushing was briefly in France in 1915 at the military hospital established at Neuilly outside Paris in the converted Lycée Pasteur, and again from 1917 to 1919 as chief of Base Hospital No. 5. Unsurprisingly, only a minimal number of patient records are available for these periods.

The first patient (1.1) included in this chapter is one of Cushing's favorites and has been discussed extensively in Cushing's books and articles. Cushing initially evaluated the patient at Johns Hopkins Hospital (Baltimore, MD) in October 1910. Through a transsphenoidal approach, Cushing completed a sellar decompression without tumor resection during two operative sessions. In September 1914, the patient met with Cushing at Brigham with the same symptoms as on his initial presentation four years before. There he underwent a right-sided subtemporal decompression (the safety of a transcranial approach to the sellar region was not established at the time). Due to the patient's continued severe headaches, his father strongly "petitioned" for another transsphenoidal attempt. Unfortunately, this attempt was unsuccessful and the patient expired shortly thereafter. At his autopsy, Cushing studied the skeletal features of acromegaly in detail; the autopsy pictures give full evidence of this. The attention to detail in the analysis of the autopsy findings is an important example of Cushing's contribution to the development of a diagnostic and therapeutic armamentarium for our discipline.

The second patient (1.2) in the following chapter suffered from acromegaly and underwent a transsphenoidal operation in April 1914. A possible error in trajectory of the sublabial corridor led to brisk venous bleeding from the sella, perhaps due to violation of the cavernous sinus. The procedure, performed in front of the members of the Society of International Surgery, was aborted. In a few days, Cushing performed a second operation to place a "radium tube" in the sella. This marked the early years of brachytherapy.[18] Following this patient's death years later in the Danvers State Hospital, an autopsy revealed a large occipital meningioma. Dr. Cushing's "lantern" slide demonstrates the arrangement of his slides for teaching purposes.

The third patient (1.3) underwent a craniotomy for "callosal puncture" to relieve his hydrocephalus. Due to a lack of localizing symptoms, signs, and skull X-ray findings, a decompression procedure (in this case ventricular drainage) was used to relieve intracranial tension. Following the patient's death, Cushing used the autopsy findings to learn more about the location and histology of the child's brain tumor, which had not been exposed at surgery. Interestingly, upon Dr. Cushing's urging, the patient's father personally brought his child's body into the hospital for postmortem examination.

The next patient (1.4) underwent left subtemporal decompression surgery by Dr. Mixter. She then presented to Dr. Cushing with an impressive protrusion at the site of previous decompression, which had been tapped on multiple occasions. Unfortunately, this patient eventually expired from a widespread bacterial infection. Although the patient was expected to die shortly after discharge, Dr. Cushing (or his research team) sent the family a letter five years later, inquiring about the patient's status. Patient 1.5 also underwent subtemporal decompression prior to admittance to Brigham. Cushing aspirated the parasellar cyst through a subfrontal approach; however, he wrote that due to "the small size of the head, it was thought inexpedient to make any further attempt to expose this field more widely so as possibly to justify partial removal of the sac wall." These statements signify Cushing's sense of caution and conservatism in surgery; these two factors no doubt were important for the attainment of positive results and favorable outcomes despite rudimentary surgical techniques during early years of neurosurgery.

In the same patient (1.5) advanced pressure symptoms made Cushing more aggressive during the next operative session (dated May 8, 1919). Most of the tumor was dislodged and the neurological condition of the awake patient was monitored intraoperatively. In this operative report, Cushing notes the possibility of enhancing the chance of gross total tumor removal by "splitting the chiasm antero-posteriorly" at the expense of leaving the patient with a permanent bitemporal hemianopsia. Follow-up visits demonstrated the management paradigm for panhypopituitarism. The last letter from the family in 1931 completed an impressive 12-year follow-up for this patient.

The operative report of Patient 1.6 demonstrates Cushing's candid disclosure of his surgical mishaps as he dictated the following note: "The removal in fact had been so complete and was so deep that Dr. Bailey cautioned the operator that he picked up by accident the 3rd and 4th cranial nerves." During the operation on Patient 1.8, attempted resection of a third ventricular glioma caused the patient to stop breathing. Cushing describes the scene:

"The field was dismantled and not being satisfied with the character of artificial respiration which some one was giving her, I took this over myself, and by gentle pressure on the thorax could get a sufficient exchange to keep the color fairly good ... after about ten minutes, she took a single deep inspiration, after about ten minutes more another. This continued for about 45 minutes, at the end of which time she began with a few superficial respiratory movements, and fairly good respirations were resumed."

Despite the removal of the lesion and the heroic resuscitation, the patient expired hours after surgery.

As intracranial surgical techniques accelerated with the introduction of electrocautery, Cushing demonstrated more radical techniques during a second attempted excision of Patient 1.12's pituitary adenoma. The details of management of panhypopituitarism for this patient are intriguing.

Patient 1.13's physician believed that the patient would "die if anyone operated on his pituitary." The patient subsequently underwent a craniotomy for excision of a pituitary adenoma by Cushing. The extrasellar portion of the tumor exposed during surgery further confirmed Cushing's belief that the transcranial and not the transsphenoidal corridor provided the best approach for complete tumor resection. We will elaborate on the evolution of this technique from transsphenoidal to transfrontal approach for the parasellar lesions in the following section.

Evolution of technique from transsphenoidal to transfrontal*

Cushing (sublabial technique) along with Oskar Hirsch (endonasal technique) popularized the transsphenoidal approach to tumor removal. Before 1922, based on his confidence in the transsphenoidal method, Cushing did not hesitate to elaborate upon his approach to pituitary tumors in his operative notes. Cushing referred to this route as his "customary transsphenoidal route." By 1929, three years before his retirement as an active surgeon, he had given up the transsphenoidal method and exclusively employed the subfrontal route. He referred to the subfrontal approach as the "transfrontal" method.

---

*The following material has been excerpted with permission from Cohen-Gadol AA, Laws ER, Spencer DD. The evolution of Harvey Cushing's surgical approach to pituitary tumors from transsphenoidal to transfrontal. *J Neurosurg* 103:372-377, 2005

While debating which of the two approaches to use, he noted in one of his operative reports in 1928:

"I have reached the stage of thinking that each of these recent transfrontal exposures is more satisfactory and interesting than the last."

The suprasellar extent of most pituitary tumors was increasingly appreciated and Cushing's "transfrontal" surgical technique allowed a more radical decompression of the chiasm with a superior and more immediate restoration of visual fields. Cushing dramatically demonstrated the transfrontal approach in his resection of a pituitary adenoma in his highly publicized 2000th brain tumor operation. He referred to this operation as an example of the progress in intracranial surgery in his lifetime.[16] Around the end of Cushing's surgical career in 1932, other neurosurgeons followed his example and transsphenoidal surgery was considered to have a minor role in the specialty. Hirsch continued to advocate and report upon the endonasal approach until the end of 1950s.[9, 10]

Cushing initially employed the transfrontal procedure for exploration of the optic chiasm in patients with "unexplained" bitemporal hemianopsia and a nonenlarged sella, many of whom had suprasellar meningiomas, craniopharyngiomas, and adenomas.[7] Through these cases, he realized that pituitary tumors may occasionally present with a normal sized sella and a large suprasellar extension. With the increasing safety of intracranial surgery, he described the relationship between the patterns of visual field deficits and the anatomical deformation of the chiasm by suprasellar lesions as observed through a transfrontal approach.[15] Importantly, non-adenomatous sellar tumors were no longer a "surprise" finding during transsphenoidal surgery. Indeed, despite the lack of modern diagnostic modalities, Cushing no longer needed to decide whether to confront the lesion from "below" or "above" because the transfrontal approach was an all-purpose technique, which allowed decompression of the optic apparatus regardless of the pathology. He mentioned in a 1926 operative note:

"Of course a transfrontal operation would have settled either question and the procedure {transsphenoidal surgery} I carried out would only have settled the adenoma."

The following patient hospital records accompanied by Cushing's hand-drawn sketches and patient photographs illustrate the operative events in the early years of caring for sellar/parasellar tumors. They are the written record of the evolution of neurosurgery.

Aaron A. Cohen-Gadol, M.D., M.Sc.
Indianapolis, IN
Edward R. Laws, M.D.
Charlottesville, VA
William T. Couldwell, M.D.
Salt Lake City, UT
Martin H. Weiss, M.D.
Los Angeles, CA

References

1. Aron DC: The path to the soul: Harvey Cushing and surgery on the pituitary and its environs in 1916. *Perspect Biol Med* 37:551-565, 1994
2. Caton R, Paul F: Notes of a case of acromegaly treated by operation. *BMJ* 2:1421-1423, 1893
3. Cushing H: Acromegaly from a surgical standpoint. *Br Med J* 2:48-55, 1927
4. Cushing H: Disorders of the pituitary gland. Retrospective and prophetic. *JAMA* 76:1721-1726, 1921
5. Fulton J: *Harvey Cushing: A biography.* New York: The Classics of Medicine Library, 1974
6. Halstead A: Remarks on the operative treatment of tumors of the hypophysis. *Surg Gynecol Obstet* 10:494-502, 1910
7. Henderson W: The pituitary adenomata. A follow-up study of the surgical results in 338 cases (Dr. Harvey Cushing's series). *Br J Surg* 26:811-921, 1939
8. Hirsch O: Endonasal method of removal of hypophyseal tumors. With a report of two successful cases. *JAMA* 55:772-774, 1910
9. Hirsch O: Life-long cures and improvements after transphenoidal operation of pituitary tumors (thirty-three patients, followed up for 20-37 years). *Acta Ophthalmol* (Suppl 56):1-60, 1959
10. Hirsch O: Pituitary tumors. A borderland between cranial and transphenoidal surgery. *N Engl J Med* 254:937-939, 1956
11. Horsely V: On the technique of operations on the central nervous system. *BMJ* 2:411-423, 1906
12. Kanavel A: The removal of tumors of the pituitary body by an intranasal route. *JAMA* 53:1704-1707, 1909
13. Kocher T: Ein Fall von Hypophysis-Tumor mit operativer Heil-ung. *Dtsch Z Chirurgie* 100:13-37, 1909
14. Liu J, Kaushik D, Weiss M, Laws Jr E, Couldwell W: The history and evolution of of transphenoidal surgery. *J Neurosurg* 95:1083-1096, 2001
15. Ray B, Patterson R: Surgical treatment of pituitary tumors. *J Neurosurg* 19:1-8, 1962
16. Rosegay H: Cushing's legacy to transphenoidal surgery. *J Neurosurg* 54:448-454, 1981
17. Schloffer H: Zur Frage der operationen an der hypophyse. *Beitr z. Klin Chir* 50:767-817, 1906
18. Schulder M, Loeffler JS, Howes AE, Alexander E, 3rd, Black PM: Historical vignette: The radium bomb: Harvey Cushing and the interstitial irradiation of gliomas. *J Neurosurg* 84:530-532, 1996

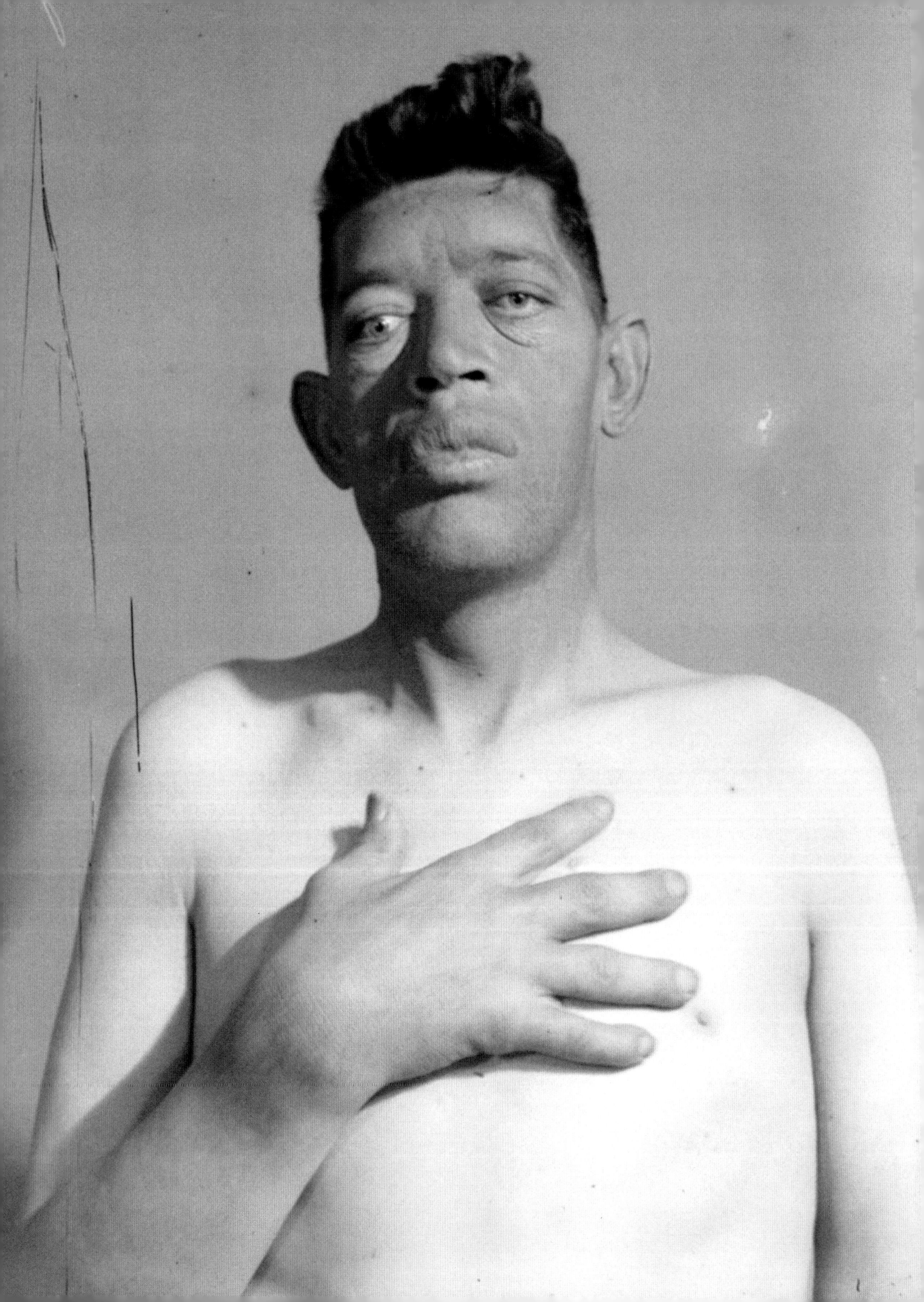

1.1 Pituitary adenoma

SEX: M; AGE: 39; SURG. NO. 1784

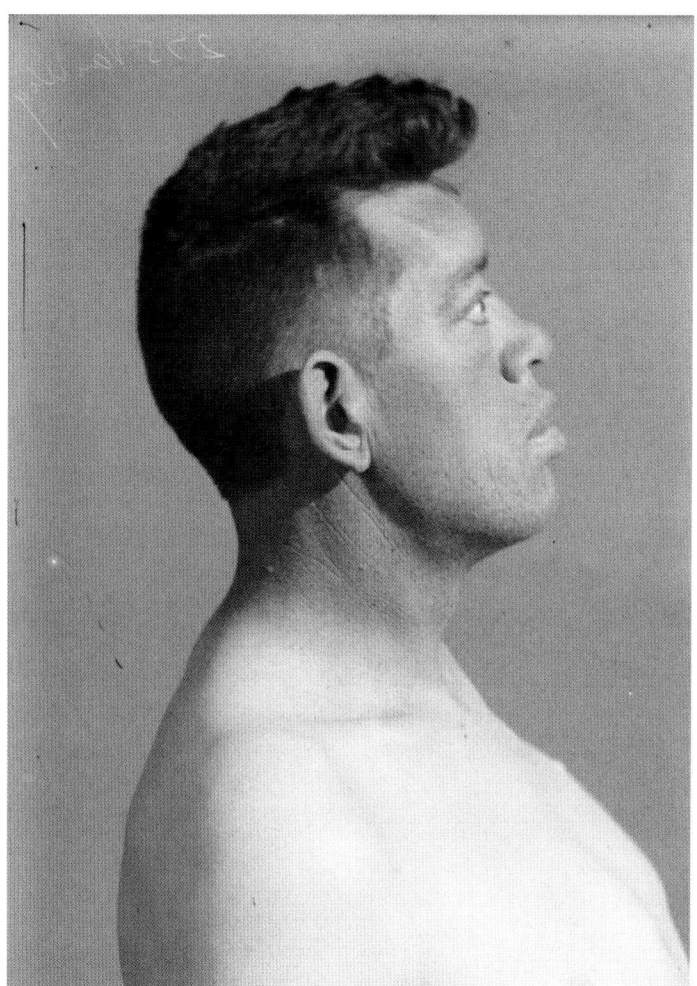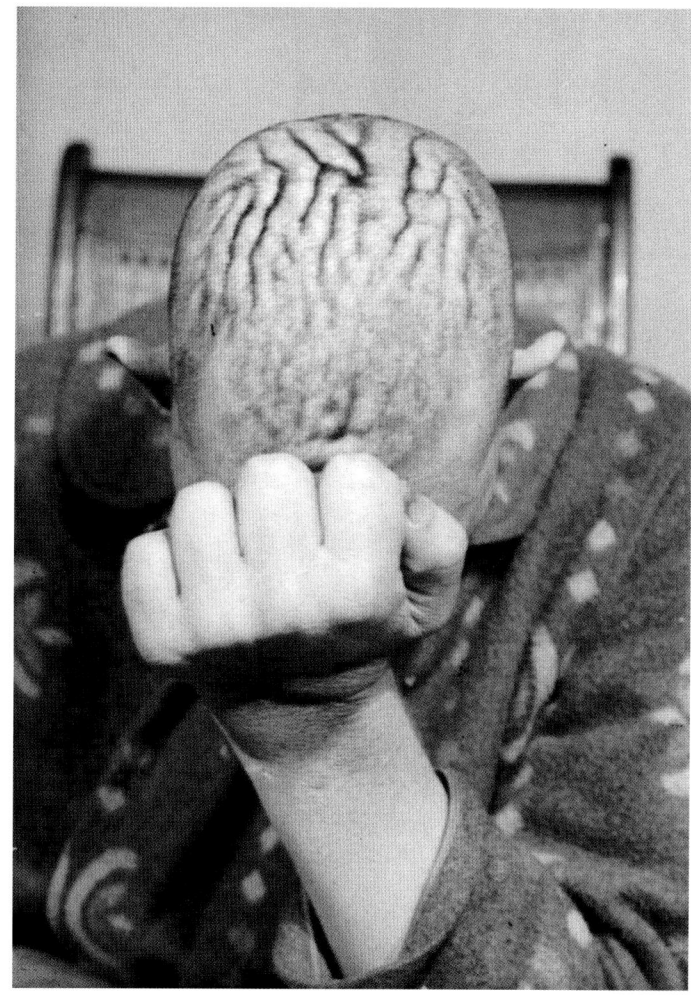

FIGS. 2 AND 3. PREOPERATIVE.

HISTORY

The patient suffered from marked acromegaly since 1904. In October of 1910, he underwent a transsphenoidal operation for sellar decompression followed by a second stage operation in January of 1911 by Dr. Cushing at the Johns Hopkins Hospital.

SUMMARY OF POSITIVE FINDINGS
September 16, 1914
Dr. Rand

SUBJECTIVE
1. Skeletal changes – marked acromegalic changes since 1904
2. Failing vision – left eye 12 years; totally blind about 5 years. Right eye about 8 years.
3. Frontal and temporal pain in the head, relieved by operation 4 years ago.
4. Asthenia, very noticeable past 10-11 years.
5. Decrease in libidosexualis – past 5-6 years.
6. Decrease in amount of hirsutes – past 4-5 years.
7. Constipation – past 10 years.
8. Difficulty in keeping warm.

OBJECTIVE
1. Weight 248 lbs; height 201 cm.
2. Patient is a man of gigantic proportions showing marked evidences of acromegaly. The hands and feet are particularly large, the bones of the skull are massive, and the jaw shows marked prognathism.

OPPOSITE PAGE. FIG. I. PREOPERATIVE.

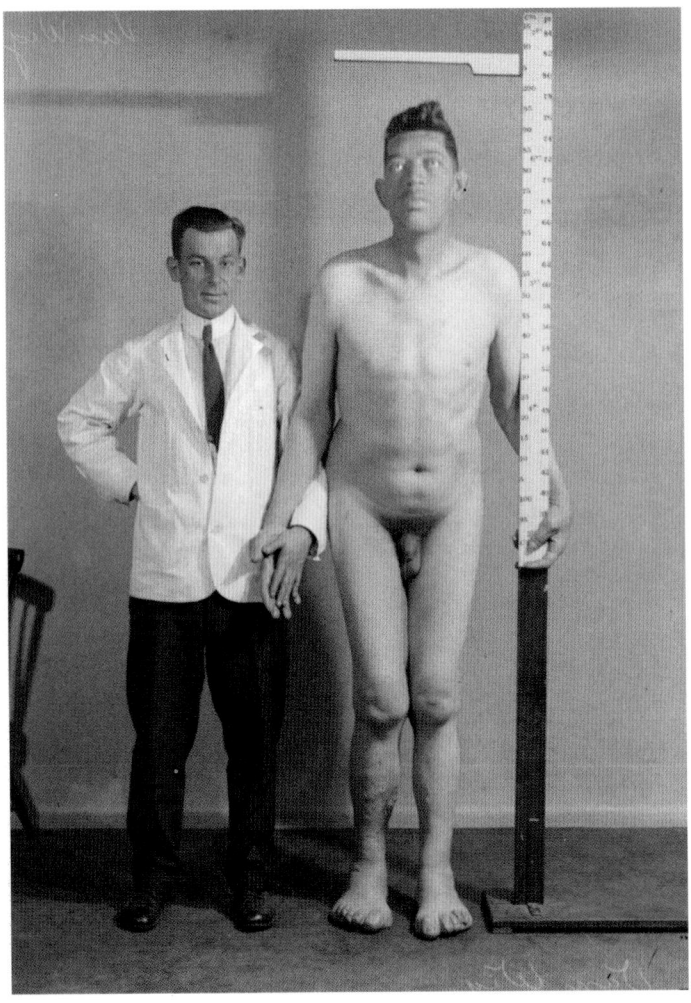
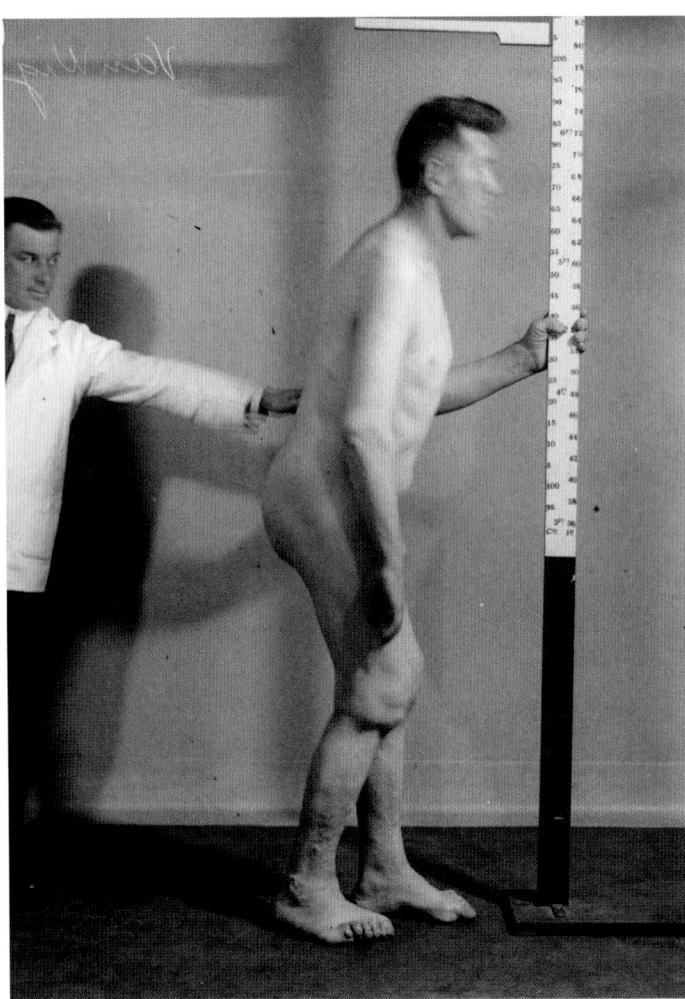

FIGS. 4 AND 5. PREOPERATIVE.

3. There is a rather small distribution of fine hair over the thighs, legs and forearms.
4. Cranial nerves
   II – optic – recognizes light from dark, otherwise no vision.
   Fundus OU – Disc level – outlines distinct. Pallor very marked. Lamina cribrosa and cupping normal. Arteries and veins not enlarged or tortuous. No new tissue.
   III – Right pupil larger than left, both regular – do not react.
   VI – Weakness of left 6th
   VII – Right naso-labial fold smoothed out.

RADIOLOGY REPORT
September 19, 1914

The examination of the skull shows thickening of the soft tissue of face and calvarium. In the frontal and parietal region the thickness of the skull is 15-18 mm. In the occipital region it is 6-10 mm. The cortex is thin, the cancellous tissue is very developed. The frontal sinus is very large in size within it are to be seen many wavy lines and considerable amount of cloudiness. The floor of the anterior fossa is considerably foreshortened. The cerebral impressions are only slightly increased. The lambdoid suture is faintly visible. The venous channels are moderately enlarged. The occipital protuberance is not enlarged, the mandible shows marked prognathism. The sella shows enormous enlargement, the antero-posterior diameter is about 40 mm, it is about 30 mm deep. The floor of the sella is below the level of the middle fossa. The sphenoidal sinus is large. The anterior clinoid processes are indistinct and atrophic. The dorsum and posterior clinoid processes are represented by a thin atrophic shadow. The fossa shows the presence of especially near the floor, a fairly dense mottling.

The skeleton of the hand is very large, the distal phalanges show hyperostosis (typical mushroom-

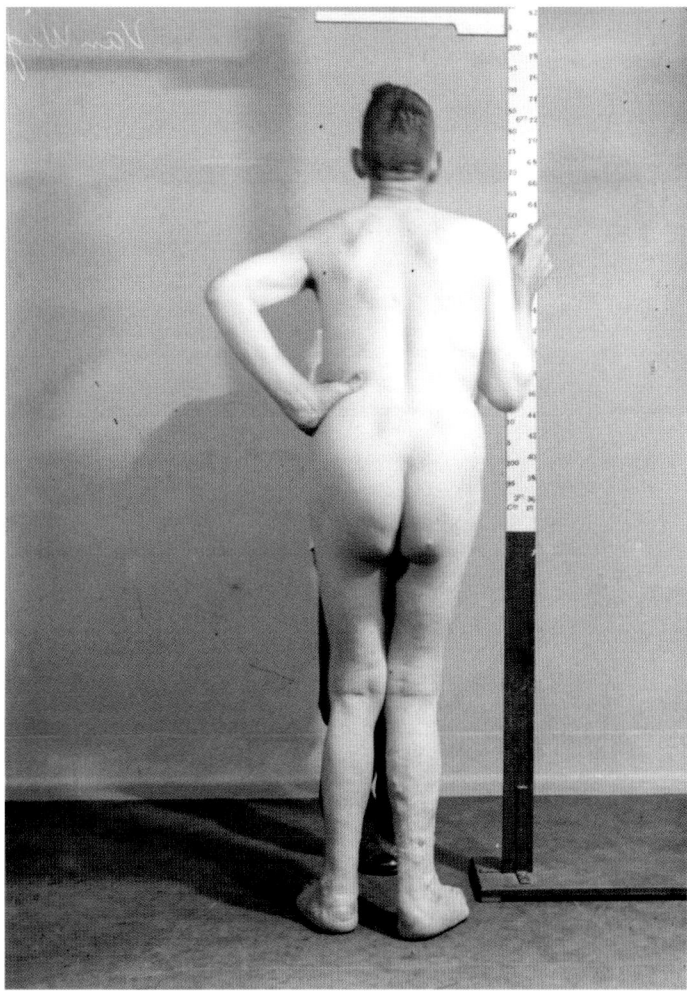 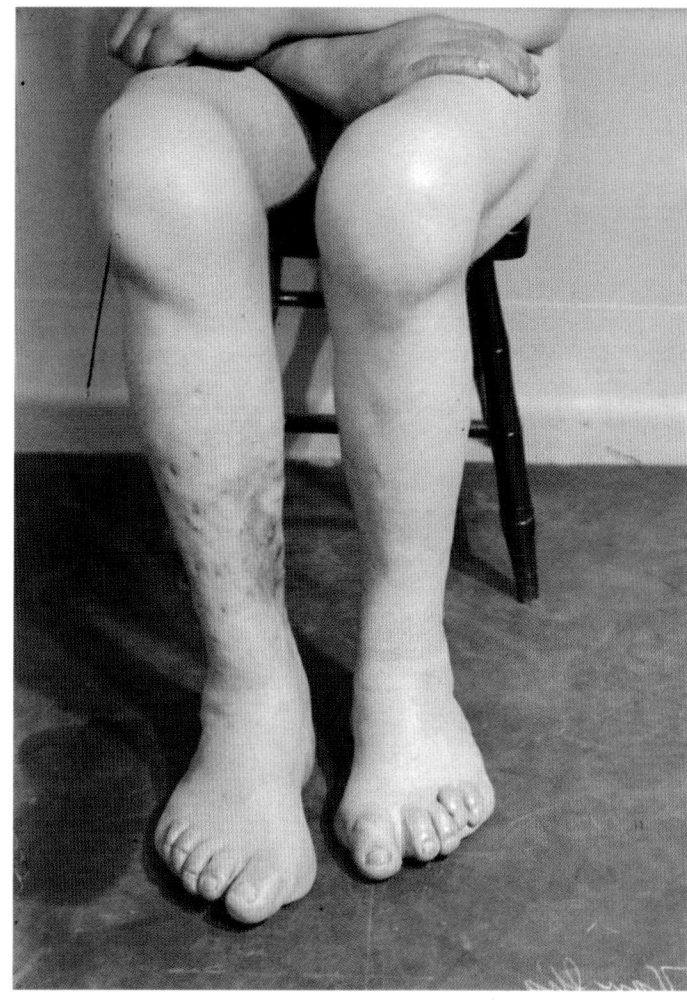

FIGS. 6 AND 7. PREOPERATIVE.

ing). A moderate amount of hyperostosis exists near the articular surfaces of the phalanges. There are no traces of epiphyseal lines in the distal end of the radius and ulna. The skeleton of the foot shows tremendous enlargement especially of the epiphyseal end of the phalanges. There is a subluxation of the proximal joint of the fifth toe.

September 23, 1914
Dr. Cushing
 Fundi: Glistening primary atrophy without any evidence of oedema. Lamina cribrosa clear and apparent. No new tissue.

IMPRESSION: from extra-cranial appearances there must be pressure. Venules in eye-lids very full. Other than for headaches, lowering of vision, increased asthenia, condition very much as in Baltimore. Asymmetry of skull with prominence of left malar bone. Greater exophthalmos left than right.

OPERATIVE NOTE
September 24, 1914
Anaesthesia – Ether – Miss Boothby

Right Sided Decompression.

Nothing unusual in the performance for the enormous field and the fact that the temporal bone was exceedingly thin. A very large defect was made and the dura was opened with an abundant escape of cerebrospinal fluid. Nevertheless, there was some tension even with this loss of fluid and I am encouraged to believe that the indications were clear for a relief of pressure by this means. It may be said that several large mastoid cells over the ear were opened and occluded with wax.

 Closure as usual in layers.

(Dr. Cushing)

POSTOPERATIVE NOTE
September 26, 1914
Dr. Rand

First dressing. Patient made an excellent operative recovery. Slightly irrational on evening of operation, and considerably drowsy the following day. This morning quite talkative; complains of headache. Temperature, pulse and respiration normal. All stitches removed by Dr. Cushing. Excellent approximation of wound margins. No reddening or injection. Silver foil and gauze collodion dressing.

December 9, 1914
Dr. Towne

It has been noticed for several days that he does not use his right arm quite as well as formerly, and on investigation it is found that he cannot put his hand on top of his head. The right deltoid muscle is very weak, and the trouble seems to be mainly here. Other motion of arm done fairly well though not as strong as left side. Visual hallucinations. These have been going on for about a week, and have just been spoken of by patient. He has been much troubled with rumbling of gas in his intestines, and frequently at this time he sees animals such as elephants, donkeys, tigers, etc., on the wall. As the story was given to the writer, three were always to patient's right, but when questioned by Dr. Cushing yesterday he said that there were not at one side particularly, that he saw them both to right and left.

February 15, 1915
Dr. Cushing

The patient has had of late recurring attacks of his severe cephalgia with vomiting and has strongly petitioned for operative relief. This, his father now has just returned from the West, also desires.

On Feb. 13, he was prepared for operation, but was in bad condition—having copious periods of projectile vomiting. Operation postponed.

OPERATIVE NOTE
February 15, 1915
Anaesthesia—Ether—Miss Boothby

Second Transsphenoidal Approach to Sella.

Impossible to Remove Sella Contents Owing to Calcareous Tissue.

The anesthetic was taken well and the approach to the sella was made with thorough removal of the medium septum. Structures were identified and the old opening in the base of the sella was opened. This was enlarged, but instead of meeting a soft struma or a cyst as had been hoped, a bony growth was found occupying the lower part of the sella with only here and there a small pocket of glandular tissue. Some small bits of this tissue were removed for study, but it was impossible with the delicate pituitary rongeurs to clean out the rest of the fossa. A study of the x-ray made it apparent that the lower third of the greatly enlarged fossa was possibly shown to be ossified or calcareous. There is a more or less definite shadow which had not been previously interpreted as the shadow of any calcareous structures.

The operation lasted an undue length of time and patient's condition at the end was rather poor. In view of the failure to secure pressure relief and in view of his previous condition, the operative prognosis is bad.

(Dr. Cushing)

POSTOPERATIVE NOTE
February 15, 1915
Dr. Towne

He made a quite well recovery. Temperature, pulse and respiration normal.

February 16, 1915
Dr. Towne

Patient became extremely restless. Pulse and temperature began to go up. Much mucus collected in throat, but drained well when he was put on side. On 1 p.m. he was sweating profusely. Temperature 107°, pulse 150 irregular and thready. Respiration with periods of apnea, but not typical Cheyne-Stokes. His color became progressively cyanotic. He died 3:40 a.m. due to respiratory arrest.

Continued on page 16.

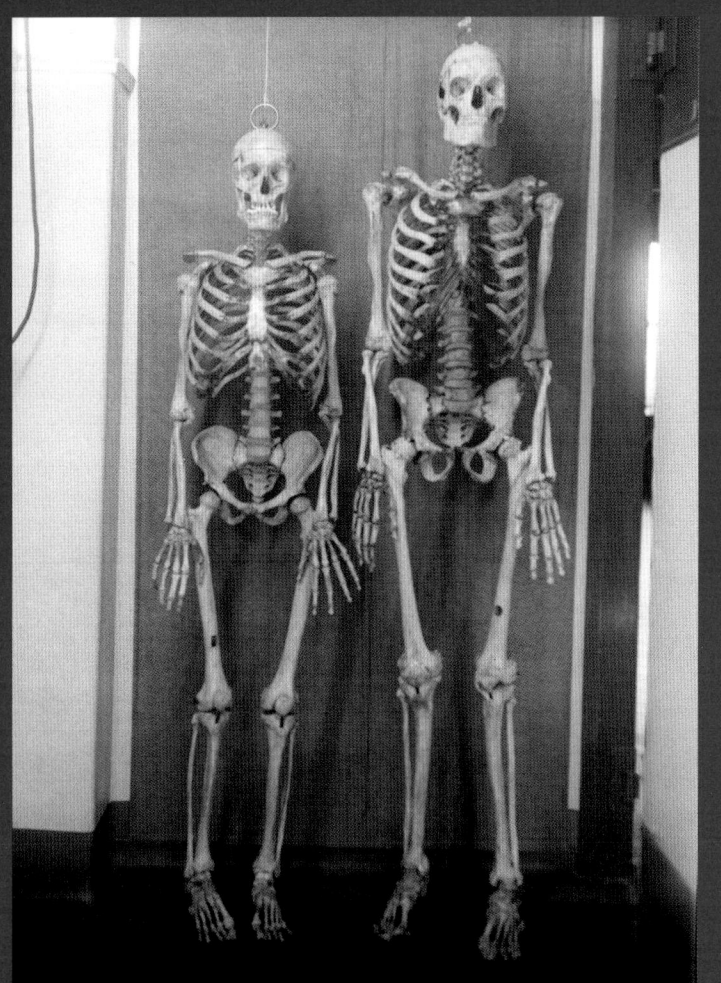
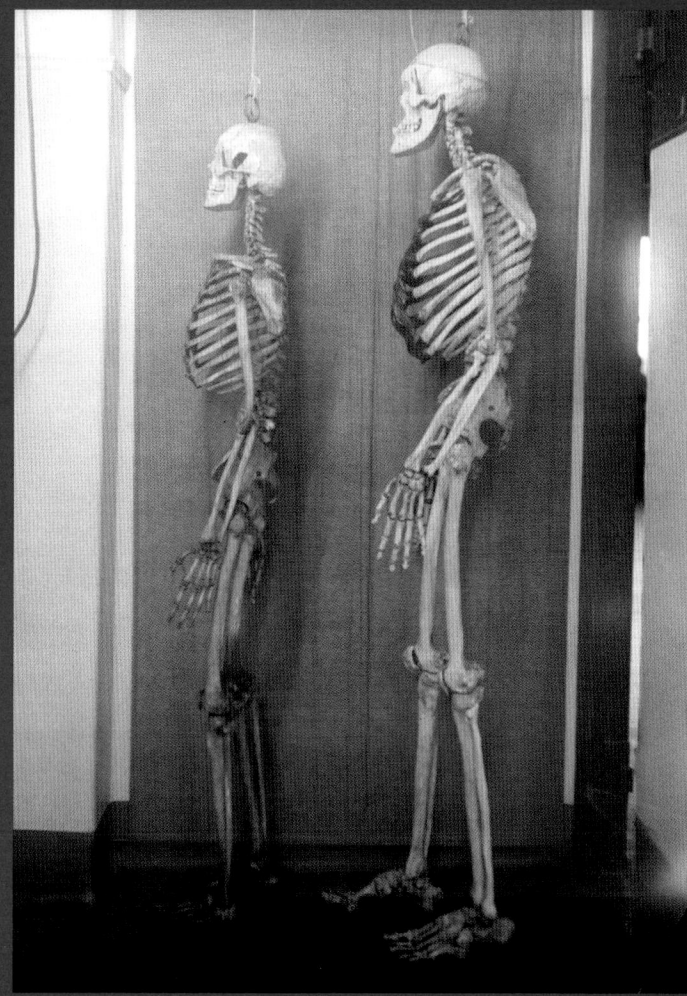

FIGS. 8 AND 9. SKELETON OF PATIENT (RIGHT, EACH PHOTO) COMPARED WITH NORMAL SKELETON (LEFT, EACH PHOTO).

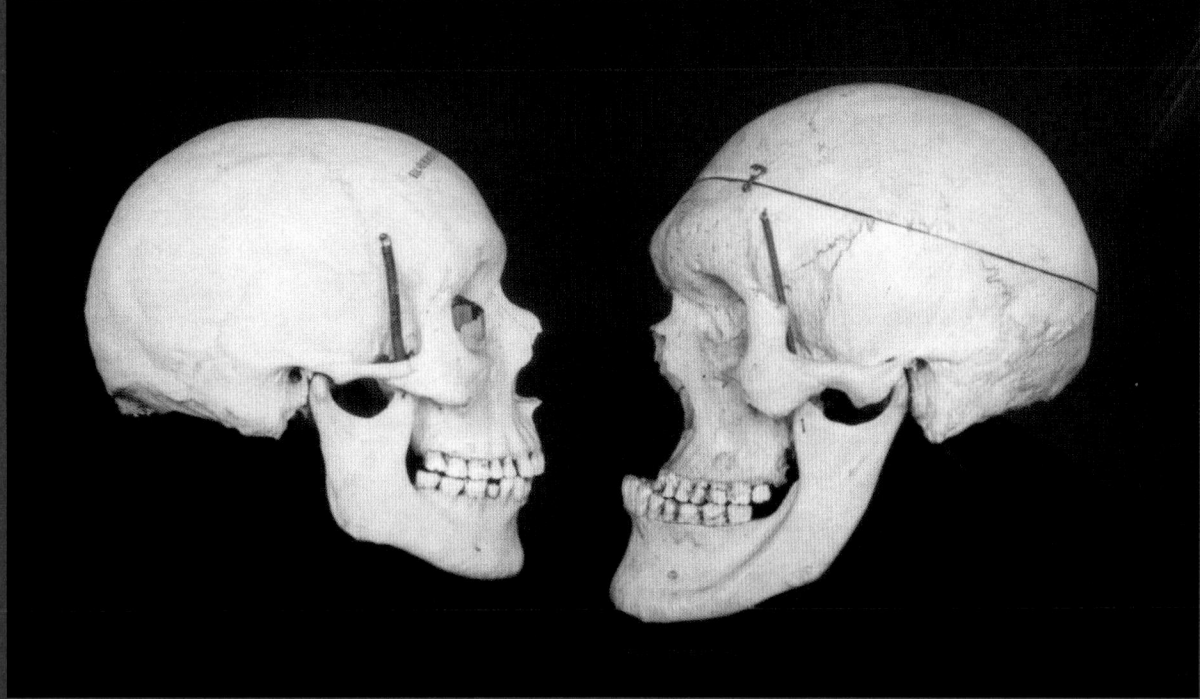

FIG. 10. SKULL OF PATIENT (RIGHT) COMPARED WITH NORMAL SKULL (LEFT).

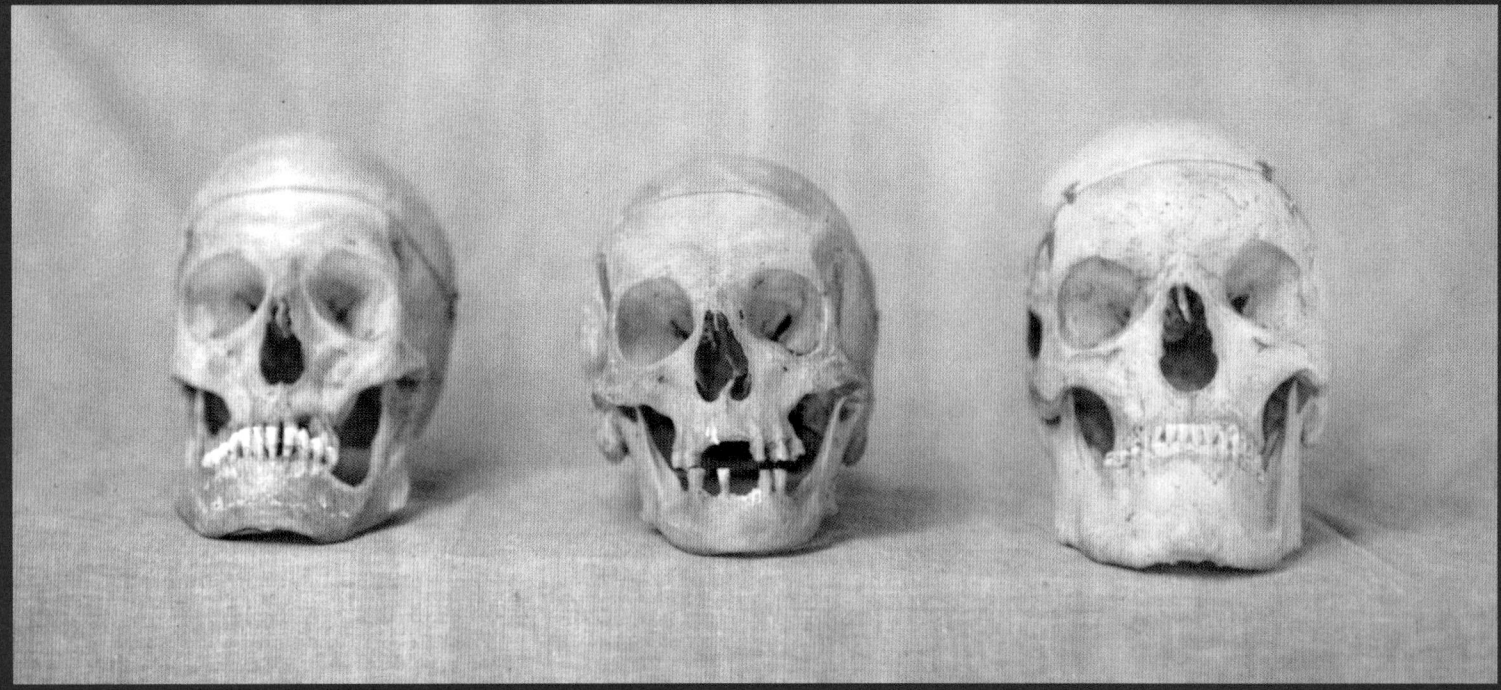

FIG. 11. SKULL OF PATIENT (RIGHT) COMPARED WITH SKULL OF ANOTHER PATIENT WITH ACROMEGALY (LEFT) AND A NORMAL SKULL (CENTER).

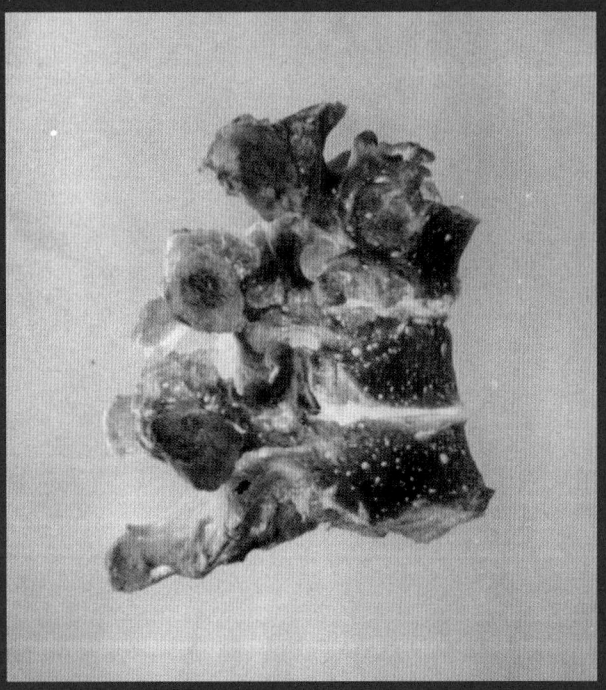
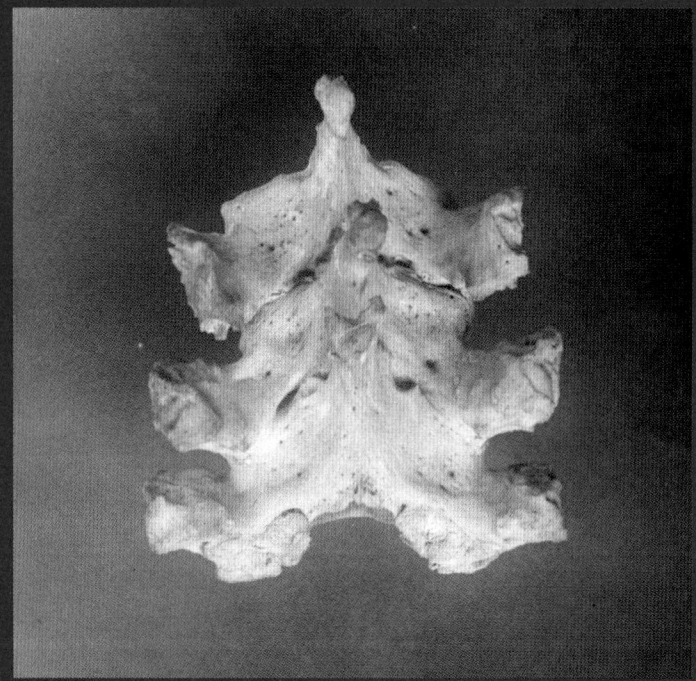

FIGS. 12 AND 13. SEBMENTS OF SPINE.

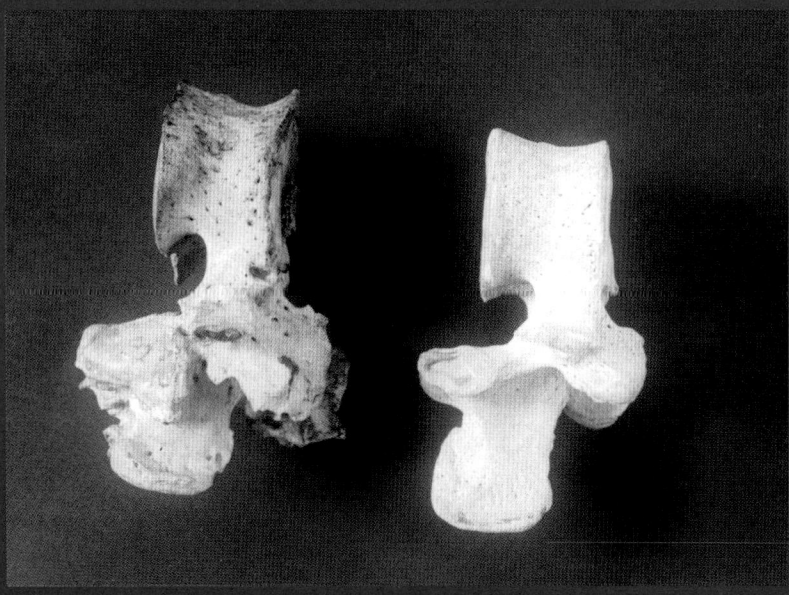

FIG. 14. LUMBAR VERTEBRAE OF PATIENT (LEFT) COMPARED WITH NORMAL LUMBAR VERTEBRAE (RIGHT).

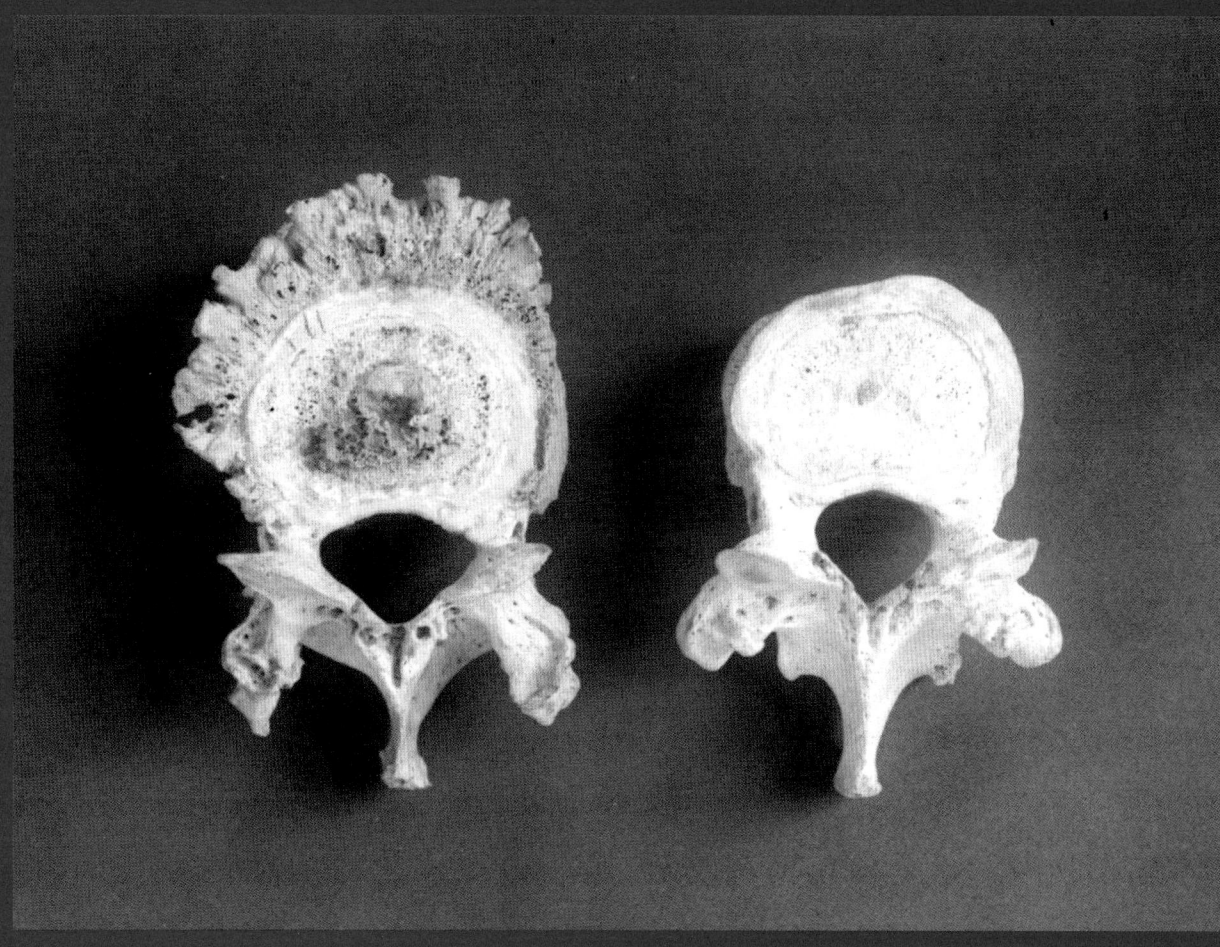

LEFT: FIG. 15. LUMBAR VERTEBRAE OF PATIENT (LEFT) COMPARED WITH NORMAL LUMBAR VERTEBRAE (RIGHT).

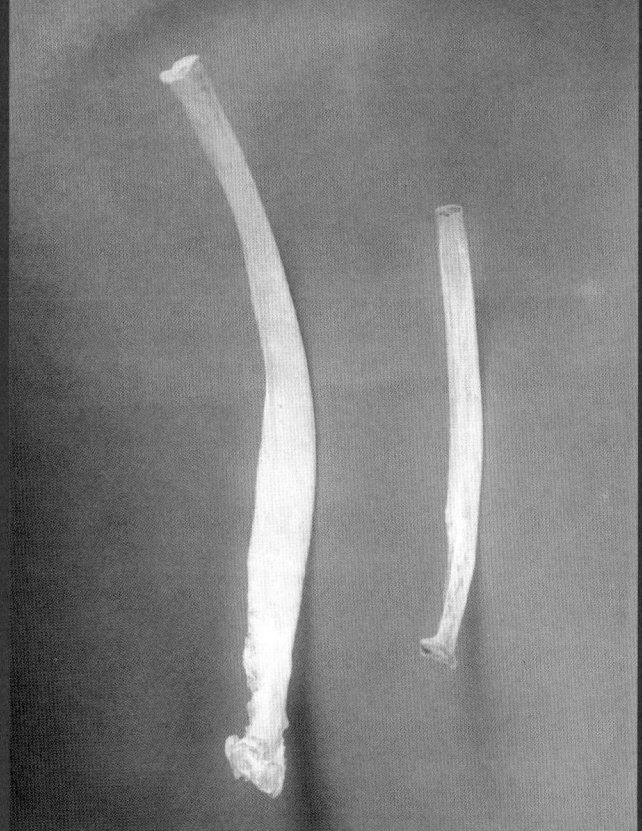

ABOVE: FIG. 16. 11TH RIB OF PATIENT (LEFT) COMPARED WITH NORMAL 11TH RIB (RIGHT).

AT RIGHT: FIG. 17. CLAVICLE OF PATIENT (LEFT) COMPARED WITH NORMAL CLAVICLE (RIGHT).

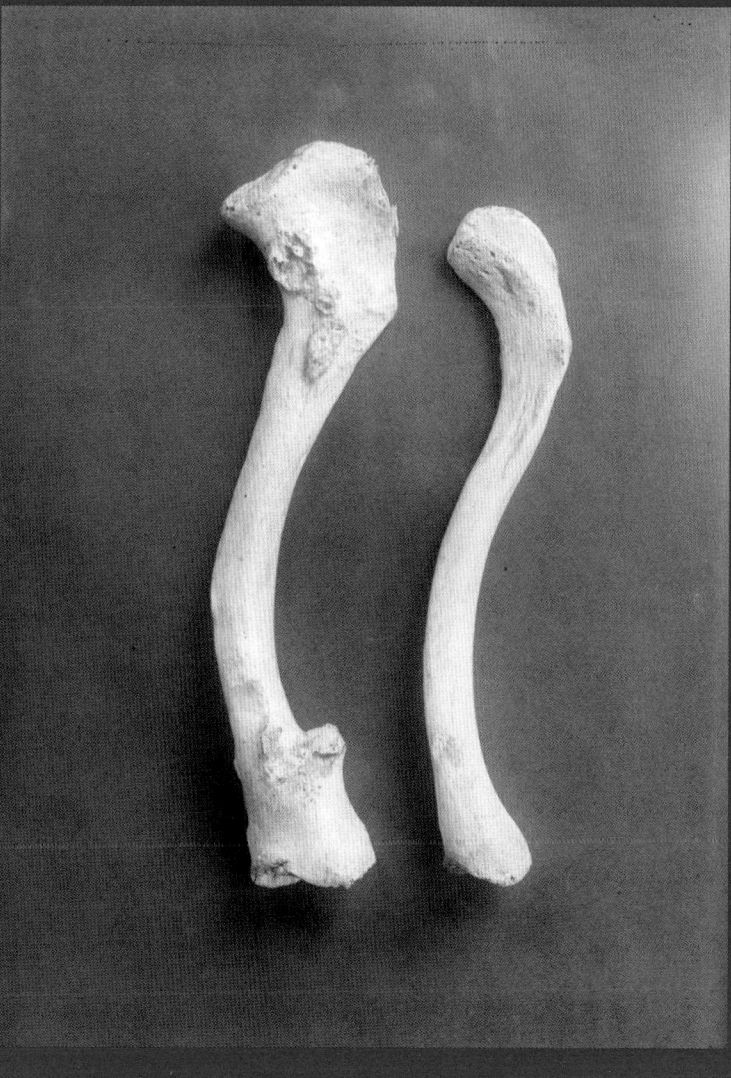

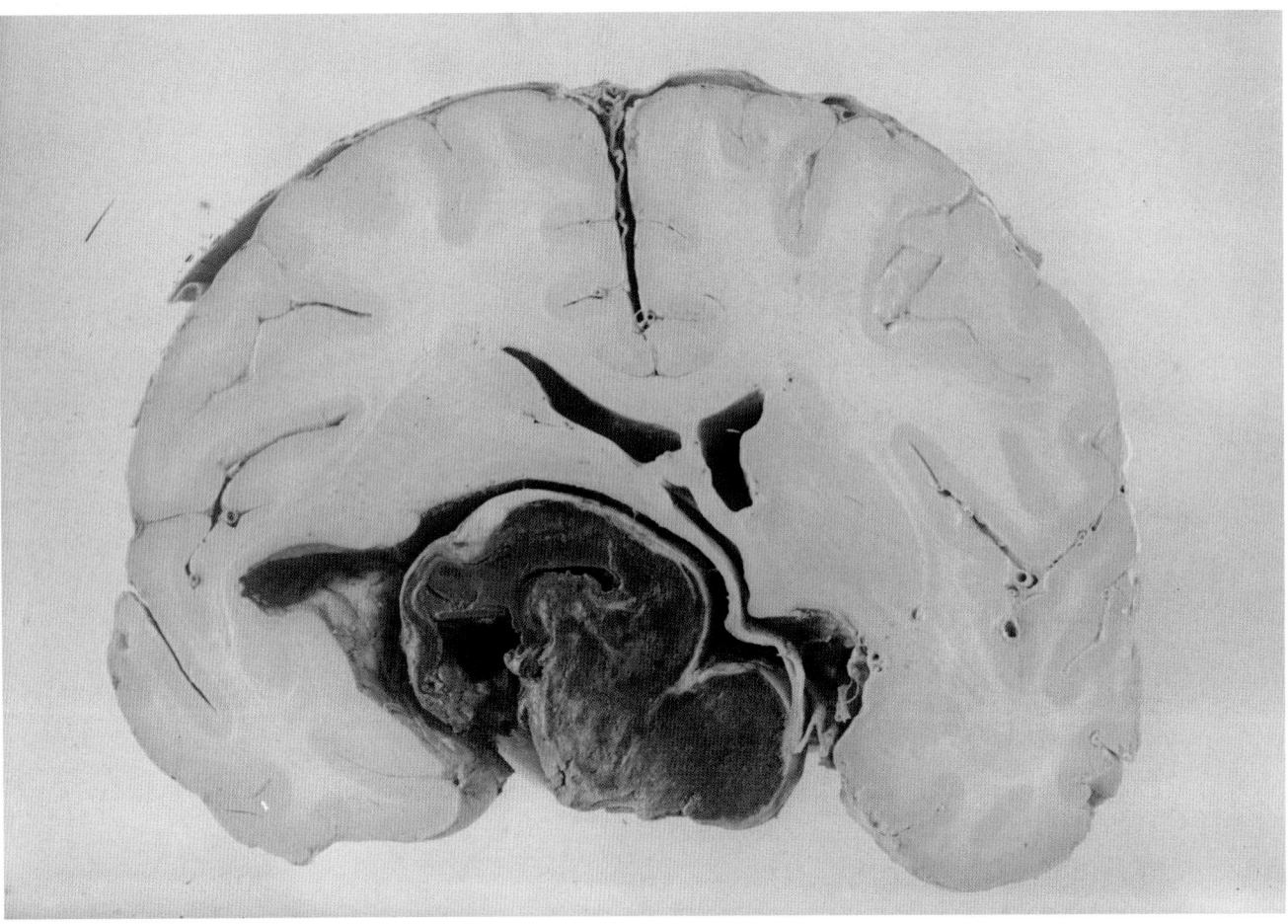

FIG. 18. AUTOPSY BRAIN SPECIMEN.

AUTOPSY REPORT
February 17, 1915

DIAGNOSES
Adenoma of hypophysis with extension to base of brain and temporal lobe.
Acromegaly.
Hypertrophy of viscera, liver, kidneys, intestines, spleen.
Fibrosis of prostate.
Fibrosis of epididymis.
Hyperplasia with active degenerative changes involving lymph nodes of neck, mediastinum, mesenteric, follicles of intestinal tract.

On removal of the brain the optic nerves were seen to extend over the mass as much thinned ribbon-like bands. They were apparently under considerable tension.

SELLA

The tumor adherent to the sella removed in fragments, in order to preserve the bony characteristics. The normal appearance of the sella is almost completely obliterated. The tumor lies in the fossa, which is 6.5 cm in breadth, as measured from the anterior clinoid processes and 5.5 cm posteriorly as measured from the posterior clinoid processes. The anterior clinoid on the left, also that on the right, seem that occasional exostosis is present, more marked on the left. The posterior clinoid processes are apparently completely obliterated on the right, remains on left. The dorsum sella is greatly enlarged and presented above the posterior clinoid process some 2.5 cm. It is markedly thinned out ... a roughened osseous mass projects along the inner aspect. In its ... portion it is perforated by numerous apertures through which a dark mass protrudes, extending through into the posterior fossa, as rather dark bulging tumors, 1 to 2 cm in diameter. In protrusion of the dorsum especially in the region of the apertures, and a little above, the mass is very much thinned and very friable. The depth of the site of the tumor varies considerably, on an average 3 cm below the level of the superior portion of the inferior clinoids. Slightly to the left of the midline a ridge extends from the olivary eminence of the ethmoid posterior to dorsum. This consists of a conglomarete mass of exostoses, giving roughened bony surface. It measures roughly 2 cm in diameter and gradually tapering as it extends posteriorly. The left carotid is seen coming through the foramen, just to the left junction of the ridge described, and the dorsum sella. Tumor extends lateral-ward from the bony mass above described. The mass projects into the tip of the temporal lobe. On the right the tumor mass extends about 2.5 cm from the median line, extending down inferiorly to the soft palate. This aperture is roughly 2 cm and its margins are roughened, due undoubtedly to operation. At one edge of the opening exostoses project upward. On this side tumor mass does not extend as far into the temporal lobe. The tumor, as removed, from the fossa above described, and as shown on photograph, is of practically uniform appearance, is dark brown (fixation), fairly firm, and suggests a mass of blood clot.

BRAIN

Section made approximately 3 cm posterior to the tips of the temporal lobe. The cut surface shows a large mass, about 5.5 cm in width, and pushing lateral ward both temporal lobes, and extending to base on the left to a level slightly below the lateral sinus, practically replacing the optic thalamus. The lateral sinus on the left is almost obliterated, on right is considerably compressed. The tumor all ways pushed the gray matter in the region of the right thalamus. The 3rd ventricle is greatly distorted. The cerebral tissue of the temporal lobes, approximately yellow, due undoubtedly to blood pigment. Section taken at the mammary bodies shows no tumor mass on the left, on the right from the median line lateral ward, running backward in the ... for a distance of about 2 cm, one sees the same characteristics. The thalamus and the external capsule above this tumor are considerably distorted.

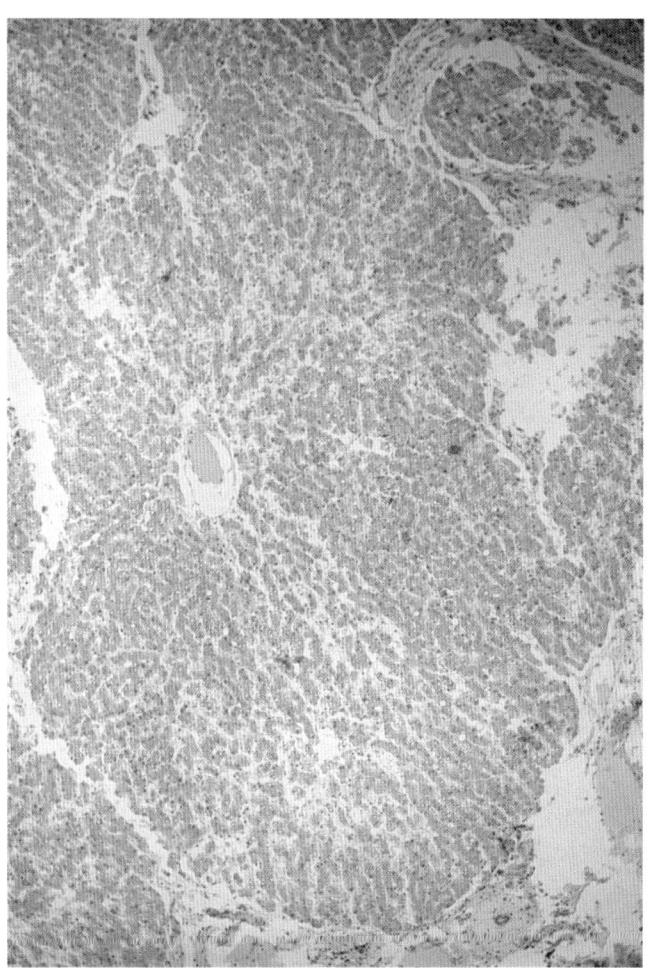
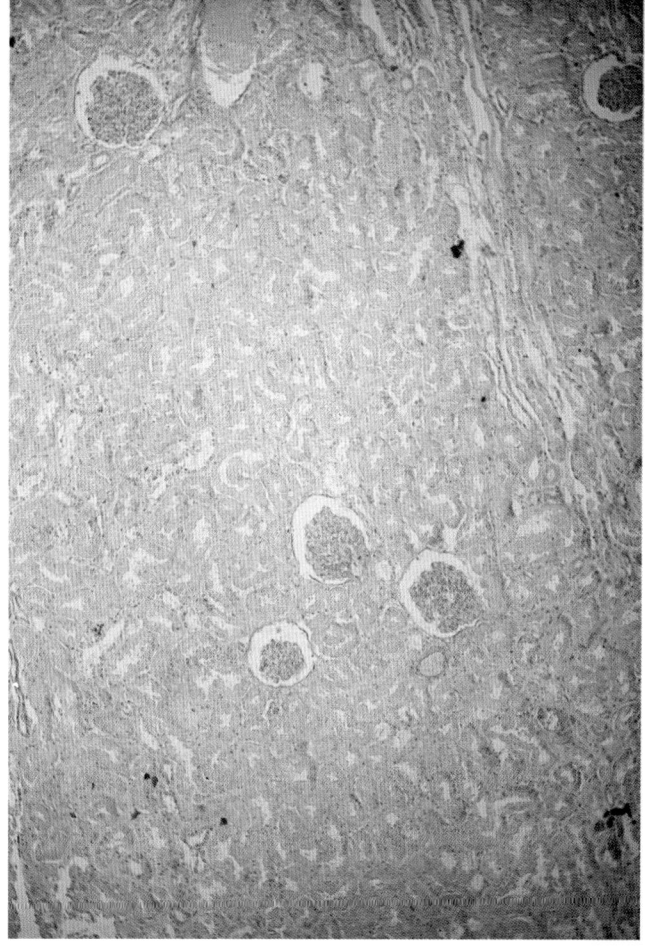

FIG. 19 AND 20. HISTOLOGY SLIDES.

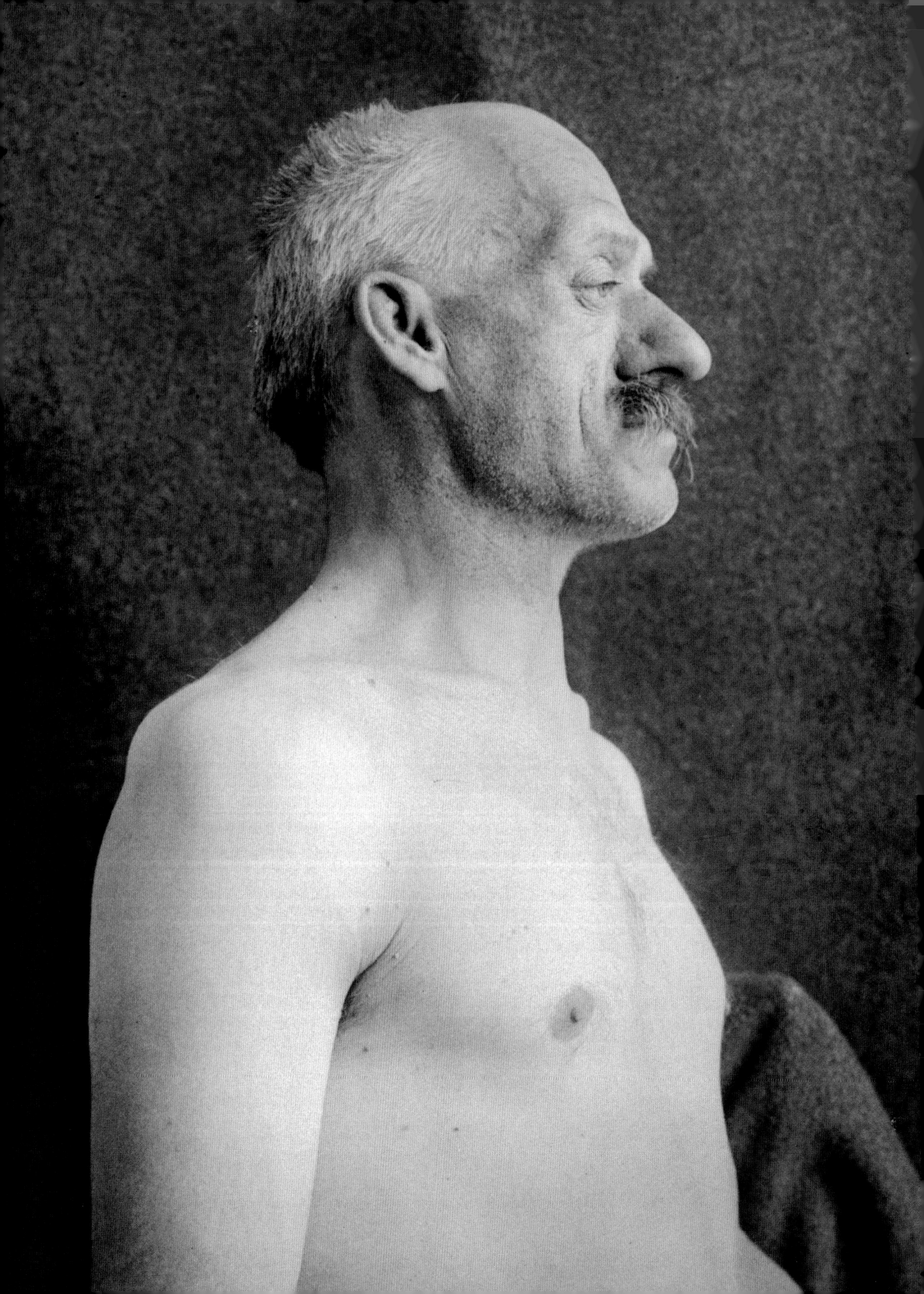

1.2 Pituitary adenoma

SEX: M; AGE: 47; SURG. NO. 1140

DIAGNOSIS: *Acromegaly, pituitary tumor.*

Transsphenoidal decompression and radiotherapy (radium implant.)

Death four years later. Autopsy revealed a large occipital endothelioma.

HISTORY

This patient suffered from "feeling of pressure" in his head and progressive acromegalic changes in his features –20 years duration.

SUMMARY OF POSITIVE FINDINGS
April 11, 1914
Dr. Rand

SUBJECTIVE
1. Feeling of pressure in head for 20 years.
2. Pain in the hands beginning 20 years ago and lasting intermittently for 10 years.
3. Skeletal changes, onset 20 years ago with enlargement of head, hands, feet, both legs and loss in height.
4. Neuralgia of right side of face for 2 years.
5. Rheumatism in right knee for 2 years.
6. Polydipsia and polyuria for 2-3 years.
7. Vomiting during the past 6 months.

OBJECTIVE
1. Changes in the skeletal configuration.
   a. General posture suggestive of Paget's disease.
   b. Skull – large calvarium, prognathism, prominence of supra-orbital ridges, malar bones, and occipital protuberance. Coarseness of features, especially nose.
   c. Hands and feet – typical spade-like appearance with increase in subcutaneous structures. Similar changes in feet.
   d. Pelvis – increase in breadth with thickening of the iliac crests and eversion of the ext. lips. Shortening of distance between lower margin of ribs and iliac crests. Protuberant abdomen.
   e. Bowing of both femora and tibiae with increase in massiveness in these bones.

RADIOLOGY REPORT
April 14, 1914

The skull shows a very high degree of thickening especially in the frontal and parietal region. The thickening of the skull is about 20 mm in the anterior aspect and 5-6 mm in the posterior aspect. The

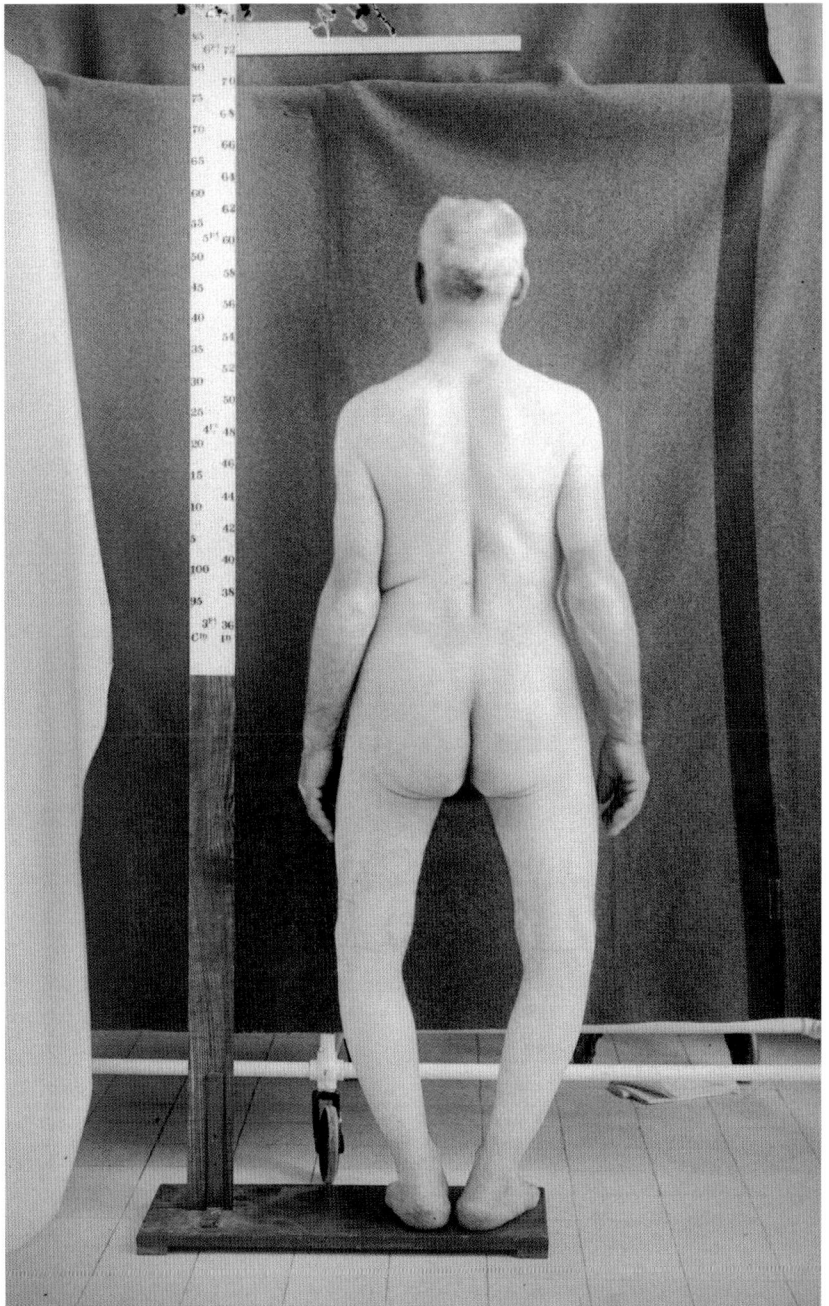

FIG. 2. PREOPERATIVE.

OPPOSITE PAGE. FIG. 1. PREOPERATIVE.

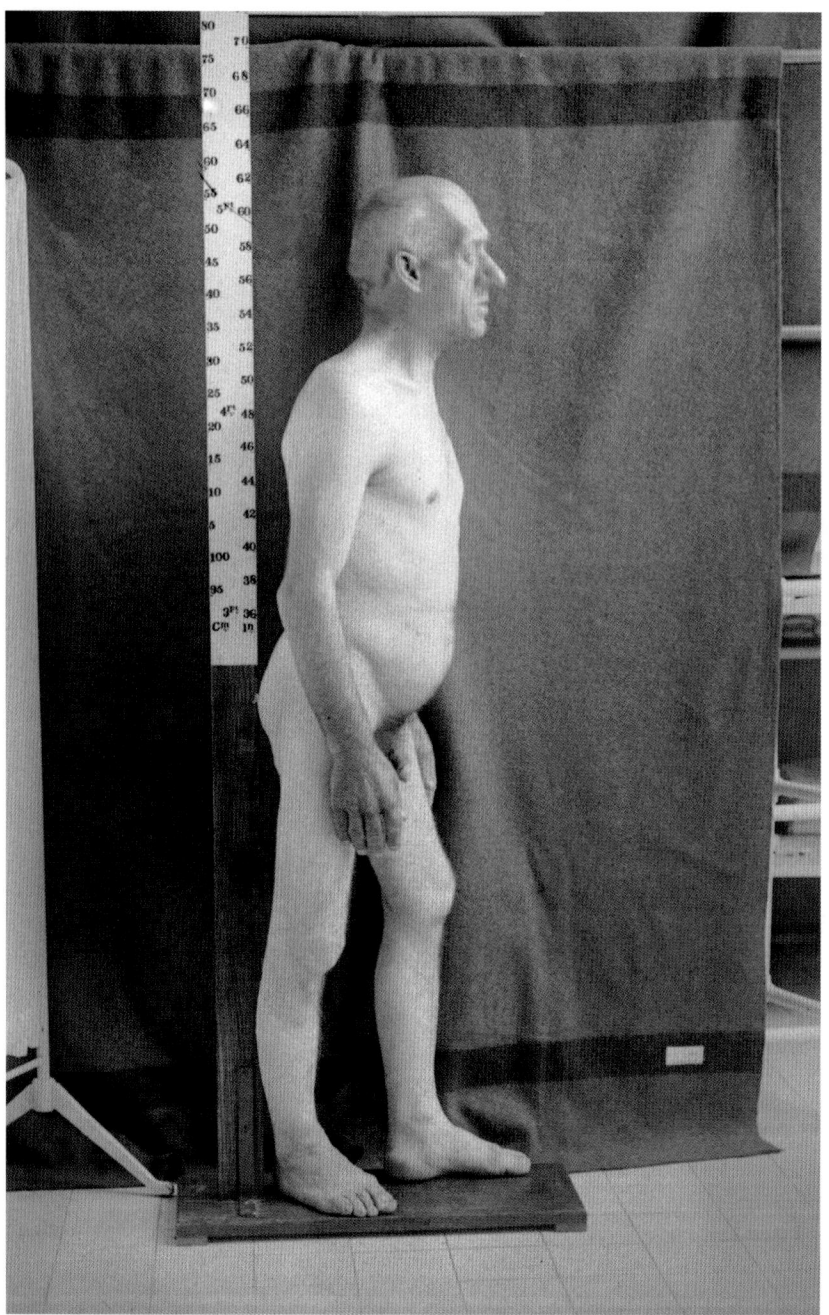

FIG. 2. PREOPERATIVE.

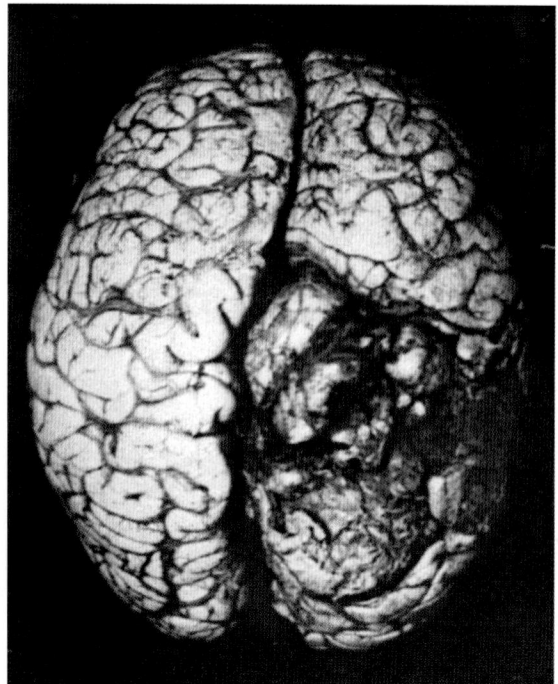

FIG. 4. AUTOPSY (MENINGIOMA)

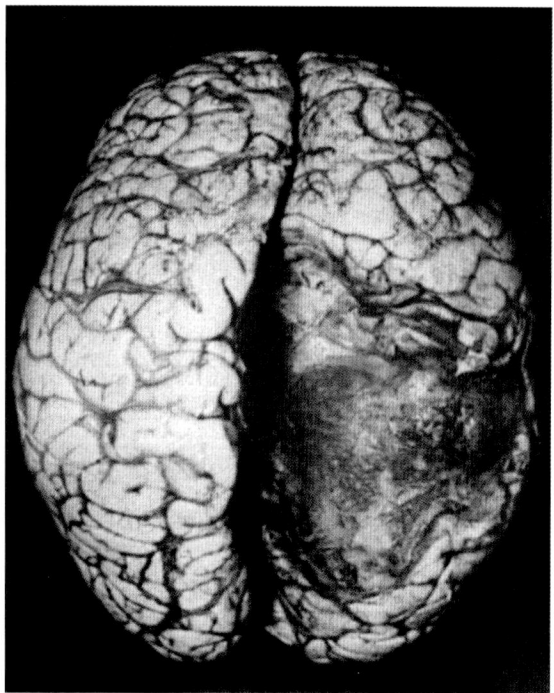

FIG. 4. AUTOPSY (MENINGIOMA REMOVED)

corticalis is rather thin. The cancellous tissue is very well developed. In the parietal region it shows definite hyperostosis. The frontal sinus is abnormally large. The inner surface of the skull is rather uneven, there are however no signs of increased intracranial pressure. The sella turcica is abnormally large. The largest anterior posterior diameter is 22 mm. The sella is shown more than 20 mm deep. The floor of the sella turcica is below the level of the middle fossa. The dorsum sella shows a very definite thickening. The posterior clinoid are indistinct. The anterior clinoid processes are well defined. There is a suggestion of calcified connection between anterior and posterior processes. The sphenoidal cells form the anterior aspect of the floor of the sella. The posterior aspect of the floor cannot be seen.

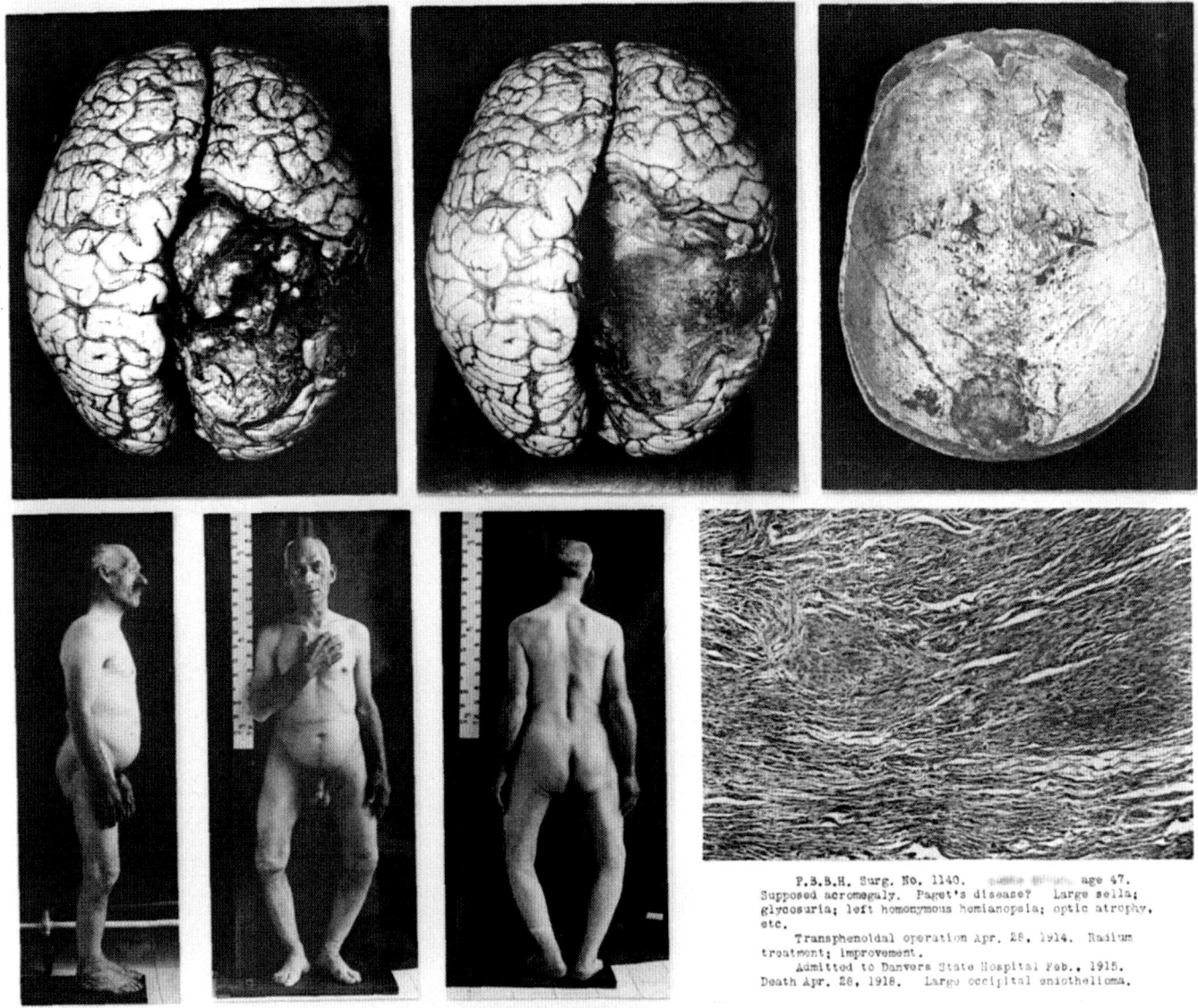

FIG. 5. CUSHING'S TEACHING SLIDE.

The hands and both feet show very definite hyperostotic changes of acromegalic type.

OPERATIVE NOTE
April 28, 1914
Anaesthesia- Ether-intratracheal-Dr. Boothby

Attempted Transsphenoidal Operation Abandoned as Decompression.

The usual sub-labial transsphenoidal approach conducted without great difficulty. The membrane on the right side was torn, but the other remained intact. The median septum was cleared away down to the ant. wall of the sphenoidal cells. An unusually good exposure of the cells was made.

The anterior wall of the cells was removed, exposing the base of a large sella turcica. The bony floor of which was intact and was removed piece-meal.

The bulging dura was incised in linear direction, but at the posterior margin a bleeding point was encountered which made further manipulation impossible. It was necessary to place a pledget of gauze on this point in order to check bleeding, as soon as the gauze was removed bleeding recurred again. A cross incision was then made in the dural capsule, but every attempt to incise the exposed gland itself led to such an amount of prompt venous bleeding that none of the tissue was actually removed for examination. It was thought bleeding might have come from a hemorrhagic cyst, but there were no cholesterin crystals in the fluid.

Wound was finally closed, a small pledget of gauze being left plastered on the aforementioned bleeding point.

Operation for the members of the Society of International Surgery.

(Dr. Cushing)

POSTOPERATIVE NOTE
April 29, 1914
Dr. Rand

Postoperative course has been favorable thus far. Nasal drains removed and patient has a good draft through each nostril. The usual boric packs have been employed and the nasal drinking cup has been put into use today. Patient has not noticed much change in his physical ability.

OPERATIVE NOTE
May 2, 1914
Anaesthesia-Ether-Dr. Boothby

The wound without difficulty was reopened and the mucous membrane on each side separated exposing the denuded floor of the struma. The small pleget of gauze which was placed at the first operation to control hemorrhage was left in situ as an attempt to remove it caused the same bleeding that had given trouble before.

An attempt to insert a radium tube loaded at its end instead of in its middle as in the case of (the name of another patient), caused bleeding every time the tube was introduced. Finally it was possible to catch it sufficiently in the substance of the gland to hold it, but the introduction was possibly less successful than had been anticipated (judging from the x-ray).

The tube was inserted at 11:00 a.m. and was removed at about 5:00 p.m.

The wound was closed as usual. No complications from the operation.

(Dr. Cushing)

DISCHARGE NOTE
May 16, 1914
Dr. Rand

Patient has been up and about the ward, perfectly himself. There has been no return of the pressure headache and neuralgia on the right side also disappeared.

Vomiting – has not recurred since operation.

Vision – Has improved wonderfully, homonymous defect now entirely disappeared.

Visual fields out to normal. Visual acuity 20/15 O.U.

Urine – He is now putting out 0.3% of sugar on limited ward diet. On admission was putting out 8%.

Patient advised to return every month for observation. Discharged.

REPORT OF DEATH
(four years later)
Danvers State Hospital

Death on April 28, 1918.

Autopsy-A large occipital endothelioma.

Attached you can find the teaching slide related to this patient used by Dr. Cushing during his lectures (Fig. 5).

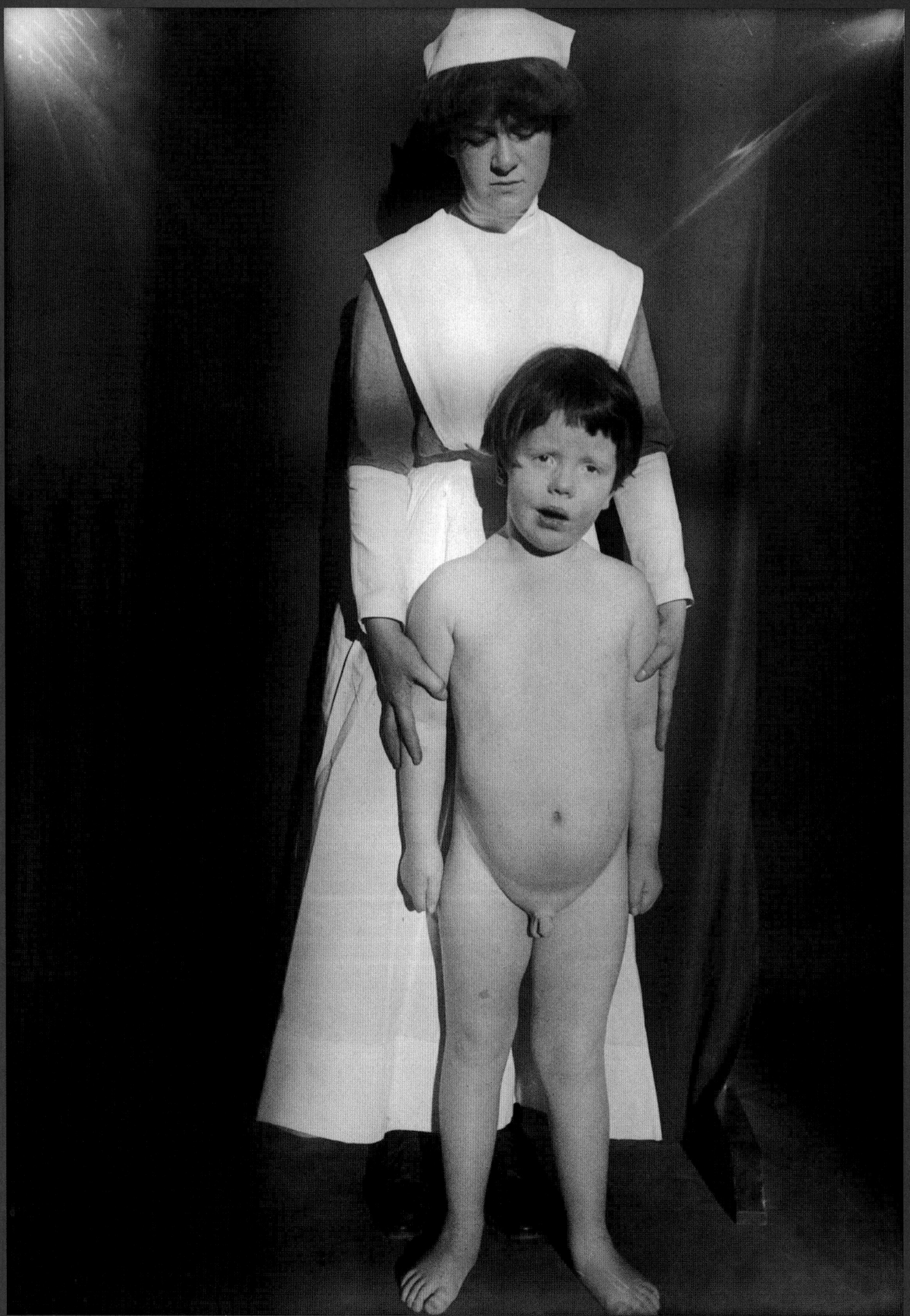

1.3 Optic chiasm glioma

SEX: M; AGE: 4½; SURG. NO. 3951

HISTORY

The child was admitted with the diagnosis of hydrocephalus (unknown etiology.)

COMPLAINT

Loss of vision, vomiting, polyphagia, polydipsia and polyuria.

SUMMARY OF POSITIVE FINDINGS
December 3, 1915
Dr. Horrax

SUBJECTIVE
1. History of malnutrition and delayed development; possible rickets; treatment with thyroid extract for past year with improvement. Mother has goiter.
2. Loss of vision during past year.
3. Polydipsia, 2 to 3 years.
4. Polyphagia, during last year.
5. Polyuria, 5 months.

OBJECTIVE
1. Large boy for his age.
2. Moderate adiposity.
3. Head large (55.5 cm) – hollow percussion noted.
4. Fundi-optic atrophy-bilateral.
5. Dilated veins – scalp and eyelids.
6. Double knock-knee – some uncertainty of gait.

RADIOLOGY REPORT
December 4, 1915

Average thickness of the skull is 3–6 mm. The convolutional impressions are increased. The largest antero-posterior diameter is 20 cm. The coronal suture is distended. The lambdoid suture is faintly seen. The sella is of normal size and shape. The antero-posterior diameter is 10 mm. It is 8 mm deep. The dorsum and clinoid processes are distinct. There are no signs of increased venous or arterial pressure. The development of the skeleton is in advance of the age, corresponding to that of a child 6–8 years. The fibulae are bowed toward the tibiae.

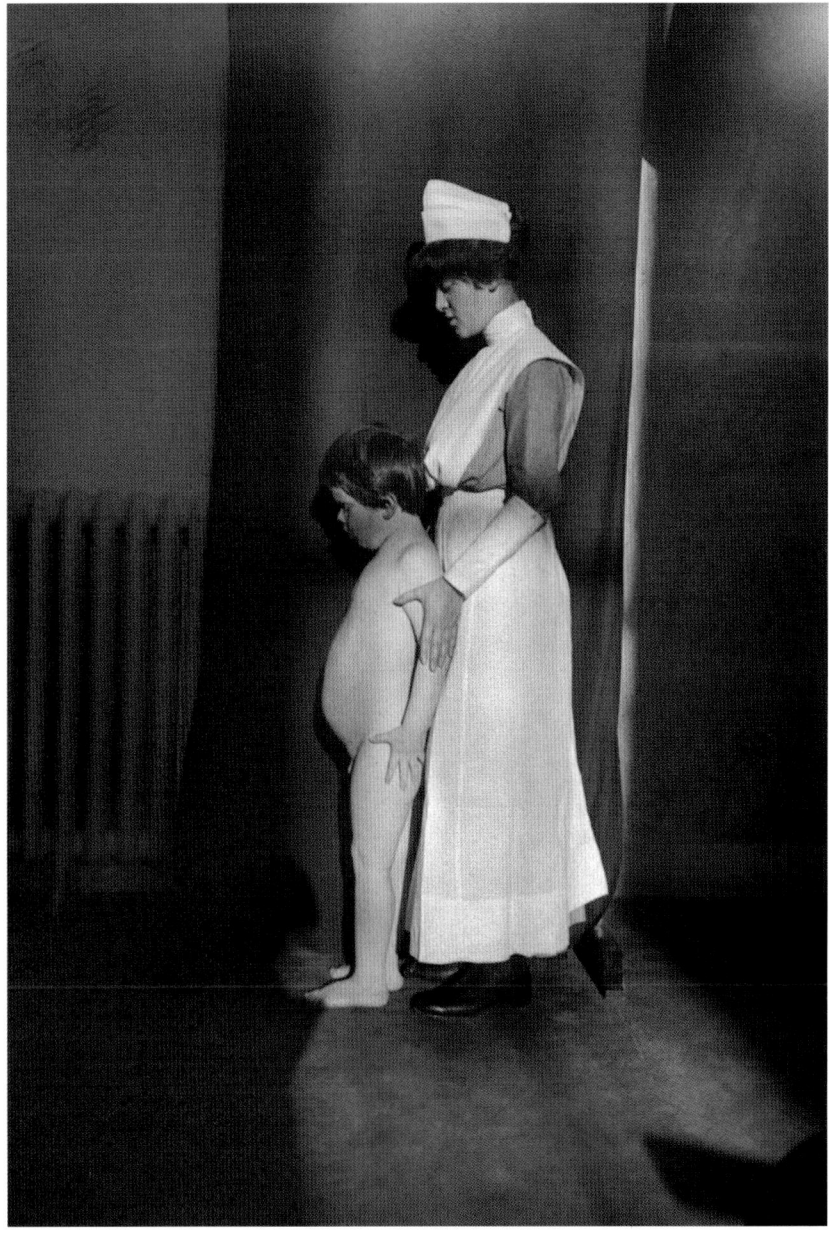

FIG. 2. PREOPERATIVE.

OPERATIVE NOTE
December 20, 1915
Anaesthesia – Ether – Miss Gerrard

Callosal Puncture. Puncture of Ventricle.

A small bone flap was reflected from the vertex of the scalp with the base towards the median line. Dura was opened concentric with the bony opening and a puncture of the right ventricle was made.

OPPOSITE PAGE. FIG. 1. PREOPERATIVE.

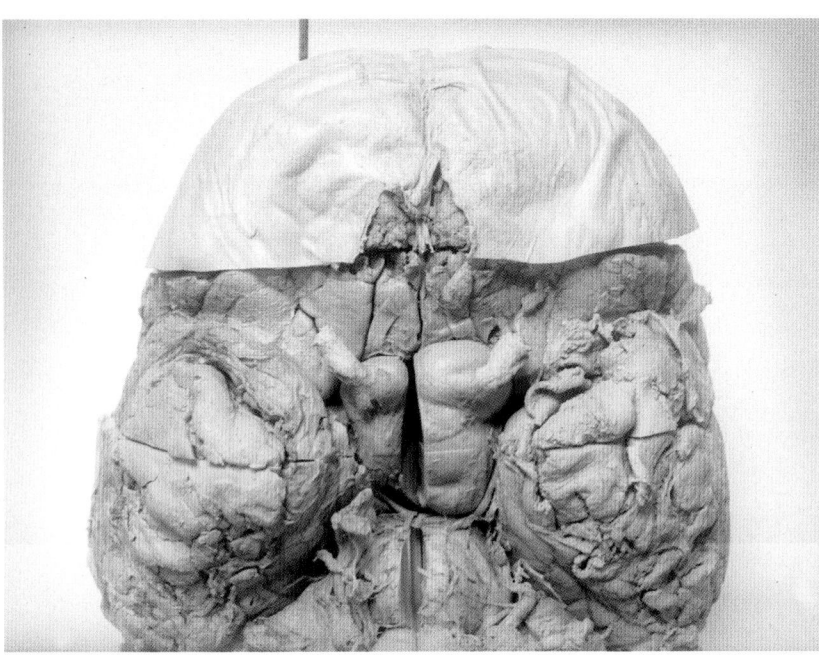

FIG. 3. AUTOPSY SPECIMEN.

It was necessary to introduce the needle a third time before fluid was encountered and then not a large amount was secured.

The straight staphylorrhaphy instrument was then introduced alongside of the falx to a depth of something over 7 cm. and was turned so as to be sure of getting a good opening. A large amount of fluid came out along side of the instrument. In order to make sure that the instrument was in the ventricle, a curved hollow brain needle was then introduced in its place with a free evacuation of the fluid.

Bone flap was replaced and the wound closed as usual in layers.

(Dr. Cushing)

January 14, 1915
Dr. Horrax

Condition unchanged since admission. He sleeps a great deal during the day as well as at night. Urine output cannot be accumulated accurately because he wets the bed frequently.

January 15, 1915

Wassermann reaction: Spinal fluid 2.0 to 0.05 negative

January 15, 1915
Dr. Horrax

Wound clean and edges well approximated. No tenderness nor swelling. All sutures removed. Redressed with silver foil and collodin strips. Patient condition in general is about same as before operation.

DISCHARGE NOTE
January 19, 1915
Dr. Horrax

Condition the same. Wound clean and well healed. Patient remains same as on admission. Discharged.

AUTOPSY NOTE
December 7, 1916
Dr. Cushing

Child's father has brought body in for postmortem examination.

Subsequent history of child after operation and discharge from this hospital. His mental condition improved greatly and he regained his use of speech from more monosyllables to the forming of words into sentences. He remained better until a month or so before death with a happy disposition and free from discomforts. His appetite was ravenous and he was active in all respects though his vision was not regained. Some weeks ago, his appetite began to fall. His mother thought this was due, however, to his tonsils as they were greatly enlarged and diseased. He had a bad fall also 10 days before death, striking his forehead. Whether from this or from his general malnutrition, he began to go down hill

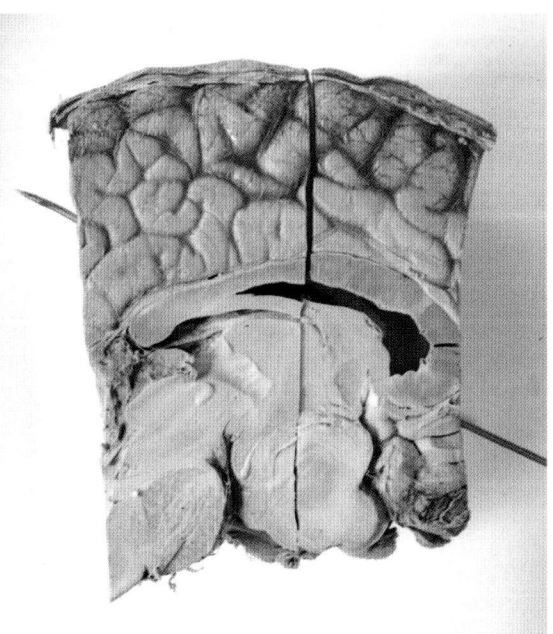

FIG. 4. AUTOPSY SPECIMEN – SAGITTAL SECTION.

and was taken to a hospital in Hanover where ten days before death, his tonsils and adenoids were removed. After this procedure, he took no nourishment that was given, up to the time he died.

PATHOLOGY REPORT
(Examination of the brain several
years later after the patient's death)
April, 1922

The external aspect of this brain, which had previously been fixed by an undertaker, shows a tumor which evidently involves the optic chiasm, particularly the chiasm on the left. There is a large, bulbous tumor mass filling the interpeduncular space, measuring about 3x3 cm, out of which the optic nerves spring, as shown in Miss Warner's sketch of the lesion.

A longitudinal section shows that the growth extends upward and is lost in the tissues comprising the third ventricle. In the lower part of the tumor thus longitudinally sectioned, one can make out all fibers of the chiasm, and above it there is evidently tumor which extends upward all the way to the mid portion of the brain. There is a moderate degree of internal hydrocephalus.

On coronal section, the tumor is lost, but it appears to extend up between the lenticular nuclei, which, however, appear intact. It would be very difficult to tell from these sections whether the tumor is primary in the chiasm and has burst through and involved the third ventricle or whether it was originally a tumor of the third ventricle which had secondary invaded the chiasm. The stalk of the pituitary body was originally apparent, or at least what was taken to be the stalk of the pituitary body lying between two masses of tumor. This has been lost on section.

(Dr. Cushing)

Microscopic report: Section is composed most entirely of neuroglia tissue, apparently traversed by bundles of myelineted nerves. The fibrils are very abundant and the cells are mostly of the spindle cell type. Many of the cells show the peculiar hyaline degeneration resulting in globoid masses of hyaline material and chains of globules. There are also rod-like hyaline bodies, evidently formed

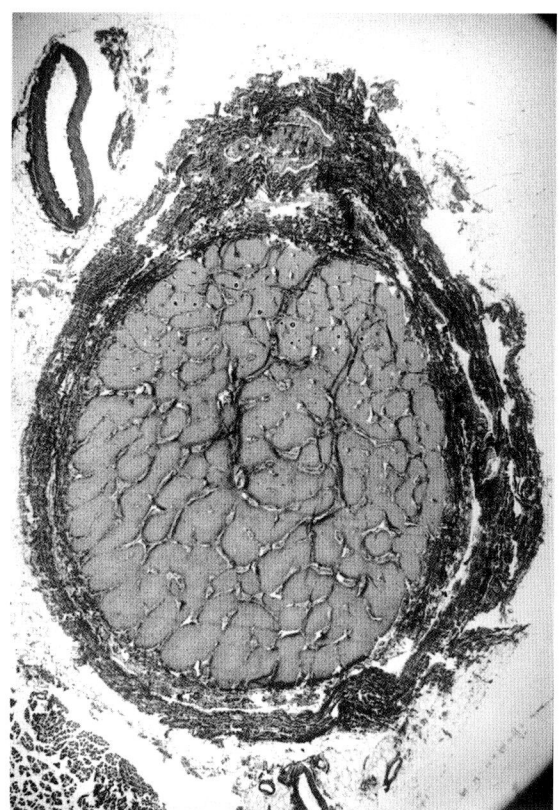

FIG. 5. HISTOLOGY SLIDE — OPTIC NERVE.

within cells with appearance such as Verhoff has described in gliomas of the orbit. From the homogeneous structure of the tissue, one must conclude that it is a glioma.

There are two cross sections of the optic nerve. In both of these sections one finds that nerves have been almost entirely replaced by neuroglia. The general structure of the optic nerve as seen in cross section is preserved, and the neuroglia at the periphery of the nerve bundles in most places possesses the normal arrangement of tangential and radial fibrils as seen on the surface of normal nerve tissue. Here and there one can make out cross sections of myelinated nerves. There are occasional corpora amylacea in the tissue. There is some irregular extension of neuroglia into the dura.

AUTOPSY DIAGNOSIS: Glioma with gliomatous invasion of optic nerve.

(Resident pathologist)

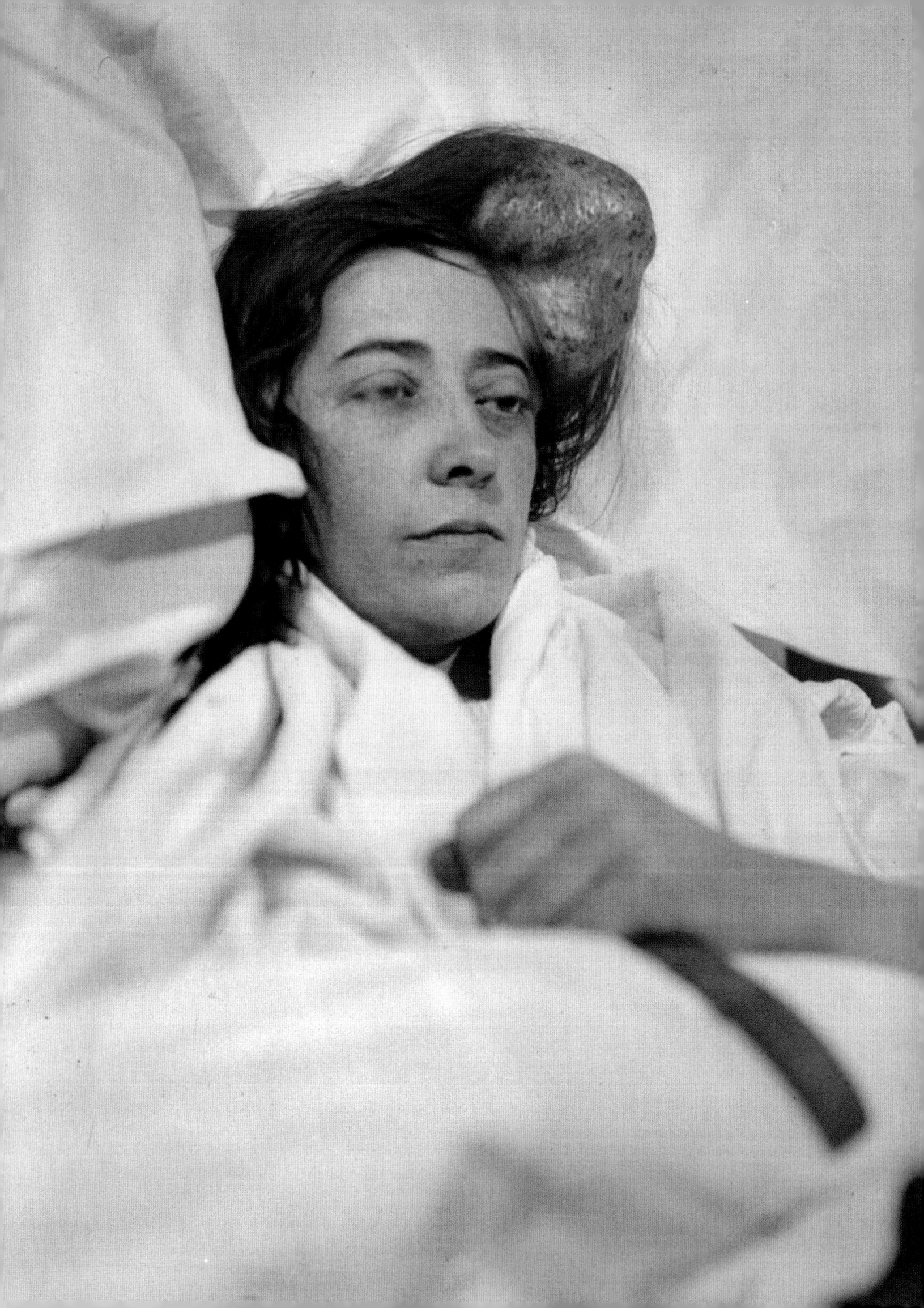

1.4 Parasellar lesion

SEX: F; AGE: 30; SURG. NO. 3883

HISTORY

The patient started to have persistent left eye pain associated with headaches since 12 years ago. She also "grew quite fat and had an enormous appetite" for the past ten years prior to admission.

By June 1911, her headaches were associated with nausea and vomiting. Her right arm became weak and a left lateral homonymous hemianopsia was diagnosed on physical examination. By June 1912, she lost her vision in the left eye. She also developed right facial weakness. She was then admitted to the Massachusetts General Hospital (MGH) for further evaluation.

NOTES OBTAINED FROM THE RECORDS OF MGH

A well developed and nourished young woman, apparently comfortable and happy. Left pupil widely dilated and immobile. Right circular and reacts to light. Ptosis of eyelids, more marked on left with some left internal strabismus. Left eye is totally blind and slightly prominent. Some tenderness on percussion over left temporal region. No adenopathy. Knee-jerks equal and active. Babinski present on right. No ankle clonus. Coordination good in left arm; less so in right. No gross defect in sensibility to touch. No asterognosis. Examination otherwise negative.

OPERATIVE NOTE FROM THE MGH
Operator: Dr. Mixter
Anesthesia – Ether – HA Porter

Exploratory Craniotomy and Decompression for Tumor Cerebri.

Dorsal position, head resting on right side. Curved nine-inch incision over left temporal region. Periosteum elevated in line of incision. Cranium opened with Hudson drill and De Vilbis forceps and osteoplastic flap turned down, exposing dura through a semi-circular opening about 2.5 by 2.5 inches. Dura appeared normal, but under considerable hypertension. Dura opened by crucial incision on director, whereupon cortex bulged immediately and distinctly more than normal brain should. Except for a large varix in the pia-arachnoid vessels nothing abnormal except the increased tension was noticed. Because of pressure of cortex against the edges of the opening, it was impossible to explore beyond them. Dura was replaced over the pia but not sutured. The osteoplastic flap could not be replaced on account of bulging brain. Bone removed. Scalp and muscle sutured into position with interrupted s.w.g. stitches to small rubber tissue wick. Dry dressing. Bendex bandage. Sent to Ward F in good condition.

Discharged unrelieved to out-patient department.

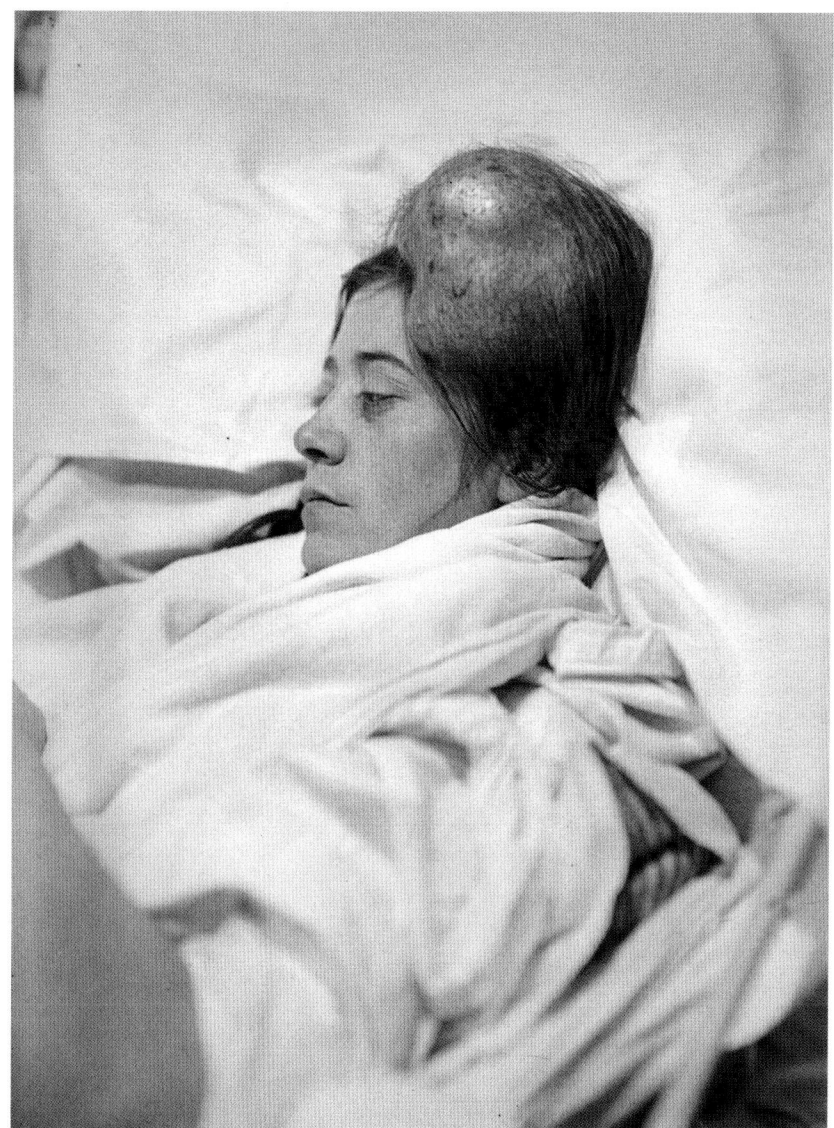

FIG. 2. PREOPERATIVE.

OPPOSITE PAGE. FIG. 1. PREOPERATIVE.

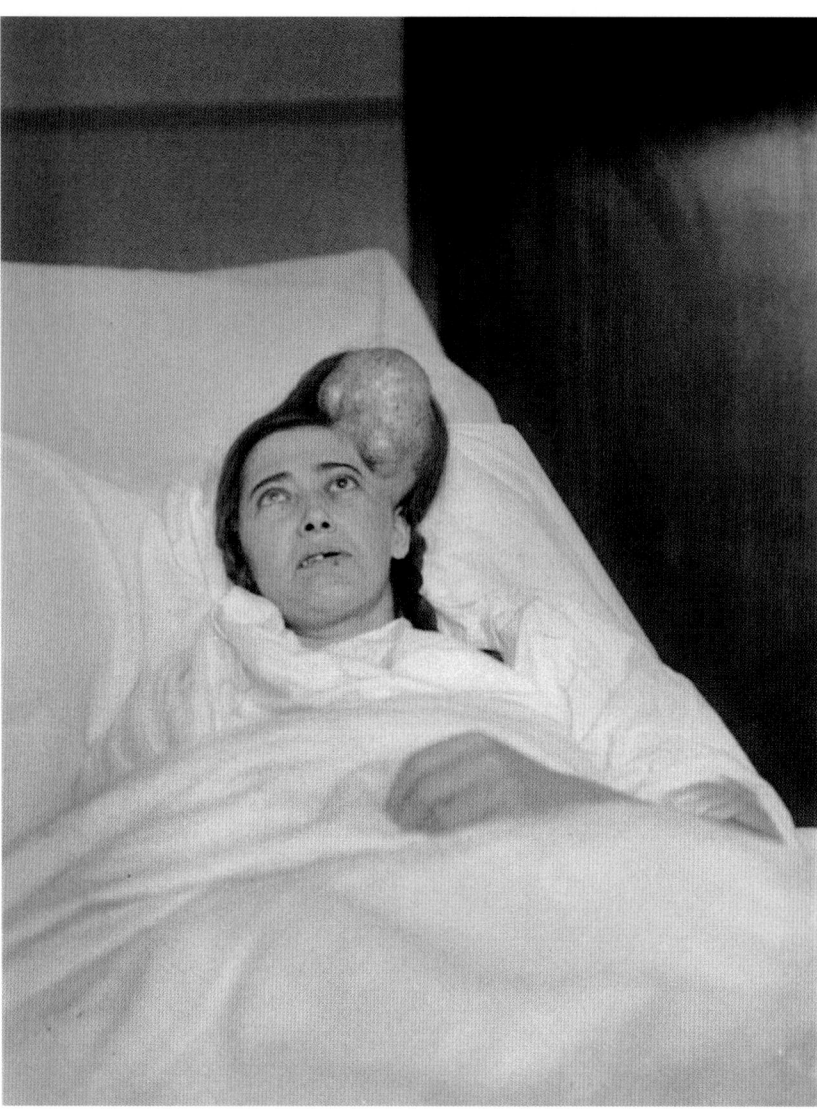

FIG. 3. PREOPERATIVE.

About four months after her discharge from the MGH, she started to have Jacksonian Epilepsy. The "lump" on the left side of patient's head also grew gradually larger, but noticeably so during the past month prior to her presentation to the Peter Bent Brigham Hospital. She was then admitted to Dr. Cushing's service.

SUMMARY OF POSITIVE FINDINGS
November 15, 1915
Dr. Horrax

SUBJECTIVE
1. History of headache.
2. Loss of vision.
3. Twitching of right face, arm, and leg.
4. Aphasia.
5. Decompression operation at MGH three years ago.
6. History of possible polyphagia.
7. Adiposity and drowsiness.
8. Amenorrhea since age of 15.

OBJECTIVE
1. Huge tumor over left temporo-parietal region at upper end of decompression scar.
2. Does not recognize odors.
3. Fundi–discs markedly pale. Outlines distinct. Typical secondary atrophy.
4. Left pupil larger than right.
5. Right hemiplegia and hemi-hypesthesia.
6. Attacks of twitching of right side of face.
7. Difficulty in talking–slurring speech.
8. Memory and orientation somewhat impaired.
9. Superficial abdominal reflexes absent on the right.
10. Deep reflexes exaggerated on the right.
11. Babinski positive on the right.

ADDENDUM NOTE
Dr. Cushing

Temporal hemianopsia of right eye 3 years ago after operation at MGH.

Impression is that the left eye shows secondary atrophy.

RADIOLOGY REPORT
November 20, 1915

The examination of the skull shows the presence of a very large, irregularly shaped, dense tumor of the soft tissue in the left frontal and parietal regions. There is a very large defect of the skull in this region. The sella is increased in size. The examination is not satisfactory because of the condition of the patient, so that further details in the skull are not seen.

December 1, 1915
Dr. Horrax

Patient has had several more right-sided attacks during the last few days, always with loss of consciousness. Administration of sodium bromide has proved to lessen their frequency. She complains of a good deal of pain in the limb and in the left thigh. This afternoon a needle was introduced at the inferior margin of the brain and 750 cc of clear, yellow fluid evacuated. Patient seemed much relieved. X-ray and photo taken individually after evacuating fluid (Please see the attached photos.)

RADIOLOGY REPORT
December 2, 1915

The sella is very much enlarged and deepened. It is 20 mm deep. The anterior clinoid processes are fairly distinct, but are irregular and show signs of atrophy. The floor is only partially seen. The dorsum and posterior clinoid processes are almost entirely obliterated. The floor of the sella has projected downward.

December 5, 1915
Dr. Horrax

The lump has almost completely refilled again. In view of the x-ray findings and the report of her condition at the MGH with right temporal hemianopsia together with her history of amenorrhea, drowsiness, polyphagia, and adiposity, it seems probable that the condition has been hypophyseal, either primarily or secondarily.

OPERATIVE NOTE
December 7, 1915
Anesthesia – Ether – Dr. Boothby

Tapping of Herniation.
Transsphenoidal Pituitary Operation.
Lumbar Puncture.

Needle was inserted into the large herniation as on a recent occasion and the same highly colored fluid as before poured from the wound. Indeed the fluid was more highly colored than on the first occasion and had a slightly reddish tinge.

A transsphenoidal operation was then performed and the floor of the sella removed. This was in immediate juxtaposition to the walls of the sphenoidal cells and a thinned out perforated shell of sella floor finally came away in one piece. This disclosed tough tumor growth fragments of which were taken for immediate examination showing probably a teratoma. A considerable amount of the tissue was removed, but owing to the character of the lesion, it bled somewhat more than usual. This bleeding was caused largely by one small spurter which finally was checked by a bit of rectus muscle from another patient.

Withdrawal as usual without injury of the mucous membrane.

About 300 cc of yellowish fluid had been removed from the herniation and with the expectation that a lumbar puncture would show clear

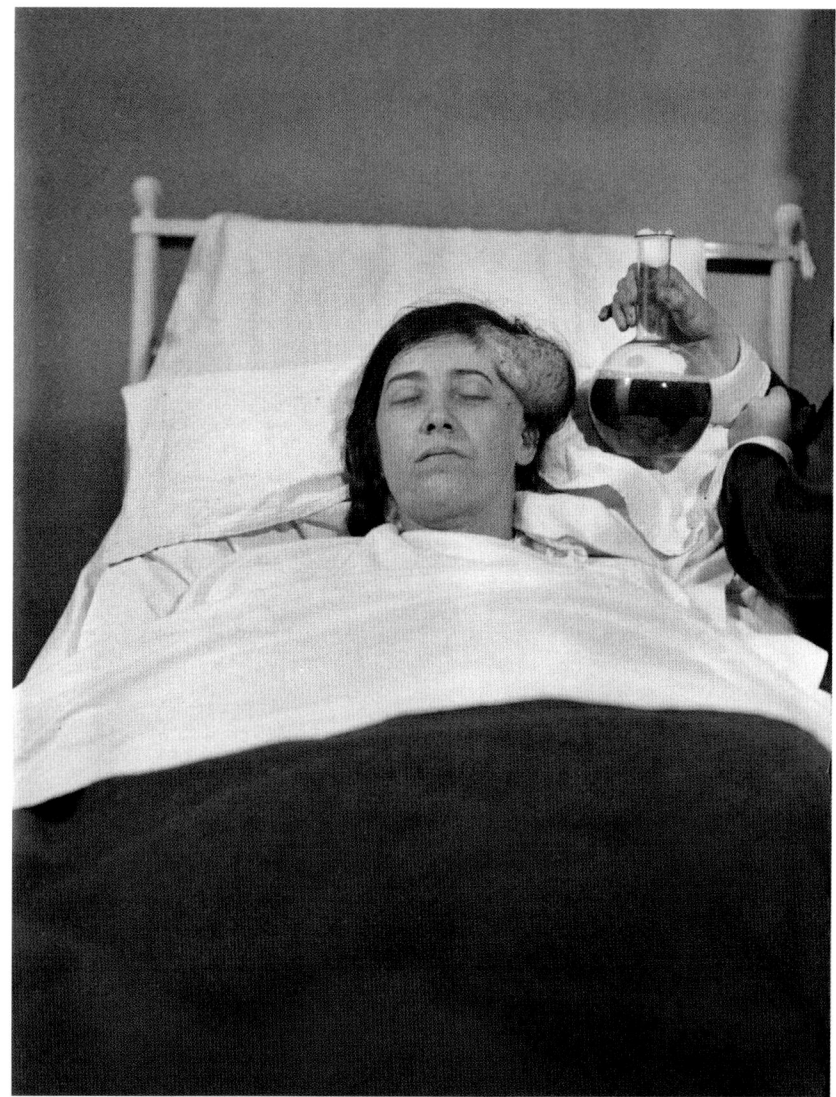

FIG. 4A. PREOPERATIVE (THE MASS DRAINED THROUGH A NEEDLE).

fluid, a puncture was made at this time. To my surprise, the fluid was of the same xanthochromic character as was found in the cyst at the first tapping. It was additionally confusing to find that a very large amount of fluid could be expelled from the lumbar region – probably about 200 cc in all were withdrawn, though it was apparent that the two fluids did not communicate for the lumbar fluid was much clearer than the fluid from the cyst.

(Dr. Cushing)

PATHOLOGY NOTE
December 7, 1915
Material: Fragments of pituitary tumor

The material consists of a mass of mucus in which there are a few pus cells and masses of round cocci,

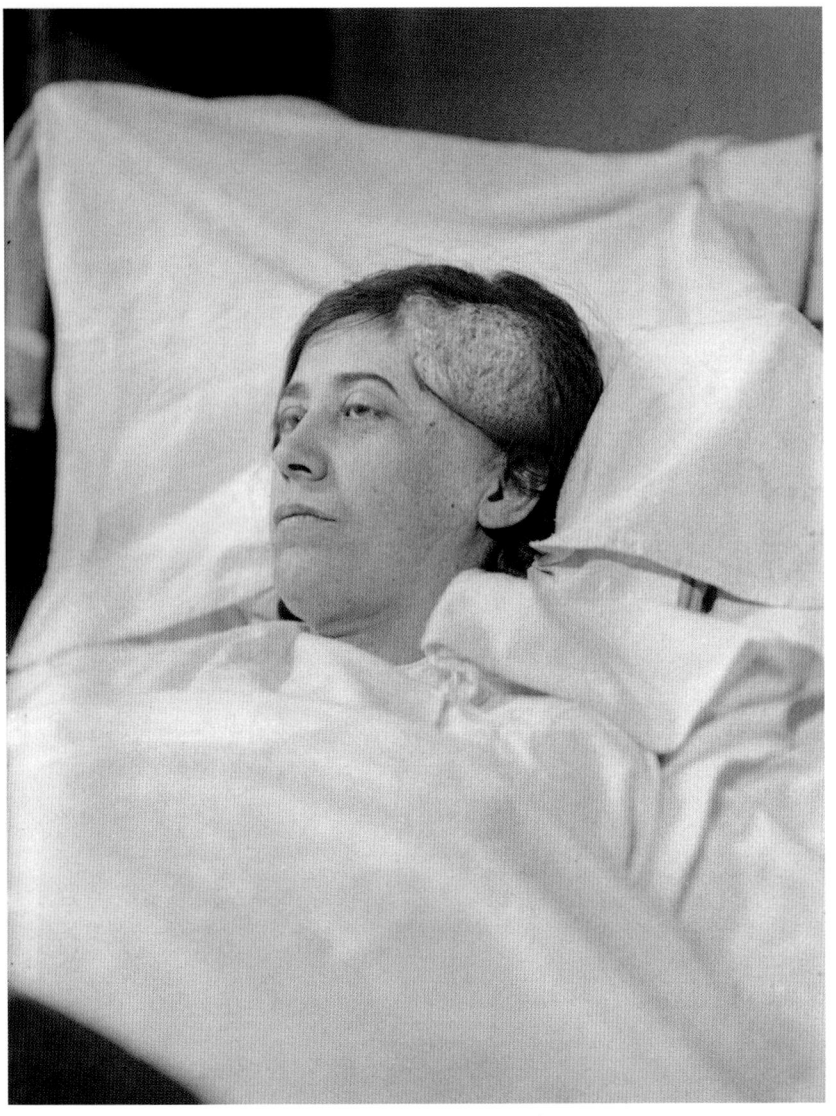

FIG. 4B. PREOPERATIVE (THE MASS DRAINED THROUGH A NEEDLE).

apparently staphylococci. The hardened section shows the same thing.

(Dr. Councilman)

POSTOPERATIVE HOSPITAL COURSE

This patient recovered from her surgery neurologically unchanged, however; the lump at the site of the temporal defect refilled again within 24 hours postoperatively. The patient also developed pus draining from multiple sinus tracts leading to the deep tissues of her neck.

January 18, 1916
Dr. Montgomery

There are now three sinuses on the left side of neck. The upper one is not discharging. The lower two have a very scant discharge. On right side of the neck just under angle of jaw there are two discharging sinuses. These are quite deep and there is a septicus discharge of thick, creamy pus. In lower part of neck there is a red hot, swelling area- a suppurating gland, which will probably break in a few days. The patient is running a slight temperature – 100-101. She still has hexamethylenamine 0.9 gms daily.

PATHOLOGY NOTE
January 21, 1916
Pus from gland of neck.

The culture on glucose agar shows numerous minute gray translucent colonies in 24 hours. Smears show a Gram-negative diplococcus which grows in chains. Smears correspond to the organisms found in the pus.

DISCHARGE NOTE
March 8, 1916
Dr. Montgomery

The cause of the patient's temperature and prostration is very apparent today. There is an intense erythema over entire face. It is very hot and edematous. The right side is much the worst. Yesterday the patient's temperature was normal. She was much improved. She had no nausea or vomiting.

This afternoon the patient had several general convulsions and passed into a semi-comatose condition. Her temperature has reached 103 at 4 P.M. today from a normal temperature this morning.

She was seen by Dr. Cushing and he advised discharge as patient relatives were very desirous of having her at home.

LETTER TO DR. CUSHING
June 15, 1921
Dear Dr. Cushing,

In reply to your request in regard to the outcome of my sister, she lived 48 hours after being discharged from the hospital. She died on the 10th of March 1916. She did not show any changes after coming home and passed away quietly without any complains although she seemed to be very itchy and seemed relieved when we rubbed her body. If there is anything else you wish to know write and I will gladly let you know. Thanking you for your attention and interest in her, I remain,

Very truly yours,
(Signed) MO

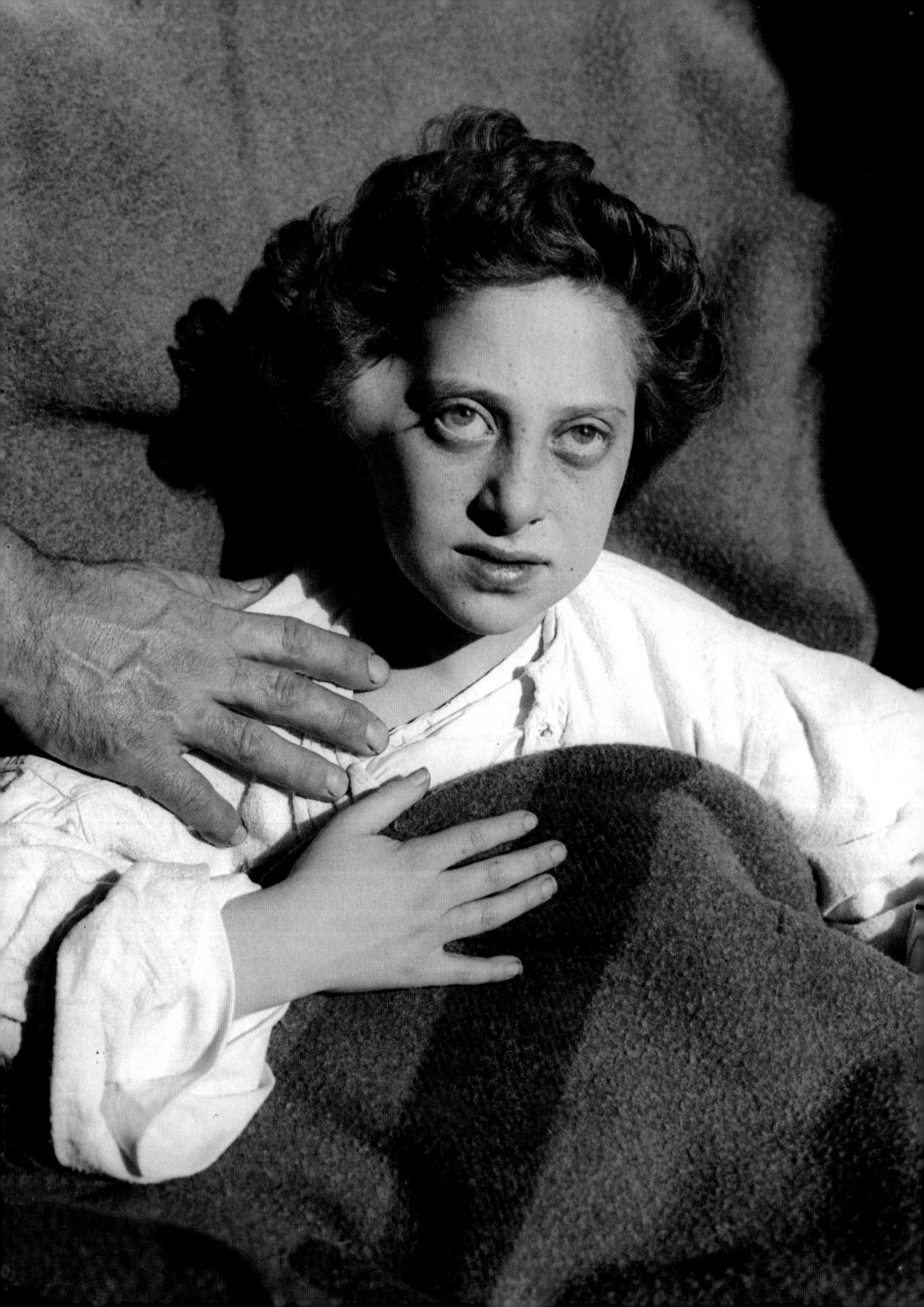

1.5 Craniopharyngioma

SEX: F; AGE: 15; SURG. NO. 10067; 10429; 16489; 29762; 34636

Multiple admissions:

Surg. No. 10067 – Diagnosis: Suprasellar tumor, pituitary group: pharyngeal pouch cyst.

Surg. No. 10429 – Diagnosis: Pituitary group with tumor: suprasellar cystic congenital tumor.

Surg. No. 16489 – Diagnosis: Suprasellar tumor: pituitary group: pharyngeal pouch cyst.

Surg. No. 29762 – Diagnosis: Pituitary group; craniopharyngeal pouch cyst, verified Hypopituitarism.

Surg. No. 34636 – Diagnosis: Pituitary group; craniopharyngeal pouch cyst, verified Hypopituitarism.

HISTORY

This 15-year-old female first complained of weekly frontal headaches and intermittent vomiting in 1917, two years prior to admission. On August 15th of 1917, she presented to the outpatient department of the Peter Bent Brigham Hospital with headaches and vomiting followed by convulsions characterized by "jumping up and down on the bed" and left-sided numbness. She was diagnosed with migraines and was administered aspirin and sodium bromides. She returned for several more treatments over the next two months. Twelve months ago after a severe attack of headaches and vomiting, she was admitted to Boston Children's Hospital where the diagnosis of a brain tumor was made. She was then sent home after two weeks to spend the next three months in bed where she was drowsy and intermittently incontinent of urine and feces. Six months ago, with failing vision, she was taken to New York where Dr. Sharp performed a subtemporal decompression. She felt better after six weeks and could walk and read large typed letters. Three weeks ago, she again became weak, unable to walk with continuous headaches, vomiting and incontinence. Her eyesight worsened and she became "irrational." She was then admitted to the Peter Bent Brigham Hospital on the service of Dr. Cushing.

GENERAL PHYSICAL EXAMINATION

She was underdeveloped and appeared to be 12 years of age. In the right temporal region was an orange size mass that pulsated with her wrist

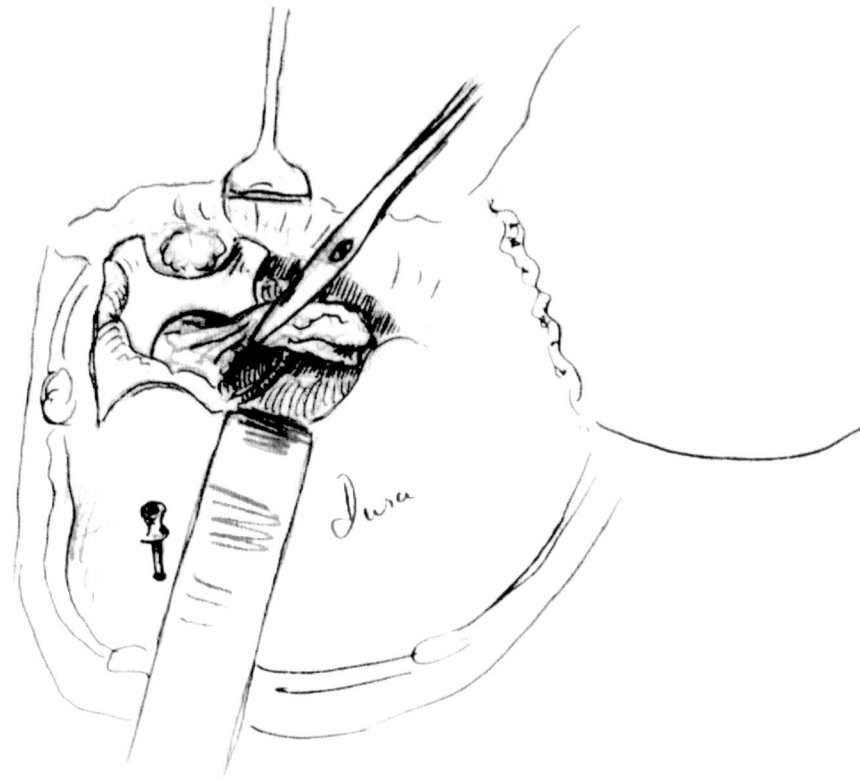

FIG. 2. OPERATIVE SKETCH.

pulse. Her pupils were irregular and sometimes reacted sluggishly to light and sometimes not at all. Fundoscopic exam showed both discs to be indistinct and pale. The reflexes were slightly more reactive on the left.

SUMMARY OF COMPLAINTS
March 4, 1919

Convulsions, vomiting, failing vision, failing memory and headache, beginning in 1917 with a subtemporal decompression 6 months after onset (Dr. Sharpe, NY).

RADIOLOGY REPORT
March 20, 1919
Dr. McCarty

Roentgen Report – In examination of the head the skull shows thinning and increase in depth of the convolutionary impressions with distention of the sutures. In temporal region is a large regular area of decreased density with indistinct borders. Out-

OPPOSITE PAGE. FIG. 1. PREOPERATIVE.

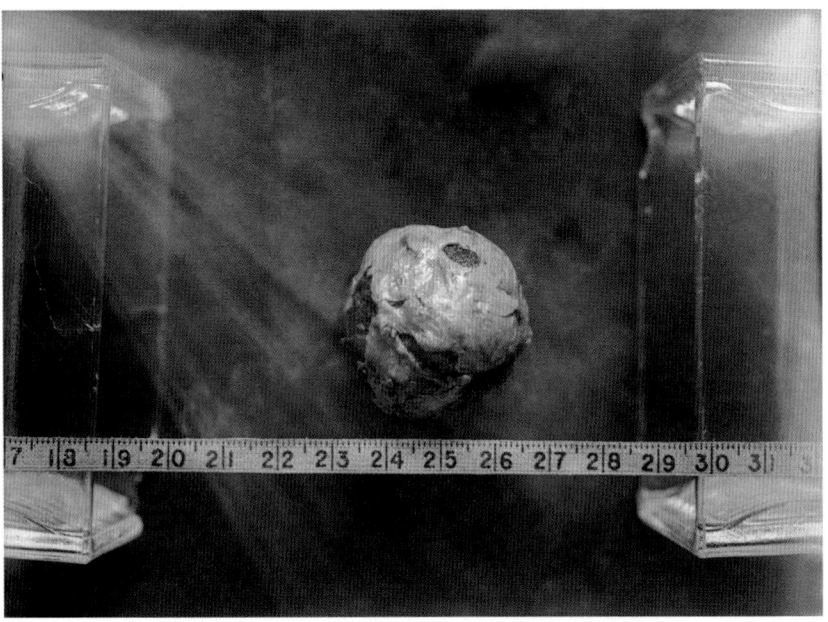

FIG. 3. RESECTED TUMOR SPECIMEN.

line of the sella is indistinct – the sphenoid cells are dense, the anterior clinoid processes appear long, apparently at the expense of the anterior upper part of the floor of the sella. There are two dense shadows near the margin of the area of decreased density, one anterior and one posterior. Frontal sinuses are absent.

DIAGNOSIS: Brain tumor involving the sella.

ANALYSIS OF PITUITARY SYSTEMS
April 1, 1919
Dr. Cushing

1. NEIGHBORHOOD

The X-ray shows a shadow of a probable tumor occupying the sella turcica.

Marked optic atrophy, probably originating as primary atrophy – though there is at present superimposed edema.

History of diplopia though lack of parallelism is present now.

Eyes are quite prominent.

2. GENERAL GLANDULAR MANIFESTATIONS

Characteristic infantilism, child 16, no secondary characteristics of sex.

Hands small and infantile.
Height – 128 cm.
No apparent record of polyuria or glycosuria.
Temperature is subnormal.
No metabolism studies made.

3. GENERAL PRESSURE SYMPTOMS

These have become pronounced with headaches for past 2 yrs. accompanied by vomiting.

Marked dilatation of the venules of the eyelids.
Extreme convolutional markings on the skull, almost as pronounced as in many cases of oxycephaly.

The child was decompressed Sept. 25, 1918 with subsequent improvement.

Decompression has become tense and headaches have become again pronounced.

There is a choked disc superimposed on the original primary atrophy with new tissue. Marked tortuosity of the veins.

4. GENERAL NEUROLOGICAL SYMPTOMS

Are somewhat confusing owing doubtless to the hydrocephalus with more or less slight exaggeration of deep reflexes and considerable static instability.

5. POLYGLANDULAR SYMPTOMS

Nothing made out.

The child has the characteristic mentality and features of infantile pituitary insufficiency. She is rather precocious mentally despite her dullness from pressure.

OPERATIVE NOTE
April 3, 1919
Anesthesia – Ether – Miss Hunt

Transfrontal Osteoplastic Exposure of Congenital Pituitary Cystic Tumor – Cyst Evacuated – Puncture of Ventricle.

Child has been having severe headaches of late and the subtemporal decompression has been at times tight. During the anaesthesia, it became excessively so, and in outlining the proposed flap on the frontal area, there was marked bleeding from many emissary vessels over the bone.

Owing to this thru one of the primary perforations, a needle was inserted into the ventricle and a large amount of fluid escaped, immediately lowering tension and immediately checking all bleeding.

There was no difficulty in turning down bone flap though bleeding occurred from the margin of dura exposed by the vertical incision with Gigli saw in the midline. Inasmuch as tension had all been removed and the dura had been more or less separated from the bone, there was considerable loss of blood necessitating rapid reflection of the flap and placement of cotton on the two bleeding points.

A very small portion of the upper wall of the orbit was removed. It was comparatively easy to strip the dura away from the roof of the orbit and to incise with the knife hook the membrane at its posterior attachment.

Good view was secured of the chiasm and the whole movable nodular, calcareous growth which showed in the x-ray protruded slightly from between the anterior legs of the chiasm.

On elevating the frontal lobe still further, the cystic protrusion was apparent between the posterior legs of the chiasm. This cystic protrusion was transparent but on the surface, there were yellowish hard flecks of deposit so characteristic of these tumors. The cyst was punctured and possibly 6 or 8 cubic cm. of turbid or granular fluid was evacuated. Some of this fluid was saved for examination.

Owing to the small size of the head, it was thought inexpedient to make any further attempt to expose this field more widely so as possibly to justify partial removal of the sac wall. Consequently, if this child does no better than other similar cases, the cyst may be expected to refill.

Bone flap was replaced and the wound closed as usual in layers without a drain, cavity having been filled with salt solution. Head was only partly shaved.

Child was left on the table and made a very prompt and satisfactory recovery from the anaesthetic.

(Dr. Cushing)

PATHOLOGY REPORT
April 3, 1919

Gross description: Specimen consists of about 6 cc of bloody fluid in which there is considerable clot. Smear shows numerous red blood cells, no cholesterin crystals seen.

(Dr. Cushing)

Microscopic report: A section of the fluid after fixing in Zenker–acetic acid shows numerous red blood cells and a few mononuclear cells but no other elements.

DIAGNOSIS: Fluid from brain tumor.

(Dr. Wolbach)

DISCHARGE NOTE
April 29, 1919

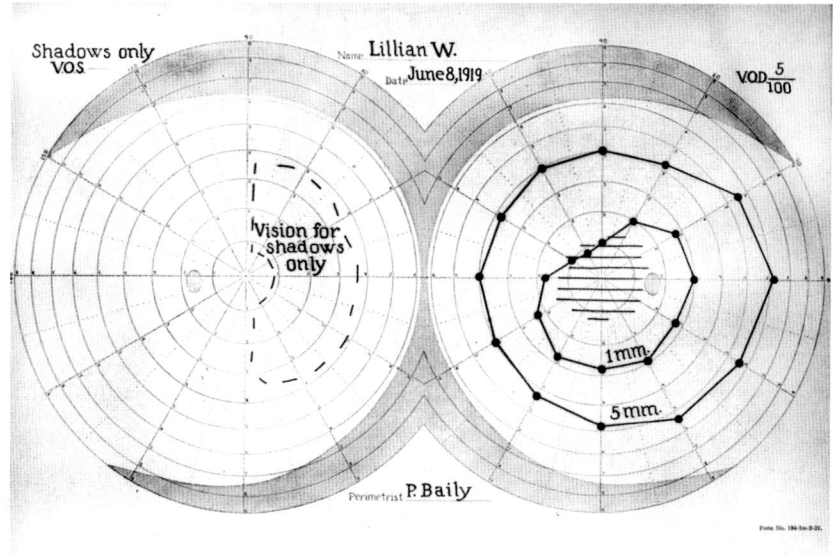

FIG. 4. ONE MONTH POSTOPERATIVE AFTER SECOND SURGERY – VISUAL FIELDS.

Dr. Parkins

The patient has been up and about the ward for 11 days. Her general condition is good. Her vision is improving considerably. Accurate estimation has not been possible. She sees well enough to be about the ward and can read one-fourth in heavy black type. She was unable to do this previous to operation. Discharged today. Discharge against advice.

SECOND HOSPITAL ADMISSION

SPECIAL NOTE
May 8, 1919

The child re-enters the hospital with not only the old original decompression extremely tense but with the bone flap bulging. Child's general condition is very dull, stuporous.

(Dr. Cushing)

OPERATIVE NOTE
May 8, 1919
Anesthesia – Ether – Miss Hunt

3rd operation for congenital pituitary cystic tumor.

The original frontal flap was reflected there being a good deal of difficulty in the procedure owing to the venous bleeding due to the great intracranial stasis. As soon as the flap was reflected, however, a needle was inserted into the ventricle and a great abundance of fluid was evacuated. Practically all

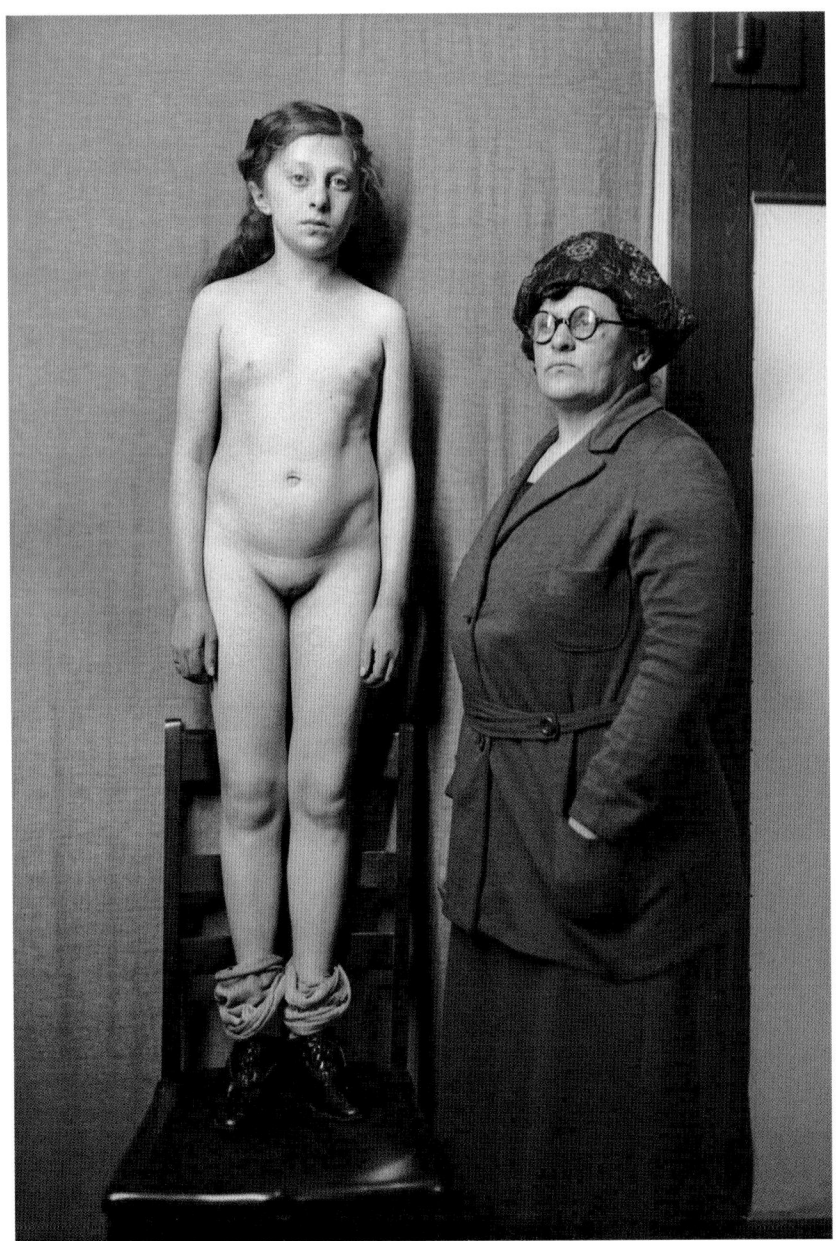
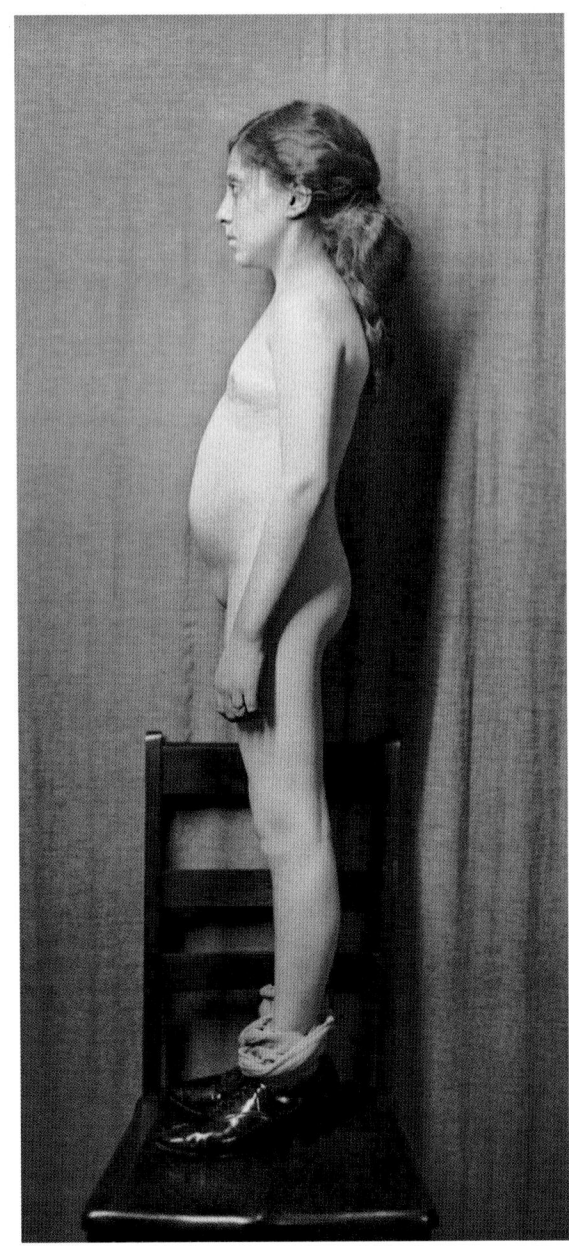

FIGS. 5 AND 6. THREE YEARS POSTOPERATIVE.

the bleeding promptly ceased. There was no extradural fluid such as had been anticipated. The dura, which had become somewhat adherent, was stripped away from the orbital plate and the old opening easily found. There was no damage or contusion to the lower part of the frontal lobe. On elevating the lobe a little more radically than was possible at the earlier operation, the greatly flattened chiasm was brought into view and the same conditions exposed that had been previously exposed. The cyst just at the posterior aspect of the chiasm was again punctured and a great amount of fluid, this time what appeared to be almost clear fluid, was evacuated. It, however, contained flecks of cholesterin such as were previously present.

It was possible, by grasping the margins of the cyst, even though but a very small part of it was exposed, to gradually pull the cyst out of its pocket above the sella and from what must have been the base of the third ventricle. Though delicate and thin, nevertheless the wall had sufficient toughness so that apparently it was completely withdrawn down its neck which passed directly into the pituitary fossa. Here the wall became somewhat thickened and the sac was finally broken off in this situation. I should judge that the sac had been about the size of a golf ball and it must have completely occluded either the foramen of Monro or else possibly the third ventricle.

After the extrusion of the sac and its dislodgement at its base, an immense amount of cerebrospinal fluid, in addition that what had already been secured, escaped leaving the brain high and dry so that the frontal lobe no longer needed to be retracted to give exposure.

During all this procedure, what caused the limitation of room was the juxta position of the anterior Willisian branch.

It is to be noted that the view obtained is not that seen in the ordinary picture of the base of the brain where the chiasm lies flat against the brain but is the view which would be obtained by turning the chiasm back and looking between it and the anterior Willisian vessels.

During all this procedure, the child's condition apparently was unaltered and no damage by bleeding appeared to have been done. The hard nodular tumor, which could be palpated between the anterior legs of the chiasm was left in situ though while tugging on the sac, it was evident that this tumor could be dislodged. It is quite probable and indeed certain that had the chiasm been split antero-posteriorly, it might have been possible to remove the tumor in its totality. I am under the impression that in the future, it might be best to deliberately do this and leave the patient with a permanent bitemporal hemianopsia but with a greater certainty that there would be no recurrence of trouble. It is hoped, however, in this case that, even though some fragment of the cyst wall may have been left, it may be many years before a complete new cyst will form, at least of sufficient size to occlude the ventricular outlets.

(Dr. Cushing)

PATHOLOGY REPORT
May, 8, 1919

Materials – wall of pituitary cyst.

Gross description – Specimen consists of 3-4 pieces of tissue. One of them is about 3 mm wide and the other is 1.3 x 6mm. Fixed in Zenker.

(Dr. Cushing)

Microscopic reports – Sections of the tissue show it to be from a dermoid cyst. It is composed of epidermal masses with a regular rounded arrangement of the peripheral or basal layer. The central portions show various degrees of keratinition and vacuolated masses of epithelium. There are many atypical "pearl" bodies of horny epithelium. In places there are areas calcified, with disappearance of surrounding epithelium.

DIAGNOSIS: Dermoid cyst.

(Dr. Wolbach)

POSTOPERATIVE COURSE
May–June, 1919

Her month long recovery from surgery was characterized by lethargy and vomiting with her subtemporal decompression site becoming tense. The pressure at the subtemporal defect was relieved by occasional lumbar or ventricular punctures. Her alertness and vision then gradually improved.

DISCHARGE NOTE
June 10, 1919

Patient discharged today in excellent condition. Her vision is not much improved but headaches are gone and the decompression is very soft.

CLINIC NOTE
April 10, 1920
Dr. Horrax

Has been in excellent health since operation and gained weight. Polydipsia and polyuria. Mother says she drinks an enormous amount of water and

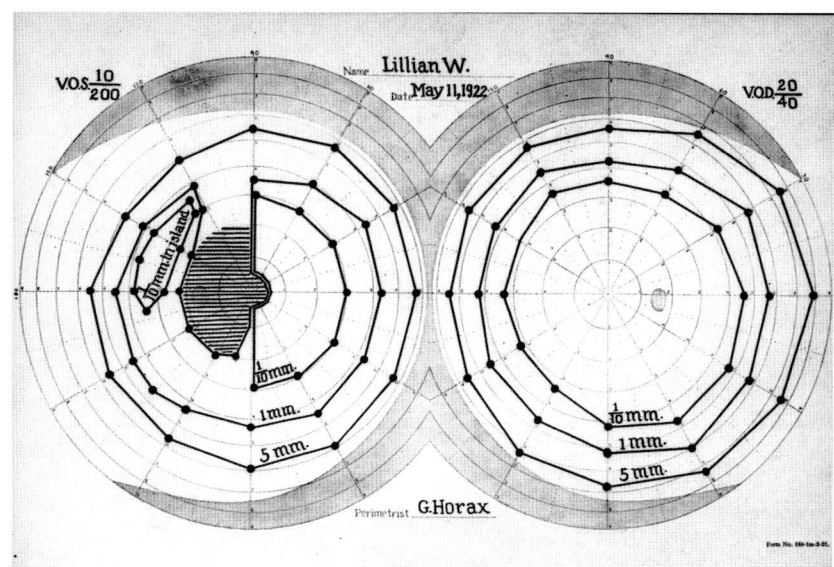

FIG. 7. THREE YEARS POSTOPERATIVE FOLLOW-UP – VISUAL FIELDS.

also passes a greatly increased amount since the operation.

Decompressed area – quite soft
Eyesight – subjectively the same.

CLINIC NOTE
May 18, 1921
Dr. Cushing

Will be 18 tomorrow. Decompression is soft, has largely disappeared, and mother says that sometimes the swelling at the decompression defect is completely gone. Subjectively her left eye is still much impaired but mother states that they are much improved. Mother states that she has an inordinate thirst; that she drinks excessively, and has to get up several times in the night not only on account of her thirst but to void.

THIRD HOSPITAL ADMISSION
April 20, 1922

She has had no headaches, no projectile vomiting, no vertigo or diplopia.

Subjectively her vision is improving, but vision in the left eye is poorer than in the right. Her gait is steady, she has gained some weight, and according to her father's measurement she has grown slightly taller. She has not been particularly troubled with thirst although she drinks a good deal of water with her meals and at times she drinks a couple of glasses of water during the night. There has been no trouble from frequency or polyuria. There is still complete amenorrhoea. The patient feels well, has no special complaint but comes in for observation upon the advice of Dr. Cushing.

RADIOLOGY REPORT
April 20, 1922

Stereoscopic films of the skull in a right lateral position show the operative defect. The sella turcica itself is not clearly defined and there seems to be some destruction of the posterior clinoids. Just within the sella turcica region there is definite calcification.

DISCHARGE NOTE

She was discharged at her own insistence following her photographs and x-rays. Her vision was slowly improving.

CLINIC NOTES

Her follow up appointments detailed stable vision. She continued to have amenorrhea, polydipsia, polyuria, and drinking 18-20 glasses of water each day.

FOURTH HOSPITAL ADMISSION

HISTORY

Patient returns to the hospital following an attack last May similar to those she had previous to her operations. The attack began with a severe frontal headache which lasted six hours. She became unconscious at four o'clock in the afternoon and regained consciousness at six the next morning. She had blurring of vision and was admitted to a convalescent home for one week.

SUMMARY OF POSITIVE FINDINGS
September 29, 1927
Dr. Courville

OBJECTIVE
1. A girl of 24 years with a physical and probably mental development of the age of 10-12.
2. Skin coarse and dry with a very marked brittleness of the hair and absence of hair in the axillae and pubis.
3. Sense of smell less acute on the right than on the left.
4. Bilateral optic atrophy, pupil smaller on the right than on the left.
5. Finger to nose test less accurately performed on the left than on the right.
6. An exaggeration of the deep reflexes on the left side.
7. X ray shows a definite calcified mass above and behind the dorsum sellae.

IMPRESSION: This patient is a definite example of a hypopituitary syndrome beginning in the pre-adolescent period. The x-ray shows a definite area of calcification above the dorsum sellae. This is probably recurrence of tumor or incomplete removal.

(Dr. Courville)

September 29, 1927
Dr. Cushing

The chief feature objectively about her is that she sleeps 12-14 hours every night. She is slower than at any time since her operation five years ago. She

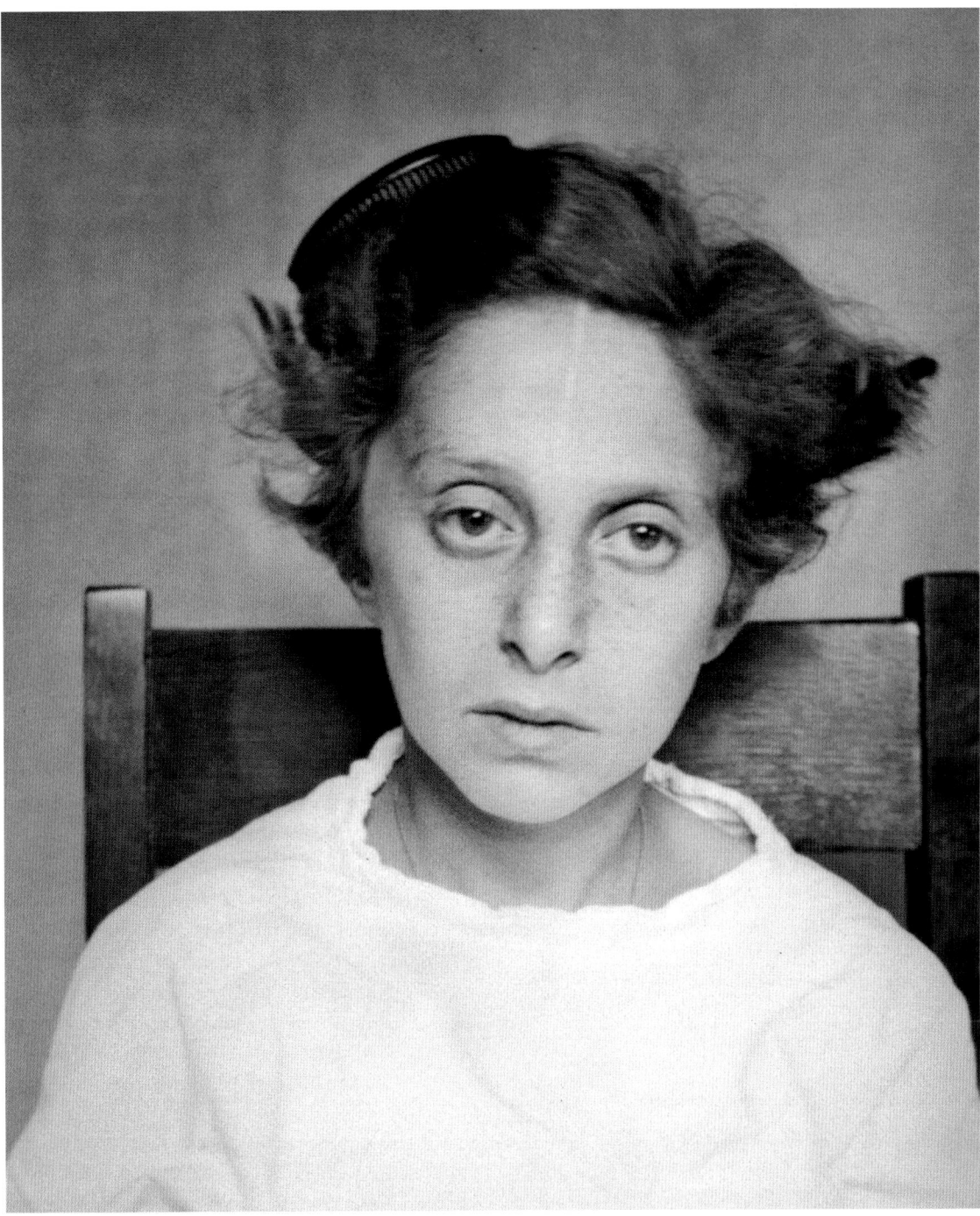

FIG. 7. EIGHT YEARS POSTOPERATIVE.

looks pale and somewhat languid. She exhibits the physical and mental attributes of a child of 10 or 12 years of age.

RADIOLOGY REPORT
September 29, 1927
Dr. Sosman

Right stereo, AP and PA of skull. There is a dense, spongy mass of calcification in and above the sella measuring approximately 1.5 x 3 cm in size and a small area of calcification in the falx.

IMPRESSION – Suprasellar cyst.

October 3, 1927

Injection of anterior lobe extract: Dr. Putnum injected 10 cc of corphyrin colored anterior lobe extract through the intraperitoneal route. She complained of "pain in her stomach."

October 5, 1927
Dr. Putnam

Dr. Cushing has advised delaying further injection until we see what course the metabolism will take following the first injection. There was no significant alteration in her height. There has been as yet no significant alteration in her weight.

October 15, 1927

Metabolism reports are very striking.
    Oct. 3rd, before 1st injection −25
        − 4th, after +3
        − 6th, −10
        − 8th, −25
        − 11th, −25

Second injection was done. Patient reacted with increase in temperature.

DISCHARGE NOTE
October 18, 1927
Dr. Oljenick

Subjectively the patient feels very well and has no complaints. Except, of course, impaired vision, which does not seem to bother her much.

October 1927
Dr. Putnam

This unfortunate little dwarf has been accurately followed for many years and has scarcely grown at all since 1919 or before. Indeed, she has lost weight. X-rays show her epiphysis still un-united while her whole appearance with a few important exceptions is that of an immature girl. Her skin is dry, sallow and slightly wrinkled like that of an old person and her eyes and cheeks are hollow. The physique, the hair, the teeth, the voice, however, are those of a young child. Her mental development is approximately normal for her age. Her operation has been unusually successful and she has had no headache or vomiting. Her vision has slowly declined. We are, perhaps, justified in regarding most of her physical disability as due to anterior lobe deficiency, mainly the infantism of bony growth and the development of sexual characteristics. The picture is, of course, not uncomplicated. The progressive visual failure and the presence of a shadow in the x-ray are present reminders of the fact that a large part of the growth remains in spite of the operation. How much of this has to do with her easy fatigability, her loss of appetite and weight is impossible to estimate at present; however, her condition has become more or less stationary and if any of her symptoms were relieved by injection of the anterior lobe extract, we might ascribe them to anterior lobe deficiency.

The changes that may be hoped for from injecting the anterior lobe extract in the first place are temporary ones upon her lower basal metabolism, her subnormal temperature, the dryness of her skin and perhaps subjective effects impossible to measure upon her ambition and energy. In optimistic moods, we might expect some permanent effects upon her stature, even an increased growth of bone, which should be demonstrable by measurements or x-rays.

With these hopes, I gave her the first injection of 10cc of free sugar sterile anterior lobe extract, the details of preparation, which may be found in the laboratory note of the surgical research laboratory on October 3rd. Dr. Fulton kept full notes. She had a fever reaching 101°, the next day had the colic and diarrhea and I believe vomiting, and complained of pains in the bones and joints, which she described as a stretched feeling. Her metabolism was increased almost to normal not only on the day when she had the febrile reaction but two days later when her temperature was normal. According to Dr. Fulton's measurements, she has gained slightly in height but I am not sure if the difference is greater than the limits of accuracy of measurements. She lost weight instead of gaining any. It is hard to say whether there is any difference in her skin. She was discouraged by the injection and was not at all sure whether she wished it repeated. She had a gastric upset probably from another cause. However, since she was feeling well yesterday, she consented to have another injection. This time, 10cc of the October 1st extract, which is somewhat more diluted but also probably somewhat freer from contaminating substances, was used intraperitoneally. The patient complained bitterly of the injection and squirmed and tossed about while it was being given so that we had fear for the safety of the needle. She complained immediately of abdominal pain and some diarrhea. This morning she had a temperature of a little over 99°, is weak and listless, and has a tender but not spastic abdomen. I cannot say that her skin is any moister than it was. She will have metabolics done tomorrow as it appears to be only confusing to determine this while she has a febrile reaction.

It is very difficult to know how much of her symptoms to ascribe to the actual hormone. She is a sensitive little thing and has always been much petted by everyone and does not bear the slightest discomfort well. She undoubtedly has less resistance than such a person as the patient (the name of another patient) who is also being treated. I am not sure that we have a single evidence of any specific action of the anterior lobe extract in this case. However, the inconvenience of the injections seem to bring her no permanent harm and the experiment may all be worth repeating even again on this case.

CLINIC NOTE
July 25, 1929
Dr. Cushing

Patient, now 26 years old, reports. She looks excellently well. Weighs 84 lbs with thin clothes on. No headaches whatsoever. Sunken decompression. Still has her polyuria for which she is having no treatment. Has taken three or four glasses of water since she has been waiting the past hour. She has had two spells of unconsciousness, apparently with convulsions: the first after she was here in February, 1928, when Dr. Putman gave her three abdominal punctures with anterior lobe emulsion. The mother is inclined to attribute the convulsions to this treatment. She had another about two months ago. Came out of a clear sky. She was unconscious over night and was taken to the Jefferson Hospital again.

I strongly advised her to enter the hospital so that I might institute a vasopressin regime, but she refused to come in. Fields taken by Dr. Scarff.

FIFTH HOSPITAL ADMISSION
August 15, 1929

Patient was admitted on August 15, 1929 to adjust her vasopressin treatment for polyuria. Discharged in a stable condition. She was to take vasopressin nasally ½ cc on cotton putty with reached intake and output at a much lower level: 1400/1200.

CLINIC NOTE
August 19, 1929
Dr. Scarff

COMPLAINT. Frequency of urination, thirst.

IMPRESSION – cranio-pharyngeal pouch tumor, congenital in origin, probably not advancing materially in size, as evidenced by the fact that the fields are probably essentially the same as at that time.

LETTER FROM FAMILY
October 7, 1931
Dear Dr. Cushing:

I have your letter of Oct. 6th and wish to express my thanks and appreciation for your kindness in asking about my daughter, (the name of the patient)'s condition at this time.

Were it possible I should be very happy to send her on to Boston for examination but due to business conditions I shall have to forego this plan until things are better.

Up to the present time for the past year (the name of the patient) has been feeling very well and has increased her weight to 91 and ¼ lbs. Stripped, her height to 54 and ½ inches in stocking feet. No headaches, eye sight fair or about the same with no apparent signs of menstruation. Intake of drinking water has decreased.

I hope that this is the information you desire and again wish to express my heartfelt thanks for your thoughtfulness.

Sincerely yours,
(Signed) (From patient's father)

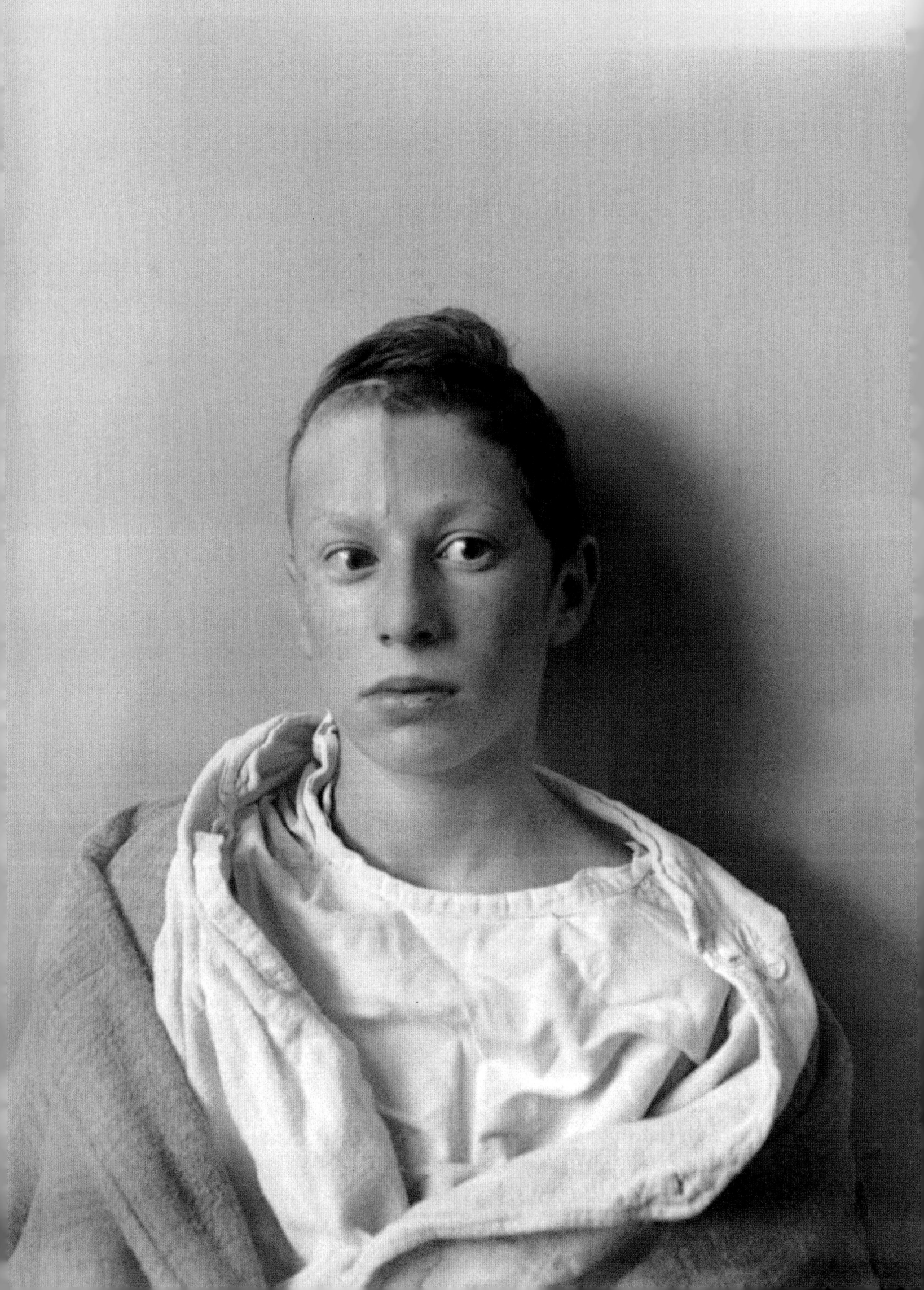

1.6 Suprasellar epidermoid

SEX: M; AGE: 13; SURG. NO. 10036; 10339; 11152

HISTORY

By March 1918, the patient noticed progressive visual changes in the right eye. In September 1918, he lost his vision in the right eye. He also noted a decrease in the vision of the left eye. He underwent a left subtemporal decompression operation, performed by Dr. Sharp at the Polyclinic Hospital in New York. Following the operation, there was no improvement in the vision of the right eye.

SUMMARY OF POSITIVE FINDINGS
February 28, 1919
Dr. Graves

SUBJECTIVE

1. Complete loss of vision in the right eye and marked impairment of vision in left eye.

OBJECTIVE

1. Fundus O.D. – optic atrophy with low grade choked disc.
   Fundus O.S. – optic atrophy with low grade choked disc.
2. Internal strabismus of the right.
3. Right pupil is larger than the left.
4. Light reflex is absent in the right pupil.
5. There is slight nystagmus on looking to the extreme left.
6. Audition is slightly better in the left ear than the right.
7. There is a temporal hemianopsia in the left eye.
8. Plantar and Tendo-Achilles reflexes are not elicited.

RADIOLOGY REPORT
March 3, 1919

Average thickness of the skull is 3-5 mm. Convolutionary impressions are increased in the anterior fossa. Dorsum sella appears atrophic. Sella appears shallow, evidence of operative interference in the left temporal region.

SPECIAL NOTE
March 3, 1919
Dr. Cushing

The patient has a small head. There is no evidence

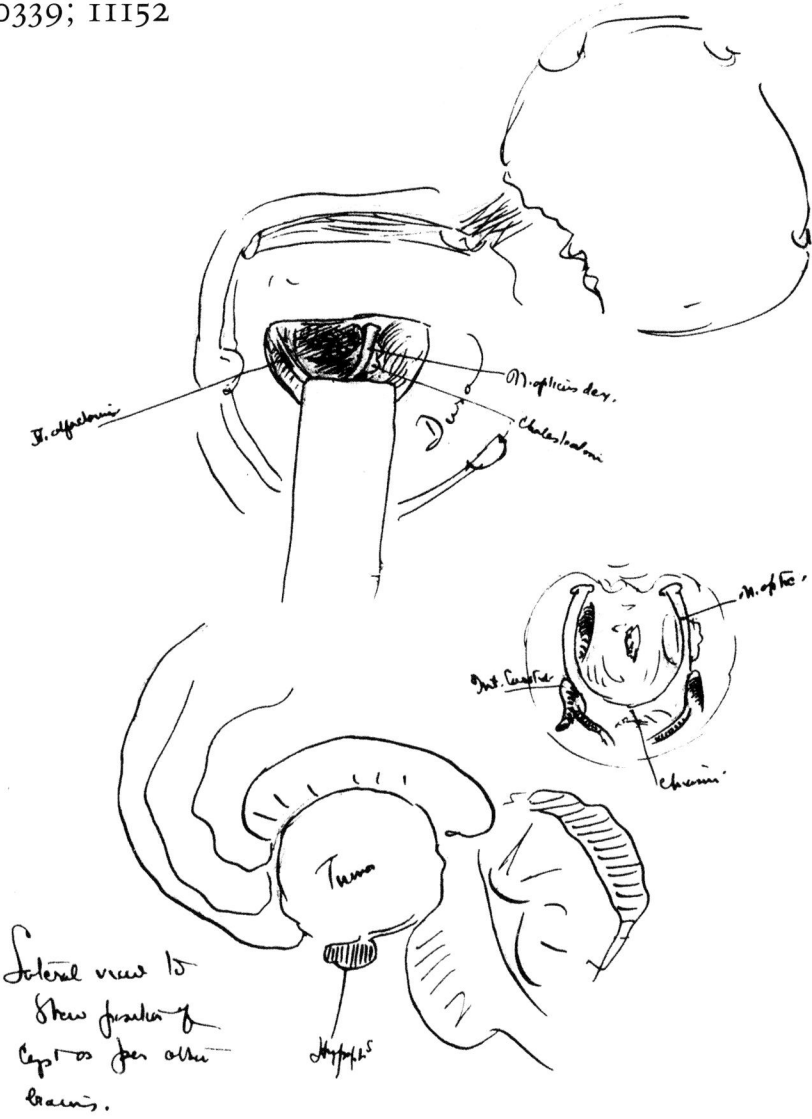

FIG. 2. OPERATIVE SKETCH.

of hydrocephalus. Some possible convolutionary absorption in the frontal region is shown in the X-ray plate. The patient seems to be below normal in size. He is well nourished but not fat. The hands are small but not typically pituitary. The genitalia show signs of early adolescence. There is certainly no evidence of dystrophy. Eyes-there is blindness on the right and apparently a temporal hemianopsia on the left. The fundus on the right shows a marked pallor of atrophy. The lamina cribrosa is sharply defined. There is marked tortuosity of the veins. Fundus on the left – condition is very similar to that just described. There is a very slight pigment ring about the disc.

OPPOSITE PAGE. FIG. 1. POSTOPERATIVE.

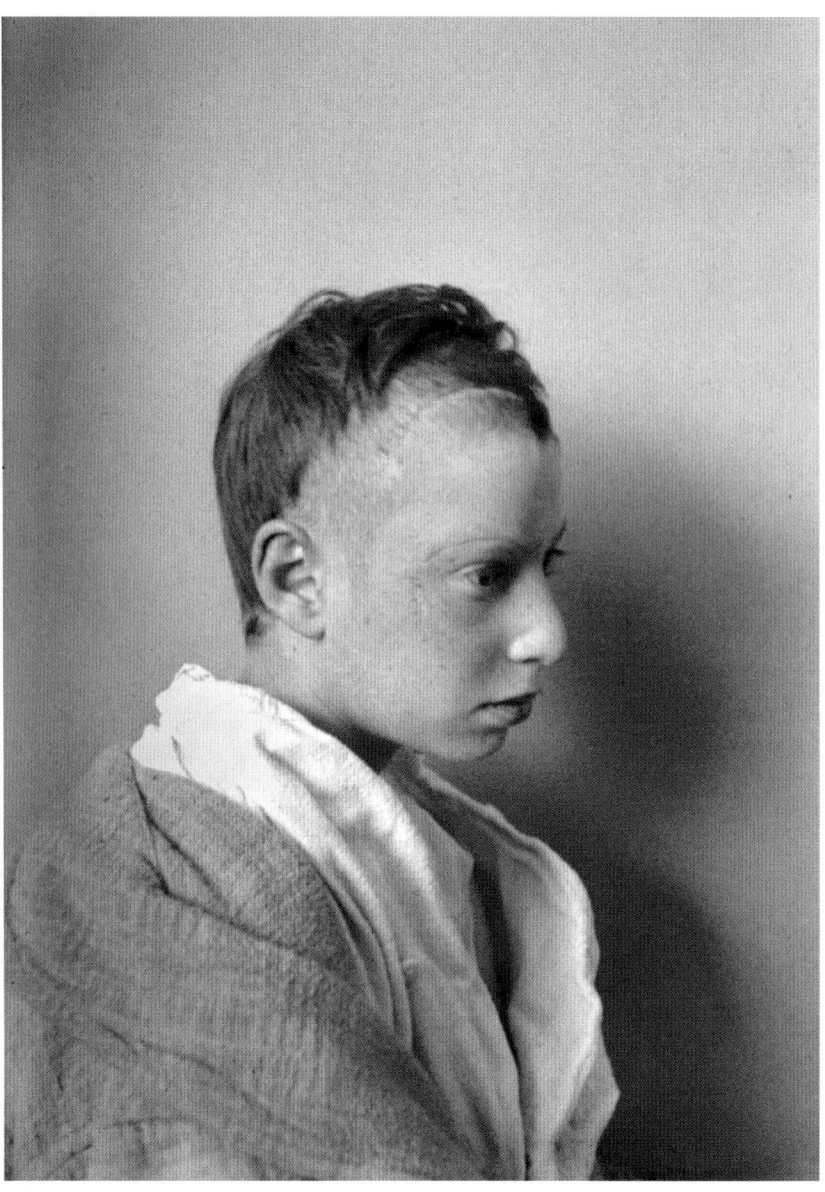

FIG. 3. ONE MONTH POSTOPERATIVE.

DISCHARGE NOTE
March 4, 1919
Dr. Graves

The patient has been up and about the ward since his admission. There has been no change in his condition. Report of X-ray plates taken of the skull is given above. X-ray plates of the hands showed no definite variation from the normal, though there is rather marked lack of epiphyseal union. The Wasserman and Von Pirquet examinations are negative. At Dr. Cushing's direction the patient is discharged today to his home with the understanding that he will return within a few weeks should his condition become worse.

SECOND HOSPITAL ADMISSION
April 21, 1919
Dr. Kababjian

The patient states that his condition has remained about the same since his discharge from the hospital and that he came back because he had received a note from Dr. Cushing telling him to come again.

DISCHARGE NOTE
April 24, 1919
Dr. Kababjian

The patient has been in the hospital 3 days. He has been up and around the ward. Yesterday he was sent to the metabolism laboratory with result of -14. Today his parents declined permission for operation and he was discharged by Dr. Cushing. Result-not treated.

THIRD HOSPITAL ADMISSION

The patient was admitted for surgical treatment. Visual acuity OD-0; OS-20/200

SPECIAL NOTE
September 20, 1919
Dr. Cushing

This boy has had practically no symptoms whatsoever except loss of vision, apparently occurring as a bitemporal hemianopsia, though since he has been seen during the past few months, it has shown itself as blindness in the right eye and temporal hemianopsia in the left. I have had many doubts as to the wisdom or propriety of operating. The sella turcica has been shown to be practically normal.

OPERATIVE NOTE
September 20, 1919
Anaesthesia – Ether – Miss Gerrard

Transfrontal Operation for Suprasellar Tumor.

Disclosing a Cholesteatoma.

The patient took the anaesthetic very badly and it was 45 minutes before he could be anaesthetized sufficiently satisfactorily to justify proceeding with the operation. I was on the point of abandoning it on several occasions for a second session. The usual low right frontal flap was made, there being much less bleeding than usual. The case was one of the type in which there are no frontal sinuses to make the outlining of the flap difficult. The dura

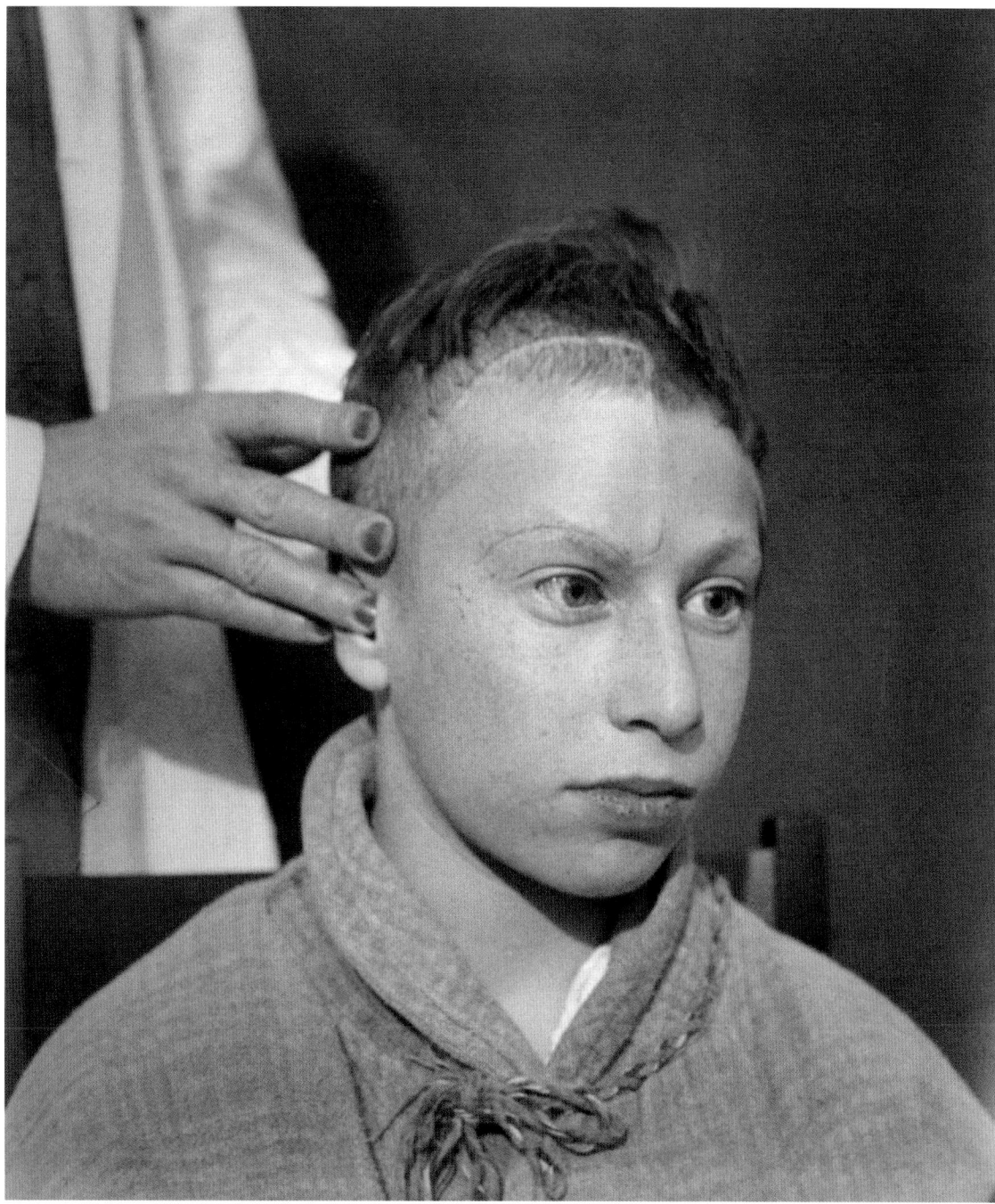

FIG. 4. ONE MONTH POSTOPERATIVE.

as exposed was not tense and after reflecting it from the roof of the orbit down to the sphenoidal edge, an incision was then made through the dura close to its line of attachment with a hooked knife. There was abundant cerebrospinal fluid which escaped. With the idea that a larger exposure would be necessary, it would be best to puncture the ventricle, an attempt was made in 3 directions to insert a needle through the frontal lobe into the ventricle without success. Probably therefore the ventricle is not dilated, nor would it have been expected to be in view of the absence of pressure symptoms. (It may be noted that the boy's decompression performed by Dr. Sharp has never given him any relief and has never been full).

After this failure of getting into the ventricle, the local region was further explored. The olfactory nerve on the right side was seen and lifted up with the frontal lobe, and before the end of the operation was probably permanently damaged,

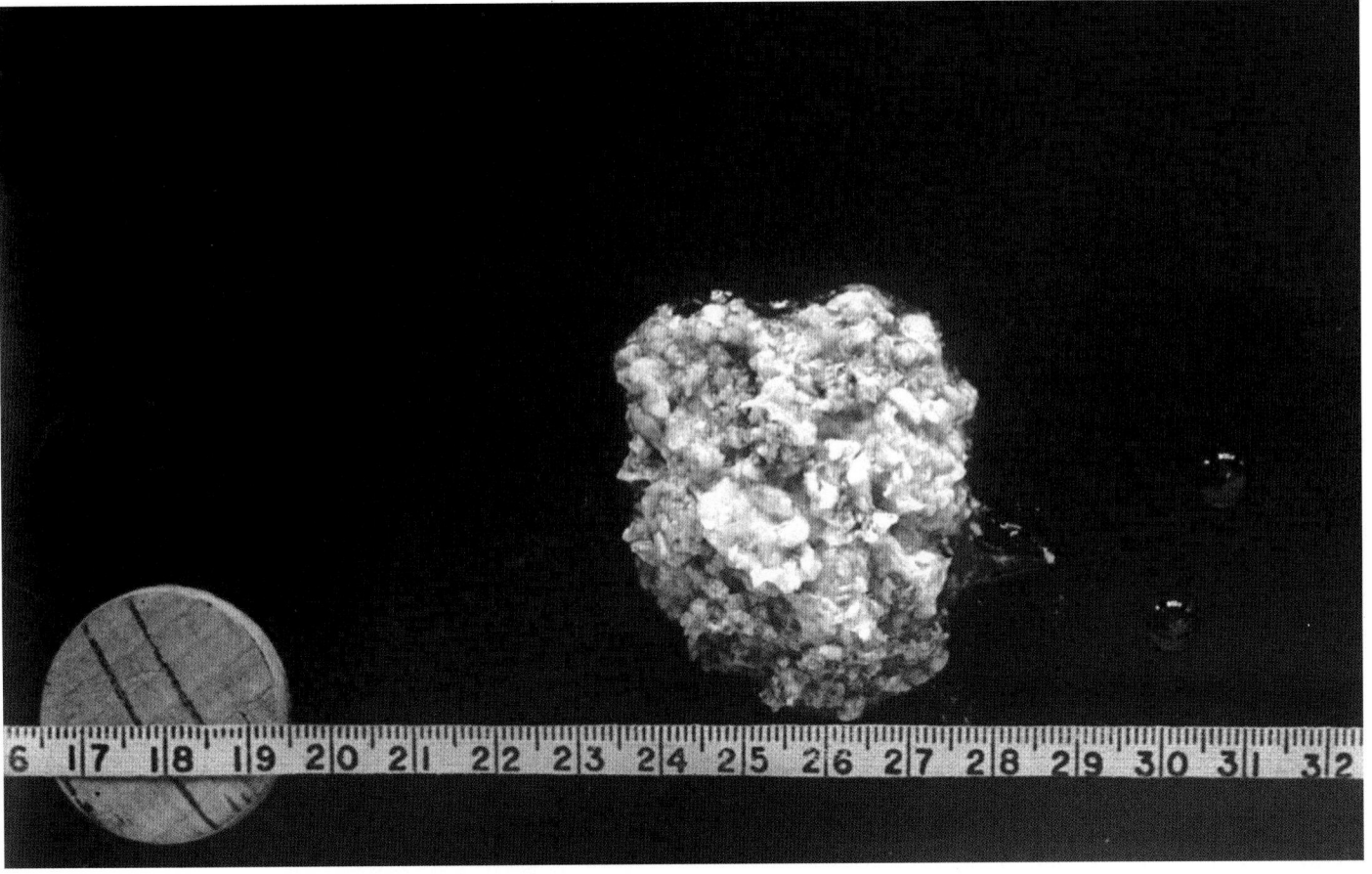

FIG. 5. RESECTION SPECIMEN.

though it was not perhaps fully divided as it often is in these operations.

The entry of the right optic nerve into its foramen was seen though the nerve where seen was reddish and appeared to be extraordinarily small. To the left of this nerve and in the space between the two clinoid processes was a grayish tangle of what appeared to be thickened arachnoid, but on entering this, the wall of a mother-of-pearl tumor was exposed with the characteristic mass of epithelial debris as its contents. With a soft pituitary spoon this material was gradually scooped out from the center of a cyst which must have been about the size of a golf ball. As the material was cleaned away, it was possible as in the case of (the name of another patient) to scoop out the contents of the cyst and to peel away a large amount of its wall, though not as completely as in the former case. This incompleteness of getting out the wall was due to the fact that the tumor had many irregularities which projected into different regions and particularly because it was very adherent to the chiasm. In fact, the two optic nerves were more or less incorporated in tumor. The nerve on the left was even smaller than the right in appearance, even though it was the only nerve which still transmitted sight impulses. After the tumor was as thoroughly cleared away as possible an extraordinary view was had of the region with the internal carotid on each side and the anterior cerebral and practically the entire Willisian circle. The removal in fact had been so complete and was so deep that Dr. Bailey cautioned the operator lest he pick up by accident the 3rd and 4th nerves. The exposure as a matter of fact must have been practically back to the pons as shown by the lateral sketch taken from a cross section of a cyst of about the same size from another case. The large cavity was filled with salt solution and the flap replaced and closed in layers without a drain.

(Dr. Cushing)

PATHOLOGY REPORT
September 20, 1919

Gross description – Specimen consistent of about 20 grm of material resembling in the color and consistency – cottage cheese. There are several flakes about the consistency of tinfoil with a characteristic mother-of-pearl appearance.

(Dr. Cushing)

Microscopic result – Tissue lost.

DISCHARGE NOTE
October 20, 1919
Dr. Bailey

Discharged to home. Mentally normal. Neurological examination negative except for eyes. Internal strabismus right eye. Bilateral optic atrophy. Complete blindness right eye and temporal hemianopsia left.

LETTER TO DR. CUSHING
October 14, 1921

Dear Dr. Cushing:

In answer to your letter of October 7th, in regards to (the name of patient) I will say that he has gained but very little since the time of his discharge from the hospital. He barely sees his way around, indoors; outdoors he seems to see somewhat better. He is attending the Perkins Institute at Watertown and shall be very glad to have you see him when I come to take him home for the Christmas holidays if you will be at the hospital at that time. He is in perfect condition, physically and it is said at the school that he does remarkably well. He had a mental test and he was the only boy at the school to pass it.

Thanking you for the interest you are taking in him, I am,

Very sincerely yours,
(signed) Mrs. MR

LAST FOLLOW UP LETTER
October 23, 1932

Patient appears fully maturated, and in excellent general health. No vision in right eye. Can see light and dark and large objects in left eye. No headaches.

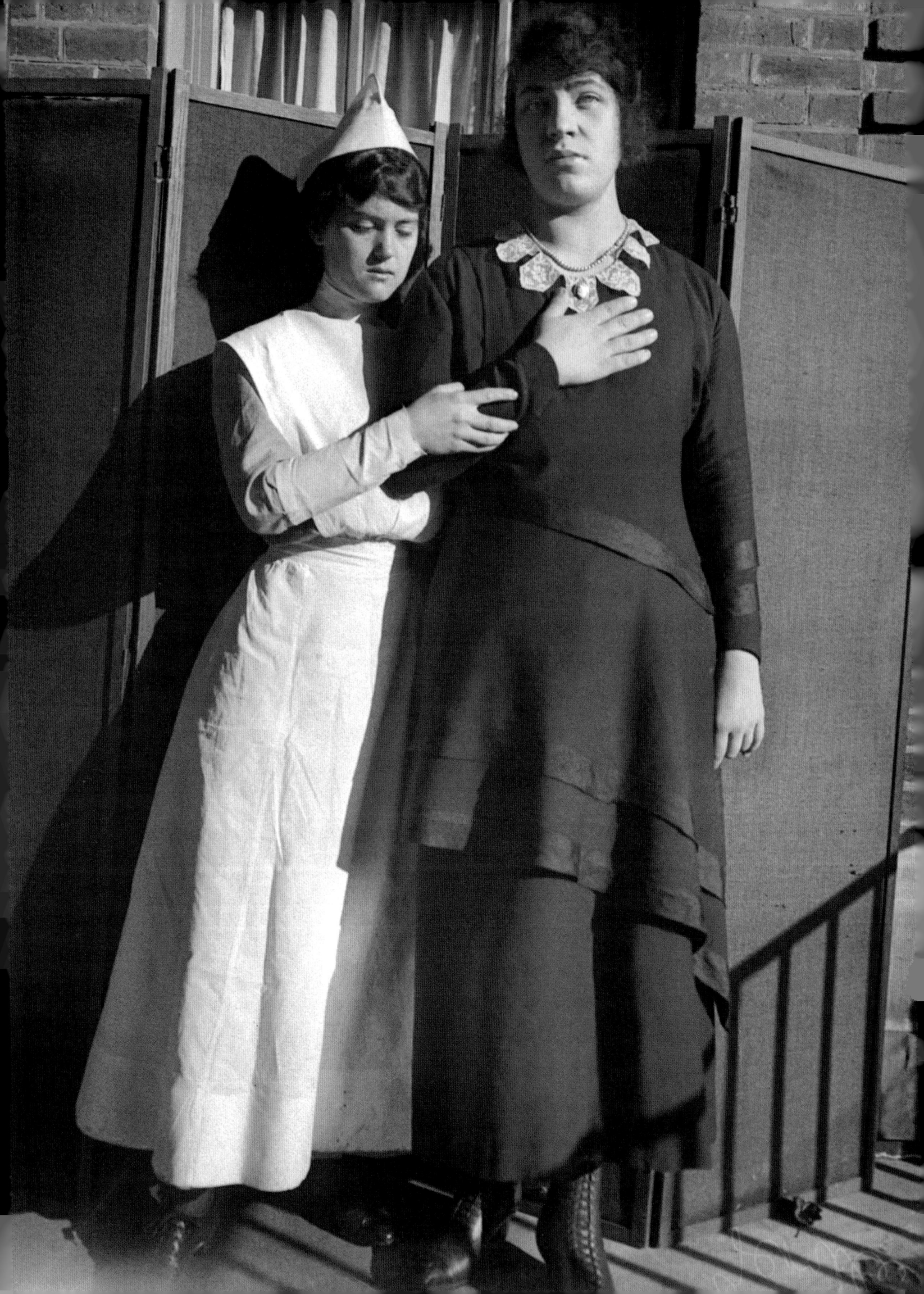

1.7 Pituitary adenoma

SEX: F; AGE: 21; SURG. NO. 11461; 11506

HISTORY

This 21-year-old woman has had a four-year history of facial flushing spells (caused by "bad odors.") Patient had coarse hands, large head, and a large protuberant lower jaw. Dr. Russell of Chicago in 1917 "gave her electrical treatment." She also received pituitary extract "by hypodermic in arm" for a couple of months. She was seen at the Mayo Clinic also in 1917 and was advised to see Dr. Cushing.

SUMMARY OF POSITIVE FINDINGS
November 10, 1919
Dr. Bailey

SUBJECTIVE
1. Impaired vision
2. Excessive size
3. Amenorrhoea

OBJECTIVE
1. Skeletal overgrowth, particularly of hands, feet and jaws.
2. The teeth are widely spaced.
3. The skin is thick, coarse grained and with excessive hairs.
4. Sella turcica enlarged
5. Homonymous hemianopsia.
6. Blood pressure very low.
7. Body temperature inclined to subnormal.

RADIOLOGY REPORT
November 10, 1919

The skull shows considerable thickening. The frontal sinuses are very large. There is no evidence of increased intracranial pressure. The sella turcica is large, having a very broad floor and there is some encroachment on the sphenoidal sinus.

DISCHARGE NOTE
November 14, 1919
Dr. Bailey

Discharged temporarily. To return for operation.

SECOND HOSPITAL ADMISSION

Patient readmitted in the hospital on November 17, 1919 for surgical intervention.

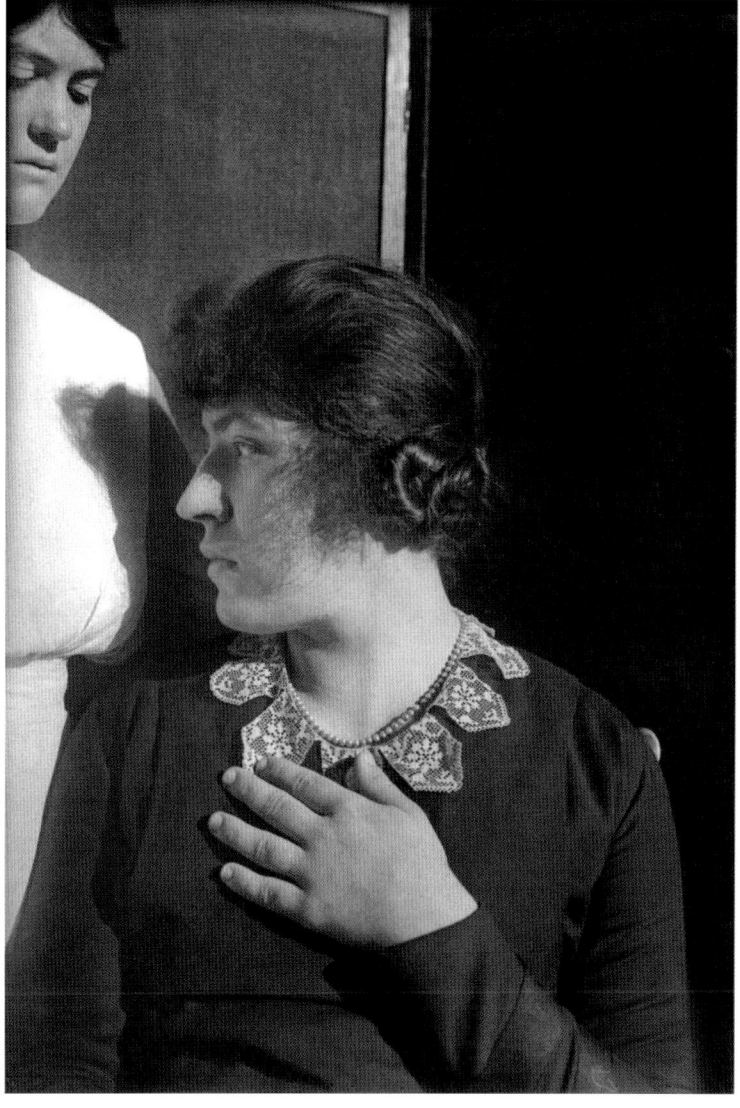

FIG. 2. PREOPERATIVE.

OPERATIVE NOTE
November 21, 1919
Anaesthesia-ether-Miss Gerrard

Transsphenoidal Approach for Pituitary Struma – Decompression with Dural Incision.

This was a difficult case owing to the great depth of the nose and to the extraordinary vascularity of the tissues. It was finally possible to separate the mucous membrane from the median septum without tearing the former except in one minute place. The exposure of the anterior sphenoidal

OPPOSITE PAGE. FIG. 1. PREOPERATIVE.

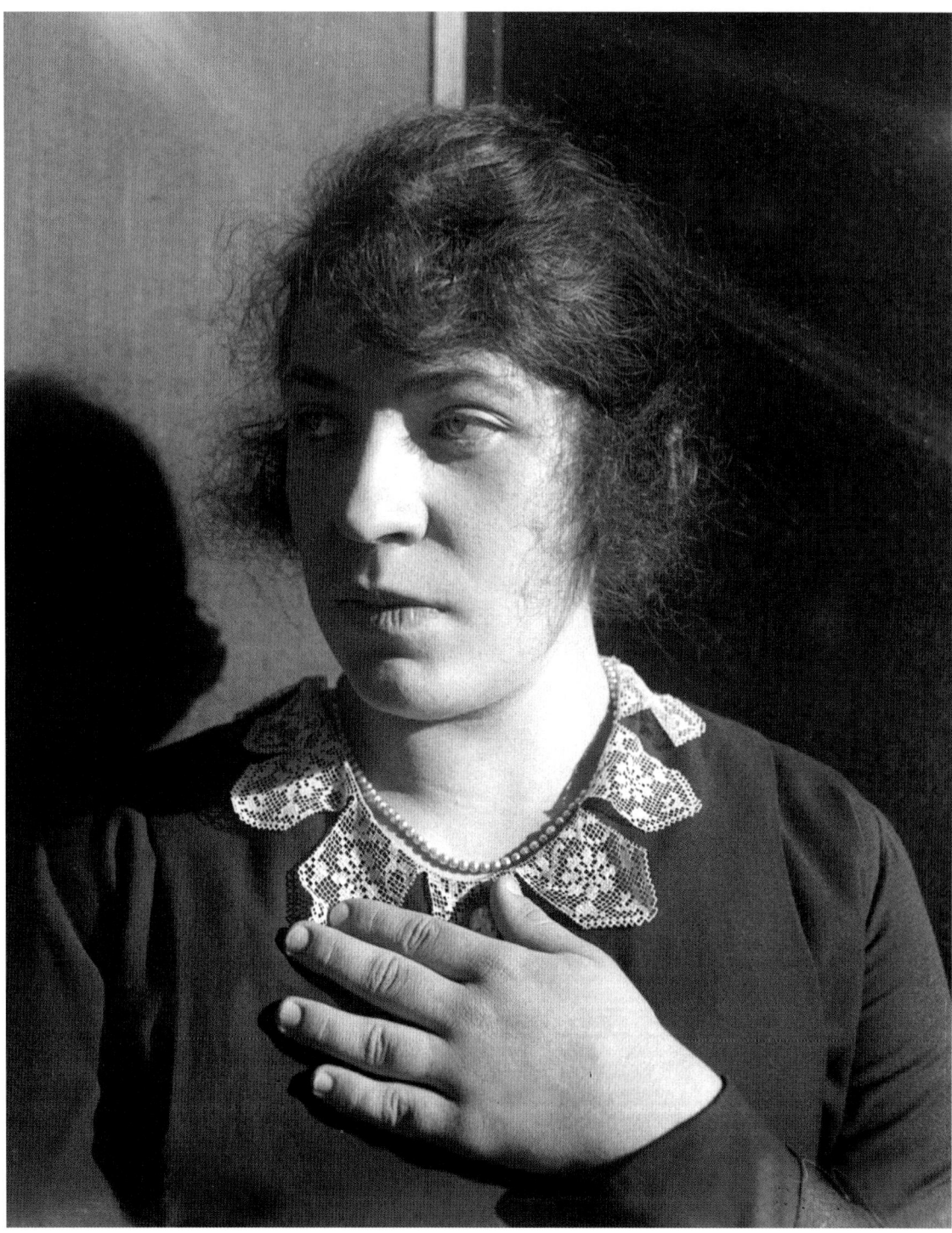

FIG. 3. PREOPERATIVE.

cells was not very satisfactory and it was found that there was a thick anterior wall of cancellous bone which had to be perforated before getting into the large sphenoidal cells. These cells, although they do not look large on the x-ray, nevertheless had great lateral extensions and from each of these extensions a huge mass of bloody mucus with mucous membrane was removed, considerable bleeding accompanying this procedure.

The floor of the bulging sellar was finally chipped away, exposing a yellow protruding tense membrane. This was incised by a vertical and then by a cross-cuts incision, a yellow, rather firm tissue turning out but not extruding as in the case of the usual soft struma. Some fragments of this tissue were rongeured away for fixation and the immediate fresh examination of some of the tissue by Dr. Horrax showed no eosinophilic granules. The operation was withdrawn from in the usual fashion.

(Dr. Cushing)

PATHOLOGY REPORT
November 21, 1919

Gross description: Specimen consists of a few very small fragments of tissue which were obtained from the region of the pituitary body by means of a small pituitary spoon.

(Dr. Cushing)

Microscopic report: Mass of tissue having the general appearance of pituitary gland tissue. Arrangement is that of pituitary gland. Some cells are seemingly larger than normal and there is preponderance of cells with eosinophilic granulations. Non-granular basophilic cells occur in groups.

DIAGNOSIS – Mixed struma

(Dr. Wolbach)

POSTOPERATIVE NOTE
November 22, 1919
Dr. Bailey

Nosal plugs removed. Subjectively well. Nose free. No cerebrospinal leak.

DISCHARGE NOTE
December 14, 1919
Dr. Bailey

Patient has been up and around the ward. Has had no more attacks. Eyes have not improved since operation.

EXTRACT OF LETTER TO DR. CUSHING
March 9, 1920

"I'm getting a little better all the time. There are times when I feel entirely free from that heavy lifeless feeling that I had all of the time before the operation. I had the nervous spells at the regular time last month. They were not quite as strong as they were the month before. It seems strange that they come regularly and still I do not menstruate.

I would feel so encouraged if I would only menstruate."

(Signed) Patient's name.

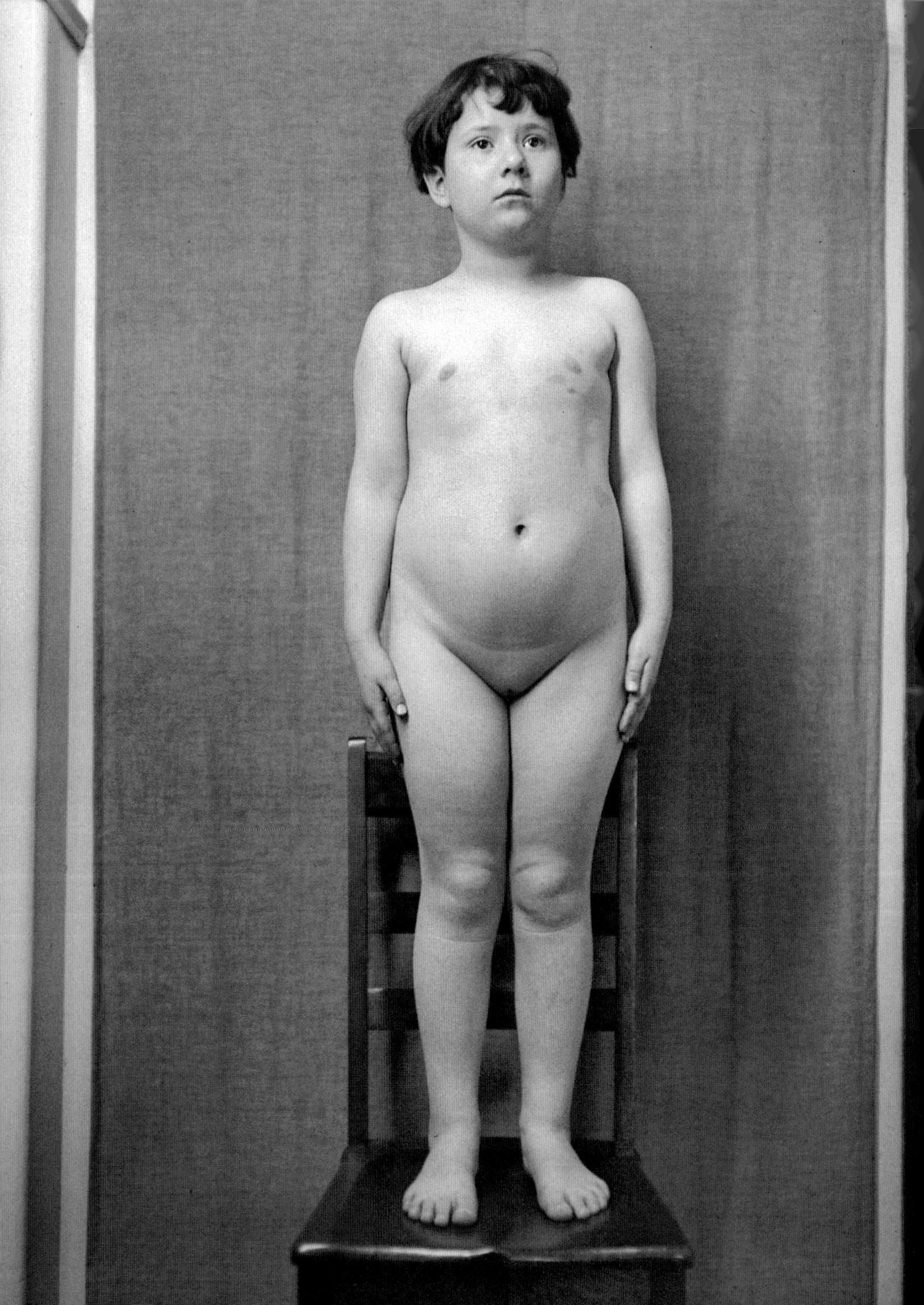

1.8 Glioma of optic chiasm

SEX: F; AGE: 6; SURG. NO. 16342

HISTORY
April, 4, 1922
Dr. Martin

Eight months prior to admission the patient "acted as if she were near-sighted, holding objects near to her face, her left eye swinging in." At the same time, she became drowsy, falling asleep at any time, and began to gain weight. Her eyesight continued to fail and she had attacks of nausea and vomiting. She became "cranky and her speech which has never been particularly clear is worse."

CRANIAL NERVES EXAMINATION
II. Optic

Subjective – History of failing vision of 8 months duration, more prominent on the left.

Objective – Fundus O.D. – Disc is of normal shape, possibly smaller than normal and of pale color, the pallor being more marked on the temporal half.

Fundus O.S. – Very similar to O.D. except that there is a discolored area of the retina along one of the vessels radiating from the disc.

PITUITARY SYMPTOMATOLOGY

NEIGHBORHOOD

2-3 attacks of headache with vomiting during the past 3 months.
  No 3rd nerve changes.
  Sella turcica-See X-ray report.
  No epistaxis or rhinorrhoea.
  No anosmia.
  No uncinate gyrus syndrome.
  Bilateral primary atrophy.
  Narrowing of fields of vision to rough test.

GLANDULAR
1. Temperature 97 to 99. Pulse 80 to 130.
2. Cerebration slow-child is very dull and has had periods of drowsiness.
3. No prominence of jaw nor offsetting of teeth.
4. Hands and feet rather short but not of acromegalic type.
5. Hair is fine, not particularly dry, of normal amount and distribution.
6. There is no precocity of sexual development.
7. No polydipsia or polyuria.
8. No increased desire for sweets.

SUMMARY OF POSITIVE FINDINGS
April, 4, 1922
Dr. Martin

SUBJECTIVE
1. History of failing vision, for 8 months.
2. History of drowsiness for 8 months.
3. History of irritability for the past few months.

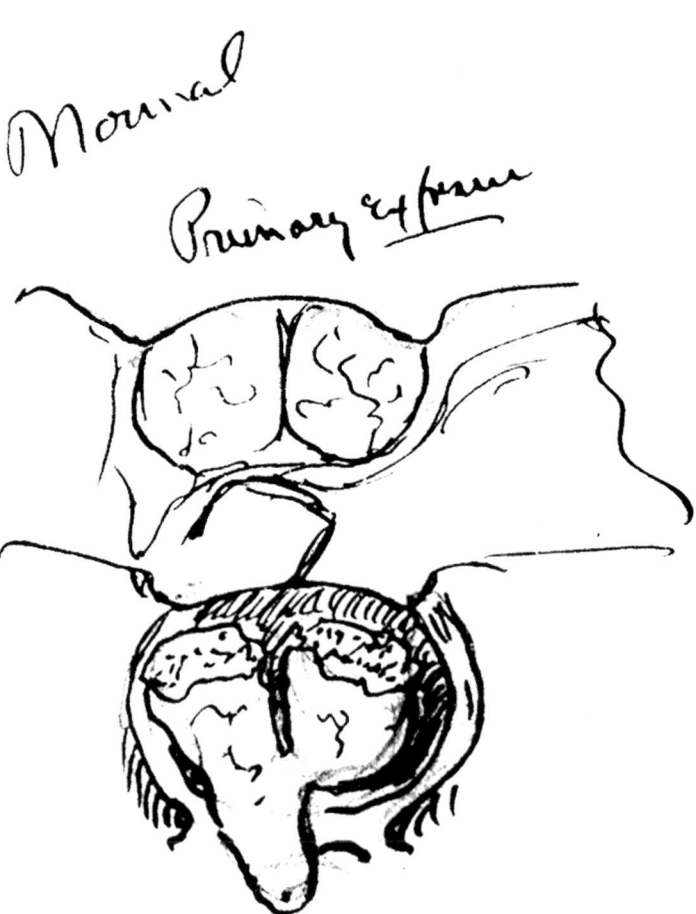

FIG. 2. OPERATIVE SKETCH.

OPPOSITE PAGE. FIG. I. PREOPERATIVE.

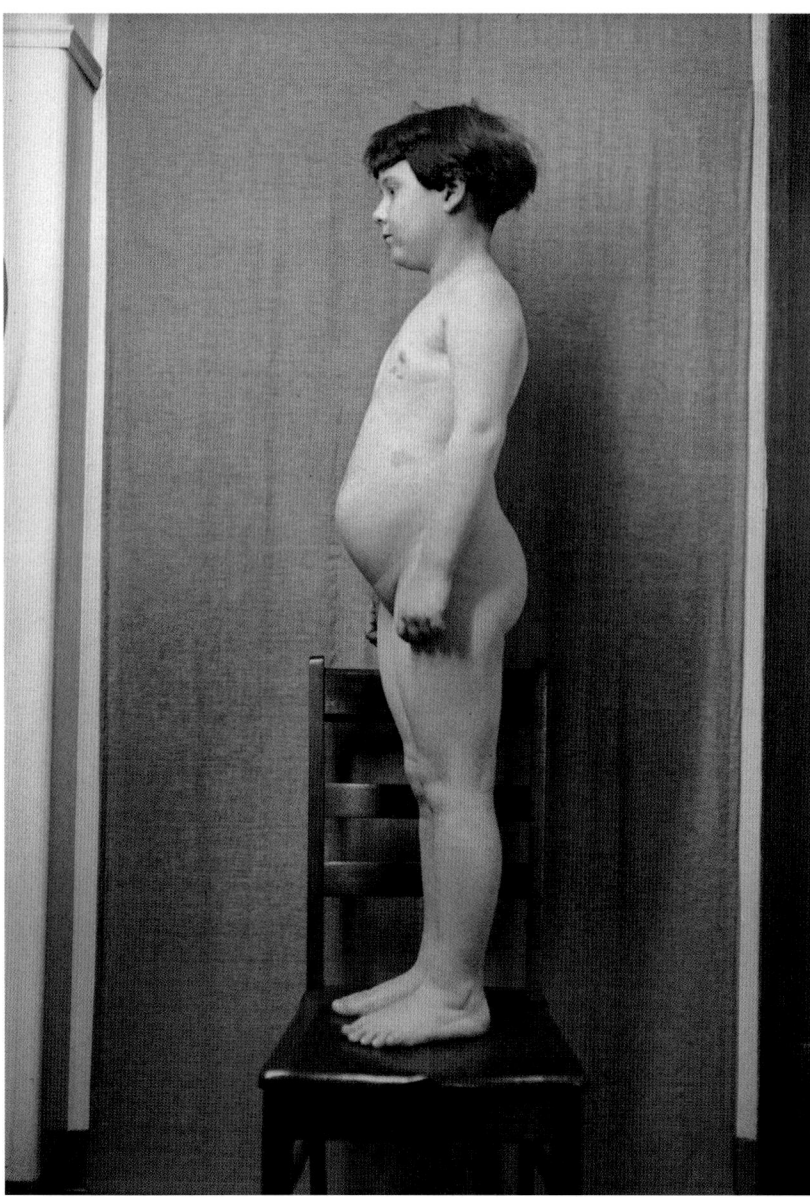

FIG. 3. PREOPERATIVE.

OBJECTIVE
    Bilateral primary atrophy.
    Obesity.
    Enlargement of the thyroid.
    Occasional tachycardia.

IMPRESSION: Dyspituitarism with tumor.

RADIOLOGY REPORT

X-ray films of the skull show some evidence of increased intracranial pressure with distortion of the sella turcica itself, the anterior clinoids are indistinctly made out but floor of the sella turcica is intact and the dorsum sella itself appears normal.

SPECIAL NOTE
April 7, 1922
Dr. Cushing

This child was supposed to have a suprasellar tumor, probably a pharyngeal pouch cyst. There was nothing about the case except her blindness with primary atrophy and a tendency to adiposity. The sella was one of the peculiar pear-shaped type of sellae shown in the accompanying sketch (Please note Dr. Cushing's Operative sketch, the upper image.)

OPERATIVE NOTE
April 7, 1922
Anesthesia – Ether – Miss Gerrard

Osteoplastic Resection of Right Frontal region.

It was possible without a primary puncture of the ventricle to elevate the lobe sufficiently to incise the dura along the sphenoidal margin in the usual fashion. There was an abundant escape of cerebrospinal fluid. Almost immediately a roundish tumor which was quite hard and which lay about in the position of the right optic nerve was exposed. My first thought was that this was a tumor projecting between the legs of the chiasm but on investigating the outer side of the tumor I could not see any sign of the optic nerve and supposed that the growth must therefore be a primary tumor of the chiasm, similar to the recent case of (the name of another patient) and a former case which had been operated upon.

On investigating further a similar mass, round, hard, so that the two looked very much like an infantile nates with a groove between them was brought into view, and I felt then almost certain that we had a tumor of each optic nerve. Dr. Wolbach and Dr. Smith were brought in to see the condition.

Fortunately, the tumor was not vascular and with a blunt dissector it was possible to scrape first the tumor on the right away from what was supposed to be the region of the optic foramen and to free it from the neighboring structures, pushing it backward. This disclosed a grayish, much distorted optic nerve which really had been in view previously but which I had taken to be the carotid artery in view of its color.

The tumor on the other side was similarly treated and in view of the fact that the growth was

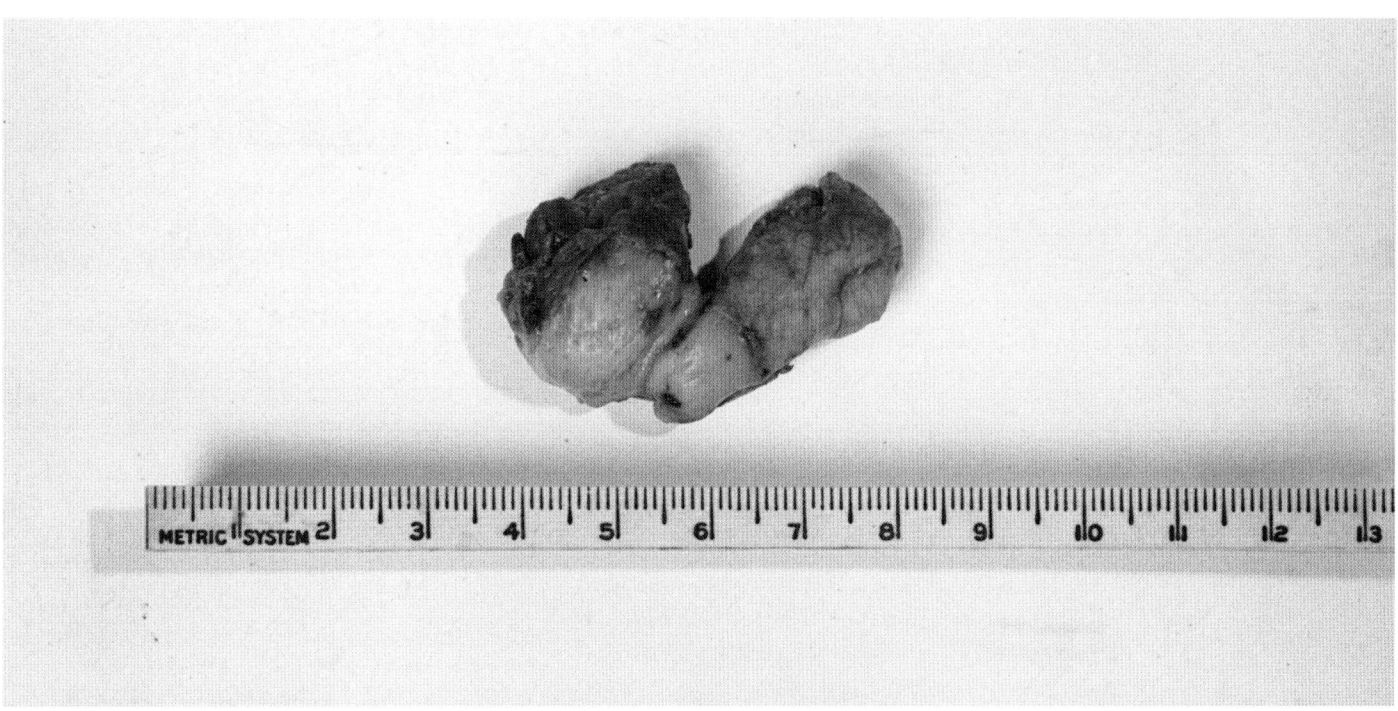

FIG. 4. GROSS TUMOR SPECIMEN.

tough and hard it could be caught with pituitary rongeurs and the whole thing began to be drawn forward. To my discomfiture, however, I notice that from the left nerve there was a prolongation which extended back for some distance, how far could not be told, and as this began to dislodge itself, Miss Gerrard stated that the pulse had become enormously slowed. I therefore desisted and it was only a moment or two when the child stopped breathing.

The field was dismantled and not being satisfied with the character of artificial respiration which some one was giving her, I took this over myself, and by gentle pressure on the thorax could get a sufficient exchange to keep the color fairly good. I did not have any idea that the child would regain spontaneous respiration. However, after about ten minutes, she took a single deep inspiration, after about ten minutes more another. This continued for about 45 minutes, at the end of which time she began with a few superficial respiratory movements, and fairly good respirations were resumed. I did not believe for a moment during all this period that there was any chance that this would occur. No further measures were instituted though there were various suggestions as to drugs, stretching the sphincter ani, etc.

Without any further anaesthesia of course the wound was then re-investigated and though I felt considerable apprehensions in doing so, the growth was again caught hold of and was completely dislodged coming away with practically no bleeding. The field was irrigated, the bone flap was replaced and closed with as great care as though this accident had not occurred. The child made a good recovery from the anaesthetic.

(Dr. Cushing)

DISCHARGE NOTE
April 8, 1922
Dr. Martin

A few hours after the operation she had not regained consciousness and at 4 p.m. her temperature was 108 degree. Her respirations were regular all through the night. Early in the morning her breathing began to be very shallow and at 7:00 a.m. she expired without having regained consciousness.

AUTOPSY NOTE

DIAGNOSES
  Glioma of optic chiasm.
  Gliosis of optic tracts.
  Normal pituitary.

Gross Specimen: The dura was incised and the brain removed in the usual manner. In removing the brain, the operative field at the base was exposed and found to contain a small amount of bloody clot. The carotid arteries are seen as thin grey bands but the optic chiasm was entirely missing. When the brain is removed the sella turcica presents a striking appearance. The pituitary body is normal in the base, in the base of sella turcica and in its fossa. Above this the sella has been greatly widened antero-posteriorly and it is now evidence that the tumor removed by Dr. Cushing at operation was a tumor of the optic chiasm, and that the portion removed at operation included the optic chiasm proper, much enlarged and destroyed. It is this tumor which has enlarged the sella turcica and has pushed into the optic foramina, enlarging its openings greatly and pushing then anteriorly. A small nubbin of tumor is found in each optic foramen and when the bone has been cleared away, it is seen that the optic nerve beyond the foramen is not enlarged.

On examination of the brain it is found that the tumor, which is very similar in appearance to that of (name of two previous patients), must have filled the entire peduncular space from which it was removed at operation. Considerable of the tumor, however, still remains and can be traced backward and superiorly for an indefinite distance along the optic tracts.

Microscopic examination: The optic tracts show marked gliosis with little increase in cellular elements. The sections taken from the floor of the third ventricle seem to represent true tumor formation with increase in blood vessels, marked increase in neuroglia fibrils and definite increase in small round and oval cells which are, no doubt, from their appearance glia cells. No mitosis are seen. The pathology is best shown in slide marked A"A. There is in this section, and to a less extent in the other sections from the floor of the 3rd ventricle, a basic staining amorphous material in masses and strands which, no doubt, represent the so-called cytoid bodies found in these tumors. There are two sections of the pituitary which show a rather large, but normal, pituitary in histology.

DIAGNOSIS – Glioma of optic chiasm.

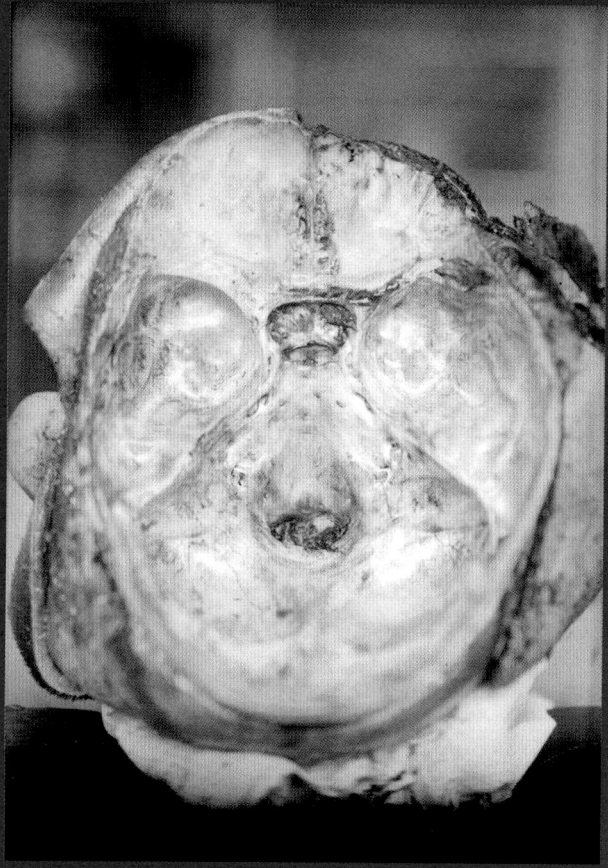
FIG. 5. AUTOPSY SPECIMEN — SKULL.

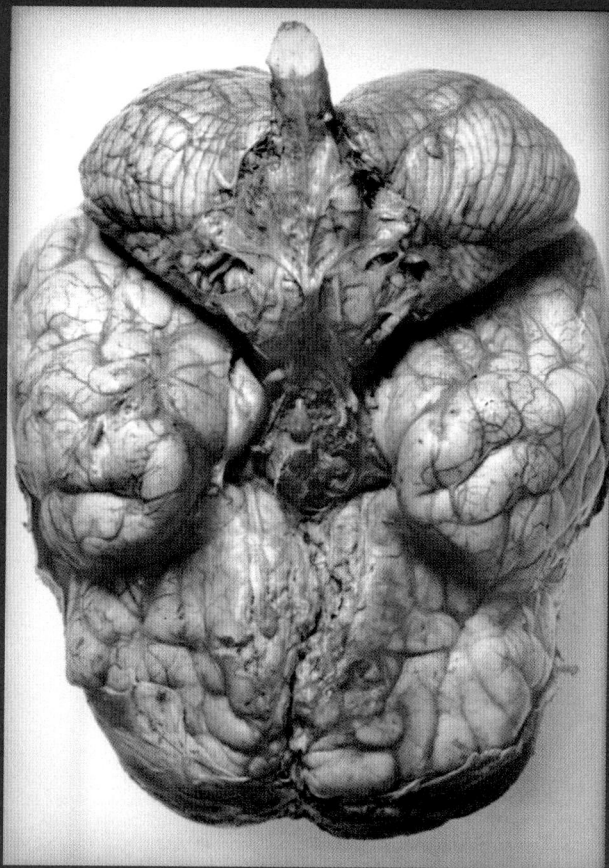
FIG. 6. AUTOPSY SPECIMEN — BRAIN (WHOLE).

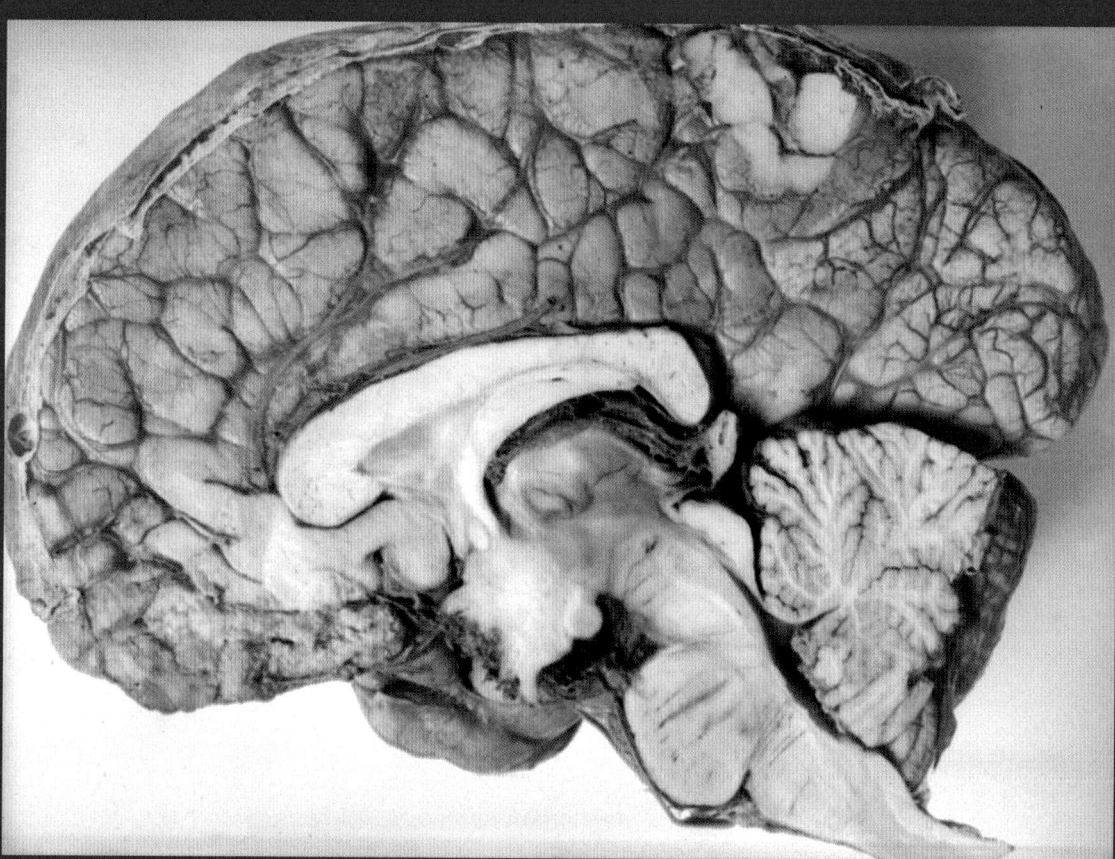
FIG. 7. AUTOPSY SPECIMEN — BRAIN (SAGITTAL VIEW).

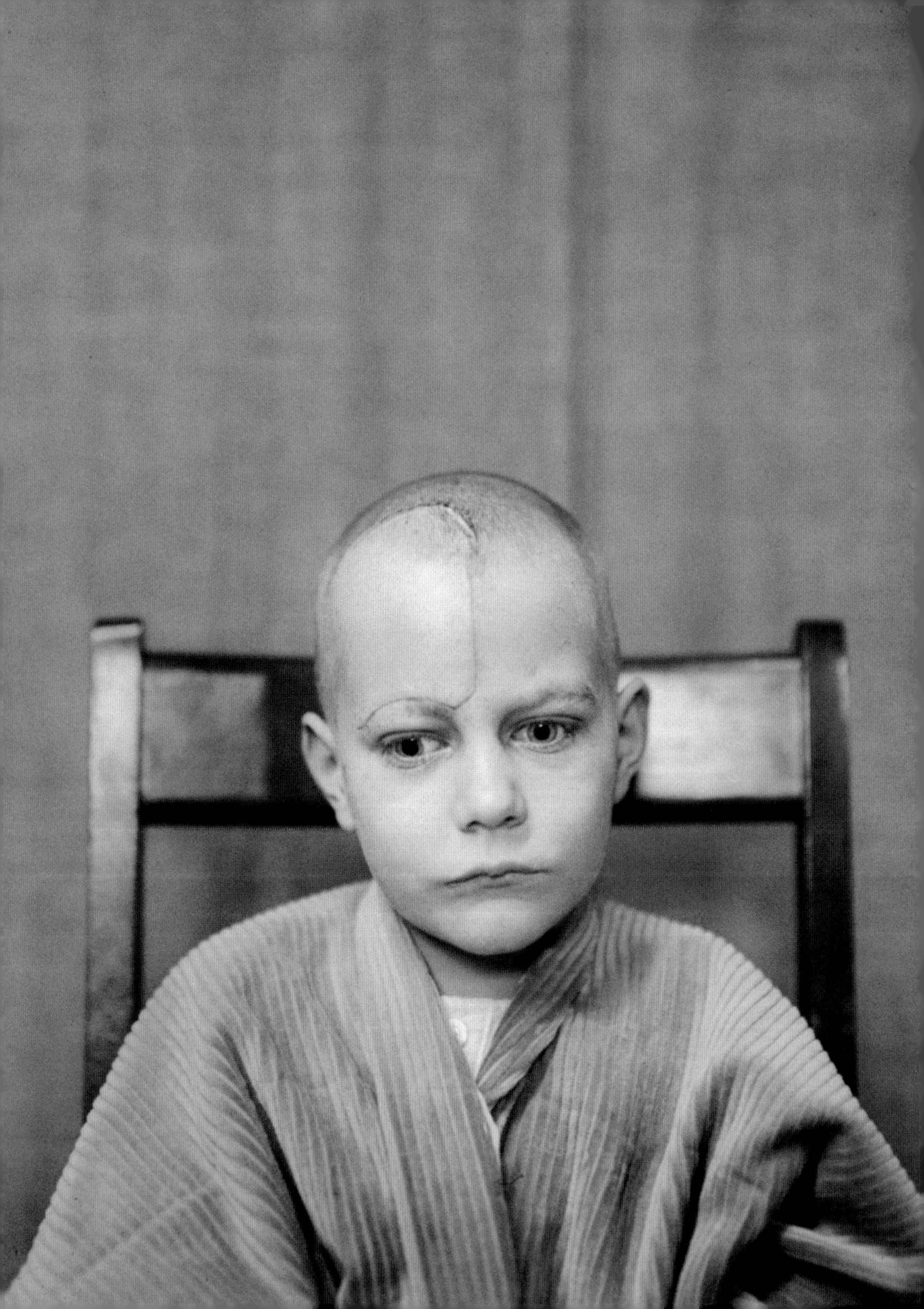

1.9 Craniopharyngioma

SEX: F; AGE: CHILD; SURG. NO. UNKNOWN

HISTORY

Six years prior to this admission, the child began to have progressive frontal headaches. She would vomit her breakfast and frequently spent the remainder of the day in bed. Two years prior this hospital entry, the right eye "became crossed and she began to hold her book closer to her eyes to read." One year ago, she could no longer read and at the time of admission was blind in the right eye and distinguishes only light and dark in her left eye.

SUMMARY OF POSITIVE FINDINGS
October 27, 1922
Dr. Bailey

SUBJECTIVE
1. Headaches for six years, mostly frontal at first, lately suboccipital and accompanied by vomiting.
2. Failing vision for the last few years, practically complete blindness now.

OBJECTIVE
1. Bilateral primary optic atrophy.
2. Right pupil does not react to light.
3. Left one reacts slowly.
4. Practically complete blindness.
5. Emaciation.
6. Some suboccipital tenderness

IMPRESSION: Suprasellar tumor.

RADIOLOGY REPORT
October 27, 1922
M.C. Sosman

Stereoscopic films of the skull in right lateral position show a small skull with marked convolutional markings. The sutures are distinct but not widened. The sella turcica is unusually wide and deep and there are multiple small irregular areas of increased density directly above the anterior clinoids and apparently in midline. Findings are strongly suggestive of suprasellar tumor.

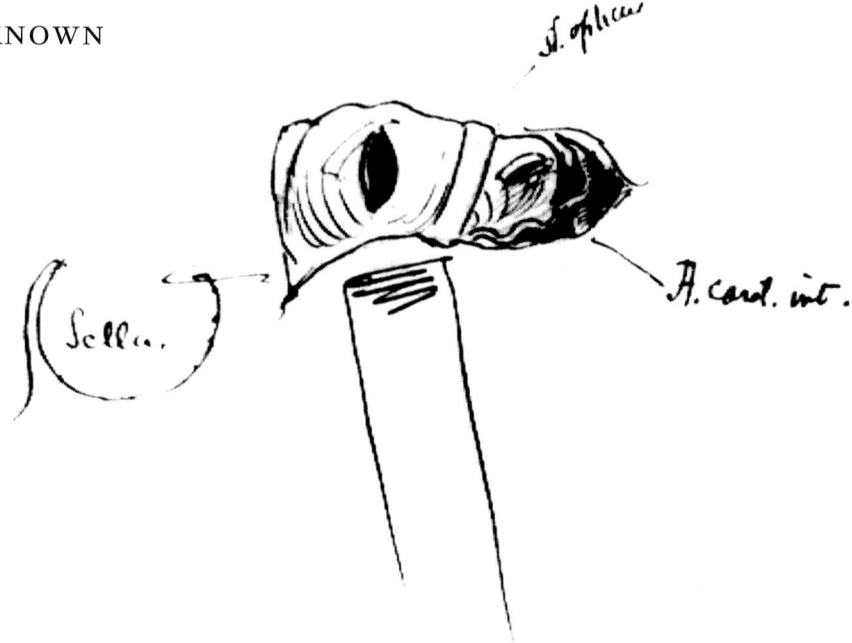

FIG. 2. OPERATIVE SKETCH.

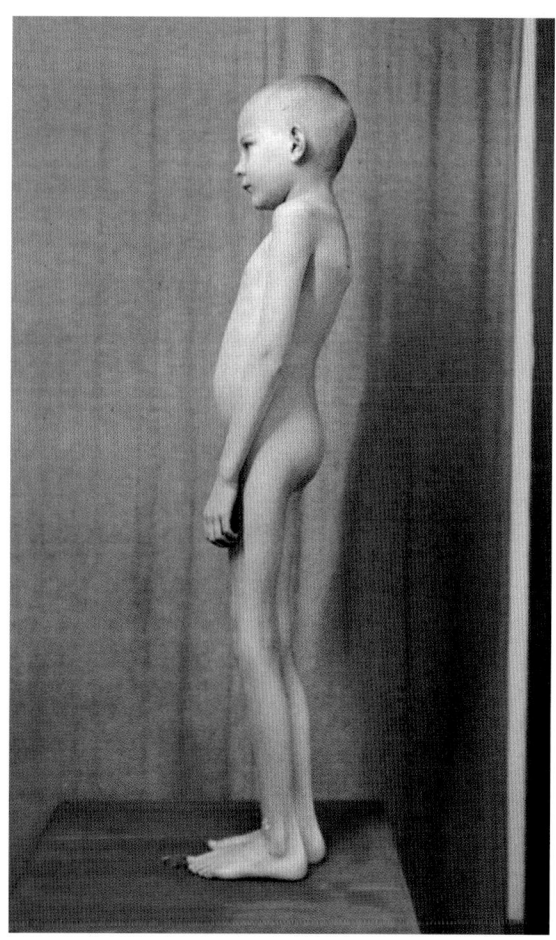

FIG. 3. THREE WEEKS POSTOPERATIVE AFTER THE SECOND SURGERY.

OPPOSITE PAGE. FIG. 1. THREE WEEKS POSTOPERATIVE AFTER THE SECOND SURGERY.

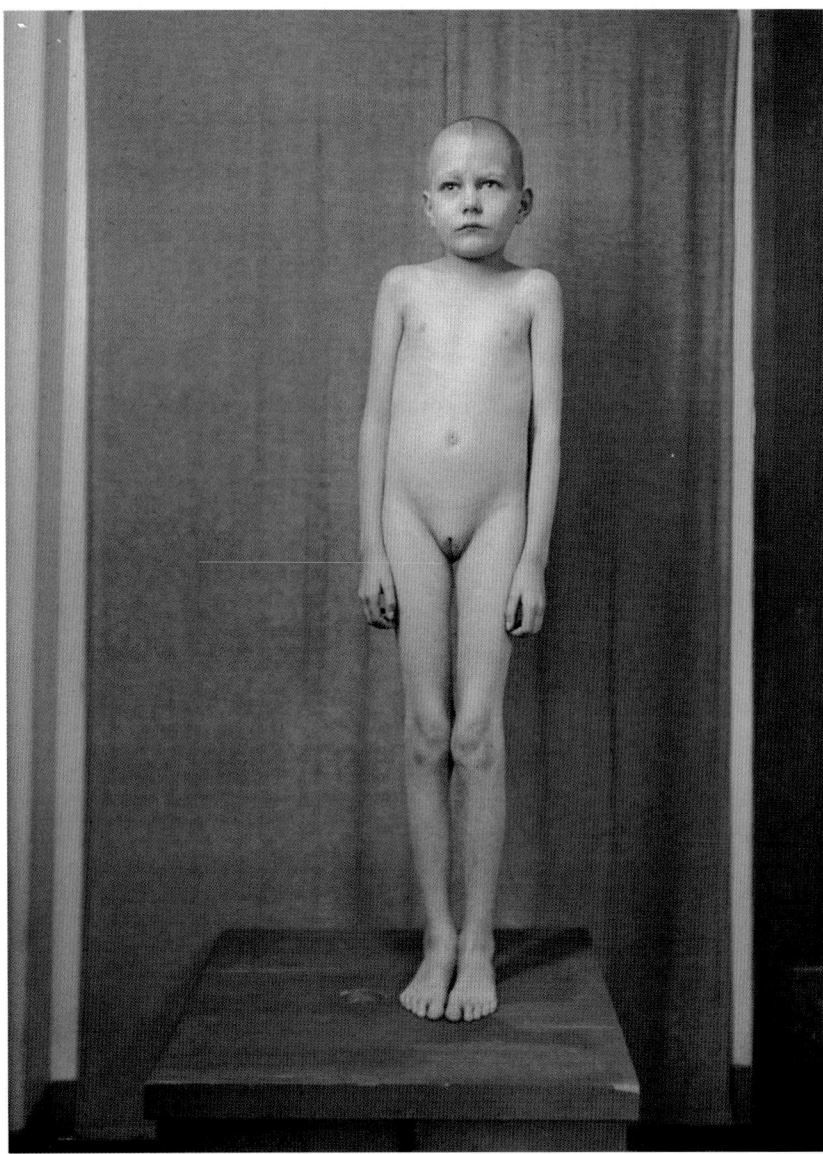

FIG. 4. THREE WEEKS POSTOPERATIVE AFTER THE SECOND SURGERY.

OPERATIVE NOTE
November 1, 1922
Anesthesia – Ether – Miss Gerrard

Transfrontal Osteoplastic Procedure with Exposure of and Evacuation of a Suprasellar Pharyngeal Pouch Cyst.

This was a very feeble blind child. Had it not been for the betrayal of the lesion by the shadows above the sella I would not have ventured to predict that she had a suprasellar lesion for she showed none of the adiposity commonly associated with this trouble. The operation was unusually simple there being no complications in elevating the flap. I had some misgivings about it and thought for a time that I would merely do a colossal puncture but finally decided upon the major procedure. A needle was introduced through the somewhat tense dura at the upper and inner angle, and two punctures in the usual direction failed to strike the ventricle. I assumed therefore there must be a good deal of distortion. The frontal lobe was elevated and the dura incised in the usual fashion bringing into view the right optic nerve flattened over a tense bluish cyst. This cyst protruded to the right of the right optic nerve. The cyst was incised and about 15 cc. of dirty brownish fluid was evacuated. The fluid contained obvious cholesterin crystals. The capsule immediately collapsed. It was thick walled and it would have been possible to deal with it perhaps at this session but inasmuch as the child was feeble, I felt it was best to let the procedure go as a simple evacuation of the cyst and to wait for a second stage. The flap was replaced and closed in layers without a drain.

It may possibly be a good thing to attempt to get in between the two hemispheres or between the hemisphere and the falx at the next session provided I can get fluid from the ventricle.

This patient had an uneventful postoperative course.

OPERATIVE NOTE
November 8, 1922
Anesthesia – Ether – Miss Gerrard

Dr. Cushing's Second Stage Operation.

The bone flap was re-elevated and an effort was made by two punctures to get into the ventricle again without success. An effort was then made by getting in between the right hemisphere and the falx to get down to what was supposed to be in view of the x-ray a large cyst, and after going in some distance below the lowest margin of the falx no cyst was encountered.

The frontal lobe was therefore again elevated. The operative field described previously was exposed, the capsule of the cyst at the point of the original incision was grasped and the cyst was finally with some dissection but without any bleeding withdrawn. When spread out it made an area of about 3 x 5 cm. The lower portion of the cyst occupying the fossa was then mildly curetted out and great masses of cholesterin came away in the spoon.

The flap was replaced and the wound closed in layers as usual.

(Dr. Cushing)

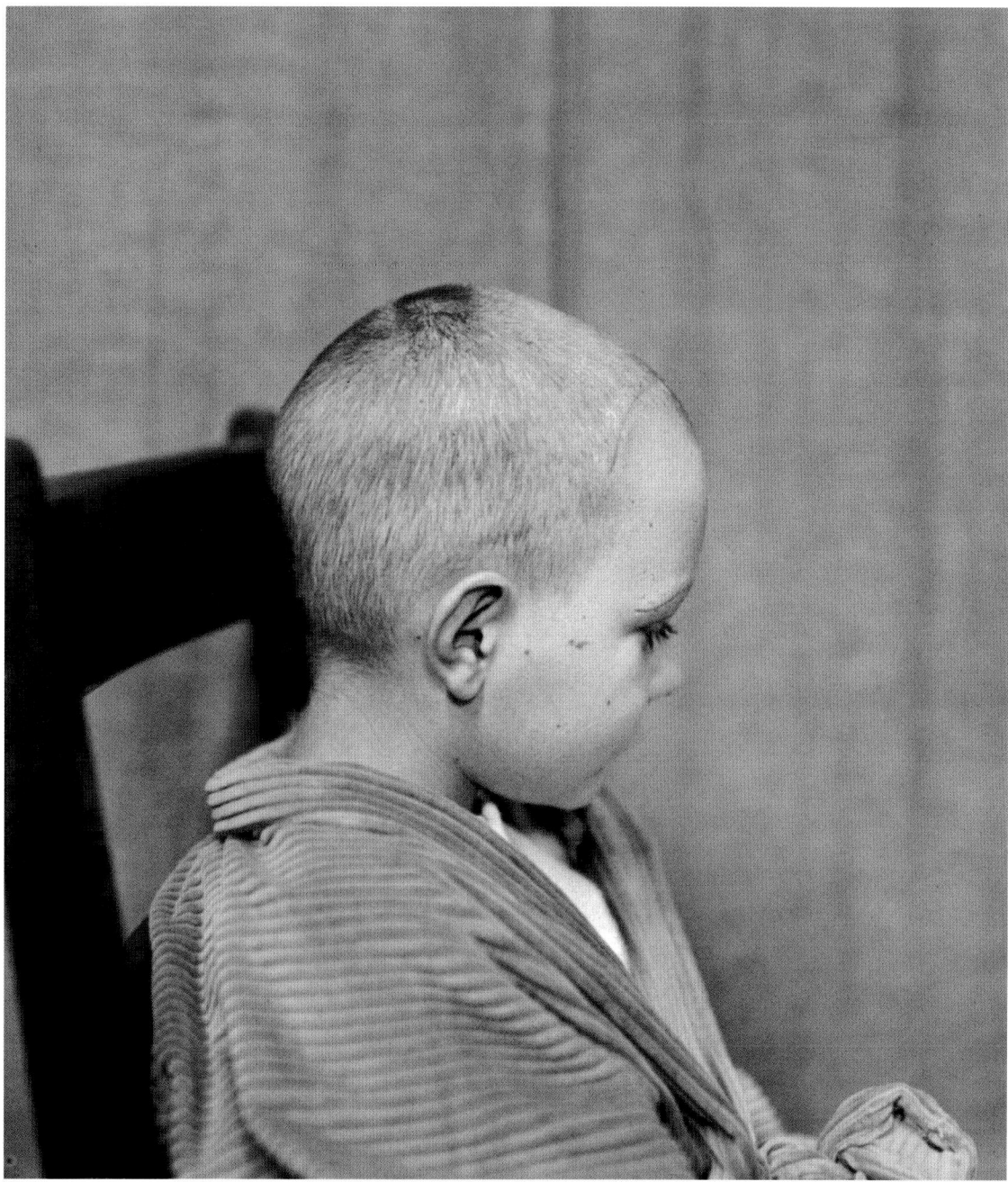

FIG. 5. THREE WEEKS POSTOPERATIVE AFTER THE SECOND SURGERY.

PATHOLOGY REPORT
November 8, 1922

Material – Cyst wall.

Description – ... This cyst wall was very tough, from 1-2 mm in thickness, the inner surface covered with calcified material and cholesterin crystals.

Microscopic – ...They show a cyst wall having numerous irregular masses of squamous epithelial cells in a stroma of fibrous connective tissue. There are also many whorls of keratinized epithelium. In areas there are large clefts which, no doubt, contained cholesterine crystals.

DIAGNOSIS – Epithelial cyst of Rathke's pouch.

HOSPITAL COURSE
November 10, 1922
Dr. McKenzie

The child has evidently acquired a marked diabetes insipidus.

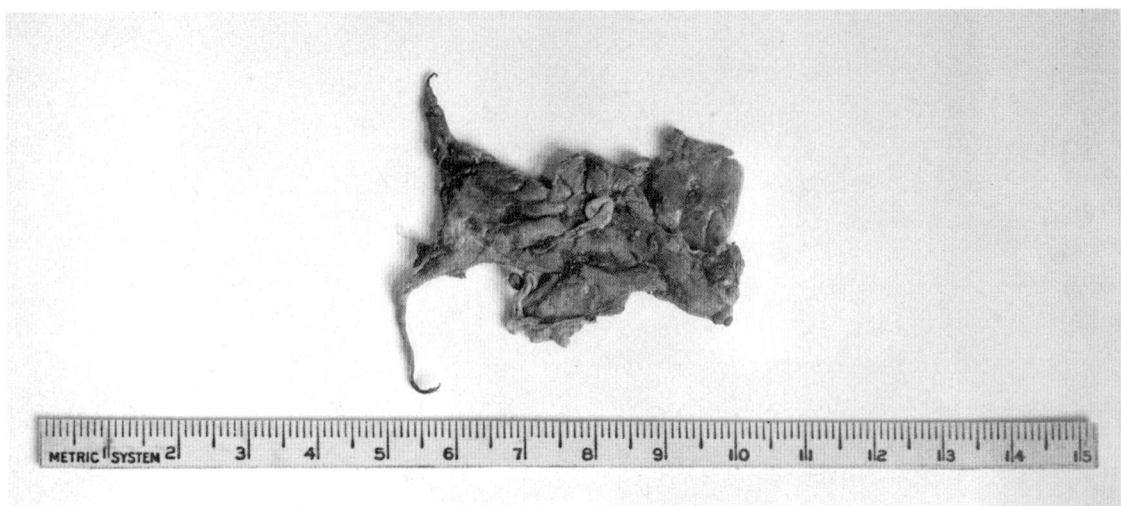

FIG. 6. RESECTED TUMOR SPECIMEN.

November 10-15, 1922

Dr. Percival Bailey, the house officer, noted that she progressed from drinking water constantly secondary to her diabetes insipidus to feeling well with practically resolved polyuria.

RADIOLOGY REPORT
November 10, 1922
M.C. Sosman

A re-examination of the skull shows an operative defect in the right frontal bone with several silver clips in the region of the dura. The calcified spots above the sella are absent. There are a few faint spots in the pituitary fossa.

DISCHARGE NOTE
November 28, 1922
Dr. Bailey

Vision unimproved. Has gained 5 pounds in weight and is much stronger than on entry. Is now very happy and lively.

LETTER TO DR. CUSHING
March 16, 1928

Dear Dr:

I am writing you in regards of your letter dated Mar. 6th that you want to know my daughter's height and weight. Well she was examined at school this morning so I know its correct. She is 4 feet ¼ inch tall and her weight 65-¼ pounds.

Well you said in your letter you wished I lived nearer that you could see her occasionally. Now Dr. if you think I could bring her up and you could take an X-ray of her head, perhaps there is something that's holding her sight back. If you think it would benefit her by bringing her back I will be glad to do so as three Drs. here claim she has vision in her eyes, Dr. Weinberger is one of them. Hoping to hear from you in regards to this, I remain,

Respectfully,
(Signed, the name of patient's mother)

OPPOSITE PAGE. FIG. 7. FOLLOW-UP IMAGES YEARS AFTER SURGERY.

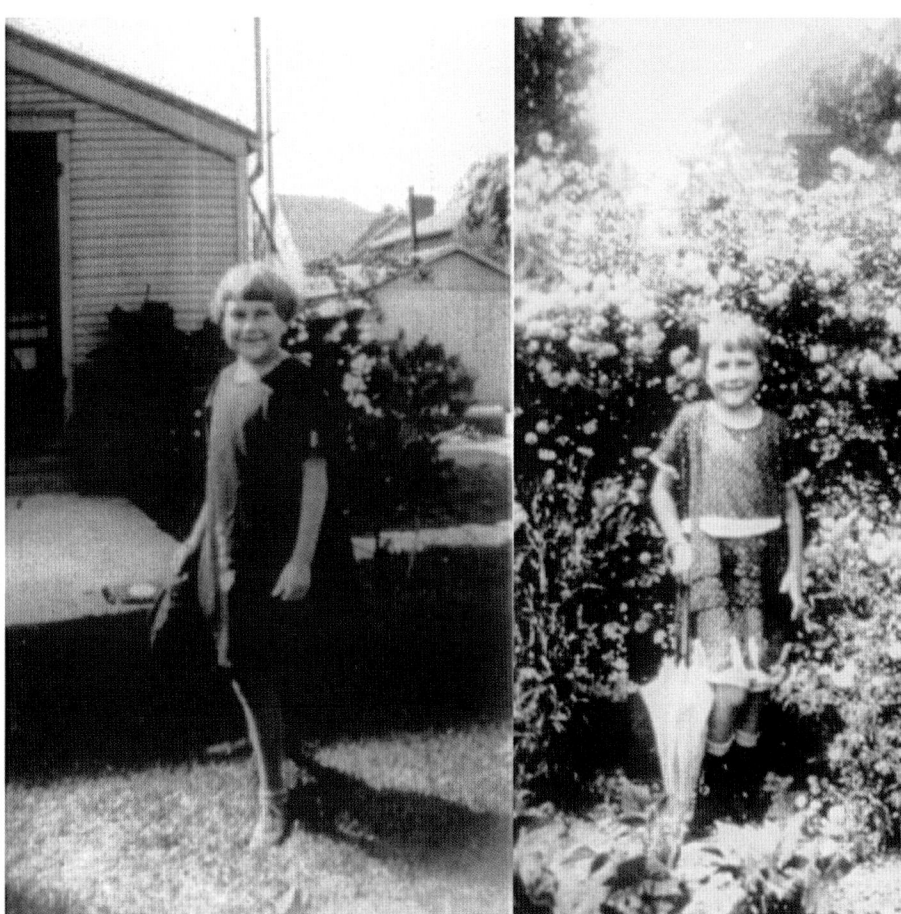

aug 19/24   July 10/23

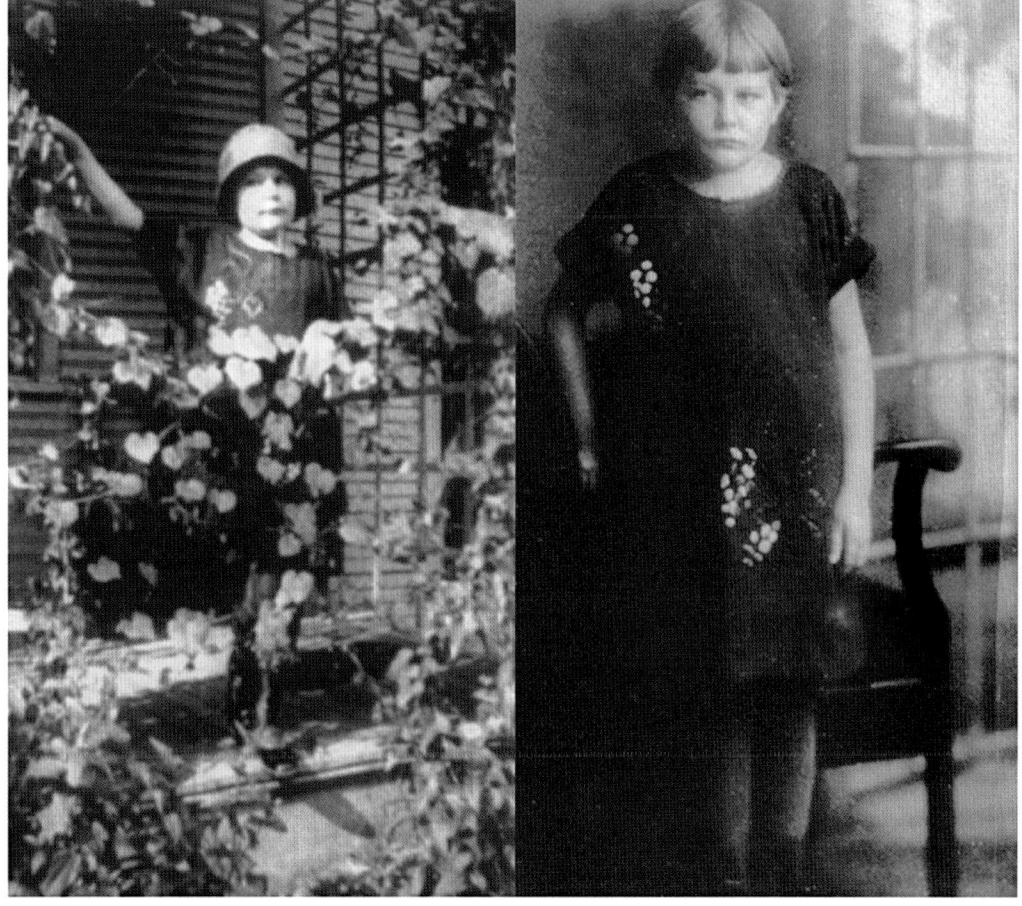

Sept 2/24

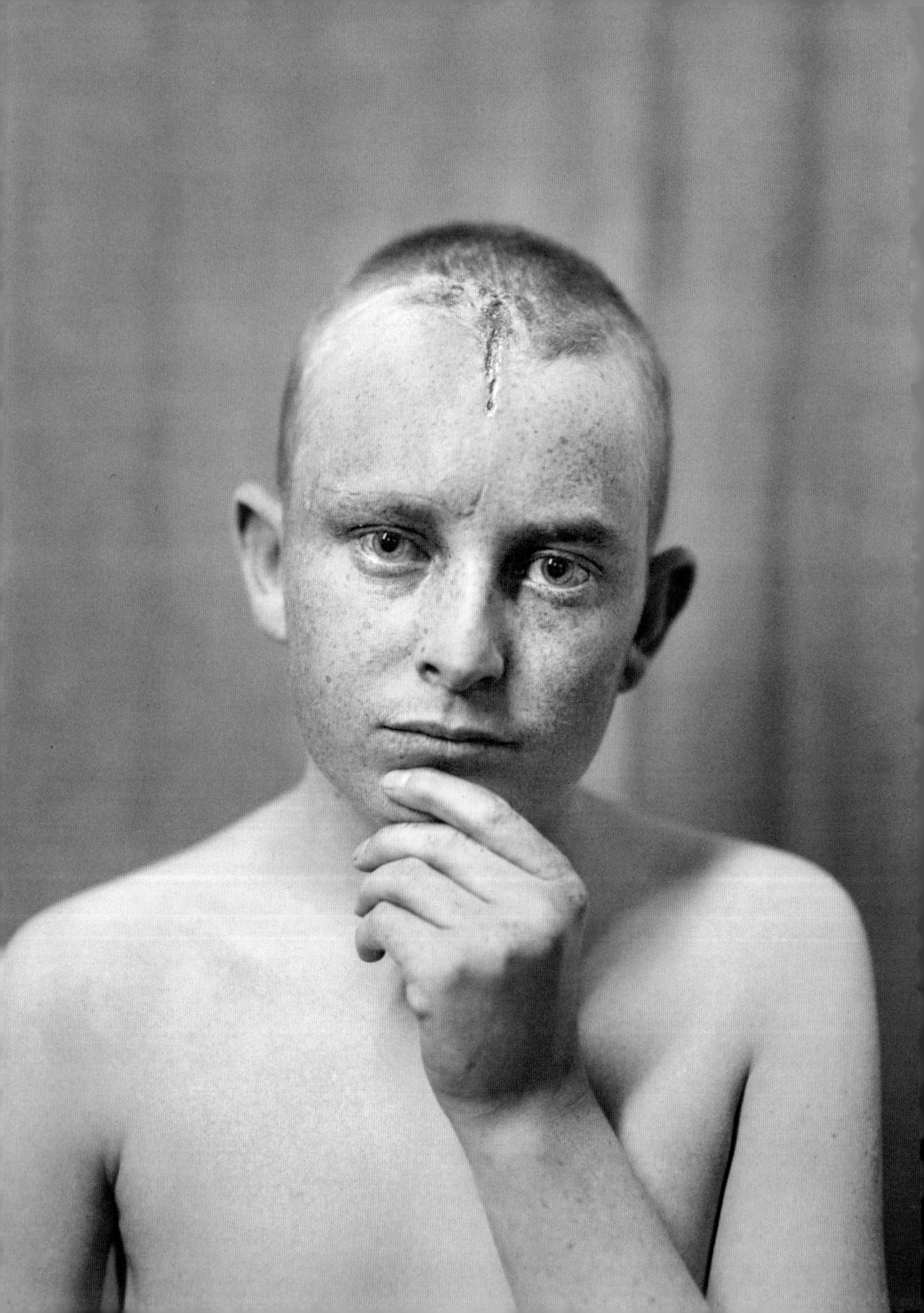

1.10 Pituitary adenoma

SEX: M; AGE: 18; SURG. NO. 18904

HISTORY

This patient suffered from frontal headaches for three years prior to his admission. His headaches came on about once a week, associated with a good deal of nausea and occasionally vomiting. Patient did not grow and did not mature during these last three years. He saw different doctors who treated him for various complaints. One and half years ago, he consulted Dr. Spearing of Cimarron who diagnosed the case, put him on pituitary gland extract, 5 grains a day. He took 500 tablets, but did not mature. About a year ago, he started to have problems with vision and five months ago his vision became so bad that he had to stop school.

SUMMARY OF POSITIVE FINDINGS
May 28, 1923
Dr. McKenzie

SUBJECTIVE
1. History of polyuria and slight nocturia for as long as patient can remember.
2. A normal individual until 15 years of age when he ceased to grow and did not mature.
3. Developed severe frontal headaches three years ago which were greatly relieved a year and a half ago by taking pituitary gland.
4. Difficulty with vision, developed a year and a half ago, becoming so severe five months ago that he had to leave school.

OBJECTIVE
1. Bilateral primary optic atrophy with bitemporal visual field defect.
2. Metabolism: --8
3. Sella greatly enlarged.
4. Small individual, smooth faced, female distribution of suprapubic hair and fat, rather small skeleton, dry, smooth skin.

IMPRESSION: Suprasellar cyst although the x-ray has not been seen yet.

RADIOLOGY REPORT
May 28, 1923

Stereoscopic films of the skull show a thin cranial vault, slightly turri-cephalic. The sella turcica is large, irregular and shows definite destruction, with a small area of increased density above the fossa. Findings are compatible with a suprasellar cyst.

SPECIAL NOTE
June 9, 1923
Dr. Cushing

I possibly should have realized that this young man had a pituitary adenoma rather than a suprasellar cyst in view of the widely dilated pituitary fossa. There was some hint that the x-rays showed suprasellar shadows, and I presume it was on this basis that the misinterpretation was made.

OPERATIVE NOTE
June 9, 1923
Anesthesia – Ether – Miss Gerrard

Right Transfrontal Exploration – Disclosure of Protruding Pituitary Adenoma. Partial Extirpation of Contents.

The osteoplastic flap was made by Dr. Horrax and the region of the chiasm exposed. I took the operation over at this juncture. Between the legs of the chiasm was a soft bulging, reddish mass which might easily have been a cyst. On grasping its walls, quite a little of it was dislodged, and I presumed that it represents an adenoma which has been through the capsule. The thin elastic wall was entered and with pituitary rongeurs and a spoon a pocketful the size of a thimble was cleaned of its adenomatous contents. There was a good deal of persistent oozing which necessitated the placement of bits of muscle taken from the subtemporal region.

There was a delay of almost an hour in this blood stilling process and then even there may possibly have been a little ooze at the time of closure.

The bone flap was replaced and closed in layers by Dr. Horrax.

(Dr. Cushing)

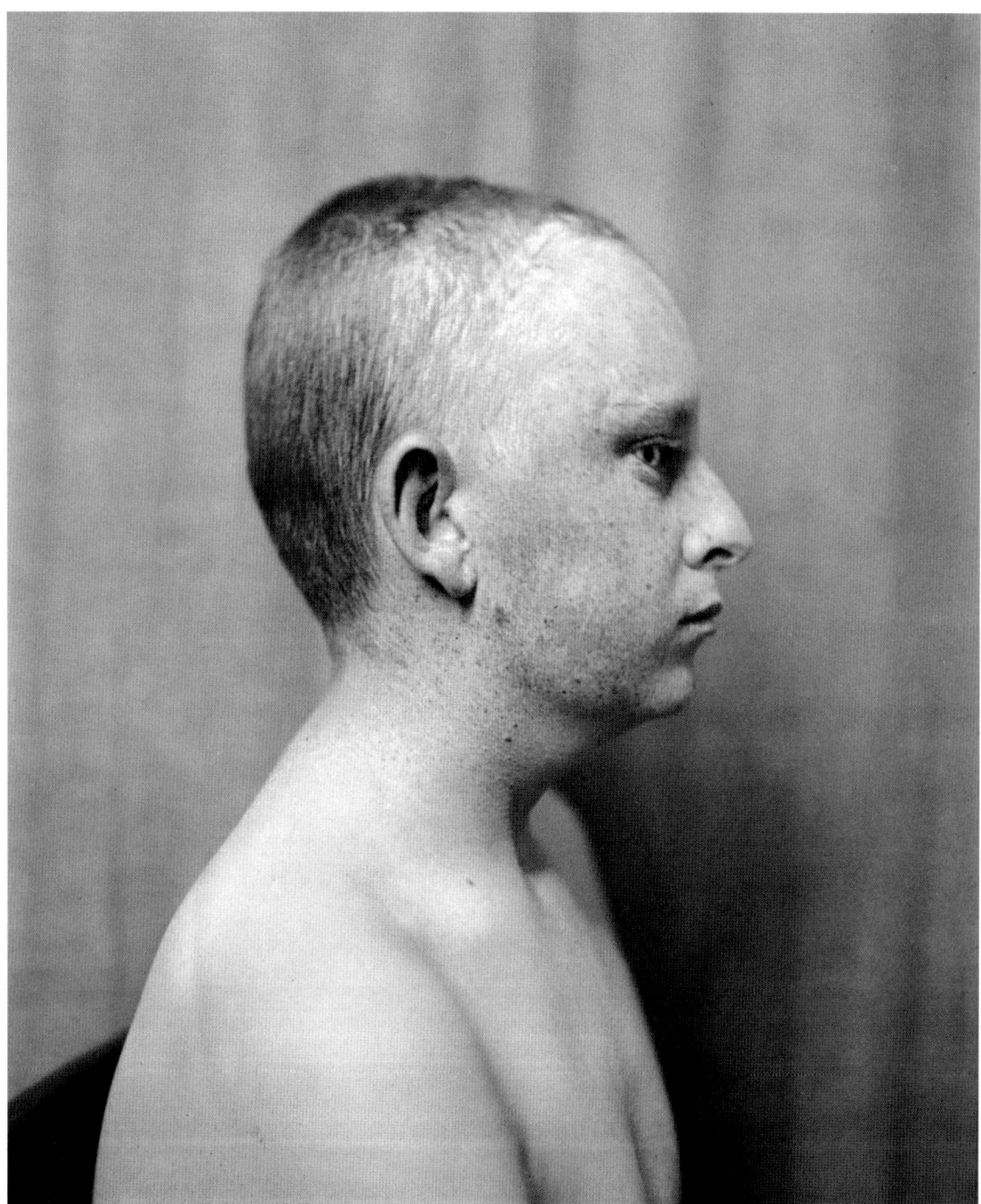

FIG. 2. THREE WEEKS POSTOPERATIVE.

PATHOLOGY REPORT
June 10, 1923

Gross description: This tissue was removed from a supposed pituitary adenoma. The whole of the tissue removed is submitted for examination. After it had been scooped out, a hole the size of a small almond was left between the two optic nerves.

(Dr. Cushing)

Microscopic result: The epithelial cells are large, granular cytoplasm and conspicuous nuclei which do not show definite mitotic figures. Some of the cells show vacuolization and cystic changes.

DIAGNOSIS – Adenoma of pituitary.

(Dr. Hansmann)

June 19, 1923
Dr. Boyd

Has complained deal of headache past few days, now much better. Yesterday, walked about ward. Wound dry. Urine output about to 2800 cc now.

June 23, 1923
Dr. McKenzie

Eye fields show marked improvement. Patient had one X-ray treatment.

DISCHARGE NOTE
July 3, 1923
Dr. McKenzie

This patient since his operation has done quite well as far as his eye fields are concerned. They have come practically to normal in the right eye with still quite a definite defect in the left. The general condition is practically the same as before operation. He still has his polyuria, which appears to be very little affected by pituitary injection or pledgets in the nose. He has been given one x-ray treatment. We felt that we would have liked to have kept him here for some time longer to see if we could not help his polyuria and also by losing a bit of weight. However, his mother insisted on taking him home. She has been told to write Dr. Cushing in a few months regarding his condition.

April 24, 1935

A questionnaire was sent to patient. The following answers were obtained: Patient is passing 48 oz of urine a day. His vision improved. He has a few spots in his left eye. His weight is 124 and ¼ lb. His height is 5' 2". There are no headaches. He is working. He is sexually active.

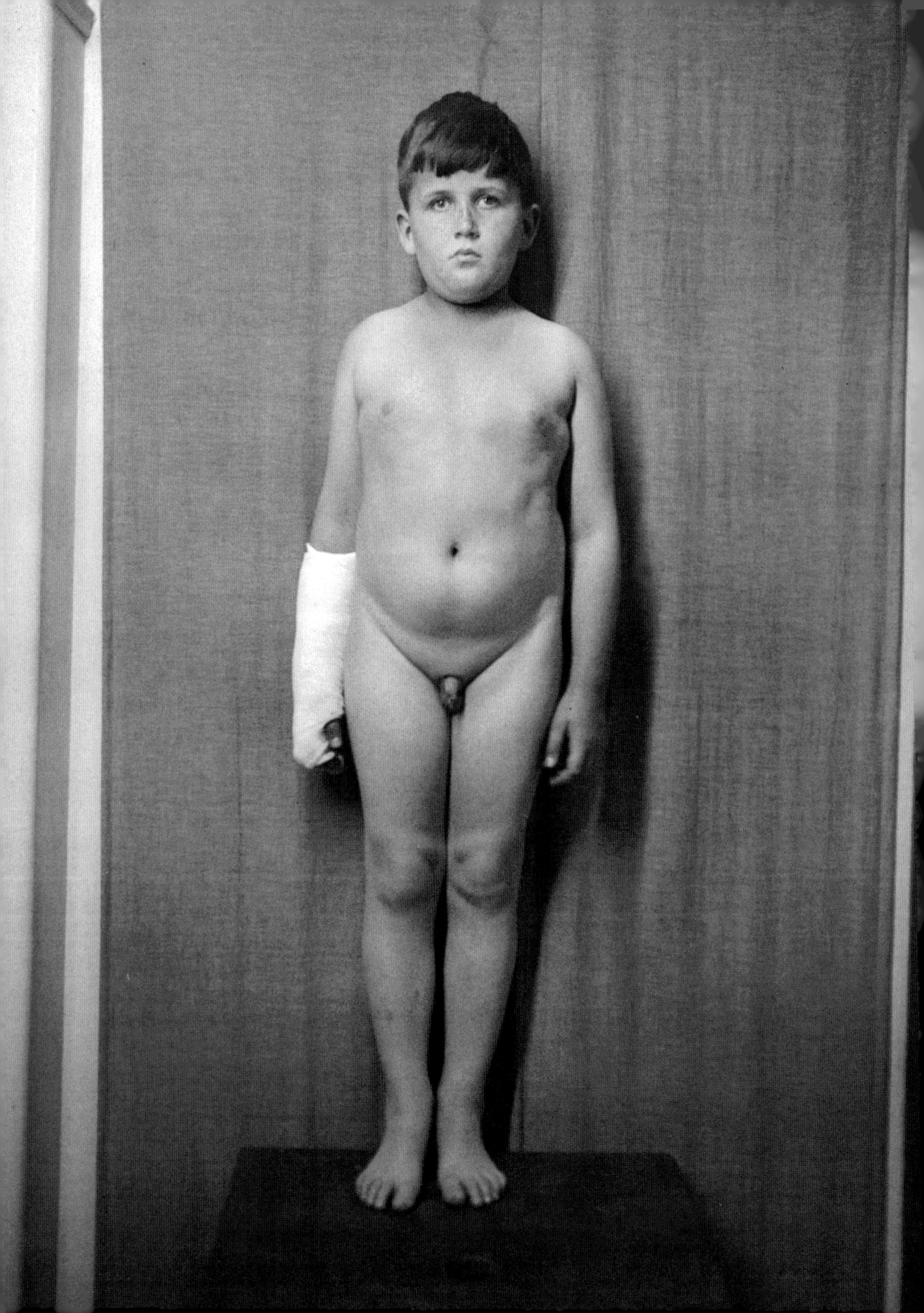

1.11 Glioma of optic chiasm

SEX: M; AGE: 9; SURG. NO. 21989

HISTORY

This patient suffered from a long-standing history of obesity, progressive mental dullness, convulsion and blindness. He always seemed "rather fat and disinclined to exertion." His development was normal until four years of age.

SUMMARY OF POSITIVE FINDINGS
August 20, 1924
Dr. Putman

SUBJECTIVE
1. Obese, lazy and irritable since birth.
2. Onset of convulsions at age of four years characterized by clenching teeth, convulsive movements, and lately falling, with only momentary loss of consciousness. A later one proceeded by aura and succeeded by sleep.
3. Primary atrophy noted shortly after onset and bitemporal hemianopsia noted since that time. Left eye more affected than right.
4. Speech has become progressively more slurred and movements of arms and legs more clumsy during the past two years.
5. Very abnormal desire for sweets, appetite very large. Some polydipsia. No polyuria.
6. Mental development much retarded.

OBJECTIVE
1. An obese, stupid, rather hyperactive child with a rather characteristic expression and habitus.
2. Bilateral primary atrophy and bitemporal hemianopsia.
3. Concomitant strabismus. Possible slight weakness of the lower part of right face.
4. Reflexes rather exaggerated.
5. Some dysmetria and intention tremor. Romberg positive. Gait unsteady but not definitely ataxic.
6. Speech nasal and slurring.

IMPRESSION: Suprasellar cyst.

RADIOLOGY REPORT
August 22, 1924
Dr. Sosman

Stereoscopic films of the skull show the cranial vault to be smooth and without signs of increased

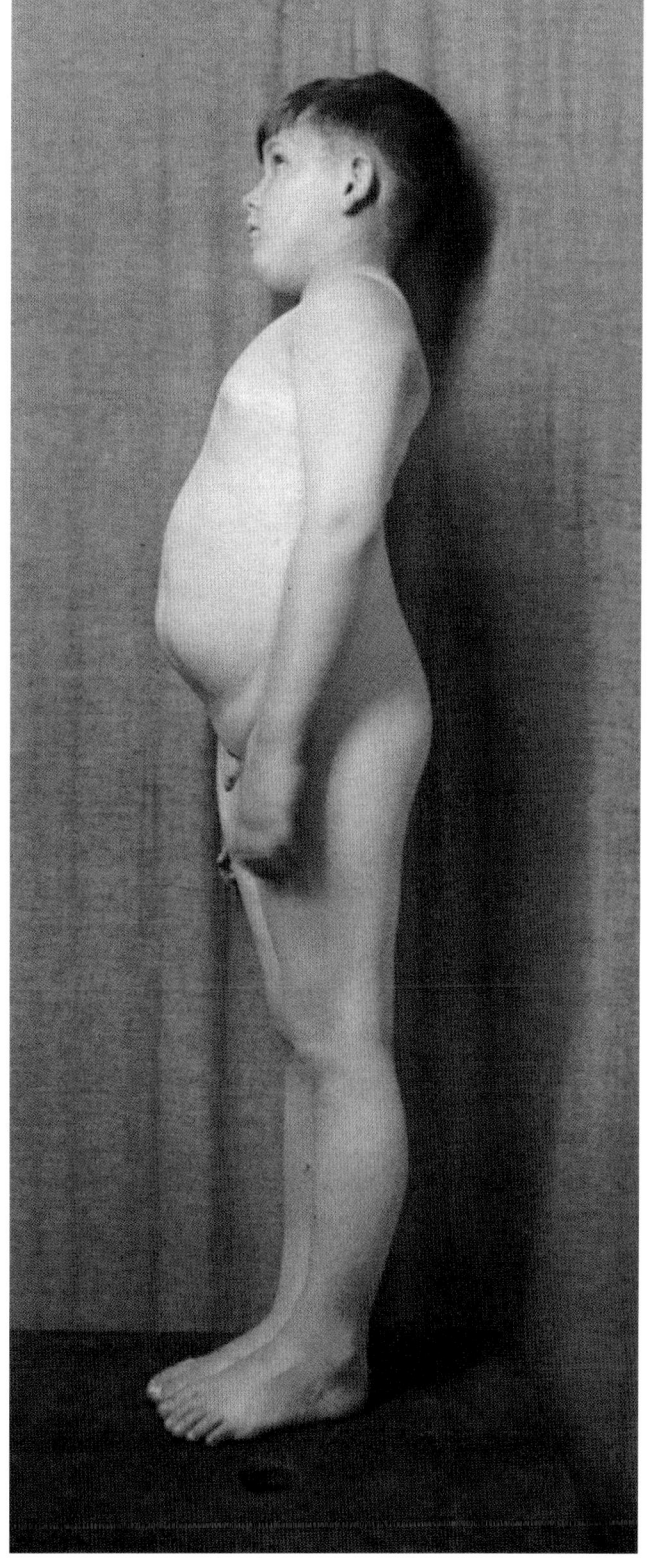

FIG. 2. PREOPERATIVE.

OPPOSITE PAGE. FIG. I. PREOPERATIVE.

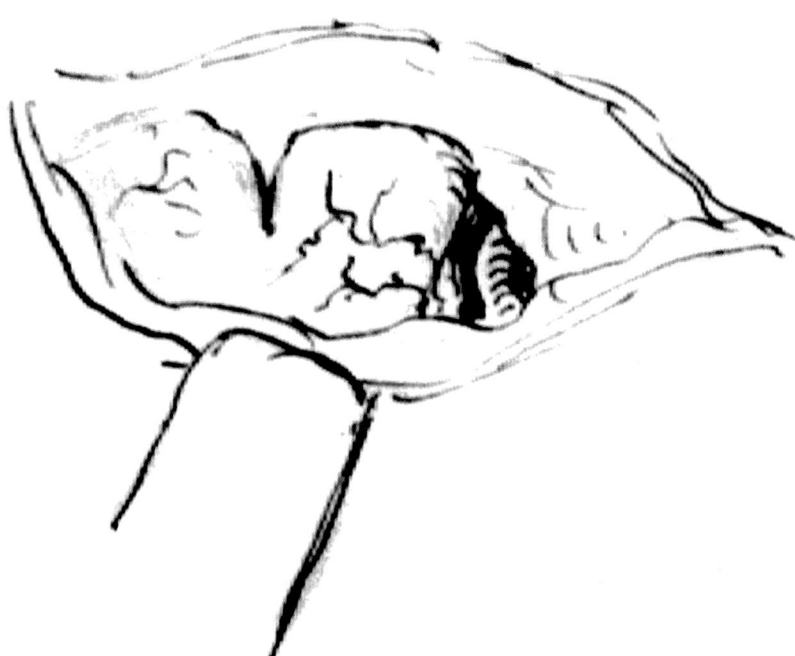

FIG. 3. OPERATIVE SKETCH.

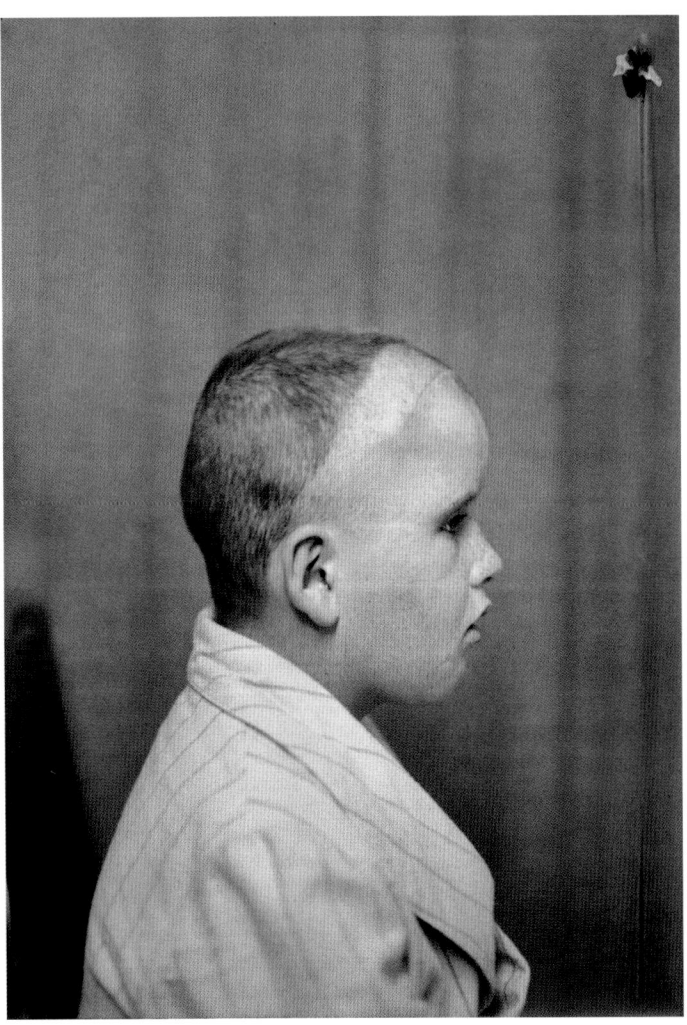

FIG. 4A. FIVE WEEKS POSTOPERATIVE.

pressure. The sella appears quite shallow but the anterior clinoid cannot be identified. No suprasellar calcification seen.

SPECIAL NOTE
August 28, 1924
Dr. Cushing

This small boy has had a long-standing history suggesting ductless gland and pituitary disorder. He has become blind in one eye and has a hemianopsia in the other with primary atrophy. X-ray, however, shows no shadow of a suprasellar cyst though it was a condition of this sort that I anticipated finding. I had no idea that we were possibly going to find a tumor of the chiasm for his secondary hypophyseal symptoms were a little too marked for this and his hemianopsia too sharply cut. It would probably be a good thing to have some x-ray exposures of his optic foramina.

OPERATIVE NOTE
August 29, 1924
Anaesthesia – Ether – Miss Moody

Right Frontal Osteoplastic Resection. Disclosure of Chiasmal Tumor.

There was no special difficulty in turning down the flap in this little boy's case though there was a funny nodular and irregular projection of bone in the middle of the flap which must have been adherent to dura for it tore away and left a hole in the dura. Moreover, a very large frontal sinus, the existence of which I did not suspect from the x-ray picture, was cut through in dividing the lower leg of the flap.

It was finally possible to get down under the frontal lobe, to open the dura, to secure a large amount of cerebrospinal fluid and finally to expose the large, succulent optic nerves which gave a picture somewhat similar to that in the accompanying sketch. There was nothing more that I could possibly do. The small hole in the dura was closed, the bone flap was replaced as accurately as possible hoping that there might not be a leak into the frontal sinus and the usual wound closure was made and dressing applied.

(Dr. Cushing)

August 29, 1924
Dr. Putman

No obvious changes in condition. Patient com-

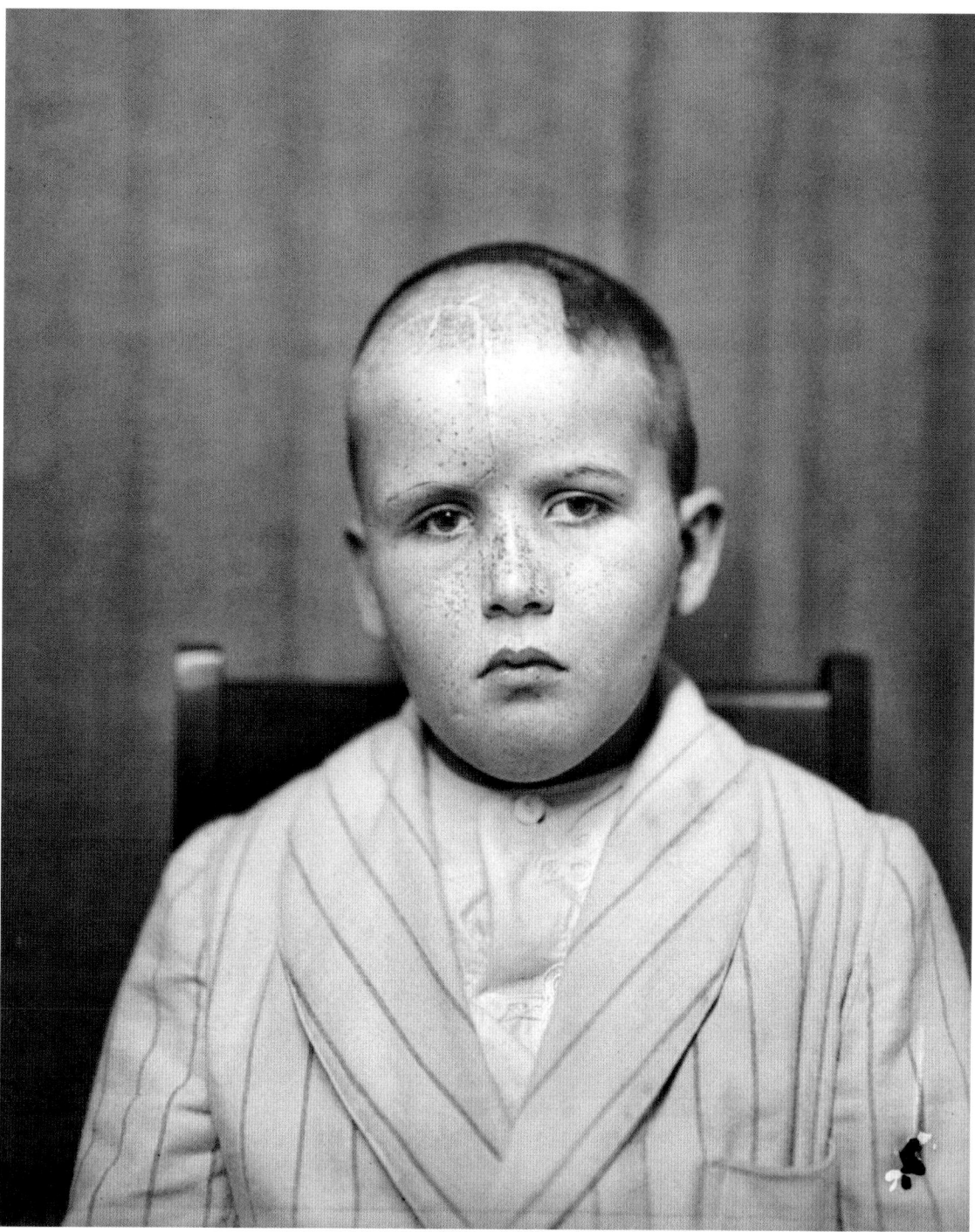

FIG. 4B. FIVE WEEKS POSTOPERATIVE.

plains of headache, sleeps a great deal, and refuses to get up.

DISCHARGE NOTE
September 1, 1924
Dr. Putman

There is no definitive change in the patient's condition since the operation.

The boy is certainly blind. No particular change in reflexes. There is still some ataxia and speech defect. Patient had one convulsion.

FOLLOW UP NOTE
January 27, 1927

The patient's condition is unchanged.

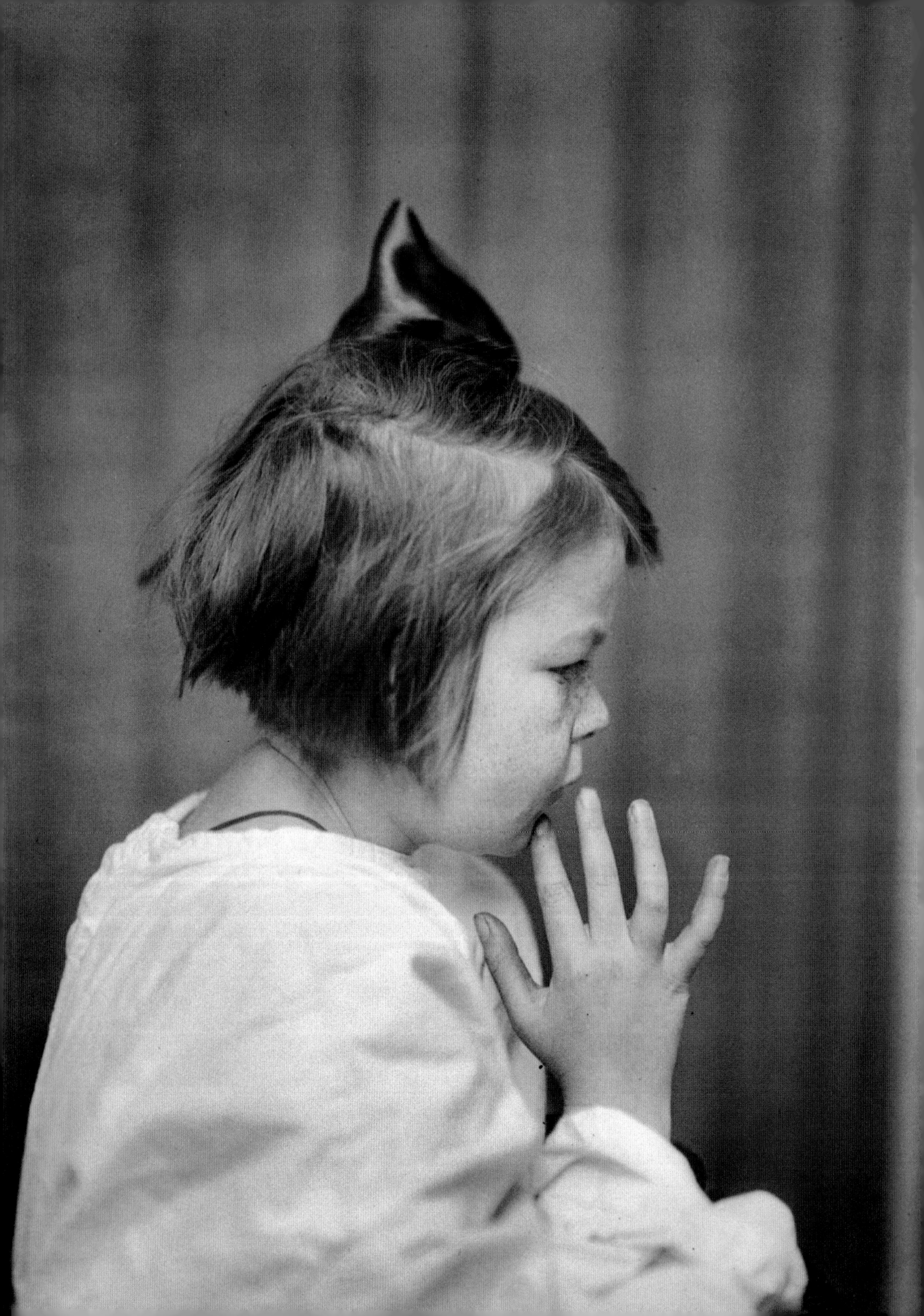

1.12 Pituitary adenoma

SEX: F; AGE: 10; SURG. NO. 22710; 35718; 39017; 40704; 41604; 42546

HISTORY

The patient suffered from headaches of six months duration. Based on her past history, she was never as active as other children. Her hands and feet always "felt cold to her grandmother." She was always bright until last year, when her teacher said "she was lazy" and she was not promoted. No subjective disturbance of vision was noticed.

SUMMARY OF POSITIVE FINDINGS
December 1, 1924
Dr. Bailey

OBJECTIVE

Regional

Sella turcica is greatly enlarged from within. There is no suprasellar shadow. There is a bilateral primary optic atrophy more marked in the left eye. Sight is reduced to movement of objects in the left eye. The right eye still has 20/70 vision. Movement is seen only in the lower nasal quadrant in the left eye and there is a temporal upper quadrant defect in the visual field of the right eye. A more accurate examination is impossible because of lack of cooperation. The eye muscle nerves are normal.

Glandular Manifestations

The patient is distinctly undersized for her age. Her skin is pale with a whitish, puffy pallor resembling that seen in nephritics. The skin, especially of the hand is finely wrinkled. There is no axillary or pubic hair, but patient has not yet reached the age of puberty. Basal metabolism – 36.

Polyglandular Manifestations

There is no enlargement of the thyroid and no signs of disturbances of the other organs of internal secretion.

IMPRESSION: Tumor of Rathke's pouch. The x-ray is suggestive of an adenoma with its enlargement from within with no suprasellar calcifications. But the age of the patient is entirely against this diagnosis, the youngest patient on whom we have found an adenoma being 14 years.

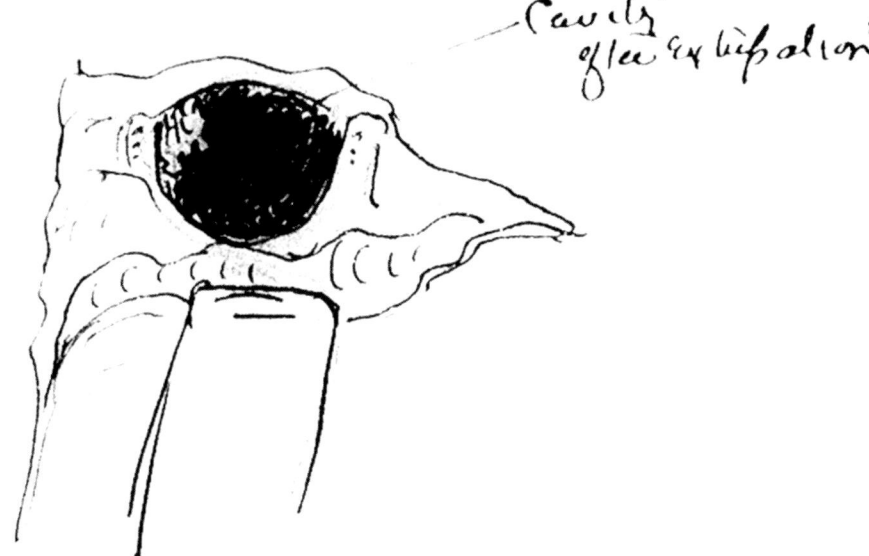

FIG. 2. OPERATIVE SKETCH.

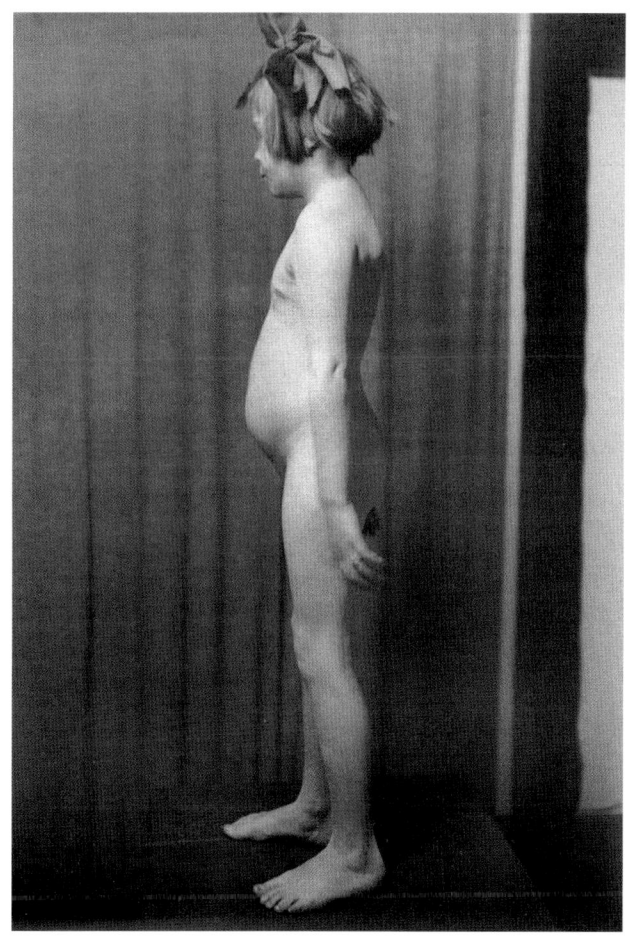

FIG. 3. PREOPERATIVE.

OPPOSITE PAGE. FIG. 1. PREOPERATIVE.

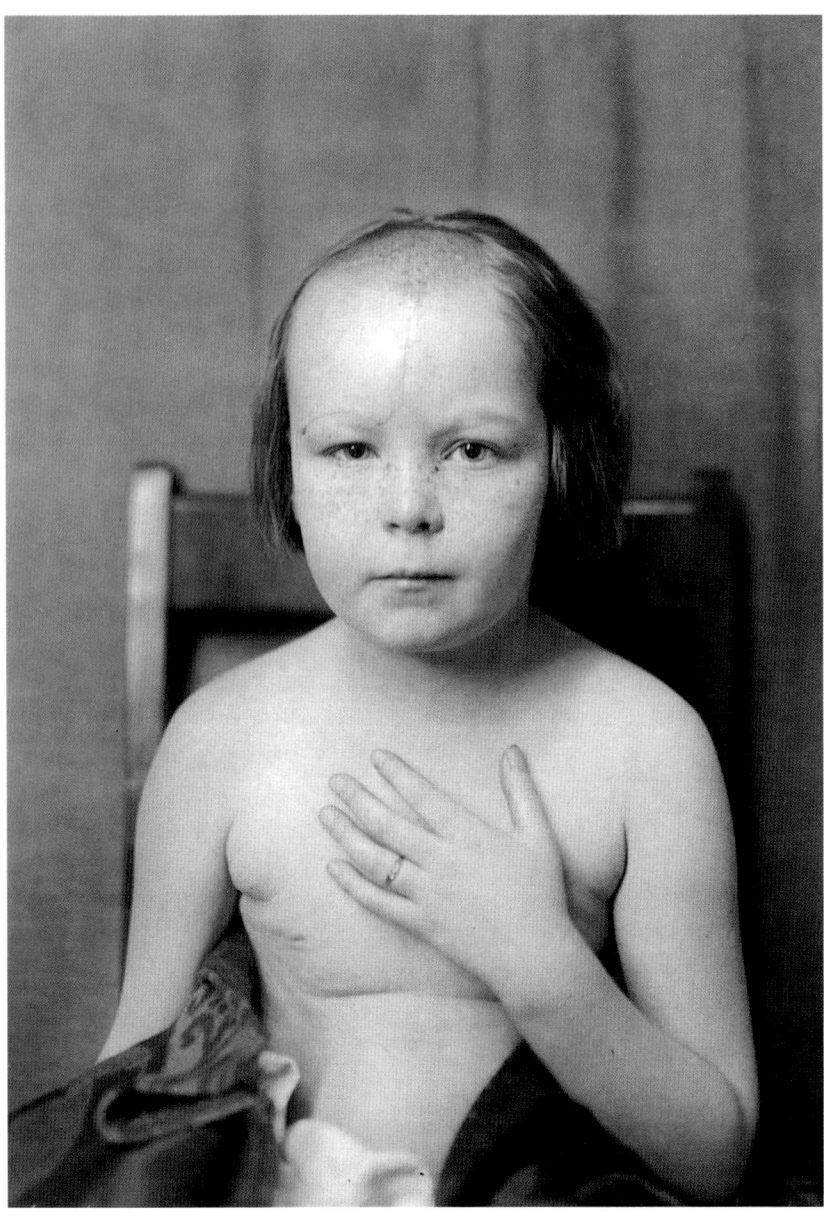

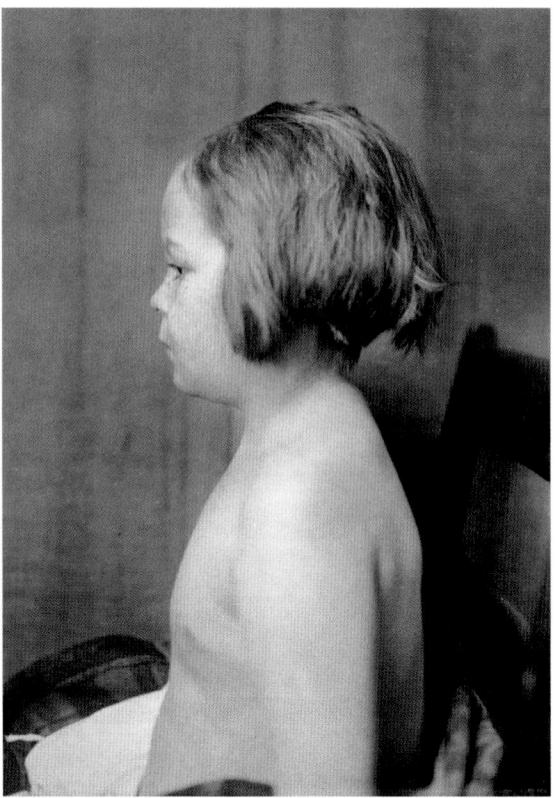

FIGS. 4 AND 5. THREE WEEKS POSTOPERATIVE (FIRST OPERATION).

SPECIAL NOTE
December 19, 1924
Dr. Cushing

This is an extremely important and interesting case – a little girl with obviously a pituitary infantilism; height 120 cm (3 ft., 11 ½ in. – normal for girl of 10, 131.5); weight 22.2 kg (i.e. 49 lbs., normal for girl of 10–64 lbs.). She had a large, ballooned sella resembling the sella of an ordinary adult adenoma except for the fact that the sphenoidal cells were underdeveloped as they often are in cases of skeletal infantilism. Obviously, the child presents an example of preadolescence hypopituitarism— pituitary cretinism it may be called, though these cases are without the mental stigma of cretins. This child was indeed like most other of these pituitary cases. She is a winning, intelligent and somewhat intellectually precocious child.

The tumor showed no calcareous deposits on the x-ray which would have practically certified it being a sellar tumor of Rathke's pouch origin. Nevertheless, it seemed probably that it must be an early one of these cystic tumors, for we have never seen an adenoma in so young of a child.

OPERATIVE NOTE
December 19, 1924
Anaesthesia – Ether – Miss Way

Transfrontal osteoplastic procedure. Disclosure of intrasellar cyst. Bulging legs of chiasm. Puncture of cyst with coffee-colored fluid. Radical extirpation of dural capsule with a large portion of tissue resembling adenoma.

This operation offered no difficulty. The flap was reflected without any loss of blood. The frontal dura was elevated and incised along the sphenoidal range. The right optic nerve was promptly brought into view and the bulging dural capsule of an intrasellar tumor brought into view. A needle was introduced through this capsule and 10 cc of a muddled, coffee-colored fluid was withdrawn. No cholestrin crystals seen to the naked eye, but many detected on microscopic examination. **The capsule had completely collapsed and the operation might have been left at this stage, but experiences have shown that these cysts refill and I was determined to attempt to extirpate the cyst, hoping that it might be a part in pressing upon the hypophysis rather than an adenoma which involved the entire gland.** Which of these two things it may have been I am not now quite sure. It was possible to clasp the wall of the cyst in clamps and to gradually withdraw it from its pocket and to tilt it out anterior to the chiasm. However, the cyst wall began to tear and although a large portion of it was removed, measuring possible 2 x 3 cm in its diameters, I am sure the lower part was left in situ. This wall was tense, though and had a glistening, oily surface and may have been little more than the upper dural diaphragm.

After the wall had been torn away in this fashion a great mass of brownish soft tissue presented, a large part of which was sucked and spooned away and put in various fixatives. A large cavity was left thereby, in the bottom of which a few further fragments of tumor of this soft, dark red adenomatous-like tissue was presenting. It might have been possible to clean out the entire fossa but I felt that we had been radical enough, if not too radical.

In this procedure, no damage was done so far as I could see, except for the pulling of the right olfactory nerve from its path.

In the bottom of the lower cavity a bit of muscle was temporarily implanted, and it apparently completely checked the oozing.

Closure as usual in layers without drainage.

It might have been said that at the last moment of suction of the cystic fluid, some blood was drawn up into the tube which completely changed the color of the fluid. Consequently, it was subsequently centrifuged and the fluid now looks to be a sort of reddish cherry color rather than the coffee color it first showed. Beneath this cherry-colored fluid is a whitish layer which presumably resembles cholestrin crystals.

As shown in the sketch at the upper left portion of the cavity, there remained a small tag of capsule. Other than for this, the upper part of the capsule was entirely removed.

(Dr. Cushing)

PATHOLOGY REPORT
December 19, 1924

Gross description: Material consists of a few small fragments of tissue removed from the region of the sella turcica by transfrontal operation. There was also the wall of cyst.

Microscopic examination: The structure is much like that of the normal pituitary gland except that it is lacking in eosinophile-staining cells. Occasional mitotic figures are seen.

DIAGNOSIS: Chromophobe adenoma.
(Resident pathologist)

December 24, 1924
Dr. Rhoads

Operation 12-19-24 Dr. Cushing. Ether. Partial extirpation of intra-sellar adenoma. Stood operation very well and returned to ward in excellent condition. ... during evening and cried out frequently, easily relieved by aspirin and pyramidon.

Complained of headache and her cast being tight. Dressing done today. Wound clear and firm. Excellent condition. Cleaned and dressing reapplied. Cast.

DISCHARGE NOTE
January 16, 1925
Dr. Bailey

She received her first x-ray treatment postoperatively. She was discharged from the hospital after an unremarkable convalescence. Her vision was improved.

FOLLOW UP NOTE
January 21, 1929
Dr. Cushing

This is I think, an extremely important case. The child differs greatly from the suprasellar cases with infantilism in that they are very lively and alert whereas she is somewhat slow and intellectually backward. She has lately been having some increase in headaches and on Wednesday had an attack of vomiting.

Fields taken; also weight (26.6 kg) and height (129.5 cm), and to be recommended to come for injections.

Visual acuity 20/200 in left eye, and 20/20 in right eye. Visual fields-marked progression of the temporal hemianopsia in left eye.

SECOND HOSPITAL ADMISSION

SUMMARY OF POSITIVE FINDINGS
January 31, 1930
Dr. Oldberg

SUBJECTIVE
1. History of previous admission to this hospital on Dec. 1, 1924, with complaint of frontal headaches of 6 mos. duration with failure in vision of at least 6 weeks' duration.
2. History of right transfrontal bone flap performed on Dec. 19, 1924, with partial extirpation at this time of a so-called cystic chromophobe adenoma.
3. History of improvement in all symptoms, particularly of vision, following the above described operation.
4. History of recent diminution in vision, most marked in the left eye, amounting to incapacitation for reading in Nov. 1929

OBJECTIVE
1. Decided retardation in physical and secondary sexual growth.
2. Scar of a well-healed right transfrontal bone flap.
3. Bilateral marked primary optic atrophy.
4. Disturbance in olfactory acuity on the right.

IMPRESSION: Recurrent cystic chromophobe adenoma.

RADIOLOGY REPORT
January 31, 1930
Dr. Sosman

Re-examination of skull show a thin vault with an old right frontal bone flap, largely united. There are no signs of increased pressure. The pituitary fossa is considerably enlarged, measuring 18 mm in depth and 31 mm in length. There is no intrasellar or suprasellar calcification visible. There is slight thickening of the anterior clinoids.

A film of the left hand and wrist shows all epiphyses open, apparently sub-development for this age.

February 3, 1930
Dr. Meagher

Pituitary symptomatology – Height 130.6 cm, weight 29.2 kilos, no polydipsia or polyuria. No increased desire for sweets. Total absence of secondary sex development at the age of 15 years. Bilateral primary optic atrophy. Temporal field defect, left.

Metabolism – 27. Total pituitary infantilism.

SPECIAL NOTE
February 19, 1930
Dr. Cushing

This child has gone now 5 years, I believe, since her former transfrontal operation. Evidently her symptoms have recently recurred. The original operation spoke chiefly of a cyst but I assume that 5 years ago we were not doing these operations nearly so radically as today. There was a small cyst in the center of the growth, and an enormous chromophobe tumor filling the large cavity. The operation was relayed with Dr. Horrax.

OPERATIVE NOTE
February 19, 1930
Anaesthesia – Novocain

Right osteoplastic re-operation for recurrent pituitary adenoma. Disclosure of bulging reformed dural diaphragm. Electrosurgical incision with radical removal by suction of soft adenoma. Coagulation of dural capsule with implantation of capsule into base of large pocket.

This little girl behaved admirably throughout the operation. Dr. Horrax had reflected the old flap when I took over the procedure and found that I could get down into the original line of dural incision, after getting an abundance of fluid. The old opening was then explored, there being exceedingly few adhesions between brain and neo-membrane.

I very soon came down upon the right optic nerve and there was a large cyst presenting, bulging between the legs of the nerves. I inserted a needle into several places but did not secure any fluid. With the electrosurgical procedure, I then made an incision into the capsule and soft tumor began to extrude. Some fragments were secured for histolog-

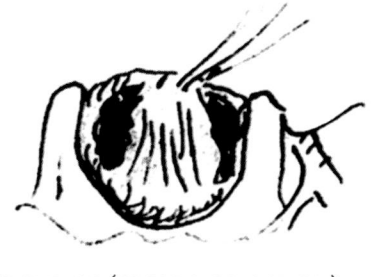

FIG. 5. OPERATIVE SKETCH (SECOND OPERATION).

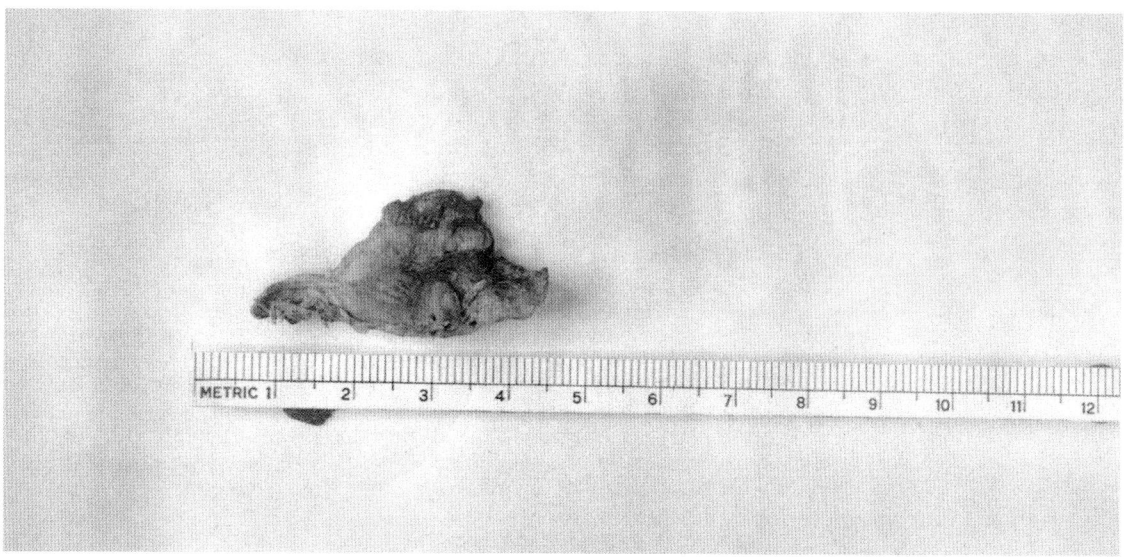

FIG. 6. RESECTED TUMOR SPECIMEN (SECOND OPERATION).

ical examination by rongeur. I finally got into a small cyst of blackish fluid just as before but this constituted a very small part of the adenoma. Bit by bit as the walls of the dural capsule were coagulated and drawn forward, I found that I could coagulate and draw in the walls of the bulging diaphragm. Step by step, I removed masses of the adenoma by dissection and by suction. There was a great deal of bleeding but this was controlled by the use of pledgets of cotton wet in Zenker's fluid. The great cavity at the end could easily have held the terminal joint of the thumb. I found, as shown in sketch II, that the posterior part of the capsule could be drawn forward and finally at the end of the operation this was implanted down into the depth of the great cavity. There was slight oozing and a small bit of gauze was left in the depth. I finally felt that the cavity was sufficiently dry to justify closure.

The operation was taken over at this time by Dr. Horrax, so that I could go into another case that he had been exposing in the next room. He completed the closure without, as I understand, a drain.

(Dr. Cushing)

PATHOLOGY REPORT
February 19, 1930

Gross description: There are fragments of recurrent adenoma, of chromophobe type in a small child, the youngest in our chromophobe series, who was first operated on 5 years ago. At this session this morning, a much more radical procedure was carried out than I would have ventured to do 5 years ago. The cavity was thoroughly cleaned out by rongeuring, suction and by coagulation of its walls. There are abundant fragments of tissue in Zenker formalin.

(Dr. Cushing)

Microscopic examination: This tumor presents an abundant vascular stroma with cells about them. The majority of the cells are chromophobe, but there seems to be a sprinkling of chromophiles among them. The cells appear in quite large sheets and masses. I can find no mitotic figures. The dense fibrous tissue in which are found some of the tumor cells, is probably due to the repair

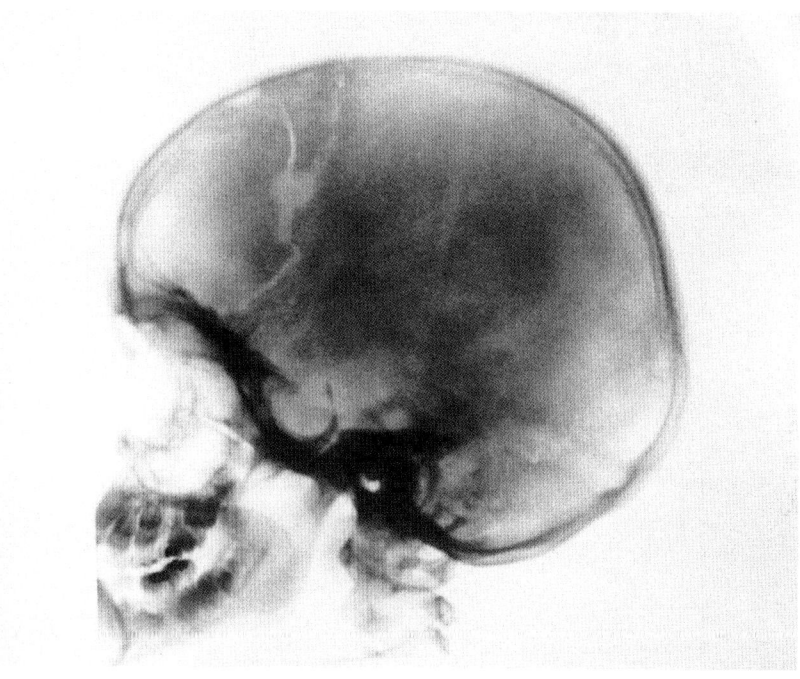

FIG. 7. POSTOPERATIVE X RAY.

process following the previous operation. Because of the abundance of stroma and preponderance of chromophobe cells, the tumor should be classified as a chromophobe adenoma.

DIAGNOSIS: Pituitary adenoma (chromophobe type)

(Resident pathologist)

The patient was comatose postoperatively and was returned to the operating room for evacuation of a large frontal hematoma on February 20th.

SPECIAL NOTE
February 22, 1930
Dr. Cushing

This child has been doing badly with high temperature, has been semi-conscious and today has become quite rigid, as though she had a decerebrate rigidity. In view of the fact that Dr. Horrax recently re-elevated the flap and found a large clot, I feared that there might be again a reformation of clot. However, there was some natural difference of opinion about this as to whether it might be edema or clot. I, however, did not dare let the matter go and so on this holiday morning, re-elevated the flap and found no evidence of clot but merely great intracranial tension.

I was unable to successfully look down into the region of the operation to see whether there might not be possibly a clot that had formed from the operative field and that was pressing in on the third ventricle.

The flap was replaced and closed again securely in layers.

I did not very well like the looks of the wound for there had been apparently no tendency to healing. The skin incision simply falling apart without any apparent cohesion.

Subsequent to the operation, I then took recourse to what we perhaps should have done before, of giving the child magnesium sulphate enemata and there were several large movements of the bowel and it was not more than a few hours before it was evident that the child's condition was improved. The improvement, however, could hardly be ascribed to the operation.

The patient had a stormy postoperative course associated with hyperthermia (reaching 106 degrees). During this time, she was given a course of six hormone injections with resultant mental status improvement.

DISCHARGE NOTE
May 4, 1930
Dr. Henderson

Visual acuity 20/200 in left eye and 20/20 in right eye. Can just detect hand movement with difficulty and cannot see light movement in left field. Patient discharged with instruction to take Armour's pituitary tablets, one grain, twice a day.

FOLLOW UP NOTE
July 12, 1930
Dr. Henderson

Still has occasional headaches but nothing like she used to have.

Vision is improving – can read easily. Still has no pep or energy – no desire to play with other children. Visual field – no change in vision. Discs – flat.

No sign of menstruation.

THIRD HOSPITAL ADMISSION

Patient re-entered the hospital at Dr. Cushing's request for study under the influence of anterior lobe extract.

SUMMARY OF POSITIVE FINDINGS
June 13, 1931
Dr. Mahoney

SUBJECTIVE
1. Hospital entries in 1924–1925 and 1930 with operations for chromophobe adenoma because of failing vision, etc.
2. Improvement of vision, disappearance of headaches but with almost no improvement in mental and physical state.

OBJECTIVE
1. Retarded physical and mental development.
2. Scar of well healed right transfrontal operation.
3. Bilateral primary optic atrophy.
4. Decreased acuity with temporal field defect, O.S.

IMPRESSION: Hypopituitarism.

DISCHARGE NOTE
June 20, 1931
Dr. Henderson

During hospital stay, injection was not done as the extract was not yet ready. She was discharged, condition unchanged after seven days of observation.

FOURTH HOSPITAL ADMISSION

This underdeveloped 17-yr.-old girl who appears very immature for her years comes to the hospital for treatment on advice of Dr. Cushing.

RADIOLOGY REPORT
March 8, 1932
Dr. Sosman

A film of hands and wrists shows all epiphyses compatible with an age of 12 years.

March 9, 1932
Dr. Thompson

Patient has had two injections today 0.2 cc subcutaneously in each deltoid region. No reaction.

March 10, 1932
Dr. Thompson

To have injections of 0.3 cc sc twice today.

Wt = 31.8 kg
Ht = 134.0 cm

March 14, 1932
Dr. Thompson

Wt = 31.3 kg
Ht = 134.6 cm

Patient is very active, offers to help with ward work.

RADIOLOGY REPORT
May 6, 1932
Dr. Sosman

Re-examination of both forearms, wrists and hands shows no changes in the epiphyses since previous examination.

May 17, 1932
Dr. Thompson

Injections continued – 3 cc per day. Patient is well and happy.

Patient continued to get injection of 4 cc extract intramuscularly daily, and showed a steady gain in weight during hospital course.

DISCHARGE NOTE
June 26, 1932
Dr. Thompson

This 17 year old girl is discharged today after 113 days in the hospital during which time she received injections of antuitrin, and alkaline salted out extract of the anterior lobe of the pituitary. She received a special diet which gave her high vitamins and fairly high protein intake.

The patient is to spend the next two weeks at home and is to return to the hospital at that time for further observation. She will not receive injections of the growth extract while at home. Her grandmother has been instructed to bring her back to the hospital at any sign of untoward disturbance.

Impression at discharge is:

Pituitary dwarfism, treated by injections of antuitrin with marked psychic improvement, gain of 5.2 kilos in weight and with questionable changes in stature and skeletal measurement.

FIFTH HOSPITAL ADMISSION

This 17-year-old girl comes to the hospital after a month at home without injections of antuitrin.

RADIOLOGY REPORT
July 26, 1932
Dr. Sosman

Films of hands wrists, ankles, shoulders and elbows show epiphyseal development compatible with 17 years of age. None of the epiphyses are closed but several of them show changes indicating maturation preliminary to closing. The middle finger has increased 5 mm in length in 2 and half years.

July 26, 1932
Dr. Thompson

Chubby girl, whose skin is very white and has numerous freckles, but whose color is fairly good, and appears retarded. Her hair is fine and dry. Face still has the contour of that of a child, although there is some definable change since her last admission I believe. Thorax and abdomen are the contour of a child with good deal of subcutaneous fat and rather prominent breasts for a child, but there does not seem to be at this time any increase in the areola or in the mammary tissue. There are no axillary or pubic hair. The legs and feet suggest the angular appearance of early adolescence. Skin is fine, and not extraordinary dry. There is no wrinkling about the face or mouth.

Weight = 34.6 kilos before breakfast.
Height = 136.8 cm
Metabolism = 27

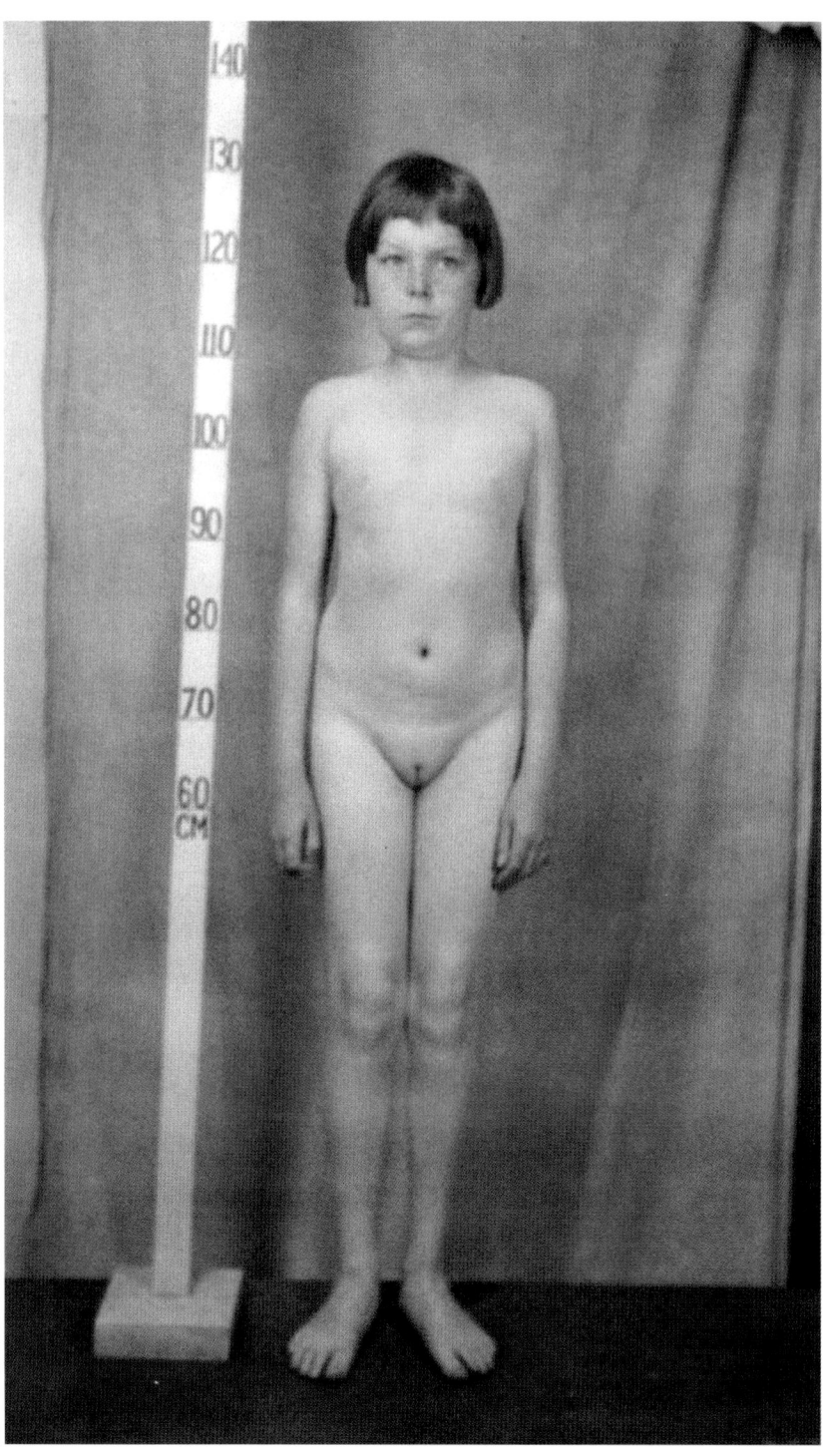
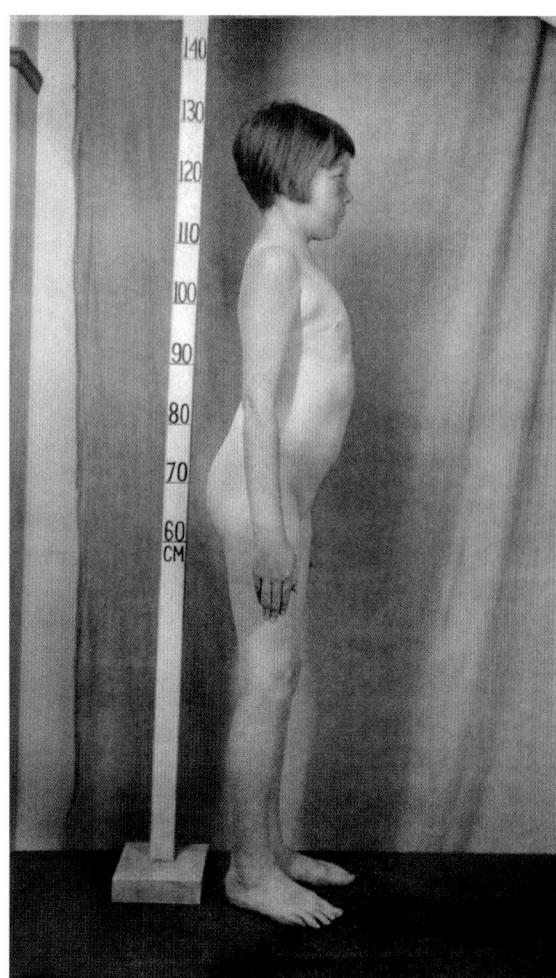

FIGS. 7 AND 8. ONE AND A HALF YEARS POSTOPERATIVE (SECOND OPERATION).

IMPRESSION: Pirtuitary dwarfism, chromophobe adenoma, postoperative; treated with injections of antuitrin with improvement. Omission of injection for one month during which time slight weight loss occurred, but increase in height and other body measurements took place.

DISCHARGE NOTE
July 30, 1932
Dr. Thompson

Patient is discharged today after 6 days in hospital, during which time she had been measured, desensitized to antuitrin, and injections have been resumed, so that she received today 5 cc of growth extract.

Yesterday she was taken to the Mast Boston Health Unit, and the superintendent became interested in her and will see that her injections are continued for several months at 5 cc a day. They will provide patient with car-fare so that she may be certain to get there each day. I visited her home, and found it to be exceedingly disagreeable and dirty, and have accordingly asked the Social Service to assist in any way they are able. The patient is to report to me at 2 week intervals for observation.

It is interesting to note that she has increased her shoe size from 2 ½ to 4 since her last admission. Her dress size has also increased two sizes since her first injections. Notes of this admission have been taken.

FOLLOW UP NOTE
December 10, 1932
Dr. Cushing

She kept on with her injections, according to her statement, at the East Boston Health Unit where a Miss White and a Miss Joyce gave her the injections. In September she was sent away to the Farrington Memorial for six weeks and had a good time there. Since then, she has had no injections.

Hg = 137.3 cm; Wt = 33.9 kg. She drinks and passes more than she should.

Dr. Thompson probably has figures of weight and so on up to that time which he has probably recorded. Without figures at hand, I would not know her present loss of weight since the time of cessation of the injections. This would be important to record, for she may possibly have gained from 35.8 kg which she weighed on June 28th at the time of her discharge. It is of course well known that cessation of injections in rats immediately leads to a marked falling off in weight with résumé of cachectic-like symptoms.

To be readmitted for study.

SIXTH HOSPITAL ADMISSION

Patient re-entered the hospital for study and continuation of injections of antuitrin G.

December 10, 1932
Dr. Thompson

Examination on this admission shows no abnormal physical characteristics except those already under study and observation. Undoubtedly her feet and hands have assumed a more adult proportion and are less the baby type than they were at her first admission. She also appears to have matured somewhat in stature and in facial expression and everyone remarks that she seems much more of a "young lady." However, she looks tired and wan and very poorly groomed. Wt = 33.4 kg; Ht = 136.2 cm.

During her hospital course, the patient was given skin tests of the drug, and injections were increased to 5 cc a day.

DISCHARGE NOTE
January 13, 1933
Dr. Thompson

Patient is discharged to continue injection at E. Boston Health unit. Family and Social Service are cooperative. To have 5 cc intramuscular each day.

Ht = 137.4 cm; Wt = 39.0 kg

FOLLOW UP NOTES
July 26, 1934
Dr. Thompson

This is my first view of the patient since July 12, 1933. She seems remarkably improved even over the last visit, and seems to be somewhat more

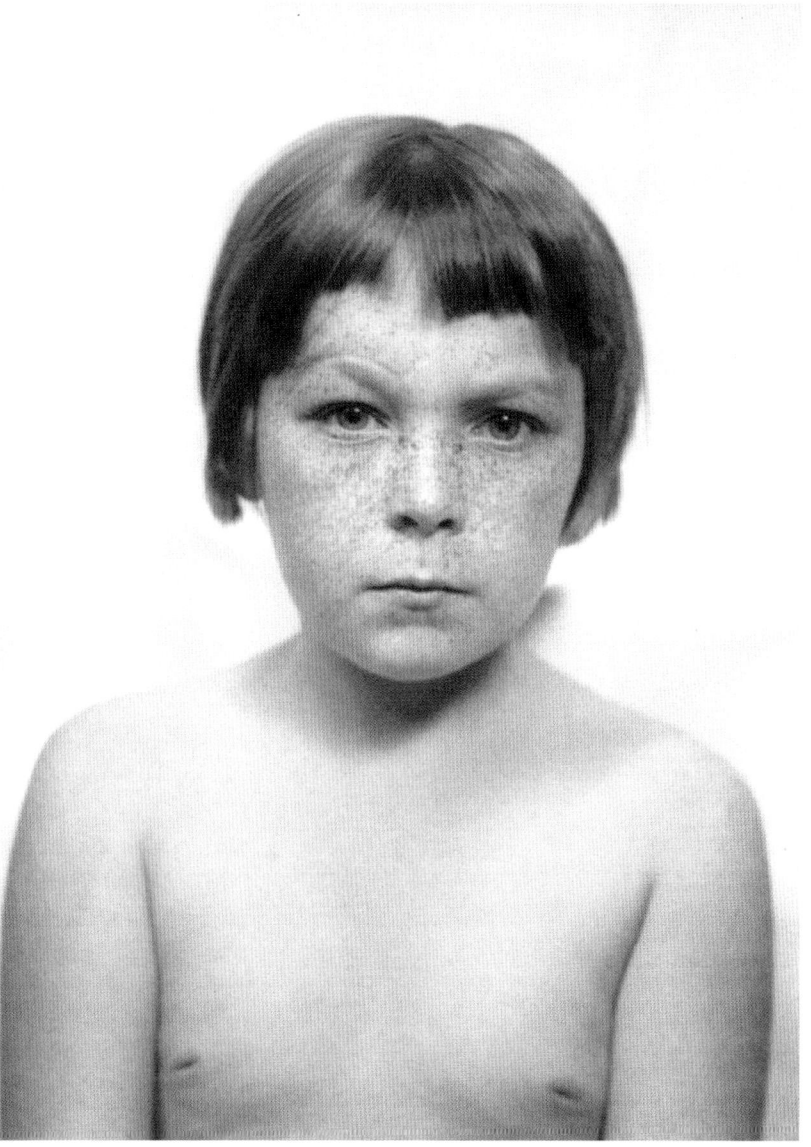

FIG. 9. ONE AND A HALF YEARS POSTOPERATIVE (SECOND OPERATION).

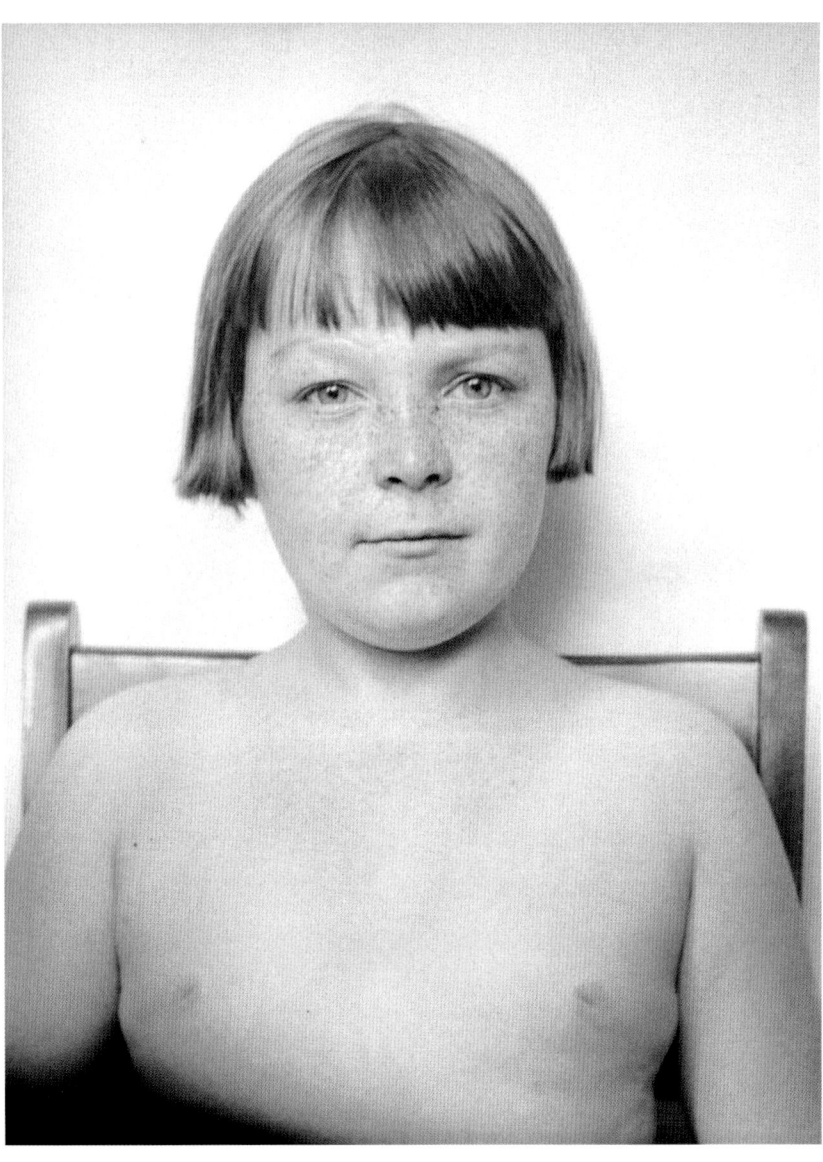

FIG. 10. TWO AND A HALF YEARS POSTOPERATIVE (SECOND OPERATION).

alert, and certainly a bit taller. She has obtained a job, and makes $6.00 a week. This is remarkable achievement when one considers what a vegetable she was a little over 2 years ago, when she first arrived for dietary and pituitary injection therapy.

She does complain now of headaches which have come on during the last 10 days, and 2 attacks of vomiting. These symptoms appear as follows: when she wakes in the morning she feels headache in her left temporal region, not severe but fairly mild, and on two occasions after arising and drinking some water she has vomited, without preliminary nausea. Yesterday she had no trouble. She has no other symptoms except a slight recurrence of the old pain she had in her left hip. The exam of her eyes is unchanged, and although I did not examine her carefully, she does not appear to have any new signs.

I suggest that she return in 3 weeks, about the time Miss Cedding returns from vacation, and then be readmitted to the Hospital for checkup of her body measurements, eyefields, etc. If in the meantime she has other symptoms which would lead to a suspicion of reactivity of an intracranial extension of her tumor, she could be readmitted at any time.

August 16, 1934
Dr. Boggs

This patient is still working and has had no recurrence of headaches. On discussion of the case with Dr. Thompson and after re-study of her case report we have decided not to admit her at this time. She will return in six mos. – Feb. 14, 1935.

February 21, 1935
Dr. Walter

Weight: 86 lbs.

Patient has no further complaints. Visual fields as on Dec. 11/32.

February 28, 1935
Dr. Walter

Weight 84 lbs.

Evidently headaches are not severe enough to warrant X-ray treatment at this time.

On May 10, 1936, the patient was admitted in the hospital with the diagnosis of acute right-sided otitis media. This 21-year-old girl had the appearance of a child of about 13 years of age; her height was 144 cm and her weight was 35.4 kg. she was taking thyroid extract.

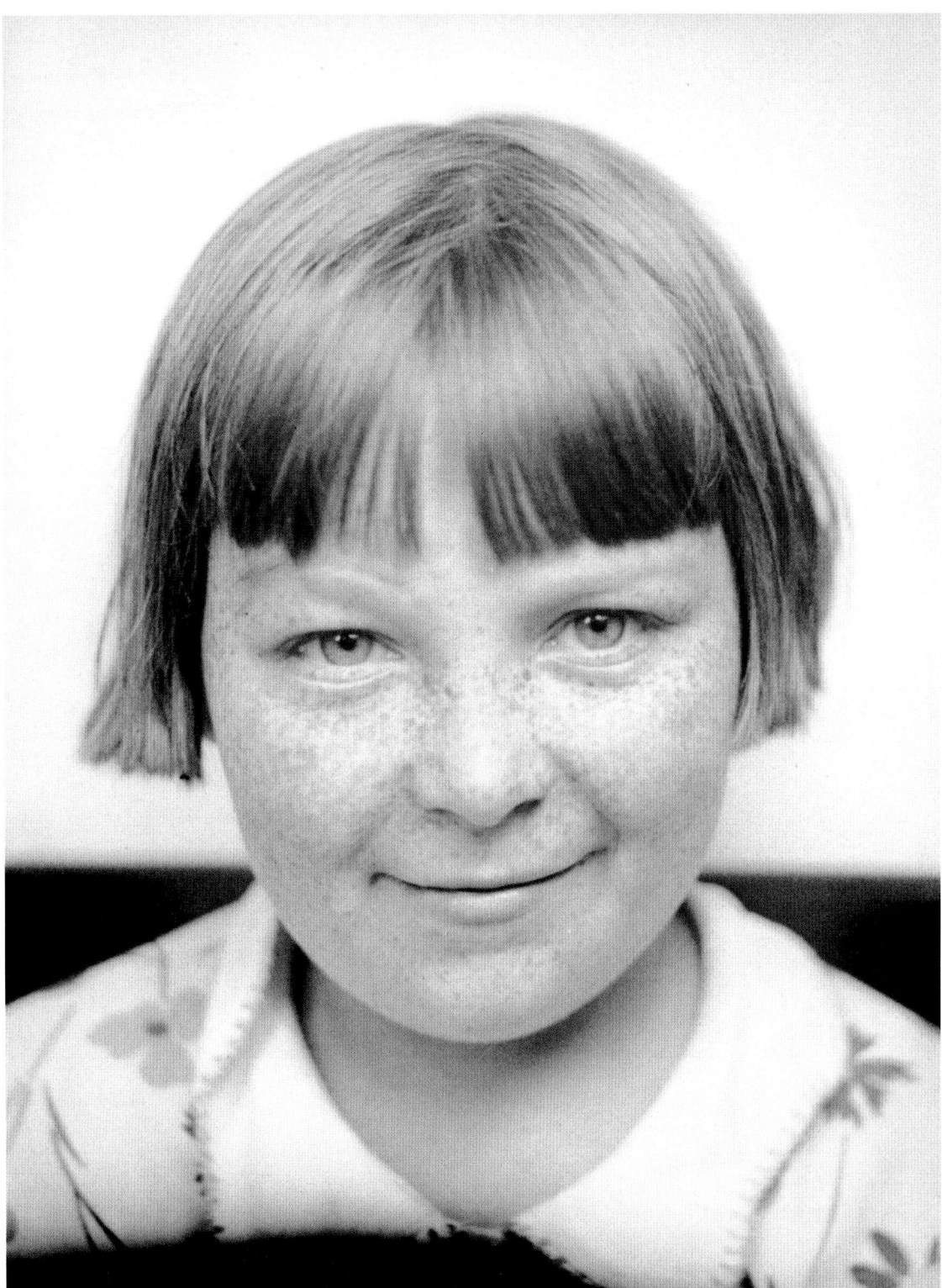

FIG. 11. TWO AND A HALF YEARS POSTOPERATIVE (SECOND OPERATION).

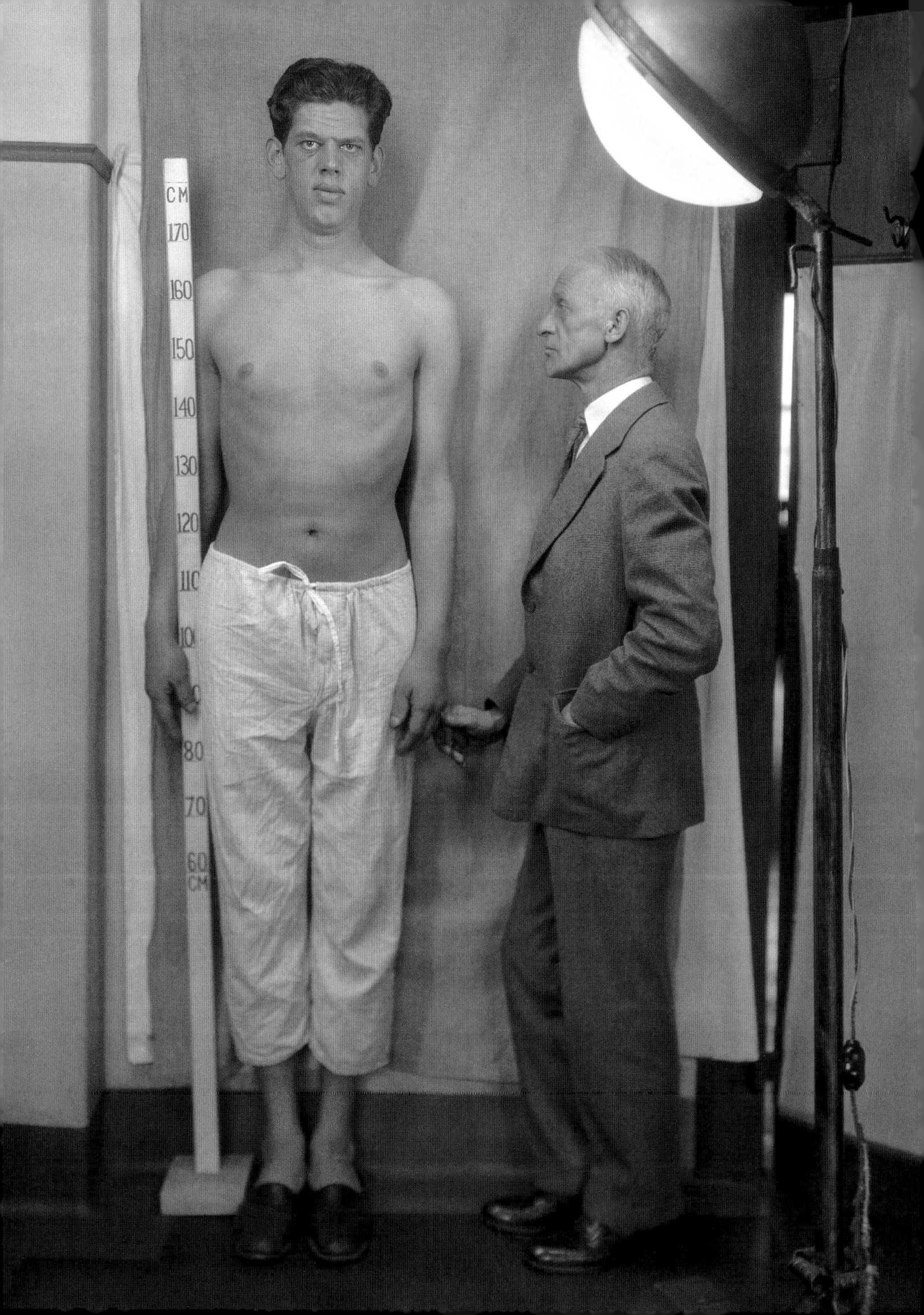

1.13 Pituitary adenoma

SEX: M; AGE: 24; SURG. NO. 37799

HISTORY

This 24-year-old patient presented with progressive visual decline and intermittent headaches. Since age 16, he was "unable to get along without women." However, he has had no interest in sex for the past 11 months. His physical exam showed a large man with somewhat "rounded features." He had large hands, head, and feet. His eye exam revealed a bitemporal field cut, more on the left. He had consulted a physician in Vancouver about his headaches. A left sinus antrum abscess was drained. **His physician also felt he had a pituitary tumor and sent him to Dr. Brodie who informed him that he would "die if anyone operated on his pituitary."** Skull x-rays revealed an enlarged sella.

SUMMARY OF POSITIVE FINDINGS
December 10, 1930
Dr. Henderson

SUBJECTIVE
1. Excessive growth beginning when the patient was 15 years of age and continuing up until about 2 years ago.
2. Progressive failure of vision with subjective temporal hemianopsia first noticed in the left eye 2 years ago which has progressed to almost complete blindness and subsequent involvement of the right eye during the last 3 months.
3. Inflammation of the left frontal sinus and antrum together with headaches beginning 9 months ago and finally relieved by drainage of the antrum 5 months ago.
4. Puffiness, tingling and numbness of the hands and feet noticed particularly during the last 6 years.
5. Very marked increase in libido, sexualis beginning when 16 years of age and continuing until about 1 year ago, when it almost entirely disappeared. He has been married 2 years and has one child of age 3 months.

OBJECTIVE
1. A typical acromegalic giant measuring 6 ft. 6 in. in height, weighting 198 lbs.

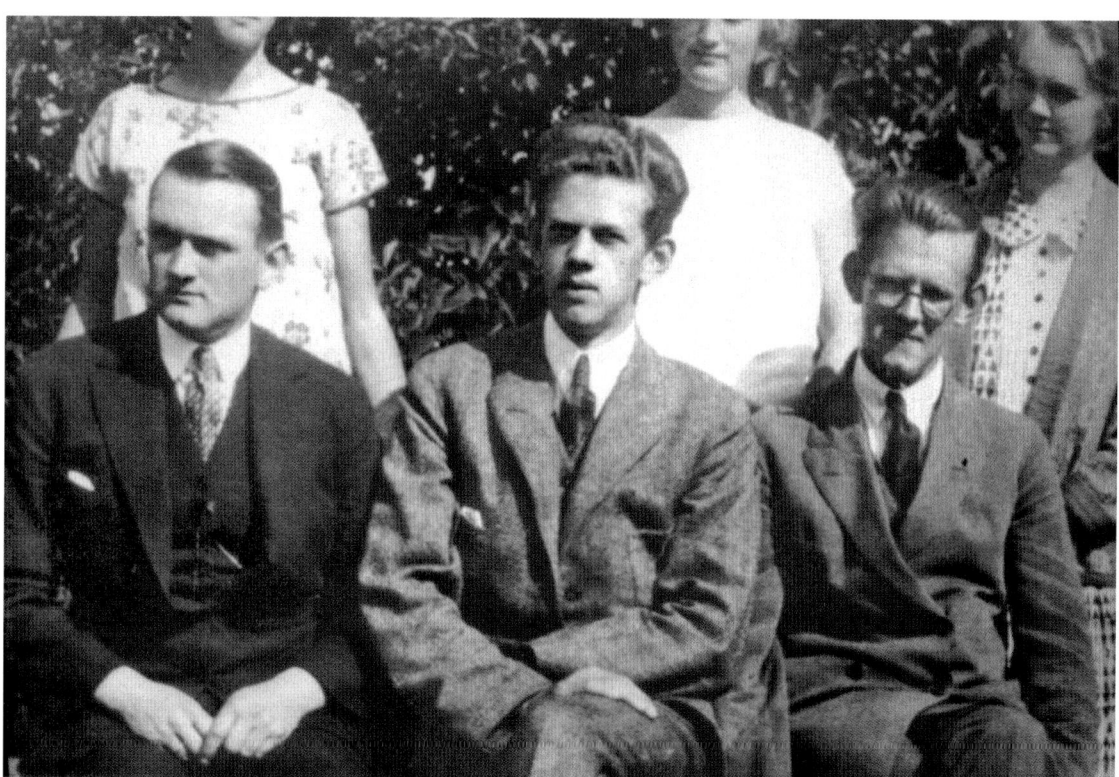

FIG. 2. FAMILY PHOTOGRAPH TAKEN YEARS BEFORE THE OPERATION.

OPPOSITE PAGE. FIG. 1. PREOPERATIVE IMAGE WITH DR. CUSHING.

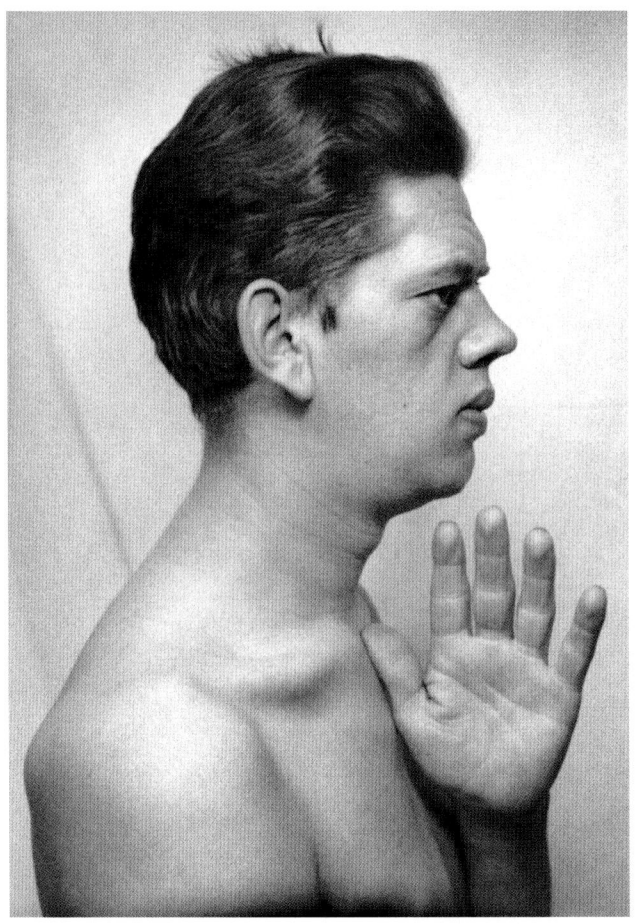
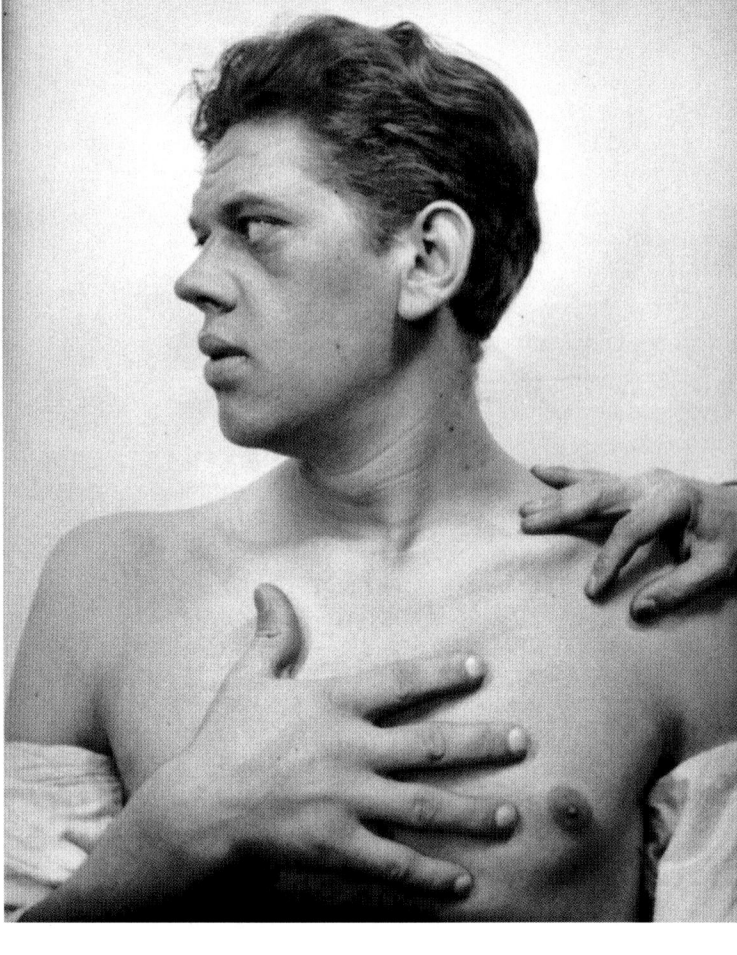

FIGS. 3 AND 4. PREOPERATIVE.

2. Typical hands, feet and facies of acromegaly together with bulldog scalp are present but not extremely marked.
3. Skin is rather coarse and leathery with increased perspiration. Hair is not abnormal.
4. There is no prognathism or off-setting of the teeth.
5. Bitemporal hemianopsia with central scotoma and 3/200 vision on the left, a spared macula with 20/25 vision on the right.
6. Slight bilateral primary optic atrophy.
7. Slight nystagmus on looking to the left.
8. B.M.R. (basal metabolic rate) +13
9. X-ray shows a large sella.

IMPRESSION: Chromophile adenoma of the pituitary with acromegalic gigantism. Operation is evidently indicated because of the serious and progressive failure of vision.

SPECIAL NOTE
December 19, 1930
Dr. Cushing

This proved a difficult and somewhat disappointing case, for I did not apprehend in the slightest that there might be an extrasellar extension of the adenoma. The man has a typical gigantism which dates back to his adolescence. He has been throughout perfectly vigorous in all respects and has been doing hard laboring work as a farmer up to the time of his hospital admission. Operation was relayed with Dr. Horrax.

OPERATIVE NOTE
December 19, 1930
Anesthesia: Novocain–Morphia

Right Transfrontal Osteoplastic Exploration; Exceedingly Bloody Flap; Difficult Exposure of Chiasmal Region; Opening of Soft Dural Diaphragm, Disclosing a Hemorrhagic Cyst with Soft Adenoma about it. Fairly

Radical Extirpation by Suction. Subsequent Disclosure of Soft Tumor Extension Overlying Left Optic Nerve. Prolonged Tedious Effort at Hemostasis. Closure with Drains.

The patient behaved fairly well throughout this long and difficult procedure. Dr. Horrax had turned down the bone flap without undue difficulty and I entered the field in time to open the dura in the usual fashion along the sphenoidal ridge. The bone of the flap was not especially thick but he had a very vascular and wide diploe.

An abundance of fluid was secured and I finally managed to elevate the frontal lobes sufficiently to get the right optic nerve in view and to see the dural diaphragm. The latter looked thin and cystic and I put a needle and suction into it without getting fluid. I then made a small incision with the electric needle and blackish blood began to extrude, evidently from hemorrhagic cyst. With the rongeurs some abundant pieces of soft adenoma were secured and removed for histological examination. I then introduced a small tube sucker and radically sucked out all the soft tumor that was within reach.

Following this procedure, the capsule collapsed markedly. There was a good deal of bleeding from the cavity but this finally was checked by placement of cotton pledges wet with Zenker.

I then endeavored to bring the left optic nerve into view and to my consternation found a bluish swelling to the left of a definite crease in the dural capsule, this swelling being just about in the position where we would have expected to find the left optic nerve. Not knowing exactly what the swelling was, I picked my way into it with the hooked knife and found it to be a nubbin of adenoma. I suppose I might have done well to have sucked at it but I was fearful of injuring the left optic nerve more than the pressure had already injured it for this was the patient's bad eye. Some of the fringes of this additional outlying nodule were coagulated and also the fringes of the opening into the main adenoma. I then went through an hour long process of hemostasis, the cavity being treated with pledgets of cotton wet in Zenker and finally a small bit of muscle was left in the cavity which was only reasonably dry.

The margins of the scalp and dura were all oozing markedly but I finally got all the bleeding points sufficiently under control to justify replacement of the flap. This was closed, the larger part of it by Dr.

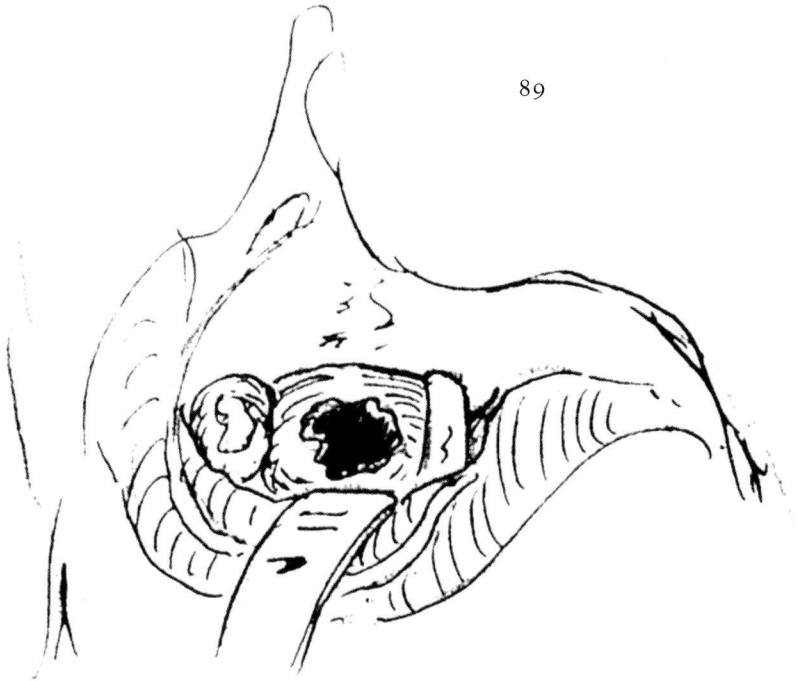

FIG. 5. OPERATIVE SKETCH.

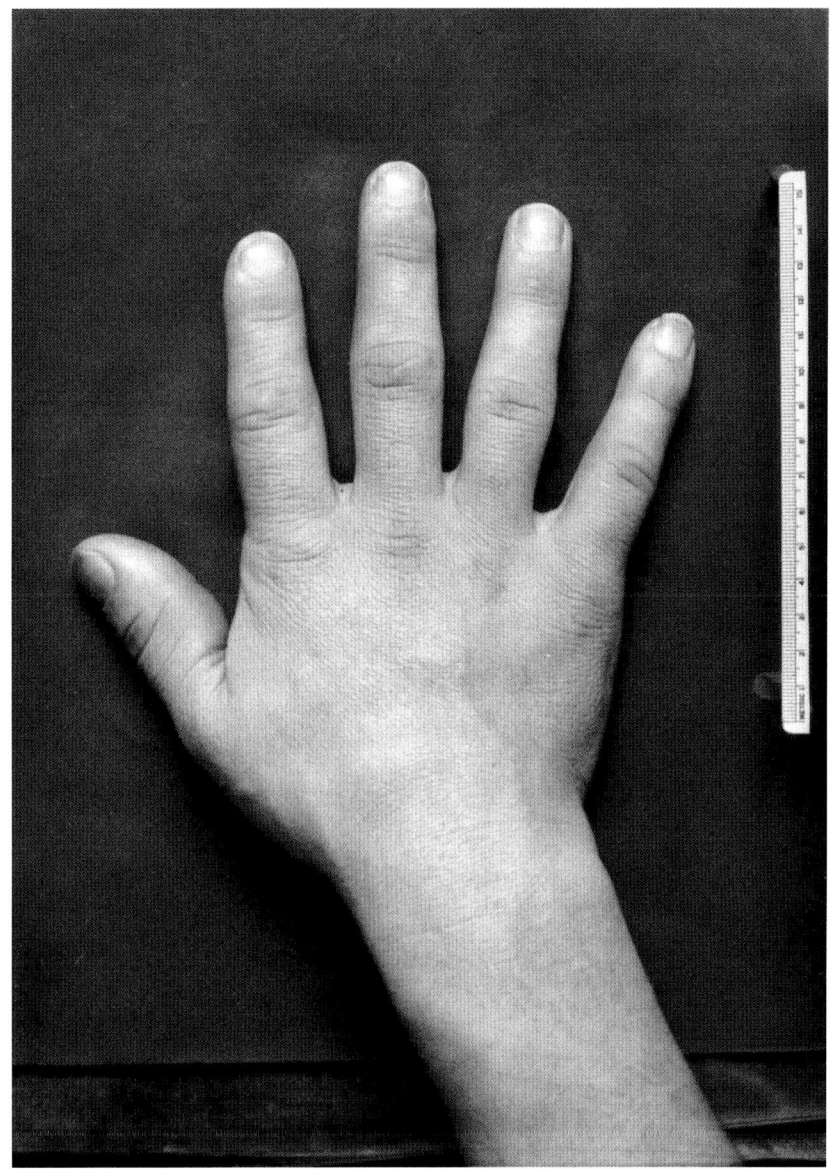

FIG. 6. PREOPERATIVE.

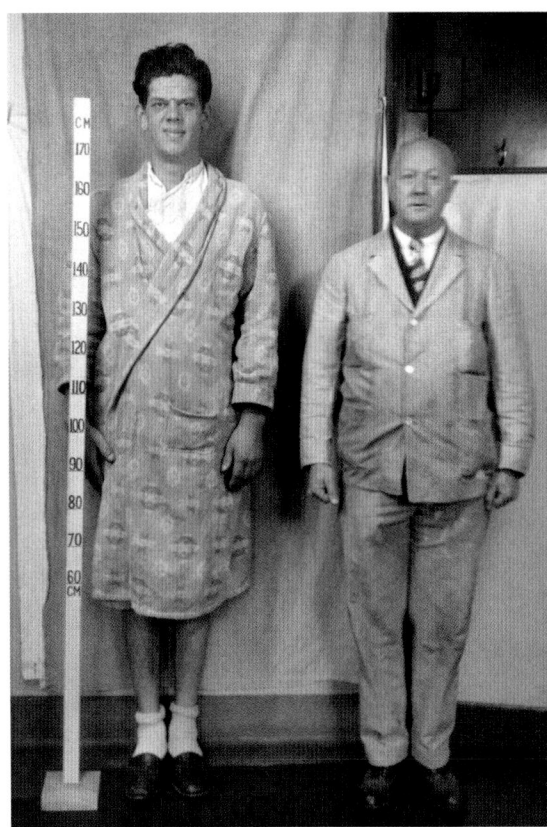

FIG. 7. PREOPERATIVE.

Horrax, drain being left in the angle of the eye and in the upper posterior angle of the incision.

(Dr. Cushing)

PATHOLOGY NOTE
December 19, 1930

There are some fragments of an extremely soft adenoma in a young acromegalic giant. The adenoma was occupied by a hemorrhagic cyst and the tissue which was removed was exceedingly soft and succulent. The major portion of it was lost down the sucker. I hope that the soft tissue represented the chromophilis adenoma and that the majority of it at least was removed.

(Dr. Cushing)

Microscopic description: This is a soft mushy fragment of tissue from an acromegalic. Examination by supravital technique shows that it consists of masses of cells packed together, with a little supporting stroma. The cells are of epithelial type, containing a round nuclei with large nucleolus. Many are multinucleated. There is some variation in the size of the cells. The cytoplasm is granular, but the granules are not so coarse, as I have seen them in other specimens from acromegalics. Some few cells had a slender ring of coarse granules at the extreme periphery, but the majority of cells have an even distribution of fine granules throughout the cytoplasm.

IMPRESSION: Pituitary adenoma.

(Dr. Eisenhardt)

December 19, 1930
Dr. Henderson

After operation the patient was fully conscious, responding well with excellent condition. Noticed no changes in vision immediately after the operation.

December 30, 1930
Dr. Henderson

There is marked improvement in vision and fields particularly of the left eye. He says he has not noticed any change in the right eye.

DISCHARGE NOTE
January 15, 1931
Dr. Henderson

Seen by Dr. Cushing and discharged home. He has 15/15 vision in both eyes. There is still slight upper temporal notching. The return of vision of the left eye has been remarkable.

LETTER TO DR. CUSHING
December 13, 1933

Dear Dr. Cushing:

I want to send the best wishes for a Merry Xmas and a Happy New Year for you. I hope that 1934 will find you in high spirits and in the best of health. I have not given up the hope to see you again some time, either in Copenhagen or in Boston or New Haven.

Last not least: Thank you so much for your wonderful treatment (scientific as personal) of me in the time past. We (my wife and myself) will always keep you in our hearts.

Gratefully yours,
(Signed)

P.S. If you have time to answer this letter, would you not give me an advice as to an operation in the future. I have read the letter through and find that the information given of myself is a terrible mixture of good and bad, please forgive that, will you not?

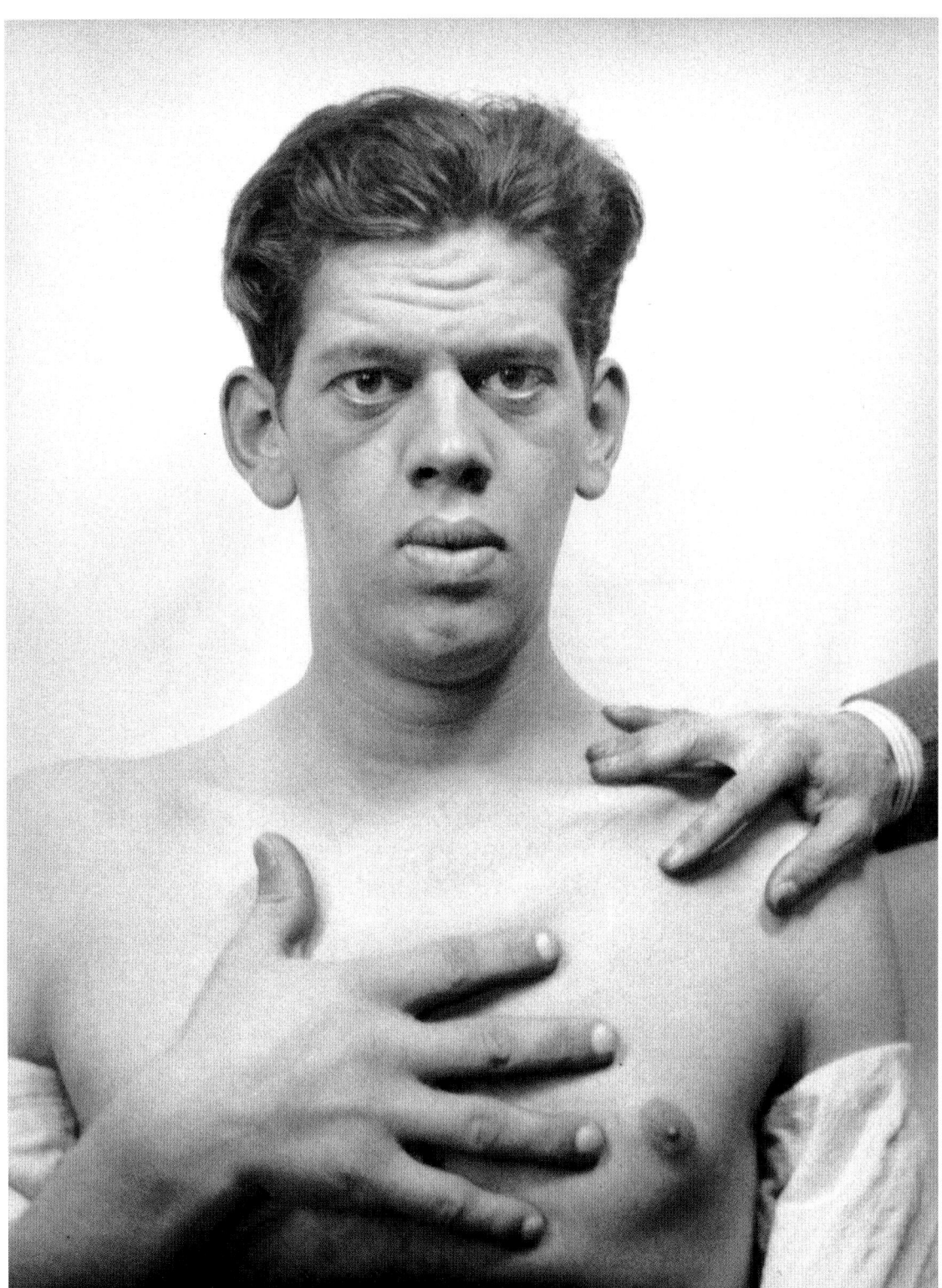

FIG. 8. PREOPERATIVE.

Chapter 2

Gliomas and other 'malignant' tumors

Introduction

"Impressed by the fact that many patients with tumors of this sort [glioma] have survived for unexpectedly long periods of time after incomplete extirpation of the lesion, it has seemed imperative that these gliomas should be reclassified and a correlated study of their clinical histories made. The information was needed not only for the sake of prognosis, but as a necessary basis for improvement in our operative procedures."

Harvey Cushing

The first reported case of glioma surgery appears to be the operation performed by Bennett and Godlee in 1884.[1] Twenty years later after this first operation, the operative mortality from intracranial surgery approached 60%. During the early years in Cushing's career (1901–1915), the high mortality rate from intracranial surgery and the poor prognosis of patients with high-grade glial tumors prompted Cushing to advocate palliative subtemporal decompression as the primary procedure for relieving intracranial pressure. By the end of his career, he operated on 862 glial tumors, representing 42.6% of all the tumors he surgically verified. Cushing may have been more aggressive about the resection of gliomas than he claimed. In fact, he operated 237 times on 158 glial tumors with an impressive 13.9% operative mortality. Subtemporal decompression and or palliative subtotal resection were followed with radiation therapy especially after 1920.

The most important contribution of Cushing to glioma care remains his classification of tumor histology and the patients' ensuing life history. In his monograph, *A Classification of the Tumors of the Glioma Group on a Histogenetic Basis with a Correlated Study of Prognosis,* Percival Bailey and Cushing described for the first time a practical categorization of glial tumors and their clinical behavior. Prior to Bailey and Cushing's classification, most brain tumors, especially those in the posterior fossa, were considered "gliomas" based on the Virchow's categorization. These tumors were thought to have a hopeless prognosis: They were not amenable to surgical resection but only to cyst drainage for short-term relief. Other contemporary surgeons of the time questioned the efficacy of surgical resection. Therefore, from the early years of neurosurgery, the aggressive course of high-grade glial tumors created both technical and ethical controversy regarding the role of resective surgery.[4]

For infratentorial tumors, Bailey and Cushing's tumor classification supported radiotherapy trials for aggressive tumors such as medulloblastomas. Cushing's favorable experience with irradiation of medulloblastomas was the first report of such success. In addition, Cushing tailored the extent of resection based on the histopathology of tumor. By 1928, Cushing would tailor his resection strategy based on intraoperative biopsy results. He would wait for Dr. Louise Eisenhardt to arrive in the operating room to announce the pathological diagnosis.

Cushing's contributions to the study of posterior fossa astrocytomas in children are also of special importance. A comprehensive review of the medical records of Cushing's pediatric patients from 1912–1932 reveals that techniques such as lateral ventricular puncture to decrease cerebellar herniation, transvermian approach to midline tumors, and electrocoagulation [6,7] were the key factors that led to his triumph in pioneering posterior fossa surgery.[2] Cushing's most important pediatric neurosurgery contribution may be his personal account of cerebellar tumor resections which appeared in *Surgery, Gynecology and Obstetrics* in 1931 titled "Experiences with Cerebellar Astrocytomas: A Critical Review of 76 Cases".[3]

In the following chapter, we present samples of patient case studies and their corresponding operative sketches and images to further illustrate the early years of glioma surgery through Cushing's practice.

In Patient 2.1, Cushing initially completed a subtemporal decompression due to a lack of localizing symptoms and signs. This patient was re-admitted to the hospital two months later with findings that allowed a more accurate lesional localization for resective surgery. The patient later underwent a re-operation by Dr. Walter Dandy. Due to the personal conflicts between Cushing and Dandy, Dandy wrote directly to Dr. Eisenhardt regarding the pathological findings. Despite the diagnosis of glioma, this patient underwent five operations. The last admission to the hospital was prompted by the husband who inserted a large trocar into the protrusion at the site of the bony decompression.

Patient 2.2 did not undergo an operation despite seven weeks of hospitalization. Although the reason for such a decision was not mentioned in the chart, the patient may have not undergone an operation due to his marked emaciation and resultant inability to tolerate surgery. This case represented another important advancement in neurosurgical science – the detailed performance of an autopsy – done routinely and personally by Cushing.

Cushing was reluctant to employ air ventriculography because he believed no tool could replace the localizing power of a thorough neurological examination. Furthermore, Cushing was compulsive about finding convincing localizing signs and symptoms so that he could perform more than just a subtemporal decompression. Curiously, despite his compulsion, Patient 2.3 underwent an exploratory craniotomy mainly based on "some tenderness on pressure just above the attachment of the pinea…" Of note, the operation was urgent as the patient was suffering from "receding choked disc" and was "rapidly advancing to blindness." Negative intraoperative findings warranted a ventriculogram and a second surgery, which was also nonrevealing. A succession of ventriculograms demonstrated an intraventricular tumor. Although the tumor was successfully approached, the patient expired about ten days later. This case illustrates the difficulties Cushing faced in the treatment of intraventricular tumors from the beginning to the middle of his career.

It is of interest to know why Percival Bailey performed the autopsy ("confined to the head") of the Patient 2.4 at the patient's home. The autopsy pictures for Patient 2.5 include those taken by Cushing and those recently taken of the specimen preserved in the registry.

The pictures of Patient 2.7 are among some of the most impressive in the collection. The patient was hospitalized for one month during her second admission. She deteriorated neurologically and expired during this admission. The final letter from the husband of Patient 2.8 reflects the letters of appreciation Cushing commonly received on the anniversary of his patients' operations.

Patient 2.9 underwent an unrevealing exploratory craniotomy. Dr. Davidoff, Cushing's resident, took pictures of the patient posturing/convulsing prior to his death. Patient 2.12 underwent multiple operations. He was only six years old and one can only admire him for singing "songs of courage" during his awake craniotomy under such underdeveloped anesthetic conditions. In the autopsy report (the description for coronal section 2), Cushing discusses his misjudgment in estimating the extent of tumor resection.

Cushing describes his "worst exhibition of a cranial operation" when he writes about Patient 2.14. This patient was restless during surgery and uncontrollable bleeding required blood transfusion. The patient expired 10 days after surgery from meningitis.

These patient records and pictures illustrate the faces of unfortunate patients who lost their lives to a surgically incurable disease. The ultimate contribution of Cushing in improving glioma care remains the development of brain tumor clinicopathological correlations. He taught us the futility of aggressive resection in providing long-term control for select tumor subtypes.[5]

Aaron A. Cohen-Gadol, M.D., M.Sc.
Indianapolis, IN

Mitchel S. Berger, M.D.
San Francisco, CA

Robert J. Maciunas, M.D.
Cleveland, OH

Joseph M. Piepmeier, M.D.
New Haven, CT

References

1. Bennett A, Godlee R: Excision of a tumor from the brain. *Lancet* 2:1090-1091, 1884
2. Cohen-Gadol AA, Spencer DD: Inauguration of pediatric neurosurgery by Harvey W. Cushing: his contributions to the surgery of posterior fossa tumors in children. Historical vignette. *J Neurosurg* 100:225-231, 2004
3. Cushing H: Experiences with the cerebellar astrocytomas: a critical review of seventy-six cases. *Surg Gynecol Obstet* 52:129-204, 1931
4. Salcman M: Historical development of surgery for glial tumors. *J Neuro-oncol* 42:195-204, 1999
5. Schulder M, Loeffler JS, Howes AE, Alexander E, 3rd, Black PM: Historical vignette: The radium bomb: Harvey Cushing and the interstitial irradiation of gliomas. *J Neurosurg* 84:530-532, 1996
6. Voorhees JR, Cohen-Gadol AA, Laws ER, Spencer DD: Battling blood loss in neurosurgery: Harvey Cushing's embrace of electrosurgery. *J Neurosurg* 102:745-752, 2005
7. Voorhees JR, Cohen-Gadol AA, Spencer DD: Early evolution of neurological surgery: conquering increased intracranial pressure, infection, and blood loss. *Neurosurg Focus* 18:e2, 2005

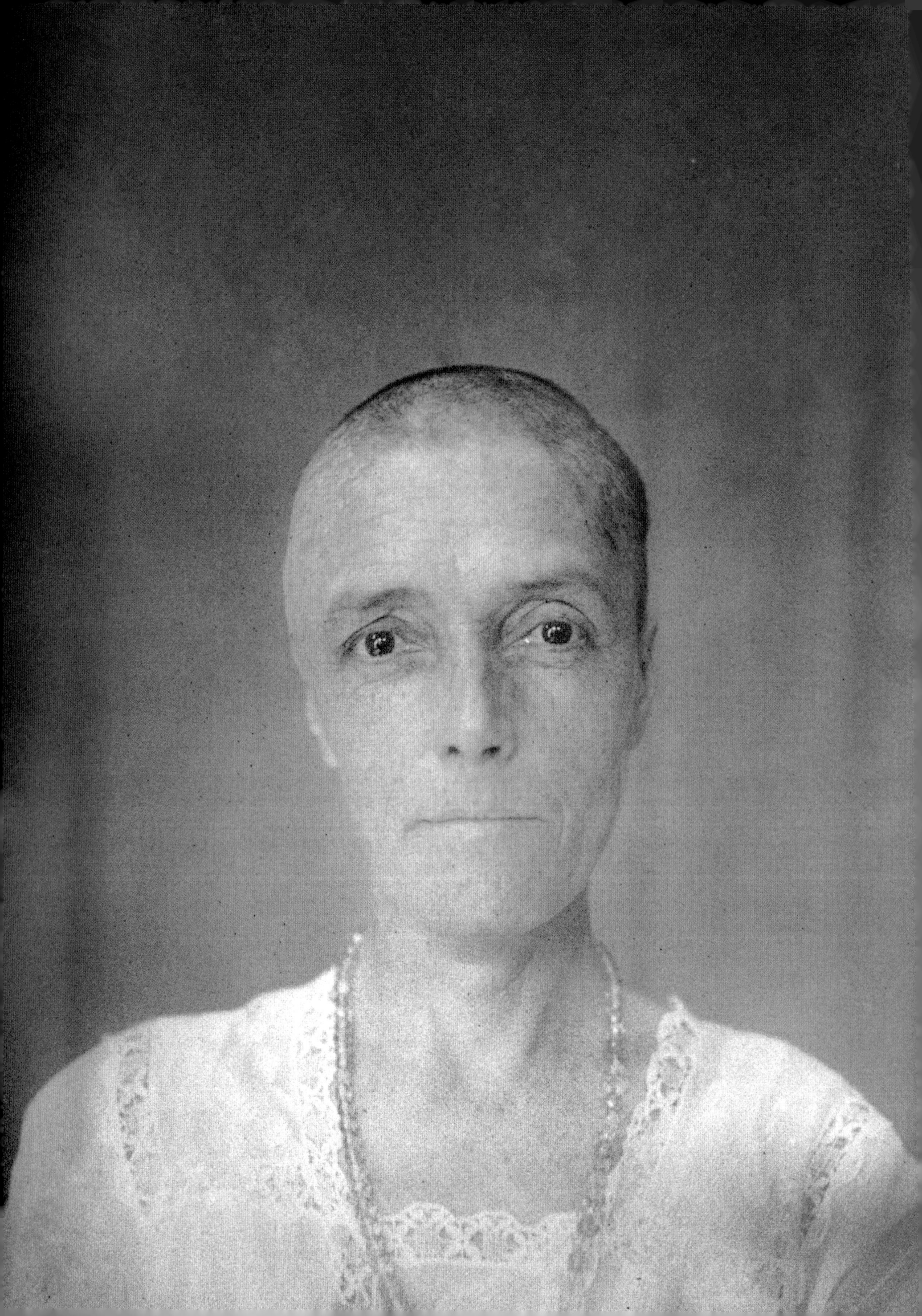

2.1 Parietal neuroblastoma

SEX: F; AGE: 42; SURG. NO. 5440; 5885; 13304; 14226; 15014

HISTORY

In 1909 and 1910, the patient had two grand mal attacks of epilepsy. Following these, she had numerous attacks of the petit mal type. Dr. Craddock prescribed sodium bromide which she took in varying amounts ever since. Six weeks previous to this entry, the patient began to have frontal headaches, blurry vision, and numbness of the right middle finger.

SUMMARY OF POSITIVE FINDINGS
September 23, 1916
Dr. Horrax

SUBJECTIVE
1. Grand mal and petit mal seizures - not focal.
2. Headaches - frontal for past six weeks.
3. Tinnitus.

OBJECTIVE
1. Slight anisocoria, R > L.
2. Fundi - very early choked disks - 3D.

OPERATIVE NOTE
September 30, 1916
Anaesthesia – Ether – Dr. Boothby

Right Subtemporal Decompression.

There were no special difficulties in this procedure which was conducted on the usual lines. The dura was very tense, but fortunately, a considerable amount of fluid was secured, relieving the pressure. A fairly wide decompression was made. An attempt at puncture of the lateral ventricle proved to secure no fluid.

Closure as usual in layers.

(Dr. Cushing)

October 2, 1916
Dr. Horrax

She made a very prompt and excellent recovery with practically no nausea or vomiting, and now taking liquids very well.

First dressing – edges well approximated – no reaction. No tension or bulging. All stitches out. Redressed with silver foil and collodion strip.

DISCHARGE NOTE
October 10, 1916
Dr. Horrax

Condition excellent. No attacks, headache or tinnitus since operation to report.

Decompressed area fairly tense and slightly bulging. Discharged.

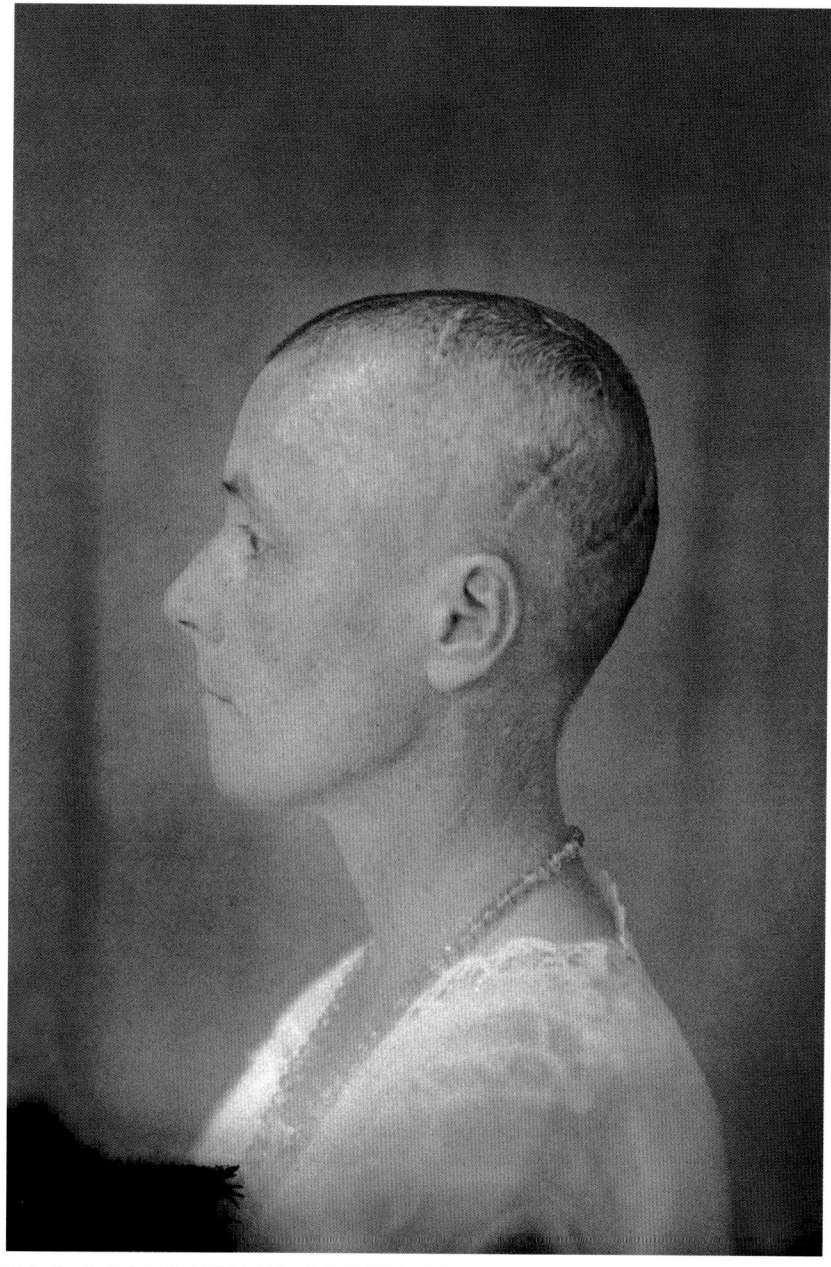

FIG. 2. POSTOPERATIVE AFTER SECOND SURGERY — FIRST RESECTION.

OPPOSITE PAGE. FIG. 1. POSTOPERATIVE AFTER SECOND SURGERY — FIRST RESECTION.

SECOND HOSPITAL ADMISSION

HISTORY

Patient returned to the hospital on December 11, 1916 having had one petit mal attack since her last entry.

SUMMARY OF POSITIVE FINDINGS
December 12, 1916
Dr. Montgomery

SUBJECTIVE
1. Petit mal – One attack since operation, not focal.
2. Vision – Some blurring in the past two to three weeks.
3. Twitching of right hand.
4. Paresthesias of right hand and forearm.
5. Weakness of right hand and arm.
6. Tinnitus on the left, only when lying on the decompression.

OBJECTIVE
1. Choked disc – 3D
2. 11th – right-sided weakness.
3. 12th – tongue protruded to right.
4. Slight weakness of right arm and hand.
5. Ataxia – very slight, left hand.
6. Biceps relatively exaggerated on the right.
7. Vasomotor – Right hand and arm cooler than left.

RADIOLOGY REPORT
December, 13, 1916

X-ray examination of the skull shows an operative defect in the right temporal and parietal region. The venous channels of the skull are somewhat enlarged, especially frontal region. Average thickness is 5 mm. The sella is of the flat type. The posterior diameter is 11 mm., it is 6 mm deep. The outlines of the fossa are not seen. The dorsum, however, is somewhat thinned and suggests a slight amount of atrophy.

OPERATIVE NOTE
December 13, 1916
Anaesthesia – Ether – Miss Gerard

Extirpation of Large Endothelioma of Left Inferior Parietal Region.

Under ether the bone flap was turned down exposing the left hemisphere somewhat anteriorly, just why I cannot now see, in view of the fact that her right sided numbness was the reason for the operation. This did not help much and there was a great deal of bleeding not only from the scalp but also from the bone. On reflecting the flap there seemed to be a marked dural process but the brain was tense. On opening the dura a little bit of fluid was fortunately secured and the membrane was gradually reflected upward and a roundish, soft, dark red tumor was partly exposed at the posterior margin of the field. The dura was slightly adherent to this tumor and consequently the dura was gradually excised corresponding to the center of the growth to which it was attached. The growth proved to be large measuring 6 cm in its surface diameter. It was fairly well affixed and did not extend at any great depth into the hemisphere. It seemed in other words, very similar to the tumor from the recent case of (the name of another patient) which also had several years history of focal attacks.

In view of the considerable loss of blood, there was some doubt as to whether the operation should be continued but the decision rested in favor of doing so. The bone had to be rongeured away posteriorly for a distance of 4-5 cm so as to expose the growth. It was then blocked out and apparently removed in toto. The brain was very soft and it was possible to clip almost all of the vessels during the process of the removal so that there was very little bleeding. The dura was then resutured except for a large defect near the posterior part of the field and the flap was replaced and closed as usual in layers.

(Dr. Cushing)

PATHOLOGY REPORT
December 18, 1916

The tumor is composed of compactly arranged polygonal cells with fairly definite outline and round or oval nuclei. Mitotic figures are fairly numerous. There is no definite architecture to arrangement of the tumor cells although these are often demarcated into islands or nests by surrounding fibrous tissue trabeculae. No neuroglia fibrillae are found. Capillaries are numerous throughout the tumor substance and there are many small hemorrhages with a few areas of necrosis. Surrounding the tumor there is extensive edema and necrosis of the brain substance.

The relation of the tumor to the dura, the compactness of the growth and the character of the cells, together with the absence of neuroglia fibrillae make a diagnosis of endothelioma seem fairly certain.

DIAGNOSIS – Endothelioma of brain.
(Dr. Goodpasture)

December 23, 1916
Dr. Harvey

Directly following the operation the patient was somewhat shocked with a very feeble pulse but soon rallied with saline per rectum so that by midafternoon she was in quite good condition. Since then there has been nothing of note in the convalescence.

First dressing. Rubber drain removed. There was not an unusual amount of drainage. Stitches all taken out. Wound healing everywhere per primum. Redressed with silver foil, gauze and crinolia.

DISCHARGE NOTE
January 12, 1917
Dr. Harvey

The condition of the patient is now normal in every respect as far as can be determined, aside from the residual of the choked disc. Bone flap is flat. The herniation is soft and receding. The wound is perfectly healed. She is discharged home to the care of her husband today.

LETTER TO DR. CUSHING
February 1, 1917

Dear Doctor:

Mrs. (name of the patient) is feeling very good in every way. She has increased seven pounds in weight since leaving the hospital. The only symptom occurred yesterday. She was unable to grasp the water faucet. At the same time a stinging sensation passed over the left operated area. About three seconds later she grasped the faucet as well as ever. We are not worrying about this at all.

I hope you are well yourself.
Yours truly,
(Signed by the patient's husband)

During the interval between February and August of 1918, attacks became more frequent and the decompression area became tight. Patient's arm became progressively weaker and there was a good deal of difficulty in writing and spelling.

August 14, 1918 – Dr. Walter Dandy of the Johns Hopkins Hospital reopened the old operative site and aspirated a large cyst.

Pathological service (Johns Hopkins Hospital): Specimen from Aug. 14, 1918 – large, irregular cells, round and oval nuclei, pale cytoplasm resembling neuroglia cells only occasionally. The larger nuclei show nucleoli and chromatin granules.

DIAGNOSIS – Glioma

August 17, 1918
From Dr. Dandy's letter to Dr. Eisenhardt:

Dear Miss Eisenhardt:

I promised to let you know about the findings in (name of the patient) case. She entered the hospital a few days ago and it was perfectly obvious that the growth was recurrent... It was perfectly obvious when the tumor was exposed that its complete removal was out of the question. It was a glioma which was very diffusely infiltrated. It contained a large cyst which was evacuated, but other than removing a piece of the tumor for diagnosis, we made no attempt at its removal.
Very sincerely yours,
(Signed by Walter Dandy)

There was therefore some confusion regarding the correct histopathological diagnosis. Following the surgery by Dr. Dandy, there was a relief of symptoms for about six months. The patient had seven radiation treatments at six weeks intervals, the last one in August 1920.

THIRD HOSPITAL ADMISSION

HISTORY

The patient returned to see Dr. Cushing with worsening of her arm symptoms and feeling of discomfort at the old operative site.

October 10, 1920
Dr. Locke

Today Dr. Cushing saw the patient and thought it advisable to open up the old incision over the tumor. This will be done just as soon as it can be arranged.

October 11, 1920
Dr. Locke

Head shows the presence of old subtemporal decompression which is bulging moderately and

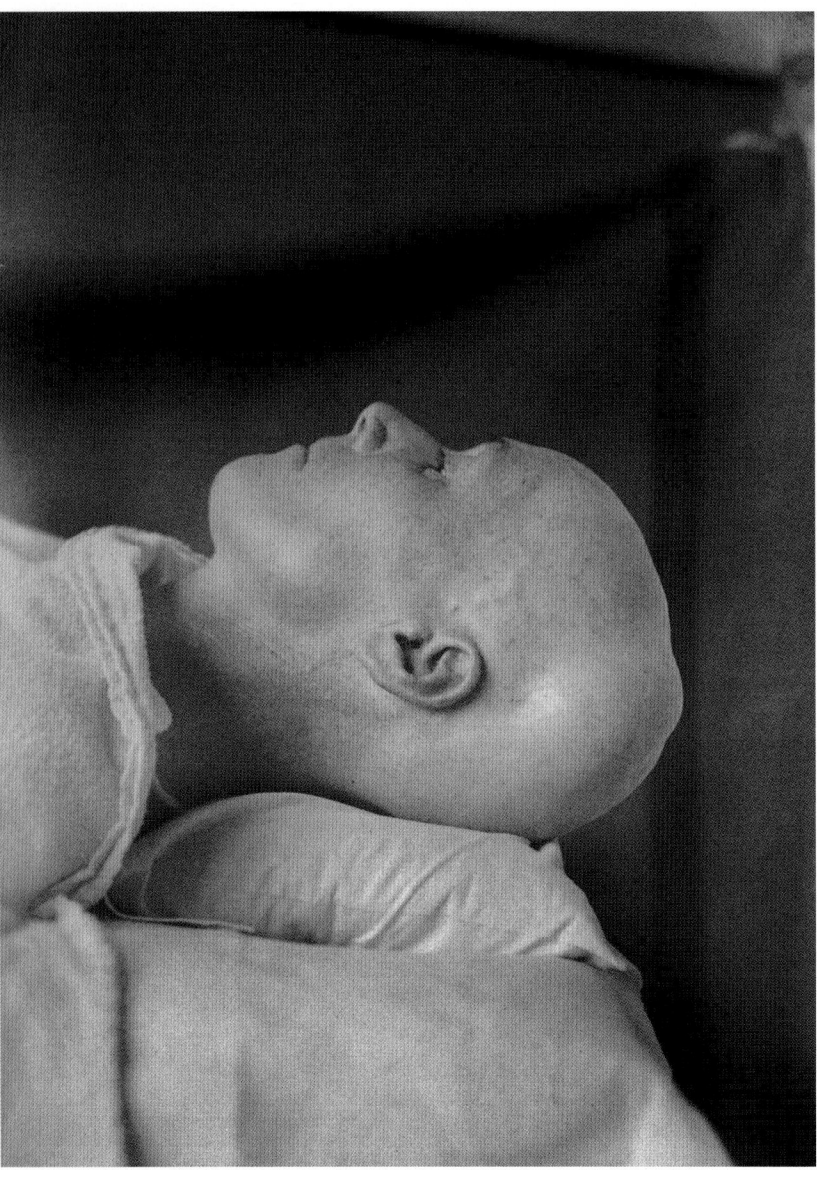

FIG. 3. PRIOR TO FOURTH SURGICAL PROCEDURE.

the protruding area is not under very marked increased tension. There is also a decompression in the parietal region. Here too there is moderate bulging. There is also the presence of the usual osteoplastic flap operative scar with the usual burr hole. Percussion note is normal except over the operative site and here there is rather a cracked note. No abnormal pulsations made out. No dilated veins seen.

October 11, 1920
Dr. Cushing

Considerable loss of muscle sense and astereognosis.

OPERATIVE NOTE
October 14, 1920
Anaesthesia – Ether – Miss Gerard

Fourth Operation for Tumor of Left Parietal Region. Partial Extirpation of Large Cystic Glioma.

This is a most interesting history in view of the confused histological diagnoses. The original operative diagnosis was endothelioma and this was supported by Dr. Goodpasture. Subsequently in Baltimore the tumor was recorded as a glioma. Dr. Wolbach on looking over the tissues considers it to be a neuroblastoma. The patient of late has been having some increase in the numbness and loss of sensory function in the right arm. The bone defect which Dr. Dandy left in correspondence with my original bone defect, though somewhat enlarged, has become the seat of considerable protrusion. Photographs were taken before the operation to show this (Please see the attached images titled "Prior to 4th surgical procedure.")

A new curvilinear incision was made surrounding the protrusion which lay at the posterior part of the old field and directly under the posterior portion of the old cicatrix. The curvilinear incision was carried down to the bone and the flap scraped away from the bone. A crescentic margin of bone was removed with a succession of bone perforations and Gigli saw. This exposed a zone of normal dura which was incised exposing an outer margin of brain, evidently overlying the tumor. The cortex was incised, the vessels being caught with clips. This exposed a large gliomatous mass and opened one large cyst, and subsequently one or two other large cysts the size of a pigeon's egg were opened and the wall of one of them was fixed with formalin and Zenker's fluid. An effort was then made to scoop out the chief mass of the tumor which became a very messy and somewhat bloody performance as the tumor was adherent to the flap and as it extended beyond the limits of the exposed field. However, a sufficient amount of it was removed to relieve the tension and to permit closure of the scalp, the wound being left reasonably dry.

(Dr. Cushing)

PATHOLOGY REPORT
October 14, 1920

Microscopic report: Mass of glia cells, most of which have round or oval nuclei. Many mitotic figures are present. In addition to the neuroglia fibrils, there is a delicate fibrillary intercellular substance. Large areas of necrosis are found in various portions. It is quite vascular, while hemorrhage, mostly recent, is an additional factor. This is a rapidly growing tumor.

DIAGNOSIS – glioma.

(Dr. Wolbach)

ADDITIONAL PATHOLOGY REPORT
(A re-review of all pathology specimens on November 8, 1920)

A slide of the original tumor, removed December 18, 1916, is restained, and in this slide as in slide from October 14, 1920, there are deeply staining, wavy fibrils connected with many of the tumor cells but in such locations as to preclude the possibility of them being neuroglia cells derived from cerebrum. One peculiarity of the tumor deserved mention as it is present in the material from both operations, that is the presence of a considerable amount of delicately staining fibrillary intercellular substance. This is particularly noticeable where the tumor has carried with it supporting connective tissue from the dura. Selected fields strongly suggest the appearance of tumor of nerve cells. While the diagnosis of glioma should be made on this tumor, it is well to keep in mind the possibility of a differentiation into both the derivatives of the neuroblasts.

(Dr. Wolbach)

POSTOPERATIVE NOTE
October 14, 1920
Dr. Locke

The patient was operated on this morning and reacted well from the anaesthetic, unusually well in fact.

October 17, 1920
Dr. Locke

Today the suture were clipped but not removed. Wound in good condition and there is no undue bulging.

DISCHARGE NOTE
October 27, 1920
Dr. Locke

Following operation there was marked increase in strength of the arm almost to normal. There was some diminishment in bulging of decompression

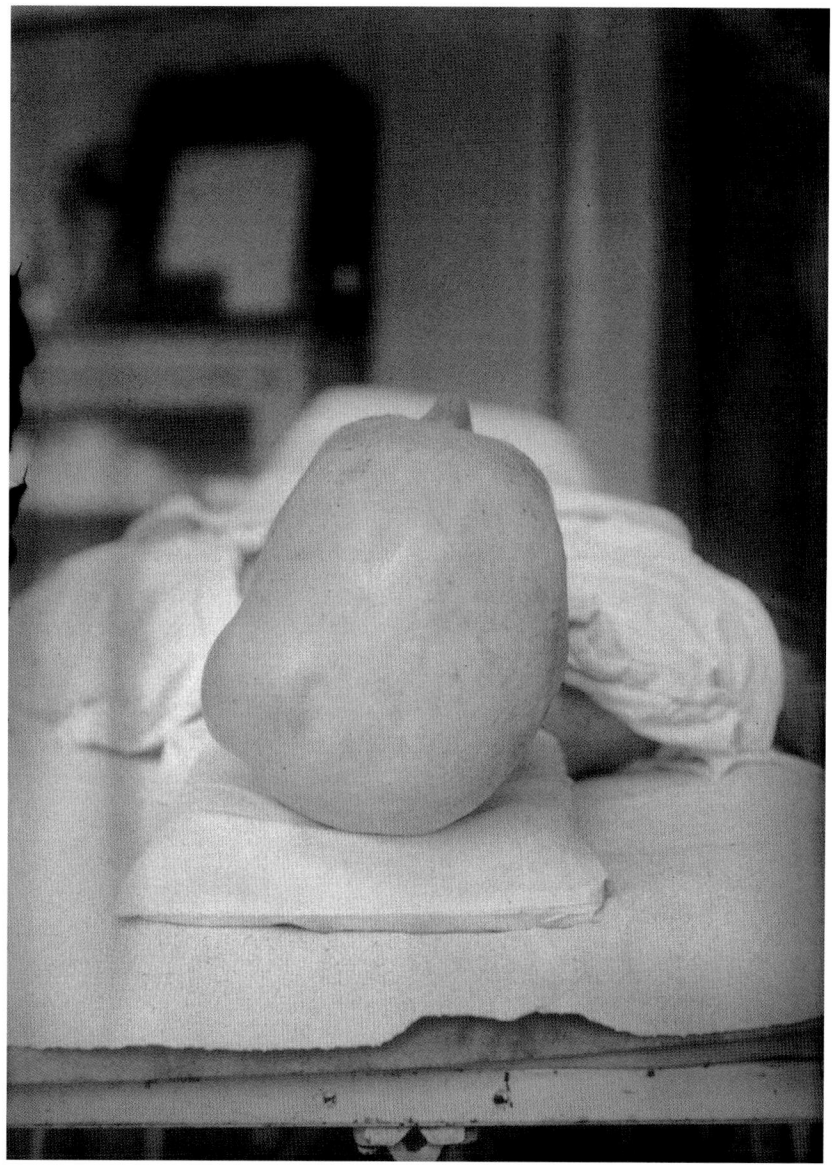

FIG. 4. PRIOR TO FOURTH SURGICAL PROCEDURE.

areas. Slight improvement in position sense and astereognosis resulted. Dysarthria continued.

FOURTH HOSPITAL ADMISSION

HISTORY

The patient re-entered the hospital with dysphasia and recurrent right upper extremity symptoms.

SUMMARY OF POSITIVE FINDINGS
March 22, 1921
Dr. Locke

OBJECTIVE
1. Head – There is the presence of a right subtemporal decompression which is slightly

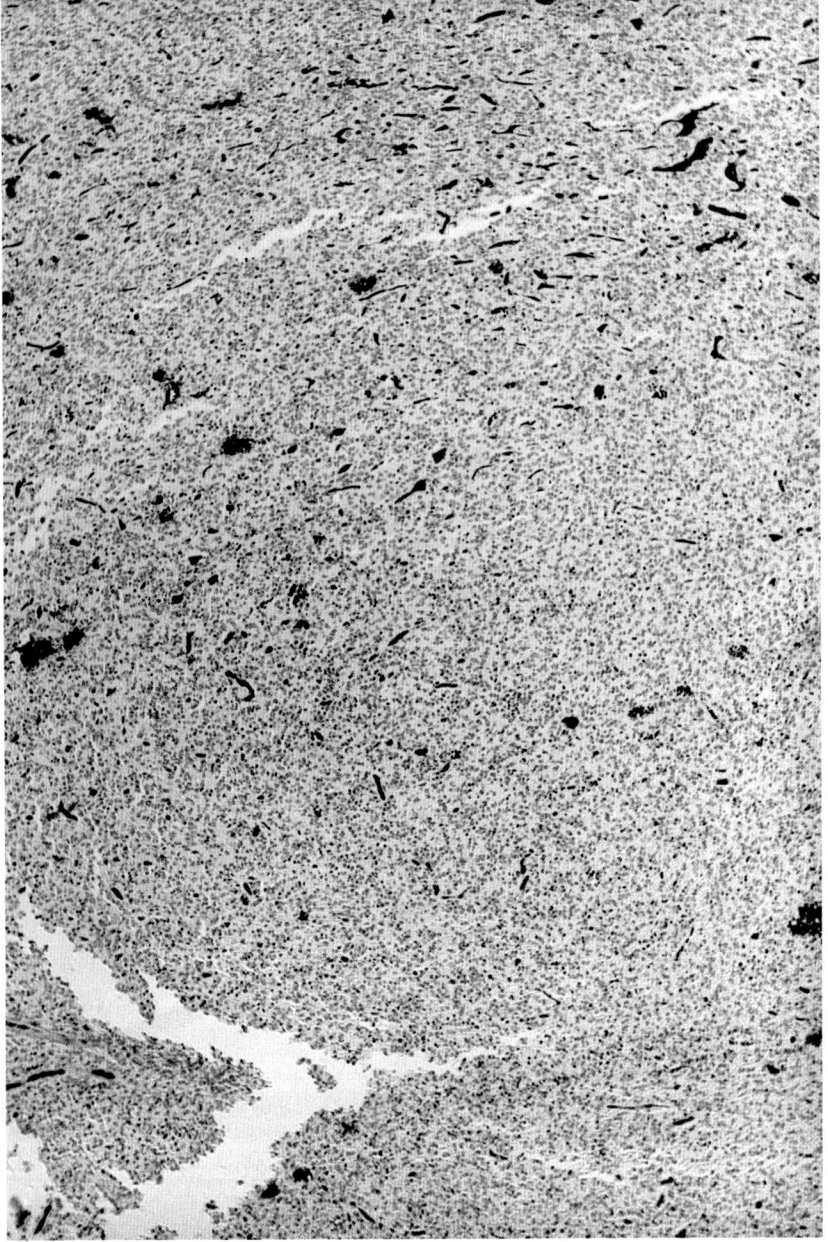

FIG. 5. PATHOLOGY SLIDE.

protruding and not particularly tense. On the left there is a scar of an osteoplastic flap operation; brain tissue is bulging slightly thru this flap but is not particularly tense.

2. Chocked disc with some new tissue formation.
3. Some aphasia, agraphia and alexia; no apraxia.
4. Marked loss of muscle sense and astereognosis, right.
5. Marked hemiparesis of right upper extremity, slight of right lower extremity.
6. Very marked impairment of sensation to touch, pain and temperature in right upper and lower extremities as well as lower half of right trunk.
7. Some deviation of tongue to the right.
8. Exaggerated deep reflexes, right with unsustained clonus.
9. Possibly a little right lower facial weakness.

OPERATIVE NOTE
March 28, 1921
Anaesthesia – Ether – Miss Gerrard

Partial Extirpation of Large Recurrent Glioma.

A flap corresponding to the last incision was reflected, solid glioma being disclosed adherent to the flap. It had been thought from palpation that the tumor would be cystic but there were no signs of cyst formation whatsoever, nor were there any indications in the gross of change due to x-ray administrations. An effort was made with the cautery to dissect out the tumor but this led to bleeding and to further fall in blood pressure. Of chart. After a delay of ten minutes, with the fingers the deep tumor was thoroughly scooped out from its bed and much bleeding points as were present at the depth were controlled either by muscle or by silver clips. The scalp was replaced, saline was given per rectum and though a transfusion was contemplated, this was not found to be necessary.

(Dr. Cushing)

PATHOLOGY REPORT
March 28, 1921

Three sections consist of a very cellular tumor in which much recent hemorrhage has occurred from many small blood vessels. The cells are of the general type of glia cell with deeply staining hyperchromatic nuclei. Mitotic figures are numerous. Glia fibrillae are abundant except where the cells are occasionally arranged in a large rosette, such as are seen in certain neurocytomas, the fibrils being few in these areas where there is a paler and more delicate fibrillary material. Bordering one section is a dense fibrous layer in which are numerous multinucleated giant cells.

DIAGNOSIS – Glioma

(Dr. Wolbach)

DISCHARGE NOTE
April 13, 1921
Dr. Locke

The protrusion in left parietal region is very marked even more than at entry. Decompression on right bulging slightly. Partial aphasia. Some confusion. Reading very poor and slow. Astereognosia on right. Tongue is midline. Exaggerated deep reflexes of upper right extremity. Numbness of right arm and slight weakness and dragging of right foot. Very slight right lower facial weakness. Fundi – OS 1D; OD 1+D. Some secondary atrophy. There is occasional slight headache. No photo.

LETTER TO DR. CUSHING
May 11, 1921

Dr. Cushing:

I wish to thank you for being so kind to us, as you certainly have been. My wife is feeling fine. She has gained several pounds, has a wonderful appetite, has no distress or discomfort of any kind. The protrusion is fairly soft. I will write you from time to time.

Sincerely yours,
(Signed) GA

FIFTH HOSPITAL ADMISSION
August 11, 1921
Dr. Cushing

Patient brought to the hospital by her husband who had inserted large trocar into the protrusion and had been distressed by the cerebrospinal fluid leak which had persisted subsequently. I do not know how many days it had persisted nor are there any details of the fact on her admission. I inserted a small needle in another portion of the protrusion and drew off enough clear cerebrospinal fluid which contained no organisms and which was sterile on culture. The collapsed protrusion was then dressed and the original leak had apparently closed the following day when she was discharged.

LETTER TO DR. CUSHING
October 6, 1921

Dear Doctor:

I am sorry to tell you that Mrs. (name of the patient) died September 28th. You did well to keep her alive and comfortable these past five years. I want to thank you again for being so kind to us both.

Sincerely yours,
(Signed) GW

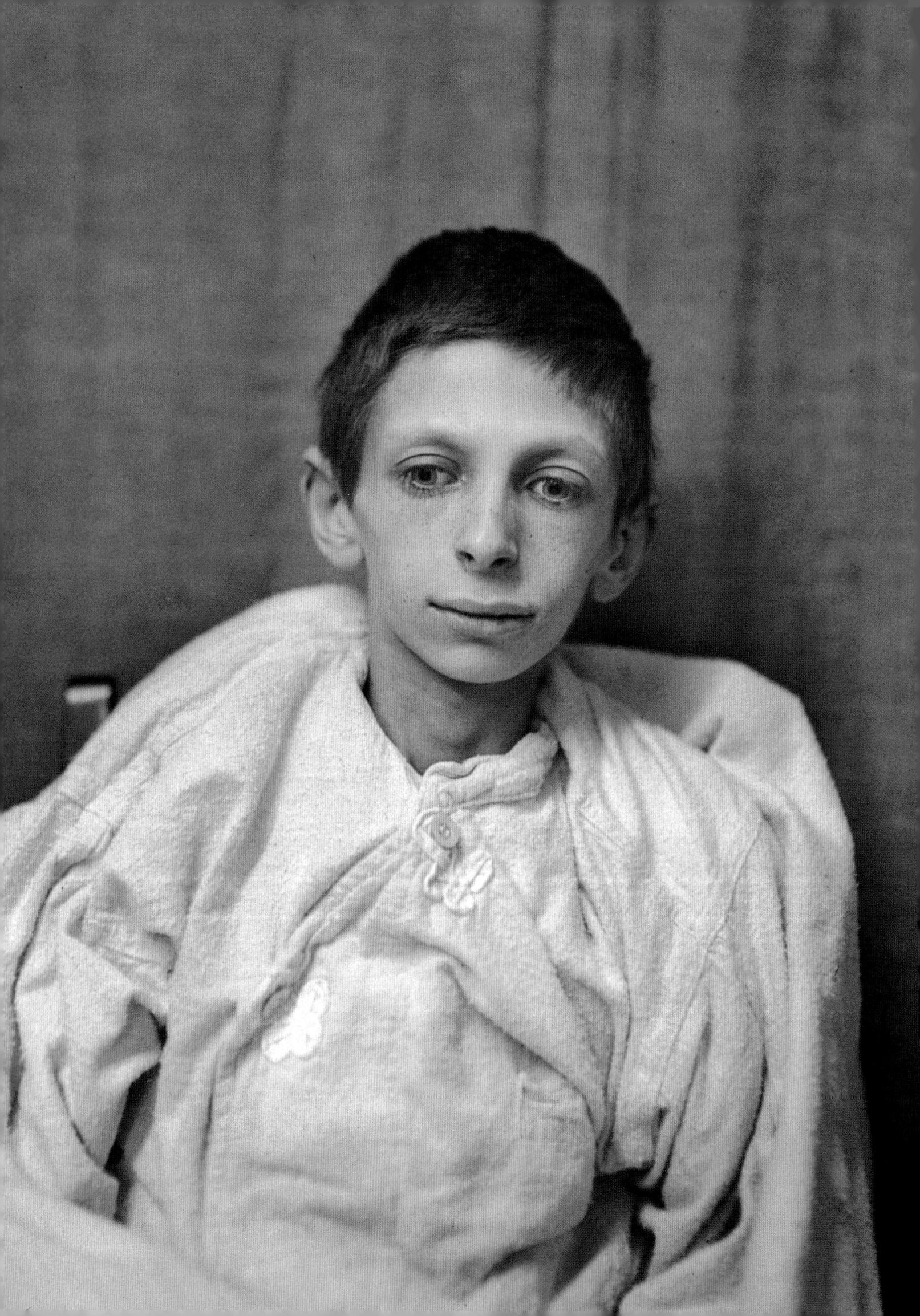

2.2 Pineal region tumor

SEX: M; AGE: 13; SURG. NO. 16012

HISTORY

The patient suffered from occasional severe headaches and polydipsia/polyuria for 1–2 years prior to presentation. Headaches became severe with onset of vomiting and blurred vision eight months ago. Bitemporal hemianopsia and changes in vision led to a right-sided subtemporal decompression three months ago followed by a left-sided subtemporal decompression two weeks later in order to save vision. Only slight improvement lasting until two weeks ago was noted when symptoms again began to worsen.

Patient's exam showed bulging bilateral subtemporal decompressions. His vision was much diminished with bitemporal hemianopsia. He was markedly emaciated with contractures of lower extremities.

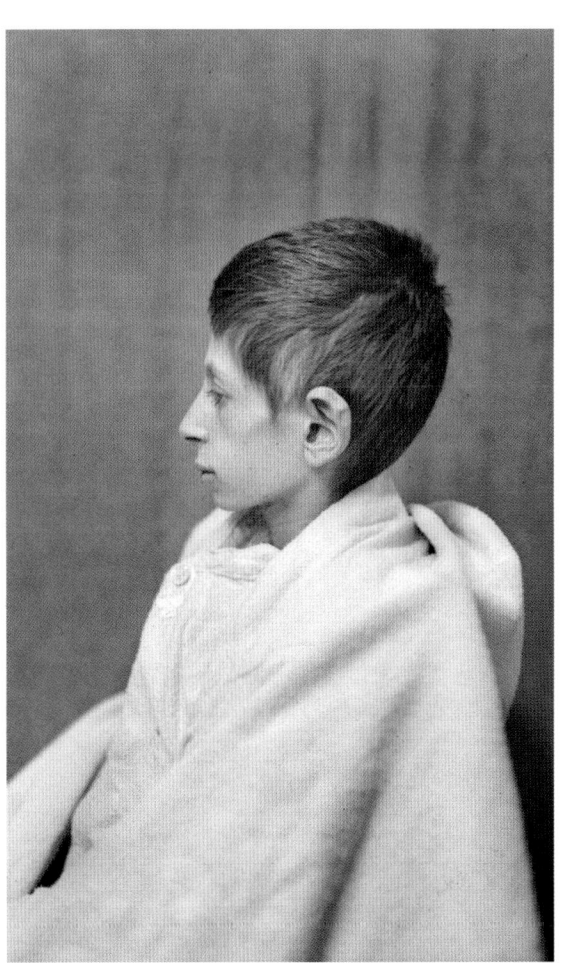

FIG. 2. AT TIME OF ADMISSION.

OPPOSITE PAGE. FIG. 1. AT TIME OF ADMISSION.

SUMMARY OF POSITIVE FINDINGS
February 1, 1922
Dr. Vickers

SUBJECTIVE
1. History of bursting type of headache, onset 2 years ago.
2. History of impairment of vision with subjective hemianopsia.
3. Onset of polydipsia and polyuria one year ago.
4. Inability to raise the eyes above the midline.
5. Loss of appetite with marked emaciation.
6. History of hair becoming coarse, dry, and straight.

OBJECTIVE
1. Bilateral temporal decompression.
2. Primary optic atrophy bilateral.
3. Bilateral trochlear nerve palsy.
4. Marked emaciation.
5. Coarse dry hair. Infantile ext. genitalia with absence of pubic and axillary hair.
6. Contracture of lower extremities.
7. Protruding upper teeth.
8. Hemianopsia.

IMPRESSION: Suprasellar tumor

RADIOLOGY REPORT
February 1, 1922
Dr. Sosman

Films show the skull to be somewhat peculiarly shaped. Convolutional impressions of the inner table are well shown. There is an operative defect on the skull in the temporal region. The sella turcica itself is normal. There is linear sticky calcification 12 mm in length of pineal, parallel to tentorium.

The patient became progressively worse as he could not take any nutrient during this hospitalization.

DISCHARGE NOTE
March 21, 1922
Dr. Macley

Patient condition was found much worse this morning and parents were called for. He passed away at 2 p.m.

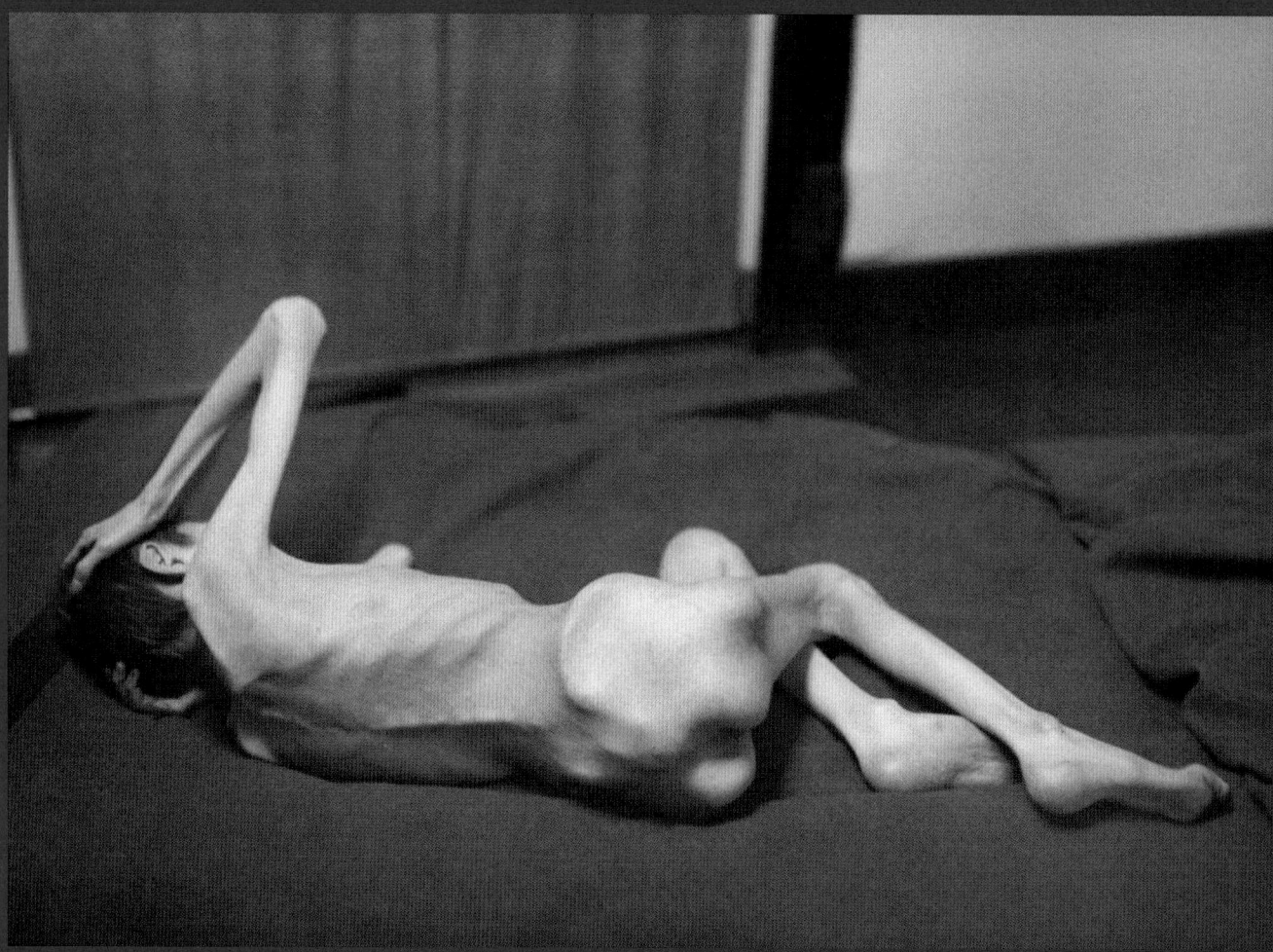

FIGS. 3 AND 4. TWO DAYS AFTER ADMISSION.

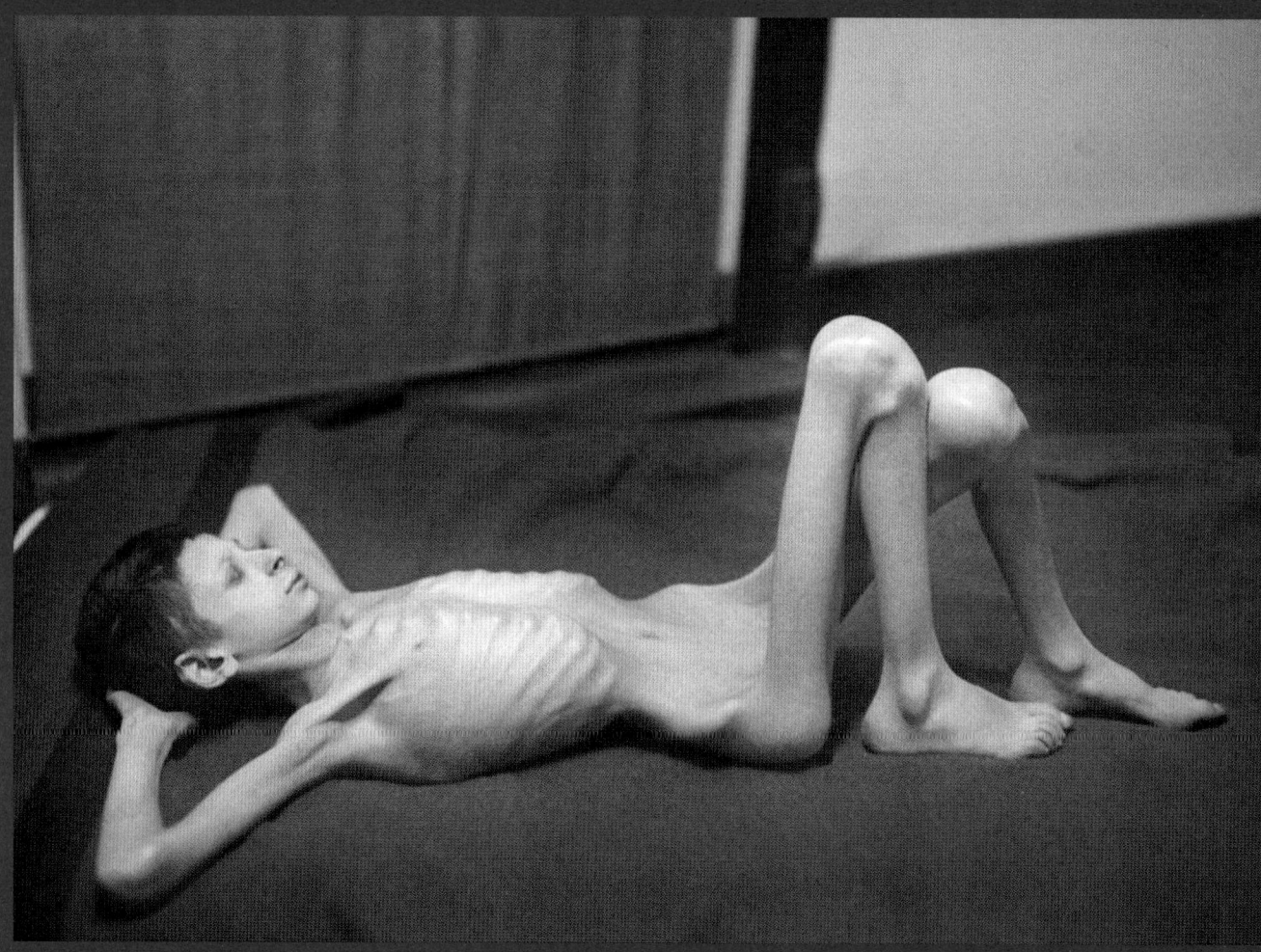

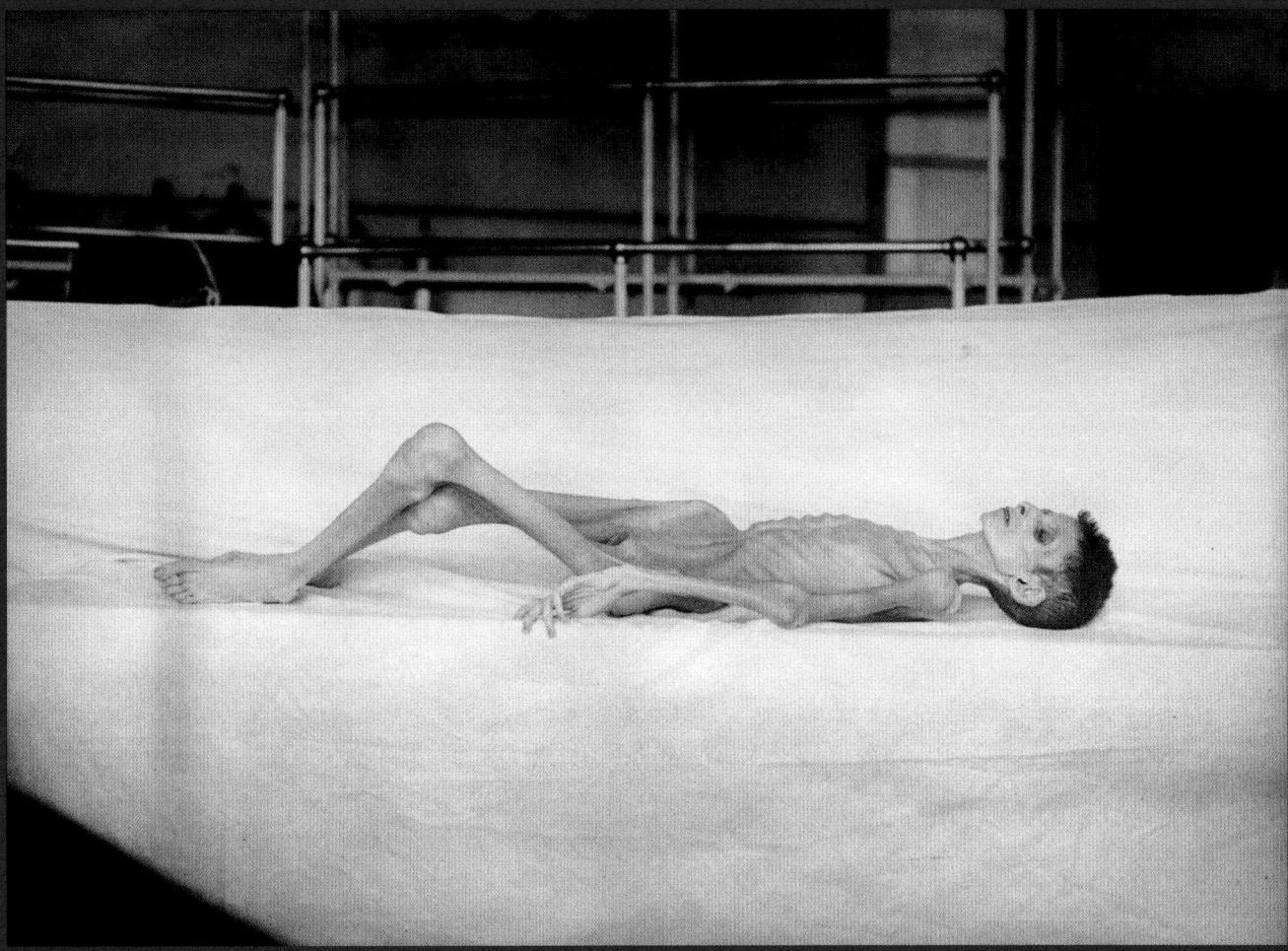

FIGS. 5 AND 6. ELEVEN DAYS AFTER ADMISSION.

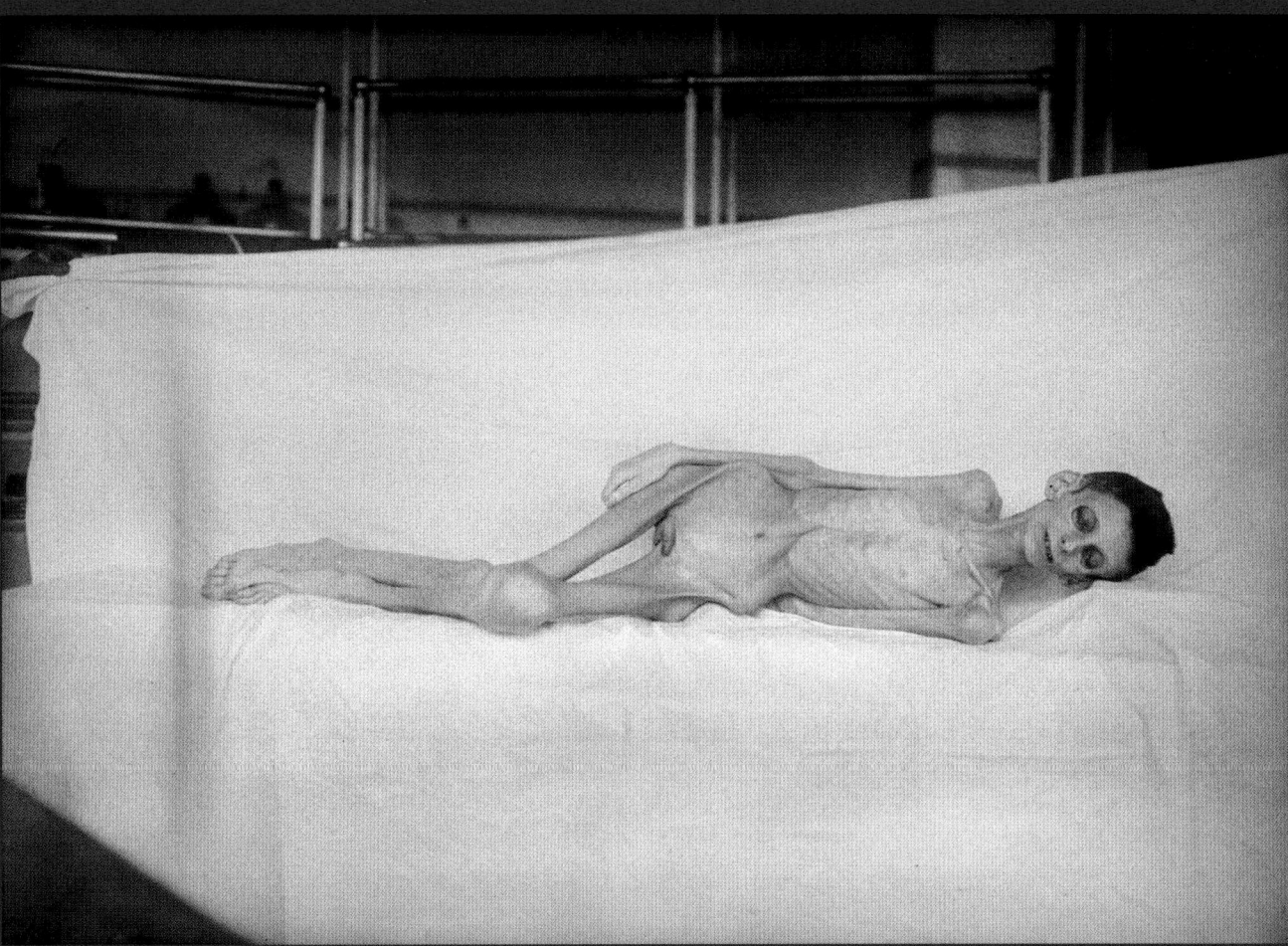

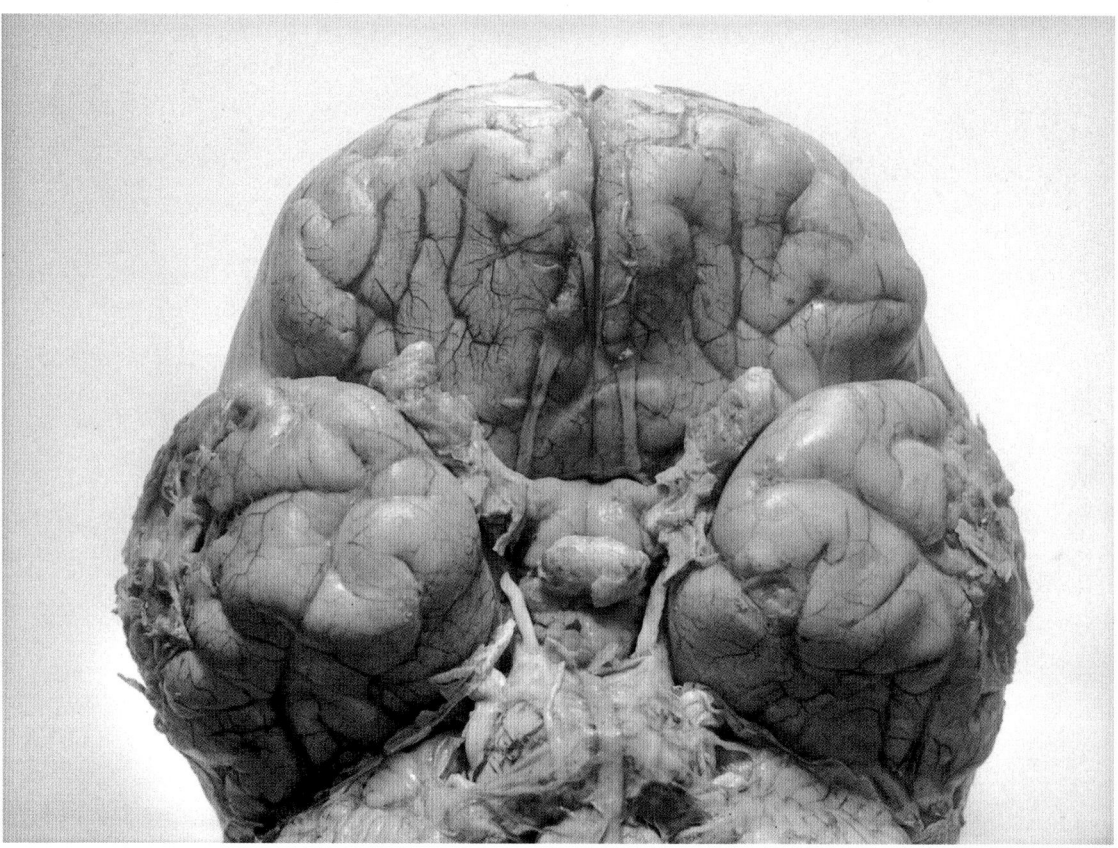

FIG. 7. AUTOPSY SPECIMEN.

AUTOPSY REPORT
March 22, 1922
Dr. Hansmann
Dr. Fremont-Smith Jr.

DIAGNOSES
    Adenoma of the pineal gland
    Tumor of optic chiasm (glioma)
    Gliosis of the optic nerve chiasm and tracts
    Tuberculosis of right lung
    Fibrous pleuritis, right
    Accessory adrenal
    Undescended testicle (left)
    Obliterated hypogastric arteries

BRAIN

The external surface of the dura presented nothing unusual. On palpation the brain is found to be plastic. On lifting the frontal lobes and exposing the optic chiasm, a pinkish grey tumor is seen occupying the position of the optic chiasm. On examining the base of the brain a tumor mass was found occupying the interpeduncular space and apparently surrounding the stalk of the pituitary body, which organ is quite normal in appearance. No trace is seen of normal optic chiasm, the whole being replaced by pinkish gray, rather soft tumor. This tumor has invaded the optic nerves to some extent and on the right a sharp line of demarcation can be seen at about the point of entrance into the optic foramen between pinkish grey tumor and white optic nerve. The tumor extends posteriorly to the mamillary bodies, in its posterior portion is very thin walled, and beneath this thin wall there is either the third ventricle or a cyst seen. The remainder of the base of the brain is normal in appearance excepting that the pons appears to be somewhat more apart than normal.

There is very little to say about the appearance of this brain on section beyond what the photographs will show. There is a large internal hydrocephalus which would appear to be due to an occlusion of the Aqueduct of Sylvius for there is a tumor mass measuring about 3.5 x 2.5 cm which lies above the pons, and must have separated the crura and which lies about between the 4th ventricle and the dilated 3rd ventricle. This tumor mass would appear to have originated perhaps from the region of the pineal gland, although there are one or two separate adjacent structures which might

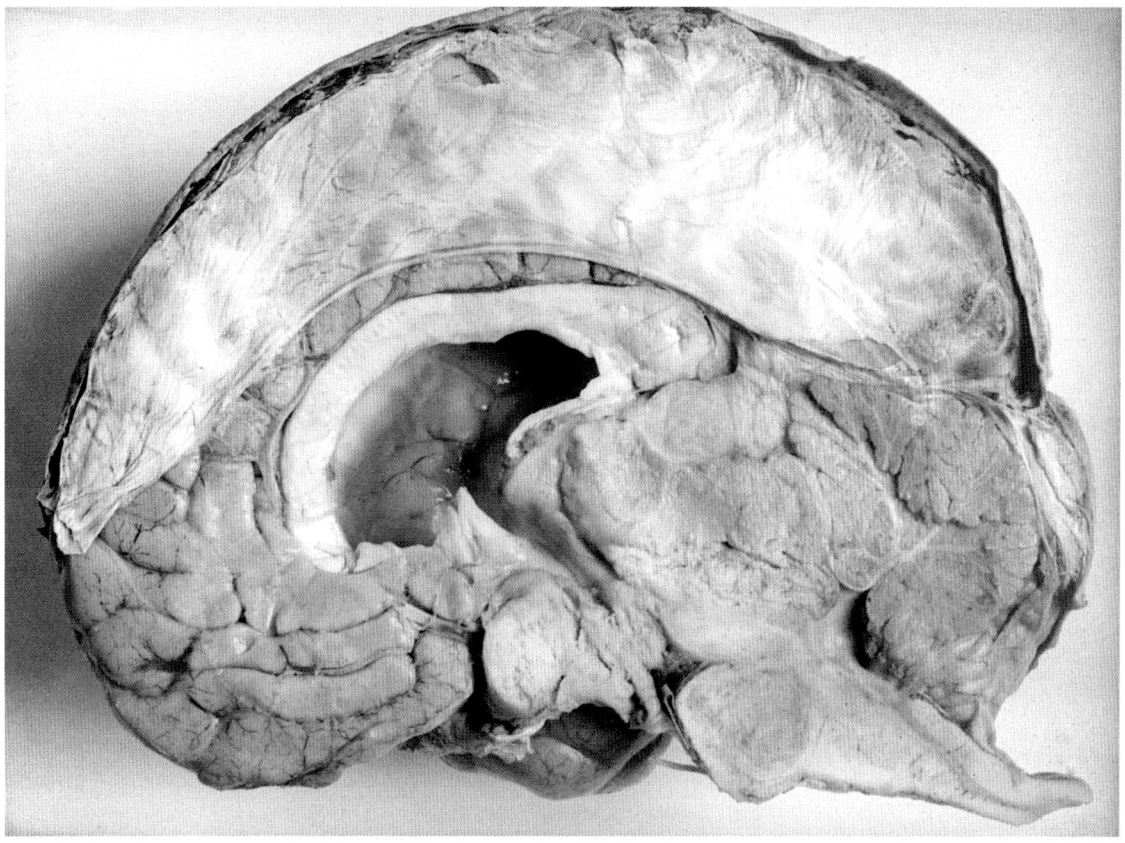

FIG. 8. AUTOPSY SPECIMEN — SAGITTAL VIEW.

possibly be sections of the pineal itself. This tumor has a pinkish, homogeneous surface, like the surface of a ripe banana. The third ventricle is greatly distorted and points backward instead of downward. At its tip, lying between its tip and what appears to be normal flattened pituitary gland, is another mass which may or may not be connected with the original tumor mass, and which probably is. This mass measures 2.5 x 1.5 cm. It is this mass which gave the appearance of spreading out into the optic chiasm and optic nerves as described in the external description of the tissue. The tumor seems to be centrally placed and must have destroyed the lower part of the third ventricle and infundibulum as well as to have obliterated the Sylvian Aqueduct.

(Dr. Cushing)

Microscopic description of the tumor: The case is one of the adenoma of the pineal gland with gliomatous optic tracts.

(Dr. Hansmann)

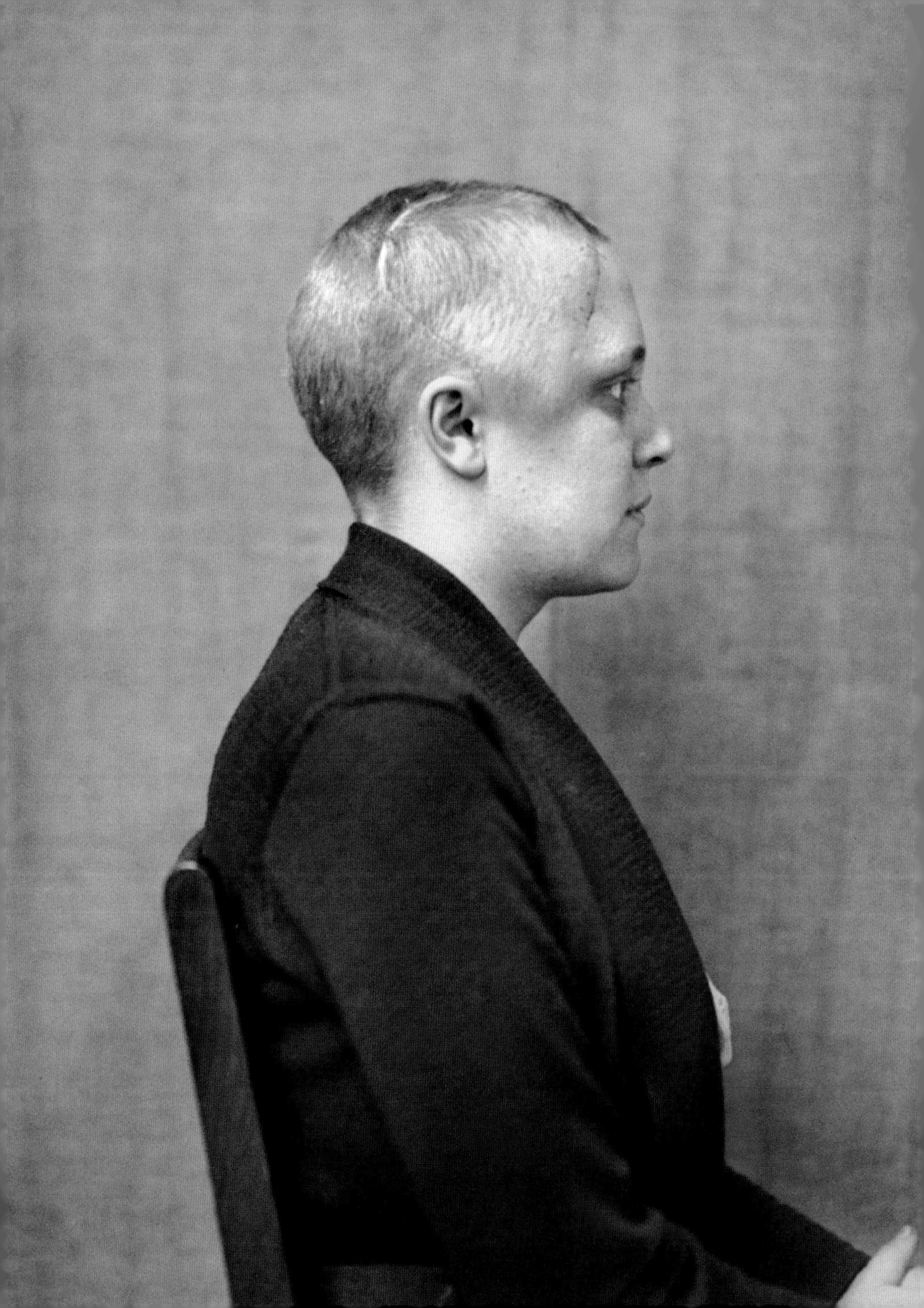

2.3 Glioma of the lateral ventricle

SEX: F; AGE: 22; SURG. NO. 15890, 18229

HISTORY

This patient presented with progressive changes in vision during the last two years. In November 1921, patient developed symptoms of increased intracranial pressure and a diagnosis of brain tumor was made. Patient was referred to Dr. Cushing with a suspected "neoplasm in the neighborhood of the hypophysis, which implicated the uncinate gyrus seizures either primarily or secondary."

COMPLAINT

Unpleasant tastes with dreamy states. Hallucinations of faces and objects. Soreness of the neck muscles. Unconsciousness.

SUMMARY OF POSITIVE FINDINGS
January 7, 1922
Dr. Wheeler

SUBJECTIVE
1. In the spring of 1919 history of transient diplopia.
2. In Nov. 1919 onset of severe girdle-like headaches extending from the frontal to the occipital region, also onset of dizziness at this time.
3. In the fall of 1919 dimness and blurring of vision.
4. In the Spring of 1921 loss of sense of taste and smells.
5. Since early fall of 1921 tendency to underestimate distance in reaching for objects.
6. Later in Oct. 1921 there has been a divergence of the right eye.
8. Since the latter part of Nov. 1921 tenderness in the right temporal region.
9. Since Jan. 1st soreness of the neck muscles.
10. Since Jan. 2nd 1922 onset of nausea and vomiting, and period of unconsciousness.
11. Jan. 4, 1922 paralysis of the left half of the face.

OBJECTIVE
1. Tenderness in the right temporal region, just in front of right ear.
2. Bilateral secondary atrophy with a residual choking disc of 1½ D.

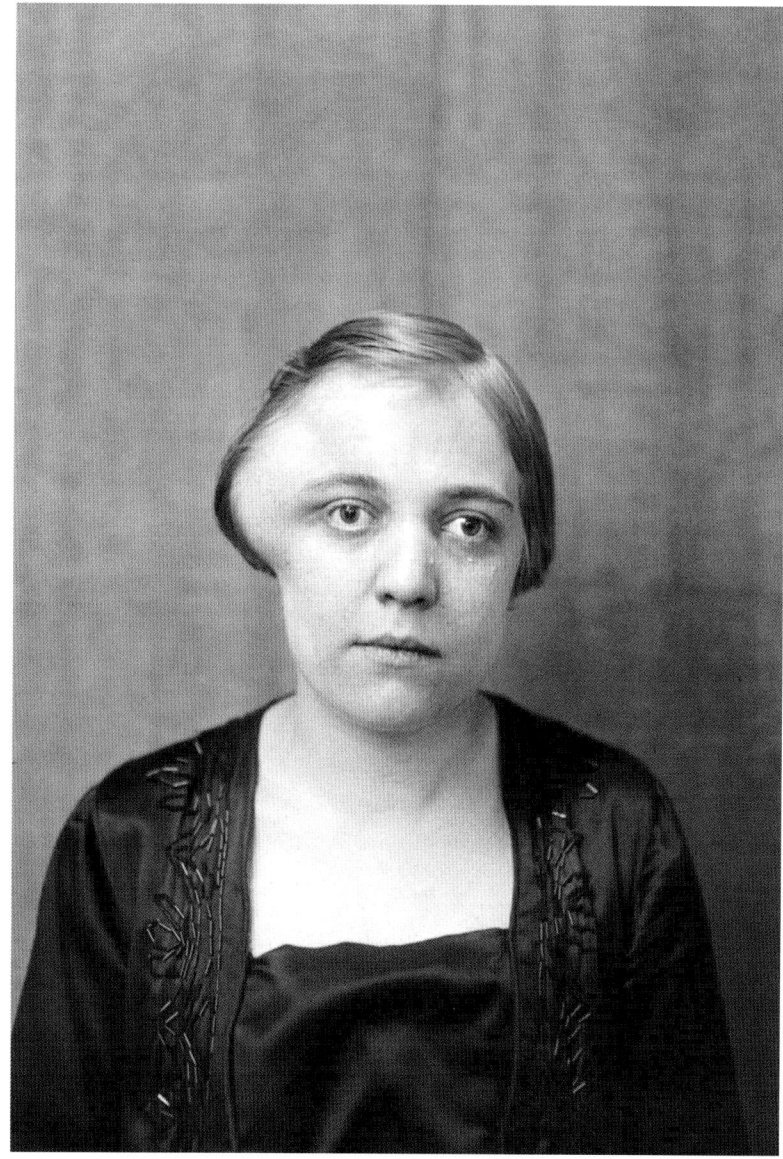

FIG. 2. ONE YEAR AFTER THE FIRST OPERATION (SECOND ADMISSION).

3. Paralysis of the right 3rd nerve.
4. Paralysis of left half of face.
5. Hypesthesia of left half of face and cornea.
6. Absence of sensation of taste and smell.
7. Nystagmus with the eyes directed to right, definite and persistent.
8. Unsteadiness of gait with staggering at the corners.
9. Inability to maintain position with hands extended on the right.

OPPOSITE PAGE. FIG. I. FOUR WEEKS AFTER THE FIRST OPERATION (SUBTEMPORAL DECOMPRESSION).

10. Definite adiadococinesia on the right.
11. Diminished abdominal reflex on the left.
12. Slightly positive Romberg.
13. Slight incoordination brought on by resistance of the hands, bilaterally.
14. Perimetric fields

RADIOLOGY REPORT
January 8, 1922
Dr. Sosman

Stereoscopic films of the skull show marked increased intracranial pressure, with displacement of the sella turcica into the sphenoid sinus, and definite calcification a little superior and anterior to the sella turcica, in a plane which passes through the channel of the middle meningeal arteries. This must be calcification in a tumor which lies in that region.

SPECIAL NOTE
January 9, 1922
Dr. Cushing

This patient entered the hospital Saturday afternoon with a receding choked disc, rapidly advancing to blindness. I did not feel justified in waiting for subsequent thorough studies and it was my intention consequently to do a right decompression today. There was some tenderness on pressure just above the attachment of the pinea so that I felt reasonably sure there was some bone thinning and that I might possibly come down on a temporal lobe tumor. She had also some slight gustatory disturbance of a severe sort. An X-ray taken this morning contrary to expectation showed a shadow deep under the temporofrontal region on the right side, which gave additional evidence of the fact that there was a tumor in this location. It may be said also that she has complete left facial palsy which I thought was peripheral and which can hardly be accounted for by her symptoms or by the operative findings.

OPERATIVE NOTE
January 9, 1922
Anaesthesia – Ether – Miss Gerrard

Right Osteoplastic Exploration with Decompression. Puncture of Ventricle Disclosing Hydrocephalus. Puncture for Tumor Negative.

A larger anterior bone flap was turned down without especial difficulty. The dura was not especially tense and there was marked thinning of the bone which was deeply digitated. Over the temporal region particularly there were many areas of thinning amounting almost to cranial tabes. An immediate subtemporal decompression was made, it being evident that there were many herniated villi through the entire temporal region. There was a good deal of bleeding from along the squamous wing which was fairly deeply removed, so that the decompression was rather frontotemporal including the Sylvian cleft.

The dura was then opened over the temporal lobe and lifted slightly upward, but not over the whole field. There was abundance of subarachnoid fluid but tension was easily reduced to zero. I made as far an exploration under the temporal lobe as I felt justified in making, finding many herniations and marked irregularity of the bone, but no evidence of tumor.

A needle was then inserted into two places, one about the 1st temporal convolution at the point corresponding to the area of greatest bone thinning. The needle apparently met some slight resistance but secured no fluid at 5 cm nor was there any bleeding. A needle was then introduced into the 3rd frontal or at its posterior portion. It also met resistance and there was slight bleeding. I did not, however, feel any calcareous masses.

A 3rd puncture was then made at the upper posterior portion of the field in the superior parietal region, and at a depth of 5 cm punctured the ventricle, and nearly 30 cc of fluid not under tension was removed by pressure.

The dural flap had not been entirely reflected and this did not seem necessary. The two lateral regions were closed with sutures and a subtemporal defect was left open. The flap was then replaced and closed in layers.

(Dr. Cushing)

January 9, 1922
Dr. Wheeler

Patient had a very easy anesthesia, after the difficulty experienced in obtaining relaxation. After operation patient rapidly regained consciousness.

DISCHARGE NOTE
February 3, 1922
Dr. Wheeler

Patient is discharged today. Decompression area is soft and … There is a definite left facial palsy and slight definitive hypoesthesia of the left half of the face. Nystagmus, more course to the right. The gait is still a little unstable. Babinski negative. No adiadococinesia. Patient fields have not changed peceptably.

SECOND HOSPITAL ADMISSION

Patient re-entered the hospital on February 8, 1923 because the bulge at the region of the subtemporal decompression was getting so large that it worried her a great deal.

SUMMARY OF POSITIVE FINDINGS
February 8, 1923
Dr. McKenzie

SUBJECTIVE
1. No diplopia during past year because no vision in right eye.
2. There have been no severe headaches in the past year.
3. Vision patient thinks has remained about the same since her discharge.
4. There has been no improvement in sense of taste or smell since discharge.
5. Divergence of right eye still present.
6. There has been no paralysis of the left half of the face during the past year.

OBJECTIVE
1. There is bilateral secondary atrophy but no elevation.
2. There is no paralysis of the right 3rd nerve.
3. No paralysis of left half of face.
4. No hypoesthesia of left half of face and cornea.
5. Absence of sensation of taste and smell present as before.
6. There is no nystagmus.
7. Unsteadiness of gait due to poor eyesight.
8. There is no adiadococinesia on the right.
9. Abdominal reflexes are equal and the same on both sides.

Head – Right decompression area is bulging, about the size of half an orange somewhat flattened. It is soft and pulsating. There is no complaint of pain in the head except when the patient overexerts the decompression area throbs. There are no areas of tenderness or other abnormal pulsation.

Ventriculograms were made on February 18, 1923.

SPECIAL NOTE
February 26, 1923
Dr. Cushing

We have been puzzled beyond words about this girl. At the last puncture of the ventricle when ventriculograms were made only one thing was definitely made out, namely that the air filled what seemed to be a normal, though dilated right ventricle, none of the air passing into the left ventricle. The natural conclusion was that there was a block at the foramen of Monroe. This made it seem more probable than before that we must be dealing with a mid-line tumor and in view of her enlarged sella turcica and the obscure calcareous shadows it seemed quite possible that there was a large suprasellar cyst, possibly of the nature of that was found in (another patient's name case).

In has been difficult to tell whether this cyst or tumor was in the right or left ventricle. Certainly she has no lateralizing symptoms except for the left facial palsy which led us astray at the time of the first operation. If there is a tumor of the left hemisphere it is extraordinary that she has not had some mental symptoms. She is an extremely well balanced young woman.

In view of the old fronto-temporal flap it was impossible to do a right sided exploration which I would otherwise have favored. This in view of the ultimate findings was fortunate.

OPERATIVE NOTE
February 26, 1923
Anaesthesia – Ether – Miss Gerrard

Left Osteoplastic Frontal Exploration. Puncture of Ventricle. Withdrawing 30 cc Xanthochromic Fluid Containing no Cells and no Cholesterin or Epithelia Elements such as might be found with a Suprasellar Cyst.

After this puncture it was easily possible to elevate the frontal lobe and to get down to the region of the chiasm. However, in this juncture certain difficulties were met with because of the fact that there were many herniations of the brain thru dura making pits in the skull. This was particularly true of the region of the olfactory groove where brain was densely adherent, evidently protruding thru defects in the skull and accounting for her anosmia.

I had some difficulty in opening the dura because of the left sided approach but nevertheless was able to get a good view finally in view of the adhesions of the frontal lobe in the olfactory groove of the ... The chiasm was small. There was no space between the anterior chiasm and the bone - in fact the chiasm lay in its normal position along tuberculum sellae. I felt that possibly there might be a cyst around the sella by projecting underneath the chiasm and I punctured thru the grayish zone in the back of the chiasm but failed to get any additional fluid or evidence of a lesion there.

Being unable to determine what more might be done I filled what I thought was the ventricle with about 15 c.c. of air and closed the wound.

It may be said that during this whole operation a needle had been inserted in the right hemisphere and about 100 cc of slightly turbid fluid was removed.

(Dr. Cushing)

Note – Patient was immediately taken to the X-ray room and the ventriculogram shows fluid in a definite cap apparently anterior to the rounded tumor projecting into or actually lying within the ventricle.

February 27, 1923
Dr. Cushing

In view of these findings it seemed best to do a second puncture if possible to get into the ventricle behind the tumor, if tumor it be. It was thought it would be desirable to do this before the air in the anterior horn of the ventricle was completely absorbed.

OPERATIVE NOTE
February 27, 1923
Anaesthesia – Novocain

Ventricular Puncture.

Patient was brought to the operating room. The old subtemporal decompression had become extremely tense during the night but nevertheless seemed to be in excellent condition. An incision was made over the left parietal region near the mid-line and an exploratory needle was inserted directly toward the ventricle and it met dense resistance into which it was introduced without bleeding and ... that there must be a tumor of the nature of an endothelioma. The needle was withdrawn but inserted again obliquely backward and at a depth of about 5 cm. Struck fluid just as was the case yesterday morning, a little resistance being felt when the needle entered ventricle. This fact was not mentioned in describing the operation yesterday for there was a definite resistance felt in introducing the needle into the ventricle, so much so that I thought I must be getting into a suprasellar cyst.

30 cc of this xanthochromic fluid immediately escaped. The needle was then put into the right ventricle again thru one of the old perforation openings and 80 cc of slightly blood tinged fluid was withdrawn completely collapsing the subtemporal protrusion.

Two syringefuls of air, about 30 c.c. perhaps, were then introduced into what I take to be the posterior horn of the left ventricle.

It may be said that the patient has had no special discomforts and the first time I have known her to complain of discomforts was when the puncture in the ventricle was made with the result of fluid spurting into the wound when she cried out with some discomfort.

(Dr. Cushing)

SPECIAL NOTE
February 27, 1923
Dr. Cushing

A succession of ventriculograms have shown that there must undoubtedly be a tumor occupying the middle of the left ventricle and that the right ventricle and left ventricle do not communicate that the right ventricle contains normal fluid whereas the left contains xanthochromic fluid both anterior and posterior to the tumor which does not completely though it nearly occludes the dilated left ventricle.

Moreover the plates have shown a fairly symmetrical disposition of air injected into the left inferior horn which had made it seem possible that there might after all be a suprasellar cyst though it seemed almost impossible that the left ventricle could be so dilated in such a way as to pass well across the midline and project into the right hemisphere. Consequently at the time of this operation, I was not at all sure but that I was going to find a large supracellar cyst the solid portion of which was represented by the aforementioned tumor. The patient last night had a considerable upset for her decompression has been exceedingly tight during the past 24 hours. She improved, however, after giving some salt per rectum.

OPERATIVE NOTE
February 28, 1923
Anaesthesia: Local

A left anterior bone flap was elevated without difficulty, the dura was incised along the mesial margin of the flap, some little difficulty with the emissary vessels being controlled because of the lowered tension brought about by tapping the right ventricle. A number of emissary vessels between the margin of the frontal lobe and the longitudinal sinus were divided between clips and it was possible to explore the falx well back to the mid-portion of the head. A large calcareous black zone in all of the antero-posterior x-rays was disclosed but aside from this the falx appeared to be normal and I hesitated to divide the corpus callosum fearing a complete apraxia. Accordingly an incision was made through perhaps the second frontal convolution and carried down to a depth of 2 cm or more where the ventricle was opened, a puff of air escaped the moment this occurred. After the fluid was removed I could see a tumor mass which owing to the dislocation I thought at first must be a tumor mass projecting upward from the pituitary region but which proved to be a mass evidently arising from the outer and lower wall of the greatly dilated ventricle. Just why the foramen of Monroe is occluded I cannot conjecture. Bulging up into the lower part of the ventricle was a thin, bladder like area which I took at one time to be a cyst and on opening it a large sac of fluid was secured. This may possibly have been the protrusion from the other ventricle but the orientation was a little obscure and I cannot be certain of this.

As the enucleation proceeded and the ventricles became completely collapsed the growth settled away toward the posterior part of the dilated ventricle and it was difficult to make sure that I had by any means completed the enucleation.

If the cerebrospinal circulation conditions are readjusted in such a way that the ventricles will not immediately refill it would be a miracle. I saw no evidence of the foramen of Monroe and it is just possible that the draining of the collection of fluid mentioned earlier in this note may in some way allowed fluid to find a new outlet.

After fairly complete blood stilling the flap was replaced and closed in layers without a drain. The patient stood the operation extremely well.

(Dr. Cushing)

PATHOLOGY REPORT
February 28, 1923

Gross description: Specimen was removed from the floor of the anterior part of the left ventricle. Exposure was made by transection of the frontal lobe. I did not get a sufficiently good look at the tumor to get any description of it in the gross.

(Dr. Cushing)

Microscopic report: There are sections, of which three are stained with methylene blue and three with phosphotungatic acid hematoxylin. They disclose a fairly cellular tumor composed of cells having a nucleus about the size of a lymphoid cell and containing a delicate network of chromatin. At times the cells are larger than a lymphoid cell and appear to have a small areas of hemorrhage intermingled with the tumor cells. Small blood vessels are fairly numerous throughout the tumor. In places the tumor cells are arranged in bands which interlace somewhat. The intercellular substance is moderate in amount and consists of delicate fibrillary processes which for the most part stain blue with phosphotungatic acid hematoxylin. Mitotic figures are infrequent.

DIAGNOSIS – Glioma

Resident pathologist (signed)

March 2, 1923
Dr. McKenzie

6 days after operation. No aphasia despite the fact that left parietal lobe was transected.

Multiple ventricular taps were necessary to relieve the tense swelling over the decompression flap.

March 6, 1923
Dr. McKenzie

Stitches out. Definite aphasia, but quite understandable. Slight CSF leak at edge of flap which is moderately riding.

March 8, 1923
Dr. McKenzie

Yesterday because of slight CSF leak along operative incision and riding of flap, Dr. Cushing punctured area of decompression. 145 cc yellow fluid removed and collodin dressing applied over flap. There has been no leak today.

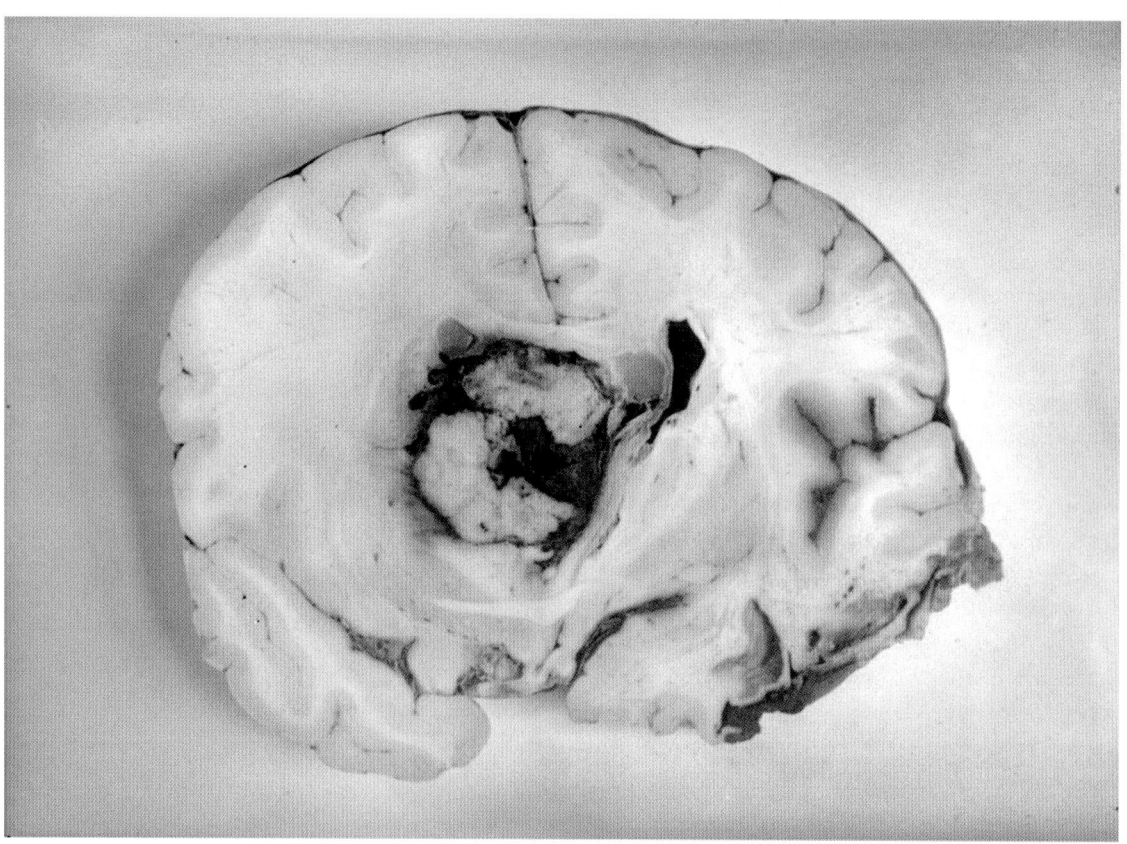

FIG. 3. CORONAL SECTION OF THE AUTOPSY BRAIN SPECIMEN.

DISCHARGE NOTE
March 10, 1923
Dr. McKenzie

In a stupor all day yesterday, ventricular puncture failed to cure her. Patient last night had a general convulsion and died.

AUTOPSY REPORT
March 10, 1923
Dr. Bailey

DIAGNOSIS – Glioma

Patient is a white girl twenty-three years of age on whom several operations had been done in an attempt to get a tumor of the third ventricle. A right subtemporal decompression had been done two years ago and decompression area is bulging markedly. The decompression is very tense. There is also a scar of a recent ventricular puncture of the right parietal region, and of a still more recent transfrontal operation in the left frontal region. A lumbar puncture needle was inserted in both ventricles through old burr holes and 20% formalin injected into each. The brain was given fifteen minutes for the formalin to act, there not being time to wait longer.

Brain was then removed with considerable difficulty because of the adhesion to the dura and the old operative incision on the right side. It was finally removed, however, fairly intact and no abnormalities were noted on the surface except a marked protrusion of the right temporal lobe in the area of the old decompression. The third ventricle was widely dilated, extending downward into the sella in the form of a sea about 7–3 mm in length and depth, 1 cm antero-posteriorly. The pituitary gland was markedly flattened and was removed for histological study. The brain was then immersed in formalin and will be sectioned later.

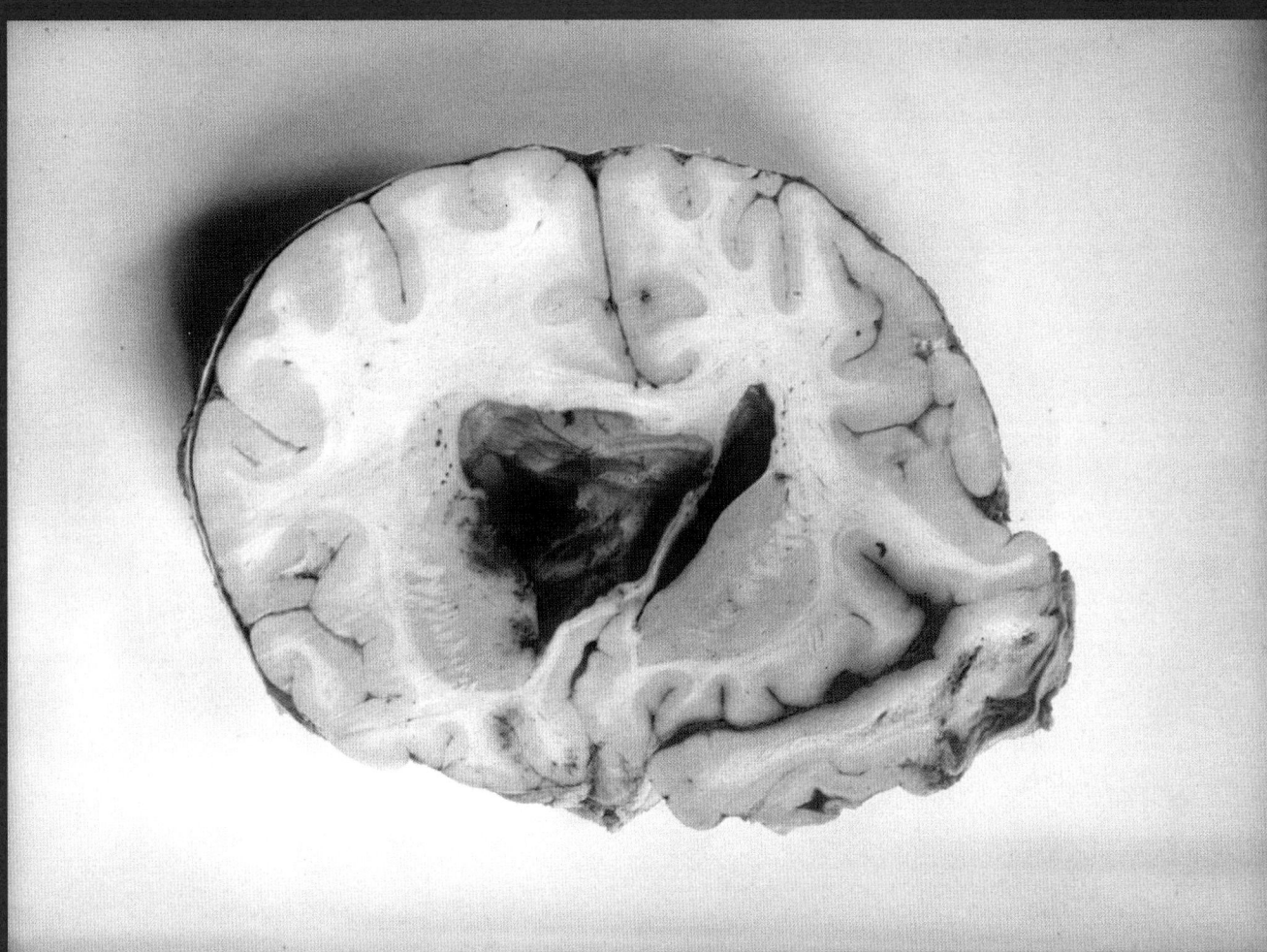

FIGS. 4–5. CORONAL SECTIONS OF THE AUTOPSY BRAIN SPECIMEN.

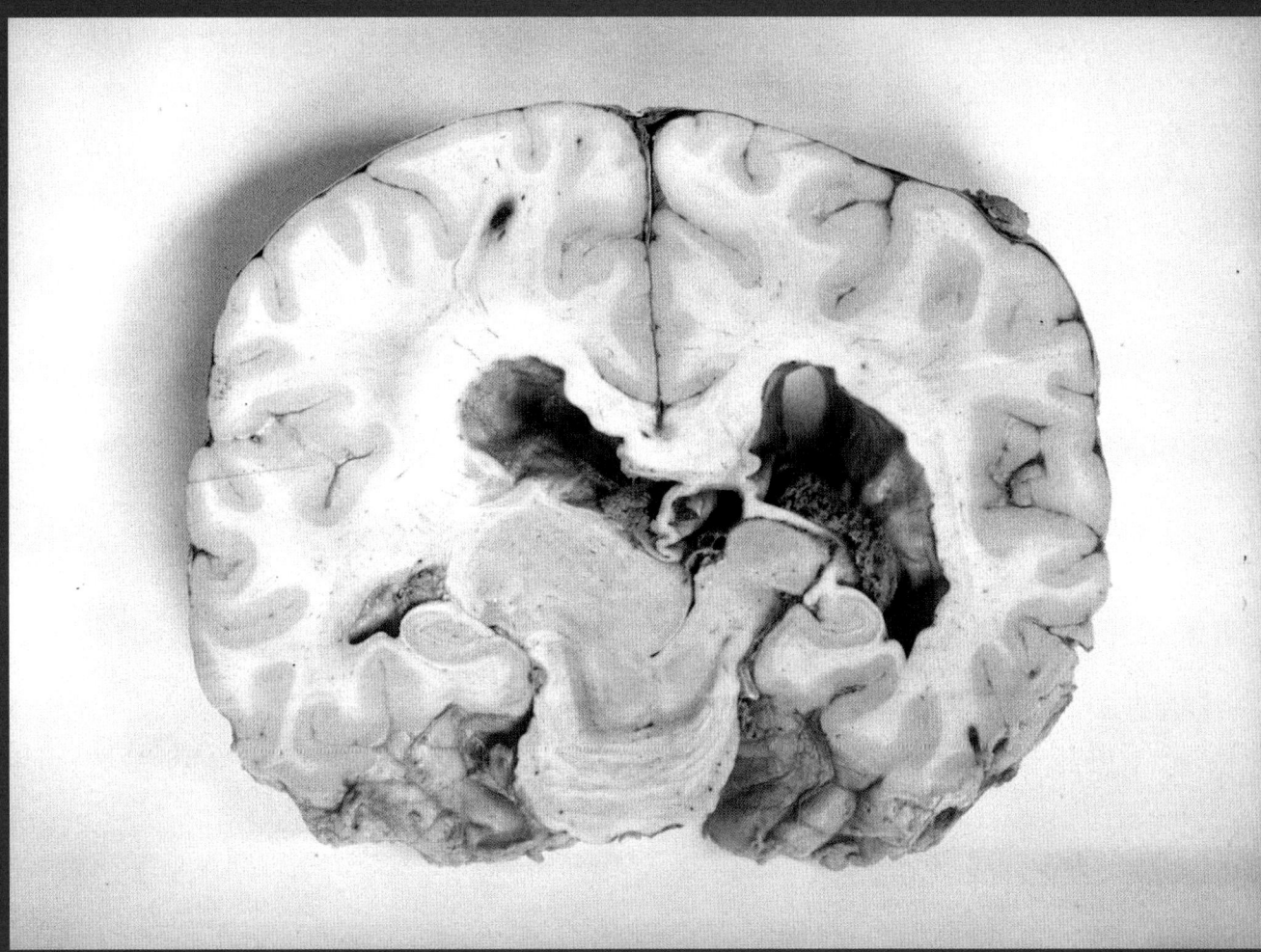

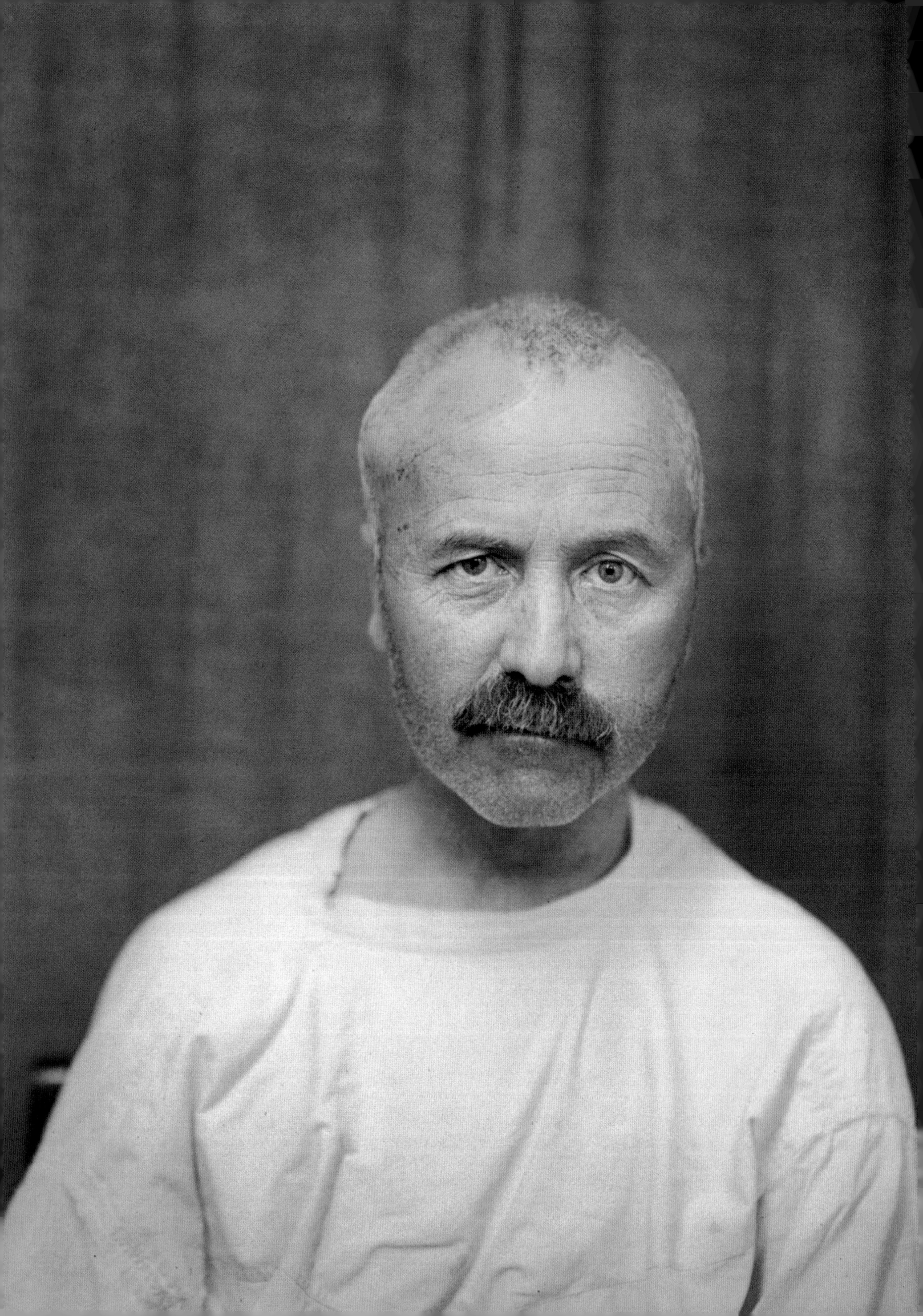

2.4 Glioma of the lateral ventricle

SEX: M; AGE: 48; SURG. NO. 17716

HISTORY

The patient presented with very obvious progressive cognitive failure.

SUMMARY OF POSITIVE FINDINGS
November 9, 1922
Dr. Bailey

SUBJECTIVE
1. Headache and vomiting.

OBJECTIVE
1. Paresis of the left facial nerve, possibly of central origin.
2. Bilateral choked disc more advanced on the right side.
3. Marked mental disturbance with loss of memory and disorientation.
4. Slight suboccipital tenderness to pressure and tenderness to percussion over the left frontal region. These, however, are not marked and not much emphasis should be placed upon them.

IMPRESSION: Glioma of the right frontal lobe.

RADIOLOGY REPORT
Dr. Sosman

There are no localizing signs of tumor.

OPERATIVE NOTE
November 13, 1922
Anesthesia – Ether – Miss Gerrard

Exploration for Right Frontal Tumor Disclosing a Large Glioma in the Region of the Right Operculum.

This man's head was shaved. There was a fairly definite prominence of the skull in the midline just anterior to the coronal suture more pronounced on the right side than the left, and I felt that there was a very great possibility that we would find an endothelioma in this region. A rescrutiny of the x-ray plates showed a very suspicious area of the bone at this point. I consequently was inclined to favor a parasagittal meningioma for a preoperative diagnosis.

A large bone flap was turned down so as to make it possible not only to expose this particular region but also to disclose the temporal lobe. There was a special difficulty in the elevation of the flap, the dura was vascular necessitating the placement of some muscle stamps. An immediate subtemporal decompression was made and an opening made over the temporal lobe. The lobe did not seem particularly tense and was so soft that I thought this was in all likelihood going to be temporal lobe cyst but on incising the dura upward and reflecting it I came down upon a soft, spreading glioma which must have been about 5 cm in diameter on the surface and which was situated just above and anterior to the Sylvian fissure. This growth was so soft that I thought it would probably be underlain by a cyst

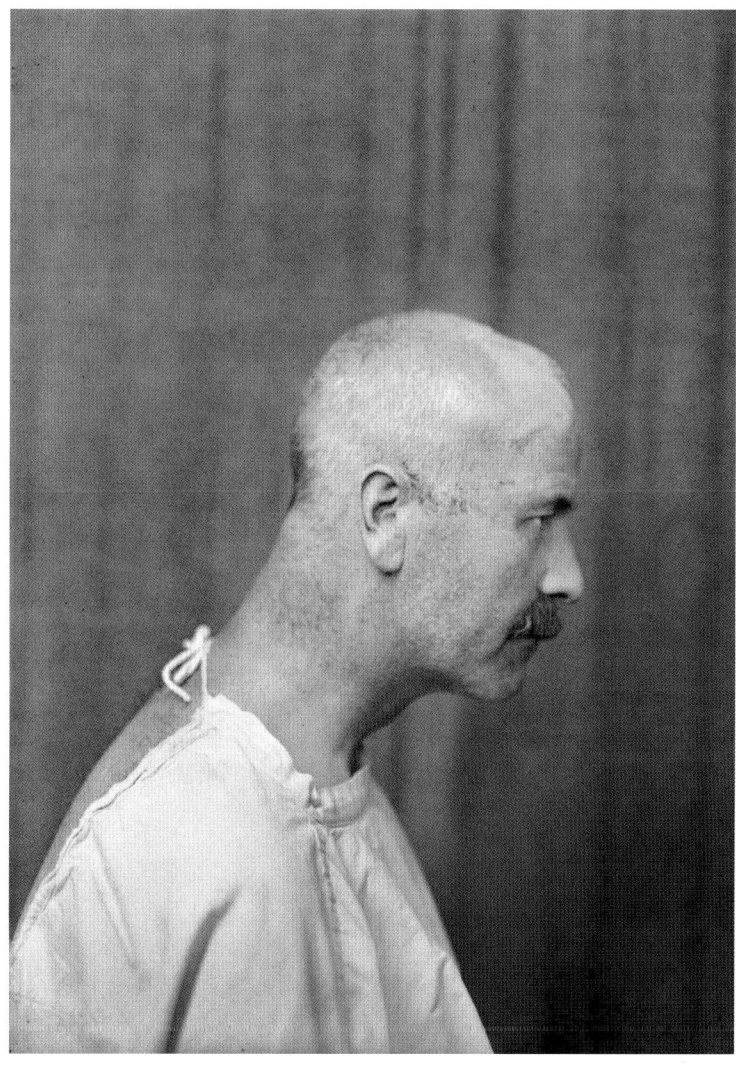

FIG. 2. TWO WEEKS POSTOPERATIVE.

OPPOSITE PAGE. FIG. I. TWO WEEKS POSTOPERATIVE.

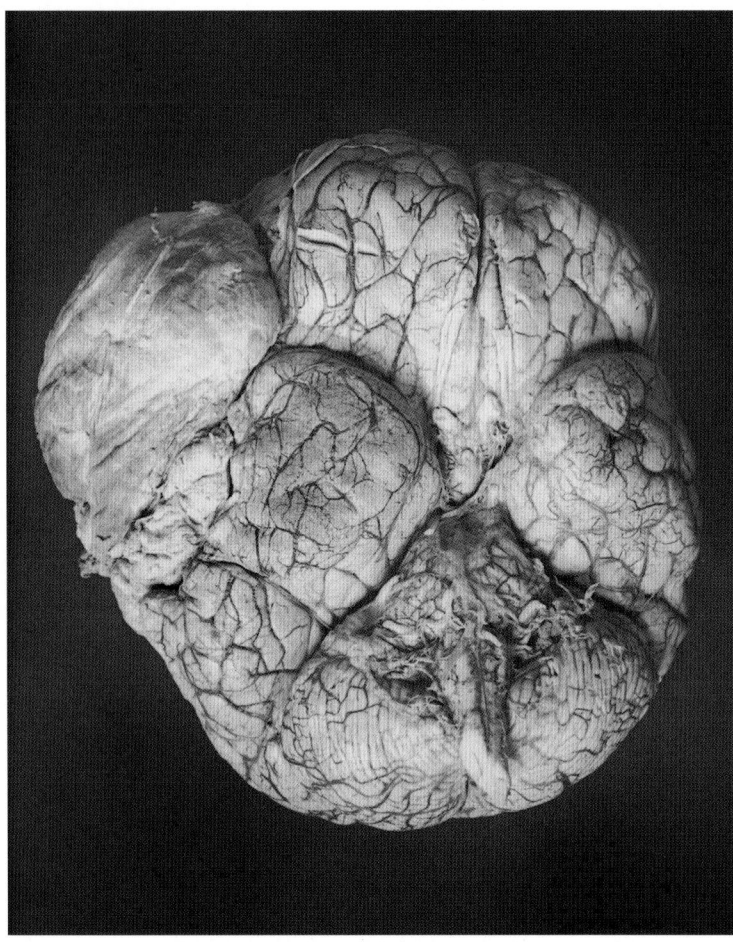

FIG. 3. AUTOPSY SPECIMEN.

and as the posterior margin of the growth had a perfectly clear and distinct edge I separated the brain from the tumor in this region down to a depth of about 2 cm without encountering fluid. Then 2-3 subsequent punctures showed that there was actually no underlying cyst – at least none was struck by the punctures.

It seemed best in view of these findings to strip off the bone entirely. The dura was resutured all but the subtemporal defect. The scalp alone was then replaced over the wound, the closure being largely done by Dr. Bailey.

(Dr. Cushing)

PATHOLOGY REPORT
November 13, 1922

Microscopic report: The sections show a tumor composed of rather large cells and very little intercellular fibrillary substance. The cells have a round or vesicular nucleus containing a network of chromatin and nucleolus. There is considerable edema as evidenced by the deposition of a finely granular acid staining substance throughout the brain tissue. Areas of necrosis and hemorrhage are also seen. Giant cells are found scattered throughout the sections. The intercellular substance is very meager in amount.

DIAGNOSIS – Glioma.

(Dr. Hassermann)

December 1, 1922
Dr. Sosman

Patient was given first X-ray treatment on this site.

DISCHARGE NOTE
December 3, 1922
Dr. McKenzie

Soft bulging (half a lemon) through sub-temporal defect. Mentally somewhat improved. Patient non-cooperative, apparently no appreciation of his condition, speaks of going back to work. Patient does not appreciate that he is totally disabled, is definitely better than before operation though. No apparent sensory disturbance. Definite muscular weakness of whole body.

FOLLOW-UP NOTE
January 29, 1923
Dr. Horrax

Patient reports for x-ray treatment. Feels quite well in general and answers questions intelligently, though still tendency to irrelevant talking. Left hand and leg still weaker than right but have fair strength.

There is an extremely marked bulging at the site of his right subtemporal decompression but although the bone flap was removed, the dura, is holding above the decompression as well as bone would hold.

Fundus O.U. Blurred margins, about 1 D elevation.

Patient died at home on May 9, 1923. Dr. Percival Bailey performed the autopsy at the patient's home.

AUTOPSY REPORT
May 9, 1923
Dr. Bailey

DIAGNOSES – Glioma

Autopsy done at home of patient and confined to head. There was a huge hernia cerebri in the right fronto-temporal region where the bone flap had been left off after an exploratory operation. It was interesting to remark that there was no herniation of the upper part of the defect where the dura had been sewn together again, although there was no bone over the dura.

An incision was made as usual, running behind the hernia, and the hernia was carefully separated off and the flaps separated, turned off and back. The skull cap was removed with difficulty, being adherent all around the edge of the hernia. The brain was removed as usual with the membranes attached and without any particular difficulty. The brain was very soft and sagged badly out of shape. It was immersed in formalin for further study.

Brain after fixation in formalin was cut in serial coronal sections, an enormous brain distorted by the presence of a huge tumor in the right frontal lobe. Bone flap had been removed at a previous operation, allowing an enormous growth to recur on the surface of the dura.

The first coronal section about 2 cm behind the tip of the frontal lobe shows a nodule of tumor about 2 cm in width x 3 cm long just under the dural surface.

The second section 2 cm back of this shows a tumor invading the greater portion of the left frontal lobe which is much enlarged, pushing the median septum far over to the right. Extending from the center of the tumor may be seen the dura which closed at the operation, leaving only a subtemporal decompression. The tumor has, therefore, grown out and through the decompression defect and then spread underneath the galea aponorodica into the frontal region.

Another section 2 cm further back shows an enormous solid mass about 8 x 5 cm, filling most of the left frontal lobe and pushing the median septum far over to the right.

The third section, 2 cm further back shows the same picture, except that the tumor has here invaded the basal nuclei on the left side and projects into the right lateral ventricle but has not broken through the ependymal surface.

Further sections show a similar picture extending as far back as the anterior surface of the pons. It is evident that the tumor does not extend much farther posterior than this section.

Microscopic examination: Six sections – Three E&B stain – three PTAH. These sections were taken

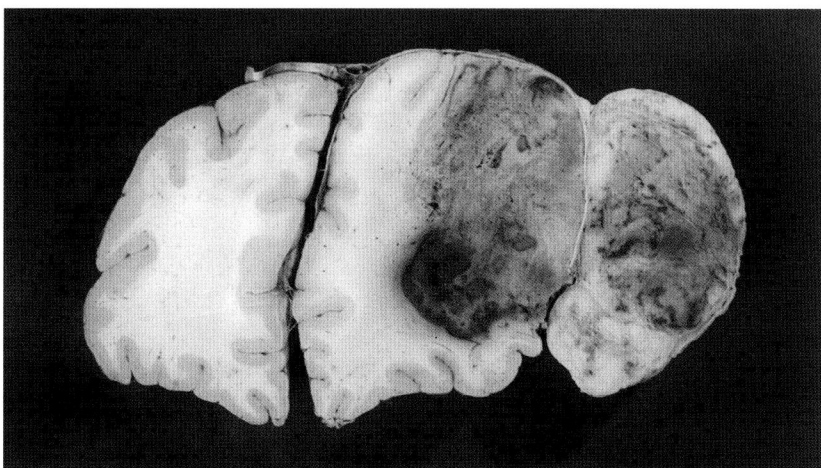

FIGS. 4–5. CORONAL SECTIONS OF AUTOPSY BRAIN SPECIMEN.

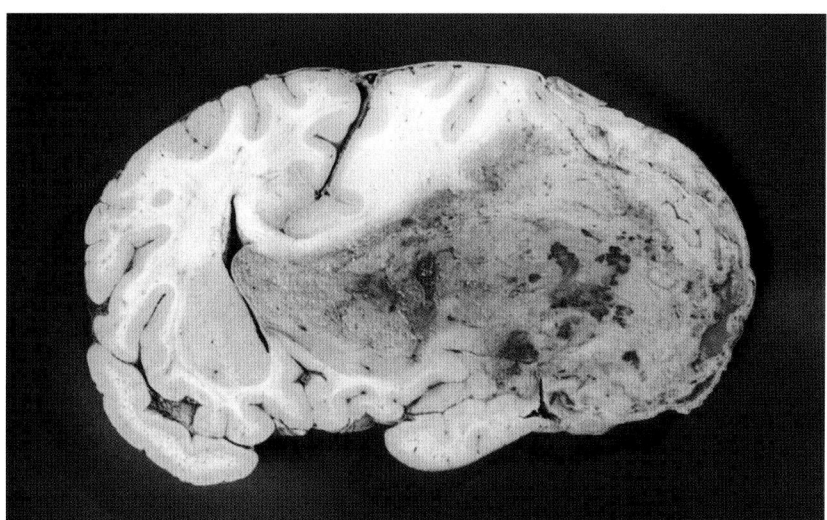

from the periphery of the tumor. They consist partly of the necrotic central mass of the tumor and partly of surrounding brain tissue with a narrow margin of tumor tissue between the two.

In this middle zone, which is really the edge of the tumor, the tissue is composed of a structureless mass of shapeless cells with rounded and irregular nuclei which vary considerably in size and shape, and chromatin content. Between them only a very few delicate glial fibrils are evident. In the edge of the tumor and the adjoining brain tissue, certain areas show a marked inflammatory reaction. There is a diffuse reaction in areas with polynuclears predominating, whereas in other regions the reaction seems to be confined largely to the neighborhood of small blood vessels. In the latter areas, the picture may be described as a perivascular lymphoid and plasma cell reaction.

(Dr. Wolbach)

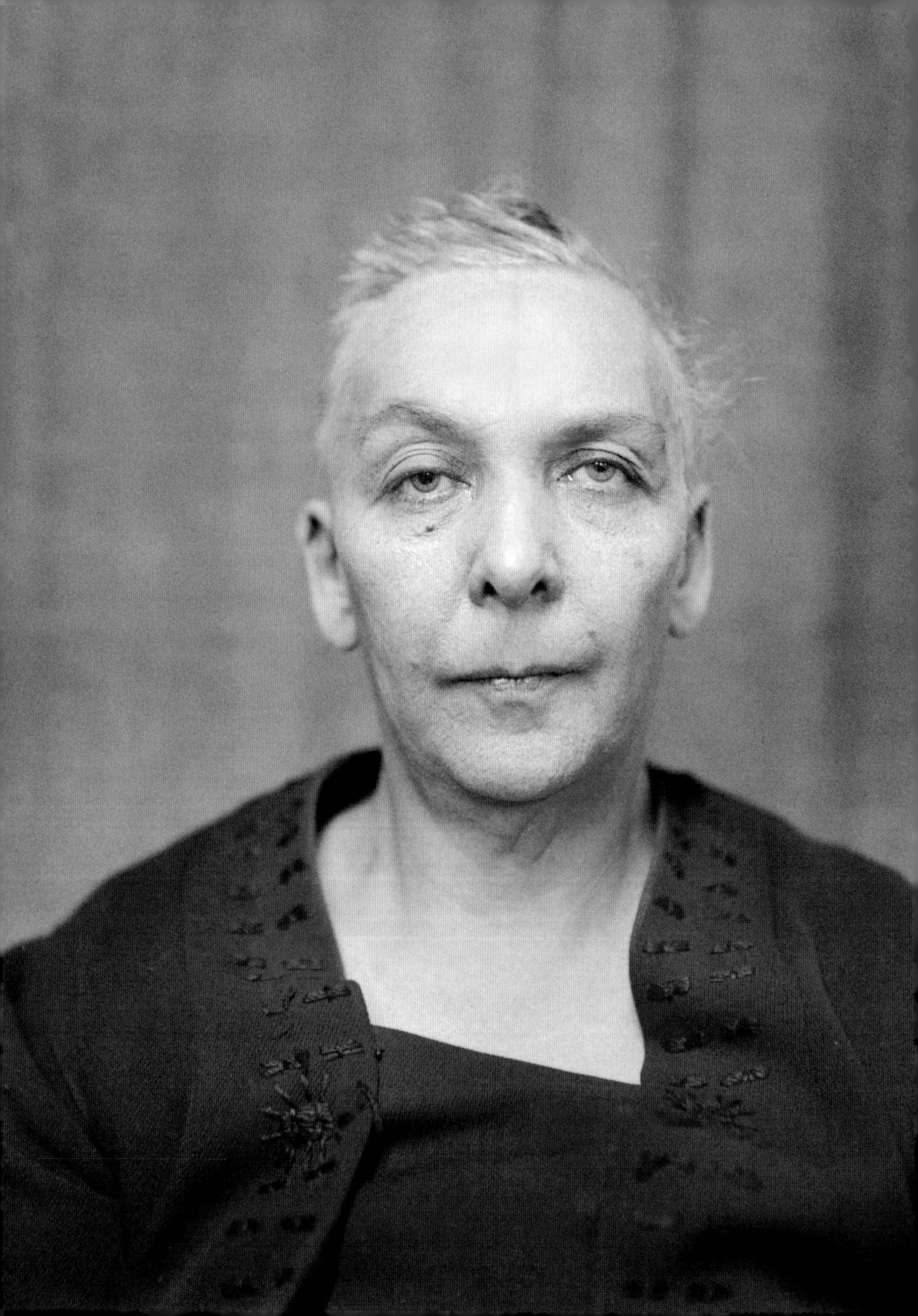

2.5 Adenocarcinoma of skull base

SEX: F; AGE: 51; SURG. NO. 17336; 17871; 18024; 18152; 18479; 18720

DIAGNOSES

Surg. No 17336 – Pituitary group, hyperpituitarism? Without acromegaly – adenoma, unverified.

Surg. No 17871 – Brain tumor, unverified. Trigeminal sheath.

Surg. No 18024 – Pituitary adenoma, unverified. Tumor of right trigeminal sheath?

Surg. No 18152 – Brain tumor, unverified. Hypophysial? Trigeminal sheath tumor, endothelioma?

Surg. No 18479 – Cerebral tumor, unverified. Trigeminal sheath.

Surg. No 18720 – Intracranial tumor, verified. Pituitary group, adenocarcinoma, verified.

COMPLAINT

Headaches and double vision.

SUMMARY OF POSITIVE FINDINGS

September 11, 1922
Dr. Martin

SUBJECTIVE

1. History of fatigue and suboccipital headaches since Jan. 1922.
2. History of diplopia coming on suddenly in June 19th. Bilateral 6th.
3. History of headaches in back of her eyes since June 1922.
4. History of difficulty in speech three months ago, lasting only a week or two. Dysarthria?
5. History of dizziness for the past two weeks.

OBJECTIVE

1. Slight pallor of both discs.
2. Right pupil larger than left.
3. Paralysis of convergence, paralysis of left and right abducens.
4. Ptosis on right.
5. Marked obesity.
6. Blood pressure 180/80.
7. Metabolism +18.
8. X-ray shows sellar absorption.

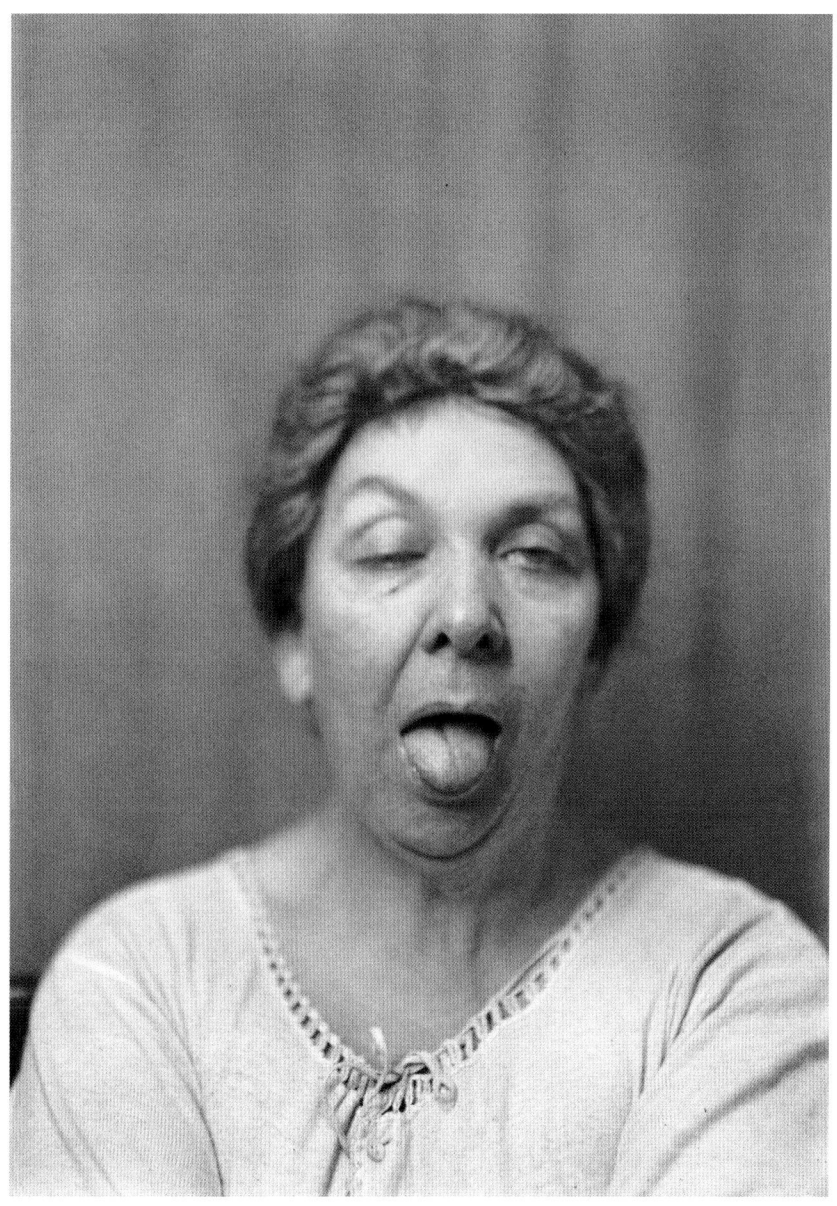

FIG. 2. TWO WEEKS POSTOPERATIVE.

RADIOLOGY REPORT

September 12, 1922
Dr. Sosman

The anterior clinoids are shown but the posterior clinoids cannot be made out. The floor of the sella does not appear depressed or destroyed. The irregularity appears to be in the region of the dorsum sellae but it is not definite due to the overlapping of the mastoids.

OPPOSITE PAGE. FIG. 1. THREE MONTHS POSTOPERATIVE.

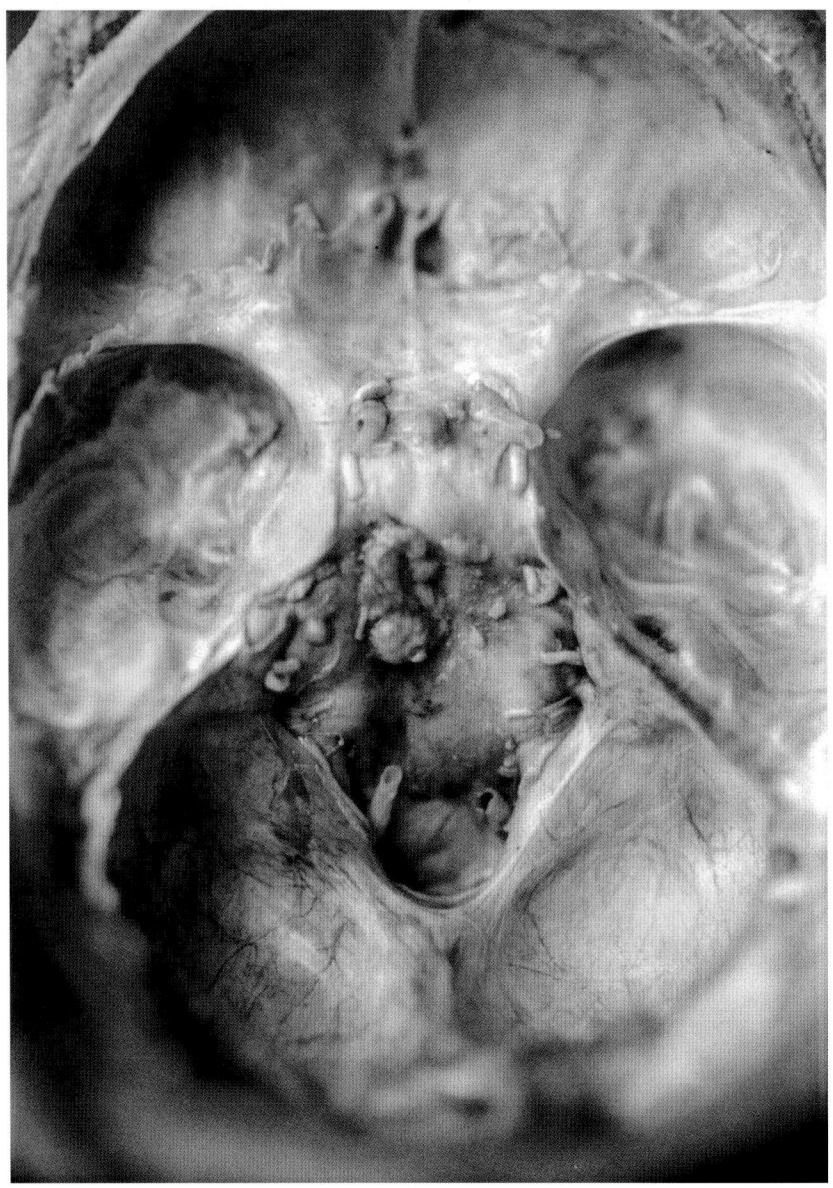

FIG. 3. AUTOPSY SPECIMEN.

SPECIAL NOTE
September 16, 1922
Dr. Cushing

This case was undertaken largely on the basis of the sellar changes. The X-rays show the unusual deformation. It was difficult for us to see how any growth in this situation could have picked out both 6th nerves without visual changes as well. To be sure, the 3rd nerve on right has also been somewhat impaired. Without the deformation shown by the X-ray we would have thought that it was probably some vascular pontine lesion.

OPERATIVE NOTE
September 16, 1922
Anaesthesia – Ether – Miss Gerrard

Frontal Osteoplastic Resection with Exploration of Sellar region.

There was no difficulty in reflection of this flap though the procedure was somewhat more "wet" than usual. The dura was a little frayed and adherent though not torn in the procedure. On reflection of the frontal lobe which could be easily done without puncturing the ventricle, and on incising the dura along the sphenoidal ridge a fairly good exposure of the chiasm was obtained. As there was no evidence of tumor this exposure was not pressed to the extent of bringing the entire chiasm into view and to such an extent that the olfactory nerve would be pulled out.

The arachnoid was greatly thickened, particularly apparent at the side of the chiasm extending up into the Sylvian fissure as a grayish membrane. It contained a very large amount of fluid and it is possible that the whole picture may be one of a chronic arachnoiditis though it is difficult to see how this could have implicated bilaterally the 6th nerves. On tearing away and opening up the arachnoid spaces to the right side of the chiasm, instead of exposing the carotid artery there was a yellowish hard projection from the side of the sella which I could not exactly identify. It is my impression that it was merely a part of a deformed sella which may indeed be a congenital deformation. The flap was replaced and closed in layers with a single protective drain.

(Dr. Cushing)

DISCHARGE NOTE
October 6, 1922
Dr. Martin

Patient had has bilateral X-ray exposure before discharge. She feels fine.

Left abducens palsy subsided. Right abducens unchanged.

SECOND HOSPITAL ADMISSION
December 7, 1922
Dr. McKenzie

Patient has returned for X-ray treatment and metabolism. Neurological examination at this time shows changes in the extra-ocular muscles of the eye and the right trigeminal nerve.

Trigeminus – There is no evidence of motor paralysis but there is definite sensory disturbances in the right trigeminal.

No evidence of cerebellar or cerebral disturbances.

Metabolism – Period I +4; Period II +8; Average +6.

RADIOLOGY REPORT
December 7, 1922
Dr. Sosman

A re-examination of the skull shows a bone flap in the right frontal region. Findings otherwise are as previously reported and appear characteristic of a pituitary tumor. A comparison of the present films with the previous films shows a distinct increase in the amount of destruction.

DISCHARGE NOTE
December 7, 1922

Patient was discharged in a good condition after X-ray treatment.

THIRD HOSPITAL ADMISSION

Patient return in hospital for a third X-ray treatment.

Admitted January 3, 1923; Discharged January 4, 1923.

At this time she developed "uncinate seizures." She felt that sensation over her right face had improved and this was not bothering her much.

FOURTH HOSPITAL ADMISSION

Patient return in hospital for radiotherapy.

Admitted January 24, 1923; Discharged January 25, 1923.

January 24, 1923
Dr. McKenzie

There has been a little change since note made 3 weeks ago, patient has returned for X-ray treatment. She feels that she is getting better. For now had 4 treatments (X-rays). There is little numbness in right face now. Eyes remain the same.

DISCHARGE NOTE
January 25, 1923

Patient was discharged after receiving X-ray treatment. Condition is stable.

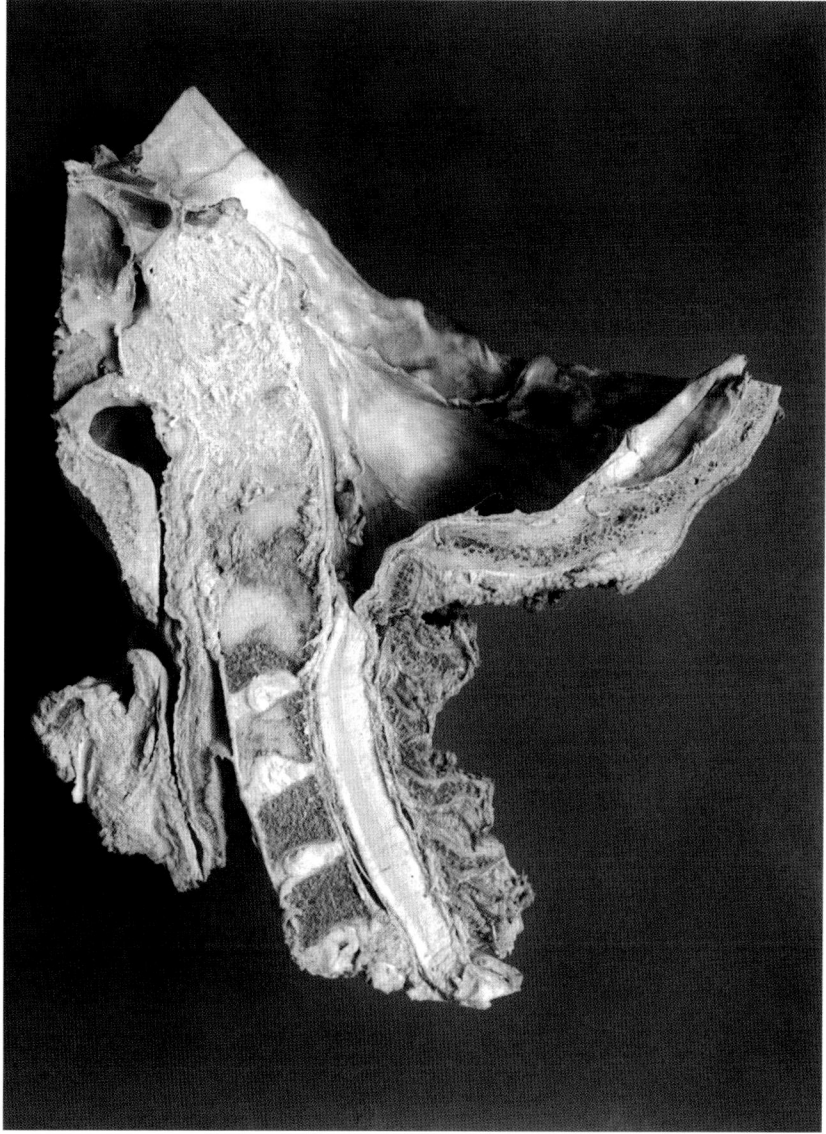

FIG. 4. AUTOPSY SPECIMEN.

FOLLOW UP LETTER TO DR. CUSHING
March 15, 1923

Dear Sir:

My sister (name of patient) does not seem to be improving steadily. She has had a few good days, but is bothered with numbness in her face and great pain in back of her neck. She has also had pain in her back but that has improved.

We did nothing for relief except rubbing back and neck and using laxatives. Awaiting an early reply as to what course to follow, I am

Sincerely,
(signed) SM

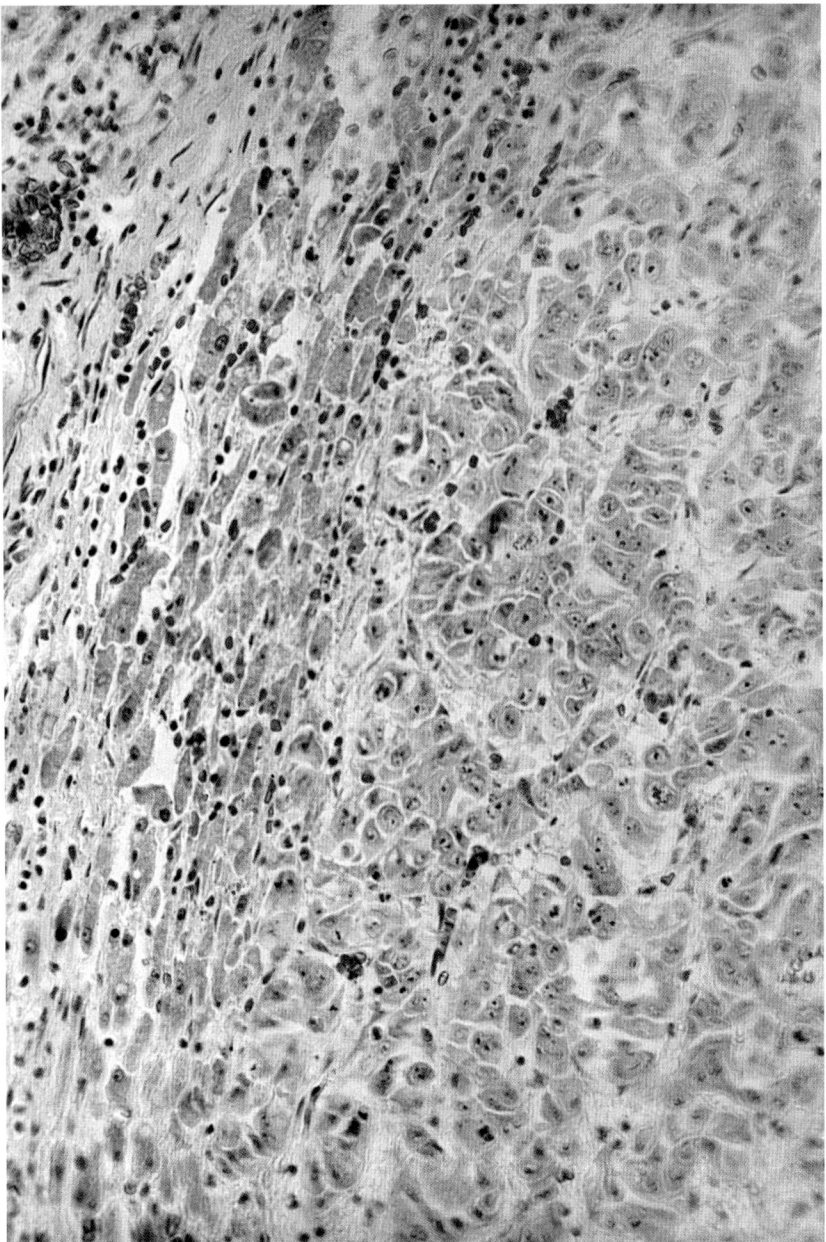

FIG. 5. HISTOLOGY SLIDE.

FIFTH HOSPITAL ADMISSION
March 24, 1923
Dr. McKenzie

There have been no further uncinate seizures for about 2 months. However, the stiffness and pain in the back of the neck is bothering the patient considerably and also feels that her right face has gotten much more numb in the last few weeks, and this is worrying her a good deal.

Complete neurological examination shows:

1st – Complete loss of smell in the right nostril. Test odors readily recognized on the left side (completely normal when first examined 6 months ago).

2nd – Discs are somewhat pale. Margins are sharply outlined. However, the veins in the left fundus are definitely full and tortuous. There is no defect in the visual field.

3rd, 4th, and 6th show definite changes.

5th – Patient complains of numbness over the 2nd and 3rd division with occasional burning over the 2nd division. Corneal reflex is definitely slower on the right and the jaw deviates very slightly to the right. The right masseter muscle does not contract as strongly as the left.

7th – There is no history of twitching of the face and there is no objective facial expressional weakness.

8th – Hearing for watch normal on each ear.

Remaining cranial nerves are quite negative except for some slight deviation of the tongue to the right. This I think is due to the loss of sensation in the right cheek.

RADIOLOGY REPORT
March 29, 1923
Dr. Sosman

Films of the skull show definite destruction of the sella turcica. The floor of the middle fossa on the right is intact as far as seen. Findings suggest a pituitary tumor.

DISCHARGE NOTE
March 31, 1923
Dr. McKenzie

Has had X-ray treatment. Metabolism: -3, 0, -1.

SIXTH HOSPITAL ADMISSION

HISTORY

Shortly after last discharge from hospital, patient commenced having difficulty in swallowing and speaking that has persisted and gradually grown worse until the present time.

April 28, 1923
Dr. McKenzie

IMPRESSION – Spreading tumor which involves the 3rd, 4th, 5th and 6th, 9th and 10th on right side and spreading over the other side. It is involving the 12th, 9th and 10th.

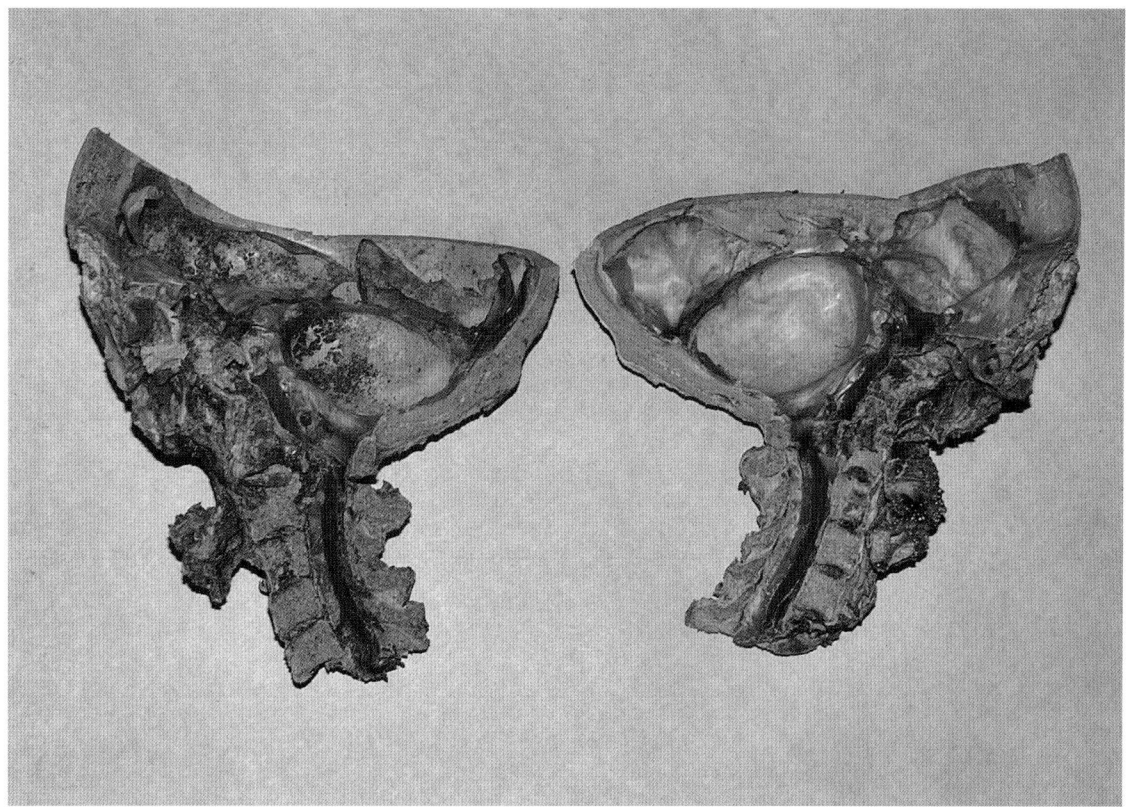

FIG. 6. AUTOPSY SPECIMENS CURRENTLY HOUSED AT THE CUSHING TUMOR REGISTRY.

HOSPITAL COURSE

Progressive involvement of cranial nerves.

May 22, 1923
Dr. Bailey

Choking of both discs, exophthalmos, right eye. Left pupil reacts to light, right does not. Corneal reflex absent on both sides. Peripheral facial palsy on left.

May 24, 1923
Dr. McKenzie

Patient died.

AUTOPSY REPORT

May 25, 1923
Dr. Bailey

DIAGNOSIS: Carcinoma of the base of the skull with extension into the spinal canal and metastasis to the liver and pyloric lymph nodes.

Bronchopneumonia.

Post mortem examination revealed an extradural tumor apparently with its center in the sella turcica, involving the basillary process of the sphenoidal bone and extending into the submucosal tissue of the nasal pharynx and deeper between the upper cervical vertebra and the dura in the anterior part of the spinal canal involving the bodies of the axis and third cervical vertebra. The spinal canal at the level of the tumor somewhat compressed antero-posteriorly. All nerves could be identified but were obviously involved in tumor. It was rather firm to palpation.

Microscopically, the tumor is an adenocarcinoma, the origin of which is obscure, but possibly from Rathke's pouch. Similar tumor masses are found in lymph nodes and left lobe of the liver.

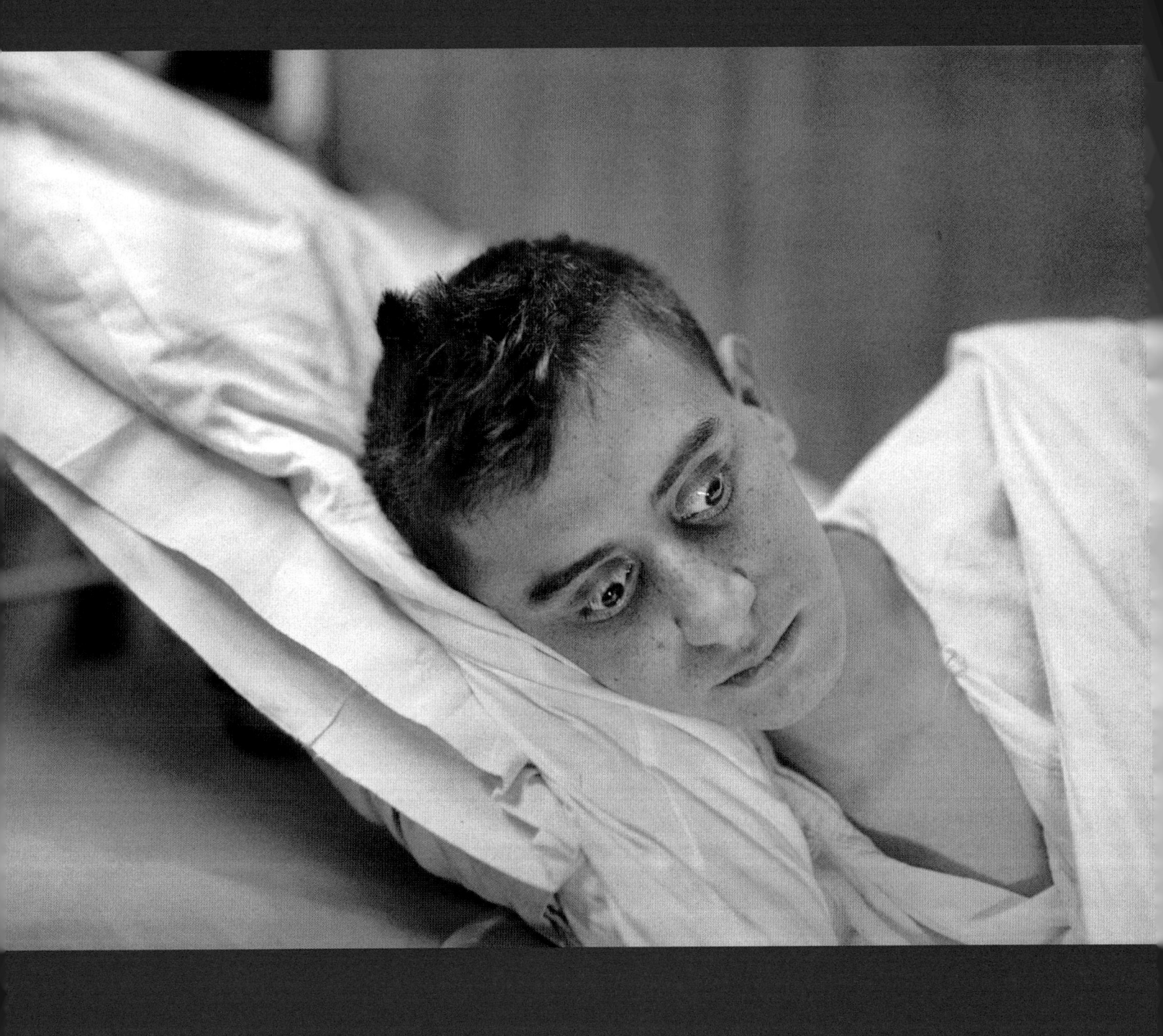

2.6 Pineal region tumor

SEX: M; AGE: 20; SURG. NO. 19214

HISTORY

The patient had a recent history of headaches, decreased visual acuity, nausea, and vomiting. He was diagnosed with diabetes insipidus and was given pituitrin at the Mount Sinai Hospital nine months ago. During the past two weeks, he has been very weak, confined to bed, totally blind, and has had continued headaches. An operation had been advised about nine months ago by his physician in N.Y. but the patient refused such treatment until the present time. His complete loss of vision, severe headaches, and weakness caused his family to bring him to this clinic to see if any relief could be afforded.

MEDICINE SERVICE
July 11, 1923
Dr. Boyd

IMPRESSION: The diagnosis of this case is not clear. It is my opinion that it lies between a tumor of the 3rd ventricle or a neoplasm in the pituitary region. Pulmonary tuberculosis?

July 12, 1923
Dr. Boyd

The physical signs in right chest seemed to indicate fluid at the base and tap for diagnosis was done under Novocain anaesthesia. A few drops of bloody fluid were obtained, dry tap, cultures and stains of this few drops. Blood negative.

RADIOLOGY REPORT
July 13, 1923
Dr. Sosman

Stereoscopic films of the skull show a cranial vault of average thickness with definite convolutional atrophy, suggesting increased intracranial pressure. The sella turcica is smooth in outline and not enlarged. The floor is depressed slightly and the posterior clinoids are quite sharp, suggesting erosion. Findings suggest a pituitary tumor with increased intracranial pressure.

Chest – diffuse clouding of the entire right side, most marked in the middle third toward the axilla where there is a triangular area of increased density with its base against the pleura. This suggests encapsulated interlobar collection of fluid or pus.

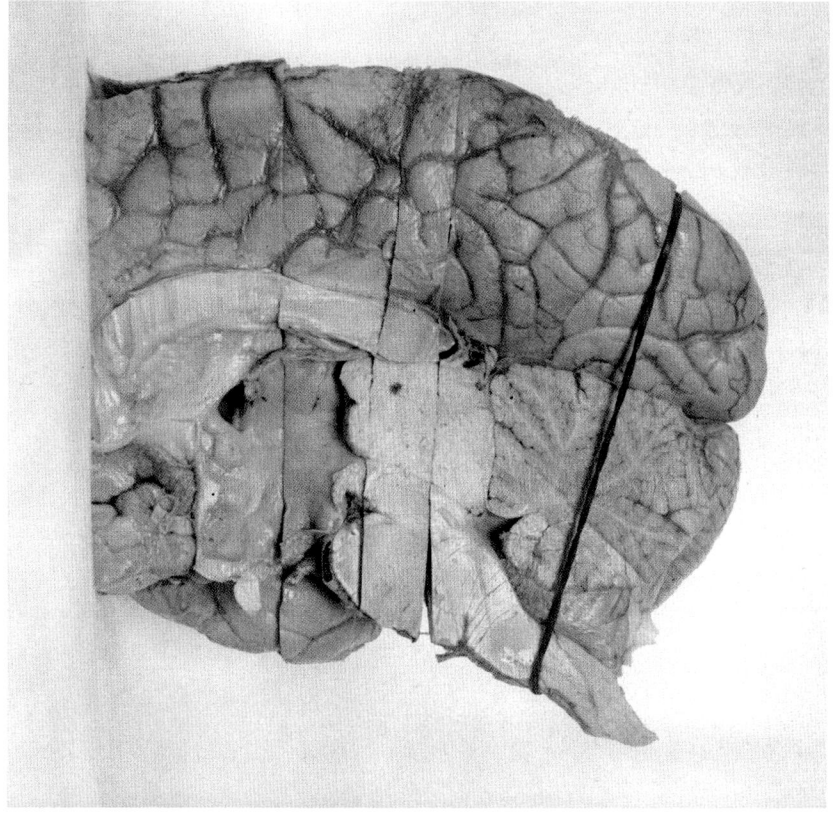

FIG. 2. SAGITTAL SECTION OF THE BRAIN — AUTOPSY SPECIMEN.

July 22, 1923
Dr. McKenzie

Patient was gone over today. There is apparently no change to be noted in his condition. Choked disc still remains 5-D. His lung condition is evidently a chronic affair. Taking everything into consideration it does not seem that there is anything possible to be done for this patient.

SUMMARY OF POSITIVE FINDINGS
July 23, 1923
Dr. McKenzie

SUBJECTIVE
1. Always rather under-sized and poorly developed. Started to shave late and only once or twice a week. Usual changes of puberty did not take place.

OPPOSITE PAGE. FIG. 1. TAKEN AT TIME OF ADMISSION.

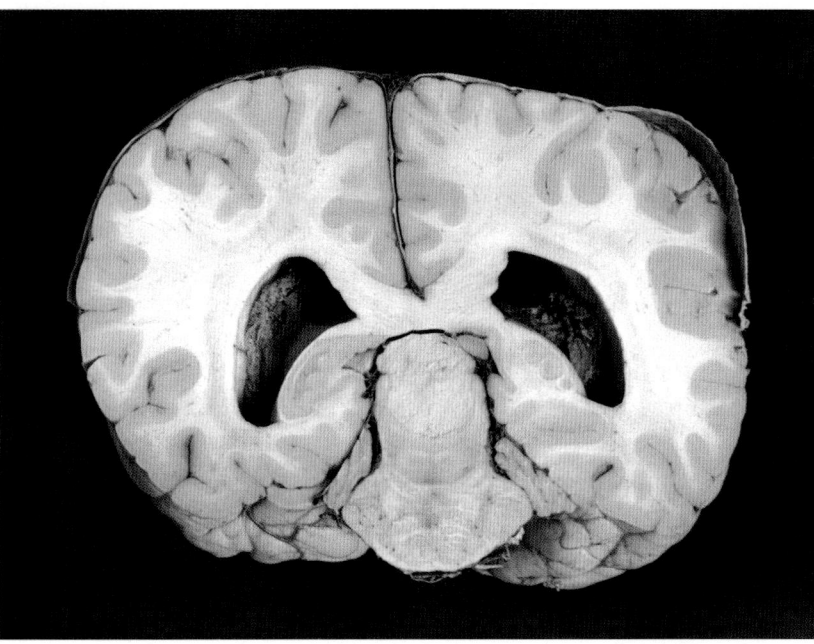

FIG. 3. CORONAL SECTION OF THE BRAIN — AUTOPSY SPECIMEN.

2. History 10 months ago of becoming weak and unable to work, having frontal headache and severe polyuria and polydipsia; also some projectile vomiting. Diagnosis of brain tumor was made at this time. Also choked disc was noted.
3. 8 months ago having had diabetes insipidus relieved by injections, he commenced having failing vision and has been blind for the past month. He was considered to have pituitary tumor at the Mt. Sinai hospital but we have been unable to obtain any record of the visual field defect.

OBJECTIVE
1. Sella is moderately enlarged, smooth in outline.
2. Bilateral choked disc, with marked secondary atrophy, 5-D.
3. Marked bilateral exophthalmos.
4. Extensive weakness of the right and left 6th.
5. Definite partial loss of upward conjugate movement of the eyes.

GLANDULAR
1. A thin, emaciated patient, with no skeletal abnormalities. Skin is not abnormal. Hair distribution very scanty on the face.
2. Marked diabetes insipidus.
3. Testicles very small.

IMPRESSION: Tumor in the region of the 3rd ventricle.

July 28, 1923
Dr. McKenzie

General condition remains unchanged, attacking the interlobar lung condition is being considered.

August 6, 1923
Dr. Boyd

Patient was again tapped, with some difficulty due to painful area from pleura and 100 cc similar fluid removed. There was apparently no reaction.

DISCHARGE NOTE TO WARD X
September 3, 1923
Dr. McKenzie

A generalized convulsion this afternoon. I saw the patient just as he had got over this. He was still unconscious, but breathing satisfactorily. 20 mins later his respirations ceased suddenly. After minutes his heart stopped beating.

AUTOPSY REPORT
September 4, 1923
Dr. Vilons
Dr. Caltoun

DIAGNOSES
Generalized military tuberculosis of lung, spleen, liver, bronchial lymph nodes.
Tuberculous pleuritis.
Hydrothorax (left)
Chronic fibrous peritonitis
Arteriosclerosis
Tumor of pineal body, probably neuron-epithelioma.

BRAIN

Brain of a patient who had been in two hospitals for some time, unoperated, with supposed suprasellar tumor, a diagnosis probably based on the evident hydrocephalus on back of secondary character or sake of history of diabetes insipidus, etc. Patient was blind with very receding choked disc and also had advanced pulmonary tuberculosis, and at the time operation seemed contraindicative. He was to be discharged when he died suddenly on the ward. It may be noted that this patient was a cousin of the small boy who had a suprasellar tumor, verified at operation.

External appearance of the brain shows no

abnormality aside from the very marked pressure cone. Coronal section at the tip of the temporal lobe shows marked dilatation of the ventricles and on looking into the greatly dilated third ventricle an irregular tumor is seen about in the region of the pineal body, projecting into the ventricle directly in the mid line. Moreover, the anterior part of the dilated ventricle shows a greatly thickened and nodular infundibulum which may in all probability be related to the patient's symptoms and perhaps account for his diabetes insipidus. Moreover, there are two nodules of tumor, evidently implanted on the anterior floor of the dilated ventricle, nodules about 7 mm in diameter which have the appearance of underlying ependyma. One of them is in the mid line in the anterior wall, the other is to the right of the anterior commissure which stands out well, owing to the dilated ventricle which lies between it and the foramen of Monroe on that side.

Section taken from the anterior part of the pons passes through the tumor which lies between the cerebral peduncles and is obviously a tumor of replacement of the pineal gland. It has projected down into the third ventricle. It is extremely friable, the color of the white matter of the brain and symmetrical in its position. The ita lies well below it as will appear in the photograph.

Section further back shows a tumor about 2 cm in diameter occupying the upper part of the pons, probably a tumor of the pineal gland.

(Dr. Cushing)

Microscopic Examination: Tissue from one block shows tumor tissue. Tissue from the other block shows pituitary which is infiltrated with tumor tissue resembling that found in the large tumor mass.

The tumor is composed of small cells of a nondescript type, strongly basophilic and arranged in cords and small, irregular groups. The general arrangement is that of small celled epithelial tumor divided into rather large acini by delicate connective tissue framework. There are occasional mitotic figures.

DIAGNOSIS – Pinealoma.

(Dr. Wolbach)

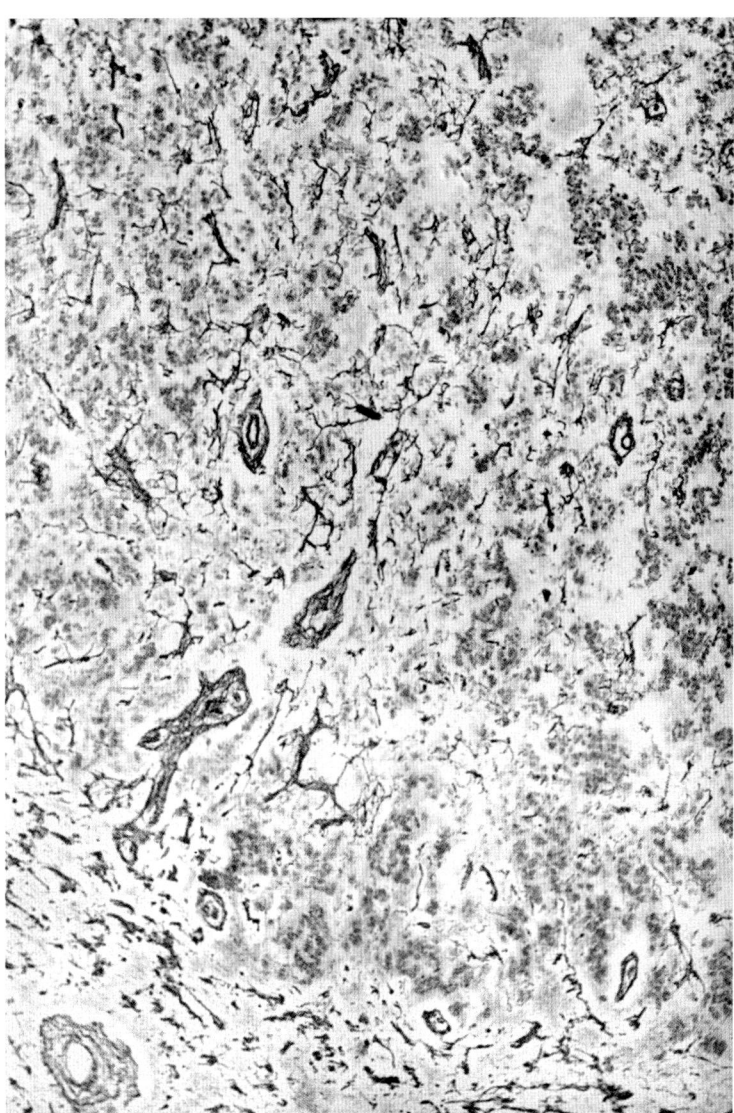

FIG. 4. HISTOLOGY SLIDE.

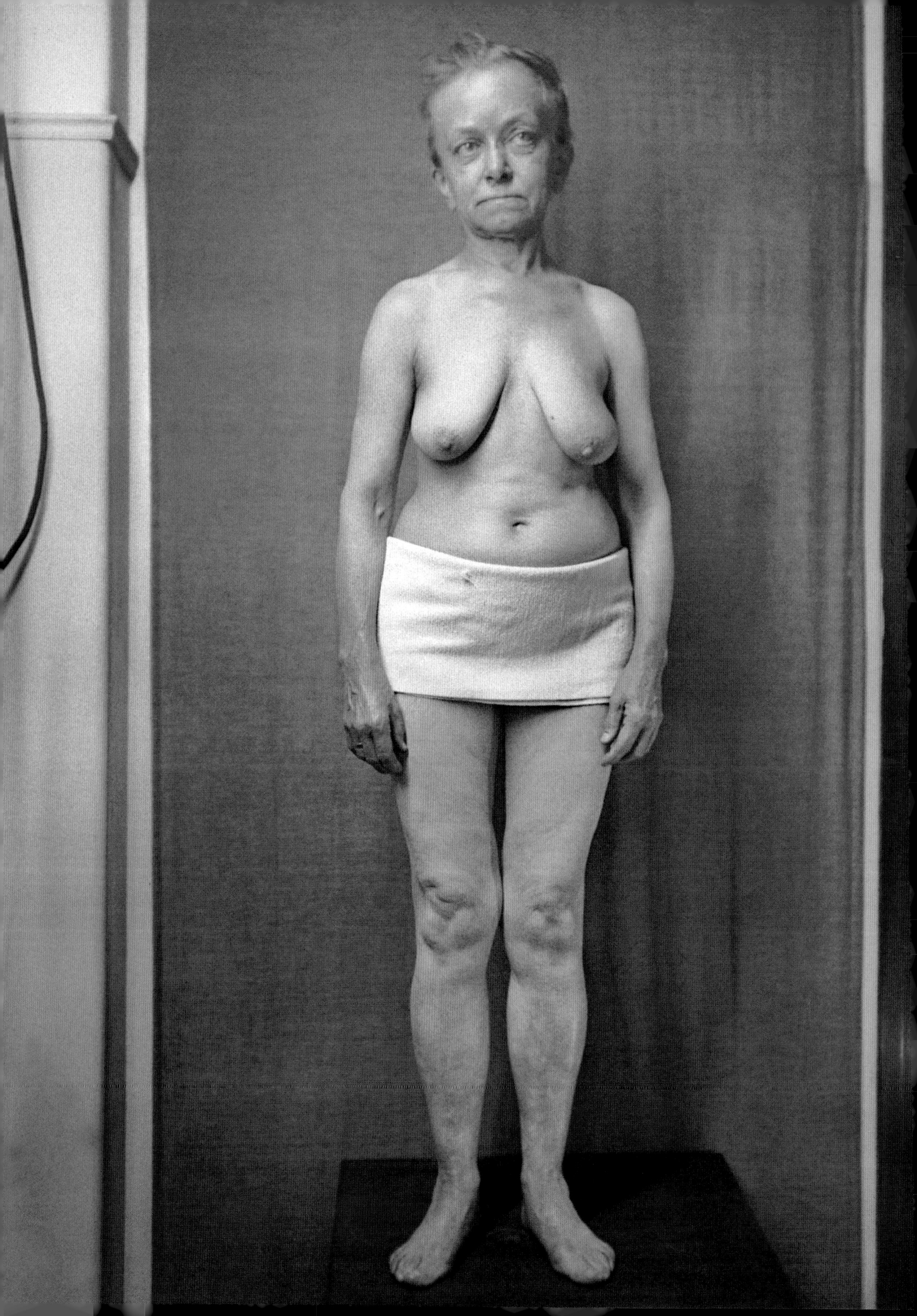

2.7 Sarcoma of calvarium

SEX: F; AGE: 66; SURG. NO. 20157, 20550

HISTORY

Thirteen years ago, her hair dresser told the patient that she "has a very tight scalp." An enlarging left parietal mass was more noticeable for the past 3–4 years associated recently with a soft swelling for the last four months.

SUMMARY OF POSITIVE FINDINGS
November 20, 1923
Dr. Bird

SUBJECTIVE
1. Mother died at 70 with an enlarged head and bowing of left lower leg.
2. Tinnitus in the left ear for 20 years, occasional shooting pain in the left ear for 6 years, a middle ear infection in the left ear 5 years ago, followed by increasing deafness, bilateral, most marked on the left.
3. Very near-sighted for years.
4. Bleeding, painless hemorrhoids 15 years.
5. About 10 yrs. ago painless nodes formed on her fingers.
6. 10 years ago a dime-sized depression was noted at the vertex of her skull.
7. 4 years before entry progressive, symmetrical enlargement of the head began.
8. 8 months ago a depression with a classic bottom the size of a dollar was felt in the left parietal region.
9. 4 months ago this began to fill, the swelling increasing rapidly, especially during the last 2 ½ months.
10. For 6 weeks a "gutter" in the right parietal region noted. 10 days before entry swelling opened by her doctor showed "blood, bony fragments and granulations."
11. X-ray of skull showed Paget's disease.

OBJECTIVE
1. Patient small, erect, 4 ft 10 ½ inches in height.
2. Arms equal in length, 44 ½ cm.
3. Right leg 79 ½ cm; left leg 78 ½ cm.
4. Sternum and costal cartilages prominent. Chest measures 77 cm.
5. Head large, fronto-occipital, 62 ½ cm

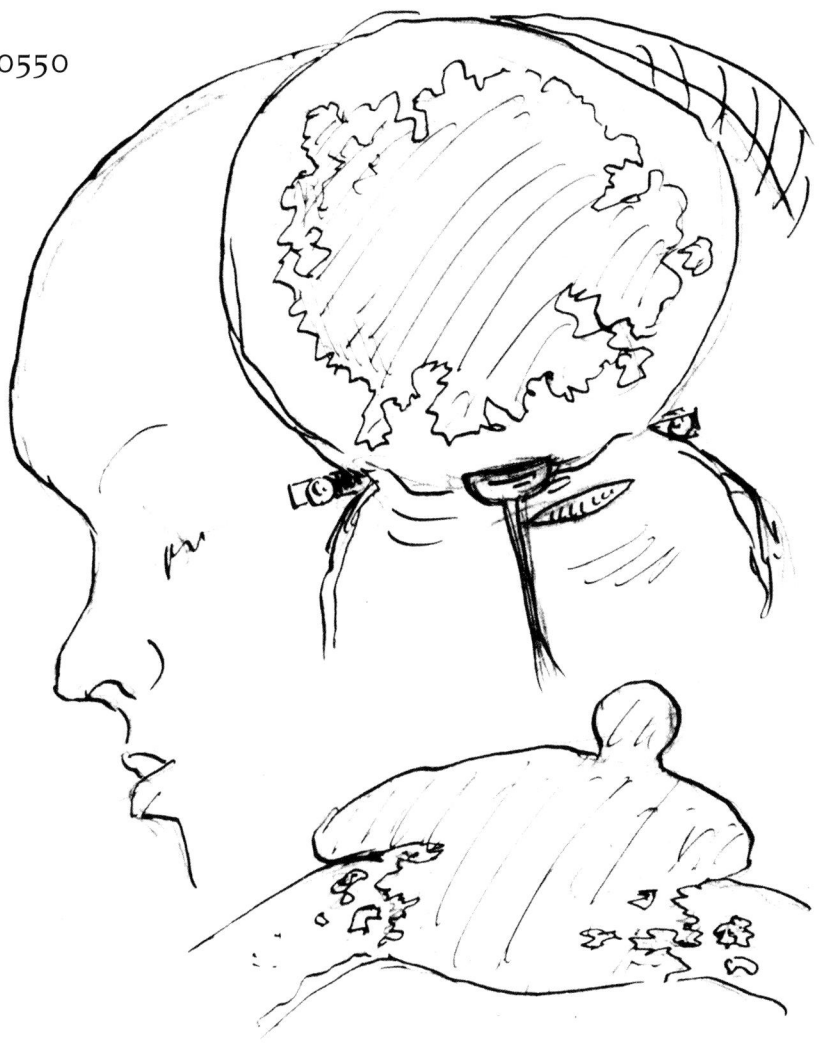

FIG. 2. OPERATIVE SKETCH.

6. Tense swelling, left parietal region, measured 12 x 14 cm, pulsating, slightly tender at periphery, with scar of recent incision 1/1/2 cm long. No bruit heard with stethoscope over the swelling.
7. Eyes very near-sighted, 18-D OD; 14-D OS.
8. Right tympanic membrane normal. Left scarred and refracted.
9. Brachial and radial vessels sclerosed.
10. Prolapsed, uninflamed internal hemorrhoids.
11. X-rays show changes of Paget's disease in skull, spine, pelvis, right femur, and of both arms and forearms.
12. X-ray shows several root abscesses.
13. Heberden's nodes on fingers.

IMPRESSION: Paget's disease, multiosseous. Sarcoma of skull, spine, pelvis. Internal hemorrhoids.

OPPOSITE PAGE. FIG. I. PREOPERATIVE.

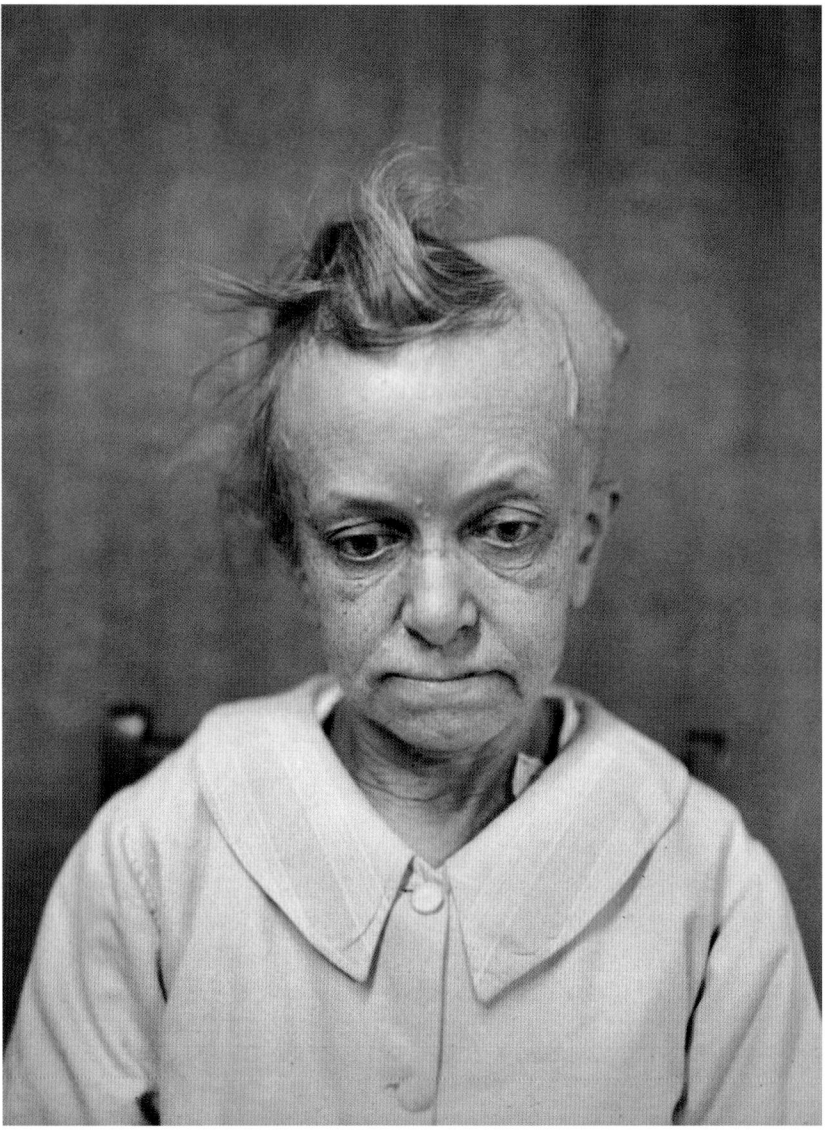

FIG. 3. PREOPERATIVE.

RADIOLOGY REPORT
November 12, 1923
Dr. Sosman

Stereoscopic films of the skull show an enormously thickened cranial vault with alternate areas of rarefaction and increased density, most marked in the left parietal region. Findings appear quite characteristic of Paget's disease.

OPERATIVE REPORT
December 5, 1923
Dr. Cushing
Anesthesia – Ether – Miss Gerrard

Partial Rough Extirpation of Massive Sarcoma of the Left Parietal Region. Implantation of Pectoralis Major from Breast Operation.

I had very little foreknowledge as to what, if anything, I might be able to do in this case. Evidently the tumor has been growing rapidly and the small fungus at the site of the recent exploratory incision has been enlarging until now it is the size of a robin's egg. After shaving the scalp and cleaning this small protrusion as well as could be a small crust was picked off from it and a spurting artery shot out a foot from the surface. This was finally controlled by a little pressure, but it gave warning of what an extreme degree of vascularity the tumor might possess. This small nodule was treated with iodine and the operation was prepared for in the usual fashion. The temporal arteries were shut off by the use of Dr. Lochs temporal clamp. Palpation of the tumor, which was soft, and gave a fluctuant feel, showed that there were spicules of bone in the growth which would crackle, and it was evident that we were going to find an exceedingly irregular edge. The condition that was found is represented in the sketches above.

I began with a 2–3 inch incision in the anterior part of the field and reflected the scalp and galea and pericranium down to the bone coming back to the irregular margin of the tumor. There was a good deal of bleeding at this juncture and I took some long strips of the pectoralis major muscle, which Dr. Cheever had removed from a patient operated upon shortly before, and stuffed these into the margin. In this way finally the entire great bulging tumor was encircled and I began to reflect the flap. I found, however, that I was going too deep and had to separate the pericranium from galea, and when this was done a perfectly smooth glistening surface over the tumor was left lying between galea and pericranium over the tumor which was intact except for one small place where the fungus occurred. This fungus was cut off at its neck and subsequently an incision shown on the inner surface of the flap in the sketch was made and the nodule tilted out, and galea here closed securely from within. I then began working first at one side then another of the tumor stuffing in muscle as the rough dissection was made. The entire margin of the bone was greatly honeycombed with tumor, and the bone which was fully an inch thick would have been difficult to handle. The patient's blood pressure was dropping off and I had not completely stilled bleeding, and it seemed best to take a large teaspoon and scoop out the great mass. Fortunately it was soft and did not bleed excessively though considerably. The whole layer of pectoralis major muscle was then laid across this wound and packed into position, and held for about 15 minutes until the fall in blood pressure reached its level. I would have been glad to have done more than this but her condition hardly justified it and moreover I had clinic impending. Consequently, the surface of the muscle was largely cut away leaving, however, a great mass of muscle implanted on the base of tumor. This was pulsating showing that we were well down the dura though I was not certain at any time of actual pulsation in the original growth as felt through the scalp.

During this procedure some fairly fresh pieces of muscle were secured for frozen sections and for perfect fixation in various ways. Also a piece of bone edge was chiseled away for decalcification and study.

It was my intent if I had been able to remove the growth a little more cleanly than this to have subjected the patient immediately to a deep radiation but I hope that this may be possible on a second session.

The scalp was reflected and sutured in place carefully in layers largely by Dr. Bailey.

Preparations were made for transfusion and blood from the case was also held in readiness there being about 500 cc of blood, containing 2 million red cells. I was glad enough to get out of things as they were even leaving muscle in place, and hope on a 2nd session it may be possible to clean out the edges of the infected bone and to leave a fairly clean cavity.

(Dr. Cushing)

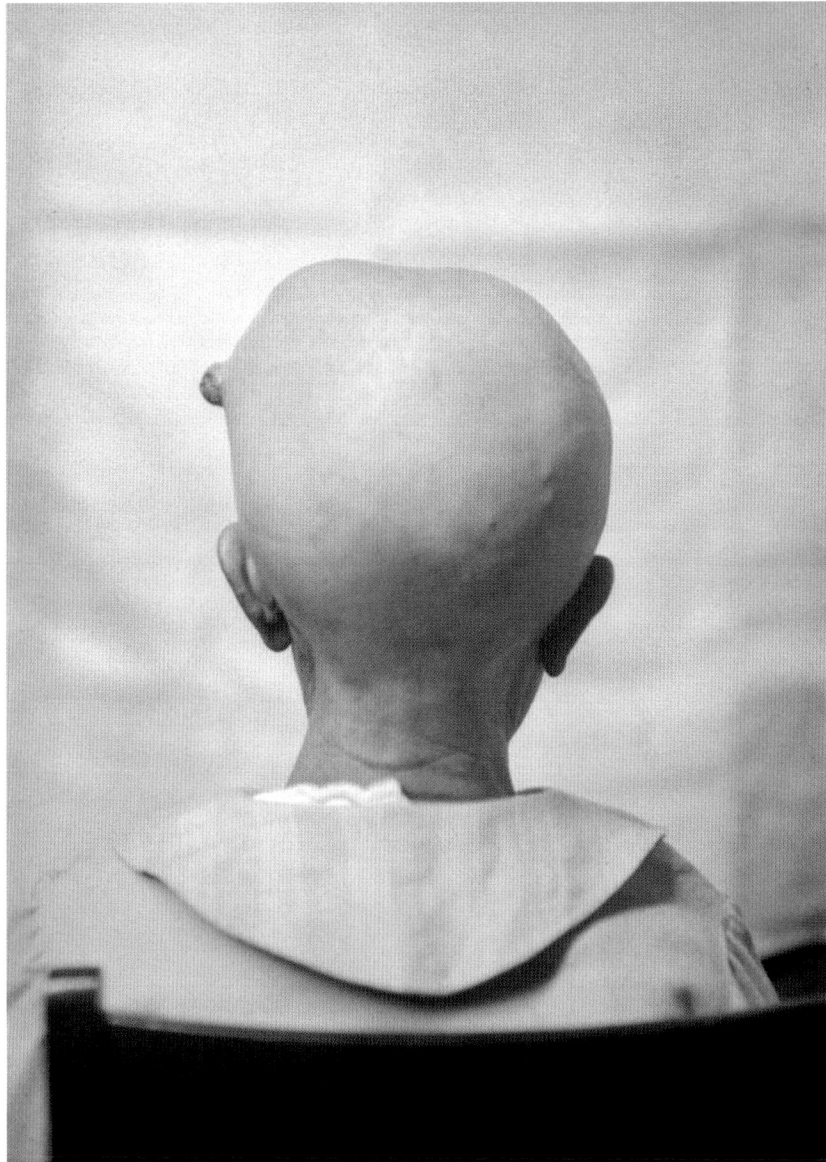

FIG. 4. IMMEDIATELY PREOPERATIVE.

PATHOLOGY REPORT
December 5, 1923

Surgical specimen consists of a large mass of tumor tissue about the size of a man's hand, removed from the skull with a spoon. The tumor had eroded the bone, completely destroyed it down as far as the dura and had produced a noticeable swelling which had projected about 3 cm above the level of the scalp. The greater mass of tumor was placed in 10% formalin and retained as a gross specimen.

(Dr. Cushing)

Microscopic diagnosis. Chondro-fibro sarcoma.

(Dr. Wolbach)

SPECIAL NOTE
December 8, 1923
Dr. Cushing

Since the last operation there has been no reaction whatsoever but the flap of scalp replaced over the wound has been getting more and more tense and I could not tell whether there had been any undue reaction around the great mass of muscle left in the pocket or not. It seems to me that it was best to again reflect the flap and to see if I could not do something a little more toward removing the ragged edges of bone which evidently were infiltrated by the lesion. The patient's greatly lowered

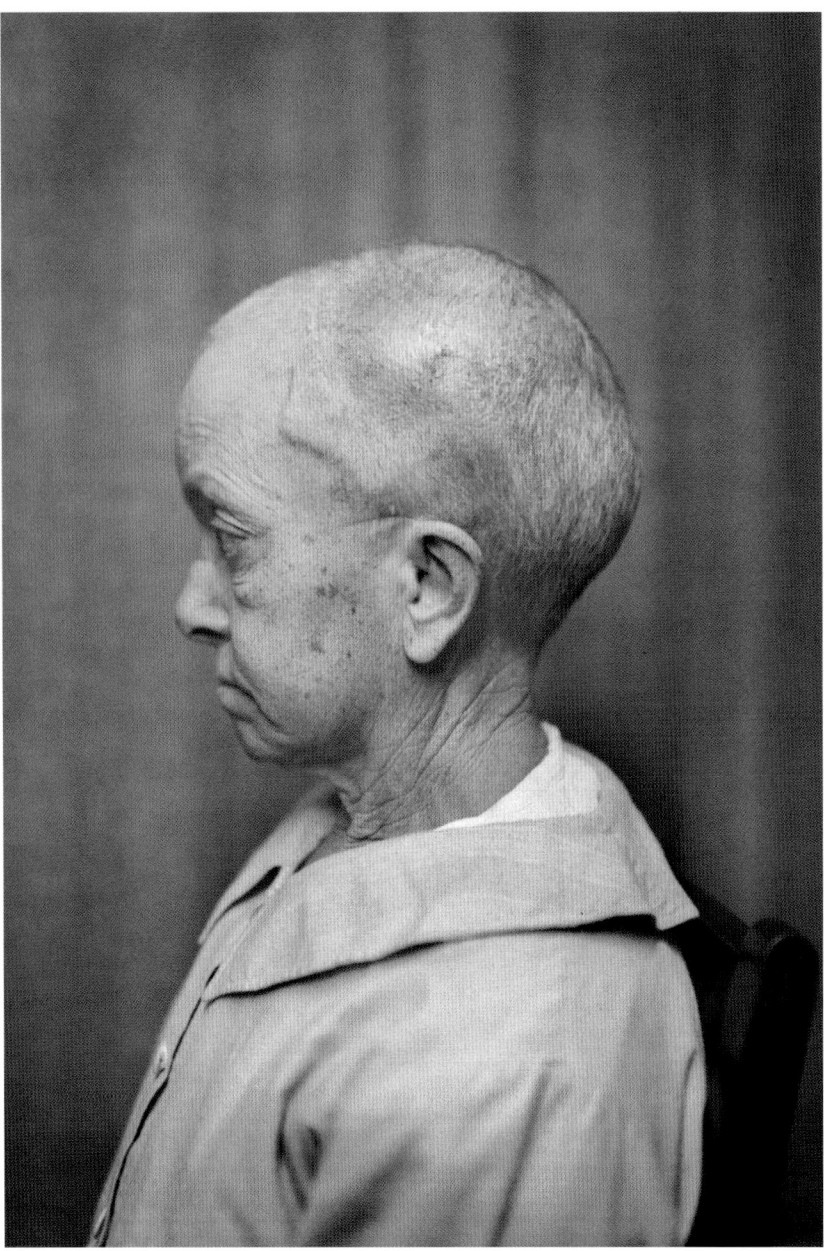

FIG. 5. THREE WEEKS POSTOPERATIVE.

blood pressure again came back to normal but her blood remained low in hemoglobin and erythrocytes though the latter were rapidly coming up – perhaps much more rapidly than if she had had a transfusion.

I hesitated to put the patient on before the Neuro-Surgical Society which was meeting here but was rather impelled to do so owing to the fact that a breast case had been done the day before and a large mass of muscle had been carefully preserved in sterile towels and put in the ice chest for an emergency such as might arise from this procedure.

OPERATIVE NOTE
December 8, 1923
Dr. Cushing
Anesthesia: Novocain

Reflection of Flap – Partial Removal of Very Vascular Margin of Defect, Infiltrated with Tumor. Re-closure of Scalp.

On reflecting the scalp there escaped a large amount of yellowish semi-gelatinous fluid evidently the reaction from the great mass of muscle. No cultures were taken. It was evident from the first that there was going to be a good deal of bleeding if I should endeavor to remove the muscle for the mere dislodgement of this attached muscle caused bleeding. However, with the rongeurs in 2-3 places I chewed away great masses of sphenoid bone, a little more than the consistency of a hard cheese, all of it seeming to be infiltrated with tumor as far as I thought fit to go. Even had there not been great bleeding which had to be checked by the placement of some of the muscle mentioned above I would hardly have been able to remove all the tumor for it would have meant taking practically the whole side of the cranium.

I consequently had to withdraw, leaving in one mass of the original muscle though some of it was cut away and in addition some other pieces which had been inserted to stop the fresh bleeding.

The patient stood the operation fairly well. Closure without a drain.

(Dr. Cushing)

POSTOPERATIVE COURSE

The patient underwent an unremarkable postoperative course. The scalp flap was tapped to relieve the fluid collection underneath.

DISCHARGE NOTE
January 2, 1924
Dr. Bailey

Appointment made for X-ray treatment and patient instructed to return at frequent intervals so that her scalp could be watched because of large amount of muscle left in wound.

SECOND HOSPITAL ADMISSION

HISTORY

She received one X-ray treatment in January of 1924.

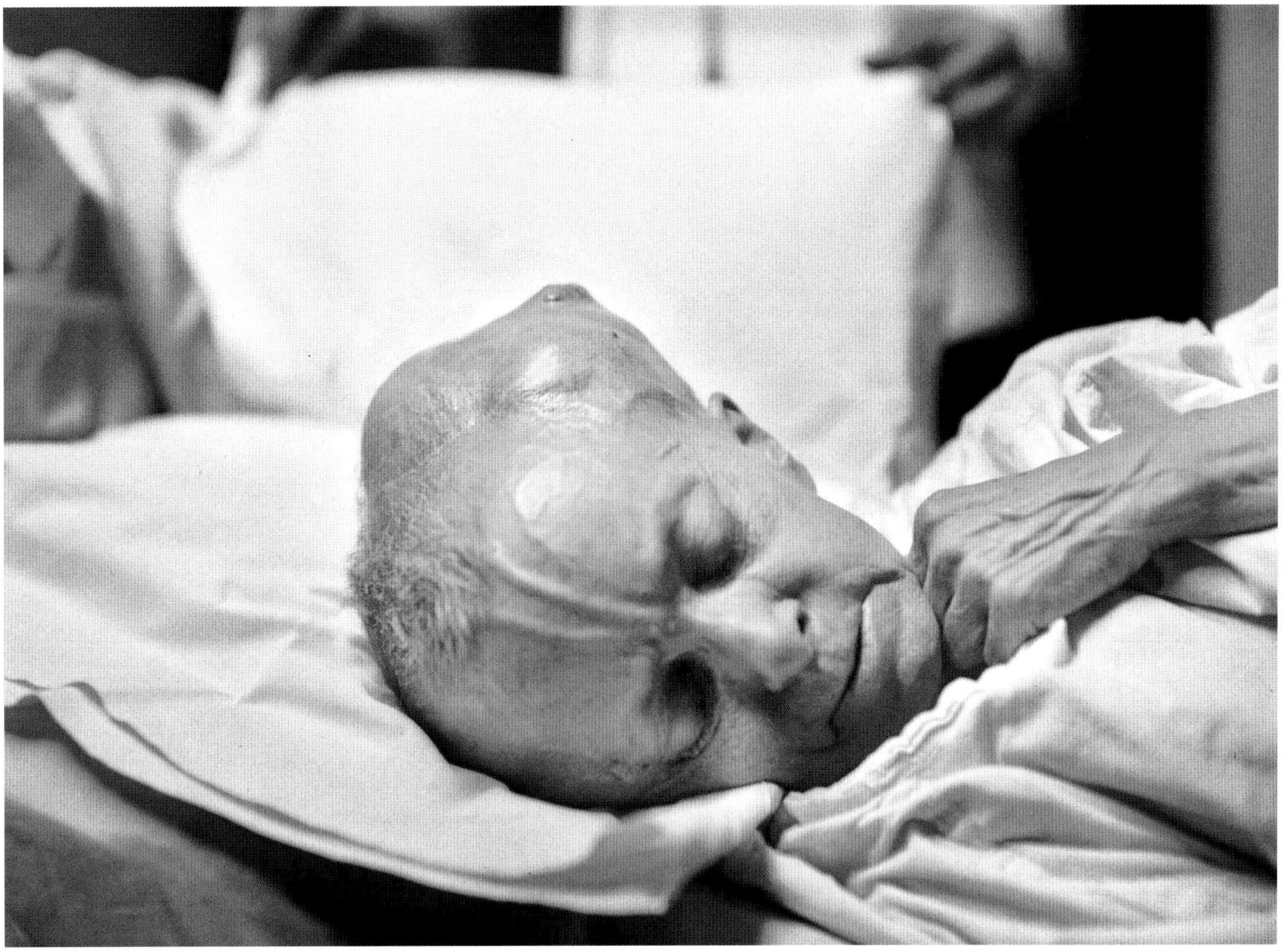

FIGS. 6 AND 7. TAKEN DURING SECOND ADMISSION.

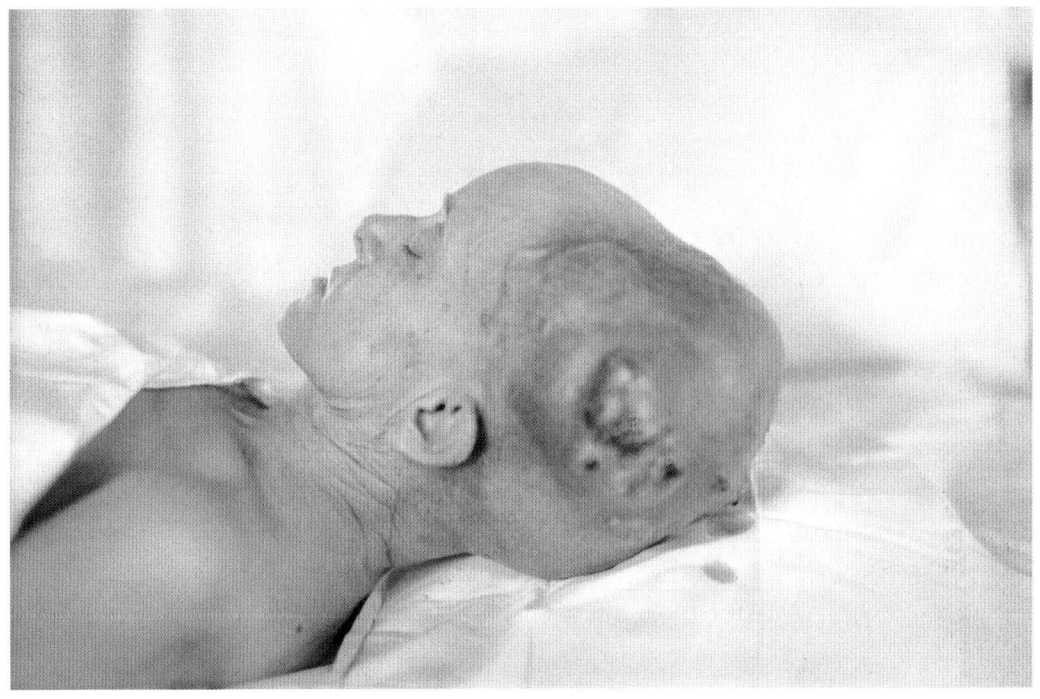

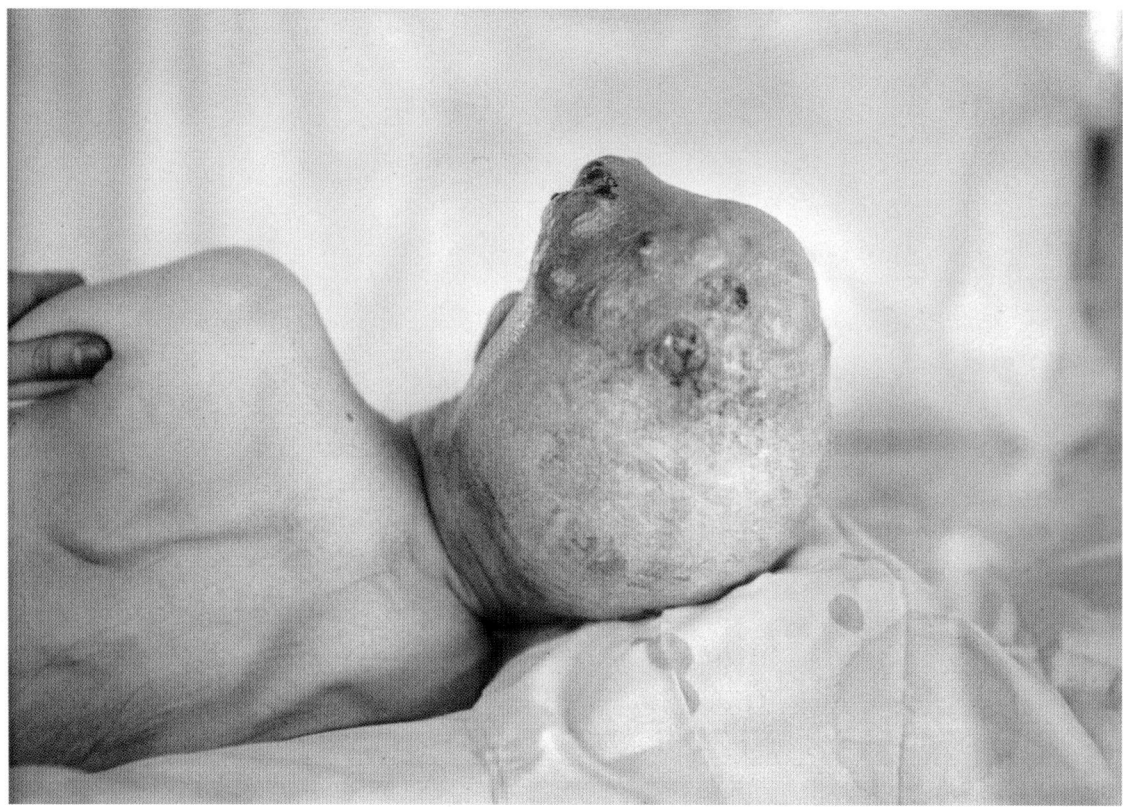

FIG. 8. TAKEN DURING SECOND ADMISSION.

COMPLAINT

Weakness, mental confusion, rapid recurrence of sarcoma of the skull, 7 ½ weeks postoperative.

January 22, 1924
Dr. Bird

The growth has grown greatly in size and has become quite tender to touch. She has noticed slight tenderness at the back and sides of the neck. She has had very little appetite but has not felt sick to her stomach and has not vomited. She has had no generalized headache. She has felt increasingly weak when she tries to walk and has felt slightly dizzy at times. There have been no visual disturbances except slight blurring with the dizziness. Patient is re-admitted because she cannot be easily taken care of at home. Ultimate disposition is to be decided.

Head: Is much larger and heavier than first examined 2 months ago. The vascularity has so increased that the whole scalp is dull, reddish purple in color. The enlarged arteries coursing over the temple region no longer stand out as they originally did because of the vascular swelling of the surrounding scalp. A large area of tumor recurrence now measures 19 x 17 cm extending from 1 to 2 cm outside the scar of her operative incision.

The growth elevates the scalp all the way. Palpation of the scalp over the growth gives a sensation of marked thinness and softness as if there were fluid beneath which was about to break thru. This is particularly true at 3 or 4 of the highest elevations. At 2 or 3 points about the edge of the growth there are firmer nodules, which are rather anaemic in appearance. These have the feeling of cartilage, in view of the nature of the growth may well be. There is an enlarged left posterior auricular node. On right side the glands are enlarged just as they are on the left. In addition, on the right, there is moderate edema of the eye lids, right side of the face and right cervical region.

IMPRESSION: Paget's disease (osteitis deformans) multiosseous. Chondrosarcoma of skull; metastasis to glands of neck and right cavernous sinus. Right cavernous sinus thrombosis. Metastases to the tibia.

HOSPITAL COURSE

No surgical treatment was offered. The skull lesion continued to grow rapidly. The patient died on February 21, 1924, during her stay in the hospital.

AUTOPSY REPORT
(Summarized)
February 21, 1924
Dr. Wilson
Dr. Bailey

DIAGNOSES
    Paget's disease.
    Sarcoma arising in calvarium with metastasis in cervical lymph nodes.
    Arteriosclerosis.
    Calcification of aortic valve and papillary vessels.
    Leiomyoma of uterus (calcified.)
    Nephrolithiasis.
    Thrombosis of inferior vena cava.
    Pulmonary thrombosis.

Arising from the left side of the head, from the region of the left parietal bone, there is a large, rounded, lobulated mass of soft tumor tissue which at the apex is ulcerated and in this region projected a deep red, granular surface. Other portions are covered with skin. This large mass of tumor tissue covers all of the parietal bone, the squamous portion of the temporal and small adjoining portion of both frontal and occipital bones. Photographs give an idea of its contour and size. On the right side of the scalp there are three small, rounded projections, each about 2 cm in diameter which present flattened, hemispherical projections in the region of the right forehead just above the supra-orbital margin. The consistency of these is soft on palpation. The scalp in all areas with the exception of one area at the apex of the large tumor mass, is covered with smooth, gray skin.

Permission for a complete autopsy with special study of the skeleton had been obtained, and for this reason the ordinary procedures were performed.

Brain-The outstanding feature as the skull is viewed before opening, is the presence of a large mass of tumor tissue projecting from the left side. This tumor mass is in a general way hemispherical in shape and at its base measured 14.5 cm in diameter. Palpation reveals the fact that it is extremely soft and for the most part friable and necrotic. It is gray with patches of red, the latter representing areas of hemorrhage. Other portions of the calvarium are smooth. In it, however, there are numerous gray areas which are easily distinguishable from the pale brown of the surrounding bone. These rounded areas measure up to 2.5 cm

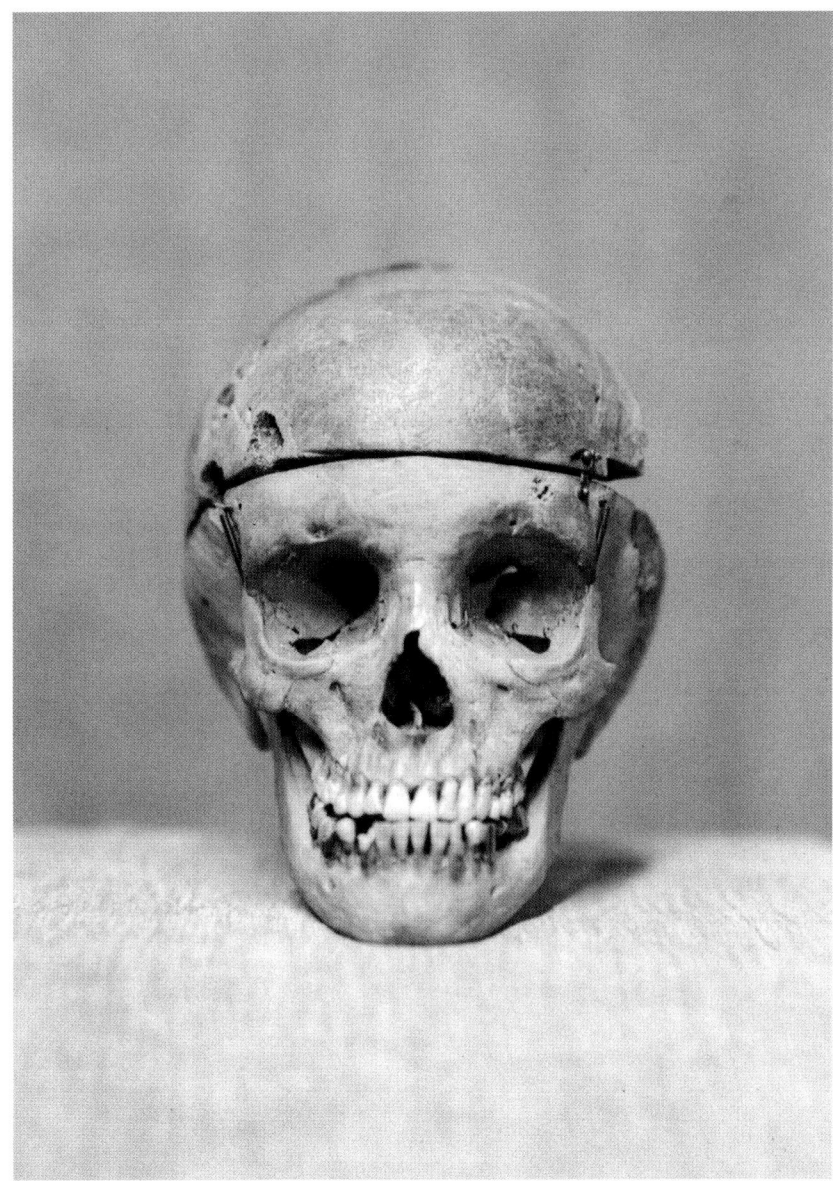

FIG. 9. AUTOPSY SKULL SPECIMEN.

in diameter. Some present a slightly concave surface. The centers of the larger mass are soft, the tissue resembling the gray tumor tissue described in the large mass on the left side.

The large tumor mass on the left pushes inward against the dura, producing a large, hemispherical mass which markedly distorts the shape of the brain. The dura is quite readily stripped from the calvarium.

The outstanding feature is the marked distortion in shape of the brain, realizing from the pressure of the tumor growth on the left side, transmitted through the dura. The left cerebral hemisphere shows a large, deep concavity immediately

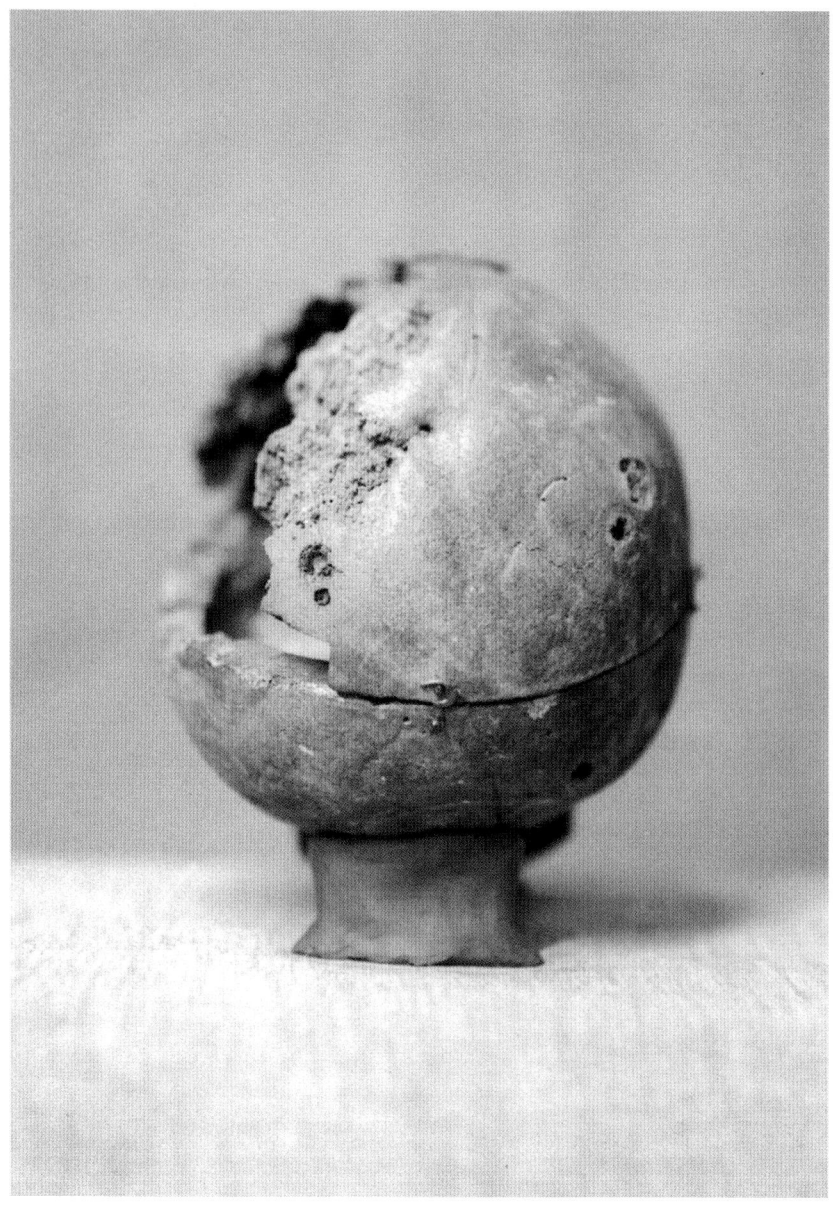

FIG. 10. AUTOPSY SKULL SPECIMEN.

beneath the tumor. At its margin the depressed area measures approximately 9.5 cm in diameter. The convolutions elsewhere show some flattening. The pia arachnoid is thin and transparent, free from exudate.

The vessels at the base show only a few atheromatous plaques. The brain will be fixed in 10% formalin and sectioned after fixation.

Microscopic examination: Three sections were taken from the calvarium and near the edge of the large tumor mass on the left side. The bone is loose textured, resembling only slightly the bone normally occurring in the skull. The spicules are very irregular, enclosing irregular marrow spaces, the latter being filled with a loose connective tissue which is supplied with a moderate number of blood vessels. Where the bone is close to the large soft tumor, these spaces are sometimes filled with tumor cells. The spicules of the bone are quite cellular. The intercellular material stains pink, has a laminated appearance, as if deposited in successive layers and through it ran, very irregularly, narrow blue lines apparently without any special purpose. Bordering many of the bony spicules are a layer of osteoblasts. Osteoclasts are fairly numerous. The picture suggests that the bone is proliferating. The proportion of bone to marrow spaces is short one and one-half to one.

Five sections. Four of these are from the large tumor on the left side of the head and one from a metastasis growth in one of the each cervical lymph nodes. The tumor in these sections varies somewhat in appearance. In some of them the tumor cells tend to be spindle shaped and produces fibrils which stain line connective tissue fibrils whereas in other sections the tumor cells resemble large mononucleated wandering cells with an extremely scanty intracellular material. Large areas of necrosis and areas of hemorrhage are numerous. In areas where tumor cells tend to be spindle shaped, they have elongated, granular nuclei and a small amount of cytoplasm streaming out from one or both ends. Between these cells there are numerous fibrils which with phosphotangetic acid hematoxylin stain pale brown. In areas adjacent to these there are groups of cells which resemble only slightly connective tissue cells. These cells vary greatly in size and shape. Their nuclei are often multiple and mitotic figures are numerous. In other areas the tumor cells are represented by a mass of cells resembling large mononuclear wandering cells supported by an extremely small amount of stroma which in some places is so scanty that the tumor cells appear to be without support. Tumor cells here are rounded, mononucleated cells which vary greatly in size from cells smaller than red cells to cells of mammoth size. They have a moderate amount of cytoplasm. Their nuclei are rounded and granular. Tumor giant cells are common and mitotic figures are numerous.

(Dr. Brown, Resident pathologist)

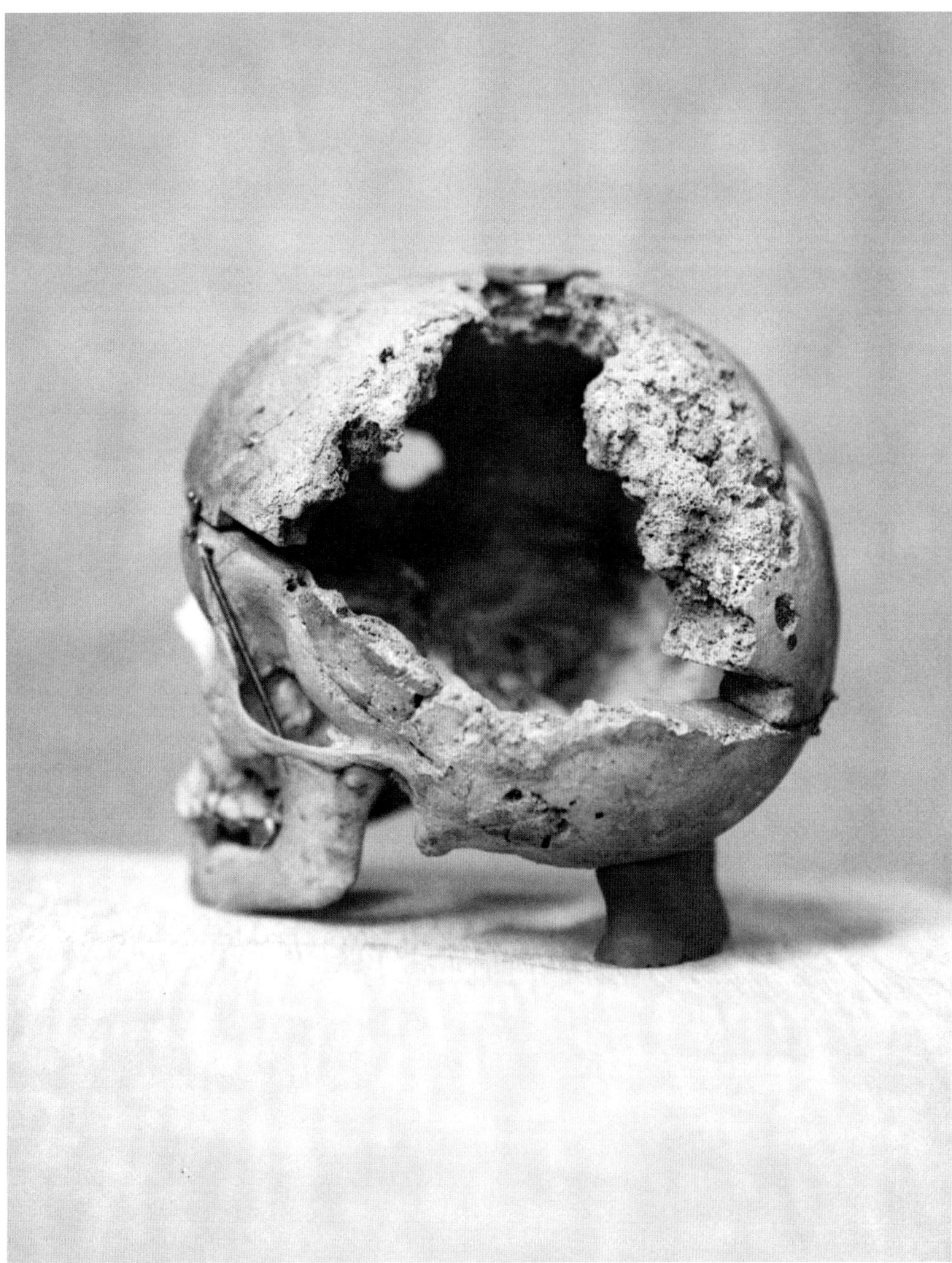

FIG. 11. AUTOPSY SKULL SPECIMEN.

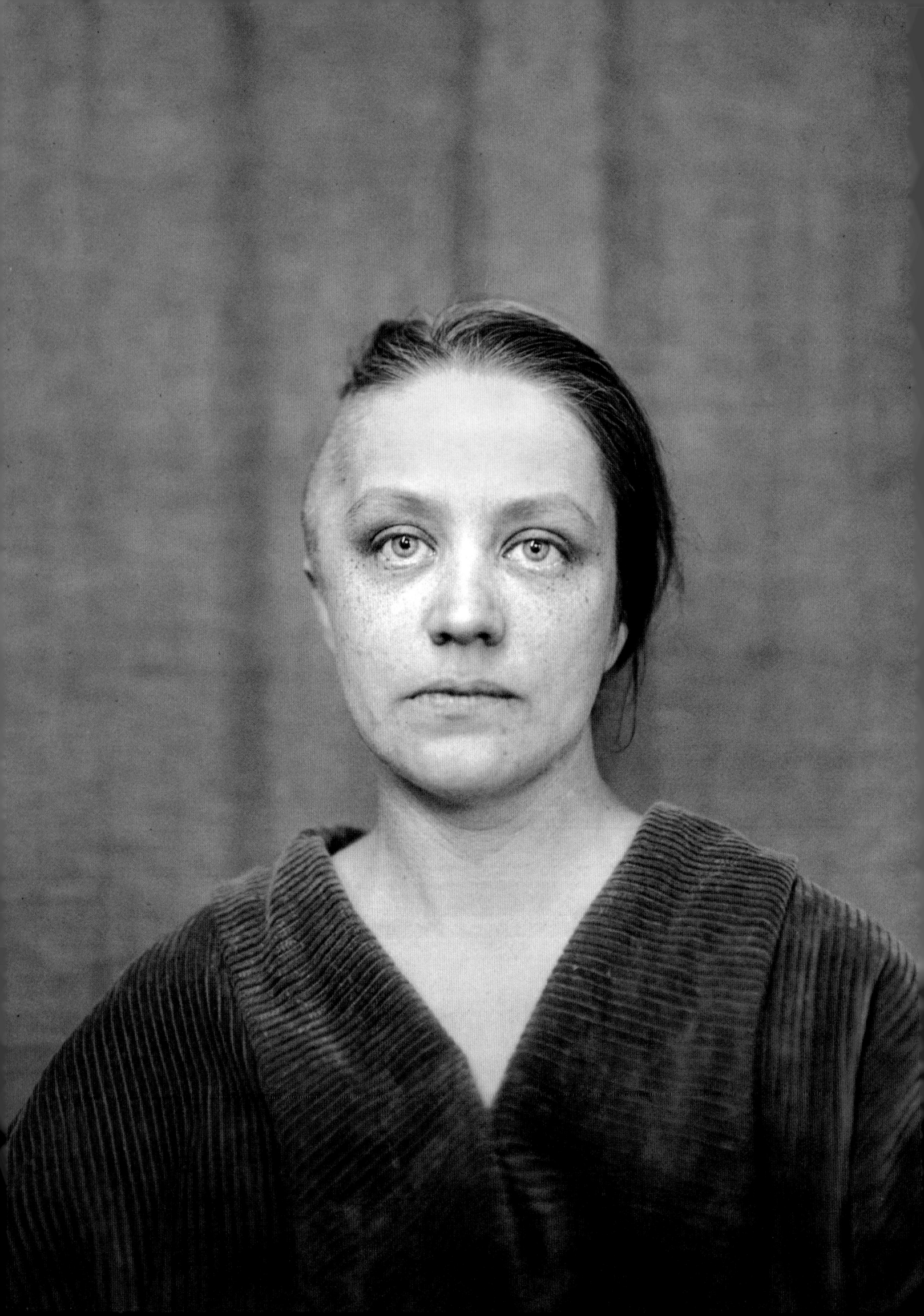

2.8 Temporal glioma

SEX: F; AGE: 35; SURG. NO. 21049, 22891

Diagnosis: Surg. No 21049 - Cerebral tumor: unverified

Surg. No 22891- Right temporal glioma: verified

HISTORY

This patient had one convulsion several months ago and was diagnosed with bilateral papilledema at the time of first admission.

SUMMARY OF POSITIVE FINDINGS
April 1, 1924
Dr. Putnam

SUBJECTIVE
1. Generalized convulsion with cyanosis and biting of the tongue in May, 1922.
2. Extreme nervousness and the expectation of further attacks ever since.
3. Some stomach trouble and belching.
4. Blurring of vision since Nov. 1923 with history of choked disc.

OBJECTIVE
1. An extremely nervous individual.
2. Bilateral choked disc, 2D.
3. Slight spasticity of left leg.

IMPRESSION: I can find no localizing signs except possibly the spasticity of the left leg. It seems to me we are again confronted with the problem of a tumor versus arachnoiditis.

RADIOLOGY REPORT
April 2, 1924
Dr. Sosman

Right lateral stereoscopic film of the skull shows a smooth cranial vault. The sella turcica appears moderately atrophic but shows no destruction. The pineal appears displaced to the right of midline.

IMPRESSION – in view of the displaced pineal, would suggest a ventriculogram.

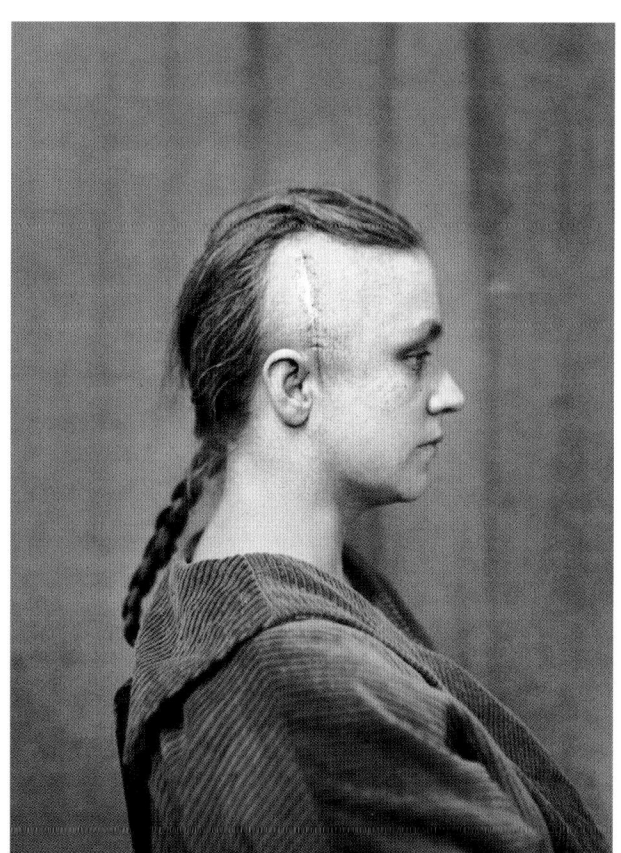
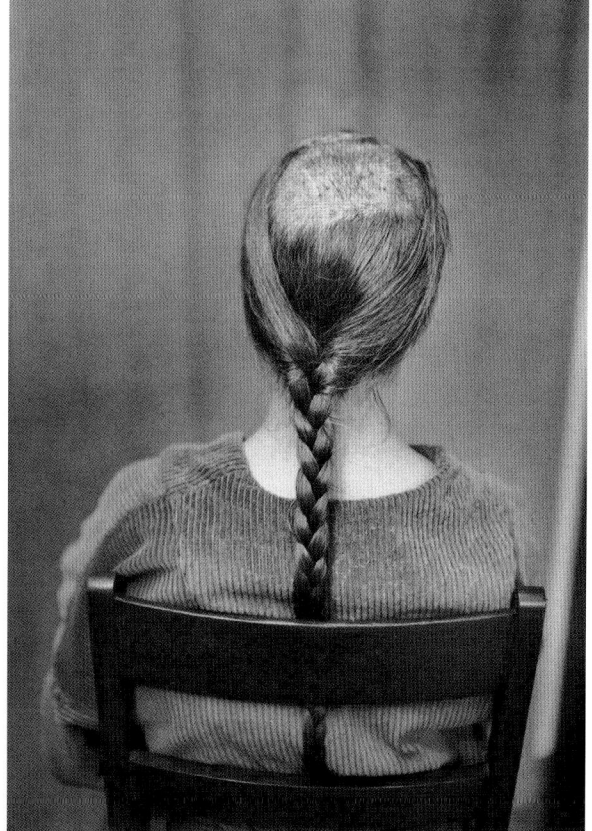

FIGS. 2 AND 3. ONE WEEK POSTOPERATIVE FOLLOWING SUBTEMPORAL DECOMPRESSION.

OPPOSITE PAGE. FIG. I. ONE WEEK POSTOPERATIVE FOLLOWING SUBTEMPORAL DECOMPRESSION.

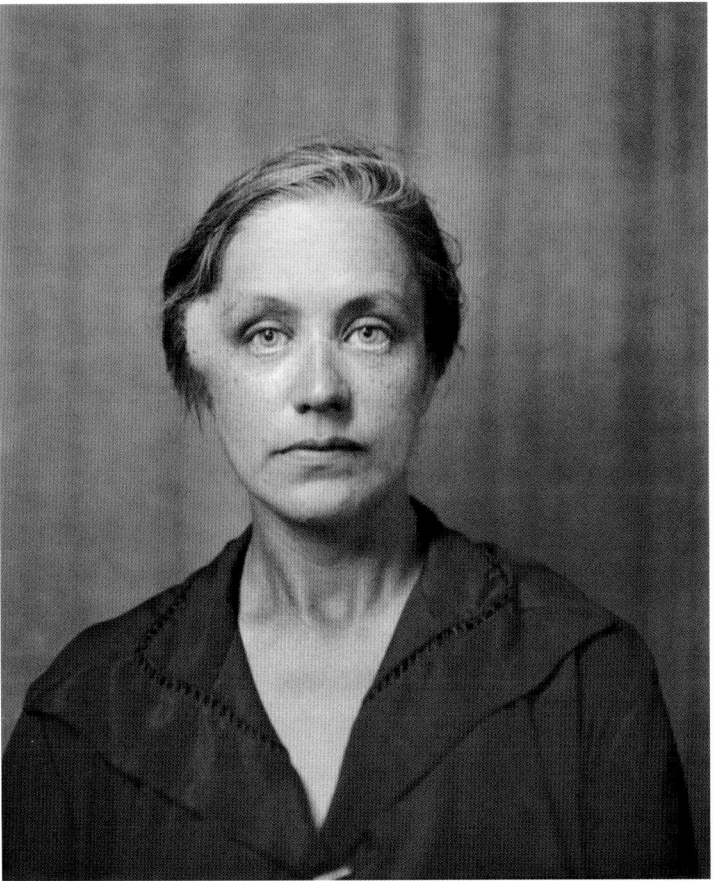

FIG. 4. FIVE MONTHS POSTOPERATIVE FOLLOWING SUBTEMPORAL DECOMPRESSION.

OPERATIVE NOTE
April 4, 1924
Operator: Dr. Horrax and Dr. Putnam
Anesthesia: Cocaine

Bilateral Ventriculogram

This was a very easy ventriculogram. The patient cooperated perfectly. Patient was placed on the table, both the head and the feet being elevated, which makes a very satisfactory position. Puncture was made, first on the right side, in the parieto-occipital region. The skull was rather thick. The needle was introduced 5 cm in a direction slightly forward and vertical. About 3 cc of fluid escaped and then no more came. Other taps did not reveal anymore fluid. The wound was therefore closed and a similar opening made on the other side. Another tap, this time at a depth of 4 cm produced about 6 cc, only a drop or two more could be obtained by moving the head. Corresponding amount of air was introduced under slight pressure and the needle withdrawn. The needle was again inserted, slightly more posteriorly, to a depth of about 5 cm and again struck a very little foamy fluid, supposedly containing the air previously injected. About 2 cc of fluid were allowed to escape and again 5 cc of air were injected under slight pressure and the needle withdrawn. A little air bubbled out along its tract.

It seems very doubtful whether this homeopathic dose of air yielded any information of value. The wet plaster show it to lie in a roughly triangular area with very funny, moth-eaten borders. Apparently none of it has crossed midline. It will probably be necessary to repeat the air injection. The patient felt no discomfort from the procedure and behaved very well.

(Dr. Putnam)

VENTRICULOGRAM
April 4, 1924
Dr. Sosman

Attempted ventriculograms show a collection of air in the left occipital lobe, very irregular in outline and multi-locular in appearance. In none of the positions is any portion of the ventricle outlined. The pineal still appears displaced to the right.

Impression – The air is probably in the brain tissue. It may possibly be in a degenerated or cystic area.

SPECIAL NOTE
April 5, 1924
Dr. Cushing

This patient has surprisingly few symptoms except for high grade of choked disc, not even any complaint of headache at the present time. There are no localizing manifestations and an x-ray, after Dr. Putnam's attempted injection, shows a very peculiar, fuzzy appearance of a small amount of air in one hemisphere which did not cross to the other.

OPERATIVE NOTE
April 5, 1924
Anesthesia – Ether – Miss Gerrard

Right Subtemporal Decompression

The dura was found extremely tense and without fluid. Convolutions were flattened. The temporal lobe bulged immediately into the wound. Palpation showed it to be tense and as though there were an underlying tumor.

I inserted a needle at the depth of about 5 cm without getting resistance. I luckily got away without further damaging the lobe.

(Dr. Cushing)

April 7, 1924
Dr. Putman

Comfortable. Right disc 4 D., Left 4 ½ D.

DISCHARGE NOTE
April 18, 1924
Dr. Putnam

Right disc about 1 ½ D, left 1D. There does not now seem to be any difference in reflexes, strength, or sensation on both sides. Decompression bulging, but not extremely tense. Excellent general condition. Comfortable. Patient will discharged tomorrow, returning in 2 weeks for observation.

SECOND HOSPITAL ADMISSION

HISTORY

The patient was subsequently readmitted to Dr. Cushing's service with gait difficulty and markedly tense subtemporal decompression flap on December 30, 1924 (Please note the accompanied images called "Before second surgery.")

SUMMARY OF POSITIVE FINDINGS
December 30, 1924
Dr. Van Wagenen

SUBJECTIVE
1. History of a right subtemporal decompression in April 1924.
2. Symptoms and signs leading to this procedure-bilateral choked disc, with unlocalizable tumor, probably cerebrum.
3. History of generalized convulsion two yrs. prior to admission.
4. Slight spasticity of the left leg as compared to the right.
5. Freedom of headache, nausea and vomiting until about a weak ago.
6. Tense, bulging decompression all the time.
7. Improvement of vision, until patient can read newspaper print.
8. Slight change in personality, becoming somewhat more irrational.
9. Extreme nervousness at times, by which is apparently meant tremor of muscles.

OBJECTIVE
1. Apparent loss of weight since last admission.
2. Bilateral fullness of the discs; secondary atrophy.
3. Absent reaction of pupils to light, with questionable reaction to accommodation.

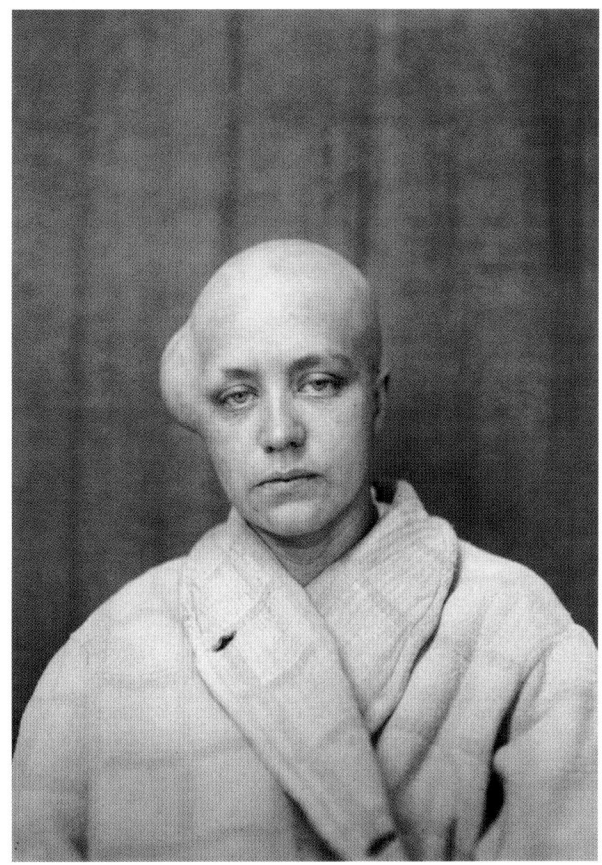

FIGS. 5 AND 6. BEFORE SECOND SURGERY.

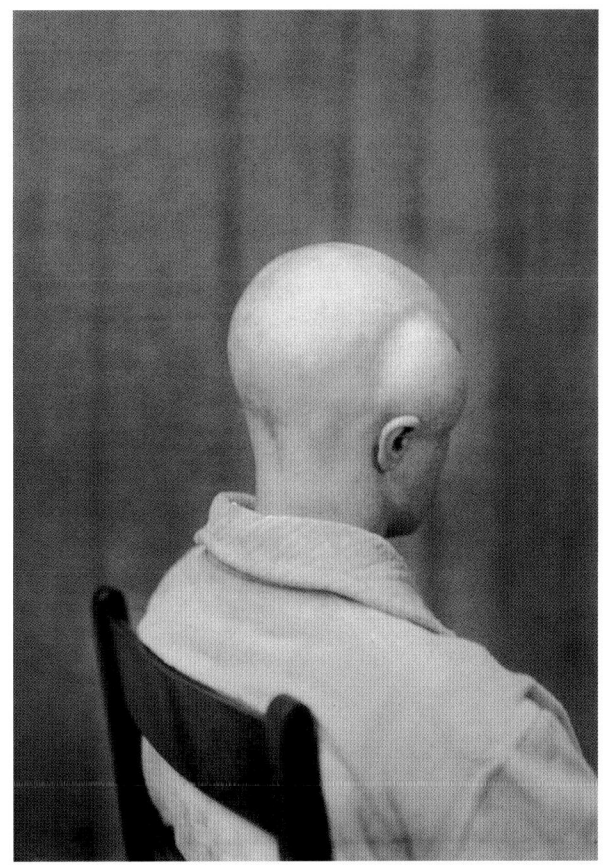

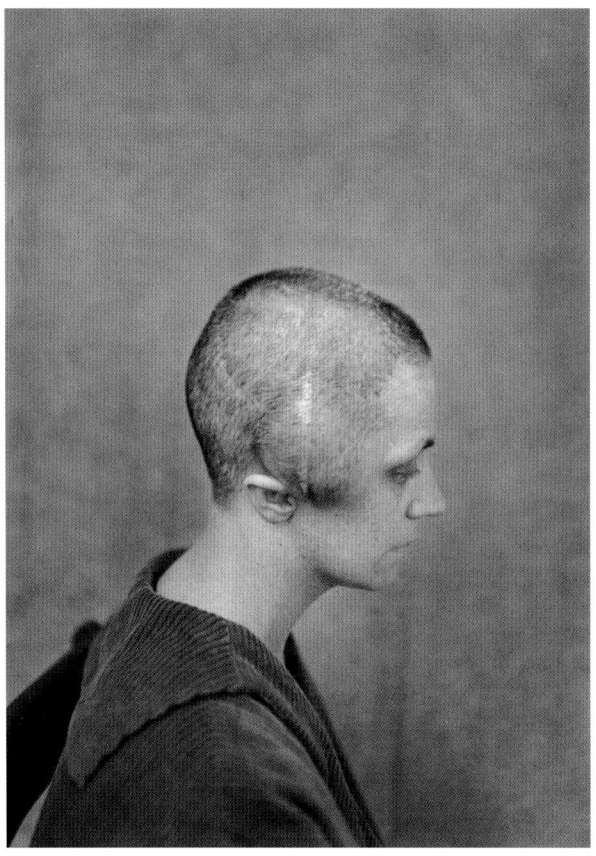

FIGS. 7 AND 8. THREE WEEKS POSTOPERATIVE AFTER SECOND SURGERY

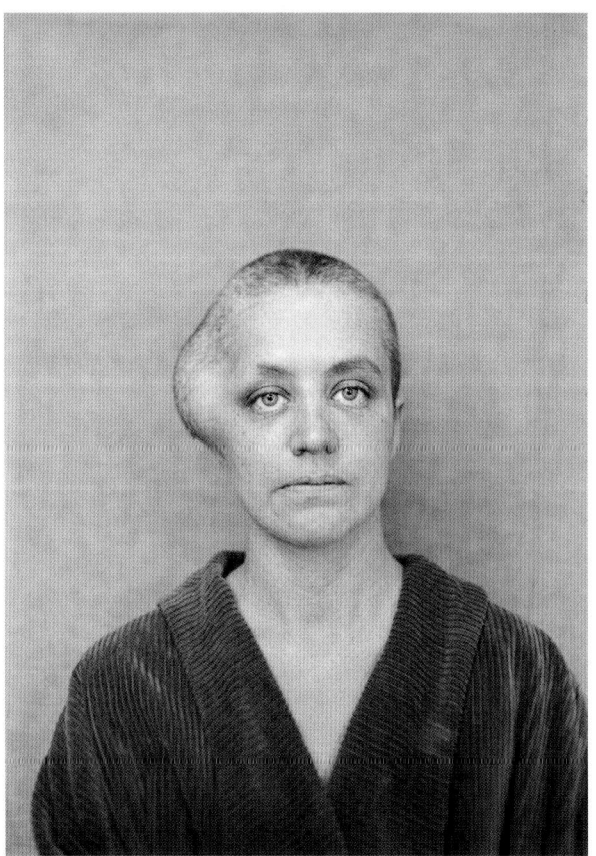

4. Deviation of the jaw to the right.
5. Staggering gait, positive Romberg, tendency to stagger to the left and backward.
6. Hyperactive reflexes, bilateral, more so on the left, – biceps, triceps, K.J. A.J.
7. Ankle clonus and patellar clonus on the left. Babinski on the left.
8. Very full, tense and compressible right subtemporal decompression.

IMPRESSION: I should be inclined to think that this was probably a tumor, very deeply situated, probably in the region of the 3rd ventricle, posterior part, or some point where it was interfering with the circulation of the cerebro-spinal fluid. It seems inconceivable that the enormous amount of tension budged by the subtemporal decompression could be caused from actual tumor substance and still produce little in a way of cranial nerve palsy or so few lateralizing symptoms. I believe that the decompression fullness is due to hydrocephalus, in turn due to some lesion above the tentorium rather than below. The few lateralizing symptoms present could well be due or associated with marked internal hydrocephalus as well as a subcortical lesion.

December 30, 1924
Dr. Wagenen

Patient has been placed on generous doses of magnesium sulphate, brisk catharsis, with limited intake of fluids. X-rays taken.

SPECIAL NOTE
January 9, 1925
Dr. Cushing

This woman had an illocalizable tumor though almost certainly a cerebral tumor in view of the findings at the time ventriculograms were undertaken. Almost certainly the peculiar ventriculogram is explained on the ground that Dr. Putnam had forced some air directly into the cerebral substance for more air was introduced than fluid had been removed according to his note.

The tumor moreover was probably on the right side owing to the persistent finding of increased reflexes on the left. Beyond this, there was nothing to go on except the fairly persistent notch in the lower right nasal field of vision. In view of what was found today, these were sufficient evidences to make a definite localization. However, I did not believe that we could depend too much upon the field of vision and aside from her general pressure symptoms the woman was really in very good condition.

OPERATIVE NOTE
January 9, 1925
Anesthesia: Novocain

Osteoplastic Exploration and Disclosure of Gliomatous Cyst in the Right Posterior Temporal Region. Replacement of Flap.

A large flap was turned down from the right hemisphere, disclosing a very tense brain. Subtemporal defect which was already a large one was increased slightly and incisions were made in its upper margin, permitting of a little more room.

The dura was extremely vascular and the bone in the upper anterior part of the field was comparatively thin. I thought that this might possibly indicate an underlying lesion. The chief vascularity was in this region and one could see through the dura some enormous dilated veins. A little more bone consequently was removed in this region and several punctures led me to think that there might be a meningioma. I presume that I must have missed my orientation sufficiently so that I had detected falx rather than tumor.

Search in other parts of the field had been negative for 2-3 openings and several attempts had been made posteriorly and anteriorly with the hope possibly of striking fluid.

I was about to close with the prospect perhaps of making a more thorough exploration of the frontal region at another session when to secure a little more relief from pressure I carried the posterior incision from the decompression area upward a little so as to expose the back of the temporal lobe. This area seemed somewhat soft and I inserted a needle, striking the ventricle and drawing off 4-5 cc of fluid. Another puncture struck a gliomatous cyst and about 5 cc of canary-colored yellow clotting fluid was removed. That this did not come from the ventricle is shown from the fact that another puncture subsequently got clear fluid from the ventricle. This leaves us without question that there is a large tumor, partly gliomatous, partly cyst, occupying the posterior part of the temporosphenoidal lobe - a tumor which has pressed upon the upper part of the geniculo-calcarine pathway and pressed somewhat upon the motor radiation.

The flap was then replaced and closed securely in layers. Patient stood the operation extremely well.
(Dr. Cushing)

During the postoperative period, the patient had a left sided hemiplegia which dramatically improved at the time of discharge. She also had a number of generalized convulsions.

DISCHARGE NOTE
January 29, 1925
Dr. Van Wagenen

The patient has done remarkably well since operation- is able to be up and about, is quite clear mentally and seems much improved to her family. Headaches nil. Nausea and vomiting nil.

The left side is a little weaker than the right and reflexes are hyperactive on that side with a positive Babinski. No hypesthesia could be demonstrated at time of discharge.

The decompression is now full and quite tense. Wound is in fair condition. Discs- secondary atrophy. First X-ray treatment given.

A LETTER FROM THE PATIENT'S HUSBAND
April 1, 1925

Patient has had her fourth X-ray treatment. The lump on the side of her head seems to have shrunk some and it is much softer than it ever has been since the first operation. She has had no sign of any convulsions since she left the hospital.

THE LAST LETTER TO DR. CUSHING
May 25, 1925

Dear Dr. Cushing,

You may think it strange to hear from me, but I feel I want to write to you and let you know I appreciate all you did for my wife, during her trouble. My wife passed away on April 29th, but I must say that considering her trouble, you certainly kept her comfortable until the end. She had a convulsion about a week before she died which left her paralyzed and blind, but she suffered no pain through it all. A few days before she died, she realized she was going to die and had no pain. She thought of you til the end and was conscious enough at that time to ask me to thank you for all you have done for her and I am writing this note to you simply to carry out her request as well as to show my own appreciation for what you have done for her.

Truly yours,
AH

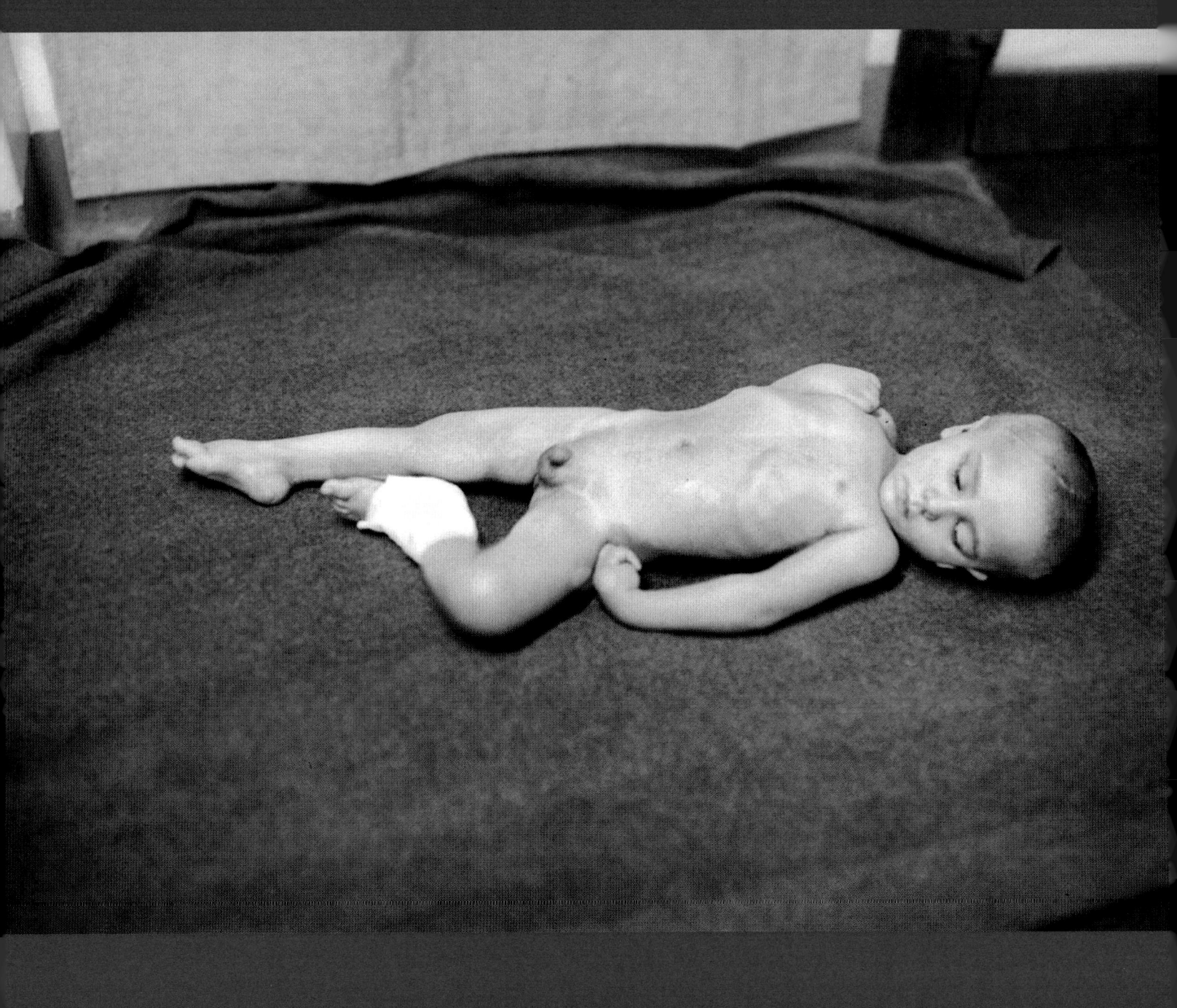

2.9 Thalamic glioma

SEX: M; AGE: 3.5; SURG. NO. 25919

HISTORY

The patient, 3 ½ years old, was a normal child at birth, breast fed for six months, and was always healthy and well. He developed progressive left sided weakness associated with headaches and nausea/vomiting since about a year before his admission to the hospital.

SUMMARY OF POSITIVE FINDINGS
March 10, 1926
Dr. Grant

SUBJECTIVE
1. In June 1925 the child began to drag the left foot.
2. In July 1925 left arm also involved.
3. Dec. 1925 onset of vomiting with headache and increase of symptoms in left upper extremity. Development of photophobia at this time.

OBJECTIVE
1. Head enlarged, separation of sutures in x-ray, cracked-pot sound to percussion, right and left.
2. Engorgement of veins of the eyelids, apparently equally on both sides.
3. Stiff neck.
4. Bilateral choked disc of at least of equally right and left. It looks like a secondary atrophy with marked increase in exudates and paling of the disc edge.
5. Left internal rectus weakness.

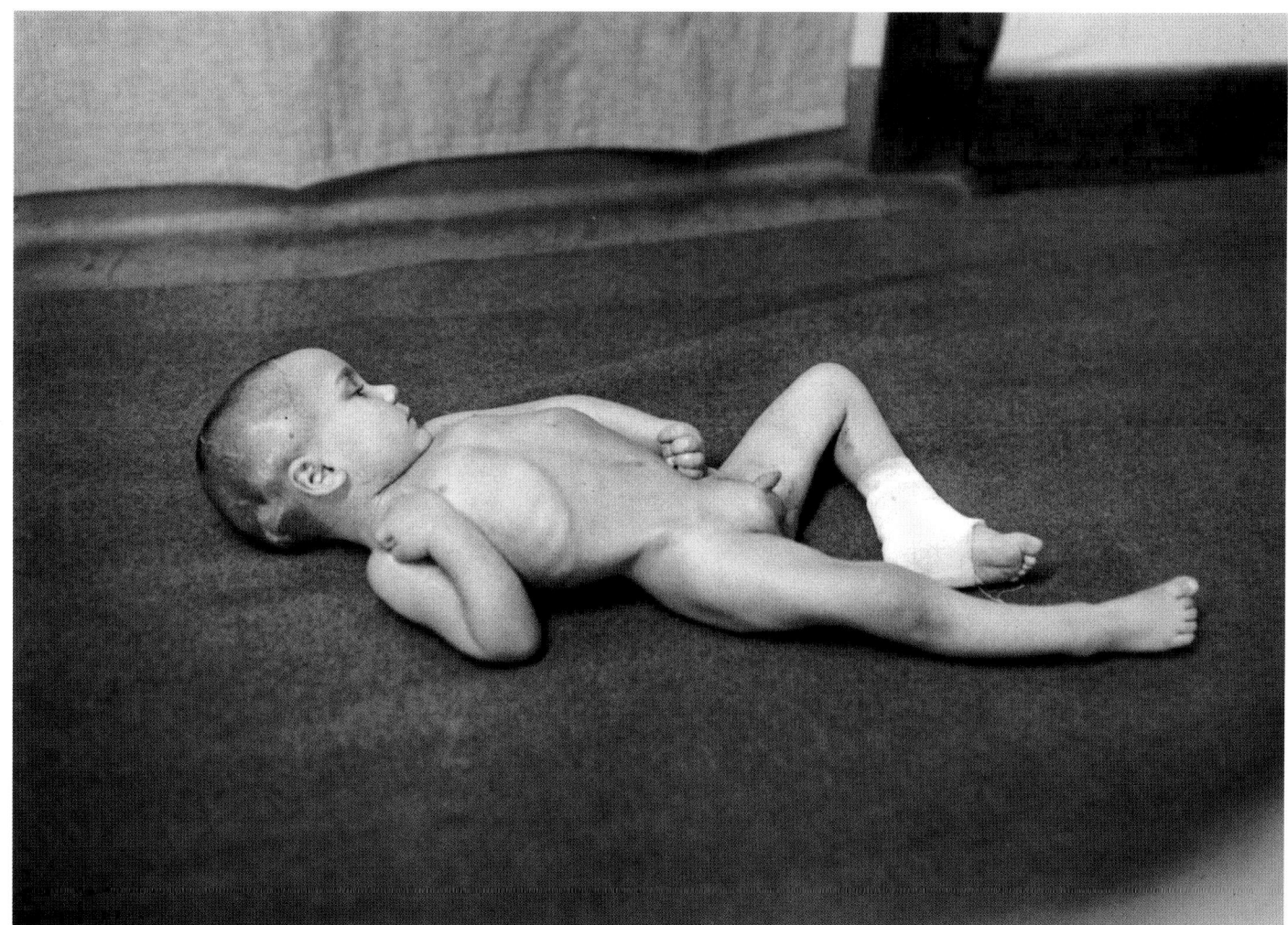

FIG. 2. POSTOPERATIVE — PATIENT "POSTURING/CONVULSING."

OPPOSITE PAGE. FIG. 1. POSTOPERATIVE — PATIENT "POSTURING/CONVULSING."

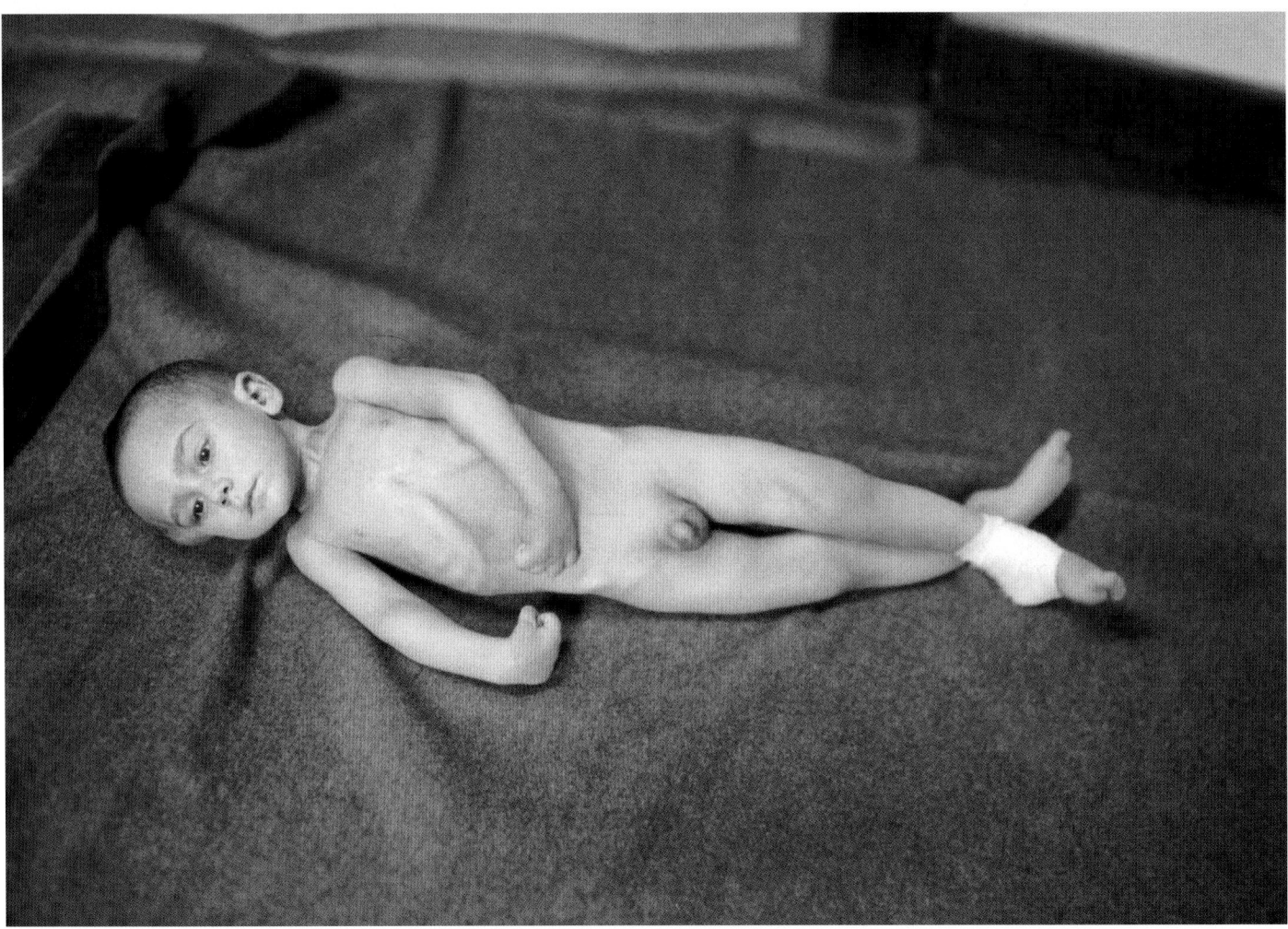

FIG. 3. POSTOPERATIVE — PATIENT "POSTURING/CONVULSING."

6. Weakness of the left face, lower division.
7. Paresis with spasticity of left upper and lower extremity.
8. Slight increase of ankle and knee jerks on the left side over the right.
9. Bilateral Babinski, more marked left than right.

IMPRESSION: Lesion of right cerebral hemisphere, probably neoplasm, although ? of abscess must be considered.

RADIOLOGY REPORT

March 9, 1926
Dr. Sosman

Right stereos and A.P. film of the skull show a thin vault with marked separation of sutures. The pituitary fossa is apparently normal. No localizing signs of tumor.

OPERATIVE NOTE
March 10, 1926
Anesthesia – Ether – Miss Way

Right Cerebral Exploration for Presumed Tumor. Finding of Internal Hydrocephalus.

It was the general opinion of all who saw this little boy that the most prominent feature of his examination was the definite weakness of his left side, and therefore, that he had a tumor, very possibly a large cyst, of the right hemisphere, as has been the case with 1-2 other similar children. At all events, no definite cerebellar signs could be demonstrated except that he did complain of considerable suboccipital tenderness and discomfort on flexion of the head.

A bone flap over the central area of the right hemisphere going well up toward the midline was turned down without difficulty, although there was rather more than the usual bleeding for a child along the upper margin. An immediate subtempo-

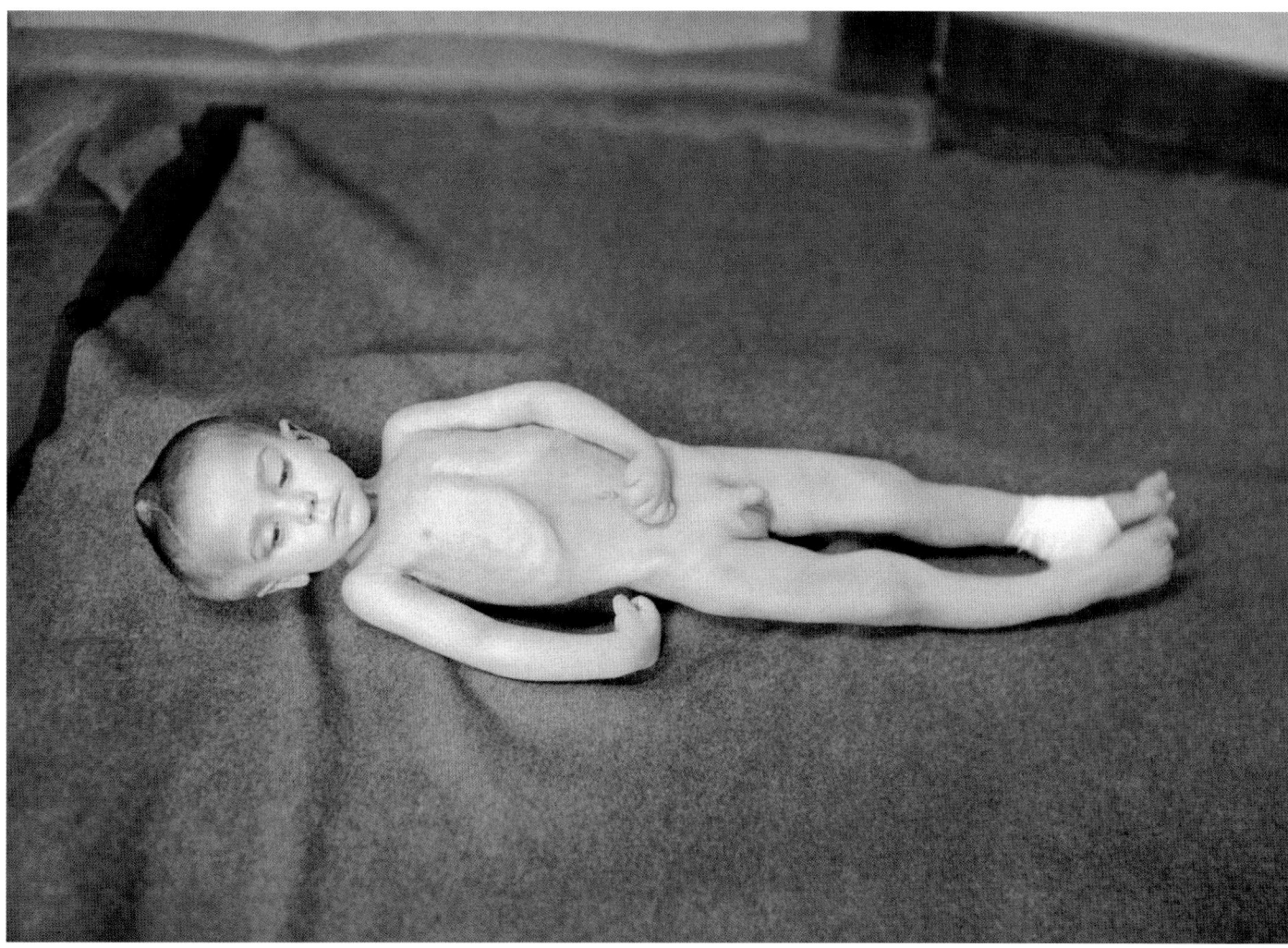

FIG. 4. POSTOPERATIVE — PATIENT "POSTURING/CONVULSING."

ral defect in the bone was made when the flap was broken up. The bone was quite thin throughout and there was considerable convolutional atrophy of the skull. The dura was under extreme tension but showed no surface abnormalities.

A nick was made in the posterior upper region of the area exposed and a needle introduced to a depth of 5 cm. reached no fluid. A needle was then introduced somewhat further forward over the upper central region of the area and at a depth of 3 cm. clear fluid in large amounts was encountered, obviously from a dilated ventricle. About 50 cc. of this fluid was evacuated at first, thus lowering tension completely, and the dura was then opened by a flap with its pedicle in the upper anterior part of the field. Upon exposing the cortex, it was noted that the convolutions were somewhat generally flattened throughout, perhaps a little more so in the post-central area than anywhere else, although this was not very striking. The whole hemisphere was fluctuant with the underlying hydrocephalus. Exploration was made beneath the dura around the whole area exposed going well up to the sinus in the median line, but no surface lesion was seen.

In view of the obvious internal hydrocephalus, it seemed sure that the child did not have a cerebral lesion but rather that his tumor, if such it be, is either pontine or cerebellar after all.

At Dr. Cushing's suggestion, the ventricle was pretty completely evacuated, about 90 cc. in all being removed and some 60–70 cc. of air replaced. This air injection was made through the upper anterior burr hole after closure had been made all the way around except over this area. Closure was made as usual by replacing the flap and stitching with fine silk without drainage. The patient stood the operation very well and was in good condition at the end. He was taken immediately to the x-ray dept. where ventriculogram studies were made.

(Dr. Horrax)

VENTRICULOGRAPHY
March 11, 1926
M.C. Sosman

Ventriculograms show markedly dilated lateral ventricles with no definite lateral displacement and no definite deformity except that the ventricles appear bumped-up somewhat as if by a suprasellar tumor. The third ventricle is not definitely seen but the air passed freely from side to side.

March 10–April 27, 1926

This patient was slightly more awake after surgery. However, he suffered from multiple generalized seizures and progressively developed "rigidity in his upper and lower extremities" (possibly posturing.) Dr. Davidoff, the house officer, took pictures of the patient while he was convulsing/posturing (Please see the accompanied photos.) Multiple ventricular taps relieved additional intracranial tension. This patient eventually died in the hospital of "respiratory failure."

AUTOPSY REPORT (BRAIN)
April 27, 1926

This is a brain of a child who died on the wards, after a prolonged illness which clinically resembles a condition of decerebration. The child was spastic and in all probability evidently had a lesion which would cut the cerebellar impulses from the body. Exploratory operation was performed with negative findings other than hydrocephalus. Brain has been removed without previous fixation so that it is greatly distorted and it is impossible to say how much this is due to the tumor, but unquestionably a large part is due to a huge tumor which obviously occupies the entire central area of the brain, chiefly on the right side. The huge tumor mass protrudes under the ventricle, pushes the chiasm off to the left and extends backwards and makes a shell of the temporal lobe and apparently extended through the region of the thalamus where a thick wall of a gliomatous cyst which has in all probability compressed the pons. The tumor has pushed the chiasm well off to the left and could it have been possible to detect the condition in so young of a child it would have certainly shown left hemianopsia. Tumor unquestionably belongs to the glioma group and is partly cystic.

A simple coronal section taken through the left part of the temporal lobe discloses a large necrotic tumor and as suggested by the description above, chiefly involving the basal ganglion on the right, but there has been at the same time dislocation into the hemisphere. The tumor measures about 6x6 cm.

(Dr. Cushing)

Blocks of tumor tissue were sent to the Harvard Medical School Museum.

The right thalamus is flattened out as a thin band along the distorted third ventricle. The corpus striatum and the internal capsule are totally destroyed. The tumor leaves the wall of the right posterior lateral horn and is covered only by a thin medullary layer.

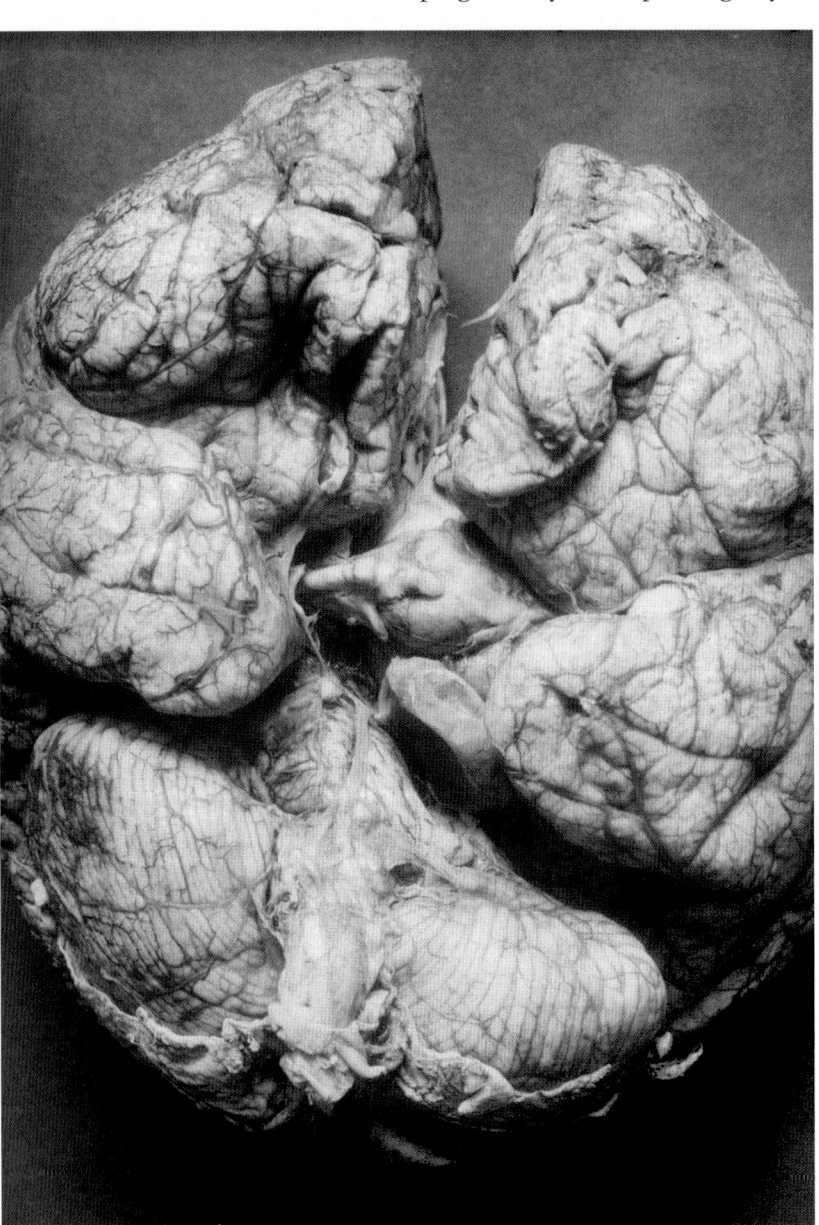

FIG. 5. AUTOPSY SPECIMEN.

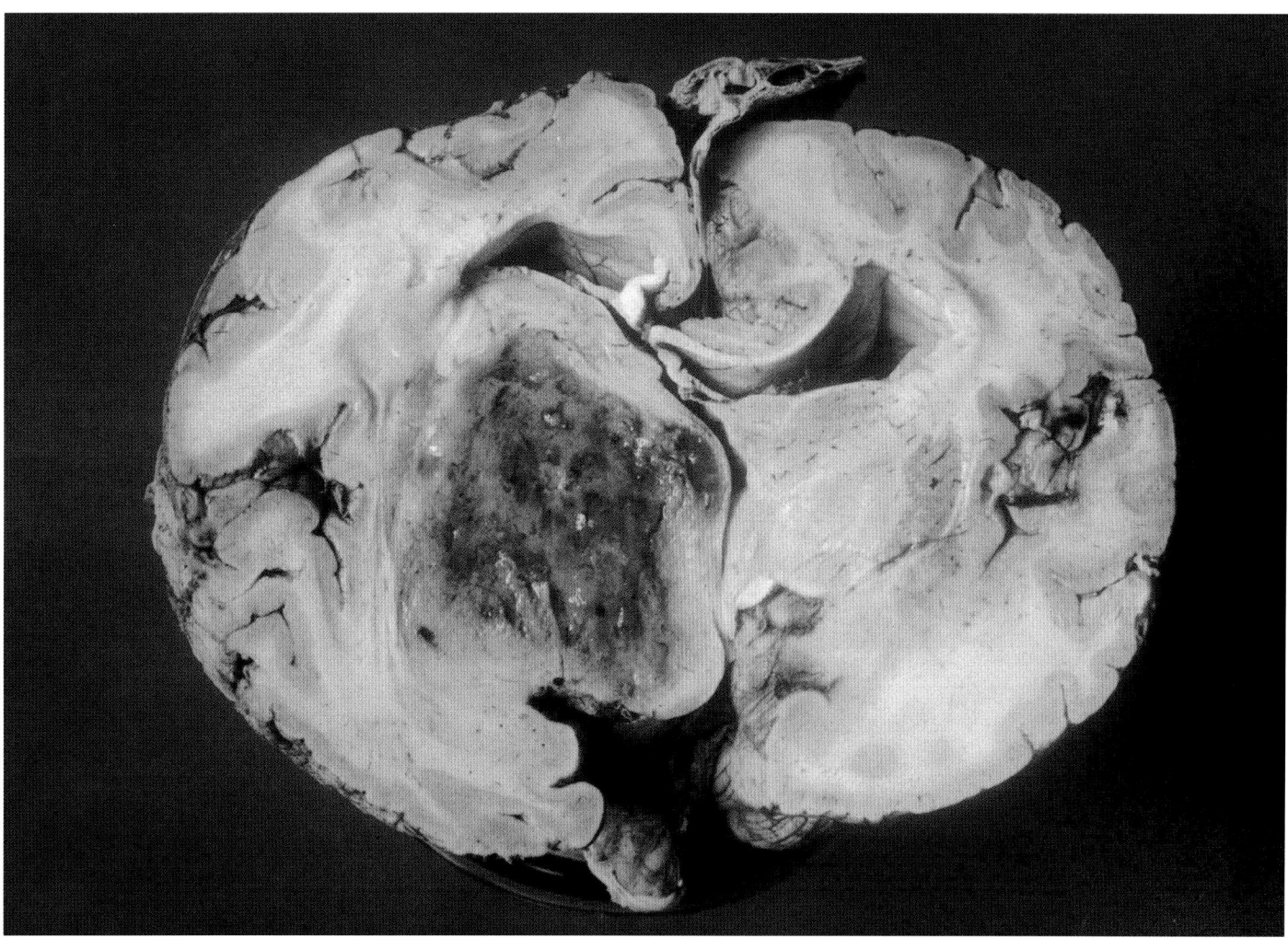

FIG. 6. AUTOPSY SPECIMEN – CORONAL SECTION.

An extraordinary dislocation caused by the tumor is well shown in section taken passing just through the anterior part of the pons. There is absolutely no sign on any of the sections of the thalamus or ventricular nucleus, though perhaps the thalamus is crowded upward above the tumor.

(Dr. Schaltenbrand)

Microscopic evaluation of the tumor was consistent with a "glioma."

2.10 Temporal fibrosarcoma

SEX: M; AGE: 19; SURG. NO. 27828; 28704

Record No 27828-Diagnosis: Cerebral tumor, unverified, right hemisphere.

Record No 28704-Diagnosis: Cerebral tumor, verified right temporal fibrosarcoma.

HISTORY

This patient presented to Dr. Horrax in December 1926 with progressive visual difficulties, vomiting, and headaches. Physical examination was remarkable for papilledema and left homonymous hemianopsia. A tumor in the right temporo-occipital lobe was suspected.

SUMMARY OF POSITIVE FINDINGS
December 17, 1926
Dr. Cairns

SUBJECTIVE
1. Failing vision for 2 months.
2. Vomiting for 7 weeks, especially in the morning.
3. Headaches for 3 weeks, mostly occipital.
4. Bumping into things on the left of him for the past 2 days.

OBJECTIVE
1. Bilateral papilledema, right possibly 6 D., left 4 D. but measurement on the right is doubtful owing to old ophthalmia with obscuration of the media.
2. Left homonymous hemianopsia.
3. Definite cerebellar signs, nystagmus, hypotonicity, more on the right side, inability to walk along a straight line, unsteadiness in the tandem position. Finger to thumb poorly performed.
4. Defect of vision in the right eye with diminished power of convergence and external squint - results of an ophthalmia at birth.

IMPRESSION: Tumor in the right occipital lobe.

SPECIAL NOTE
December 17, 1926
Dr. Bailey

It was a very great surprise to me to find the field defect when doing the visual fields. Without this finding I would have not entertained any diagnosis but that of cerebellar tumor. In view of the tenderness in the right occipital region and the absence of intimate seizures or any involvement of the right pyramidal tract, I think that the right optic radiation is affected in the occipital region. An inquiry should be made as to whether there have been hallucination of sight.

There was a question whether he had an occipital tumor or possibly one in the temporal lobe which is extending inward sufficiently far to reach the external geniculate body and possibly even deeper than this in the midbrain.

RADIOLOGY REPORT
December 18, 1926
Dr. Sosman

Right stereo, A.P. and P.A. of skull show thin cranial vault without localized changes. The pituitary fossa is normal. The mastoids are clear. The sinuses are also clear. No evidence of tumor or disease.

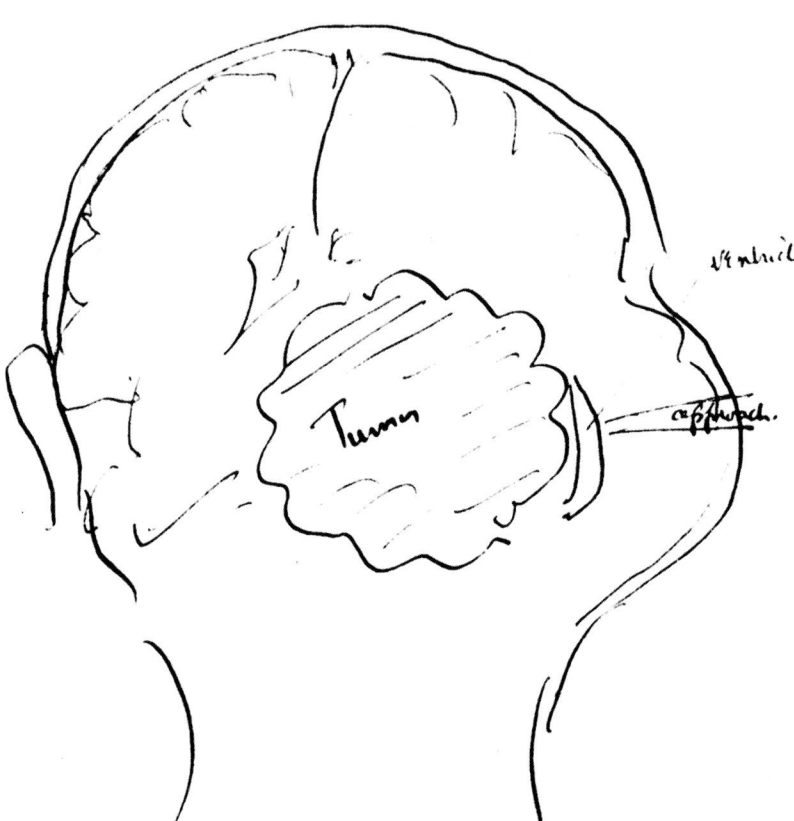

FIG. 1. OPERATIVE SKETCH.

appearance is that of fibrosarcoma and I believe it would be so regarded without hesitation if it presented in any other part of the body.

DIAGNOSIS – Fibrosarcoma (probably of meningeal origin)

(Dr. Wolbach)

SPECIAL NOTE
May 18, 1927
Dr. Cushing

This boy has not been doing well, owing undoubtedly to filling up of blood clot in his wound. The flap had been elevated and on 2–3 occasions bloody fluid has been sucked out from under it. He has been having stiffness of the neck and Mr. Cairns feared that he might have set up a meningitis. Remembering that we had completely shut off the temporal wound from the upper portion of the flap by suturing dura to upper edge of the old subtemporal decompression, I felt that we perhaps ought to re-explore the wound and am very glad that we did so.

OPERATIVE NOTE
May 18, 1927
Anesthesia – Ether – Miss Melanson

Reflection of Flap of Recent Operation. Disclosure of Soft Hemorrhagic Condition of the Temporal Lobe at the Site of Operation. Removal by Suction of Immense Amounts of Edematous Tissue with Great Fragments of Tumor and also Many Large Black Clots.

So soon as this flap had been reflected and the sutures above the subtemporal defect were divided, great masses of degenerated brain substance extruded into the wound and were removed by a sucker. So soon as the bulging temporal lobe was fully exposed, clots and degenerated brain poured into the wound and also many large fragments of degenerated tumor which had evidently been pushed outward by dislocation. It will be recalled that the first operation was somewhat bloody and had been conducted at a very great depth. I must have had some bleeding backward into the surrounding tissues. Many large black clots were finally sucked out as they presented themselves in the wound.

The tension was ultimately relieved and the flap was replaced and closed as usual in layers.

(Dr. Cushing)

May 25, 1927
Dr. Putman

Dressing changed. Wound is in good condition. Decompression bulging but soft.

General condition excellent. Able to sit up and has weak left arm and leg.

Left disc 1½ D., right impossible to measure.

DISCHARGE NOTE
June 5, 1927
Dr. Putman

Going home tomorrow. There is weakness and hypoesthesia on the entire left side of the body. All types of sensation are impaired on left. Deep reflexes exaggerated, ankle clonus on left. Left Babinski; left abdominal reflex absent. But patient walks without assistant. Patient will have X-ray treatment given at home.

FOLLOW UP NOTE
September 15, 1927
Dr. Putnam

Patient has had 10 X-ray treatments.

LETTER TO DR. CUSHING
April 21, 1928

(The name of the patient) died Thursday, his father would not consider autopsy.

Very truly yours,
Dr. Daniel McCann

Attached you can find Dr. Cushing's teaching slide illustrating the case of this patient.

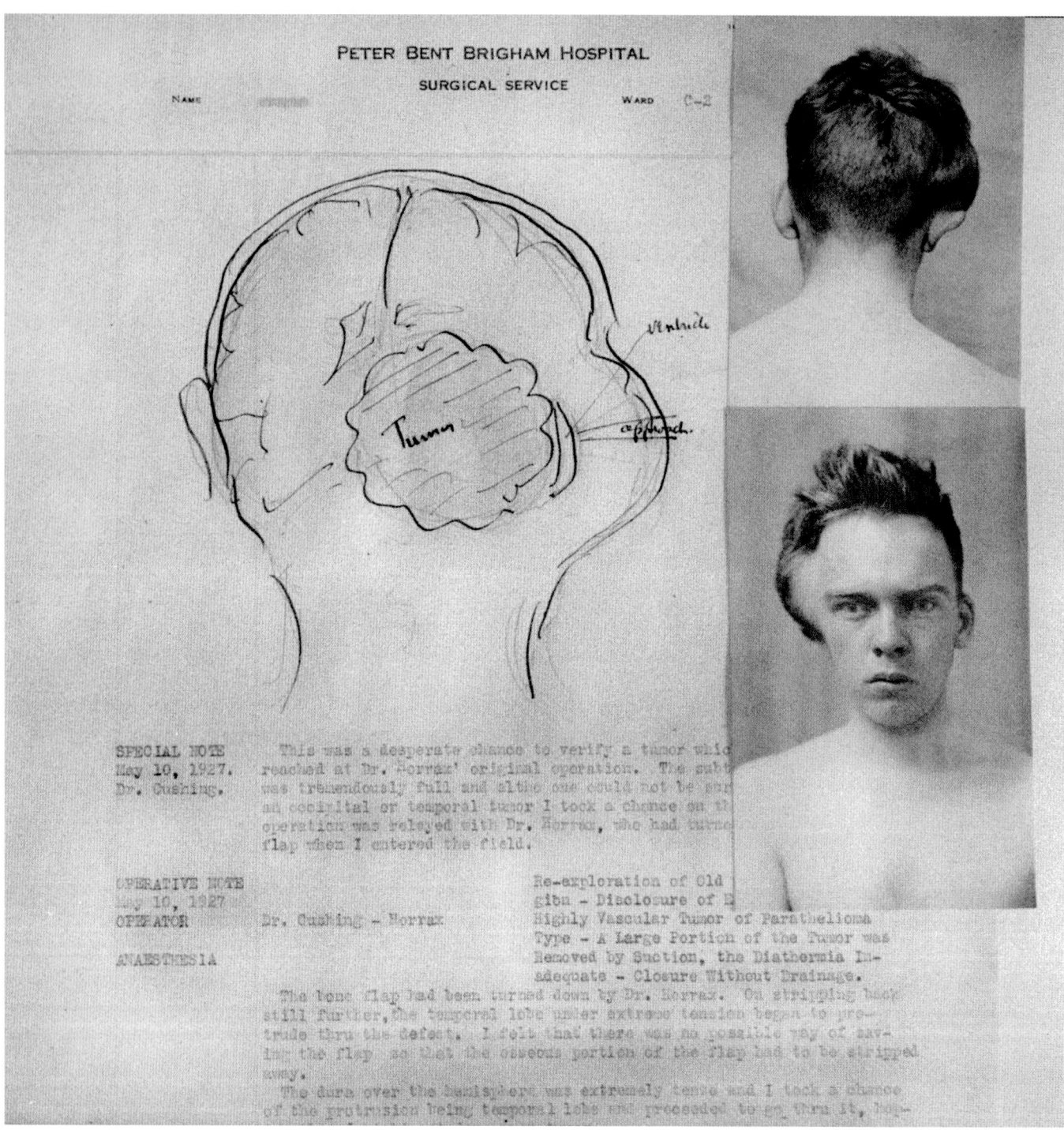

FIG. 4. CUSHING'S TEACHING SLIDE.

dure would be to turn down the flap once more and see if more of the tumor has not tumbled into the wound and shown a tendency to extrude itself. It is quite possible that in this way, we will make a fairly complete extirpation of what I take to be at the worst a comparatively innocent lesion – a blood vessel tumor, I presume.

(Dr. Cushing)

PATHOLOGY REPORT
May 10, 1927

There is a slight tendency to whorl formation in a few areas. In areas of beginning degeneration, the tumor cells are markedly vacuolated. The formation of collagen like intercellular substance is one of the characteristics of this tumor. The general

2. Discs slightly elevated, the left to 2 D.
3. Left-sided hemiparesis, almost complete, and hemihypesthesia, for all sensations.
4. Exaggerated deep reflexes on the left.

IMPRESSION: Tumor of the right occipital and temporal lobes.

RADIOLOGY REPORT
May 2, 1927
Dr. Sosman

Re-examination, right stereo, and A.P. of skull shows a bone flap in the right posterior parietal region with decompression at the inferior edge of the flap. There is a large soft tissue mass bulging thru this area and the bone flap is definitely elevated. The sella appears atrophic as if due to pressure. There are no localizing signs of tumor.

SPECIAL NOTE
May 10, 1927
Dr. Cushing

This was a desperate chance to verify a tumor which had not been reached at Dr. Horrax's original operation. The subtemporal region was tremendously full and although one could not be sure whether it was an occipital or temporal tumor I took a chance on the latter. The operation was relayed with Dr. Horrax, who had turned down the bone flap when I entered the field.

OPERATIVE NOTE
May 10, 1927

Re-exploration of Old Subtemporal Region – Disclosure of Enormously Deep, Highly Vascular Tumor of Parathelioma Type – A Large Portion of the Tumor was Removed by Suction, the Diathermia Inadequate – Closure without Drainage.

The bone flap had been turned down by Dr. Horrax. On stripping back still further, the temporal lobe under extreme tension began to protrude through the defect. I felt that there was no possible way of saving the flap so that the osseous portion of the flap had to be stripped away.

The dura over the hemisphere was extremely tense and I took a chance of the protrusion being temporal lobe and proceeded to go through it, hoping that I might get down upon tumor.

The diathermia loop was tried and I came across a number of sulci which I thought, as Dr. Horrax had done at the previous operation, might be tumor. A portion, indeed, was sent to Dr. Bailey for examination but it was nothing but cortex.

I then proceeded to go somewhat more deeply into the protruding hemisphere and at a depth of about 2 cm got into a large cavity of a greatly dilated ventricle. On stripping open this cavity, I saw what represented the inner surface of a highly vascular tumor, covered by blood vessels.

I cut away most of the huge protruding temporal lobe and finally got the surface of the tumor fairly well exposed. I hoped that I might be able to take it with the diathermia loop and removed one or two specimens for histological study but there was such bleeding that it was evident that this was not the right way to go about the extirpation.

I found fortunately that the growth was soft enough to remove by the sucker and so I proceeded to excavate it, getting a good deal of bleeding. I feared that we might need a donor and one was prepared and Dr. Horrax removed a large piece of muscle from the leg which I finally used in temporarily checking the bleeding.

As the tumor was cored its walls kept falling in so that I had nothing more than a channel to work through. Ultimately, there were a number of large pieces representing the surface of the tumor for it was quite enucleable and pulled up into the wound and were withdrawn. Had it not been for the bleeding and for the depth of the growth, I could certainly have taken out the entire lesion in this way. As it was, I must have removed fully ⅔ of the growth until tension was largely reduced.

There must have been still some bleeding at the bottom of the tumor but I did not see how I could control it and so left muscle and pledgets of cotton in the bottom of the cavity for some little time until I could try again.

Each time this maneuver was practiced, more tumor had fallen into the deep cavity and I was working fully at a depth of 6 or 7 cm below the level of the intact dura – consequently must have been well across the median line.

Patient's pressure began to fall off and he vomited so that I felt I had better withdraw.

The flap was then replaced, the galea was sutured to dura so as to confine the subtemporal part of the wound, the scalp was replaced and closed by Dr. Horrax.

Should this man have a postoperative filling up of the cavity with blood, I think the proper proce-

HOSPITAL COURSE

On December 26, 1926, Dr. Horrax performed a right ventricular tap and right temporo-occipital craniotomy/exploration; however, extreme brain herniation through the craniotomy defect limited the extent of the exploration to a subtemporal decompression and biopsy of the abnormal brain. The results of the biopsy showed no evidence of tumor or gliosis.

The patient made a satisfactory convalescence.

January 14, 1927

Patient received one X-ray treatment

DISCHARGE NOTE
January 16, 1927
Dr. Cairns

He was discharged improved. He had 2D. of choking in the left disc, was free from headaches and felt very well. There was a very slight weakness and hyper-reflexia on the left side. His visual field findings were unchanged.

SECOND HOSPITAL ADMISSION

HISTORY

The patient re-entered the hospital with increasing numbness and weakness of the left side. He noted a rapid swelling of the subtemporal decompression.

SUMMARY OF POSITIVE FINDINGS
April 30, 1927
Dr. Putnam

SUBJECTIVE

1. Onset of numbness of entire left side of body except face immediately after the operation.
2. Onset of weakness of left leg one month after the operation.
3. Weakness of left arm began about the middle of March and it has progressed rapidly until the arm is now entirely paralyzed.
4. Clonic convulsions of the left foot on two occasions during the past month.
5. Subjective improvement in vision with retention of crude visual hallucinations.

OBJECTIVE

1. Swelling of decompression with elevation of bone flap.

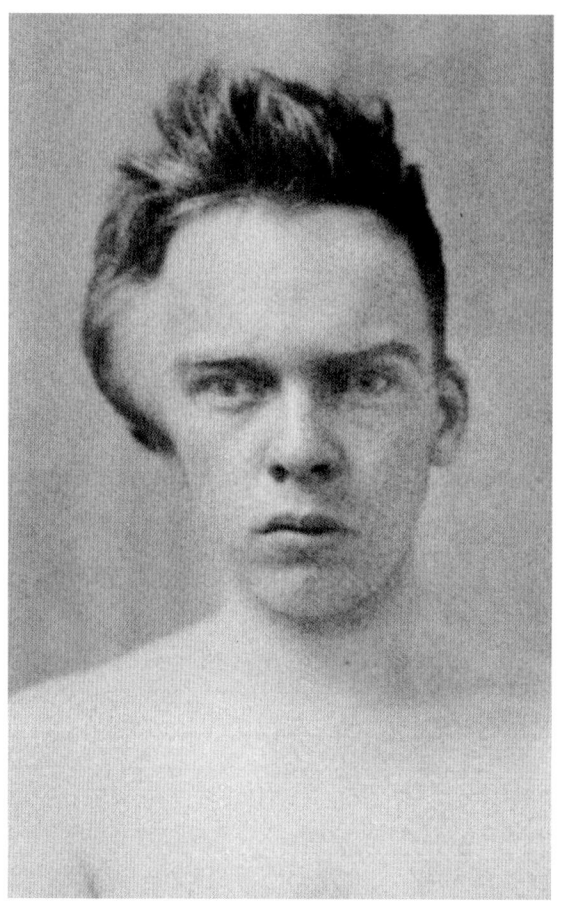

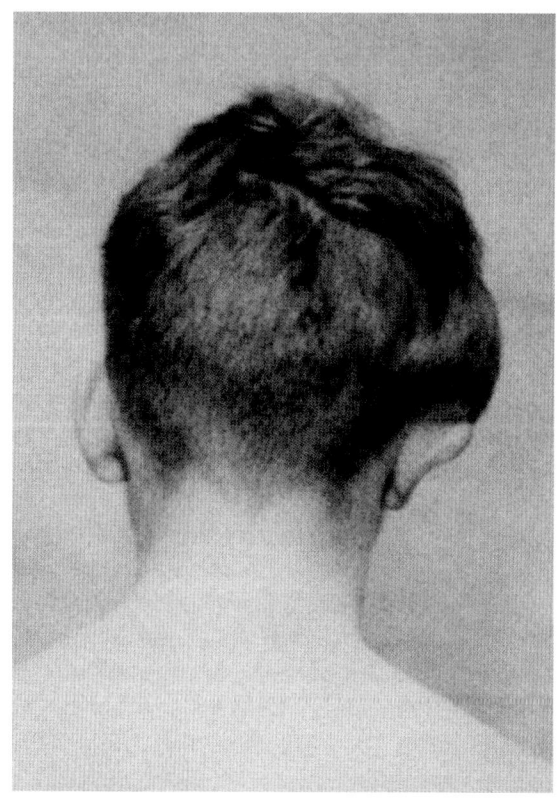

FIGS. 2 AND 3. PREOPERATIVE – BEFORE SECOND SURGERY

2.11 Pineal region tumor

SEX: M; AGE: 17; SURG. NO. 25286; 25737; 26935; 27053; 29664

FIRST TWO HOSPITAL ADMISSIONS

HISTORY

The patient started to suffer from excessive thirst and urination six months prior to this admission. He drank 4–5 gallons of water everyday. He was treated by pituitrin hypodermically twice a day without affecting his thirst significantly.

Owing to patient's continued emaciation, friends of family convinced the patient's mother that the boy had a tapeworm though on two occasions the medical service had informed her that there was no evidence of such infestation. However, the mother gave him a large dose of Dr. True's Elixir, together with the male fern and this was followed by two large doses of Epsom's salts, all on the day of discharge. The next day a third dose of salts was given with an enema and in the midst of this the boy collapsed and was taken back to the hospital.

During the second admission, the patient's exam showed an emaciated boy with acute abdominal distress, moaning and clutching his stomach. He recovered from his acute diarrhea and was discharged three days later taking 1 c.c. of surgical pituitrin subcutaneously every morning and 0.13 gm. of whole gland twice a day by mouth.

THIRD HOSPITAL ADMISSION

COMPLAINT

Loss of appetite, vomiting and severe pain in the stomach.

SUMMARY OF POSITIVE FINDINGS
August 9, 1926
Dr. Schaltenbrand

SUBJECTIVE
1. Development of polydipsia and polyuria in 1924.
2. This polydipsia and polyuria did not react to pituitrin injections.
3. It was cured by himself, by not drinking any more.
4. Rapid recovery of the patient after this.
5. On the 3rd of July patient got a severe psychic shock, his mother being struck by a drunken policeman and himself being knocked unconscious by this man.
6. Since that time severe stomach ache, vomiting and loss of appetite.
7. Metabolism (-20)

IMPRESSION: This patient seems to be not a neurosurgical case. Gastric ulcer ought to be ruled out. I have the impression that this boy is a psychopath with abnormal emotional reactions.

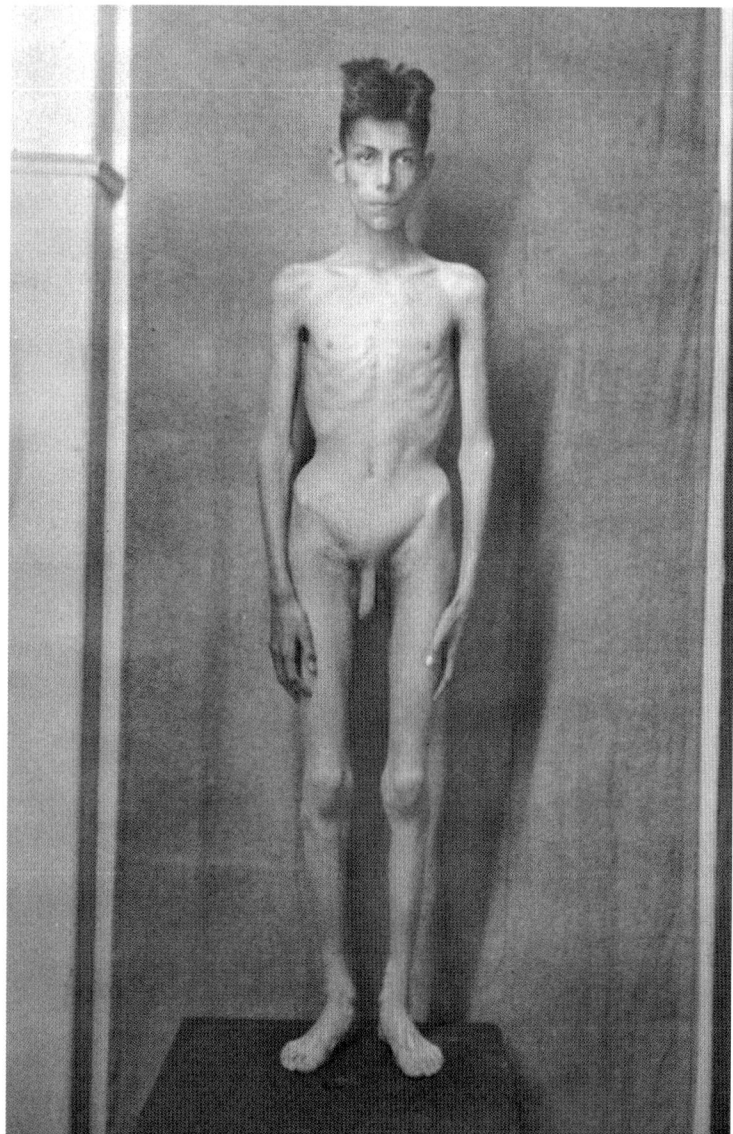

FIG. 1. TAKEN DURING FOURTH HOSPITAL ADMISSION.

RADIOLOGY REPORT
August 8, 1926
Dr. Sosman

Right stereos of skull show no localized changes in cranial vault except that the channel for the meningeal artery is larger than usual for this age. Pituitary fossa small and the sella is rather rugged. The pineal is in midline at the lower edge of normal.

DISCHARGE NOTE
August 11, 1926
Dr. Bailey

Patient was seen by Dr. Cushing who felt that he was not a neurosurgical case and advised transfer to medical service.

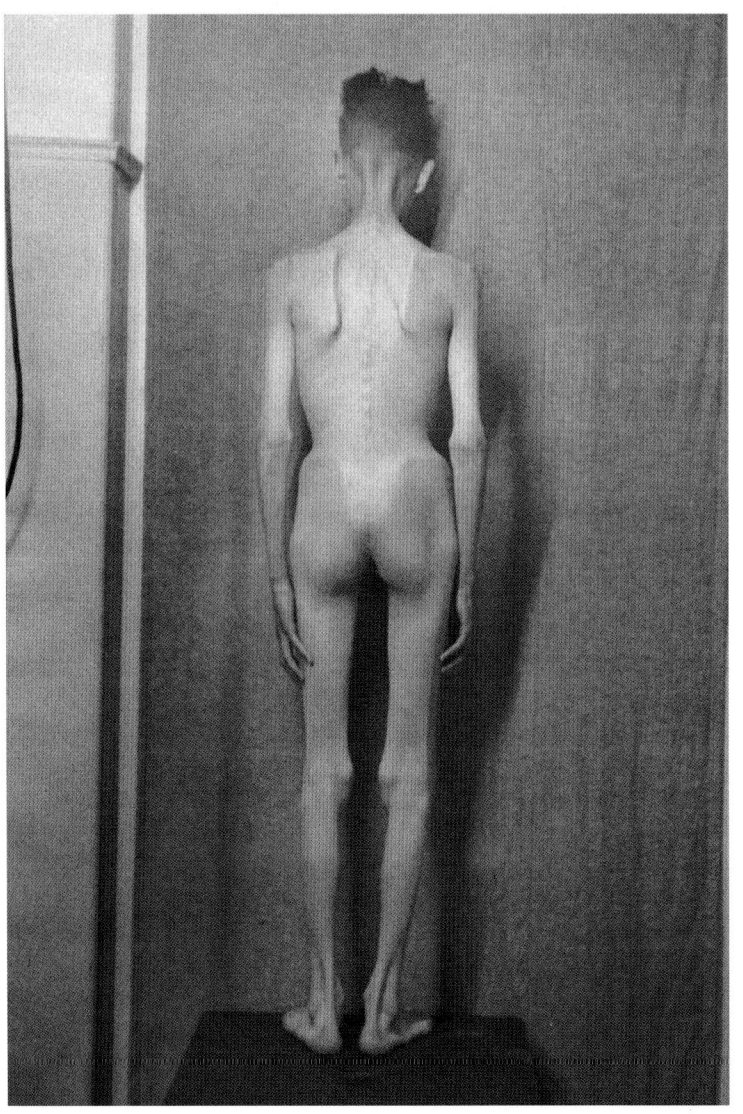

FIG. 2. TAKEN DURING FOURTH HOSPITAL ADMISSION.

FOURTH HOSPITAL ADMISSION

COMPLAINT

Vomiting and loss of weight.

ADMISSION NOTE
August 23, 1926
Dr. McLean

A neurotic boy of 17 with a negative F.H. and P.H. of "diabetes insipidus" which did not yield to pituitrin, and of which he "cured himself" by "will power," is re-transferred from the medical service for ventriculograms, a 3rd ventricle tumor suspect. Patient's exam is negative except for emaciation, vomiting and constitutional psychopathic inferiority.

IMPRESSION: Constitutional psychopathic inferiority.

DISCHARGE NOTE
August 24, 1926
Dr. Bailey

The patient was already in the operating floor, for ventriculogram, when he began to cry and refused absolutely any expective interference. Discharged.

FIFTH HOSPITAL ADMISSION

COMPLAINT

Headaches, failing vision and irrationality.

SUMMARY OF POSITIVE FINDINGS
September 18, 1927
Dr. Fulton

SUBJECTIVE

1. Three years ago the patient, then an alert and unusually precocious boy of 15, began to develop exceptional thirst with polyuria. He soon began to consume 4-6 gallons of water every 24 hours.
2. Entered this hospital on the medical service Feb. 6, 1925 and was treated for 2 1/2 months without improvement.
3. He re-entered this hospital a year and half later because of persistent nausea and vomiting. He believed then that he had cured his diabetes insipidus, by gradually diminishing his water intake voluntarily. X-ray, neurological and ophthalmological examinations completely negative at that time.
4. Gradual failure of vision, one month.

5. Excruciating headache, one month.
6. Persistent headache, one month.
7. Diplopia, three weeks.
8. Gradual loss of suprapubic hair during past year.
9. Periodic attacks of drowsiness during past three weeks.

OBJECTIVE

1. Bilateral primary atrophy with absent cupping, fullness of veins, and possibly slight elevation suggesting superimposed choking.
2. Bilateral hemianopsia.
3. Greatly reduced visual acuity, more left than right, probably 20/200.
4. Periodic attacks of narcolepsy, 4-5 times a day.
5. Left internal strabismus.
6. Periodic attacks of striking and yelling, apparently irrational but possibly due to headache.
7. No increased thirst.

IMPRESSION: The boy certainly has an organic lesion above his sella. As the latter is normal or possibly somewhat smaller than usual, a suprasellar cyst seems unlikely. However, X-ray appears to show early separation of the sutures but no suprasellar calcification. A suprasellar cyst certainly cannot be excluded. The periodic narcolepsy with the history of diabetes insipidus certainly suggests a tumor of the hypothalamus, possibly a glioma. In view, however, of the atrophy, the superimposed pressure symptoms a suprasellar cyst seems somewhat more probable.

RADIOLOGY REPORT
September 16, 1927
Dr. Sosman

A.P., P.A. and right stereos of the skull show a smooth vault with some slight separation of the lambdoid suture and probably slight signs of increased pressure. The sella appears normal. There is no calcification seen. The mastoids are clear. No localizing signs of tumor.

DISCHARGE NOTE
September 19, 1927
Dr. Fulton

The boy was seen by a night supervisor at 3:30 A.M. and was thought to be in good condition. He

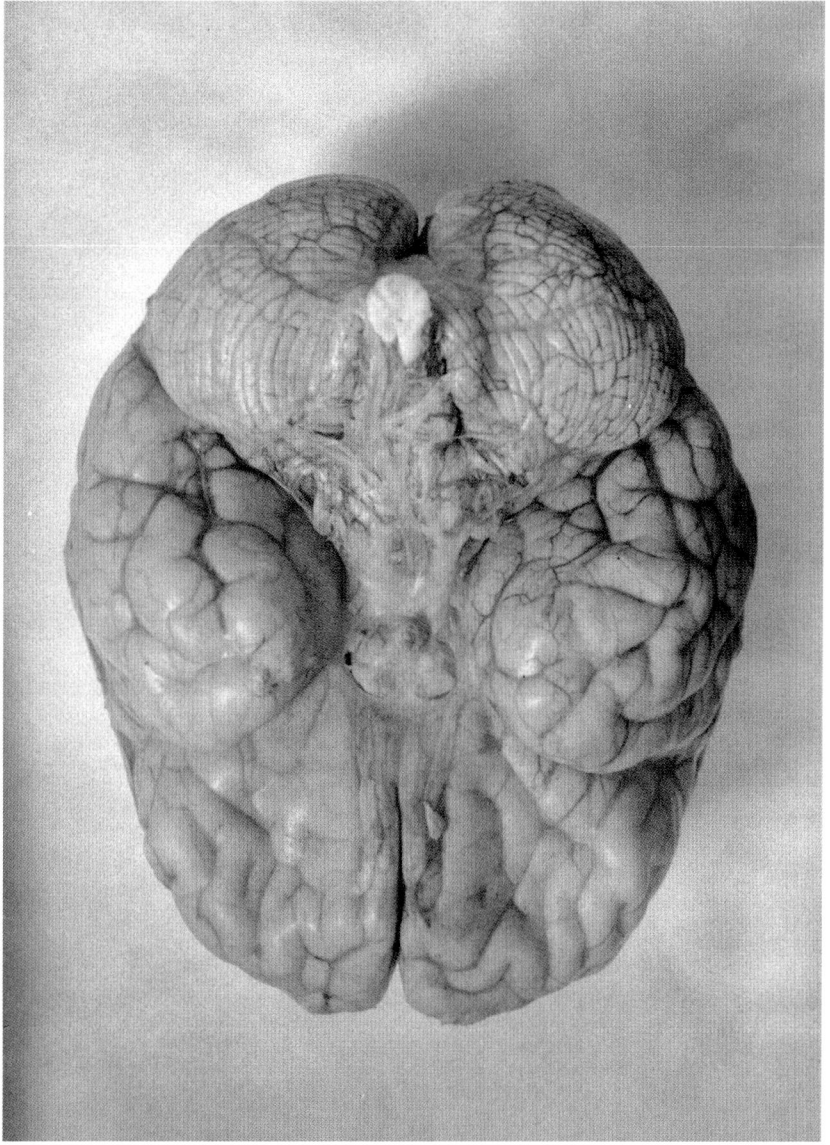

FIG. 3. AUTOPSY SPECIMEN.

was asleep but breathing quietly and she did not attempt to disturb him. At 5:30 a nurse looked at him again when it was noticed that he was not breathing. Seen by Dr. Cairns a few minutes later he was already in rigor, most marked in his right upper extremity; there were no signs of violence. There were no relatives present and he was not on the D.L.

Permission for autopsy was obtained by Dr. Cushing this morning with some difficulty.

AUTOPSY REPORT
September 19, 1927
Dr. Bailey
Dr. Schulz

Diagnosis: Malignant tumor. Pinealoma.

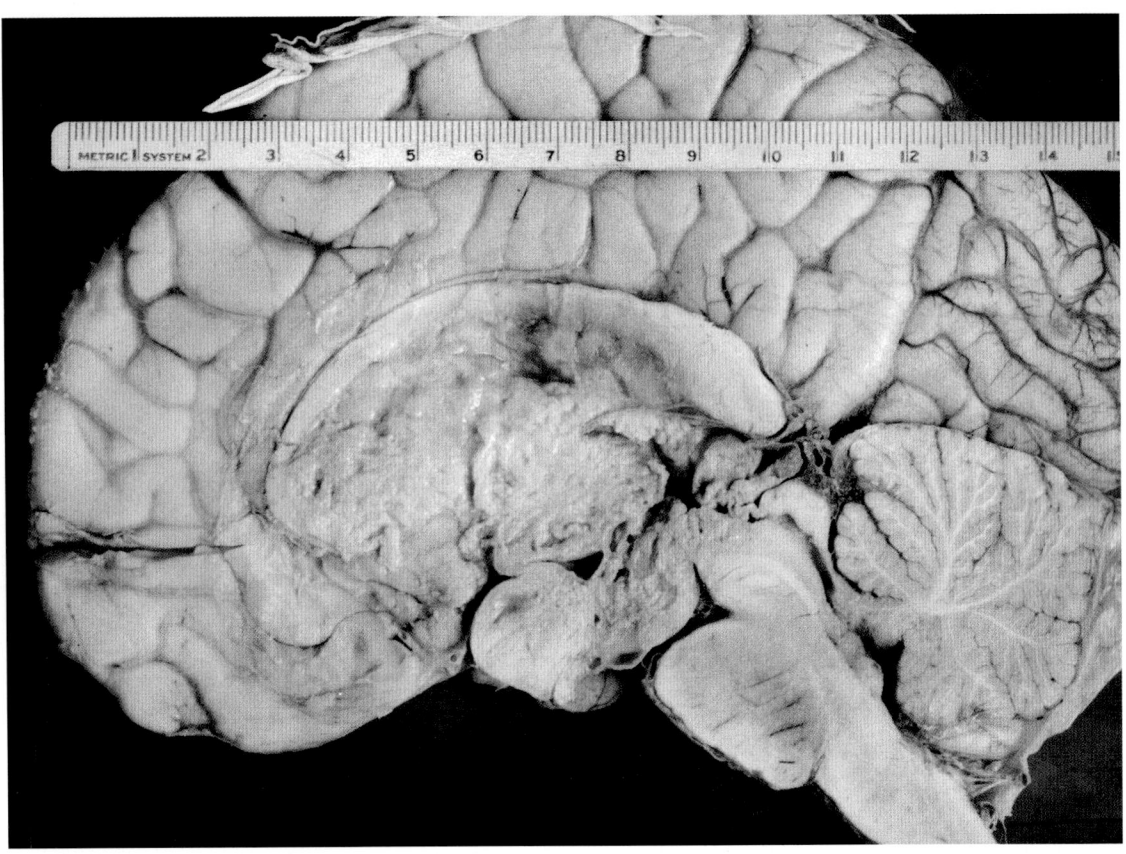

FIG. 4 AND 5. SAGITTAL SECTIONS OF THE BRAIN.

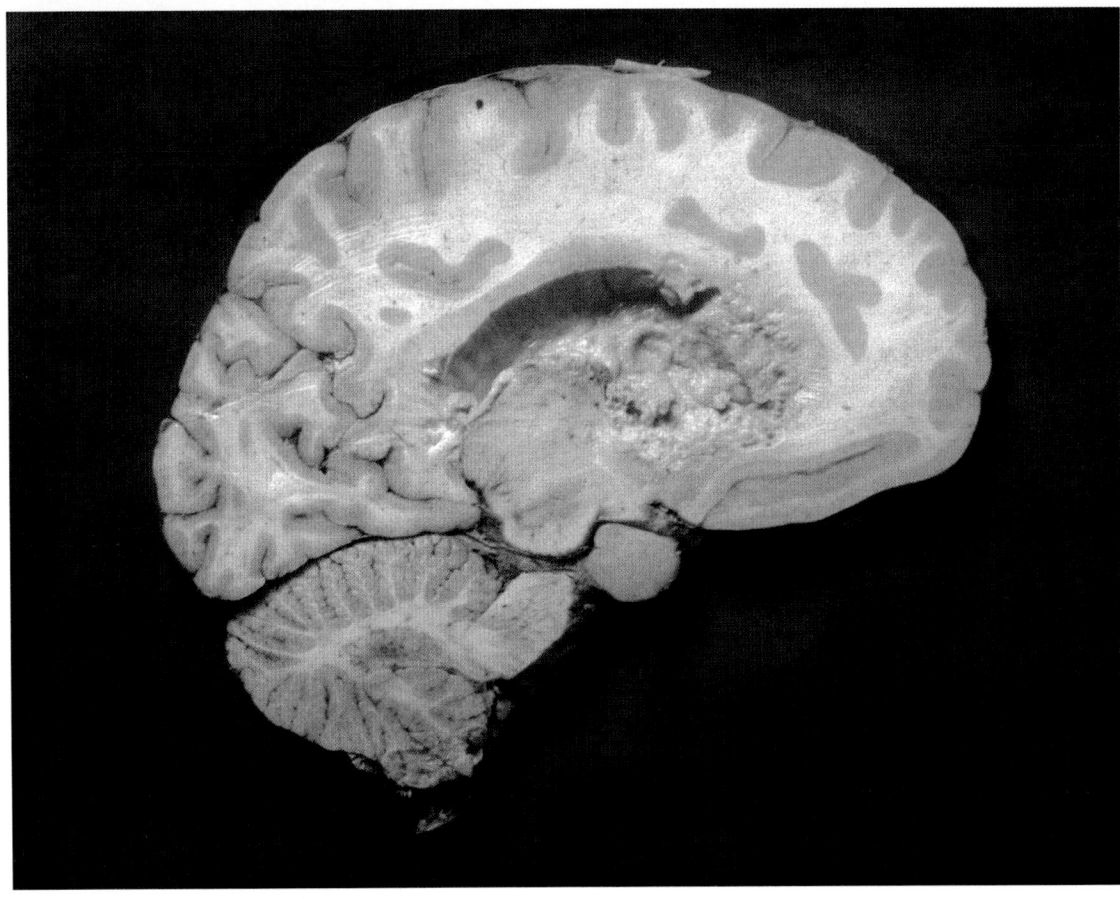

From the gross appearance of the other tissue of the body there is no pathology other than an apparent decrease in the size and consistency of the adrenal gland.

Exteriorly the brain shows a flattening of the cerebral convolutions and a grayish white tumor mass in the region of the 3rd ventricle covering and enclosing the optic chiasm. There is a little nubbin of tumor which compresses the central part of the pituitary body.

The middle ear cavities and accessory nasal sinuses as well as the sinuses of the dura are free from signs of any pathological changes.

The meninges are quite thickened and opaque around the region of the hypophysis and the optic chiasm. It was quite evident that the optic nerves after entering the optic foramen, spread out suddenly into a tumor mass 2 1/2 x 2 cm in diameter which occupied the region of the optic chiasm and to the under surface to which is attached the stalk of the hypophysis.

When the brain was sectioned by median, sagittal sections however, there was disclosed in addition to a more or less pedunculated mass a couple of cm in diameter which had been seen on the under surface of the brain that the entire 3rd ventricle is filled with a soft grayish red, avascular mass of tumor, which completely filled the third ventricle. The septum lucidum was no longer visible and the tumor seems to invade somewhat the under surface of the corpus callosum. There could also be seen nodules of tumor in the floor of the 4th ventricle. The aqueduct of Sylvius however is free. From its medial surface it was thought that the tumor was probably a glioma of the septum pellucidum and shows a nodule which was calcified, about 5 cm in diameter in the position of the pineal body, the normal structure of which could not be recognized.

Sagittal sections were made of each hemisphere, disclosing a dilation of the lateral ventricles and showing also that the walls of the ventricles were covered with nodules of the same grayish tumor. The choroid plexus of the lateral ventricles seems to be quite filled with tumor growth. Blocks of tissue were taken from the posterior portion of the 3rd ventricle, including the splenium of the corpus callosum, pineal body and corpora quadrigemina and another was taken from the tuber cinereum including the optic chiasm and stalk of the hypophysis.

Examination of the microscopic specimen shows the tumor to be a typical pinealoma, the characteristic association of large cells with large vesicular nuclei, containing heavy nucleoli and long strands of lymphoid around the vessel, being quite characteristic of this growth. The tumor was therefore of pineal origin and it is as very likely, as has been apparent in other cases of my experience that a fragment of tumor broke off and fell into tuber cinereum and growing, gave rise to a diabetes insipidus.

Other cells or masses of cells found their way into the lateral ventricles and down into the 4th ventricle, undoubtedly other cells were found by lumbar puncture in the fluid removed on such occasions for the clinicians are puzzled by the number of cells which they found, the number being too great to correspond with the other fluid findings. The minute examination of these cells was not made but it is very likely that they were tumor cells, considering the wide spread metastases present in the ventricular system.

(Dr. Bailey)

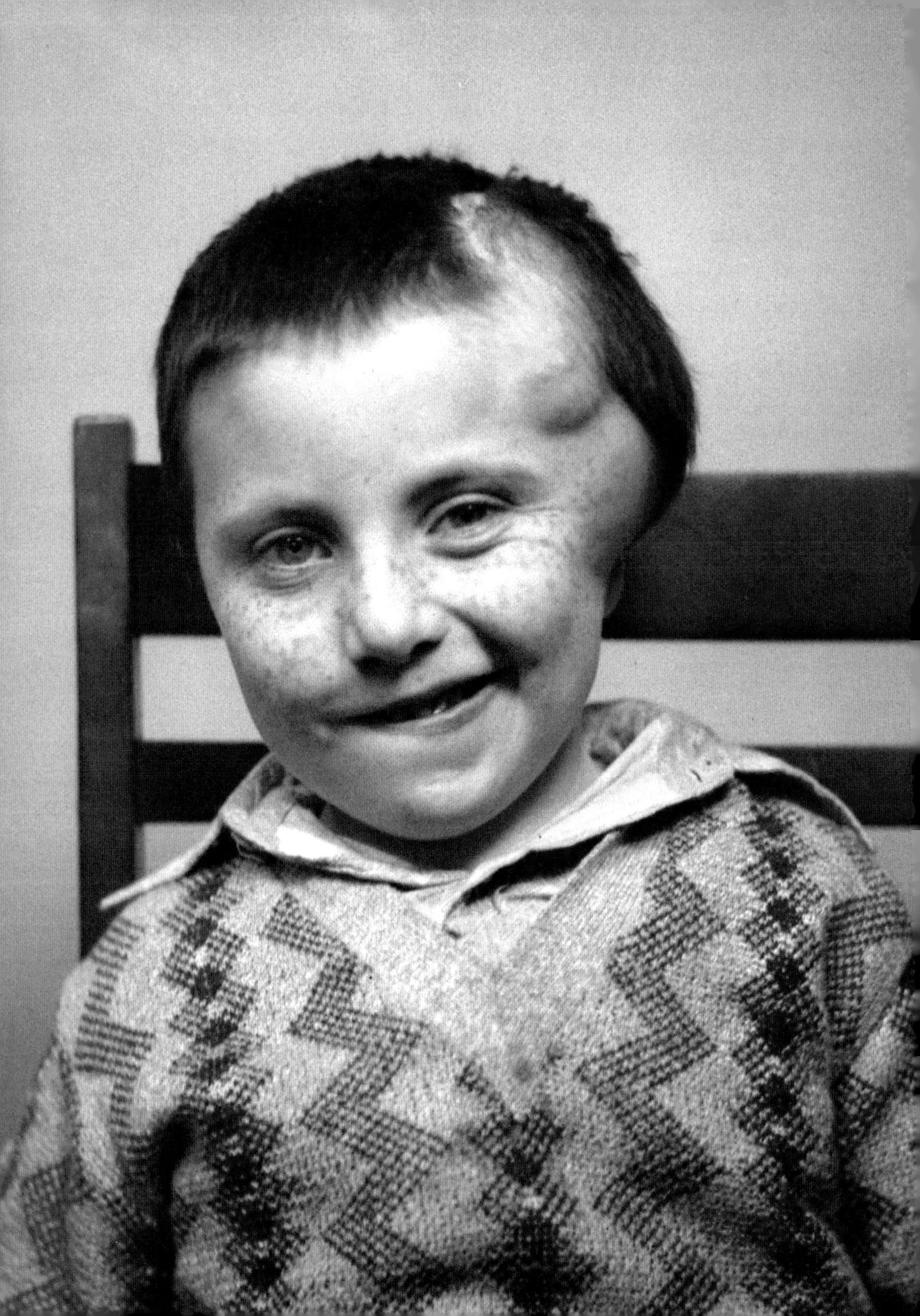

12 Left fronto-temporal medullablastoma (Radium bag)

SEX: M; AGE: 6; SURG. NO. 35201, 35660, 36443

Diagnosis:

Surg. No: 35201 – Glioma? Craniopharyngioma?

Surg. No: 35660 – Astroblastoma

Surg. No: 36443 – Medulloblastoma, verified.

HISTORY

This six-year-old boy was admitted to the hospital with a four-month history of frontal headache, nausea and vomiting.

SUMMARY OF POSITIVE FINDINGS
November 10, 1929
Dr. Oldberg

SUBJECTIVE
1. History of peculiar transient swelling in front of the right ear since April 1929.
2. History of nausea and vomiting since April 1929.
3. History of frontal headaches since July 1929.

OBJECTIVE
1. Bruit heard in the right orbit.
2. Bilateral acute choked discs, 5 D on right, 4½ D on left.
3. Marked right lower facial weakness of central type.
4. Slight spastic paresis of left arm and leg.

IMPRESSION: Left cerebral lesion, most likely tumor. Possibility of abscess must be borne in mind. Ventriculograms indicated.

RADIOLOGY REPORT
Dr. Sosman
November 12, 1929

The sella appears normal and the mastoids are clear. No localizing signs of tumor.

SPECIAL NOTE
November 22, 1929
Dr. Cushing

This boy is said to have nothing to show clinically except a high grade choked disc, and a slight weakness of the left face. He had a high grade choked

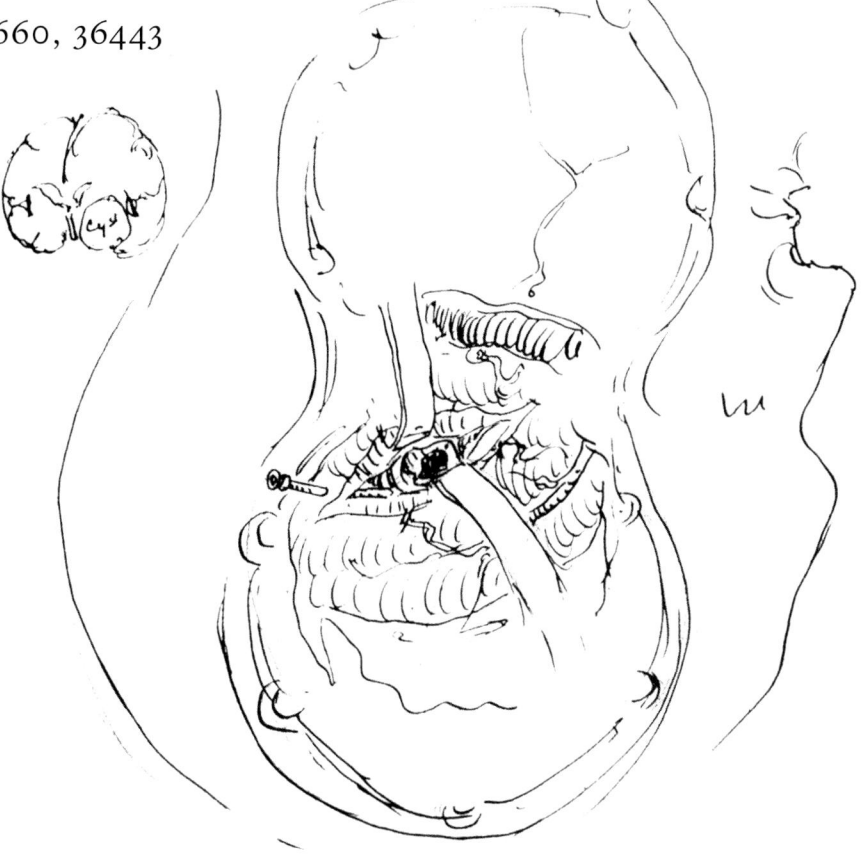

FIG. 2. OPERATIVE SKETCH (FIRST OPERATION).

disc and operation was therefore scheduled as an emergency. Not being quite sure where the growth would lay, a preliminary ventriculogram was made.

VENTRICULOGRAPHY
November 22, 1929
Dr. Horrax
Anesthesia – Novocain

The needle was introduced into the right ventricle, and a small amount of fluid, under tension was secured. Air was introduced, and x-ray showed definite distortion of the ventricles to the right side with what appeared to be a probable large tumor in the temporal lobe to the inner side of the ventricular horn.

RADIOLOGY REPORT
November 22, 1929
Dr. Sosman

Ventriculograms show fairly marked displacement

OPPOSITE PAGE. FIG. 1. PREOPERATIVE BEFORE SECOND SURGERY.

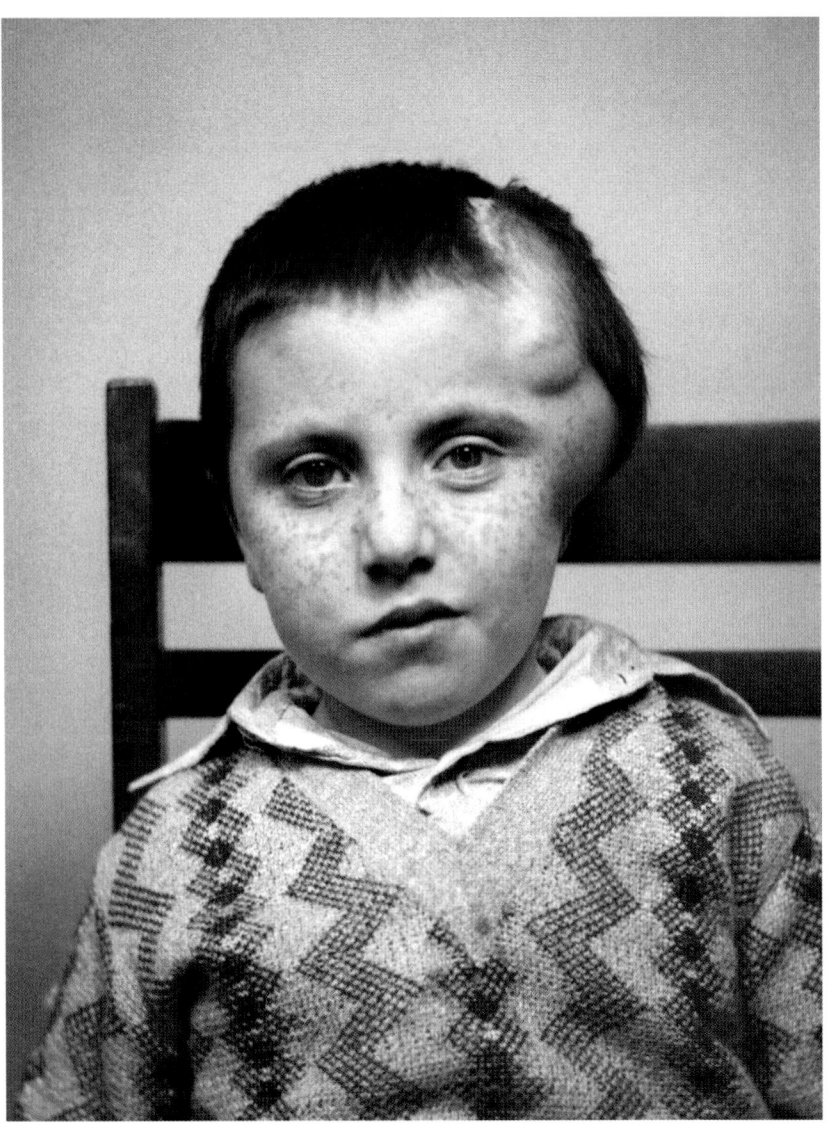

FIG. 3. PREOPERATIVE BEFORE SECOND SURGERY.

of both anterior horns to the right of the midline and the left ventricle appears displaced slightly upward in addition. The left ventricle is not filled in the lateral stereos. The P.A./view shows distortion of the left ventricle with lateral displacement of the temporal horn. Both ventricles are displaced slightly to the right of the midline. The findings indicate a deep left temporal lobe tumor.

SPECIAL NOTE
November 22, 1929
Dr. Cushing

It should be stated that this boy had some slight fever, and leukocytosis, and Dr. Horrax was under the impression that he might have an abscess. Nevertheless it seemed best to me to turn down a bone flap, for the symptoms had been present for a long time, and were it an abscess we might conceivably have extirpated it by electrosurgical methods.

The operation was relayed with Dr. Horrax.

OPERATIVE NOTE
November 22, 1929
Anaesthesia – Ether – Miss Keach

Reflection of Left Central Osteoplastic Flap with Subtemporal Decompression. Exceedingly Tense Dura. Series of Punctures, One of These Striking a Deep-Seated Xanthochromic Cyst, Probably Containing 30 cc of Fluid. Transcortical Electrosurgical Excision with Fragmentary Removal of Tissue from Cyst Wall for Verification.

Dr. Horrax had turned down the bone flap in this case and made the decompression when I entered the field. The dura was exceedingly tense. It was opened and reflected. A tense, dry brain protruded. There was no surface indication on palpation where the lesion might lie. The Sylvian veins were not pushed forward. On the chance of finding a temporal lobe lesion, I inserted a series of three needles in the left, and came down twice upon resistance at a depth of 2–3 cm. As events turned out, this resistance was merely due to dislocated gyri which I encountered. Each of these punctures bled slightly. A third puncture was made in the situation indicated in the sketch, and entered a cyst at a depth of about 6 cm. Probably 2 cc of highly xanthochromic fluid escaped.

With the needle still in place, I made a transcortical incision, as shown, having some difficulty in doing so, as I had to go across some gyri. Finally at a depth of fully 5 cm, I came down upon a cyst which was fully evacuated, but as it was collapsed markedly it was extremely difficult to determine the nature of its walls, for I was unable to look freely into it. A small fragment of tissue was removed from the wall over the cyst, said to be cortex. After wiping out the cyst I got another small piece of tissue which showed tumor.

The edges of the incision were drawn together, dura laid back in place without suturing, and the flap replaced, and closed by Dr. Horrax.

(Dr. Cushing)

PATHOLOGY REPORT
November 22, 1929
Dr. Eisenhardt

The first specimen submitted was cortical tissue.

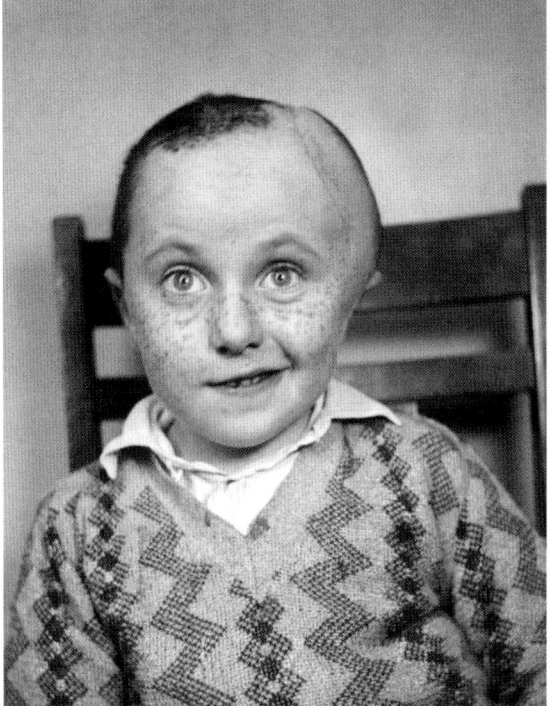
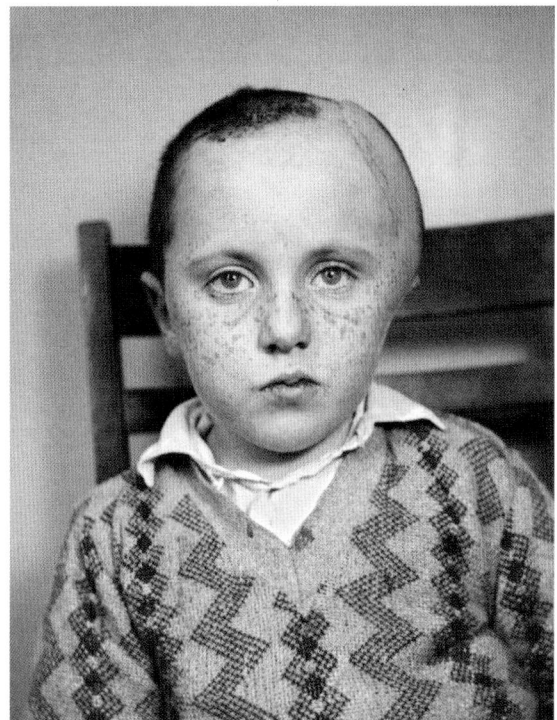

FIGS. 8 AND 9. FOUR WEEKS AFTER SECOND SURGERY.

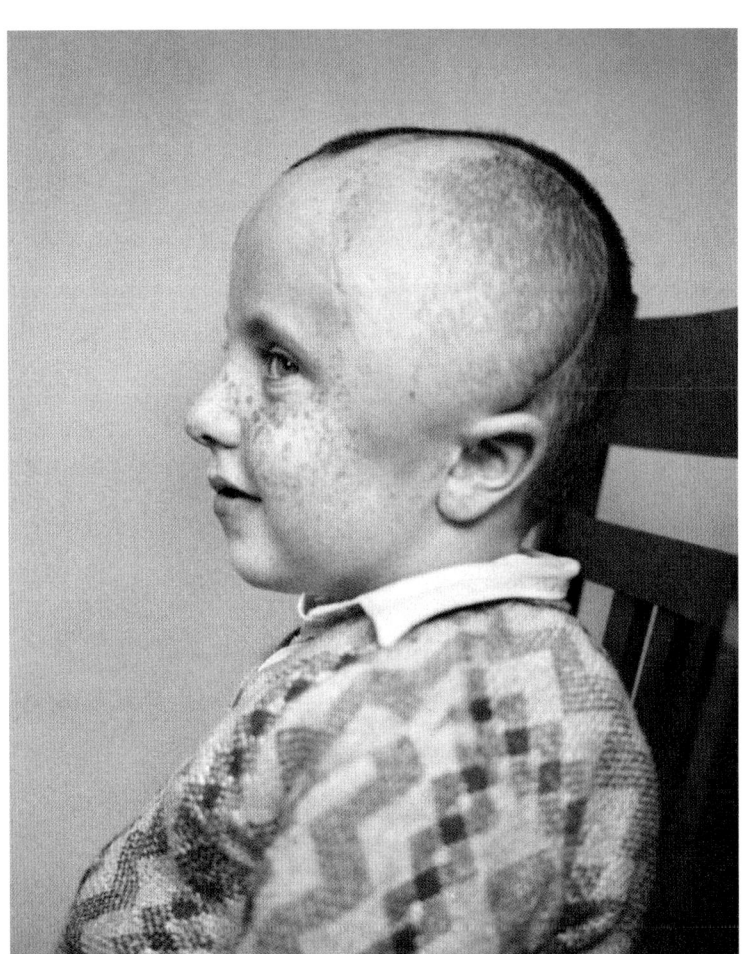

FIG. 10. FOUR WEEKS AFTER SECOND SURGERY.

The thin shell of frontal lobe tended to flop into the cavity but this was held up by a spatula during the latter part of the operation. One could easily have put a fist into this huge cavity. Dr. Meagher prepared a ball of radium and it was so small that it was simply lost in the cavity and he then made another about the size of a lemon which was put into the sac and the flapping part of the brain was replaced and closed in 2-3 layers, Dr. Horrax taking over the latter part of the procedure.

(Dr. Cushing)

PATHOLOGY REPORT
February 11, 1930

Microscopic diagnosis – Astroblastoma.

SPECIAL NOTE
February 15, 1930
Dr. Cushing

This boy has now gone for four days with a large rubber sponge ball containing radium that has been implanted. Each day, owing to tension, I have had to puncture the wound and cerebrospinal fluid has begun to accumulate and lead to a permanent leak. I would otherwise have left this to go over for two more days, but it seemed best to remove the radium today.

flap at the anterior lower angle where there had been a bulge in the soft tissues, I got into a cyst which in this position was very superficial and sucked out of it 200 cc of the same reddish fluid that was described at the time of the taps.

With the flap not fully turned back, owing to discomforts on the boy's part, I proceeded to make an incision through dura which had not previously been incised, namely around the anterior part of the field. I came down on to cortex of the frontal lobe which I then incised electrically and soon entered the huge cyst. The incision was then carried around as shown in the sketch so that it communicated with the point where there had been a leak in the cyst.

I then had an excellent view into the huge cavity and could see a great mass of tumor bulging forward into the cavity.

After removing some fragments for histological examination, I then began with the sucker to clean out this huge cavity by primarily transsecting most of it, meanwhile holding forward the anterior shell of the growth into the cavity. The tumor appeared to be of several qualities. Some of it was excessively soft and suckable, like a medulloblastoma. Other parts of it were hard and almost cartilaginous. There were, moreover, many areas where there was evident necrosis and I must have gotten into one of these areas in my original tap for I could see no reason from anything that was encountered today why there should have been so much cholesterin.

I kept pursuing this tumor, coagulating the base of it as we proceeded with pledgets in Zenker's fluid, until I came down to a perfectly extraordinary depth, measuring from the anterior edge of the bone flap 15 cm which must have carried me well back to the proper position of the pineal body. The depth indeed from the surface of the flap across to the opposite side of the tumor must have been almost as great, namely about 15 cm.

Then as a last step in the operation, I removed the anterior section of the tumor which laid open the huge cyst, the wall of which evidently was everywhere covered by a layer of granular reddish tumor.

I think that this tumor must be more or less encapsulated for certain fragments of it began to strip away from around in the region of the frontotemporal part of the field, that is, along the Sylvian region and I had a little difficulty there for a time with bleeding which I feared might be from the Sylvian vessels.

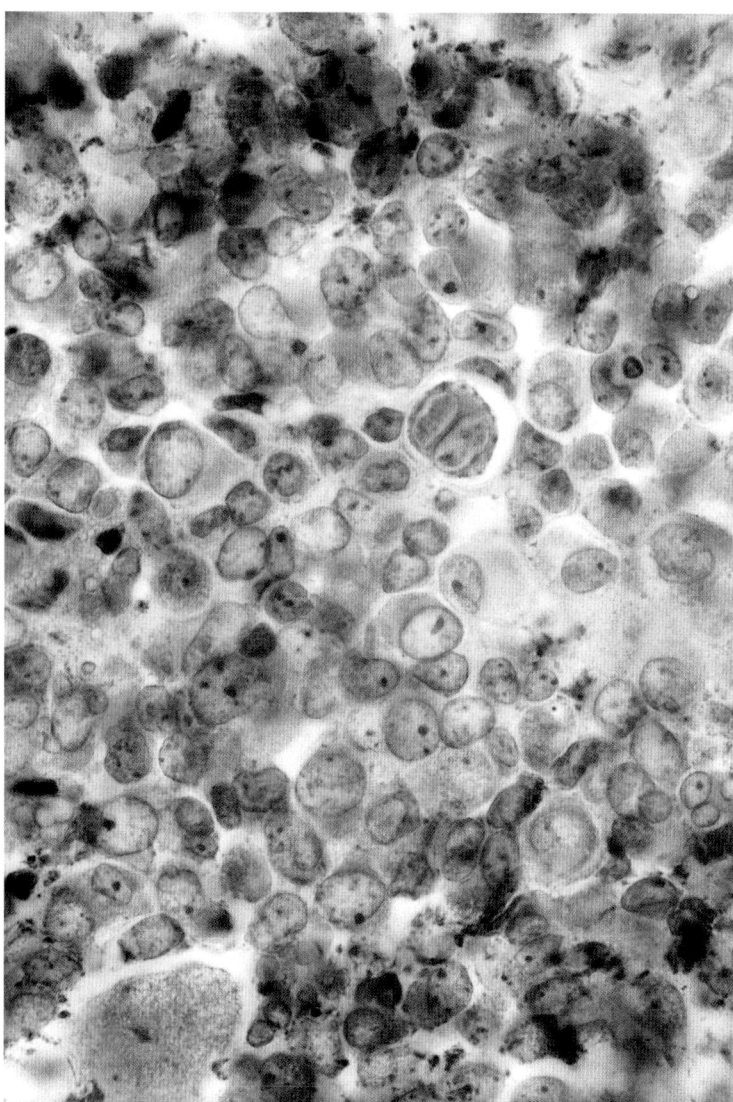

FIG. 6. HISTOLOGY SLIDE FROM SECOND SURGERY.

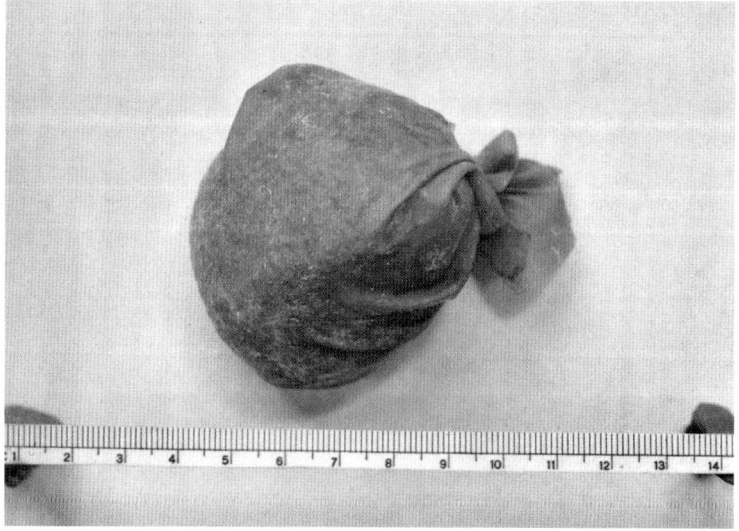

FIG. 7. RADIUM SAC IMPLANTED DURING SECOND SURGERY.

February 4, 1930
Dr. Cushing

Puncture thru parietal margin of flap. Removed at 5 cc of bloody cystic fluid to the amount of about 200 cc sucked out and replaced by 150 cc of air.

RADIOLOGY REPORT
February 4, 1930
Dr. Sosman

Fourth examination of the skull after injection of air in the cyst, shows a large cavity 10 ½ cm in A.P. diameter and 7 cm. in vertical, and 6 cm in transverse diameter. Anterior, upper and medial walls were all smooth and sharp in outline, but the base and portion of the lateral wall showed rough irregular projections suggesting a nodular tumor. Medial wall of the cyst just across the midline and the lateral wall had apparently ruptured and communicated with the subtemporal decompression. No abnormal calcification was seen in this region.

Impression – Cystic tumor, left temporofrontal.

SPECIAL NOTE
February 11, 1930
Dr. Cushing

The operation this morning on this little boy's case served to untangle those mysteries and yet leaves the exact nature of the tumor and its point of origin still undecided. From the general situation of the great central block of tumor which was largely enveloped by cyst, I assumed that the growth must have come from the pineal region which accounts for the boy's hydrocephalus and lack of general paralytic symptoms. In other words, it has been a huge, slowly growing central tumor, possibly teratomatous, which has enlarged chiefly up to the left side owing to the tremendously bulging bone flap which he has had.

Since the taps and the cystogram which had been made within the last few days, he has been in good condition with less tense flap than heretofore. The taps as well as the ventriculograms made it evident that there was a huge cyst near the surface of the temporal and frontal regions with the great mass of tumor behind it. The operation was relayed with Dr. Horrax.

OPERATIVE NOTE
February 11, 1930
Anesthesia – Novocain

Reflection of Old Bone Flap; Transcortical Incision into Cyst, which Contained 250 cc of Collected Fluid and Probably a Good Deal More that was Lost. Removal Chiefly by Suction of Huge, Partly Necrotic Tumor Mass which must Have Centered about in the Middle of the Brain. The Entire Cyst Lined by Tumor. Implantation of Large Radium Bag in Cavity. Closure without Drainage.

The little boy behaved admirably throughout this operation. Dr. Horrax had begun to turn down the bone flap when I took over the operation and completed this procedure electrically so as to get as little bleeding as possible. As shown in sketch I (Please note the sketch for the second operation, middle image) there was a large denuded area of brain under flap for the dura at the first operation had not been closed. In the process of elevating the

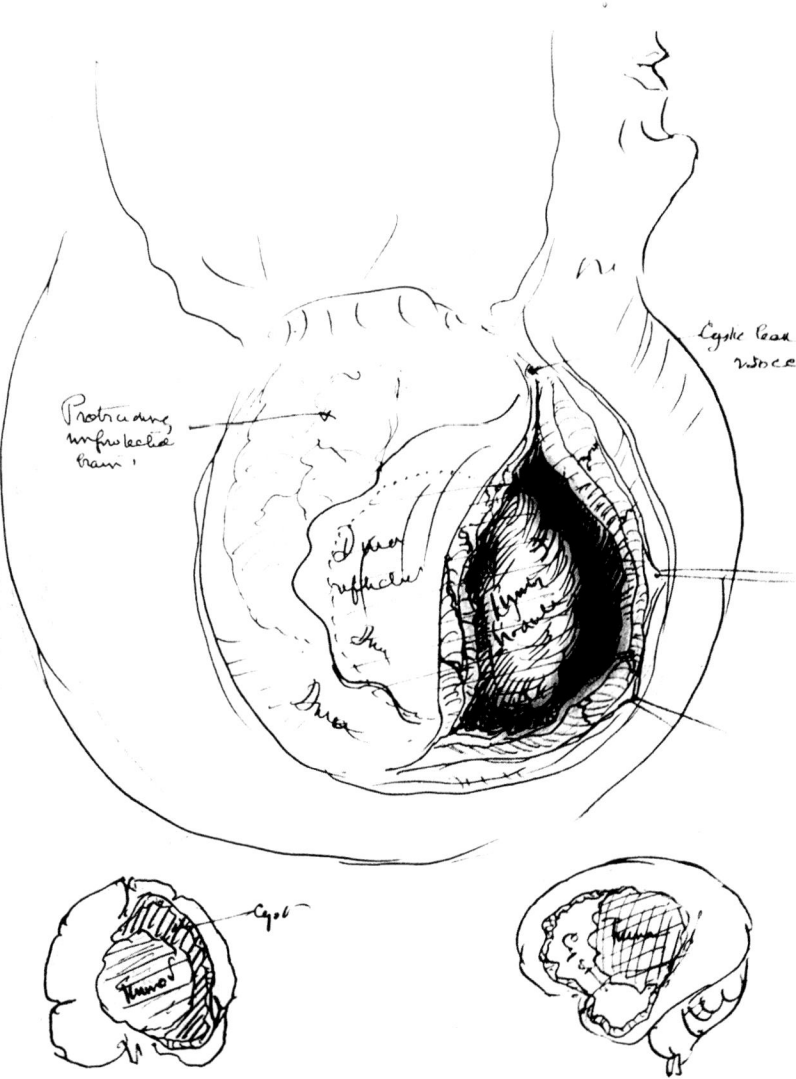

FIG. 5. OPERATIVE SKETCH (SECOND OPERATION).

Another piece sent down later and examined by supravital technique showed free blood, many clasmotocytes (a), some with neutral red dye inclusions, and masses of epithelial cells with round or oval nuclei and clearly defined cytoplasm. Some of these cells are multinucleated (c).

Where this tissue came from is not clear, but the cells are certainly like epithelial cells.

Microscopic diagnosis – Glioma?

HOSPITAL COURSE

Following the operation, the child suffered from some speech difficulty and a slight diminution in the grip strength of the right hand. These deficits cleared quickly.

DISCHARGE NOTE
December 16, 1929

The patient was discharged in good health and spirits with "flat and non-edematous discs."

FOLLOW UP NOTE
January 11, 1930

The flap over the decompression defect was found to be very tense. The patient reported to have occasional attacks of vomiting.

SECOND HOSPITAL ADMISSION

HISTORY

The patient was admitted to the hospital due to "refilling of the intracranial cyst" one month after discharge.

SUMMARY OF POSITIVE FINDINGS
January 18, 1930
Dr. Oldberg

SUBJECTIVE
1. History of previous admission to this hospital with 7 months history of nausea, vomiting, and headache, and positive findings of bilateral choked disc of 5D and right facial weakness of central type.
2. History of operation performed at this hospital on November 22, 1929, a deep left central cyst containing xanthochromic and cholesterin filled fluid being evacuated.
3. History of subsequent improvement in health with loss of headache, nausea and vomiting, and subsidence of the choked discs.

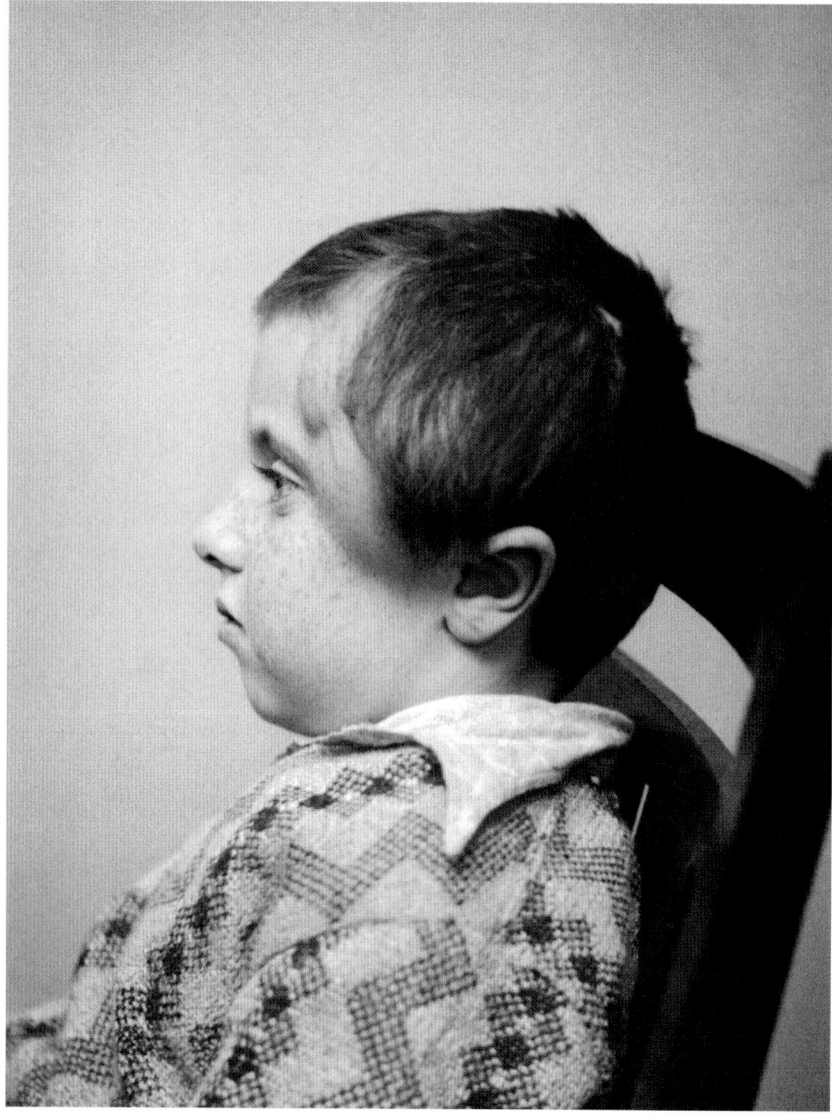

FIG. 4. PREOPERATIVE BEFORE SECOND SURGERY.

4. History of sudden return of headache, nausea and vomiting with sudden great increase in tenseness of the left decompression occurring approximately January 10, 1930.

OBJECTIVE
1. Left subtemporal decompression, with left bone flap, the decompression being extremely tense and the flap being riding.
2. Bilateral choked disc of 3D with beginning secondary atrophy on the left.
3. Pronounced right facial weakness of central type.

IMPRESSION: Recurrent deep left temporal cyst, possibly the cyst of a cranio-pharyngioma.

OPERATIVE NOTE
February 15, 1930
Anesthesia – Novocain

Re-elevation of Flap. Removal of Radium Ball from Cavity. Suction of Fringes of Rotten Tissue. Re-closure with Drains.

This most cooperative little boy, who has a song of courage which he sings on persuasion during his operation, went through the performance today with noteworthy fortitude and cooperation.

On elevation of the flap I found that there was quite an extradural hematoma that had formed, of which I had had no inkling. This mass of clot which I assumed might have an abundance of clasmatocytes in it was submitted for histological study.

On re-opening and reflecting the dura, the ball of rubber began to extrude itself, and was finally dislodged. There was a large amount of necrotic and soft tissue around it which I put in a test tube for histological examination believing it to be largely composed of clasmatocytes.

On getting a good view into the huge cavity I found that there was still tumor posteriorly, but as this was were I got bleeding at the other operation I did not venture to interfere with it. I started to suck out some of the rotten looking tissue, but got bleeding, which necessitated temporary packing and placement of additional clips.

I would be very glad to have an X-ray taken of this boy's head before long so that we can see the position of these clips in place, for they will doubtless serve to give us some idea whether the tumor is growing owing to change of position, I could see that the nodular tumor that lined the anterior wall of the cyst was still in position and had not been softened. I might have taken some fragments of it for histological examination, but I feared to set up bleeding. In as much as we did not have tissue from this particular part of the cyst wall for comparison I saw no reason for taking some now as a histological test of the activity of our radiotherapeusis.

In the act of sucking the cavity at its great depth, where I could see that there was a lot of necrosis tissue, I got into the ventricle and clear fluid began to pour in the wound. It is curious that I had not done so before. It is quite possible indeed that this tumor may have come from the ventricle and may indeed prove to be an ependymoma after all. If the growth had not been of such enormous size, and if this mass in the posterior part of the field had come to be dislocated forward instead of

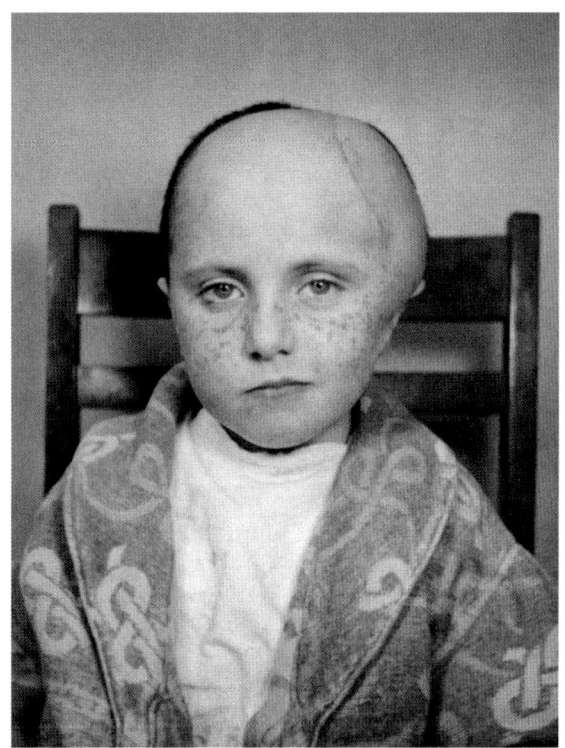
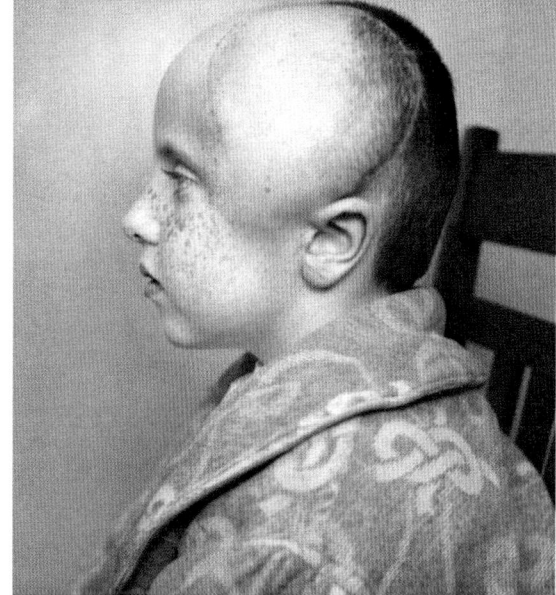

FIGS. 11 AND 12. FIVE WEEKS AFTER SECOND SURGERY.

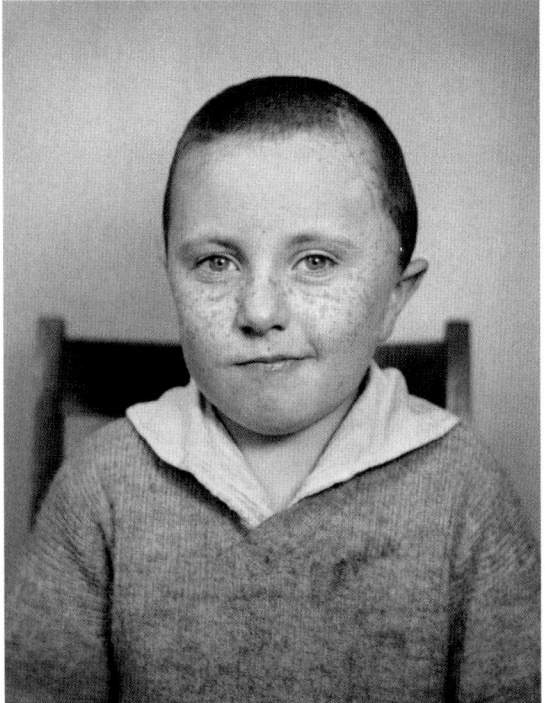
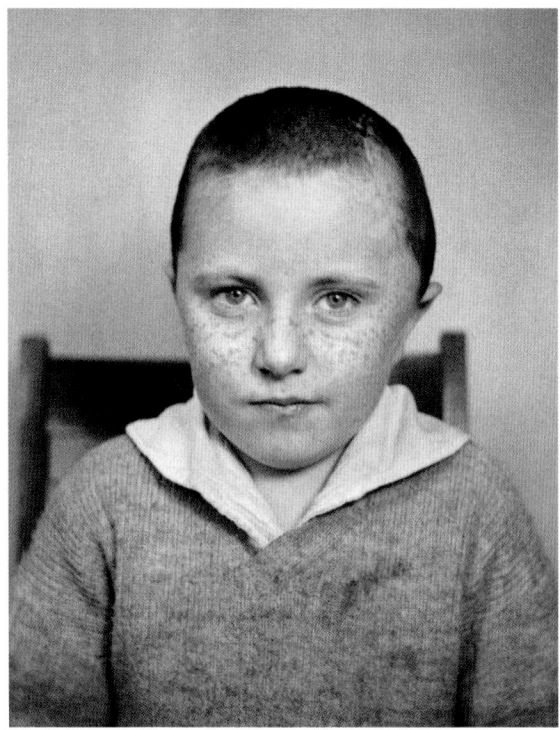

FIGS. 13 AND 14. NINE WEEKS AFTER SECOND SURGERY.

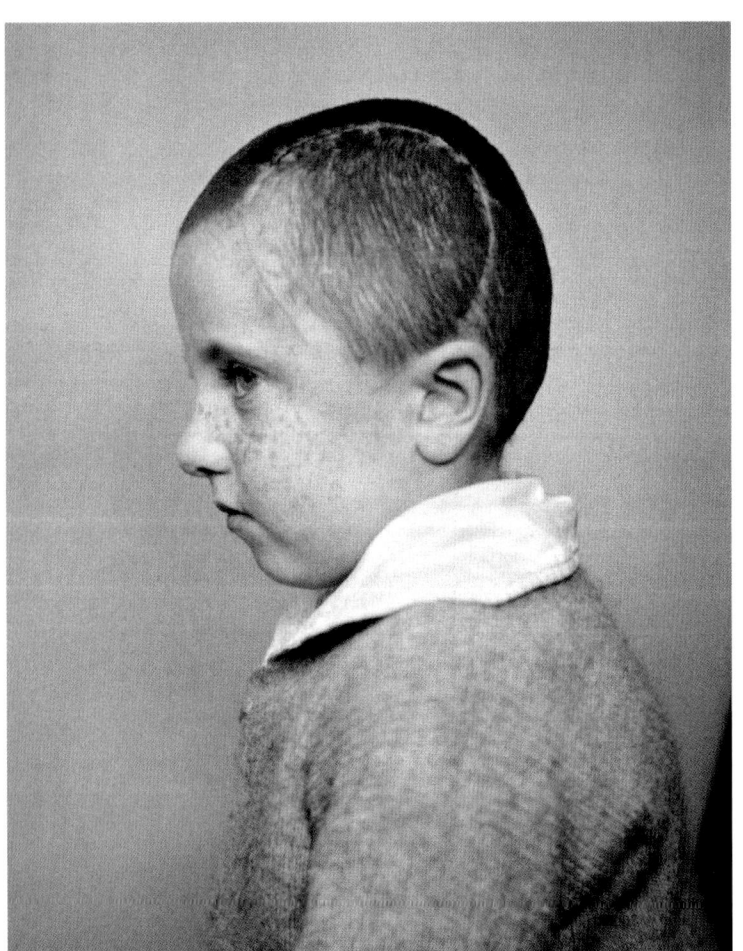

FIG. 15. NINE WEEKS AFTER SECOND SURGERY.

being held in its position at the back of the field I might conceivably have encouraged to remove it. Even so, this would not have served to modify the activity of tumor which still lines the inner anterior part of the cyst.

After careful hemostasis I put a rubber catheter through a puncture opening and led it obliquely forward under the dura, and also put a gutta percha drain through another perforation, this being led directly into the cavity. I suppose that there will be an abundant discharge of cerebrospinal fluid.

(Dr. Cushing)

RADIOLOGY REPORT
February 24, 1930
Dr. Sosman

Fifth examination of skull shows the left temporoparietal bone flap which is bulging considerably. ... beneath the anterior margin there is a large spongy shadow, 8 in diameter, in the center of which there is a capsule of radium. This is just above and slightly behind the posterior of the left orbit. The edge of the sponge is 2 cm from the bone. There are several silver clips quite a bit deeper than the edge of the sponge. The radium is lying almost transversely. The edge of the sponge is about 1 cm from the midline. Its lateral surface is 3 cm from the inner table of the bone flap.

HOSPITAL COURSE

Following the operation, the patient ran a fairly smooth postoperative course although he had developed a complete paresis of the right arm. It was noted nearly 3 weeks after operation that he had lost his hair in a fairly well demarcated line due to X-ray treatment. He had a series of sudden unexplainable transient temperature rises.

April 25, 1930

Has taken out of bed and walked fairly well.

DISCHARGE NOTE
April 27, 1930

Dr. Cushing allowed the mother to take the child home, and asked her to bring him once a week to this clinic for further observation. No changes in condition.

FOLLOW UP NOTE
May 3, 1930
Dr. Henderson

Seen this afternoon. No great change but is getting along satisfactorily. Decompression soft. Told to keep up movements of right hand.

THIRD HOSPITAL ADMISSION

HISTORY

During the week before this admission, the patient became much worse, and frequently vomited. The decompression became markedly tense and bulging. He was readmitted.

Multiple taps of the fluid underneath the subtemporal flap was performed to relieve intracranial hypertension. The fluid continued to re-accumulate. The patient suffered from convulsions.

June 4, 1930

Died on ward. The terminal stages of his illness were essentially those of an increase of intracranial tension and a gradual increase in signs indicative of unrelieved pressure.

AUTOPSY REPORT
June 4, 1930

DIAGNOSES
    Brain tumor (Medulloblastoma).
    Pneumonia (hypostatic)
    Atrophy of musculature, right

The report from the pathological department on

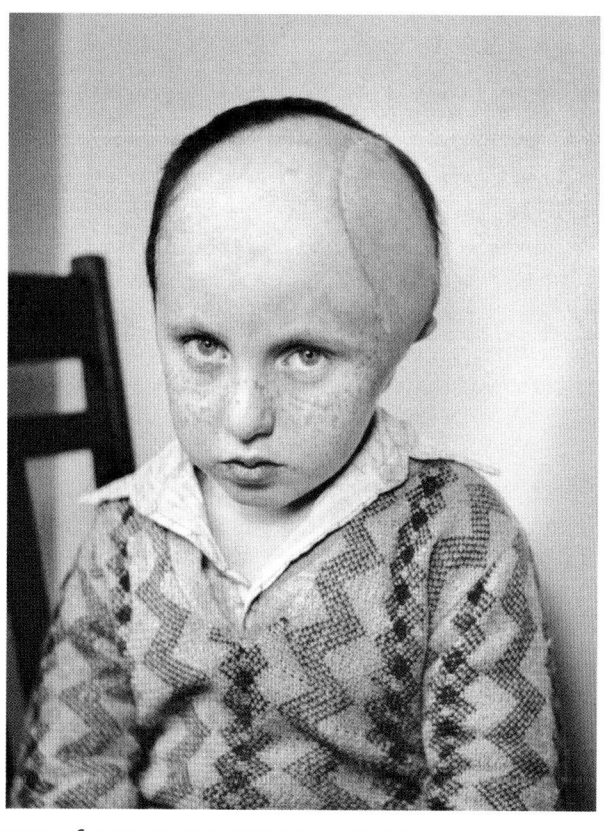
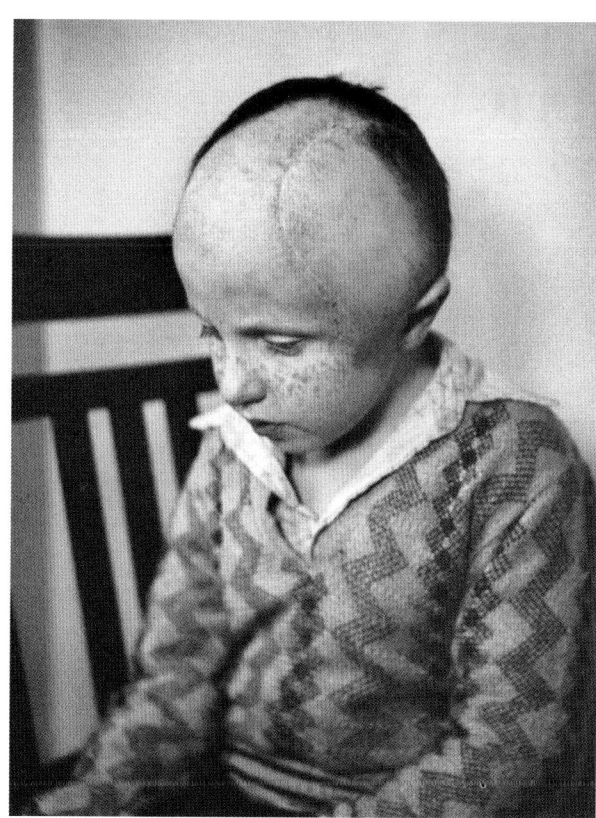

FIGS. 16 AND 17. TEN WEEKS AFTER SECOND SURGERY.

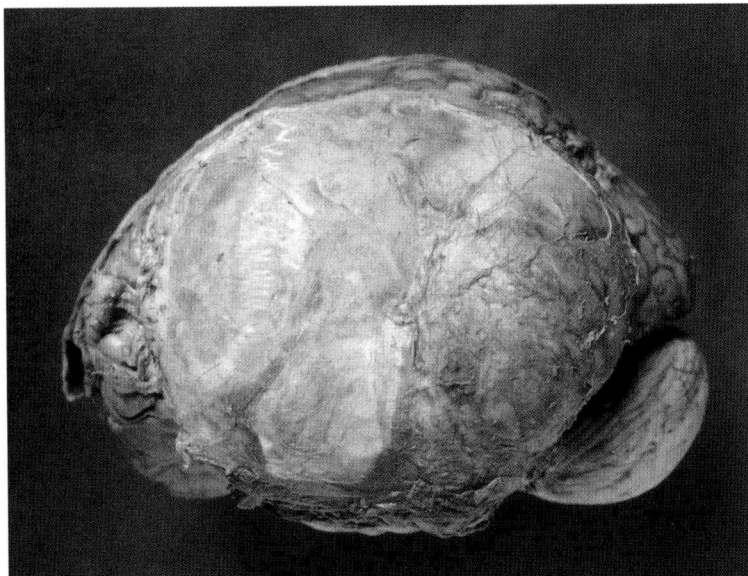

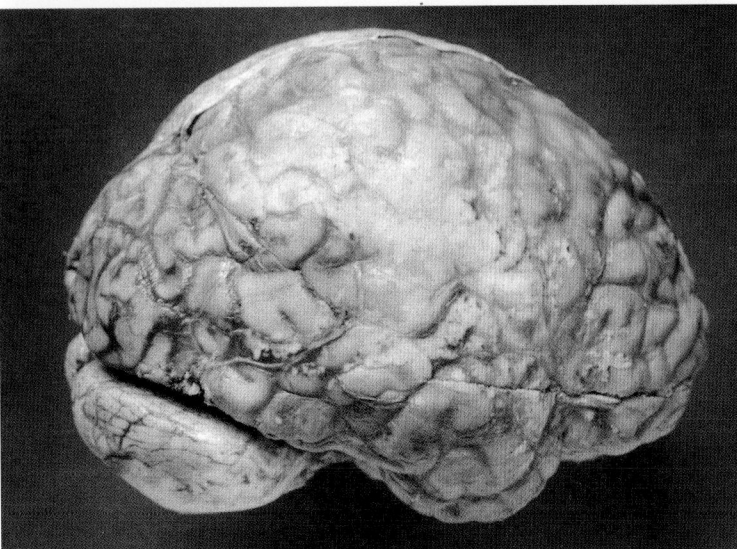

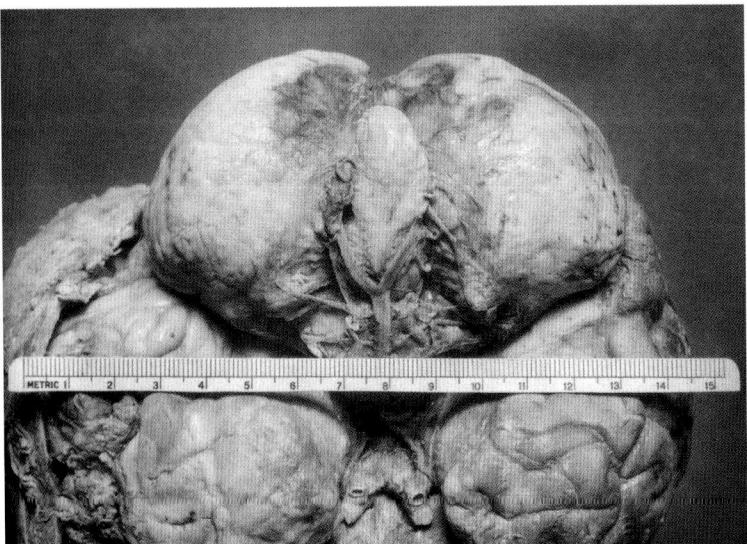

FIGS. 18, 19 AND 20. AUTOPSY SPECIMENS.

sections removed from the tumor at operation are in one case a question of glioma and in another case astroblastoma. At autopsy, however, the local findings in the left temporal lobe, the tumor in the cerebellum and in the right temporal lobe, together with the presence of tumor in the meninges and along the spinal cord, are suggestive of medulloblastoma.

The brain was removed together with the protruding bone flap.

The flap shows that tumor itself has begun to extrude through the old subtemporal decompression where there is a bluish mass about 6 cm in its vertical diameter and certainly 10 cm in its anteroposterior diameter which protrudes 1 cm or so above the level of the skull. There has been a marked extrusion, also due to tumor of the brain underlying the bone flap.

The striking feature of the brain, however, is the fact that this particular highly malignant tumor has gone into the deeper meningeal spaces and both cerebral hemispheres are covered with it as though they had been painted with an ivory colored paint, so that the convolutions are most wholly concealed. It is evident in the subarachnoidal spaces. The posterior cistern is grayish and thick walled but does not seem to be involved. There is no herniation of the tonsils. A similar whitish patch of evident leptomeningeal involvement spread up in a fan from the Sylvian fissure over the right hemisphere, its width being 5-6 cm vertically and the full extent of obvious involvement being easily 10 cm. I think one can say that here this involvement lies in the arachnoid spaces and the convolutions are elevated. There are other isolated areas in the arachnoidal spaces that one can see islands of invasion. It is strange that there is less evidence of this superficial implantation.

The usual coronal sections are made:

1. At the tips of the temporal lobes shows an enormous hydrocephalus and if I remember correctly, at the time of the major operation the left ventricle was widely opened.

2. Next section goes through what remains of the tumor and from the appearance of it I regret greatly that I did not immediately go in and try and clean it out for the tumor is evidently quite well encapsulated and extends in a cone from the mesial portion of the left lateral ventricle outward to the surface of the brain where it had protruded into the decompression.

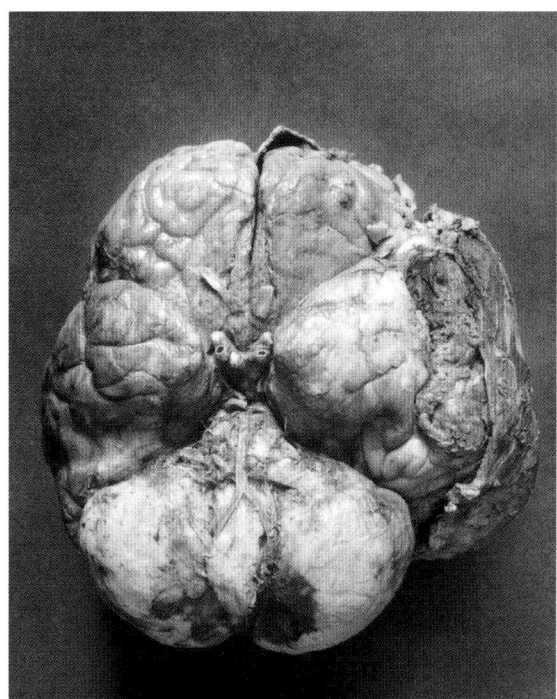

FIG. 21. AUTOPSY SPECIMEN.

3. The next section passes through the more posterior part of the tumor and here, too, one sees this enormous, massive growth which lies in alveolated spaces. This section enables one to look into what was evidently the old cavity there, I take it, radium had been planted but it does not at all explain why the ventricles should be so dilated. I assume that we will find an occlusion of the aqueduct. They, as well as the lateral ventricles, are dilated.

4. The next section through the occipital lobes shows still this huge dilatation of the ventricles which here, as elsewhere, are stained by a bluish substance. The aqueduct is a little dilated so that the occlusion, wherever it is, lies further back. It can subsequently be studied for that is not the essential part of the story. A block is taken for pathological study through the zone of the leptomeningeal implantation of the growth over the left hemisphere and also a section of the soft tumor tissue itself.

(Dr. Cushing)

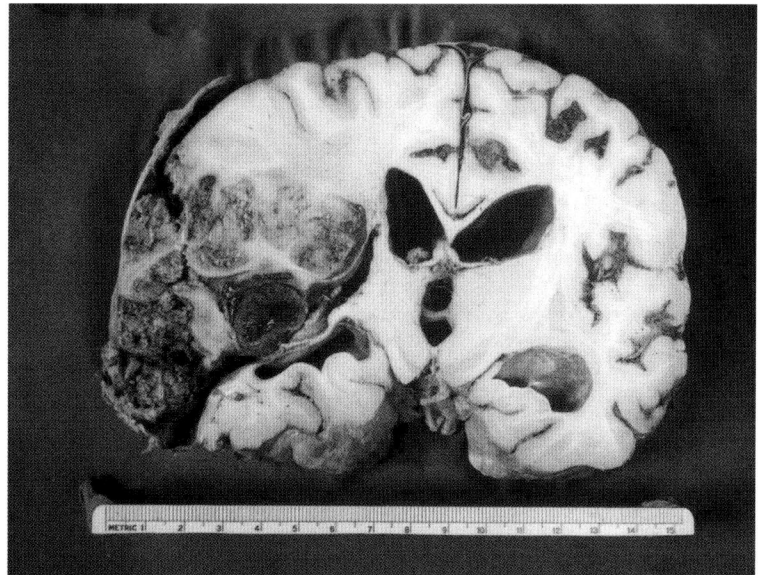

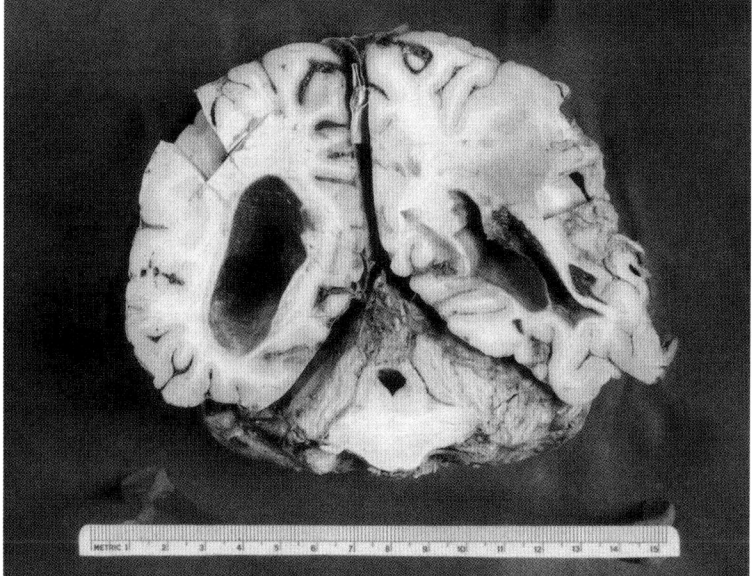

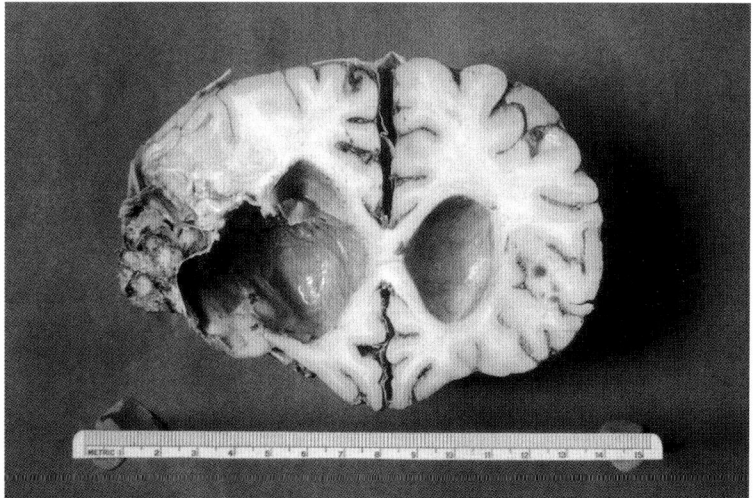

FIGS. 22, 23 AND 24. AUTOPSY SPECIMENS.

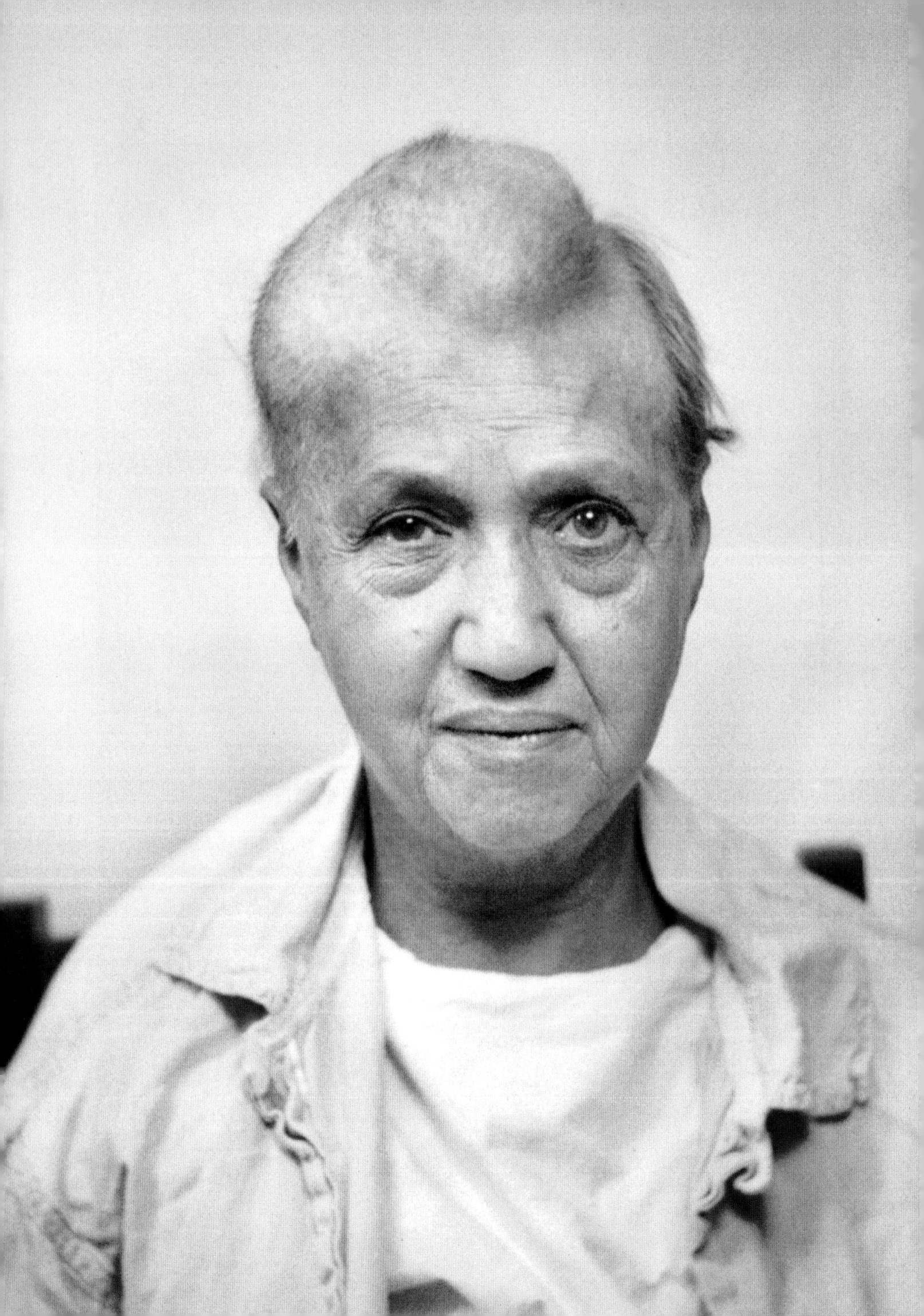

2.13 Myeloma of the frontal bone

SEX: F; AGE: 62; SURG. NO. 3721

COMPLAINT

Swelling on top and front of head of two months duration.

SUMMARY OF POSITIVE FINDINGS
September 10, 1930
Dr. Oldberg

SUBJECTIVE
1. History of rapidly increasing lump on the head of 6 months duration.
2. History of gradually increasing left hemiparesis of 3 months duration.

OBJECTIVE
1. Large mass in the right fronto-temporal region, extending across the midline somewhat on the left side and apparently consisting mostly in soft tissue.
2. Slight left lower facial weakness of central type.
3. Moderate left hemiparesis with slightly increased deep reflexes on left side.

IMPRESSION: Neoplasm of skull, probably not a meningioma.

RADIOLOGY REPORT
September 4, 1930
Dr. Sosman

Right and left stereos, A.P. and P.A. of skull show a smooth vault except in the frontal bones where there is a marked increase in the density of the posterior half of the frontal bone, particularly on the right side, but apparently extending almost to the midline. The bone has a mottled, worm-eaten appearance at this point, and there is irregular thickening of the inner table. The sella is slightly atrophic, but there are no general signs of increased pressure. There is no definite increase in vascularity. The pineal is displaced to the left of

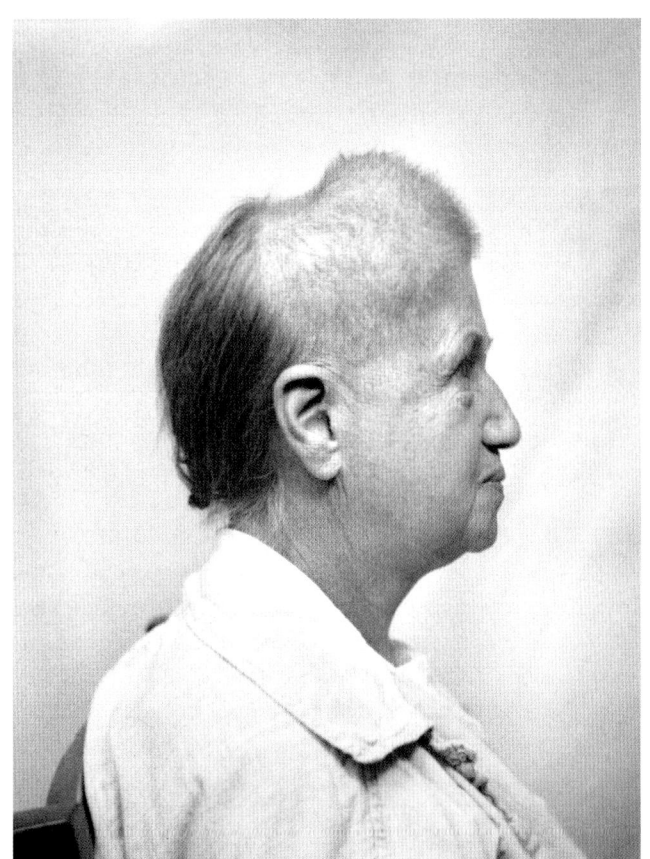
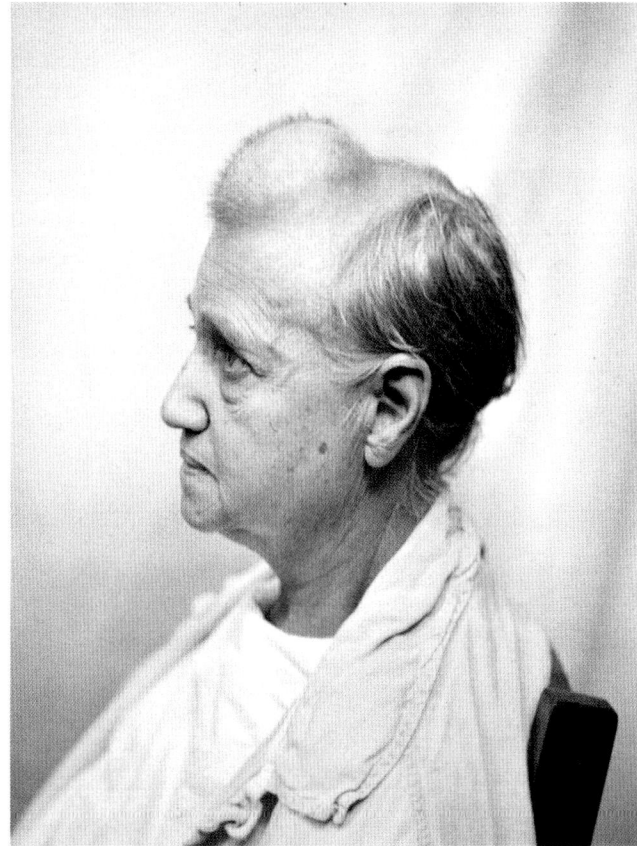

FIGS. 2 AND 3. TAKEN AT TIME OF ADMISSION.

OPPOSITE PAGE. FIG. 1. TAKEN AT TIME OF ADMISSION.

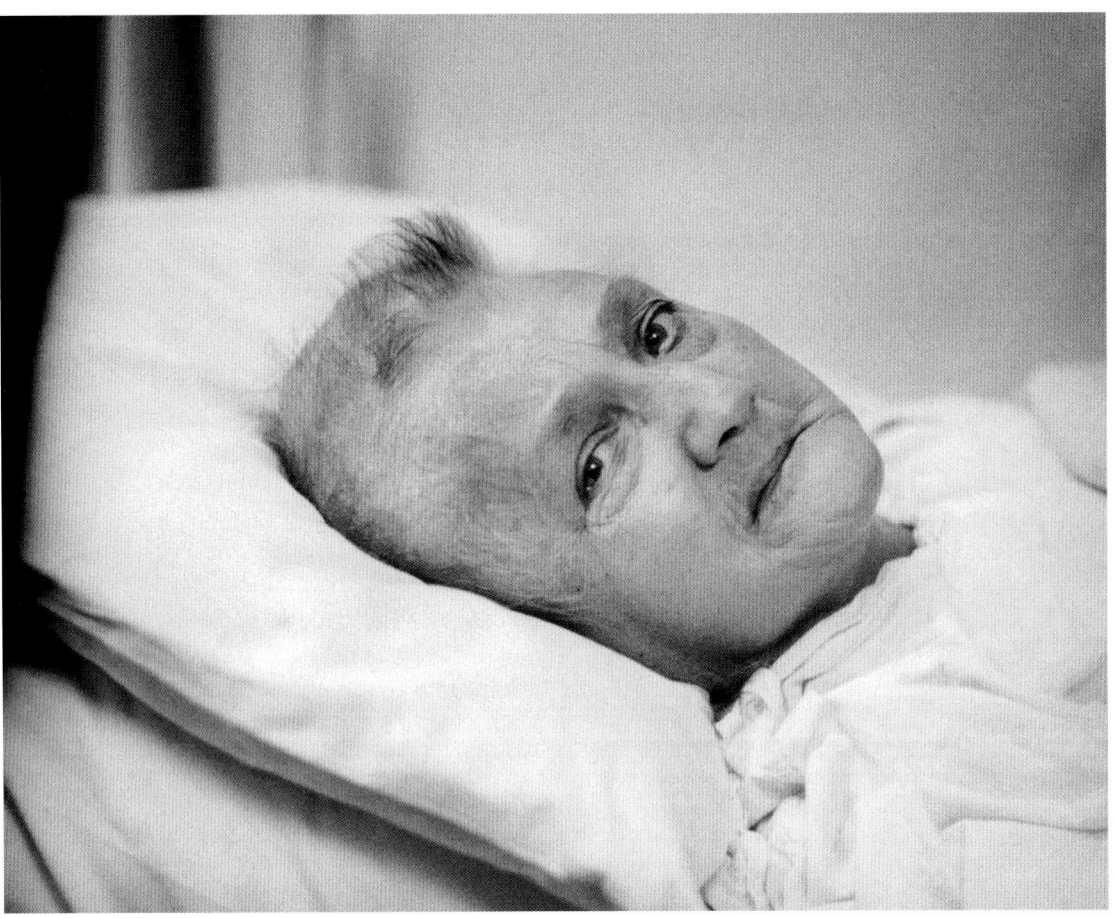

FIGS. 4 AND 5. TAKEN AT TIME OF DISCHARGE.

September 13, 1930
Dr. Cushing

The temporal arteries are unduly big. However, the lesion is so rapidly growing and in the want of more characteristic X-ray findings I think the lesion is more likely osteosarcoma. Advise against exploration. Since the tumor is actually in the scalp any kind of biopsy or exploration would be fool-hardy.

September 18, 1930
Dr. Hoen

Patient had a generalized convulsion this afternoon observed by the nurses involving both arms and face, the arms being flexed and fists clenched: all the muscles twitched convulsively. The convulsion lasted a few minutes and following it the patient was slightly more stuperous than usual.

September 26, 1930
Dr. Hoen

Continues down her course. Completely disoriented. Right facial weakness more marked.

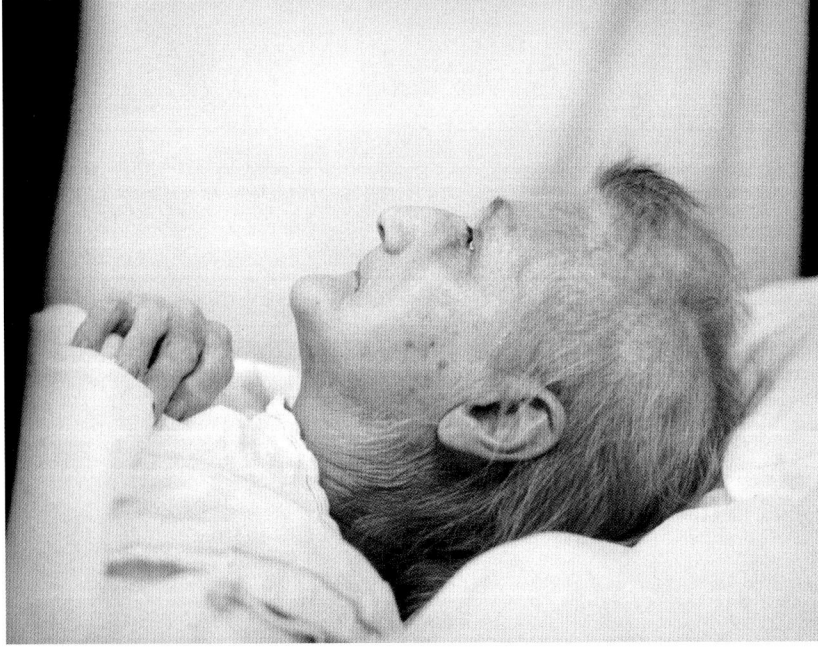

midline, and by measurements is at the posterior and inferior limits of normal. The findings probably indicate a meningioma. A gumma or a metastasis cannot be excluded.

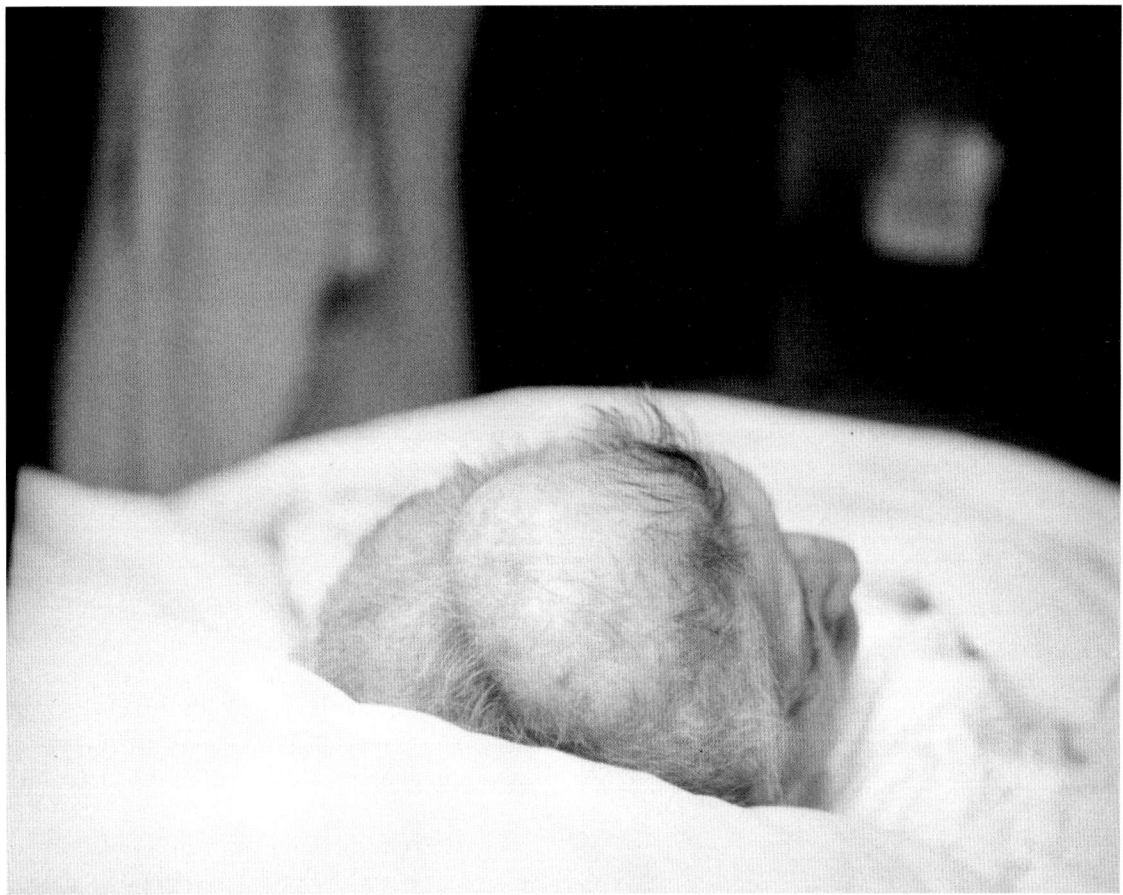

FIG. 6. TAKEN AT TIME OF DISCHARGE.

October 3, 1930
Dr. Hoen

Surface of tumor is quite reddened and surface temperature much elevated. General condition about the same.

RADIOLOGY REPORT
October 14, 1930
Dr. Sosman

Film of the chest shows the lungs to be clear. The ribs appear rather porous, but no definite metastasis can be seen.

DISCHARGE NOTE
November 7, 1930
Dr. Hoen

The condition of the patient has remained the same for the last month, except that tumor has visibly increased in size. No changes in neurological picture. She is discharged to nursing home in Providence by ambulance. Relatives will communicate per her condition.

FOLLOW UP
November 11, 1930
Dr. Eisenhardt

Telephone message from Social Service Department of Rhode Island Hospital reported death of patient last night. Permission obtained for necropsy of head and Dr. Schulz and I are off to Providence to do it.

AUTOPSY REPORT
November 11, 1930

Diagnosis: Myeloma myelocytic.

There is a definite protruding frontal mass, slightly more prominent on the right side but extends well beyond the mid line to the left frontal eminence. The tumor feels somewhat soft with no evidence of calcium deposit. It is slightly irregular in outline beginning as a slight elevation of the forehead and ending over the mid coronal area as a rather large, ledge like mass of tumor extending 3 cm beyond the surface of the skull. There is no indication of

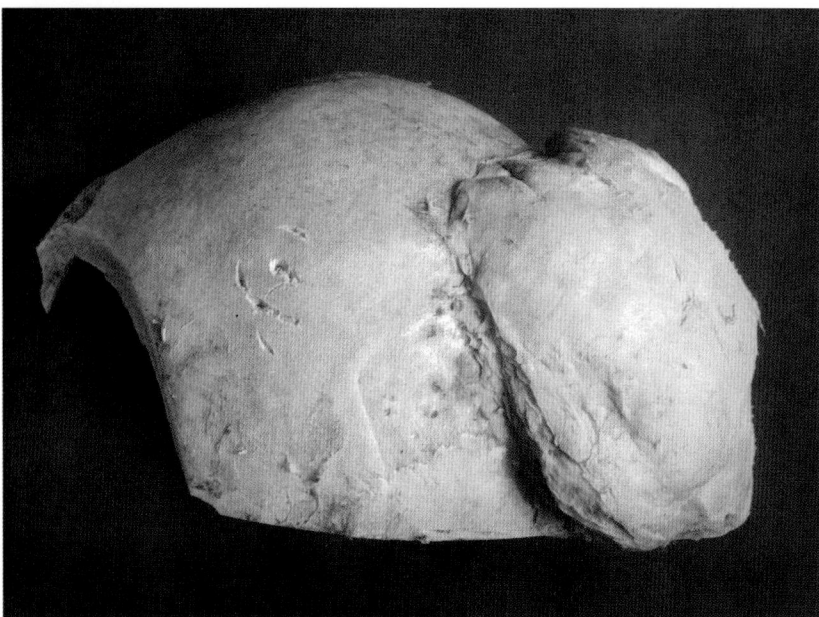

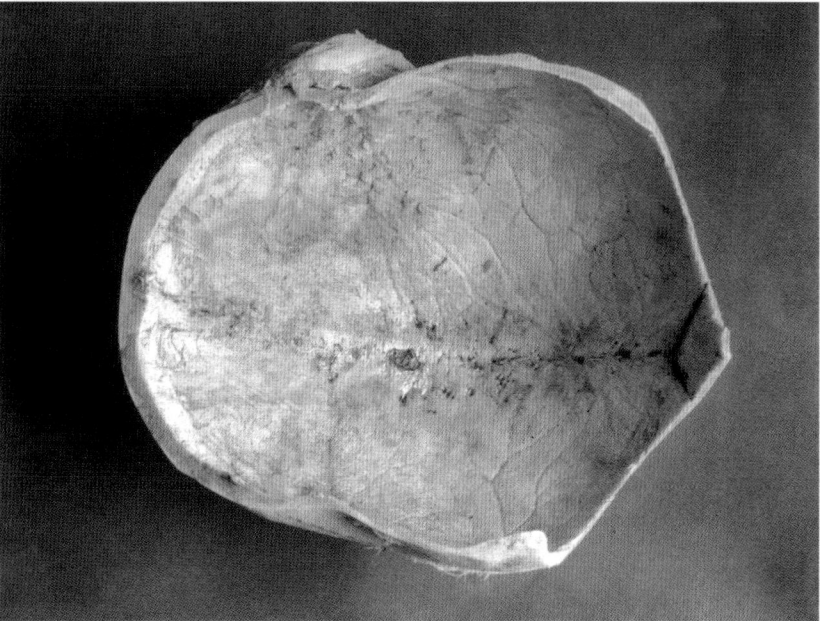

FIGS. 7 AND 8. AUTOPSY SPECIMENS (SKULL).

bone beneath this portion of the tumor although this phase will have to be determined from further section. The axillary, inguinal and epitrochlear lymph nodes are not enlarged.

On the anterior frontal surface the tumor radially rises until the vertex is reached, where there is considerable lipping or overhanging of the tumor. The tumor is however, somewhat nodular with a number of somewhat irregular prominences. The necrotic areas present a considerable amount of yellowish gray discoloration such as one finds in necrosis. The other portions of tumor are more of a grayish pink color, appear to be very cellular, although containing a fair amount of fibrous tissue. It is definitely invasive and has invaded to a good extent the temporal muscle and also the bone. The calvarium is next sawed, the dura however is only stripped for a short distance in an attempt to find the relation of the tumor to the dura. Great difficulty was encountered in this area and for that reason the dura is incised, cranial nerves and blood vessels cut and entire brain, dura and calvarium removed in one piece. Further exploration is not made as the entire specimen is to be preserved in Formalin for subsequent study by the Neurological Department.

(Dr. Schulz)

The vessels are normal. The arachnoid is not particularly thickened. The convolutions are normal. Over the frontal bone and extending backward on the parietal particularly on the right side is a flat tumor mass which measures in the mid line 10 cm in its antero-posterior diameter and extending up about 2 cm above the level of the skull. The chief mass of growth extends over to the right where it is probably 3 cm above the level of the skull and it extends down practically into the temporal region. On stripping the galea off free of its wall it is evident that the tumor has extended into the galea which has been more or less separated by it. It moreover has infiltrated into the pericranium which curiously enough can be peeled off in 2-3 layers and between two layers of pericranium a block of tumor shown as a flat disk has been submitted for section. The entire width of the growth on the curved surface is about 17 cm in its greatest width, over the right frontal region, about 13 cm. One curious thing that is observed on freeing the tumor from its pericranium in the fact that it overlies normal bone without attachment and this came out over the pericranium without attachment to the bone. In other words the growth is toward the median line and lies between galea and pericranium and does not involve bone. The longitudinal sinus almost certainly is invaded by growth and probably for a distance of 4-6 cm about back to Rolandic point. It is quite possible that her sudden accession of symptoms when in the hospital may have been due to occlusion action, and the pathological diagnosis that I could think, almost certainly is osteosarcoma of bone invading the intracranial chamber and causing parasagittally, small

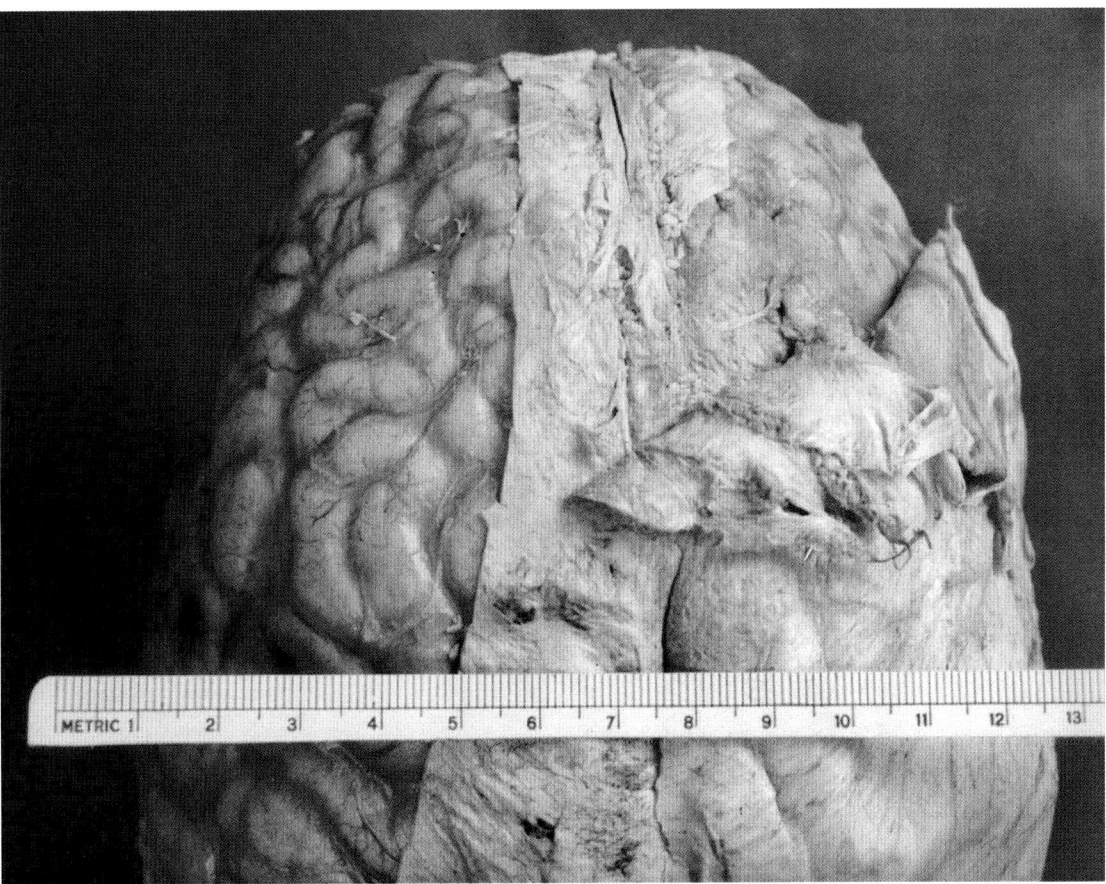

FIG. 9. AUTOPSY SPECIMEN (BRAIN).

tumor extending and bridging the right frontal lobe with a tumor of the anterior third of the longitudinal sinus. The tumor has a distinctly fibrous appearance quite unlike the appearance one sees from a meningioma though this might perhaps not have been apparent in the flesh.

(Dr. Cushing)

Microscopic report: Three sections are of an invasive tumor replacing muscle, fibrous tissue and fat. The cells in many instances bore the appearance of young myelocytes. Many of the cells, however, are in an indifferent stage, and it is impossible to accurately place them. Many mitotic figures are present. Nowhere in the section is there evidence of osteogenic sarcoma, nor is the cell type that, found in multiple myeloma, or plasma cell myeloma. The histology is rather poor, apparently due in part to the long time post mortem, without adequate cooling. It would be interesting to have a section showing relation of tumor to bone as possibly such study would make the diagnosis more certain. As far as can be determined from the material at hand, it corresponds more closely to the myelocytic myelomas and will be so catalogued.

DIAGNOSIS – Myelocytic myeloma

(Dr. Schulz)

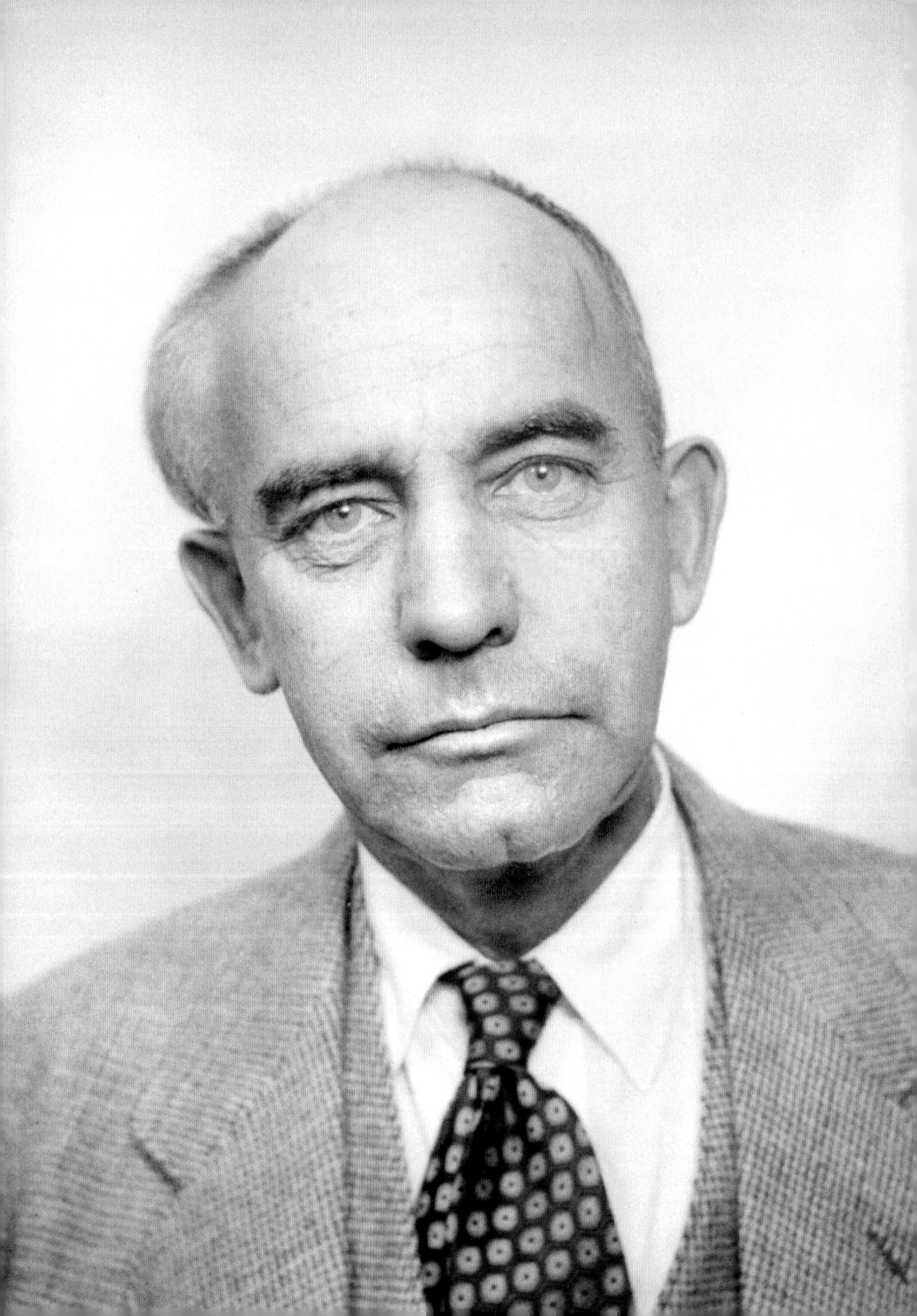

2.14 Occipital glioma

SEX: M; AGE: 56; SURG. NO. 37408

HISTORY

The patient presented to Dr. Williams of Rochester (NY) in July of 1930 with right-sided headaches, vomiting, and a left homonymous hemianopsia. Dr. Williams performed a right occipital craniectomy and decompression without tumor resection in August. During the last two weeks before admission to the Peter Bent Brigham Hospital, the patient noticed slight unsteadiness particularly when looking down, with a slight tendency to go to the right.

SUMMARY OF POSITIVE FINDINGS
October 7, 1930
Dr. Henderson

SUBJECTIVE
1. History of two severe attacks of right-sided headaches accompanied by marked vomiting in July and August of this year, together with slight occasional confusion.
2. Admission to the Clifton Springs Sanitarium in August where left homonymous hemianopsia was discovered, a diagnosis of right occipital tumor made.
3. Operation on August 29th by Dr. Williams of Rochester, in which a right occipital flap was turned down, the bone sacrificed, a dural decompression made without exposing the tumor.
4. General improvement in symptoms following the decompression.

OBJECTIVE
1. Well healed scar of a right, very markedly bulging temporo-occipital bone flap from which the bone has been sacrificed. Decompression is fairly tense.
2. Slight recent choking of discs without measurable elevation.
3. Slight lowering of the visual acuity with a left homonymous hemianopsia.

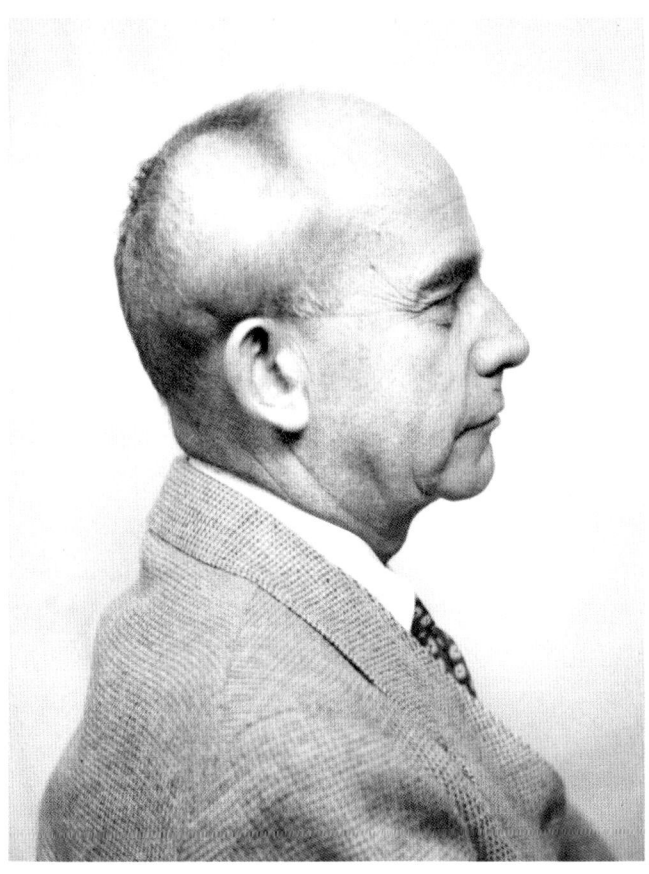
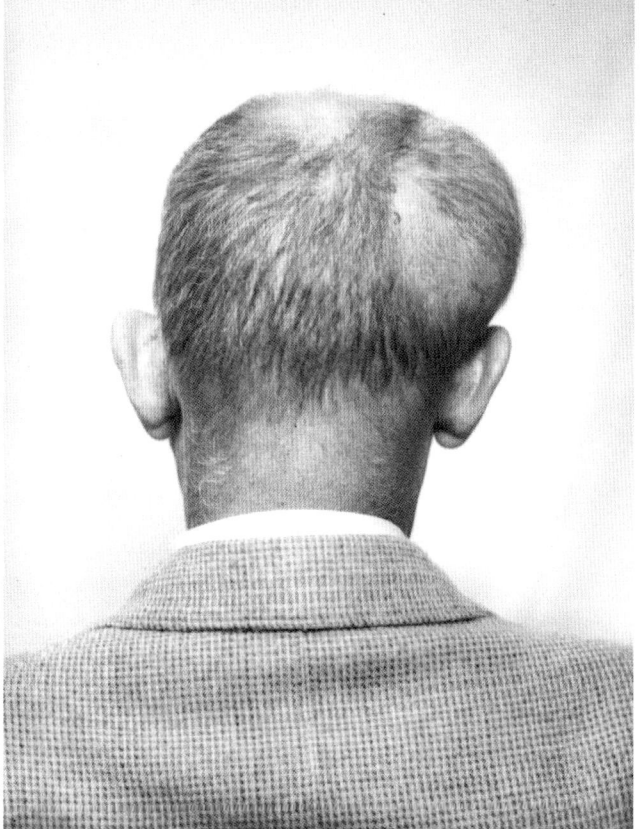

FIGS. 2 AND 3. TAKEN BEFORE RESECTIVE SURGERY.

OPPOSITE PAGE. FIG. 1. TAKEN BEFORE RESECTIVE SURGERY.

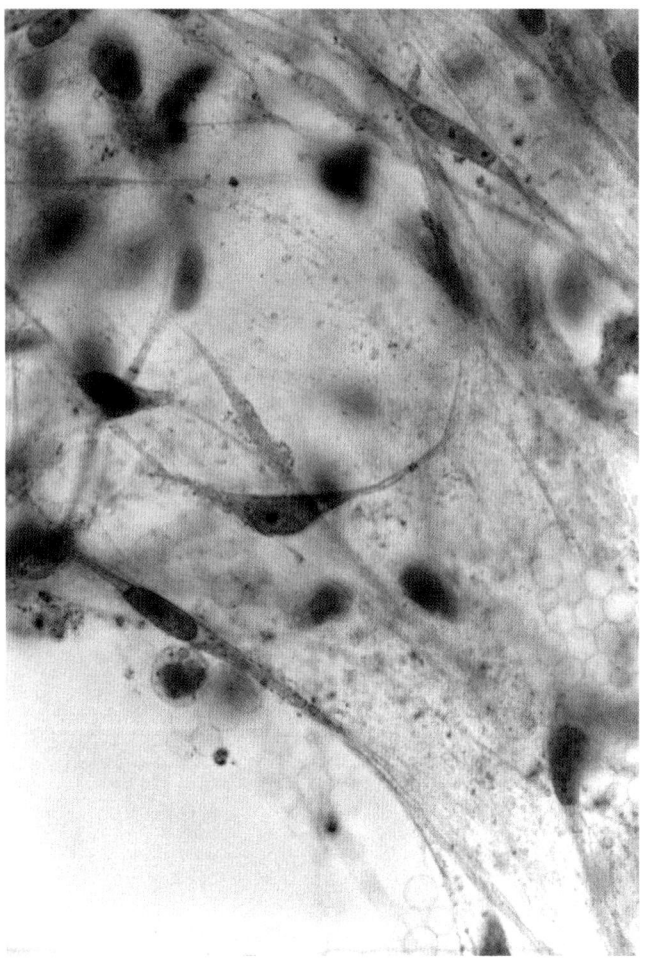

FIGS. 4. HISTOLOGY SLIDE.

4. Slight diminution of thermal sensation over the left side of the body.
5. Astereognosis in the left hand, with a marked diminution in deep muscle sense of the left hand and foot.
6. Absent abdominal reflex on the left.
7. Slight bilateral and equal ataxia on finger to nose test.
8. The patient is naturally left handed, but shows no sign of aphasia.
9. X-ray shows the operative bony defect; no calcification.

IMPRESSION: Right occipital tumor.

VENTRICULOGRAM
October 18, 1930

Ventriculograms show both ventricles displaced to the left of the midline in spite of the large right occipital bone flap which has been sacrificed. The right occipital horn is displaced upward and forward, including the adjacent portion of the right temporal horn. The left ventricle is not deformed. The findings indicate a large right occipital tumor lying about opposite the lower edge of the bone flap.

SPECIAL NOTE
October 18, 1930
Dr. Cushing

This has been about the worst exhibition of a cranial operation that I can remember. The man in the first place had a very huge recurrent glioblastoma multiformae in the occipital region which had been operated upon in another hospital without tumor verification and with a huge protrusion. He had a hemianopsia and we could not tell whether his lesion underlay his occipital protrusion or may possibly have been further forward.

Consequently, ventriculograms were made by Dr. Henderson before operation and they showed a forward dislocation of the occipital horn as though there were an underlying lesion, in other words, a low occipital lesion extending forward in the temporal lobe. Operation went badly from the beginning. The patient's head was in such a poor crutch that he kept complaining and the anaesthetist did not seem to know how to get it into a better position. I finally gave him an extra 10 mgms of morphia and then found it necessary to give him an anaesthetic but there seemed to be difficulty about this and after prolonged primary stage he kept coming out of partial anesthesia and all told it was a most difficult and poor exhibition. Finally, the great mass of tumor was gradually sucked out with bleeding and fall in B.P. and a transfusion was undertaken. I felt from the man's general condition and his activity that he could scarcely be exanguinated, and a transfusion was attempted in his popliteal region with the cross incision in the skin which I think is on an entirely wrong principle, so that blood could not be introduced after the vein had been finally dissected out and exposed. **Incidentally, there was a Harvard and Army football game on today which everyone wanted to go to and this too may perhaps have hooded the procedure.**

OPERATIVE NOTE
October 18, 1930
Anesthesia – Novocain

Reflection of Old Occipital Flap with Great Bleeding. Final Partial Exposure of Occipital Lobe. Electrical Transaction of Lobe, Soon Coming down upon Huge

example, the reflex examination included knee and ankle jerks, triceps, supinator, flexors and extensors of the arm, and superficial responses of the abdomen.[29] Thomas commented that he knew "of no case in the hospital records that has been worked up so carefully as this."[98]

The reason for this sudden wealth of detail is uncertain. Despite claims that Cushing's patient records stood out even during his internship,[102] they were actually quite comparable to those of his contemporaries.[85] We examined patient records from all cases of acute appendicitis admitted to Cushing's surgical service at the MGH. Although Cushing's admitting histories were slightly longer on average than those written by other house officers, they were within a common range. Note was made of the white blood cell count (then on the cutting edge of diagnostic technology) in 50% of Cushing's cases and in 48% of cases worked up by other house officers. It was probably the unique combination of personalities among the JHH attending staff during Cushing's residency, added to his own innate drive for perfection and complete collections of every sort, that fostered this change.

Regardless of its source, Cushing's taste for detailed examinations was apparent throughout his earliest neurosurgical work. Notable sensory examinations occur in his work on sacral nerve root distributions[39] and spinal cord lesions, including his first meningioma patient.[31] His most careful examinations were reserved for his trigeminal ganglionectomy patients. Light touch was tested with a horse hair mounted "like a von Frey aesthesiometer," pain with a sharp pin on a cardboard handle, and temperature sense with a camel's hair brush dipped in ether and a warmed test-tube.[42] He conducted the examinations alone with the patient in quiet surroundings, with "observations invariably deferred when evidence of even a slight degree of fatigue was given." A series of articles was the result.[33,42,46,47]

The requirement for accurate and detailed histories and examinations was immediately impressed upon his trainees. Kenneth McKenzie was told on his arrival from Canada in 1922 that he "was to make sure that [Cushing] would never look up one of my case histories in future years and find it inadequate." All histories were checked by Cushing himself on Saturdays.[88] Another resident said it was easy to keep Cushing happy: "simply have all the visual fields done, all the records up to date, know the condition of every patient when he called, and be available every moment."[76]

By the late 1920's, a typical chart of one of Cushing's patients contained a typed history and physical examination by his resident (the "special" examination), five single-spaced, legal-sized pages long; residents dictated the notes which were typed by stenographers from the wax dictaphone cylinders.[63] It is from these notes that the neurological examinations contained in the Cushing Tumor Registry case summaries presented in this book were extracted, typically limited to just the positive findings. The full "neurological examination" in the original hospital chart included descriptions of the skin, hair, head, neck, cranial nerves I–XII, visual fields, cerebral function (frontal, temporal, precentral, paracentral, postcentral, and occipital lobes), cerebellar signs, reflexes, vasomotor findings, sphincter function, peripheral findings, and pituitary symptomatology.[8,89] The "general" examination, conducted by a surgical intern, addressed the rest of the body; this tended to be shorter than for other surgical attendings' patients. Cushing relied primarily on his own hand-picked trainees to gather critical data rather than on the general surgery house officers.

The part of the examination that Cushing made his own special province was the visual fields. As early as 1902 we find him examining the eye grounds in trauma patients,[15] probably having learned the use of the ophthalmoscope during his trip to Europe in 1900-1901. By 1908 he reported "observations on choked disc" in 200 cases,[10] and experimental work followed.[50] Systematic formal perimetry began in 1905 (only 3 of 42 cases of brain tumor seen in the preceding 15 years had perimetry, compared to 123 of the next 200 patients, the remainder being blind, too young, or unconscious).[54] Fields were plotted for multiple colored targets (white, blue, red, and sometimes green) and observations were correlated with the appearance of the optic disc.[21] Again, a series of publications resulted.[20-22,38,54-56,103] Of these, the most important was the description of visual field changes resulting from temporal lobe tumors.[22] He won the Knapp Prize in Ophthalmology for his work on tuberculum sellae meningiomas and was elected an honorary member of the American Ophthalmological Society.[51,92]

Before the introduction of ventriculography, changes in the visual fields often provided the best guide to a cerebral tumor's location. But the ritual of ophthalmoscope and perimeter served another purpose in Cushing's clinic: it was a rite of initiation for his house officers which they apparently never forgot. William Sharpe wrote about the experience 41 years after his 1911 internship.[93] The day Dr. Cushing borrowed his ophthalmoscope – and broke it – stood out in Thomas Hoen's memory two decades later.[68] Kenneth McKenzie arrived at the Peter Bent Brigham Hospital (PBBH) having never seen a patient with a brain tumor; weeks passed before he could use the ophthalmoscope properly; the examination, including perimetry, took hours.[88] Percival Bailey spent long nights reading articles to learn the use of the intricate perimeter, since the inventor had gone to California.[1] The last man to work alone as Cushing's assistant, Eric Oldberg, recalled that formal visual fields were to be recorded for every patient, even spinal cases; optic disks were to be examined on every patient at least every 48 hours.[76] The medical student on the service later remembered Oldberg as "the most exhausted man in white he ever saw."[96]

Cushing's relentless pursuit of seemingly trivial detail certainly paid a dividend when he looked back over his meningioma experience. He was able to piece together coherent clinical syndromes for meningiomas of the olfactory groove, suprasellar region, optic sheath, sphenoid wing (lateral, middle, and medial thirds), convexity, parasagittal, and falx tumors, and tumors of the cerebellar convexity and cerebellopontine angle.[52] It was probably his recognition that these clinically consistent syndromes were primarily based on tumor location, paired with the favorable prognosis shared by most histological subtypes of meningiomas if completely excised, that led him to coin the term "meningioma" in 1922 to cover the range of distinct pathological variants of dural-based tumors.[32] He offered the new omnibus term almost apologetically, but adopted it immediately himself for published writings. Patient 3.6 offers an interesting window into this semantic shift – Cushing refers to the tumor as a meningioma in the operative note and as an endothelioma in the pathology report. Perhaps he briefly entertained using different terms for the clinical and pathological entities.

Operative Technique

Cushing's contributions to neurosurgical technique have been previously described.[77,81] These included, among many other technical points, the systematic use of decompressive subtemporal craniectomy,[24] the midline suboccipital craniectomy,[24] and closure of the galea.[77] In a broader sense, his training at JHH as a resident by William Halsted – a slow, painstaking operator who emphasized gentle handling of tissues and absolute hemostasis – resulted in a careful approach to surgery that was radically different both from his early training in Boston[4] and from the slapdash technique he saw Horsley employ in London.[67] "I am a little disappointed in Victor Horsley," he had written to his father. "His place is in the laboratory doubtless ... The technique of all these men is execrable from our standpoint and they must have many septic wounds" (HC to HKC, 7/7/1900; Yale University Library).[74] Cushing, in contrast, was a very slow surgeon by contemporary standards.[68]

Hemostasis was an aspect of neurosurgery to which Cushing made key contributions.[82] "In few surgical operations is a critical loss of blood so likely to occur" as in a meningioma operation, Cushing wrote,[52] and he customarily had prepared blood donors available, as well as experimenting with autotransfusion of blood recovered from the suction.[58] He frequently applied crushed raw muscle (from the patient's thigh or from another operating room) to stanch venous oozing, as in most of the patients in this chapter,[52] and prompted two of his residents to work on fibrin preparations for local hemostatic use.[72,73] Other measures he introduced or popularized included a pneumatic tourniquet around the scalp to reduce scalp bleeding (1904),[40] the silver clip for occluding small cerebral or tumor vessels (visible on his surgical specimens as early as 1910, and on most of the specimens illustrated in this chapter),[18,52] and the celebrated introduction of the Bovie electrocautery to intracranial surgery (1926; see Patients 3.8–9, 3.11–12).[70] Although others had used electrocautery for the removal of cerebral tumors, including Sir Rickman Godlee in the first brain tumor operation ("galvanocautery"),[7] Cushing's persistent use of the Bovie device enabled him to attack meningiomas he had previously dismissed as inoperable. At first there were problems with the new instrument: During its first use, on a tumor thought to be a meningioma, Cushing's medical student fainted and his assistant Hugh Cairns, newly arrived from England, had to be replaced by a more experienced surgeon.[63,70,89] There were induced seizures, ether explosions, and occasional grounding of the current through Dr. Cushing.[23] More serious was the transient increase in operative mortality that was noted as Cushing called back cases he had been afraid to tackle, such as the second operation on Patient 3.8.[52] "The Chief is sailing very near the wind these days," Cairns wrote in 1926, "attempting more and more each time."[63]

When the Bovie was in use, disaster was as close as the nearest major blood vessel, and Cushing's next-to-last meningioma patient died on the operating table when he burned a hole in the supraclinoid carotid artery, "a surgical tragedy which made the senior author feel that these delicate procedures were not ones for a highly strung sexagenarian."[52] It was the tenth intraoperative death in his meningioma series.[52] An oral tradition passed on in Boston held that as the operating room slid into chaos on this occasion, Cushing bent over to the patient – who was awake – and whispered that in a short time she would feel very much better.

Despite such setbacks, Cushing successfully developed the basic procedure of electrosurgically coring out the center of the meningioma, followed by dissection of the capsule from the brain, which is still in use today. This was an adaptation of his previously developed technique for subtotal removal of acoustic neurinomas[49] with the addition of removal of the tumor capsule after the central debulking. Originally, Cushing had attempted to remove convexity and parasagittal meningiomas en bloc, and occasionally attributed late recurrences to his having violated the tumor capsule at the initial surgery.[52] He proposed and sometimes achieved a procedure in which the bone flap was allowed to remain attached to the affected dura, and the tumor, dura and bone dislodged as a single specimen (Patient 3.11) – reminiscent of the fatal procedure he had witnessed as a medical student.[52] The many photographs of bulky, intact meningiomas from his resections bear witness to the effort this principle must have cost him at the operating table. Cushing described the technique:

"The actual tilting out of a tumor is largely a one-man performance, and the operator's left hand is necessarily occupied in holding and guarding the tissue in process of separation. The manipulations meanwhile are carried on by slow, blunt dissection with the right hand, while an assistant keeps the field clean by the careful use of wet cotton pledgets. During the progress of the measure, particularly in the case of a deeply-seated tumor, vessels may be encountered passing from brain to tumor ... Under these circumstances the silver "clips" ... may be found to be useful."[18]

It is tempting to trace the concepts behind Halsted's en bloc resection of breast carcinoma through radical mastectomy in this meningioma technique, which Cushing only slowly abandoned for the advantages of a careful dissection of the capsule of a centrally debulked tumor away from surrounding structures. In fact, the first time he debulked a convexity tumor centrally was as a measure of desperation (see operative note, Patient 3.9) because he was afraid of being unable to close the scalp over a bulging tumor and brain. In his last meningioma case, in 1932, he described removing the central core of the tumor electrosurgically for hemostasis, and then the "remaining cup-like shell was cleanly dislodged from its nest" by "brushing it away from the surface of the brain with wet cotton pledgets."[52]

Whether Cushing systematically tried to divide the blood supply to meningiomas before debulking or removing them, as we often do today, is a harder question to settle. Certainly postoperative films show the site of convexity meningiomas surrounded by a ring of silver clips on the dural margin, as seen in Patient 3.12. Cushing's illustrations of his technique for skull base tumors do not seem to show a division of the tumor from the skull base as a separate step preceding central debulking. He typically removed the bulk of olfactory groove meningiomas before attacking the vascular central attachment to the anterior fossa floor as the final step.[52] For "globular" pterional meningiomas, with which he faced his greatest challenges, he allowed that a preliminary ligation of the external carotid could be helpful (see Patient 3.9).[52] Cushing had no experience with diagnostic arteriography, which was found useful by later workers in delineating the vascular supply of meningiomas preoperatively, and his single headlight and lack of operative magnification would have made devascularizing many skull base tumors a formidable task.

Greenblatt[71] has written that Cushing's ability to understand, and control, intracranial pressure (ICP) was his paradigmatic contribution to neurosurgery. Two methods of controlling ICP are mentioned in operative notes in this chapter. The first method, employed by von Bergmann as early as 1888,[45] was puncture of the lateral ventricle, attempted unsuccessfully in patient 3.1. Although Charles Frazier's name is linked with an occipital burr hole for lateral ventricular puncture placed during posterior fossa exposure, in 1905 he stated that resection of the lateral cerebellar hemisphere was a preferable means of improving exposure during cerebellar operations: "The former method [ventricular puncture] we disapprove of on the grounds that it is so fatal in its tendencies. The alternative [cerebellar resection] on the other hand is attended by very different results."[65,66] Cushing found the technique useful and by 1908 had punctured the lateral ventricles in about 40 patients.[45] He always acknowledged the danger of ventricular puncture, particularly when followed by injection of air or contrast material (Dandy's ventriculography), and spoke out strongly against the unnecessary use of these imaging techniques.[19] He often performed ventriculography in the operating theater with preparation for immediate subsequent craniotomy, as described in some glioma patients in this volume.

By 1921, when Patient 3.2 was operated, the use of intravenous hypertonic saline to reduce brain swelling had entered Cushing's practice. Based on experimental work by Lewis Weed,[105,106] a former research fellow of Cushing's at JHH, Frederick Foley introduced the clinical use of hyperosmolar therapy at Cushing's clinic in 1920 using salt per rectum or intravenously[53,61,62] and Ernest Sachs reported a similar experience.[91] It seems doubtful that Cushing relied on this technique for very long, as it is mentioned in only one later patient's summary in this chapter (Patient 3.6, 1923); one glioma patient in this book received salt per rectum with "improvement" in 1923.

Cushing's contributions to anesthetic technique are perhaps less well known. These include the precordial stethoscope[48] and the development of regional anesthesia.[28,36,37] Although Cushing did not invent the anesthesia chart, he certainly popularized it and introduced it from Boston to Baltimore.[4,6] His most important contribution to anesthetic monitoring, and arguably to medicine as a whole, was the importation of the Riva-Rocci sphygmomanometer on his return from Europe and its immediate adoption for all intracranial cases at JHH.[37] Cushing was soon able to demonstrate the rise in blood pressure that accompanies temporal lobe elevation and the manipulation of the Gasserian ganglion, even under a general anesthetic.[37] Blood pressure monitoring during operations was quickly adopted in other clinics, especially for operations on the brain.[64]

Cushing changed the anesthetic regimen for his meningioma cases more than once during his career. Between 1901 and 1902, after discovering that chloroform anesthesia (as recommended by Horsley and Elliot) was uniformly associated with hypotension, he discarded it in favor of ether.[37,46] He later switched to local anesthesia for the great majority of cases, even in children, since this technique was thought to avoid the increase in intracranial pressure sometimes associated with general anesthetics. Cushing had performed operations under local anesthesia during his internship in 1895[85] and second-stage craniotomies on conscious patients as early as 1907, allowing the patient to awaken from general anesthesia after the skin and bone flaps had been reflected.[34,99] His shift to local anesthesia for all cases has been attributed to the influence of Thierry de Martel, the French neurosurgeon who used local anesthesia for craniotomies during the first World War.[17,35,59] Cushing had recommended novocaine to the American Red Cross in 1916 as an essential medical supply, but only for dental use.[74] Within days of his arrival at the front in 1917 he was grumbling over

"The unusual experience for me of operating alone on heads with a strange anaesthetist using chloroform ... of course too much loss of blood, poor if any X-ray, practically no neurologic study."[74]

Two months later he was conducting "enormous operations" under local anesthesia, presumably in reaction to the lack of a skilled anesthesiologist on his team. But on his return to his own operating rooms in Boston he immediately reverted to general anesthetics. Six years passed before the first year in which half of his meningioma cases were performed under local anesthesia (1925).[52] Although the desire to avoid explosive volatile anesthetics once electrocautery was in frequent use may have hastened the switch to novocaine, Cushing was already using local anesthesia for a significant fraction of cases by that time.

End-Results

The details of Cushing's postoperative ritual have not stood the test of time as well as his preoperative routine and painstaking operative technique. We no longer use the silver foil dressing that he allowed to remain in place for two weeks, or the elaborate crinoline hood, resembling a full-head Minerva cast, for suboccipital incisions.

But in one aspect of postoperative care Cushing remains the nonpareil: his pursuit of complete and accurate follow-up on all cerebral tumor cases. This habit began in Boston and persisted beyond the end of his active surgical career. His MGH records contain careful notes on follow-up, sometimes obtained through notes from the Waverly Convalescent Home or by sending letters to his patients after discharge.[35,102] This habit probably reflects his close friendship with Emory Codman, the pioneer in studying "end-results" in American surgery;[13] it was an early lesson that Cushing took to heart. During his tenure at the PBBH, it was Cushing's custom to send a letter to each patient on the first anniversary of their operation, requesting a progress report. Replies were transcribed or bound directly into the patient's hospital record.[41,89] Of 313 consecutive patients with verified meningiomas in his personal series, only one had an "unknown" duration of postoperative survival.[52] Much of the credit for this remarkable record belongs to Dr. Louise Eisenhardt, Cushing's assistant from 1915 on, who began to collect survival data prospectively on Cushing's tumor patients in 1922.[69] In lieu of the computerized database which might be selected today for such a task – more than 2000 patients, of whom some 800 were still living in 1946 – Dr. Eisenhardt used a "little black book."[14,69]

Shortly after his retirement to New Haven, Cushing established a Brain Tumor Registry to continue follow-up on his patients as well as to serve as a consulting center for neuropathological enigmas.[67] Many of his cases "survived ... as long and, as it turned out, longer than their surgeon (as cases will)."[79] Even after Cushing's death, Eisenhardt continued to accrue information on his tumor patients, apparently as late as 1963.[60]

This invaluable information on postoperative survival was conscientiously used to the full. Many of Cushing's assistants were encouraged to publish comprehensive follow-up studies using his records and, later, the Brain Tumor Registry. These reports might be written immediately after the assistant's year with Cushing[11,84] or several years later ("end-results").[12,57,75] Another characteristic project was the comprehensive study of a particular histological type of tumor. This might form a lengthy journal article (e.g., cerebellar astrocytomas,[26] oligodendrogliomas,[2] and medulloblastomas[27]) or a book (e.g., acoustic neurinomas,[49] gliomas,[3] and meningiomas[52]) These communications were often so detailed that Kaplan-Meier survival curves can today be plotted based on the data they contained (Figure 1).

Extended follow-up on brain tumor patients was quite unusual in Cushing's day, although not entirely unique; most surgeons limited their published reports to postoperative mortality statistics. Cushing not only recorded survival, but often included data on quality of life, which he considered to be more important than "the mere statistical enumeration of the dead and the living"[101] – a perspective that is regaining ground in brain tumor treatment today. In 1905, he wrote that "the mere lengthening of a patient's months or years without making them more livable is ... no justification whatsoever of an operative procedure."[43] As results improved with passing time, Cushing's standards for "useful" survival rose. Follow-up reports from the 1930's emphasized "usefulness, both social and economic, of the patients who survived."[12,57,101] Hugh Cairns stated that "the great desideratum ... [was] not only to alleviate suffering, but if possible to restore the patient's 'Arbeitsfähigkeit' [ability to work],"[12] and these reports used the criterion of return to former work or level of activity as their yardstick in determining useful survival.

Although Cushing's occasionally ungenerous behavior toward his contemporary competitors, such as Walter Dandy, has received much attention since his death, one senses clearly from his writings that his ultimate competition was with himself alone. "Games are hardly worth playing

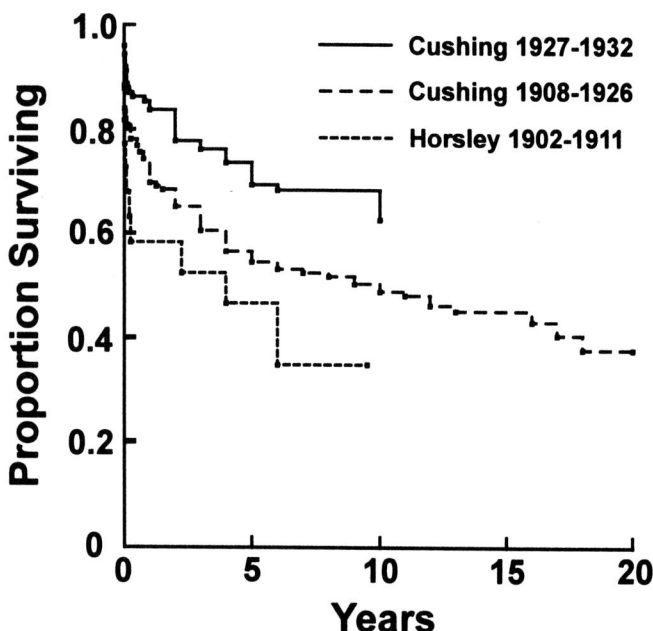

FIGURE 1. KAPLAN-MEIER CURVES ILLUSTRATING SURVIVAL AFTER INITIAL OPERATION FOR MENINGIOMA PATIENTS OPERATED BY HORSLEY[100] AND BY CUSHING, BEFORE AND AFTER THE INTRODUCTION OF ELECTROSURGERY.[52]

unless one keeps a score," he wrote in 1932.[30] Geoffrey Jefferson felt that this was an important motive for Cushing's frequent reviews of his results:

"From his earliest days he made a practice of publishing his operative mortality. He did this first because it was necessary for him to prove to an incredulous world that neuro-surgery was not beset with a depressing and terrifying mortality, but he did it, too, because of his deep faith that he could continuously better his performance. He was almost frightening in his belief that whatever the lesion was (unless hopelessly malignant) he could always show vastly better results in the next five-year period, frightening because such confidence seemed to invoke the wrath of the gods. Yet time proved that he was right."[80]

Popular biographies of Cushing characterized his contribution to neurosurgery as reducing the mortality of a "brain operation" from 90% to 10%.[86] With modern statistical techniques we can derive a more impartial estimate (Figure 1). Cushing's meningioma patients before the introduction of electrosurgery (1908-1926) had an overall risk of mortality 47% lower than Sir Victor Horsley's meningioma patients (1902 - 1911) (Cox proportional hazards model; $P = 0.035$). Cushing's patients first operated upon after the introduction of electrosurgery (1927–1932) enjoyed an additional 41% reduction in overall mortality (Cox model; $P = 0.006$). Hyperbole aside, this 69% overall reduction in mortality represents a true therapeutic revolution, one which took place within the span of a single career and was largely due to the work of a single man.

Cushing's Patients

Much has been written about Cushing, and about meningiomas, and so little about his patients. The processes by which his 300 meningioma patients found their way to him remain largely obscure, as do the economics of how his patients paid for their care and what happened to those who could not pay.[9] Certainly to seek out an operation for a brain tumor in the early years of Cushing's career bespoke considerable fortitude. One of Cushing's first meningioma patients was a household word for courage in early 20th century America: General Leonard Wood, one of Theodore Roosevelt's "Rough Riders," in 1910 the senior general officer in the US Army, and President Taft's chief of staff.[83,87,90] Wood had undergone a previous extracranial procedure for a right frontoparietal skull-based mass; fibrosarcoma was diagnosed. Intractable left-sided seizures compelled him to seek an operation for the intracranial portion of the tumor; he wrote President Taft that "As I have nothing especial to do ... I have decided to go to Johns Hopkins tomorrow and have Doctor Cushing look the thing over."[87] Cushing had never "looked over" anything quite like this before – it was his third intracranial meningioma – but he undertook what proved to be a harrowing removal. During the long case Wood's personal physician, Arthur Cabot, shuttled between the operating room and the patient's wife, constantly praising his courage and stamina but unconsciously using the past tense, as it was inconceivable he should survive. Wood's recovery and prolonged survival was later credited with winning Cushing the appointment as Surgeon-in-Chief at PBBH, where Wood later died after Cushing resected his recurrent tumor in 1927.[52,87]

Cushing's patients came from the full range of Progressive Era American society's spectrum, including its extremes. Patient 3.2 was a well-to-do lawyer and Patient 3.3 a Pullman porter. In an era before Medicaid, Medicare, or widespread health insurance, the inequities in complex health care delivery could be severe.[95] Yet Cushing's practice appears to have been largely immune to economic pressures. For example, three of his 18 meningiomas treated at JHH were African American in an era when Southern private neurosurgeons treated no such patients.[52] Cushing personally supported a private nurse to care for indigent brain tumor patients at PBBH[9] and performed all postoperative dressings personally, impartially for private and public ward patients.[68] When one former patient's glioblastoma recurrence made him unable to work and economic collapse threatened, Cushing returned his $500 fee from the operation a year before.[68]

Although Cushing's contributions to operative technique were notable, the impact of his beliefs regarding pre- and postoperative care represented a still greater advance over the methods of his forerunners and contemporaries. He systematized the preoperative diagnostic process, kept the pathological interpretation of brain tumor specimens under close personal supervision, and raised the standards by which neurosurgical outcome should be judged to a new level.

Many of these innovations sprang from Cushing's choice to keep every aspect of his patients' care under his own control. As early as 1902, he wrote of the surgeon who wished to undertake cranial cases that

"He must be neurologist and physiologist as well, for the sphere of the true surgeon in contradistinction to that of the operator does not begin and end with the incision and closure of the wound. He himself must direct the procedure, must interpret its indications and consequences. Valuable as consultations are the surgeon who can hold his neurological consultation with himself alone is able in case of necessity to intelligently direct his otherwise aimless manipulations ..."[74]

He continued to express this sentiment throughout his career. For a "brain surgeon" to operate only under the direction of a neurologist always seemed to Cushing to be an invitation to disaster, perhaps because of his memories of Elliot's operations at the MGH. The neurosurgeon "must make his own diagnoses and must have an intimate knowledge of neuro-pathology if he is to know what conditions are amenable to surgical therapeutics."[44] Today, this viewpoint seems natural, even a truism; but at the time it "lashed the neurological physicians into a frenzy."[79] Osler wrote in a letter that "from all I hear you are getting the Neurolog[ist]s of the country by the filum terminale."[74] But despite this temporary ruffling of feathers, Cushing's system quickly took hold throughout the English-speaking world and beyond. The dire rituals of initiation to which his trainees were subjected seem only to have strengthened their conviction that the Chief's way was the right way, and probably the only way. His belief that surgeons could be adequately trained to be the best judges both of therapy and of postoperative results persists today as a fundamental neurosurgical tenet, as witnessed by surgical training programs in fields such as stereotactic radiosurgery and interventional neuroradiology. It is reasonable to assume that the philosophy which has brought neurosurgery so far since Cushing's day will continue to be a useful one in the future.

Fred G. Barker II, M.D.
Boston, MA

Stephen B. Tatter, M.D., Ph.D.
Winston-Salem, NC

Acknowledgments

The authors gratefully acknowledge the generous assistance of Dr. Peter McL. Black, Mr. Richard Wolfe and the research staff of the Francis A. Countway Medical Library at Harvard Medical School, Boston, MA, and the staff of the Manuscript and Archives Department of the Yale University Library, New Haven, CT.

References

1. Bailey P: Pepper pot, in Bucy PC (ed): *Neurosurgical Giants: Feet of Clay and Iron*. New York, Amsterdam, Oxford: Elsevier, 1985, pp 73-89
2. Bailey P, Bucy PC: Oligodendrogliomas of the brain. *J Pathol Bacteriol* 32:735-751, 1929
3. Bailey P, Cushing H: *A Classification of the Tumors of the Glioma Group on a Histogenetic Basis with a Correlated Study of Prognosis*. Philadelphia: J.B. Lippincott Co., 1926
4. Barker FG, 2nd: The Massachusetts General Hospital: early history, and neurosurgery to 1939. *J Neurosurg* 79:948-959, 1993
5. Barker LF: Henry M. Thomas, M.D. 1861-1925. *Arch Neurol Psychiatry* 16:78-81, 1926
6. Beecher HK: The first anesthesia records (Codman, Cushing). *Surg Gynecol Obstet* 71:689-693, 1940
7. Bennett AH, Godlee RJ: Case of cerebral tumour. *Med-Chir Trans* 68, 1885
8. Black PM, Tyler HR, Khoshbin S: Cushing and the Peter Bent Brigham Hospital medical records, in Black PM (ed): *The Surgical Art of Harvey Cushing*. Park Ridge, IL: American Association of Neurological Surgeons, 1992, pp 7-34
9. Bliss M: *Harvey Cushing: A Life in Surgery*. New York and Toronto: Oxford University Press, 2006
10. Bordley J, Jr., Cushing H: Observations on choked disc. With especial reference to decompressive cranial operations. *JAMA* 52:353-360, 1909
11. Cairns H: A study of intracranial surgery. *Med Research Council Special Report* 125:1-89, 1929
12. Cairns H: The ultimate results of operations for intracranial tumors. *Yale J Biol Med* 8:421-492, 1936
13. Codman EA: Report of results in nontraumatic surgery of the brain and spinal cord. Observations upon the actual results of cerebral surgery at the Massachusetts General Hospital. *Bost Med Surg J* 153:74-76, 1905
14. Cushing H: Address by Dr. Cushing, in *Harvey Cushing's Seventieth Birthday Party*. Harvey Cushing Society, 1939, pp 32-38
15. Cushing H: The blood-pressure reaction of acute cerebral compression, illustrated by cases of intracranial hemorrhage. *Am J Med Sci* 125:1017-1044, 1903
16. Cushing H: Concerning a definite regulatory mechanism of the vasomotor centre which controls blood pressure during cerebral compression. *Johns Hopk Hosp Bull* 12:290-292, 1901
17. Cushing H: Concerning operations for the cranio-cerebral wounds of modern warfare. *Milit Surg* 38:601-615; 39:22-30, 1916
18. Cushing H: The control of bleeding in operations for brain tumors. With the description of silver "clips" for the occlusion of vessels inaccessible to the ligature. *Ann Surg* 54:1-19, 1911
19. Cushing H: Discussion [on paper by Dandy on ventriculography]. *Trans Am Neurol Assoc* 1922:69-74, 1922
20. Cushing H: Discussion on perimetric methods. *Br J Ophthalmol* 4:467-470, 1920
21. Cushing H: Distortions of the visual fields in cases of brain tumor (Second paper). Dyschromatopsia in relation to stages of choked disk. *JAMA* 57:200-208, 1911
22. Cushing H: Distortions of the visual fields in cases of brain tumor (Sixth paper). The field defects produced by temporal lobe lesions. *Brain* 44:341-396, 1922
23. Cushing H: Electro-surgery as an aid to the removal of intracranial tumors. *Surg Gynecol Obstet* 47:751-784, 1928
24. Cushing H: The establishment of cerebral hernia as a decompressive measure for inaccessible brain tumors; with the description of intramuscular methods of making the bone defect in temporal and occipital regions. *Surg Gynecol Obstet* 1:297-314, 1905
25. Cushing H: Ether Charts. Francis A. Countway Library of Medicine, Harvard Medical Library, Harvard University, Boston, MA, 1895-6
26. Cushing H: Experiences with the cerebellar astrocytomas. A critical review of seventy-six cases. *Surg Gynecol Obstet* 52:129-204, 1931
27. Cushing H: Experiences with the cerebellar medulloblastomas. A critical review. *Acta Pathol Microbiol Scand* 7:1-86, 1930

28. Cushing H: Exploratory laparotomy under local anesthesia for acute abdominal symptoms occurring in the course of typhoid fever. *Phila Med J* 5:501-508, 1900
29. Cushing H: Haematomyelia from gunshot wounds of the spine. *Am J Med Sci* 115:654-683, 1898
30. Cushing H: *Intracranial Tumors: Notes Upon a Series of Two Thousand Verified Cases with Surgical-Mortality Percentages Pertaining Thereto*. Springfield, IL: Charles C. Thomas, 1932
31. Cushing H: Intradural tumor of the cervical meninges. With early restoration of function in the cord after removal of the tumor. *Ann Surg* 39:934-955, 1904
32. Cushing H: The meningiomas (dural endotheliomas): their source, and favored seats of origin. *Brain* 45:282-316, 1922
33. Cushing H: A method of total extirpation of the Gasserian ganglion for trigeminal neuralgia. By a route through the temporal fossa and beneath the middle meningeal artery. *JAMA* 34:1035-1041, 1900
34. Cushing H: A note upon the faradic stimulation of the postcentral gyrus in conscious patients. *Brain* 32:44-53, 1909
35. Cushing H: Notes on penetrating wounds of the brain. *Br Med J* 1:221-226, 1918
36. Cushing H: Observations upon the neural anatomy of the inguinal region relative to the performance of herniotomy under local anesthesia. *Bull Johns Hopkins Hosp* 11:58-64, 1900
37. Cushing H: On the avoidance of shock in major amputations by cocainization of large nerve-trunks preliminary to their division. *Ann Surg* 36:321-345, 1902
38. Cushing H: The perimetric deviations accompanying pituitary lesions (preliminary note). *J Nerv Ment Dis* 40:793-794, 1913
39. Cushing H: Perineal zoster, with notes upon cutaneous segmentation post-axial to the lower limb. *Am J Med Sci* 127:375-391, 1904
40. Cushing H: Pneumatic tourniquets: with especial reference to their use in craniotomies. *Med News* 84:577-580, 1904
41. Cushing H: *Report of the Surgeon-in-Chief, in Peter Bent Brigham Hospital, Boston. Sixth Annual Report, for the Year 1919*. Cambridge, MA: Harvard University Press, 1920, pp 54-150
42. Cushing H: The sensory distribution of the fifth cranial nerve. *Bull Johns Hopkins Hosp* 15:213-232, 1904
43. Cushing H: The special field of neurological surgery. *Cleveland Med J* 4:1-25, 1905
44. Cushing H: The special field of neurological surgery after another interval. *Wis Med J* 19:501-520, 1921
45. Cushing H: Surgery of the Head, in Keen WW (ed): *Surgery: Its Principles and Practice*. Philadelphia and London: W. B. Saunders Co., 1908, Vol 3, pp 17-276
46. Cushing H: The surgical aspects of major neuralgia of the trigeminal nerve. A report of twenty cases of operation on the Gasserian ganglion, with anatomic and physiologic notes on the consequences of its removal. *JAMA* 44:773-778, 860-865, 920-929, 1002-1008, 1088-1093, 1905
47. Cushing H: The taste fibres and their independence of the N. trigeminus. Deductions from thirteen cases of Gasserian ganglion extirpation. *Bull Johns Hopkins Hosp* 14:71-78, 1903
48. Cushing H: Technical methods of performing certain cranial operations. *Surg Gynecol Obstet* 6:227-246, 1908
49. Cushing H: *Tumors of the Nervus Acusticus*. Philadelphia: W. B. Saunders, 1917
50. Cushing H, Bordley J, Jr.: Observations on experimentally induced choked disc. *Bull Johns Hopkins Hosp* 20:95-101, 1909
51. Cushing H, Eisenhardt L: Meningiomas arising from the tuberculum sellae. *Arch Ophthalmol* 1:1-41, 168-206, 1929
52. Cushing H, Eisenhardt L: *Meningiomas. Their Classification, Regional Behaviour, Life History, and Surgical End-Results*. Springfield, IL: Charles C. Thomas, 1938
53. Cushing H, Foley FEB: Alterations of intracranial tension by salt solutions in the alimentary canal. *Proc Soc Exp Biol NY* 17:217-218, 1920
54. Cushing H, Heuer GJ: Distortions of the visual fields in cases of brain tumor. Statistical series. (First paper). *Bull Johns Hopkins Hosp* 22:190-195, 1911

55. Cushing H, Walker CB: Distortions of the visual fields in cases of brain tumor (Fourth paper). Chiasmal lesions, with especial reference to bitemporal hemianopsia. *Brain* 37:341-400, 1915
56. Cushing H, Walker CB: Distortions of the visual fields in cases of brain tumor (Third paper). Binasal hemianopsia. *Arch Ophthalmol* 41:559-598, 1912
57. Davidoff LM: A thirteen year follow-up study of a series of cases of verified tumors of the brain. *Arch Neurol Psychiatry* 44:1246-1261, 1940
58. Davis LE, Cushing H: Experiences with blood replacement during or after major intracranial operations. *Surg Gynecol Obstet* 40:310-322, 1925
59. de Martel T: Surgical treatment of cerebral tumors. *Surg Gynecol Obstet* 52:381-385, 1931
60. Eisenhardt L: Discussion, in *Second International Congress of Neurological Surgery: abstracts and descriptions of contributions to the scientific program*. Amsterdam: Excerpta Medica, 1961, p E 10
61. Foley FEB: Clinical uses of salt solution in conditions of increased intracranial tension. *Surg Gynecol Obstetrics* 33:126-136, 1921
62. Foley FEB, Putnam TJ: The effect of salt ingestion on cerebro-spinal fluid pressure and brain volume. *Am J Physiol* 53:464-476, 1920
63. Fraenkel GJ: *Hugh Cairns. First Nuffield Professor of Surgery, University of Oxford*. Oxford: Oxford University Press, 1991
64. Frazier C: Remarks upon the surgical aspects of operable tumors of the cerebrum, in Mills CK, Frazier C, Spiller WG, et al (eds): *Tumors of the Cerebrum. Their Focal Diagnosis and Surgical Treatment*. Philadelphia: Edward Pennock, 1905, pp 1-46
65. Frazier C: Remarks upon the surgical aspects of tumors of the cerebellum, in Mills CK, Frazier C, de Schweinitz GE, et al (eds): *Tumors of the Cerebellum*. New York: A. R. Elliott Publishing Co., 1905, pp 39-85
66. Frazier C: Remarks upon the surgical aspects of tumors of the cerebellum. *New York Med J* 81:272-280, 332-337, 1905
67. Fulton JF: *Harvey Cushing: A Biography*. Springfield, IL: Charles C. Thomas, 1946
68. Fulton JF, Ray BS, Davidoff LM, Hoen TI, Scarff JE, Bagley C, Jr., et al: Harvey Cushing as we knew him. A symposium. *Bull New York Acad Med* 2s 30, 1954
69. German WJ: Dr. Louise Eisenhardt. *J Neurosurg* 26:285-288, 1967
70. Goldwyn RM: Bovie: the man and the machine. *Ann Plast Surg* 2:135-153, 1979
71. Greenblatt SH: Harvey Cushing's paradigmatic contribution to neurosurgery and the evolution of his thoughts about specialization. *Bull Hist Med* 77:789-822, 2003
72. Grey EG: Fibrin as a haemostatic in cerebral surgery. *Surg Gynecol Obstet* 21:452-454, 1915
73. Harvey SC: Fibrin paper as a haemostatic agent. *Ann Surg* 67:67-70, 1918
74. Harvey Williams Cushing Papers, Department of Manuscripts and Archives, Yale University Library, New Haven, CT
75. Henderson WR: The pituitary adenomata. A followup study of the surgical results in 338 cases (Dr. Harvey Cushing's series). *Br J Surg* 26:811-921, 1939
76. Heyl L: A selection of Harvey Cushing anecdotes. *J Neurosurg* 30:365-376, 1969
77. Horrax G: Some of Harvey's Cushing's contributions to neurological surgery. *J Neurosurg* 1:3-22, 1944
78. Horsley V: On the technique of operations on the nervous system. *Br Med J* 2:411-423, 1906
79. Jefferson G: Harvey Cushing, in Jefferson G (ed): *Selected papers*. London: Pitman Medical Publishers, 1960, pp 170-187
80. Jefferson G: Harvey Cushing (1869-1939). *Br J Surg* 27:442-445, 1940
81. Light RU: The contributions of Harvey Cushing to the techniques of neurosurgery. *Surg Neurol* 35:69-73, 1991
82. Light RU: Hemostasis in neurosurgery. *J Neurosurg* 2:414-434, 1945
83. Ljunggren B: The case of General Wood. *J Neurosurg* 56:471-474, 1982
84. Locke CE: A review of a year's series of intracranial tumors. *Arch Surg* 3:560-581, 1921
85. Massachusetts General Hospital South Surgical Service Records (1895-1896), Francis A. Countway Library of Medicine, Harvard University, Boston, MA

86. Match R: Father of modern brain surgery. *Reader's Digest* 52(2):76-80, 1948
87. McCallum J: *Leonard Wood: Rough Rider, Surgeon, Architect of American Imperialism.* New York and London: New York University Press, 2006
88. McKenzie KG: Harvey Cushing. 1869-1939. *Am J Psychol* 96:1001-1007, 1940
89. Peter Bent Brigham Hospital Surgical Records (1912-1932). Brigham & Women's Hospital, Boston, MA
90. Rolak LA, Rolak B: Leonard Wood: the physician who was almost President of the United States. *J Med Biogr* 6:35-38, 1998
91. Sachs E: The use of saturated salt solution intravenously during intracranial operations. *JAMA* 75:667-668, 1920
92. Samuels B: Harvey Cushing, M.D. 1869-1939. His contributions to ophthalmology. *Arch Ophthalmol* 23:633-640, 1940
93. Sharpe W: *Brain Surgeon.* New York: Viking Press, 1952
94. Shrivastava RK, Segal S, Camins MB, Sen C, Post KD: Harvey Cushing's meningiomas text and the historical origin of resectability criteria for the anterior one third of the superior sagittal sinus. *J Neurosurg* 99:787-791, 2003
95. Starr P: *The Social Transformation of American Medicine.* New York: Basic Books, 1982
96. Sweet WH: Harvey Cushing: author, investigator, neurologist, neurosurgeon. *J Neurosurg* 50:5-12, 1979
97. Taylor EW: Two cases of tumor of the brain, with autopsy. *Boston Med Surg J* 134:57-60, 1896
98. Thomas HM: Comment on H. Cushing, "Haematomyelia from gunshot wound of the cervical spine." *Bull Johns Hopkins Hosp* 8:196-197, 1897
99. Thomas HM, Cushing H: Removal of a subcortical cystic tumor at a second-stage operation without anesthesia. *JAMA* 50:847-856, 1908
100. Tooth HH: The treatment of tumours of the brain, and the indications for operation. *Trans XVIIth International Congress of Medicine,* London Section VII, Part 1:203-299, 1913
101. van Wagenen WP: Verified brain tumours. End results of one hundred and forty-nine cases eight years after operation. *JAMA* 102:1454-1458, 1934
102. Viets HR: Notes on the formative period of a neurological surgeon, in *Harvey Cushing's Seventieth Birthday Party.* Harvey Cushing Society, 1939, pp 115-125
103. Walker CB, Cushing H: Distortions of the visual fields in cases of brain tumor (Fifth paper). Chiasmal lesions, with especial reference to homonymous hemianopsia with hypophyseal tumor. *Arch Ophthalmol* 47:119-145, 1918
104. Washburn FA: *The Massachusetts General Hospital. Its development, 1900-1935.* Boston: Houghton Mifflin Co., 1939
105. Weed LH, McKibben PS: Experimental alterations of brain bulk. *Am J Physiol* 48:531-555, 1919
106. Weed LH, McKibben PS: Pressure changes in the cerebro-spinal fluid following intravenous injection of solutions of various concentrations. *Am J Physiol* 48:512-530, 1919

3.1 Cerebellar meningioma

SEX: F; AGE: 58; SURG. NO. 1836

HISTORY

The patient presented with frontal headaches associated with intermittent nausea during the last two years. She also complained of dizziness and balance problems during the last several months.

SUMMARY OF POSITIVE FINDINGS
September 26, 1914
Dr. Grey

SUBJECTIVE
1. Headaches – 2 years.
2. Nausea – 3 years.
3. Stiffness of joints of hands – 6 months.
4. Dizziness – 7 months
5. Disturbance in gait – 6–7 months, falling to her right.
6. Vision affected – 2 years.
7. Tinnitus in both ears – one year – none recently.

OBJECTIVE
1. Nerve II – Bilateral choked disc.
2. Nerve V – Taste disturbed on anterior part of tongue.
3. Nerve VIII – Hearing – BC and AC slightly less well on left.
4. Nerves IX and X – Tendency for liquids to regurgitate – some vomiting.
5. Strength – An equal moderate decrease.
6. Deep reflexes hyperactive.
7. Gait – Very much disturbed.
8. Ataxia – Very little, if any, visible.
9. Barany finger to finger test – Deviation of right hand.
10. Caloric – Normal right. Negative left.
11. Balancing body – Trunk falls to left.
12. Suboccipital discomfort – Some on left.
13. Nystagmus – Slight on looking to right.

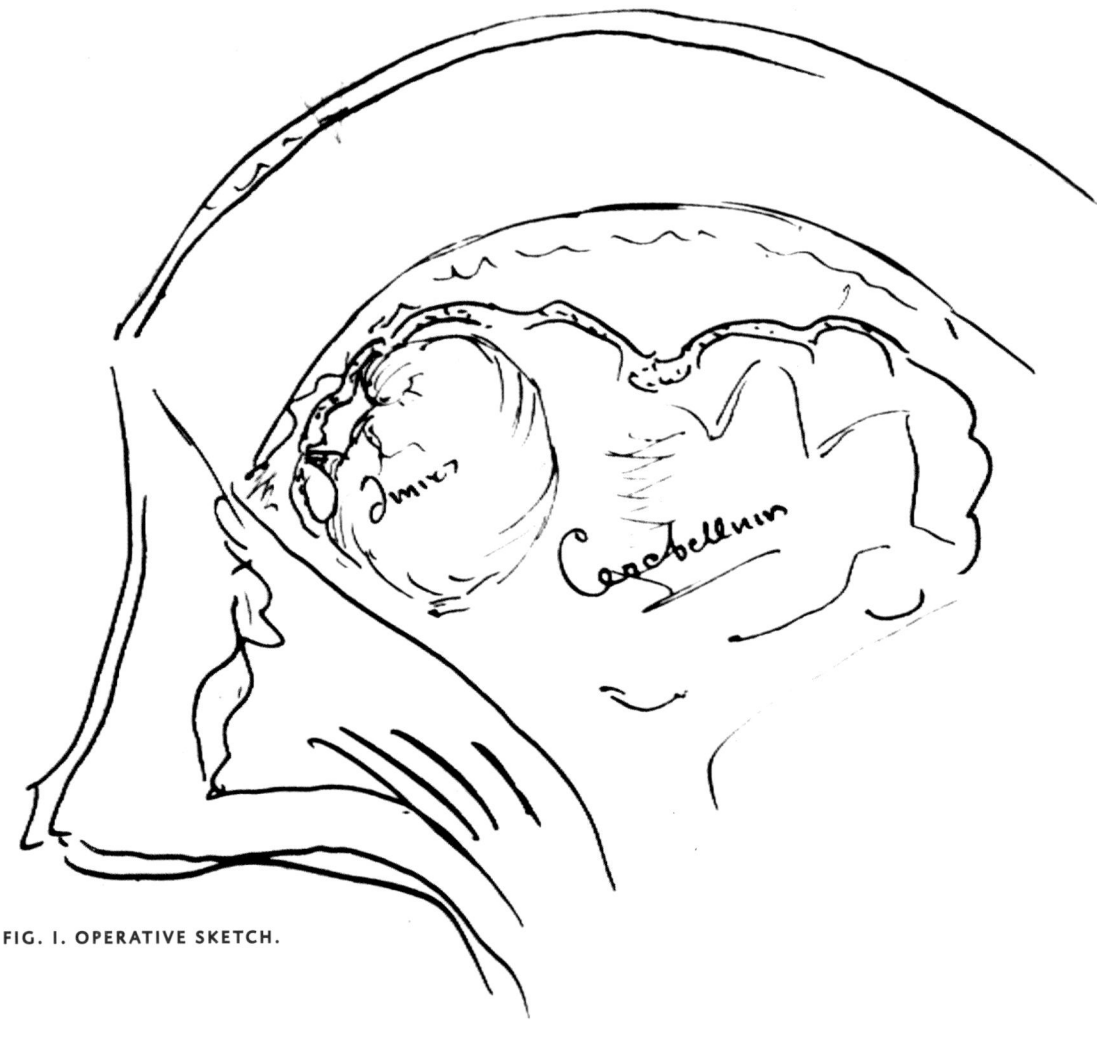

FIG. 1. OPERATIVE SKETCH.

RADIOLOGY REPORT
September 28, 1914
Dr. Carr

Average thickness of the skull 6–8 mm. The cerebral impressions are increased, especially in the frontal and anterior parietal regions. The venous channels are slightly enlarged. The sutures are faintly visible. The antero-posterior diameter of the sella is about 25 mm. It is about 12 mm deep. The anterior clinoid processes are distinct. The dorsum is vertical in direction, distinctly atrophic, and shows signs of destruction. The posterior clinoid processes are indistinct, atrophic, less so than the dorsum, however, and partially destroyed.

OPERATIVE NOTE
October 2, 1914
Anesthesia – Ether – Boothby

Exploration of an Endothelioma from Left Cerebellar Hemisphere

The diagnosis in this case pointed toward left cerebellar lesion, possibly in the posterior portion of the cerebellum.

The usual cross bow incision was made and a fairly large bony opening secured. The posterior half of the foramen was removed. The dura on the left showed a very evident discoloration and shining of the membrane suggesting the presence of underlying lesion. There had been considerable hemorrhage and attempt was made to puncture the left ventricle without success – four or five different punctures being made without getting fluid.

It was necessary therefore to progress without lowering tension by this means. The dura was opened and there was marked cerebellar protrusion. A tumor, evidently endothelioma, was disclosed as shown in the sketch. It was adherent to the left side of the fossa at the situation of the sigmoid sinus probably. The tumor was finally tilted out, most of it coming away in one large piece, though subsequently a considerable fragment of the capsule was separately dissected away and some of the remaining growth was scooped out with a spoon from the place of its dural attachment.

The conditions were almost exactly the same as those in the case of (another patient's name.)

There was considerable bleeding, but it was controlled without great difficulty and the wound closed in layers.

(Dr. Cushing)

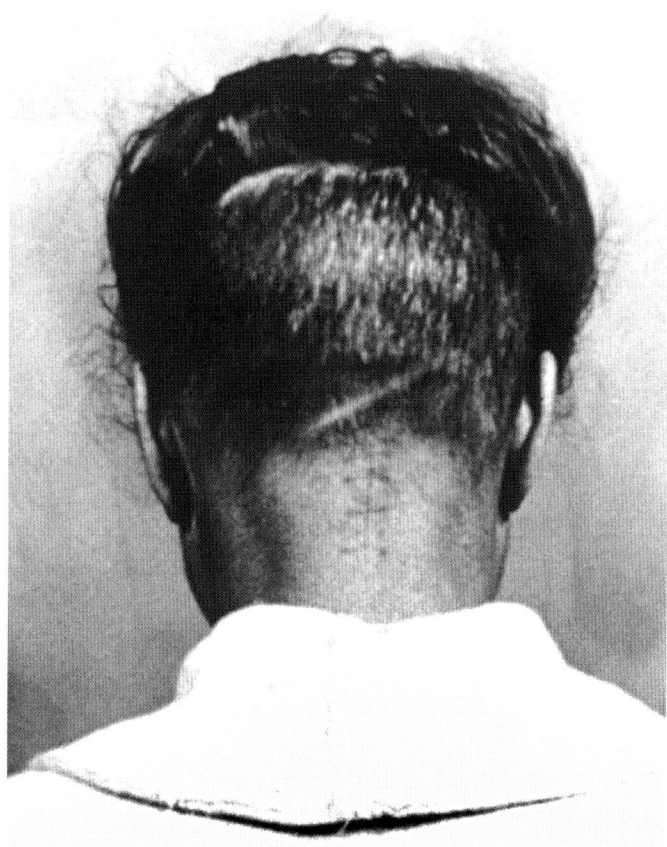

FIG. 2. POSTOPERATIVE.

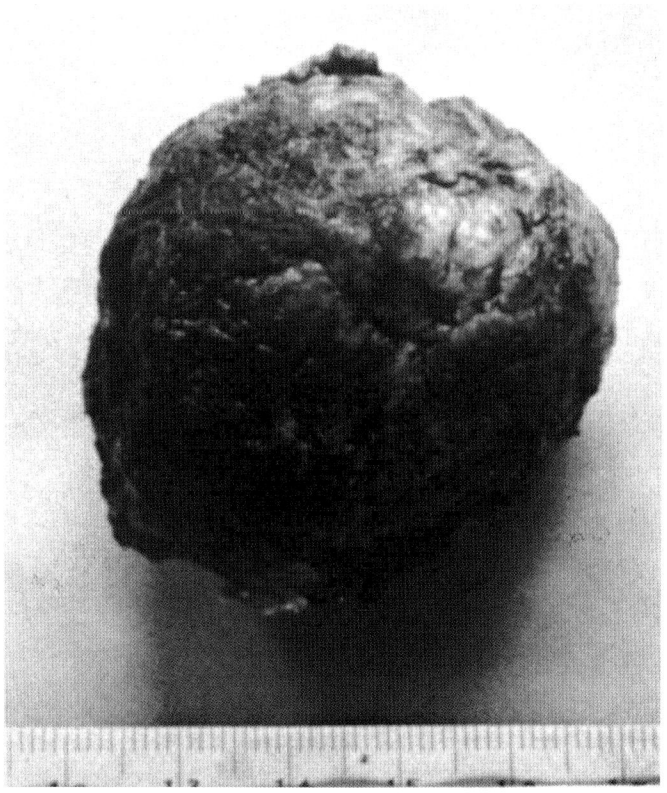

FIG. 3. RESECTED TUMOR SPECIMEN.

PATHOLOGY REPORT
October 2, 1914

The tumor is a typical endothelioma with whorls and spindle cells and with large operation hemorrhage.

    Diagnosis – Endothelioma

(Dr. Councilman)

POSTOPERATIVE NOTE
October 6, 1914
Dr. Rand

Patient has had a relatively uneventful course since operation. For first day or so, temperature was elevated from 99.6° to 101° but this has gradually gone down. She is very quiet, almost drowsy at times and has a tendency towards being irrational. General condition at present good, 6th day after operation. Dressing not yet removed.

October 13, 1914
Dr. Grey

First dressing. The cast was removed without difficulty and the wound found to be in excellent condition. Healing had taken place p.p. throughout. In only one stitch hole was there a minute trace of material resembling a purulent substance. This, however, may have been due to a very slight maceration. The balance of the stitches were removed leaving swollen base behind. The wound was washed with alcohol and a sterile gauze dressing applied. General condition of the patient is excellent. She is free from pain and appears cheerful.

DISCHARGE NOTE
November 4, 1914
Dr. Grey

SUMMARY OF POSITIVE FINDINGS AT DISCHARGE

SUBJECTIVE
1. Headache – None since operation
2. Nausea – Much less frequent
3. Has vomited a few times.
4. Stiffness of joints of hands – None since operation though one joint is slightly tender.
5. Dizziness – None.
6. Gait – Is just beginning to walk herself.
7. Vision – A little better perhaps.
8. Tinnitus – None.

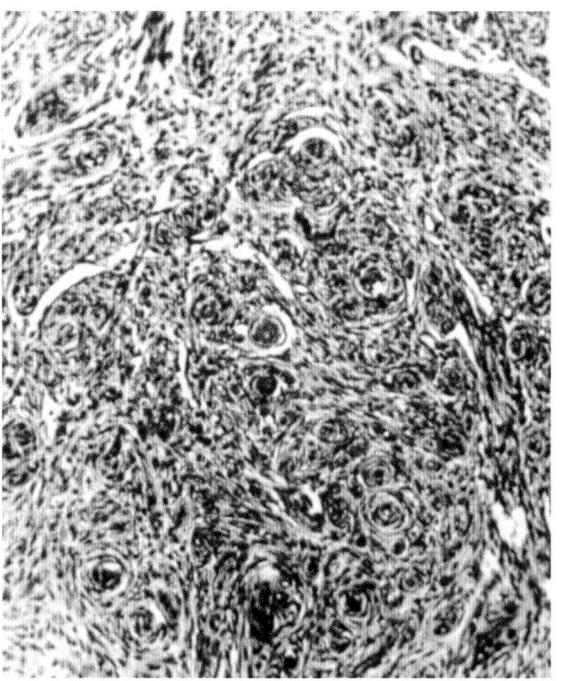

FIG. 4. HISTOLOGY SLIDE.

OBJECTIVE
1. Nerve II – Fundi show complete obliteration of discs with considerable rather white new tissue. Cups entirely filled. Vessels rather tortuous – No fresh hemorrhage. Neither eye a picture of acute recent changes.
   VA R.E. 20/70
   L.E. 20/70
2. Nerve VIII – Hears nearly equally well on the two sides.
3. Nerves IX–X – No regurgitation of fluid.
4. Strength – Has increased throughout body.
5. Ataxia – Very slight in both arms still.
6. Barany finger to finger test – Fairly performed both sides.
7. Nystagmus – Moderate on looking to either side. Jerks continue slower and coarser on looking to left.
8. Sub-occipital discomfort – Only occasionally when lying on her back. No appreciable tenderness.

LETTER TO DR. CUSHING
February 21, 1917

Dear Sir:

It has made me very happy to hear from you, and to know you have been thinking of me for so long. I have been very well since I saw you and if you are

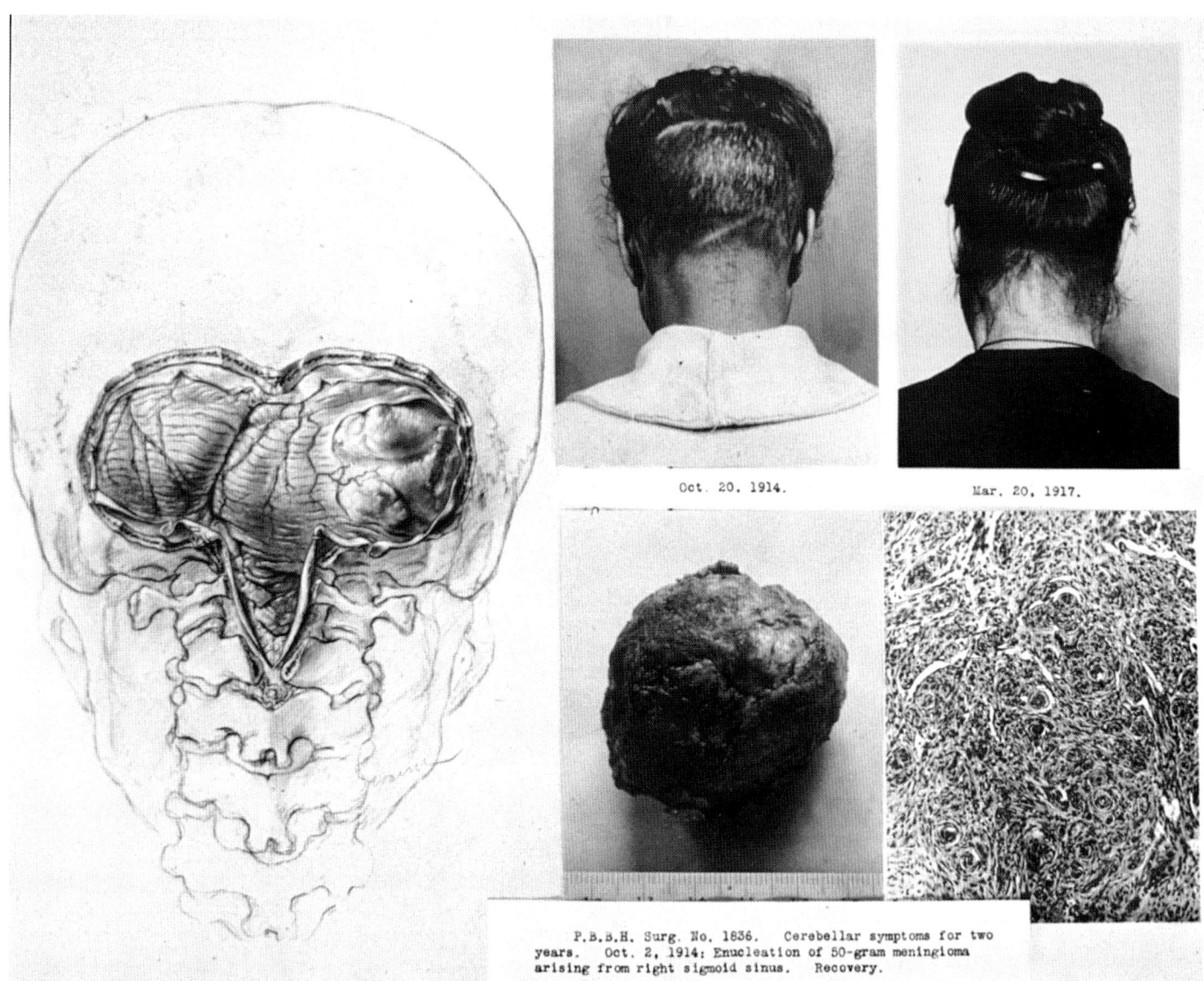

FIG. 5. TEACHING SLIDE.

not so busy I would love to go over to the hospital some day next week, and let you see how well I am and what your operation has done for me.

Hoping to hear from you again, I am

Yours sincerely,
(Signed) AC

LETTER TO DR. CUSHING
December 14, 1929

Dear Doctor:

During the early part of October I called at the hospital but was informed that you were in Europe. I regret that I was unable to see you at that time. During the past year I have felt very well except during the summer when I was bothered with rheumatism in my knees. I am now living in Flushing, New York, and if I am in Boston in the near future I will call to see you. With kindest personal regards, I am,

Yours very truly,
(Signed) AC

The patient died on December 7, 1932 (No autopsy report was available in the chart.)

Attached you can find Dr. Cushing's teaching slide describing this patient's condition.

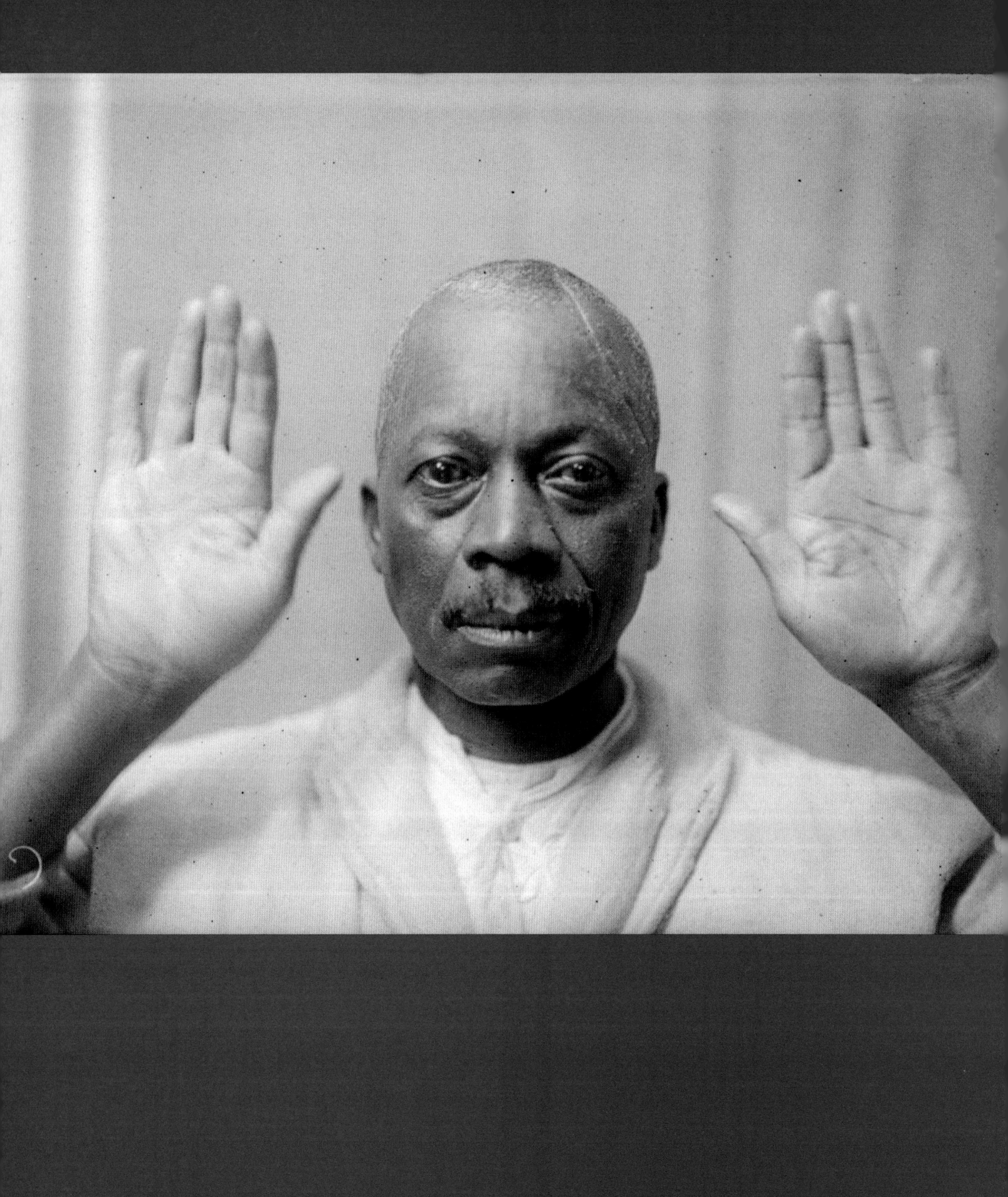

3.2 Convexity meningioma

SEX: M; AGE: 53; SURG. NO. 14371; 27326; 30123

HISTORY

The patient was admitted to the hospital (medical service) on April 6, 1921 with speech difficulty of one month duration with a presumed diagnosis of cerebral ischemia. Further work-up made such a diagnosis less likely. He was then transferred to the surgical service on April 15th with a diagnosis of "cerebral tumor."

SUMMARY OF POSITIVE FINDINGS
April 20, 1921
Dr. Foley (Medical Service)

SUBJECTIVE
1. Weakness of right facial muscles beginning March 25th.
2. Numbness of right side of face and right hand beginning March 22.
3. Speech difficulties beginning March 25th.
4. Slight frontal headache.
5. Recently dragging of right foot.
6. History of head trauma 14 years ago.

OBJECTIVE
1. Deviation of jaw to right on closing mouth.
2. Obliteration of naso-labial folds on right and right 7th nerve paresis.
3. Marked hypesthesia over sensory right 5th particularly 2nd and 3rd divisions.
4. Marked diminution of right corneal reflex.
5. Dysarthria, alexia, and aphonia, apraxia.
6. Right hemiparesis and hemianesthesia, most marked in upper extremity.
7. Deep reflexes increased in right arm.

IMPRESSION: Thrombosis of branches of right cortical vessels.

RADIOLOGY REPORT
April 22, 1921

Stereoscopic plates of the skull in a right lateral position show the skull to be normal in contour with a normal frontal sinus. There is no evidence of intracranial pressure, the sella turcica itself being normal in outline.

OPERATIVE NOTE
April 21, 1921
Anesthesia – Ether – Miss Gerard

Left Cranial Exploration for Supposed Lesion Involving Arm Center.

A fairly large bone flap was outlined and the approach was made with some difficulty and

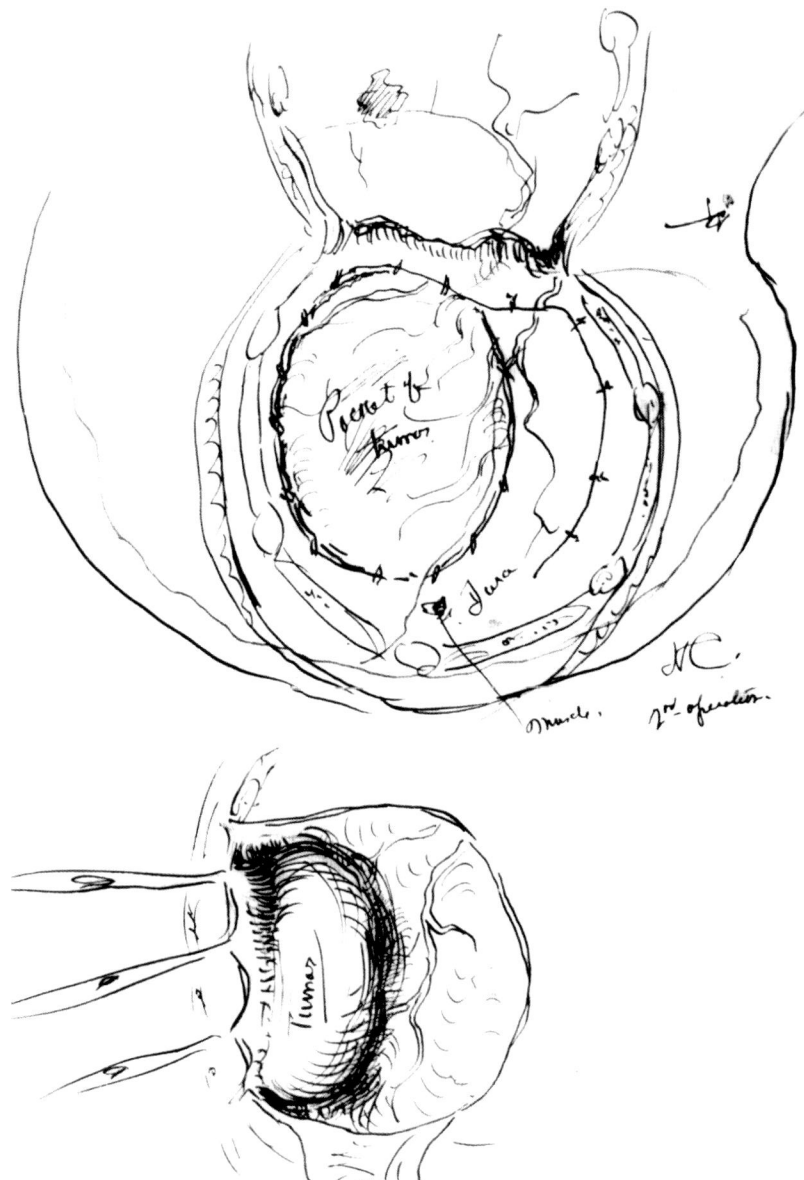

FIG. 2. OPERATIVE SKETCH.

OPPOSITE PAGE. FIG. I. THREE WEEKS AFTER FIRST SET OF OPERATIONS.

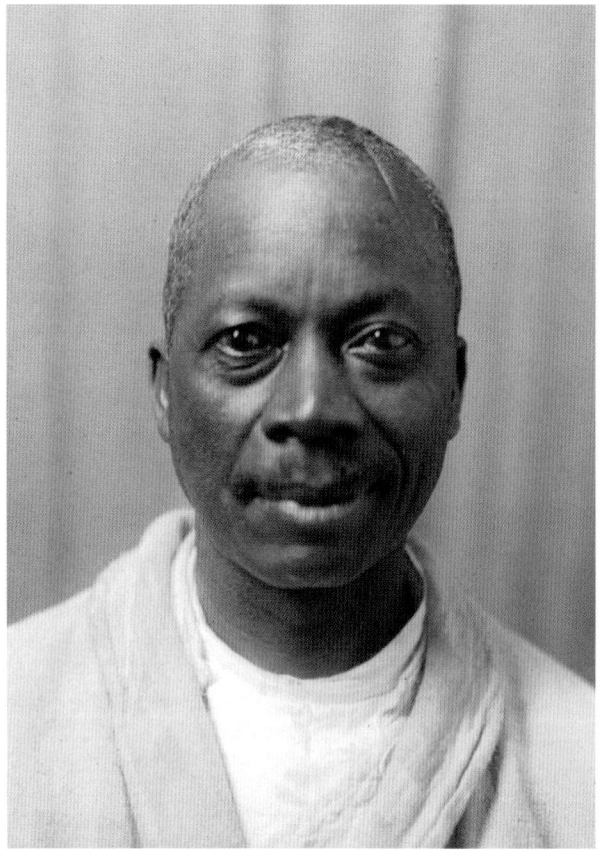

FIGS. 3–4. THREE WEEKS AFTER FIRST OPERATIONS.

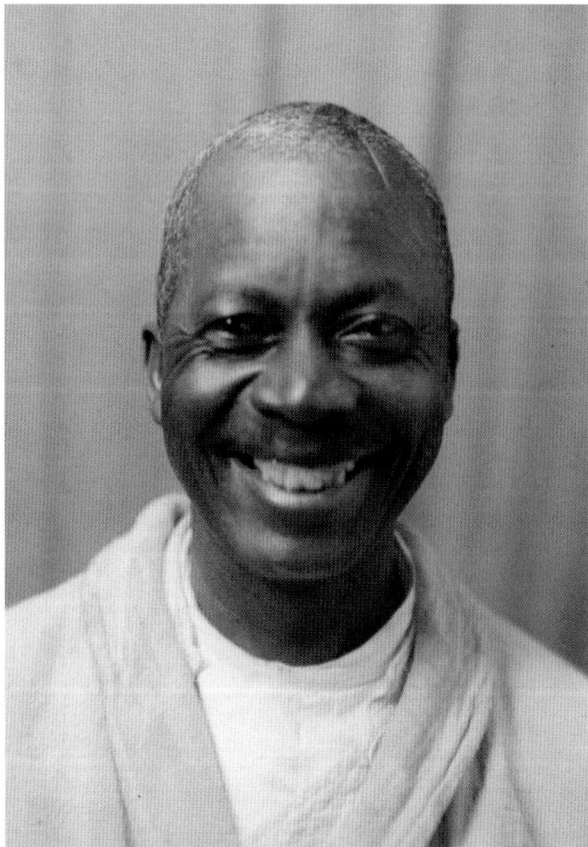

rather more bleeding than usual on account of the very great general thickness of the skull. There was no evidence of any special localized thickening but upon breaking up the flap the meningeal was found to have grooved the bone in the central region and was broken off and the meningeal channels in the flap were very deep. There was also one place over the posterior and inferior portions of the flap which was somewhat eroded and it was thought that possibly the underlying pathological change might be found at this place. Palpation of the dura revealed no very great tension. Needle was introduced at the anterior portion of the dura about over the base of the second frontal convolution. No fluid was obtained up to a depth of 5½ cm. The dura was now opened widely beginning at the anterior portion of the field and lifting the flap upward with its pedicle at the top. After cutting across the meningeal vessel at the base and carrying the incision further posteriorly for a little way a tumor was exposed which was lying probably just above the superior temporal convolution and perhaps a little forward of the supramarginal gyrus. It was adherent to the dura and was seen to have a very definite capsule and edge, leaving little doubt but that it was a dural endothelioma. As the operation had already been prolonged and the patient's blood pressure had fallen off somewhat it was deemed wise to do the enucleation in a second session so the dura was closed without great difficulty and the bone flap put back into place without leaving a decompression. A rubber tissue drain was left at the upper margin of the wound being brought out through a stab wound in the scalp about an inch above the flap incision. Closure was made as usual in layers with fine silk. Patient took his anesthesia very well and was in very fair shape at the end.

(Dr. Horrax)

POSTOPERATIVE NOTE
April 21, 1921
Dr. Locke

Patient has a slight temperature reaction. No change in signs or symptoms.

OPERATIVE NOTE
April 23, 1921
No anesthesia (Morphia).

Enucleation of Typical Endothelioma from Postcentral and Supramarginal Region as per Diagrams.

The bone flap made by Dr. Horrax at the previous operation was relifted, the patient having been given a dose of morphia. There was considerable blood clot and a good deal of oozing which, however, during the course of the operation was gradually controlled. Particularly at the upper margin, at the end of the operation, it was necessary to place a good many fragments of muscle which were taken from the patient's temporal muscle. The dural incision made by Dr. Horrax was re-elevated and the tumor located. It was then possible to surround the growth as it was gradually tilted out to cut the dura close to the attachment of the tumor. There was a small defect in the bone about the center of the tumor which showed in the reflected flap but did not show in the x-ray. The tumor fortunately had a very smooth surface and was gradually tilted out, the pia arachnoid being brushed from its surface without injury to vessels. As the growth was finally almost completely removed and the dura divided close to the margin of the bony opening, it was found that the growth here was somewhat irregular on its surface and there were attachments between pia arachnoid and tumor which had to be divided between clips. Aside from this, there was no damage to the cortex.

The small area of dura which could be preserved was then resutured and a long slow process of hemostasis was carried out so as to obviate if possible any subsequent filling up of the cavity from oozing. Oozing continued from the bone flap for a very long time and was not completely checked at the end of the procedure. A circle of dura defect corresponding to the tumor was demarcated with clips so it could be certified by the x-ray subsequently.

(Dr. Cushing)

PATHOLOGY REPORT
April 23, 1921

Gross description – Tumor is endothelioma weighing 70 gms, on one surface of which is an area of dura 6 x 4 cm, the tumor is entirely free of brain tissue and there appears to be no adherent pia arachnoid.

Microscopic – A section consists largely of long spindle cells arranged in many twists and whorls, often about a small central blood vessel. These cells are of the type usually found in dural endotheliomas but are slightly larger than ordinarily, stain deeply and one mitotic figure is seen.

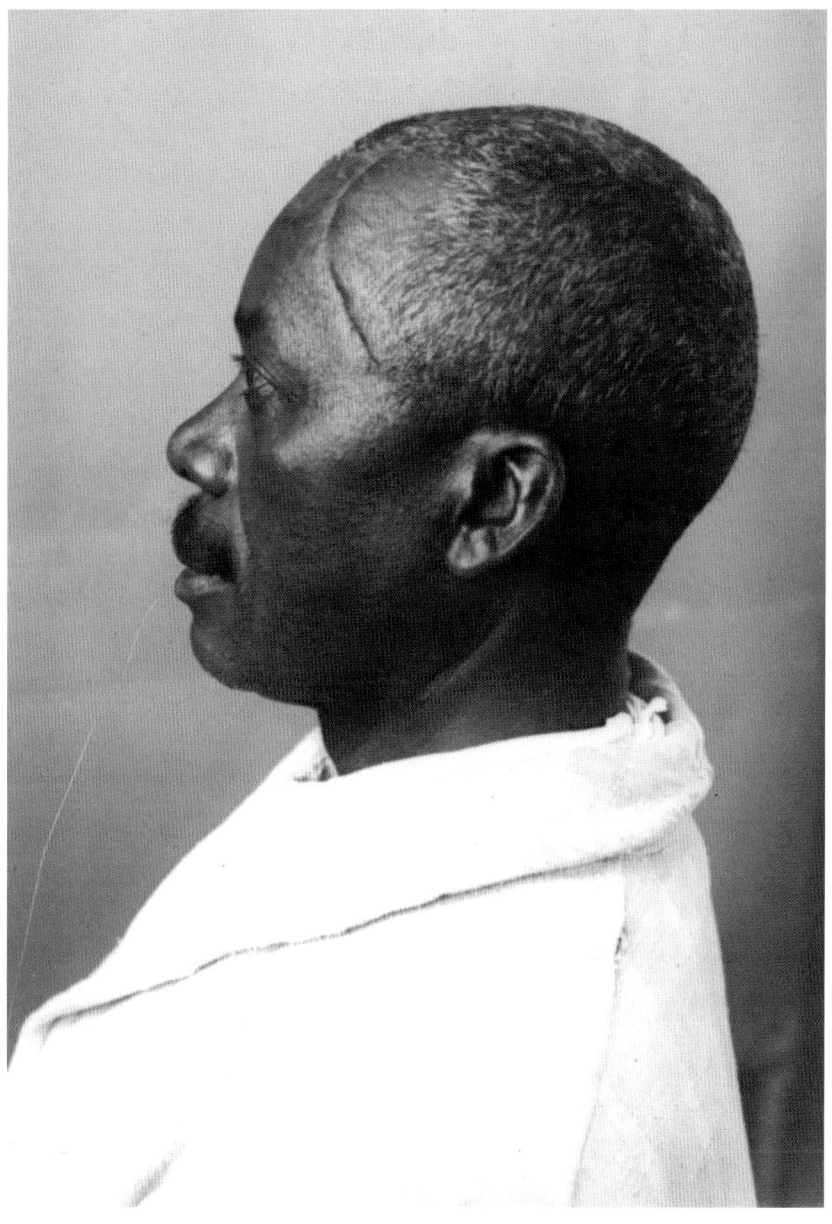

FIG. 5. THREE WEEKS AFTER FIRST OPERATIONS.

Larger blood vessels are present here and there amid tumor cells are a few collagen fibers.

Diagnosis: Dural endothelioma

(Dr. Wolbach)

POSTOPERATIVE NOTE
April 23, 1921
Dr. Locke

There is a very definite astereognosis on right. Normal plantar response on right and left. No apraxia.

This evening speech is very much better. Patient can tell his age, where he was born and his occupation without hesitancy. The date of his

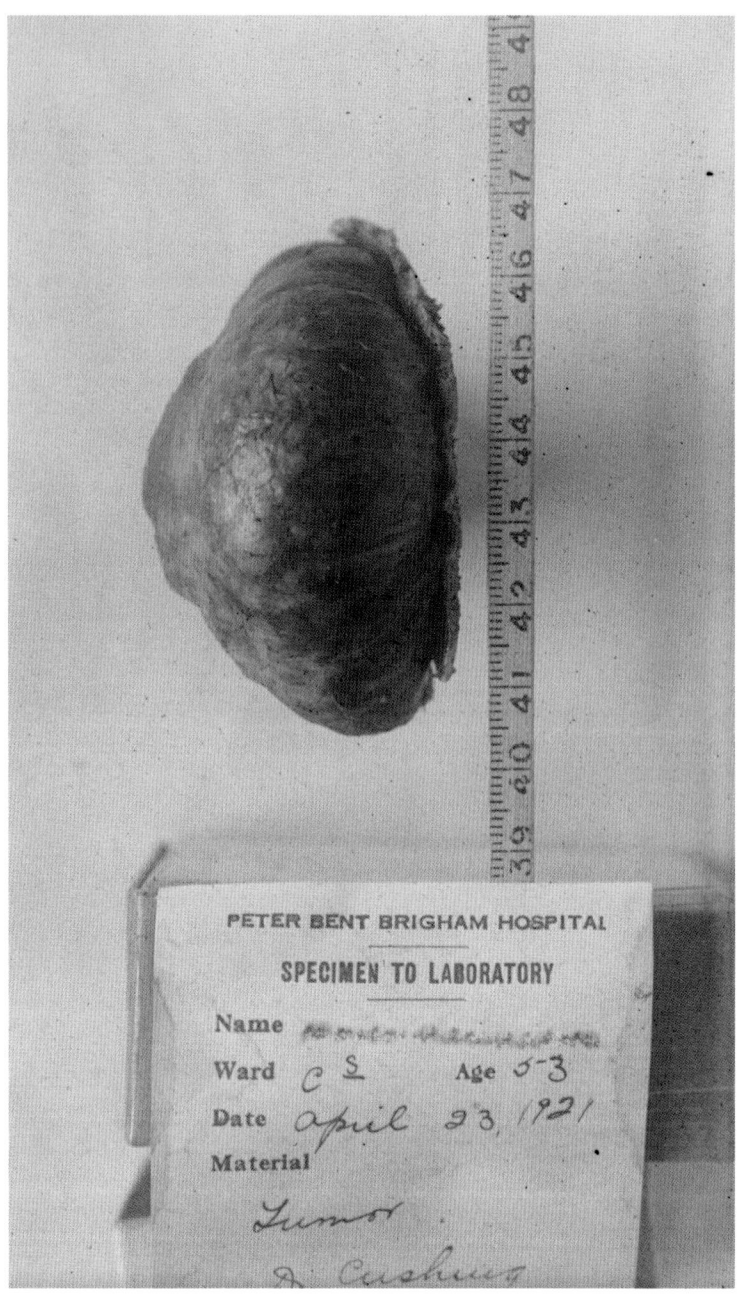

FIG. 6. TUMOR SPECIMEN.

Dressing done today and wound in excellent shape. Flap elevated, very slightly, and evident only on palpation but not on inspection. Sutures removed. Drain entirely removed. The dressing was delayed longer than usual because Dr. Cushing was anxious to see it.

DISCHARGE NOTE
May 13, 1921
Dr. Locke

The recovery of the patient has been most spectacular. He came in a hemiplegic and aphasic in appearance, and he now goes out as an alert entirely normal man. He shows by his actions that he can well hold down his job as railroad porter on one of the limited New York–Boston trains. There is absolutely no aphasia and no astereognosis and no apraxia. No sensory changes to cotton and pin. Strength normal in right arm and leg. Reflexes, triceps, biceps and radials slightly exaggerated, right arm. No changes in deep reflexes of lower extremities. Gait normal. Slight lower facial weakness on right and jaw deviates very slightly to left. Fundi are entirely normal. Corneal reflexes equal and normal. No headaches. Flap and wound in excellent condition and no subjective paraesthesias. Discharged. Photos already taken.

FOLLOW UP NOTE
November 2, 1925
Dr. Horrax

Has had seizures since operation about 3–6 weeks apart. Some are very simple but others are severe, though never with loss of consciousness. Face twitches. He is aphasic. Last seizure Oct. 8, 1925. Given luminal October 24, 1 tablet (grs.1 ss) per day. Bone flap not elevated. Fundi normal.

SECOND HOSPITAL ADMISSION

HISTORY

Patient remained perfectly well, except suffering from Jacksonian attacks. The initial preoperative symptoms recurred 3–4 months prior to this admission.

COMPLAINT

Difficulty in talking, weakness of the right hand and foot.

wife's death he hesitated over a little. No hemianopsia to rough tests now.

April 27, 1921
Dr. Locke

No astereognosis. No sensory changes and no apraxia. Patient is very bright and talking without hesitation. He reads the paper easily. He wrote a letter yesterday and spelled correctly, and wrote fairly quickly.

SUMMARY OF POSITIVE FINDINGS
October 2, 1926
Dr. Cairns

SUBJECTIVE
1. History of injury of left side of the head 14 years ago.
2. Right hemiparesis in April 1921 followed by successful removal of the left dural endothelioma.
3. Recurrence of symptoms 3–4 months ago, the symptoms follow almost identically those which appeared before the operation.

OBJECTIVE
1. Motor aphasia.
2. Right hemiparesis and hemi-anaesthesia to pin prick with loss of postural sensibility and loss in the right hand of vibration sense.

IMPRESSION: Recurrent dural endothelioma of left hemisphere, producing symptoms almost identical with those which occurred before the first operation. Apparently this time the paralysis is more marked in the leg than in the face whereas on the previous admission the reverse was the case.

RADIOLOGY REPORT
October 2, 1926
Dr. Sosman

Films of skull show a large area of bone destruction involving the lower posterior ⅔ of the bone flap and apparently crossing the operative line posteriorly. The edges of skull defect are irregular and show bone formation in spicules. **The silver clips have practically all been displaced medially, as compared with the previous examination 4 years ago. Findings indicate a meningioma, recurrent.**

SPECIAL NOTE
October 9, 1926
Dr. Cushing

This poor fellow unfortunately has gone a year without reporting in spite of the fact that an evident recurrence has been present with thickening of the bone and a tender swelling occupying fully a third of the posterior part of the old flap, in spite of the fact that he has kept at work until a few days before this admission although he has had periods of difficult speech and weakness on the right side. I knew what I was in for, a difficult job, but I hardly realized so difficult.

It is quite evident too from all history that in the lower posterior part of the field we were very little … We consequently outlined a flap keeping to the old incision except for perhaps a 5 cm wider space posteriorly. It is very curious that the whole bone should have been so greatly involved.

I am not at all sure but that the entire flap was involved though I do not think tumor had spread thru the scar, in fact I am quite sure that tumor had not spread thru the scar into adjacent bone outside the old flap.

OPERATIVE NOTE
October 9, 1926
Anesthesia – Ether

Reflection of Scalp. Removal of Major Portion of Old Bone Flap by Outlining in Around the Central Tumor Area. Excision of Dura with Tumor and Scalp, Leaving Denuded Brain Over an Area 9×8 cm in Diameter. Gutta Percha Tissue Covering. Closure of Scalp Alone.

The operative note was not quite readable. The readable portions have been summarized below:

"In operation it appeared that practically all of the old bone flap was invaded. Bone involvement was more extensive than dural involvement. In the center of the flap there was adherent tumor, which was brushed away from the cortex. There was a great deal of bleeding." Dr. Cushing resected and sacrificed the old bone flap and excised a large portion of tumor together with a cyst which apparently represented an "outpocketting of the original tumor." It was a difficult and bloody operation and the denuded brain was covered with gutta percha tissue."

PATHOLOGY REPORT
October 9, 1926

Gross description – There are the tissues of a recurrent meningioma which cannot be very malignant for it is five years since the original operation. It is a pity that the case should have been allowed to drift so long for the bone had become extensively involved. I would like to have some of the bone decalcified and cut for study and will select the pieces of tissue myself. It will be of importance to study this tissue in connection with that of the first operation to see whether to show any changes of type though I rather doubt whether it will do so.

(Dr. Cushing)

Microscopic description – Sections representing 2 blocks of tissue show tumor tissue composed of anastomosing bundles of spindle cells. Typical whorls, about blood vessels are seen in many areas. The cytoplasm of the cells appears to be drawn out at each end into a long fibrillary process which stains blue with P.T.A.H.

Those fibrils are more prominent than in the usual tumor of this type. A few collagen fibrils are also present, both around the blood vessels, and mixed in with the tumor cells. No mitotic figures are seen, nor are there other evidences of unusually rapid growth.

Diagnosis – Meningioma

(Dr. Pinkerton)

A second operation was necessary to remove a large clot which was superficial to the protective sheet (Gutta Percha.)

POSTOPERATIVE NOTE
October 11, 1926
Dr. Cairns

More difficulty with speech. Second dressing shows a large hematoma.

Second operation by Dr. Cushing. A large clot superficial to the protective. This clot was removed. Beneath the protective there were a small collection of blood.

October 12, 1926
Dr. Cairns

Speech better. Second dressing by Dr. Cushing. Aspiration of 80 cc of bloody fluid. Patient talking well and gripping strongly with right hand.

October 14, 1926
Dr. Cairns

Wound inspected by Dr. Cushing. Nothing done. Cast reapplied.

DISCHARGE NOTE
October 23, 1926
Dr. Cairns

Patient has made an excellent recovery. Strength in hand has returned. Some weakness of the right face and hand. Sensory disturbance now located to very slight numbness in the right foot. Sensation had returned to normal in the right arm, but postural sense is still diminished. Speech quite recovered, but still some difficulty in speech.

No more headaches. Wound perfectly healed. No tension. Discharged.

FOLLOW UP NOTE
November 9, 1926
Dr. Putman

Speaks gradually well. Decreasing strength in the right hand. There is also deafness and tinnitus in the right ear and a slight soreness over the decompression.

THIRD HOSPITAL ADMISSION

Patient continued to do well until about two months before the third admission (September 1927) when his old symptoms again recurred. He started to work in January 1927 and worked steadily until his hand gave out a week ago.

COMPLAINT

Weakness of the right hand.

SUMMARY OF POSITIVE FINDINGS
November 17, 1927
Dr. Fulton

SUBJECTIVE
1. History of injury to left side of head 20 years ago.
2. Right hemiparesis in April 1921 followed by successful removal of left meningioma.
3. Recurrence of symptoms 14 months ago with removal of recurrent meningioma with cyst.
4. A second recurrence of symptoms characterized by speech difficulty, hemiparesis and hemihypesthesia.

OBJECTIVE
1. Verbal aphasia.
2. Right astereognosis, with diminution of muscle, pain, pressure and temperature sensibility in right hand.
3. Decompression sunken in. No obvious evidence of recurrence to palpation.
4. Head – There is a circular, depressed defect in the left fronto-parietal region. There is a tenderness at the lower margin of this defect. There is no tenderness to palpation in the center of the defect. Over the midline very nearly in the center of the cranium there is a very small area tender on percussion.

IMPRESSION: There is no gross evidence of recurrence at this time but the intensive collapse of the decompression suggests adhesions between the

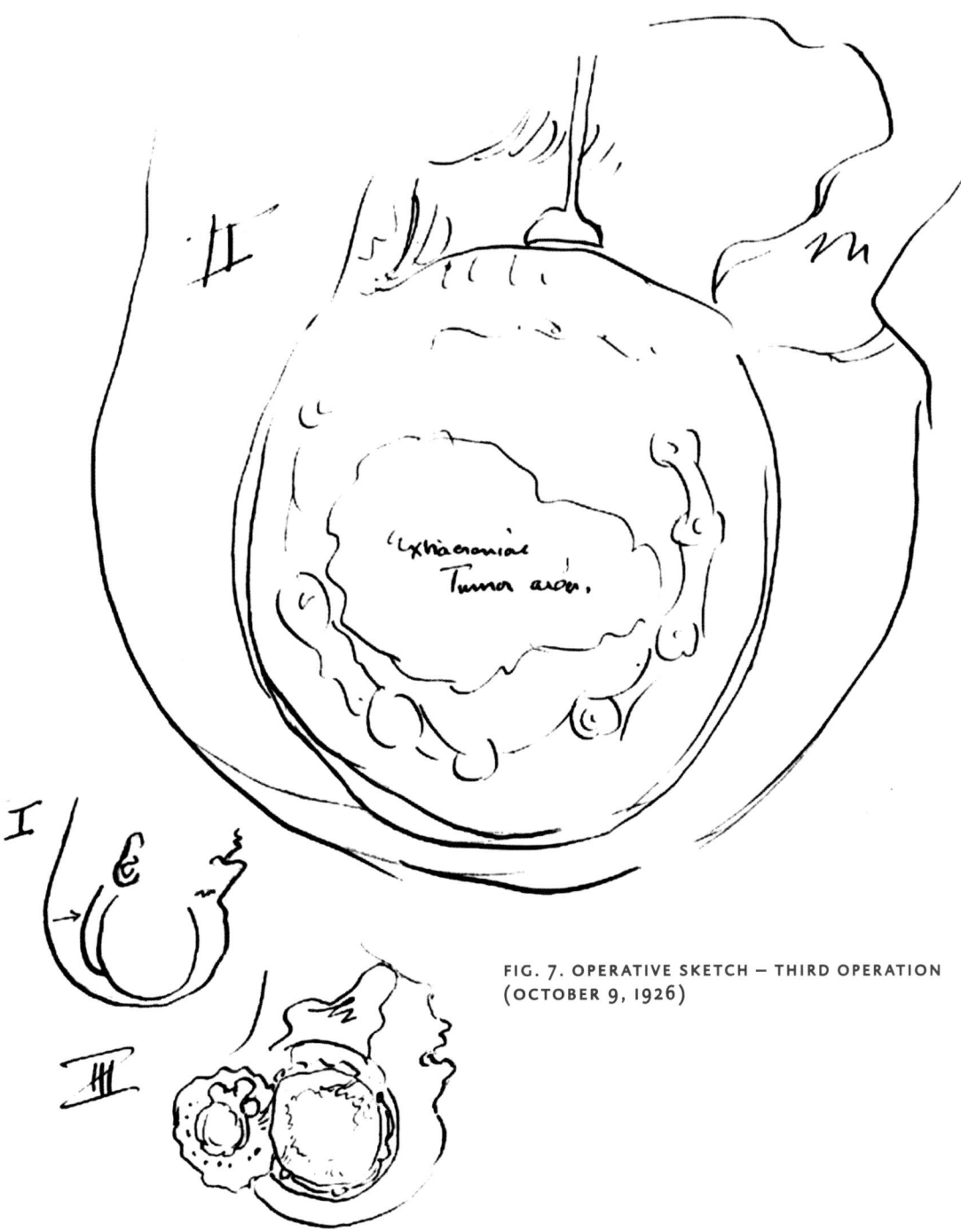

FIG. 7. OPERATIVE SKETCH – THIRD OPERATION (OCTOBER 9, 1926)

expected surface of the brain and the scalp. I suspect that his present symptoms are due rather to scar tissue than to return of his meningioma.

DISCHARGE NOTE
December 7, 1927
Dr. Fulton

Seen by Dr. Cushing, who feels that this time there is no evidence of recurrence, no operation indicated. Discharged.

FOLLOW UP ADMISSIONS

The patient's neurological status had largely remained unchanged up to April 1936. There was no evidence of recurrence of meningioma. Patient had multiple medical problems related to bilateral inguinal hernia and rectal adenocarcinoma with metastases to liver. A sigmoidectomy was done by Dr. Branch on April 15, 1936 under spinal anesthesia. Patient died in April 26, 1936, on the 10th day after surgery, due to pulmonary edema. The postoperative period was complicated by bilateral bronchopneumonia.

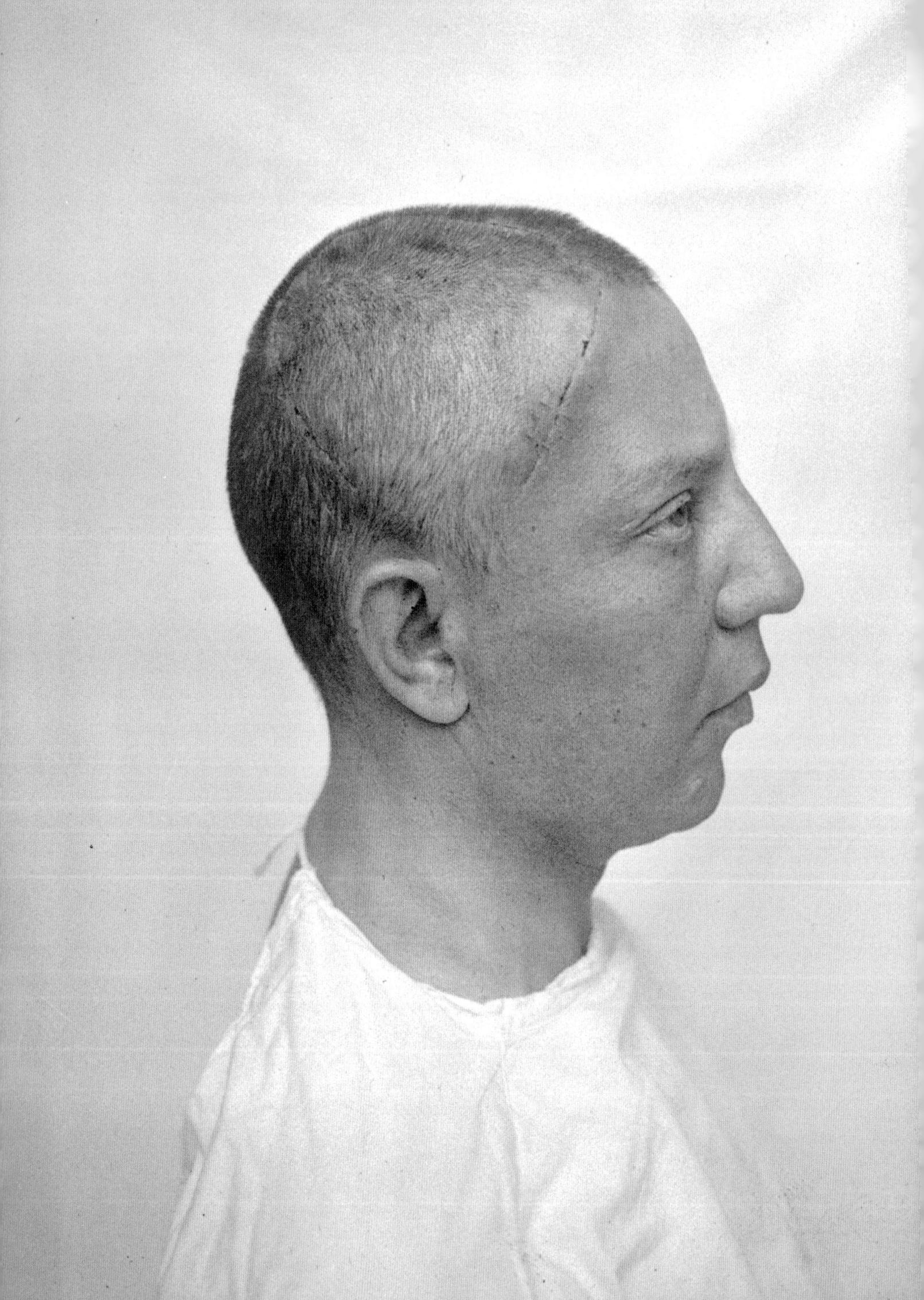

3.3 Parasagittal meningioma

SEX: M; AGE: 41; SURG. NO. 14684; 29622

COMPLAINT

Headaches, dimness of vision and a lack of concentration.

SUMMARY OF POSITIVE FINDINGS
June 15, 1921
Dr. Wheeler

SUBJECTIVE
1. April 1920 onset of continuous frontal headache with drowsiness and lack of concentration, and cooperation in the business.
2. In June 1920 lost control of urine and rectal sphincter.
3. In Oct. 1920 drooping of the left corner of the mouth was noticed by the brother.
4. At this time, the left hand would tremble and shake.
5. In Mar. 1921 the left foot began to shake and tremble with foot drop.
6. Later in Mar. 1921 onset of difficulty in finding words.
7. Also complained of some stiffness of the throat causing difficulty in swallowing.
8. In April 1921 lack of neatness and loss of power of concentration.
9. In June 1921 onset of dizziness with swaying and weakness of the left side.

OBJECTIVE
1. Suboccipital tenderness and rigidity on the right.
2. Left corneal reflex sluggish.
3. Weakness of upper and lower left facial.
4. Bilateral sluggish pupils.
5. Deviation of lower jaw to the right.
6. Tongue protrudes to the left.
7. Deep reflexes exaggerated on the left.
8. Choked disc of 2D, temporal margins clear.
9. Ankle clonus on left.
10. Questionable slight hypesthesia of left arm and leg.

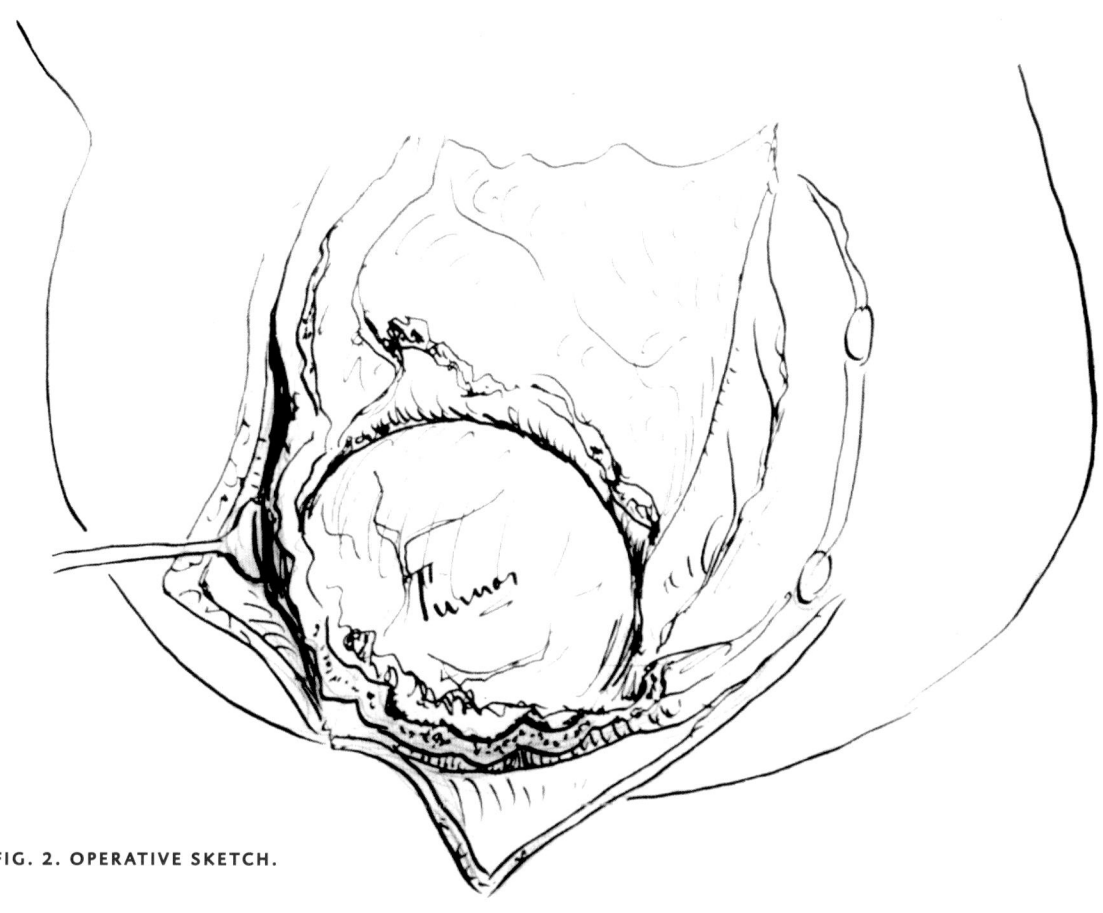

FIG. 2. OPERATIVE SKETCH.

OPPOSITE PAGE. FIG. I. THREE WEEKS POSTOPERATIVE.

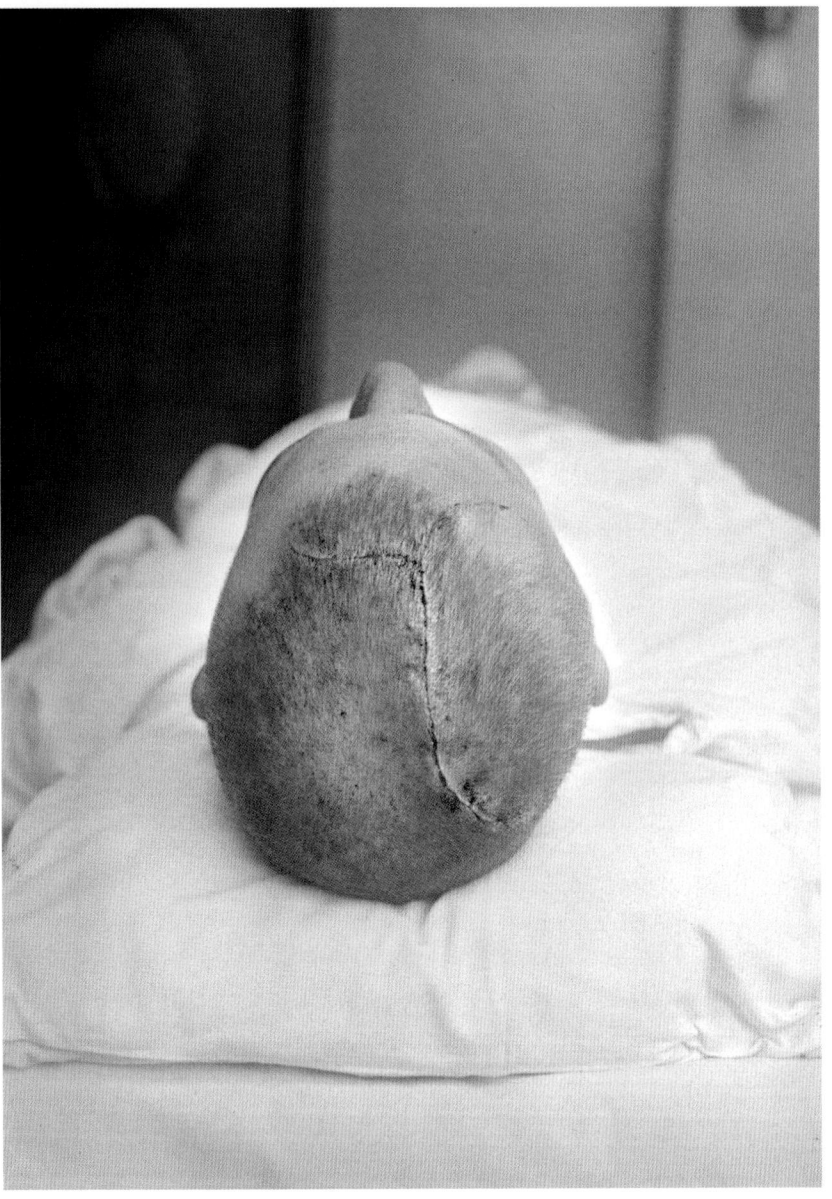

FIG. 3. THREE WEEKS POSTOPERATIVE.

SPECIAL NOTE
June 15, 1921
Dr. Cushing

The difficulties in this case have lain in the fact that this man had an homonymous hemianopsia which, if the findings can be relied upon, clearly indicates a right cerebral lesion.

He had, however, definite nystagmus, some instability, suboccipital headaches which would have suggested a suboccipital lesion were it not for the perimetric findings. In my study of temporal lobe cases, many of them showed these cerebellar symptoms. Hence, I would have favored a temporal lobe lesion. I had some doubts as to the advisability of turning up a flap rather than doing a simple decompression for I anticipated finding an internal hydrocephalus. It may be said that there were some frontal symptoms and some left-sided motor disability, no more, however, than one sees in posterior lesions.

OPERATIVE NOTE
June 14, 1921
Anesthesia – Ether – Miss Gerrard

Osteoplastic Exploration of Right Hemisphere – Negative Findings Except for Tension – A Right Frontal Tumor Suspect.

Owing to the comparatively new team this was a very difficult procedure but was carried through without any upset despite continued oozing during the closure. The bone was smooth, vascular and an immediate subtemporal decompression was made. The temporal bone was very thin but at this stage, I felt fairly confident that I would find a temporal lesion. The exposed dura was tense and in order to determine whether there was a dilated ventricle before opening the dura, I made a puncture toward the ventricle in the upper posterior part of the field. The tap was negative. The dura was then opened over the temporal lobe which bulged markedly and which had a certain elastic feel. A puncture was made in two places to a depth of 5 cm without striking fluid nor causing bleeding.

Two punctures were then made in the upper anterior part of the field and to my surprise, the needle met with resistance at a depth of a little more than a cm unless it was forced through this resistance when some bleeding was occasioned. A vertical incision as shown in the sketch was then made in the hope of exposing a margin of the tumor, possibly a parasagittal endothelioma. A considerable area of bone in the upper anterior part of the field was rongeured away. This bone was very vascular and the exposed dura was likewise necessitating the placement of some muscle.

At the juncture it was felt that further procedure was unwise and the wound was closed as usual in layers.

It might be said that the flap was made rather low owing to possibility of finding a temporal rather than a high lesion.

(Dr. Cushing)

SPECIAL NOTE
July 28, 1921
Dr. Cushing

This has been a very confusing case, a patient obviously with a lesion in the right hemisphere owing to a relative left-sided palsy. He had in addition a right homonymous hemianopsia. At the first operation with a low flap it was expected that there would be a tumor somewhere involving the visual pathway. An attempted exploration of the ventricle met with resistance as though from an endothelial tumor in the right frontal region. Purely on the basis of this chance finding, this second stage operation was undertaken.

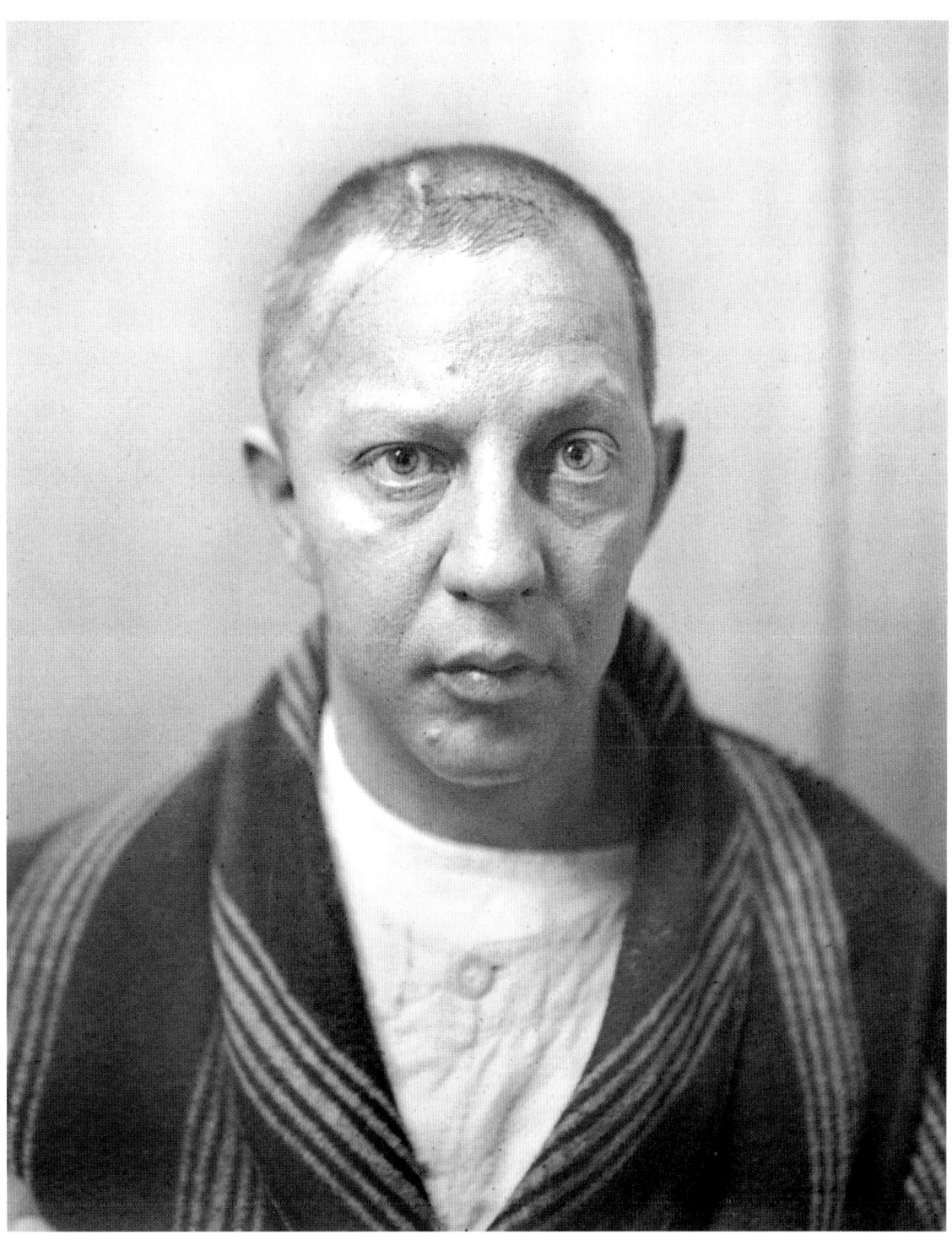

FIG. 4. SIX WEEKS POSTOPERATIVE.

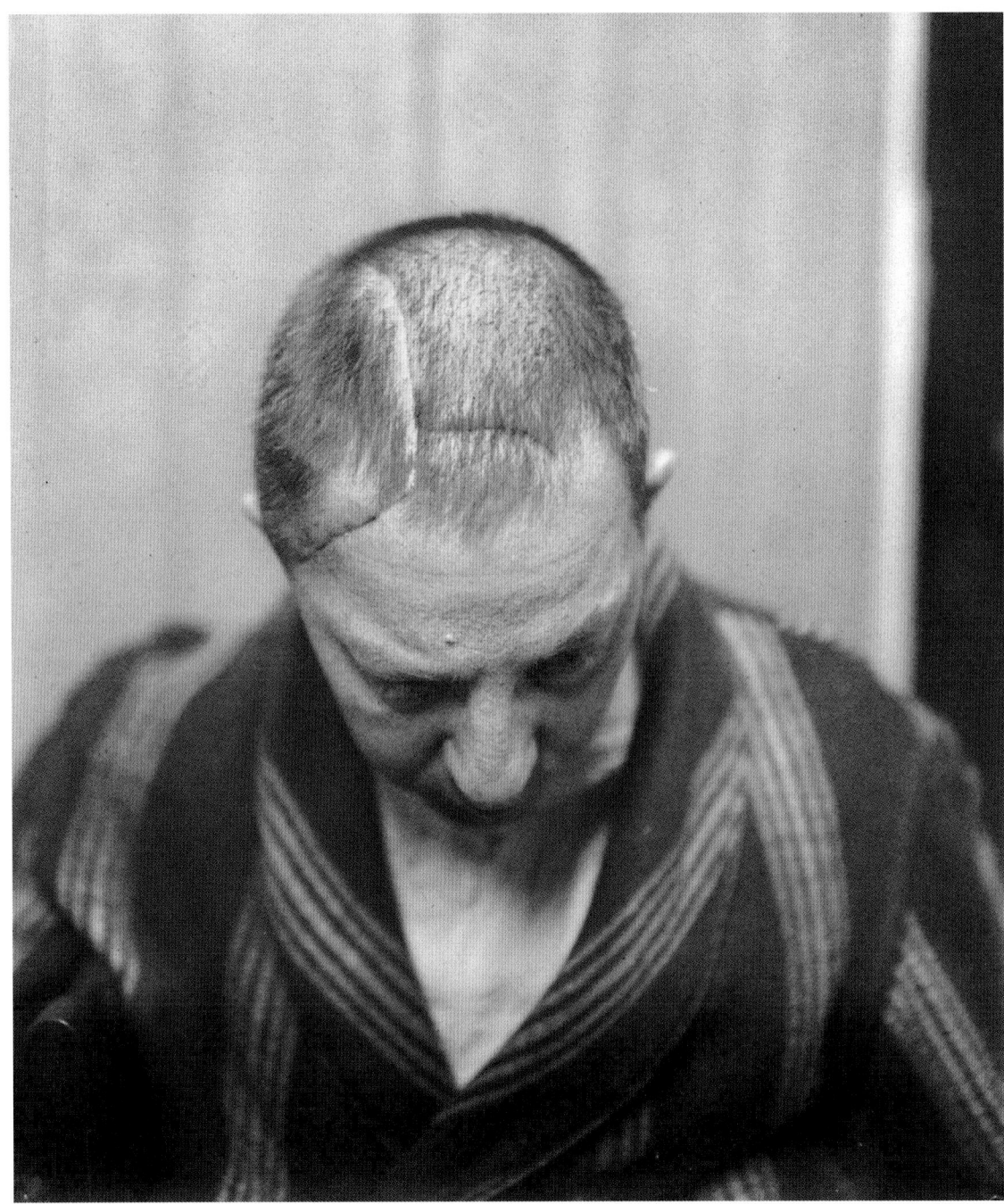

FIG. 5. SIX WEEKS POSTOPERATIVE.

OPERATIVE NOTE
July 28, 1921
Anesthesia – Ether – Miss Gerrard

Second Stage Extirpation of Large Right Frontal Endothelioma.

The attempt was made to carry out this procedure without anesthesia. The patient was given 1/3rd gr. of morphia beforehand and in view of his marked tension Dr. Foley gave him 150 cc of hypertonic salt solution intravenously. Probably both of these procedures were unwise as well as unnecessary for he insisted on having an anesthetic before the bone flap was reflected.

There was a good deal of bleeding in reflecting the flap and a good many clamps had to be put on the scalp margin. The temporal lobe protruded markedly through the subtemporal defect and the dura was opened with a good many misgivings. This was done in the line of the preliminary incision made at the last operation and connected up with the subtemporal defect. The entire hemisphere dislodged itself outward markedly.

A small incision was then made in the cortex at the situation of the earlier puncture opening and came down at a depth of about 1 cm upon the smooth surface of an evident endothelioma.

At this juncture, the bony opening was considerably enlarged and a lateral incision from the original horseshoe-shaped flap was made and carried to the midline. The bone was removed practically to the midline as shown in the sketch.

It was not possible to detect the tumor free of the surface and it had the appearance of being entirely subcortical. An incision was made through the cortex of the frontal lobe downward toward the Sylvian region and crossed backward so that two large flaps of cortex were turned back. The tumor which proved to be a large one of possibly 150 gm in weight gradually began to be exposed. It was necessary to place a good many clips on dural margin and on the margin of the divided hemisphere.

The tumor was finally exposed as thoroughly as possible under the awkward situation which the wound developed and finally the growth was tilted out intact. Luckily it had a very small point of attachment evidently to the longitudinal sinus and there was pretty sharp bleeding which was controlled by the pressure fingers and subsequently by a large muscle stamp taken from the patient's leg. A huge cavity gradually filled in and the bleeding was checked without any great difficulty.

By slow, careful effort the flaps of brain were replaced in position and the dura was completely re-sutured except for the subtemporal defect.

It may be said that a quite serious accident happened during the closure for I found that over the entire frontal lobe there was quite a large clot, evidently a recent clot which had formed during the process of the enucleation. In an attempt to lift this clot out, a small emissary vein between cortex and dura was ruptured and there was quite a little troublesome bleeding which gave me a good deal of anxiety. It, however, appeared to have been stopped by placement of a piece of muscle and in the end this muscle was withdrawn. The scalp was reclosed as usual in layers without a drain.

(Dr. Cushing)

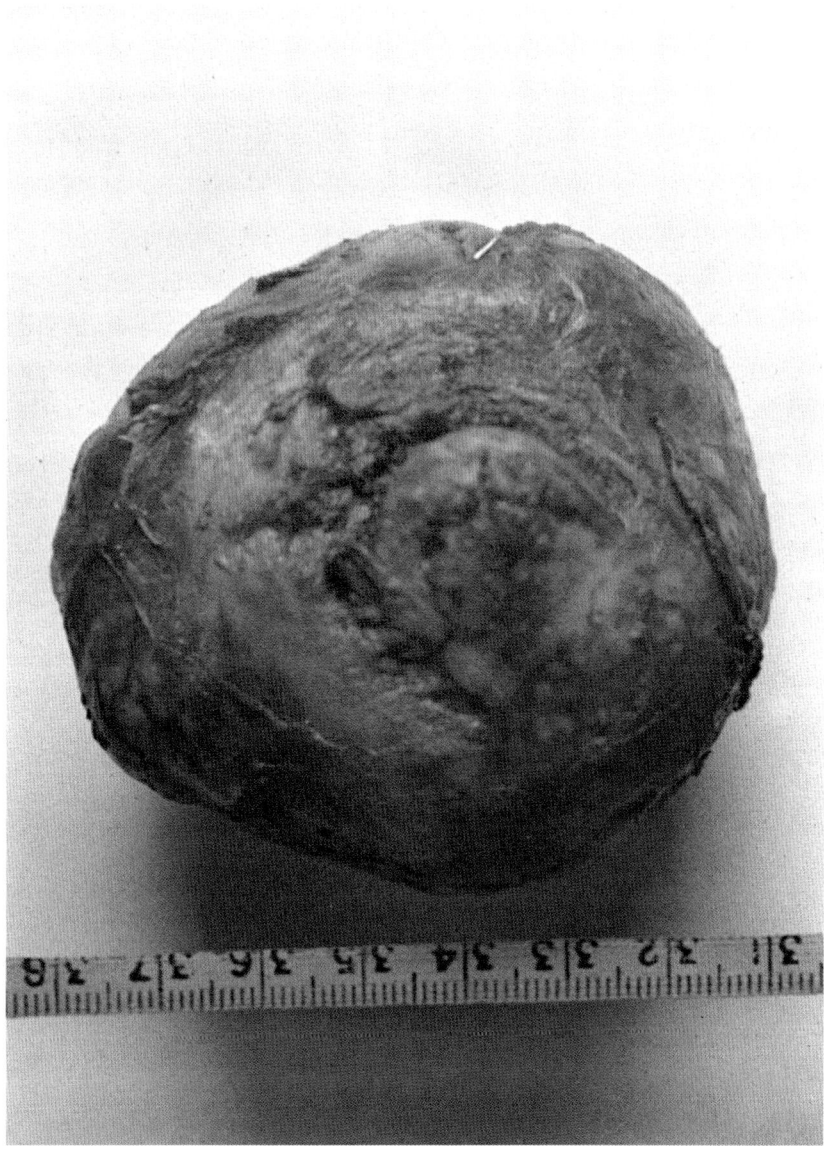

FIG. 6. GROSS TUMOR SPECIMEN.

PATHOLOGY REPORT
July 28, 1921

Gross description: This specimen consists of a rather large nubbin of tumor, weighing of 146 gms, and with it a portion of the cyst wall from which it was taken.

The cyst was a rather large, intracerebral one containing a pale yellowish fluid.

Microscopic report: The sections show a typical endothelioma with well formed whorls, with markedly compressed cells at their periphery. The growth is relatively avascular. Cells vary considerably in size and shape, the shape varying from spindle to round. Mitotic figures are not seen. A portion of the meninges involved by the tumor is present in the section. The portion of the tumor near the meninges shows many brown staining fibers in the region of meninges.

Diagnosis: Endothelioma

Postoperative course was complicated by infection of the wound.

August 6, 1921
Dr. Wheeler

Dr. Cushing made a slight incision over the small abscess at the back of the original incision. A few c.c. of thick yellow necrotic material was irrigated out with Carrel–Dakin solution. Bichloride dressing. Grey cap applied.

SPECIAL NOTE
August 12, 1921
Dr. Cushing

This man's wound has done perfectly well and I have been a little fretful about his remaining in the hospital so long. His persistence in staying has been fortunate, however, for a short time ago there was a small point of infection in the wound such as might have occurred from a poorly placed suture. This was opened and some sterile pus with flecks of debris was wiped out. Scalp promptly closed again and I felt that there must be something behind this which was undisclosed and consequently reopened a portion of the wound.

OPERATIVE NOTE
August 12, 1921
Anesthesia – Gas – oxygen

The upper portion of the V shaped incision was reopened, disclosing a long sinus which led from the posterior corner where recently a small incision was made as stated and after cleaning out the tract of its granulation tissue there was disclosed a small sinus which led thru what seemed to be otherwise intact dura. On investigating this and pulling out the granulation tissue there was a slight discharge of pus and immediate smears showed a few large, rod shaped organisms. This opening was then enlarged with some hesitation as it was in this situation that some silver clips had been left at the previous operation. The sinus lay, it may be added, directly alongside the longitudinal sinus. On enlarging the opening there was a gush of pus which had rather an offensive odor and also a good many necrotic flecks of tissue so that for a moment I supposed that it might have been the discharge of the old fragments of muscle.

The cavity which really represented an abscess about the size of a pigeon's egg was emptied and cleaned and its walls scraped and alleged to collapse, a protective drain containing cotton pledgets being left in the cavity so that it would close slowly. The rest of the wound was closed with sutures.

(Dr. Cushing)

POSTOPERATIVE NOTE
August 12, 1921
Dr. Wheeler

Dr. Cushing opened the incision more extensively today. A large amount of sterile pus was removed. Patient recovered quickly from the gas–oxygen.

OPERATIVE NOTE
August 26, 1921
Anesthesia – Gas – oxygen

Closure of Granulating Scalp Wound.

The old abscess is completely healed and there has been a small oval wound in the scalp which has been granulating but in the hope of accelerating its closure it was cleaned, the edges of the scalp separated and loosely reclosed.

(Dr. Cushing)

DISCHARGE NOTE
September 14, 1921
Dr. Wheeler

After 96 days in hospital patient was discharged to his home. The scalp incision had entirely closed. Fundi O.U. – apparently normal except for slight haziness of the discs outlines. The right and left arms have no difference in strength or sensation. Reflexes slightly more active on the left. No clonus. Patient is alert and accurate in judgment.

Photo taken.

FOLLOW UP NOTE

Since December of 1921 patient started to have seizures. He was advised to take luminal.

FOLLOW UP NOTE
July 24, 1922
Dr. Cushing

Patient reports in excellent condition. Thinks his left side is better than his right because he has had a little sub-deltoid bursitis on the right. Has had three convulsive attacks, the last one occurring recently after three weeks omission of luminal. Advised to continue with luminal in small doses daily, particularly as he is spending his time fishing in a tipping boat. Has gained greatly in weight and seems in perfect condition.

SECOND HOSPITAL ADMISSION
September 1927

COMPLAINT

Seizures with loss of consciousness every 2–3 months since removal of right frontal meningioma 6 years ago.

SUMMARY OF POSITIVE FINDINGS
September 12, 1927
Dr. Fulton

SUBJECTIVE

1. 7 years ago patient began to have severe frontal headaches, failure of vision to the left side, left hemiparesis and hemihypesthesia.
2. Six years ago Dr. Cushing did a 2-stage operation, removing a large frontal meningioma attached to the longitudinal sinus on the right side.
3. Since then patient has had convulsive seizures lasting 10–30 minutes with complete loss of consciousness every 2–3 months.
4. Enters hospital now for going over. No new symptoms from seizures.

OBJECTIVE

1. Both discs slightly full with possibly ½ D elevation.
2. Visual acuity 20/30. Fields full and normal.
3. Generalised hyperactivity of deep reflexes.
4. Absent right abdominal and right scrotal reflex.
5. Enlarged prostate with frequency of micturition.

RADIOLOGY REPORT
September 13, 1927

X-ray – defect apparently does not bulge. There is no evidence of calcification and no definite evidence of increased pressure.
   Impression – postoperative skull.

DISCHARGE NOTE
September 16, 1927
Dr. Fulton

Dr. Cushing does not think there is a recurrence. Has advised a regular course of luminal.

The last letter from the patient dated April 13, 1934, is not available in the chart.

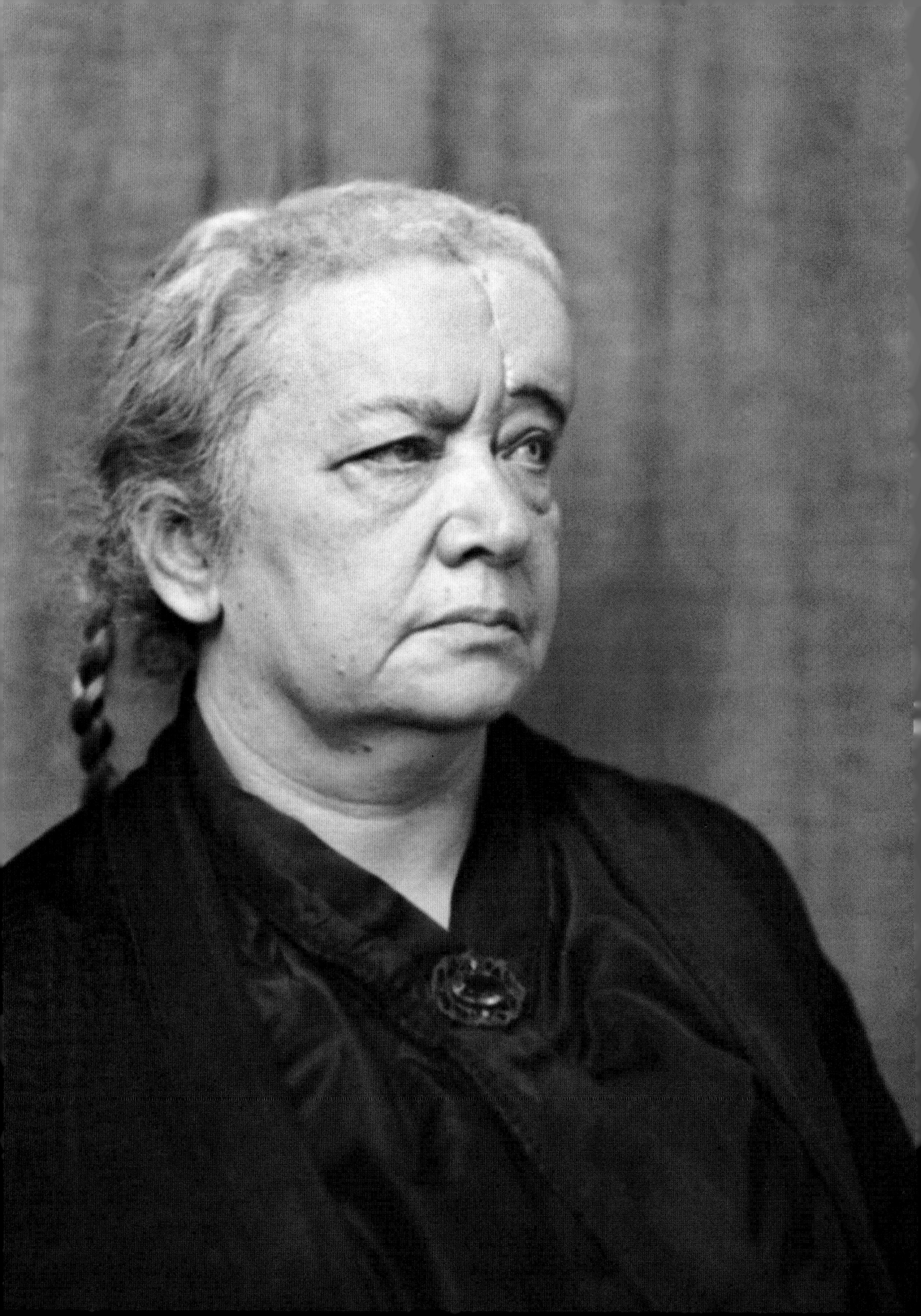

3.4 Olfactory groove meningioma

SEX: F; AGE: 62; SURG. NO. 15922; 17955; 22364; 28758

HISTORY

The patient was suffering from headaches and progressive loss of vision during the last 1.5 years. She was practically blind on admission. There was also a loss of smell and progressive mental status changes.

SUMMARY OF POSITIVE FINDINGS
January 13, 1922
Dr. Wheeler

SUBJECTIVE
1. Since fall of 1920 patient has had some frontal headache which has not been very severe.
2. Since January 1921 there has been a gradual diminution of vision.
3. About January 1921 first noticed impairment of power of smell.
4. Since January 1922 patient is euphoric, uncooperative and mentally confused.

OBJECTIVE
1. Peculiar primary atrophy of fundus O.S. There is secondary atrophy with 1D. of swelling in O.D.
2. Bilateral anosmia.
3. Uncooperative euphoric condition.

RADIOLOGY REPORT
January 13, 1922

Films of the skull in a right lateral position show no evidence of erosion of either table of the skull. The sella turcica itself is quite large and somewhat deeper than usual. There is no evidence of generalized increased intracranial pressure, and the pineal gland shows calcification.

Films of the skull in A.P. position show some erosion of the wing of the left sphenoid.

SPECIAL NOTE
January 13 1922
Dr. Cushing

This has been an unusually difficult case, there being nothing to show except her optic atrophy and beginning mental changes. There was a slight exophthalmos and a little edema of the left eye.

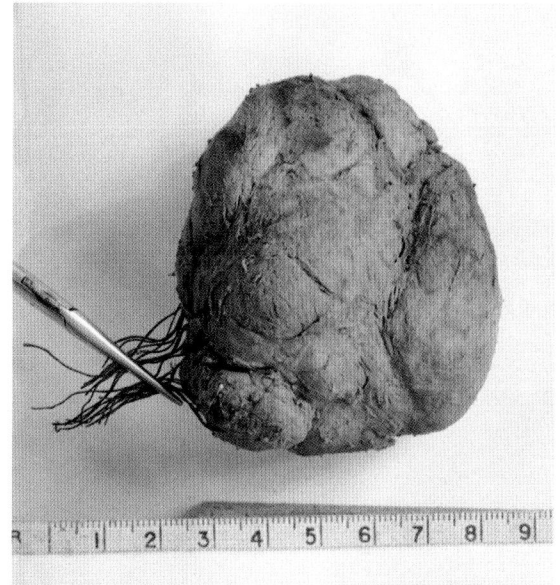

FIG. 2. RESECTION SPECIMEN.

This made me feel that we ought to have very careful x-ray studies and one of the plates which she brought with her showed some absorption of the sphenoidal ridge. Stereotactic plates also showed on subsequent study that there must be some absorption of the orbital plate on the left. In view of this and in view also of her anosmia, the diagnosis seemed reasonably certain of an endothelioma, possibly rising from the olfactory groove, particularly on the left side.

OPERATIVE NOTE
January 3, 1922
Anesthesia – Ether – Miss Gerrard

Osteoplastic Left Frontal Flap Carried Down in the Temporal Region. Demonstration of Tumor by Brain Puncture. Negative Puncture of Ventricle. Closure for Second Stage Operation.

There was no special difficulty in turning down this flap which was made in the position of the usual transfrontal pituitary procedure though the outer legs of the incision were carried down farther into the temporal region so as to give a wider view. The bone, particularly, in the lower part of the field in the orbital region was much more vascular than usual as might be expected with an

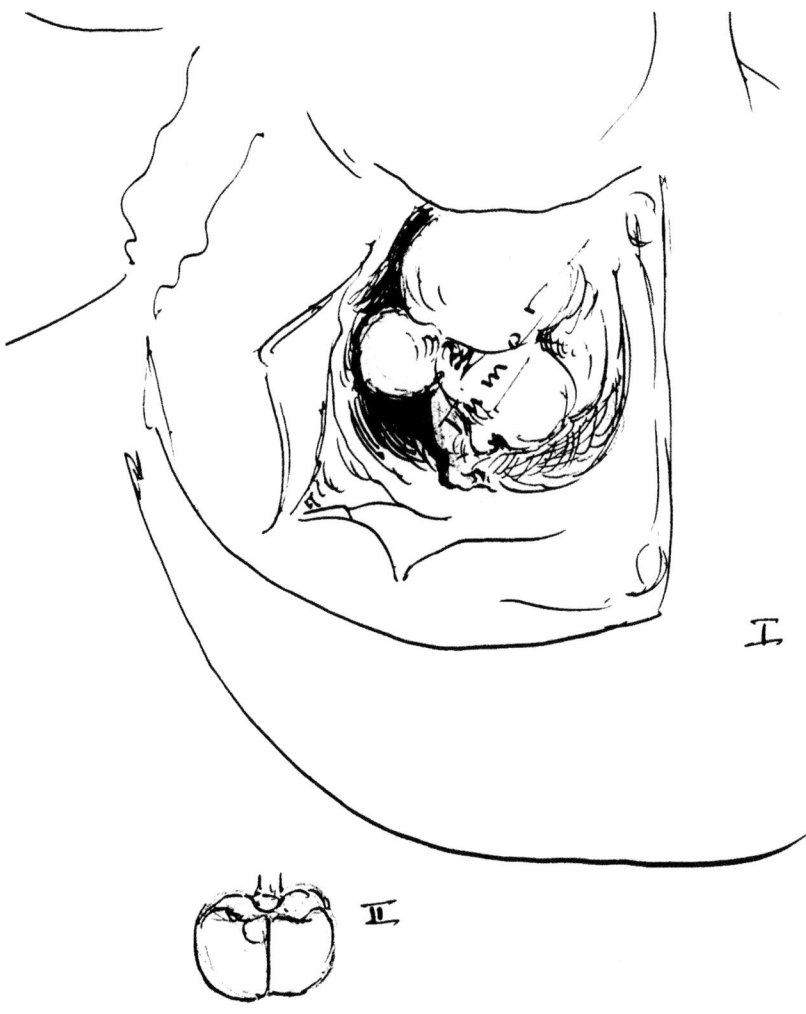

FIG. 3. OPERATIVE SKETCH (SECOND OPERATION).

lioma, probably of the mesial type rising from the ethmoid gutter. The bone flap was replaced and closed as usual in layers preparatory for subsequent operation.

(Dr. Cushing)

OPERATIVE NOTE
January 28, 1922
Anesthesia – Ether – Miss Gerrard

Second Stage.

The bone flap was again reflected disclosing a dura not under particular tension. An incision was made in the dura close to the bony margin of the median incision and this came down directly upon tumor, which therefore on an anterior view of the brain was directly under dura and slightly adherent to dura at the very inner and lower tip of the left frontal lobe. See sketch II (Operative Sketch 1, the inferior small image). The brain was easily brushed away from this and a larger and larger endothelioma which proved unfortunately to be very nodular was finally brought into view. As the brain was brushed away from the growth, large individual nodules as big as the end of the thumb were brought into view in the crevasses. Between these nodules were many vessels and in several places difficulty was experienced in checking bleeding from these vessels which were sinusoidal in character, some of them. Apparently the very anterior portion of the tumor was quite distinct from the rest and this could be freed and could be fairly well grasped in the fingers and fairly well handled. However, after this anterior mass was fairly well freed, a still larger posterior mass of tumor was brought into view. There was no possible way of dislodging this without an enormous damage to the frontal lobe; indeed a good deal of damage had already been done by this time. I finally hit upon the only possible way it seemed to me of attacking such a lesion with any reasonable prospect of removing it, namely by practically the same method used in the acoustic tumors. Consequently with this anterior portion of the tumor well in hand, a deep cup-shaped incision was made into the growth which proved to be exceedingly tough and resistant, but by good fortune comparatively nonvascular. As this circular cup was completed the free margins of the tumor were then grasped in a series of Kelly clamps and the tumor was drawn upon. A second procedure of the same

endothelioma and required a great deal of wax. On reflecting the flap an immediate subtemporal decompression was made and the dura was not opened. The dura of the frontal lobe was tense and there were many protruding villi. An effort was made to elevate the frontal lobe from the orbital plate but this could not be carried back very far on account of bleeding and tension.

The needle was inserted into the ventricle and only a few drops of fluid secured, evidently the ventricle was collapsed. Palpation of the frontal lobe disclosed a good deal of hardness of the lobe in the lower and mesial portion of the field. A needle was inserted through the dura in its lower angle and met dense resistance, evidently of a hard tumor at a depth of a few mm. Another puncture farther out and nearer the middle of the field met the same resistance at a depth of about 1 cm. There is evidently a large tumor, doubtless an endothe-

sort removed another large cup shaped block of the growth and the edges were again caught and drawn forward. It was quite evident that in this way the growth could be largely dislodged though of course the vascular attachment of it had not as yet been approached, and that is the place where the chief trouble may be expected.

On one occasion after there had been a little loss of blood only controlled by placement of some muscle, the patient's pressure fell off markedly and I was about to desist from further manipulation. However, she picked up again and the second stage of the enucleation was carried out as described.

This it seemed to me was about as much as she was likely to stand and I hit upon the device of closing the cavity by sewing up the tense capsule to which the clamps were attached and thus checking all bleeding from the center of the excavation and at the same time reducing the size of the protruding mass much as in the old thyroid operations the capsule used to be drawn together to check bleeding.

I have little doubt but that there is a much larger portion of tumor still remaining. I suppose that what was removed may perhaps weight little more than 50 grams. If this is the case, the tumor itself will probably weigh well over 100 grams in its entirety.

Even with the growth treated as it was and with the tumor removed that I have described, there had been a sufficient amount of swelling of brain and dislodgement of tumor to make replacement of the bone flap out of the question. In spite of the ugly deformity which was the result if it is permanently removed it was stripped away and the scalp replaced over the area, a layer of protection having been left over the tensed brain and tumor.

The patient was pulseless at the end of this procedure and she was given some blood, 300 cc. Whether this was a necessary procedure I do not know. Curiously enough in spite of her low pressure, the pulse remained slow throughout.

It is to be expected that a very marked mental degradation will follow this procedure. Whether a third session will be required during which this same procedure that I have mentioned can be carried out more fully it is impossible to foretell. The bone flap has been preserved with the idea that it may conceivably be replaced after healing, though I have never attempted the replacement of such a large portion of skull which would act as a foreign body.

(Dr. Cushing)

PATHOLOGY REPORT
January 28, 1922

Gross description: Specimen consists of about 79 gms of nodular endothelioma removed from the left frontal region at operation. This tumor was perhaps as large as a closed fist with three or four nodular projections a little smaller than the ordinary hen's egg. The fragments removed at the first operation were removed by incision by scalpel rather than the ordinary method of scooping out. The tumor was so fibrous that the ordinary clamps would go right through the tissue rather than grip it, and finally the capsule which was dense and fairly resistant had to be clamped and used for traction. This tumor was only partially removed at the first operation, the capsule being sewed, closed and long threads left in situ to mark the side of the removal.

(Dr. Wheeler)

Microscopic report: All the sections show the same type of tumor, which is an endothelioma. It is composed of large masses of round or polyhedral cells which tend to form whorls. The nuclei are round and oval and stain a deep blue and contain small particles of chromatin.

The cytoplasm is rather abundant and stain pink. Along one margin is dense fibrous tissue which undoubtedly is dura. Among this tissue is found masses of cells similar in appearance to those described above. There are many vacuoles in the section which look like fat cells. Under high power many large mononuclear cells which evidently have been engorged with fat are seen.

Diagnosis – Endothelioma

(Signed) Resident pathologist

SPECIAL NOTE
February 6, 1922
Dr. Cushing

This woman had a stormy convalescence after her 2nd stage procedure at which time a block of tumor weighing 78 grams was removed and as stated in my previous note the cup-shaped defect was closed bringing the sutures in so they could be utilized at the other session. As stated, the bone flap was sacrificed and even so tension became so great

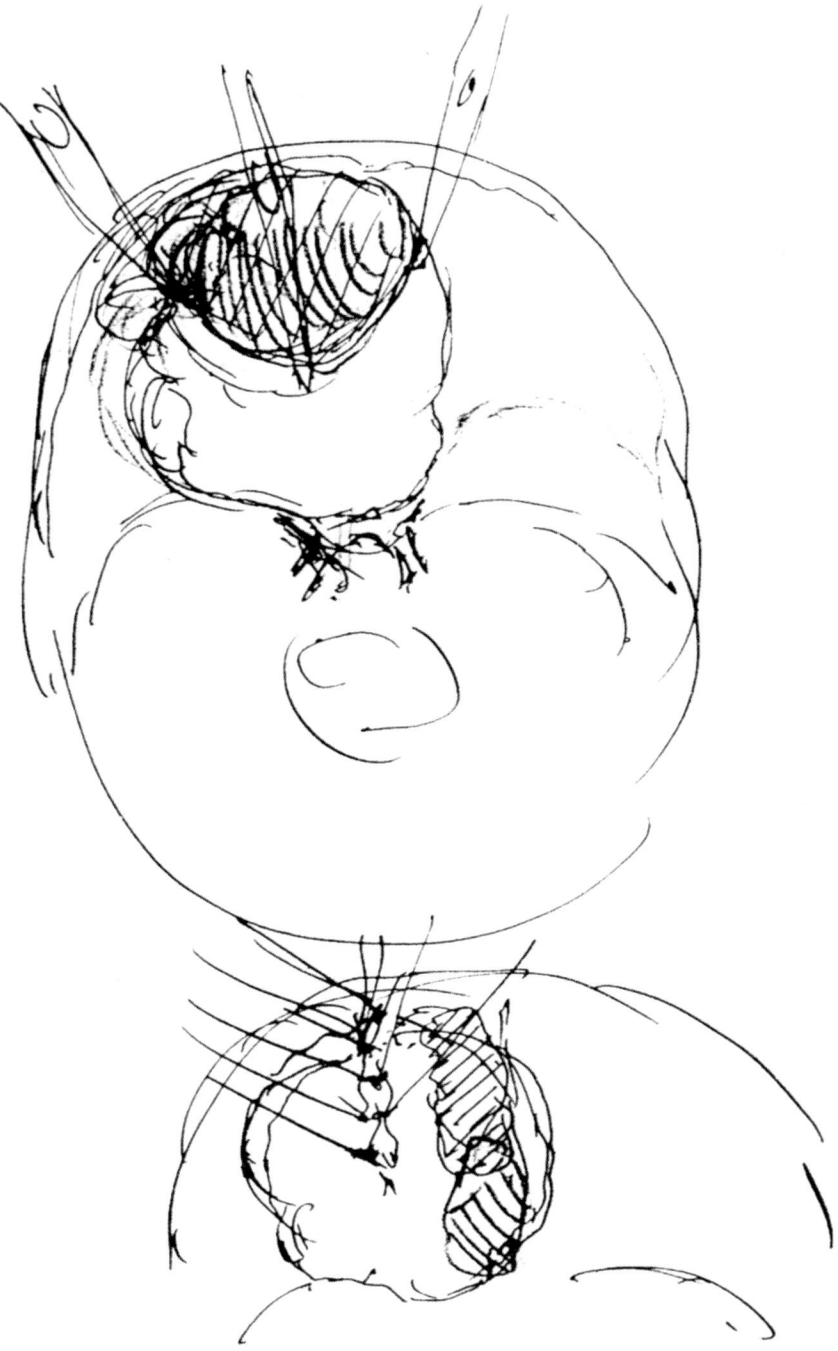

FIG. 4. OPERATIVE SKETCH (THIRD OPERATION).

OPERATIVE NOTE
February 6, 1922
Anesthesia – Ether – Miss Gerrard

Removal of 126 Gram Remaining Fragment of Endothelioma. Its Base of Attachment Being in the Anterior Olfactory Groove.

On reflecting the flap and drawing back the protective covering which had acted perfectly in the way intended the tumor was disclosed very much further forward than before so that it evidently tilted forward with its attachment anterior rather than posterior as I had suspected in view of her optic atrophy and the changes shown in the x-ray.

It was a fairly simple procedure by drawing on the row of sutures which had been left in place and by the customary use of pledgets to brush the brain away from the tumor and to dislodge it markedly, and then to sweep some pledgets under the base of attachment so that the growth became free and was easily removed. There was a little bleeding from the area of attachment which could not have been more than the anterior half of the olfactory groove, but this was controlled by a large muscle stamp secured from another patient. Subsequently after the bleeding had become stilled this stamp was removed and a small bit of muscle left in position on the one suspicious point.

I had hoped to be able to replace the bone flap. The brain was so edematous that when it was gradually molded back into position filling the great defect which had been left it would hardly have been possible to put the bone flap back. If this is to be done indeed it ought to be done within a few days, and I probably made a bad error in not leaving another sheet of protective in position preparatory to such a procedure. However, I was glad enough to get out of a difficult and ticklish task as well as we did. It was easily possible to resuture the upper and lower legs of the incision, but where the wound had been beginning to break down it was necessary to cause a good deal of overlapping in order to get galea together. This has left a very ugly median wound which probably will need repairing.

At one stage of the operation there was a considerable fall in blood pressure but she promptly began to improve and there was very little subsequent bleeding.

(*Dr. Cushing*)

that the mid-vertical incision has gradually begun to give way and I did not wait longer in view of this fact fearing a fungus. Fortunately under the portion of the incision which did give way the brain was protected by a protective sheet. For the past several days, she has begun to improve considerably in her mentality though it is unquestionably far less good than on her admission. She is irritable and tends to strike other people if they annoy her.

PATHOLOGY REPORT
February 6, 1922

Gross description: The remaining fragments of the endothelioma described in N–22–9 were removed in toto by gradually separating the cortex away from the definite capsule. The tumor apparently was attached to the falx near the frontal sinus or perhaps more definitely along the olfactory groove. Here the tumor was broken off from its stalk. Only one half of the tumor was very vascular, the remainder being very dry and fibrous. The tumor weighed 126 gms.

(Dr. Cushing)

DISCHARGE NOTE
April 24, 1922
Dr. Wheeler

Mental state rather better than on admission. Patient talks quite intelligently. She is able to walk with very little support. Vision better than on admission. She is able to read large text. No motor or sensory changes. Fundi are unchanged.

SECOND HOSPITAL ADMISSION

Patient has returned to hospital on account of local bulging in the line of the old operative scar.

December 5, 1922
Dr. McKenzie

At the present time discloses practically nothing. No motor or sensory disturbances.

Cranial nerves are all normal, excepting the 1st and second. Patient's sense of smell is somewhat deficient. There is marked improvement in her eye sight. No change in the left eye, but in the right her vision is 10/70 to about 1/200 before operation. Reflexes are normal and equal. There is local bluish bulging in the line of the old operative scar. This is the size of a pigeon's egg, quite soft and the skin appears very thin.

Diagnosis – Meningocele.

SPECIAL NOTE
December 6, 1922
Dr. Cushing

This woman had a return of a protrusion in the middle of the scar of the forehead at the point where the former hernia took place. The protrusion resembles a small meningocele, being about 3 cm in its longitudinal and 2 cm in its lateral diameters. It is bluish, has a thin membrane over it, evidently contains fluid. I with some hesitation decided that it would be best to excise this and hoped that I might be able to close the wound though I was not certain that I could do so.

OPERATIVE NOTE
December 6, 1922
Anesthesia – Ether – Miss Gerrard

Excision of Meningocele.

The meningocele sac was excised by a spindle shaped incision and it was possible to treat it just as one would treat a spina bifida by dissection up from its lateral walls of the film of dura and

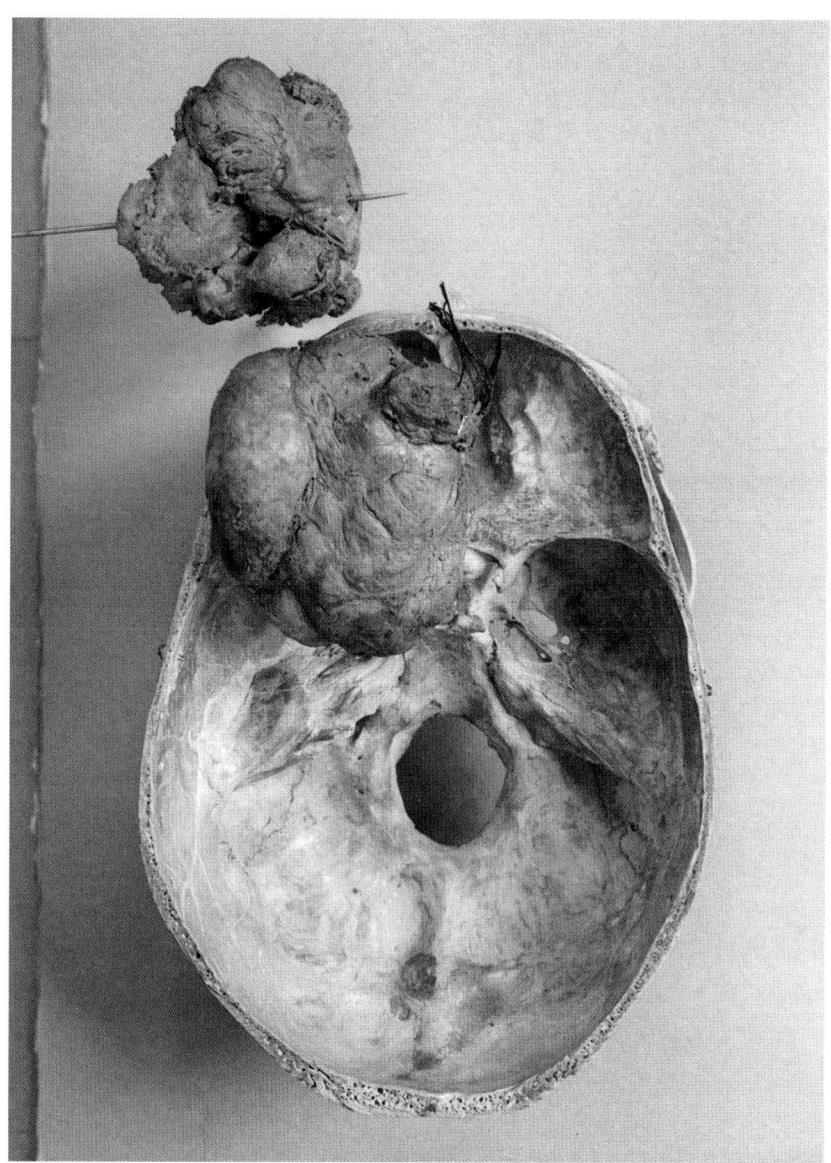

FIG. 5. SIZE OF THE TUMOR IN COMPARISON WITH THE CRANIAL VAULT.

fibrous tissue which was subsequently closed as securely as possible in double layers. So far as I could see the sac was really an arachnoid cyst, which behaved like a meningocele though it is possible that it may have communicated with the cerebrospinal spaces. There was a secondary film which overlay the brain which I did not disturb. Patient was completely relieved and after closing the dura securely in two layers I was unable to close the scalp up and dissected flaps back for some distance on each side and got a fairly good approximation – as good that it was not necessary I thought to place skin sutures. The wound was covered with silver and collodin dressing applied. There was some leaking of blood from the wound owing to the patient's vomiting.

(Dr. Cushing)

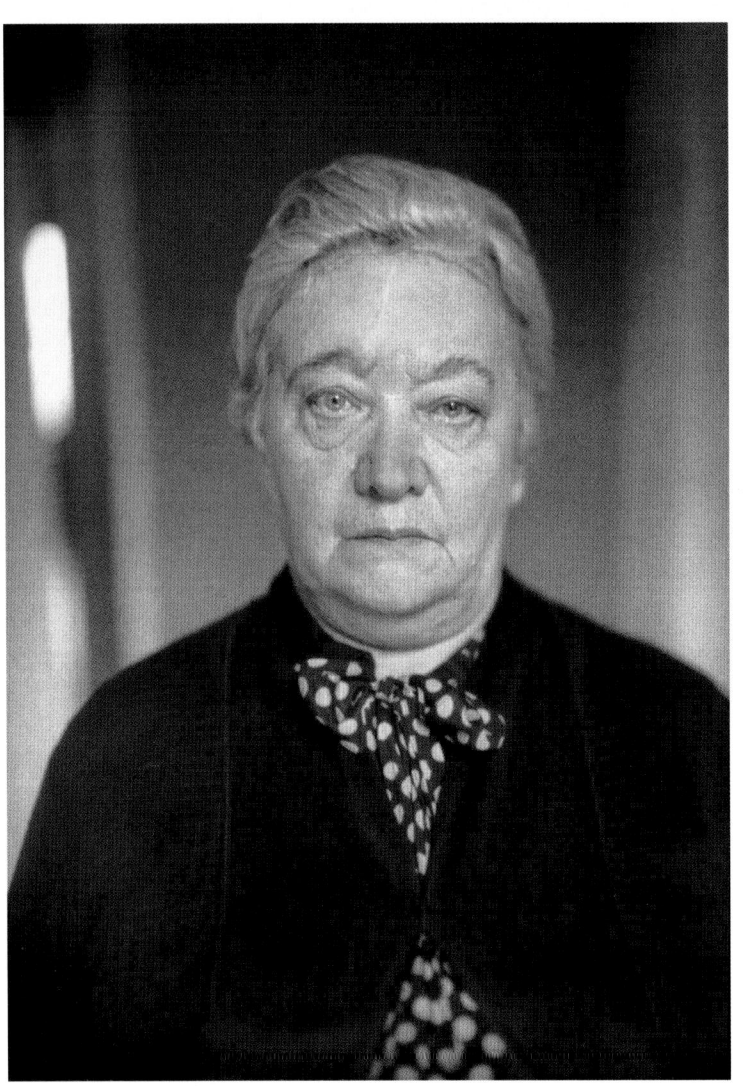

FIG. 6A. PHOTO FROM MAY 1927, PRIOR TO RESECTION OF THE SCALP NODULE

December 10, 1922
Dr. McKenzie

Postoperative 4 days. Temperature is remaining normal and patient doing well.

DISCHARGE NOTE
December 18, 1922
Dr. McKenzie

Excellently healed; inspected by Dr. Cushing who ordered her discharge.

THIRD HOSPITAL ADMISSION

October 12, 1924
Dr. Van Wagenen

Since discharge from the hospital some 2 years ago the patient has been steadily improving as regards to her eyesight. Mentally she has been clear. She has been up and about the house all the time, has gained about 70 lbs in weight. 3 days ago she was seized with a feeling of numbness in the right side of the face, the right face and right arm twitched; she sank rather quickly to the floor and had a generalized convulsion, lasting some 45 minutes. She did not lose control of urine or feces. Following this there was a ptosis of the right eyelid and a slight drooping of the right side of the face. Patient's exam shows a very obese woman lying in bed rather difficult to examine, but extremely jocular, good natured, and very grateful for what has been done. There is the scar of a left frontal and fronto-temporal osteoplastic flap. On palpation it is found that the bone flap has been left out. However, the skin and subcutaneous tissue are up flush and full as the other side. On general inspection one would never suspect that the bone flap had been left out.

DISCHARGE NOTE
October 14, 1924
Dr. Van Wagenen

The patient was seen by Dr. Cushing who considered that the attack might have been due to G.I. indiscretion. She was advised to go on an obesity diet, take daily doses of magnesium sulphate, and have a new pair of glasses fitted by Dr. May in N.Y. She was discharged the next day after admission.

LETTER TO DR. CUSHING
January 23, 1925

Dear Dr. Cushing

Once again I want to take advantage of your kindness and ask for your advice. Yesterday morning mother woke up with a cold in her head and clear fluid (like water) ran from the right nostril, almost continually while she sat up but stopped when she laid down. And the swelling on her forehead fell in considerably. This morning the swelling on her forehead has filled up again and it now looks the same as always. But her nose still continues to run when she sits up. She is taking aspirin and has no temperature. We would be very thankful if you advise us what you think of this.

Most gratefully yours
Signed (daughter of patient)

A response letter was not available in the chart.

FOURTH HOSPITAL ADMISSION

Patient was doing well until the end of 1926 when a small lump formed in the antero-internal angle of the operative incision. This lump gradually increased in size.

OPERATIVE NOTE
May 7, 1927
Anesthesia – Novocain

Excision of the Nodule of Recurrent Meningioma in the skull.

Plastic Operation.

Under Novocain anaesthesia Dr. Cushing excised the nodule with the overlying skin. The nodule went down as far as dura and may possibly have passed thru dura tho there was no definite evidence of this. In removing the nodule on one or two places the excision had of necessity been carried rather close to the nodule, and tumor was encroached on once or twice. Eventually, however, it appeared that all the tumor had been removed. There was some difficulty in bringing the skin and galea together afterwards, the sutures being rather tight.

(Dr. Cairns)

PATHOLOGY REPORT
May 7, 1927

Gross description. Specimen consists of a small nodule of tissue 1.5 cm in diameter together with

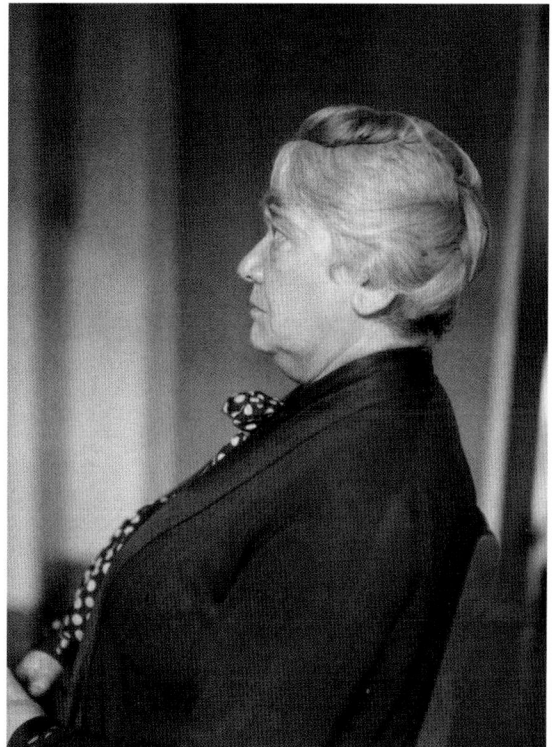

FIG. 6B. PHOTO FROM MAY 1927, PRIOR TO RESECTION OF THE SCALP NODULE

the overlying and attached oval fragment of skin. The nodule is sharply defined, where it is cut into. It had a soft, moist, glistening white anterior surface.

(Dr. Cairns)

Microscopic report: Irregular area of tumor tissue is composed of spindle cells arranged somewhat concentrically in the form of small islands. These islands are interaction with dense connective tissue. The tumor cells themselves do not appear to be forming any intracellular substance.

Diagnosis–Meningioma

May 11, 1927
Dr. Cairns

A cast was applied and left on for 3 days. At the end of that time the stitches were cut and the wound appeared to be healing very well. A collodin dressing was applied.

DISCHARGE NOTE
May 11, 1927

The patient was discharged from the hospital in a good condition.

Last follow up letter was in April 9, 1931. (The letter is not attached in the chart.)

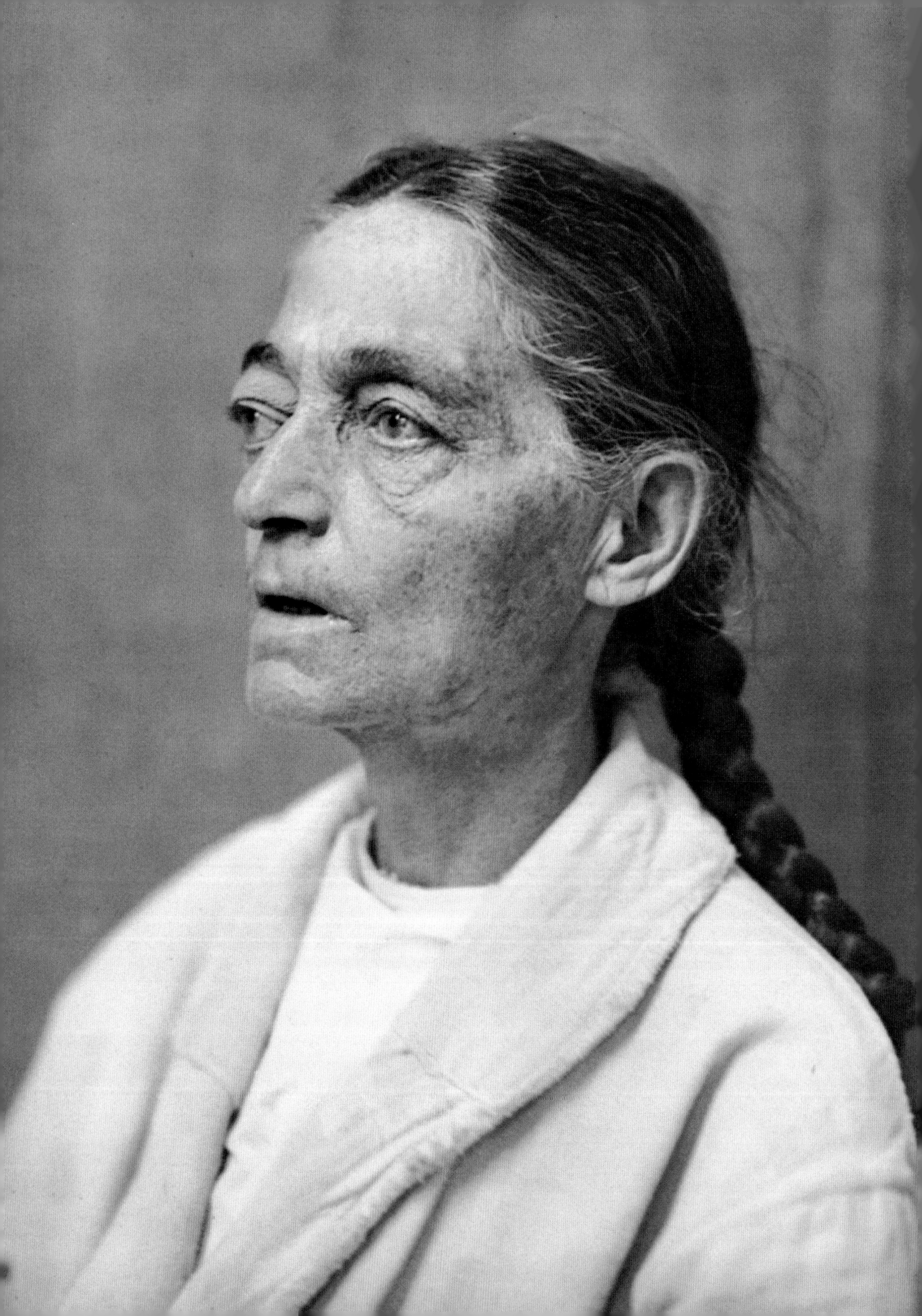

3.5 Sphenoid wing meningioma

SEX: F; AGE: 64; SURG. NO. 18997

HISTORY

This patient reported protrusion of the right eye for four years. She also complained of progressive mental deterioration, fainting spells, dizziness, unsteady gait, and diplopia.

SUMMARY OF POSITIVE FINDINGS
July 15, 1922
Dr. Bailey

SUBJECTIVE
1. Mental derangement, patient complaining that her thoughts do not go right; also poor vision.

OBJECTIVE
1. Marked exophthalmos of the right eye.
2. Weakness of the right masseter muscle.
3. Right corneal reflex weak.
4. Weakness of right platysma.
5. Slight exaggeration of the left radial reflex.
6. Weakness of the optic discs without actual elevation.
7. Marked mental derangement consisting of disturbance in orientation, moody for recent events, and lack of power of concentration.

IMPRESSION: Endothelioma in the region of the right sphenoidal ridge.

Since the patient had a history of "heart disease and atherosclerosis" Dr. Cushing was cautious about offering the patient an operation. The family, however, was very interested in their surgical option despite the risks. Medical consultation recommended the use of digitalis postoperatively if necessary.

X-rays revealed changes along the right sphenoid wing suggestive of a meningioma.

OPERATIVE NOTE
July 28, 1922
Anesthesia – Ether – Miss Gerrard

Low Osteoplastic Exploration in Right Temporal Region. Extradural Rongeuring Away of Bone Down to the Clinoid Process. Closure.

Contrary to expectations the patient took her anaesthetic beautifully. On reflecting the flap I

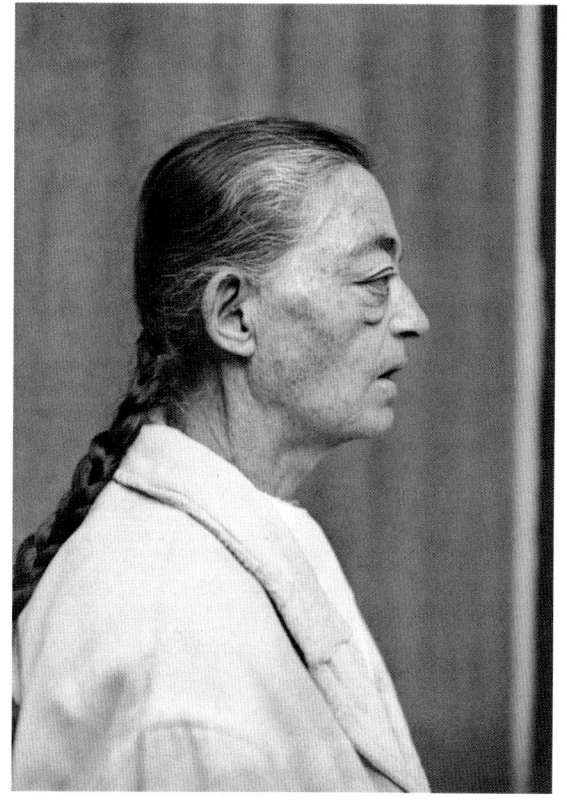

FIG. 2. PREOPERATIVE.

came down low in the orbital region upon bone which was greatly channeled, thickened and evidently the seat of endotheliomatous invasion. I had some difficulty with the meningeal which channeled the thickened bone, but apart from this there was no difficulty in rongeuring and burring away the bone more thoroughly than I have ever done heretofore. The entire outer side of the orbit was cleaned away down to and including the orbital foramen. In this process I detached what looked to be the superior oblique muscle.

There is obviously a dural endothelioma but how large a one could not be determined. The dura was thickened and the seat of tumor into the anterior tip of the temporal lobe. The dura was not opened.

As complete blood stilling as possible was carried out and the flap was replaced and closed with a single protective drain.

(Dr. Cushing)

OPPOSITE PAGE. FIG. I. PREOPERATIVE.

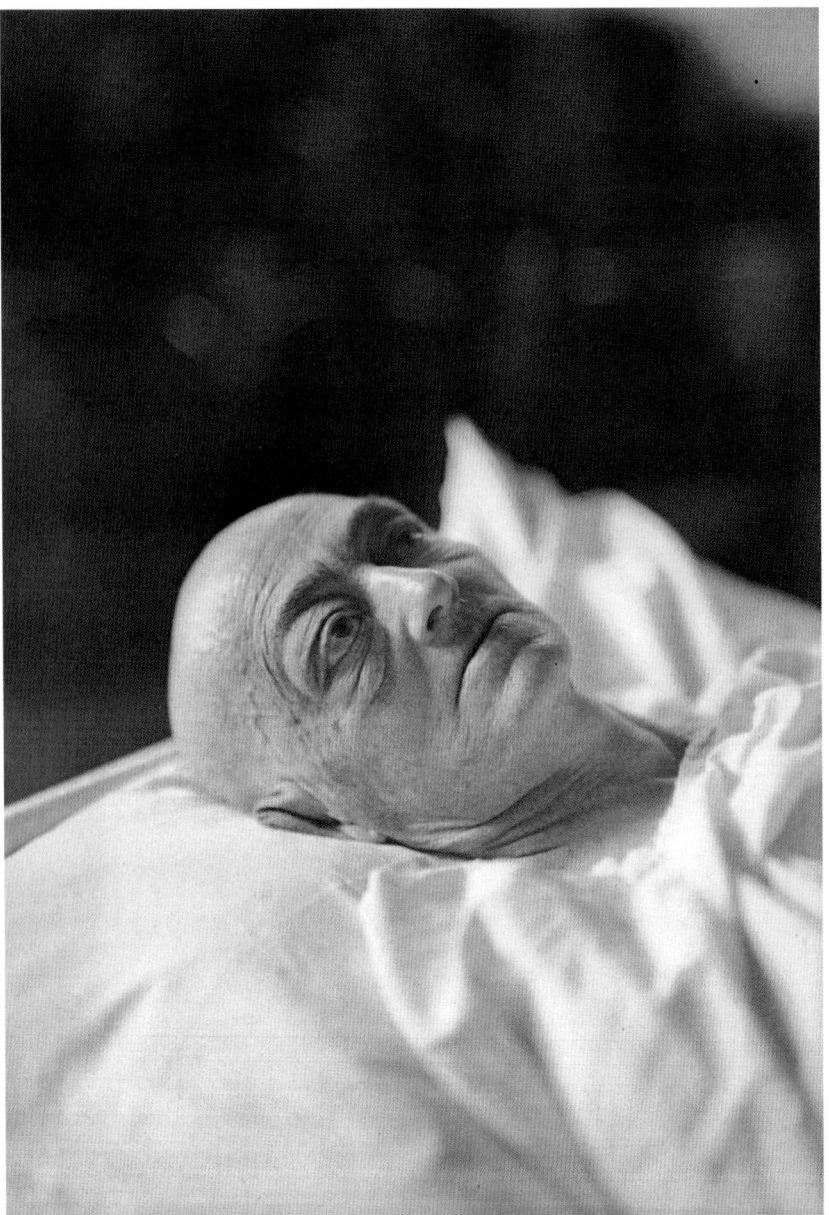

FIG. 3. PREOPERATIVE, JUST BEFORE SURGERY.

PATHOLOGY REPORT
July 28, 1922

Gross description: Specimen consists of many fragments of bone removed from the right temporal region of the skull, which markedly thickened, consisting of soft, cancellous bone apparently from gross appearance filled with tumor tissue. Fragments were removed with a sharp curet and submitted in Zenker's.

Microscopic report: Sections show bone tissue being invaded by a tumor growth. The tumor cells are arranged in irregular masses between the spicules of bone. Some of the cells are vesicular and tend to have a whorl-like arrangement around blood vessels. Others of the cells are flattened almost spindle in shape and are arranged somewhat in parallel rows. The nuclei for the most part are hyperchromatophilic. Some mitotic figures are seen. Interfibrillar substance is fairly numerous and for the most part stains brown with phosphotungatic acid.

Diagnosis: Endothelioma, invading bone.

July 31, 1922
Dr. Bailey

Patient has not recovered consciousness since operation. Constant Cheyne–Stokes respiration. Marked edema and exophthalmos around right eye.

August 1, 1922
Dr. Bailey

Marked spontaneous nystagmus to left. Left hemiparesis with tendency to clonus in right ankle. Babinski positive.

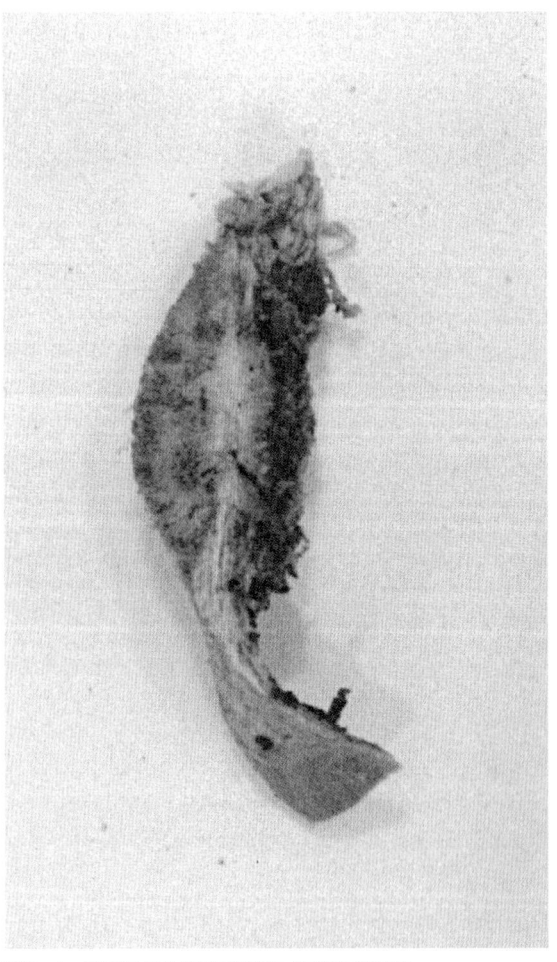

FIG. 4. PIECE OF RESECTED SPECIMENS.

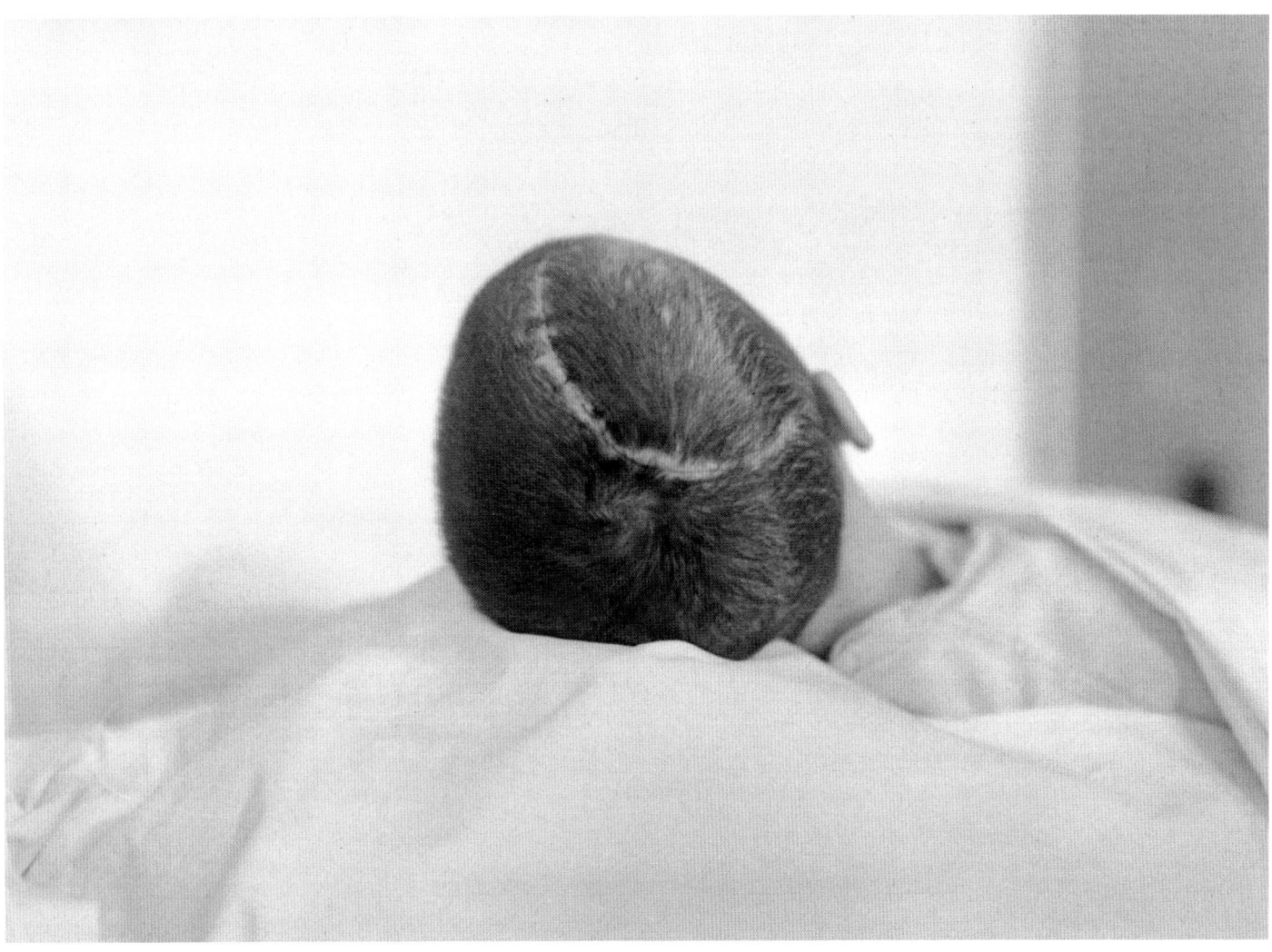

FIG. 4. THREE WEEKS POSTOPERATIVE.

ing was made in the bone with the rongeur, so as to give a circle, which it is hoped may suffice for tumor removal. This was replaced and closed in layers by Dr. Horrax.

(Dr. Cushing)

POSTOPERATIVE NOTE
48 hours postoperative
January 28, 1923
Dr. McKenzie

Sutures removed. Wound inspected by Dr. Horrax. Dressings had stained through. Coagulation time must be increased in this patient.

OPERATIVE NOTE
January 30, 1923
Anesthesia – Novocain

Second-Stage Extirpation of Right Parasagittal Meningioma.

Under local anaesthesia the flap was again reflected there having been no formation of blood clot. Working fore and aft from the original small nick made in the dura disclosing the edge of the tumor, a curvilinear incision exposing a comparatively small part of the hemisphere was then made about as in the accompanying sketch. The tumor proved to be much larger than anticipated, and it was evident that it was going to be difficult to remove it through the small field. It is possible that I should have placed more emphasis than I did upon the symptoms which she had in her foot, but I thought that we were probably going to find a small enucleable tumor largely limited to the arm area. Encircling the field in which the next of the tumor lay was a large vein which finally had to be clipped though the margin of the cortex was not split. The enucleation would have been a simple affair had it not been for the fact that the tumor was found to

3.6 Parasagittal meningioma

SEX: F; AGE: 26; SURG. NO. 18144

HISTORY

There was a two-year history of "twitching of left arm." The attacks were very often accompanied by an abnormal sensation of drawing and tingling in the left side of the face. There was also a progressive decrease in vision during the last six months, starting from the left eye, followed by involvement of the right eye.

SUMMARY OF POSITIVE FINDINGS
January 23, 1923
Dr. Bailey

SUBJECTIVE
1. Failing vision.
2. Weakness of left leg.
3. Convulsive attacks in the left hand with sometimes attacks of paraesthesia in the same hand and in the left side of the face.

OBJECTIVE
1. Bilateral optic atrophy, more advanced on the left side with greater choking.
2. Left facial paresis.
3. Exaggeration of the tendon reflexes in the left arm with very slight motor weakness and diminution of acuity of perception of pain stimulation.
4. Exaggeration of tendon reflexes in the left leg with slight motor weakness of the flexor muscles.
5. Positive Babinski with clonus at the knee and ankle.

IMPRESSION: There must be a glioma of the right cerebral hemisphere which has probably broken down and become cystic.

OPERATIVE NOTE
January 26, 1923
Anesthesia – Ether – Miss Gerrard

Right Osteoplastic Resection – 1st Stage. Disclosing Tumor. Presumably Endothelioma.

Under anesthesia a large right osteoplastic flap was reflected without incident, disclosing a tense dura. The flap was so made as to exposure the arm center but was probably too low for the very

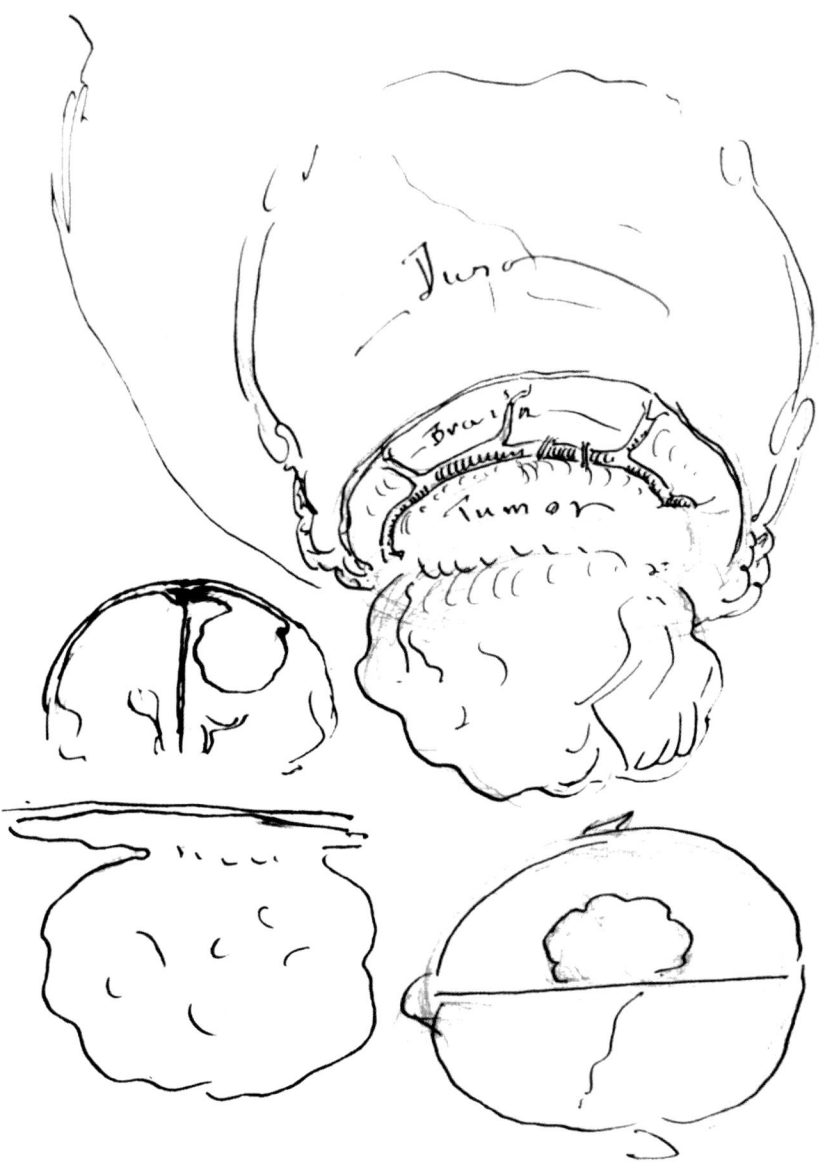

FIG. 3. OPERATIVE SKETCH.

upper margin of the bone incision, and slightly thickened dura was observed. Palpation showed this area to be somewhat more tense than elsewhere and there was a slight thickening of bone, indicating what was evidently the center of an endothelium. In order to verify its presence an incision was made in the dura to the outer margin of what might be tumor about 3 cm below the central point of indentation. The incision came down directly upon the margin of tumor which was slightly reddish and granular. An extra open-

OPPOSITE PAGE. FIGS. 1 AND 2. FOUR DAYS POSTOPERATIVE – FUNGUS CEREBRI.

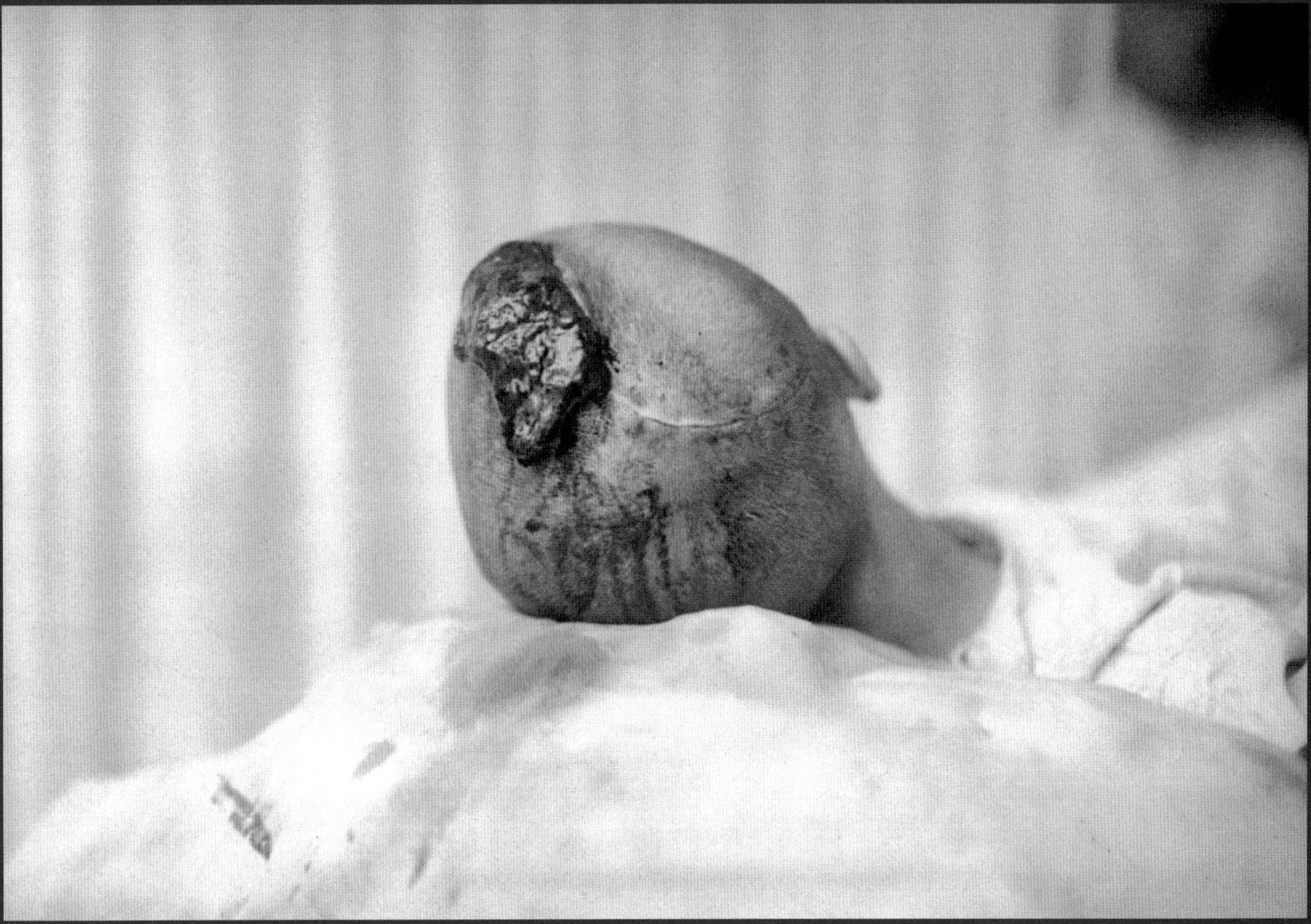

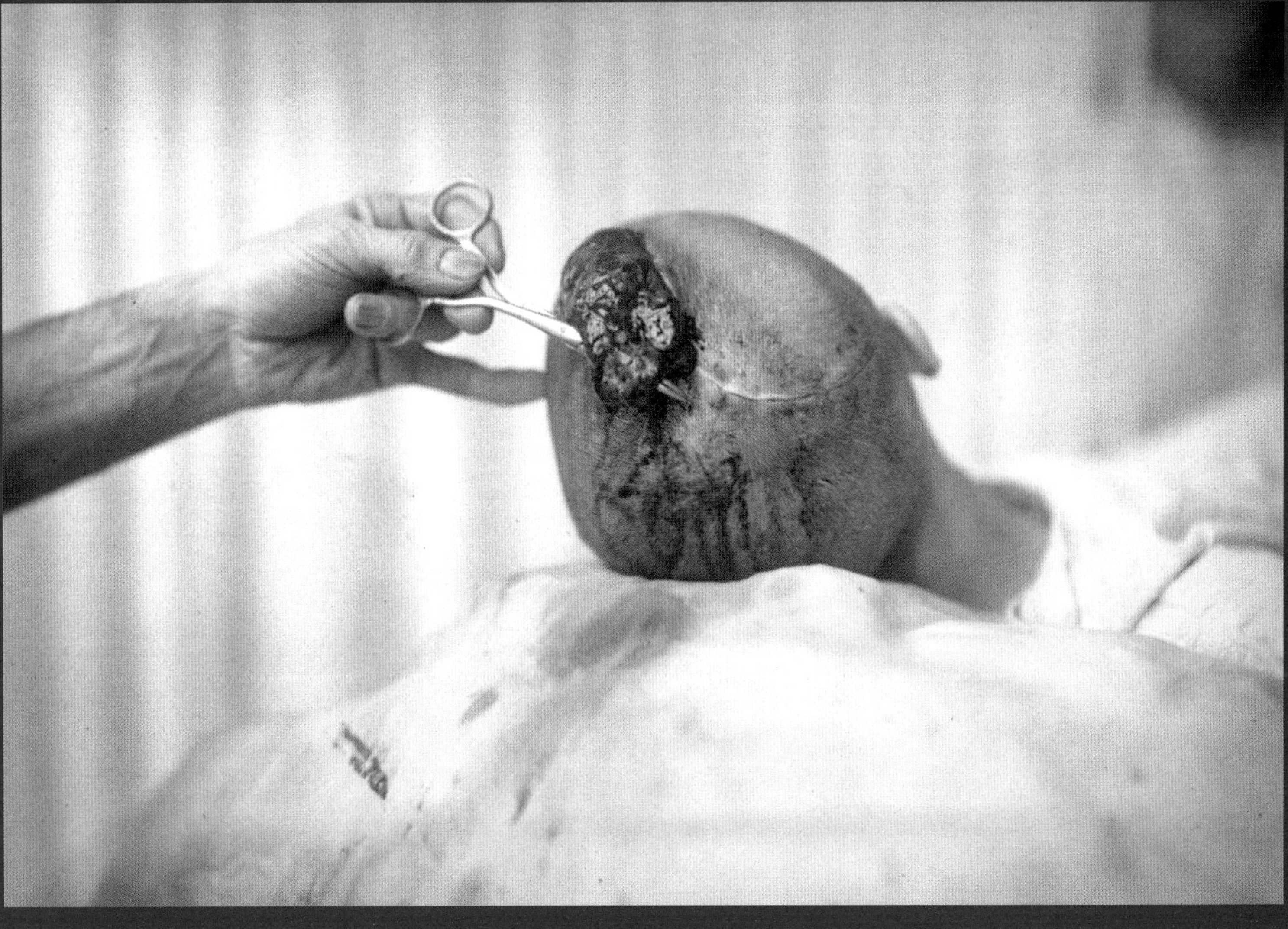

DISCHARGE NOTE
August 3, 1922
Dr. Bailey

Patient has failed gradually. Cheyne–Stokes respiration. Patient developed ventricular fibrillation and bronchopneumonia, attempts at nasal feeding unsuccessful because of profound coma. Death.

AUTOPSY REPORT
August 3, 1922
Dr. Martin
Dr. Bailey

Diagnosis: Dural endothelioma

This brain has been removed without fixation. It shows on the surface a very extraordinary degree of arteriosclerosis. The basilar and vertebral arteries are thickened and atheromatous, and also the internal carotids, evidently the explanation of the patient's postoperative symptoms which led to her death. The dura corresponding to the bone flap shows at the place where it had been palpated an area of thickening, which, however, is astonishingly small. It had been assumed that her mental symptoms might possibly be due to tumor rather than to arteriosclerosis, though her atherosclerosis was recognized clinically. The bone of the orbit was involved in an endotheliomatous process producing exophthalmos. Specimens had been sent down from the Operating Room.

The tumor which was palpated at operation in the Sylvian cleft does not even protrude on the inner surface of the dura. There can be no question, however, but that it is an endothelioma, at least within the layers of the dura which are greatly thickened. As the brain was not fixed, it is hard to tell whether there was any corresponding indentation of the brain. A small section of the tumor is taken for histological study.

(Dr. Cushing)

Microscopic examination: Sections all present a tumor of the dura which is considerably thickened. The tumor apparently is involving all layers of the dura and from appearances has extended through the dura and involving the bone tissue. There are small, irregular nests of cells with a perivascular

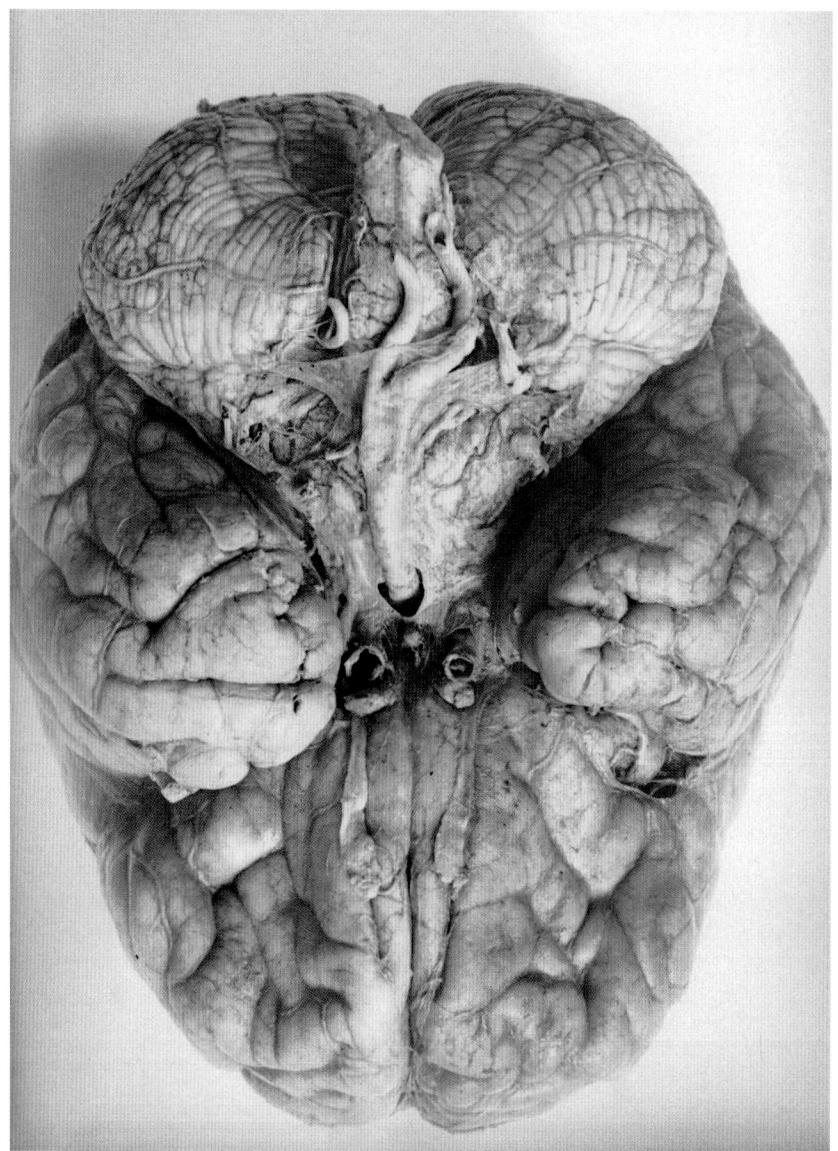

FIG. 5. AUTOPSY SPECIMEN.

arrangement. The cells are fairly large with a vesicular nucleus and a small amount of cytoplasm. Many of cells have hyperchromatic nuclei. Small blood vessels are frequent throughout the sections. With the phosphotungatic acid hematoxylin stain a considerable amount of fibrous connective tissue is seen in the dura. There are no areas of hyalinization or calcification in the tumor.

Diagnosis: Dural endothelioma.

Resident pathologist (signed)

have a flat expansion which carried its margin to the edge of the falx. It was necessary to rongeur away considerably more bone even though the flap was made quite high and although there was a little loss of blood which caused a lowering of blood pressure. It was possible by the placement of Kelly clamps along the margin as the flat portion of the growth was tilted out to control bleeding with the subsequent placement of a few bits of muscle and some clips.

There was an unusual degree of tension and the tumor practically extruded itself. At the end of the operation to from the fossa from which it had been removed had filled up completely, and I fear indeed that there may be some subsequent edema. Over the raw surface of brain a layer of protective was left in position to encourage an endothelial lining.

The flap was replaced and closed with a single layer of sutures in the galea though I am not at all sure at this writing that it would not have been better to have placed some sutures in the scalp for there may possibly be some danger of herniation. This gutta percha tissue must be removed in about 10 days.

(Dr. Cushing)

PATHOLOGY REPORT
January 30, 1923

Gross description: The specimen consists of an endothelioma, the configuration of which is best shown by the accompanying photographs. The tumor was removed from the right hemisphere. It has the usual nodular form of epithelium which has ... sheath with extension, carrying it along underneath the dura. The dura over the growth is very greatly thickened and the fragment for study done from both dura and underlying tumor.

(Dr. Cushing)

Microscopic description: The sections presented a ... tumor arranged in irregular concentric masses around small blood vessels. The cells are round or spherical and contain relatively little ... materials. The intracellular substance consists of fine, delicate fibrils.

Diagnosis – Dural Endothelioma

(Dr. Hansmann)

OPERATIVE NOTE
February 3, 1923
Dr. Cushing

I made a very bad technical error in this case by trusting to a layer of buried sutures in the galea alone without supplementing them with skin sutures. The wound came together very well and on the first dressing after 48 hours looked perfect in all respects. Just what could have happened to have increased her tension and led to a rupture I cannot tell. Something in the ward, perhaps straining at stool or an attack of vomiting would be sufficient to produce the wound

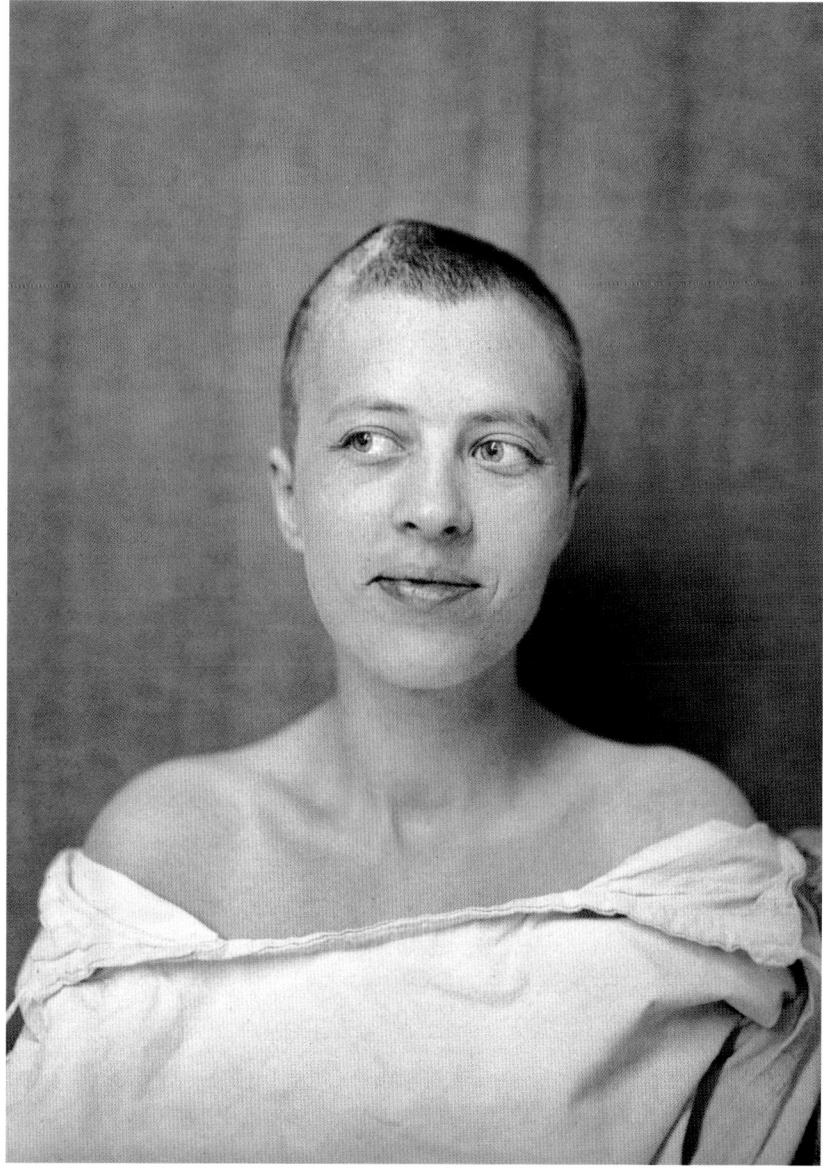

FIG. 5. FOUR WEEKS POSTOPERATIVE.

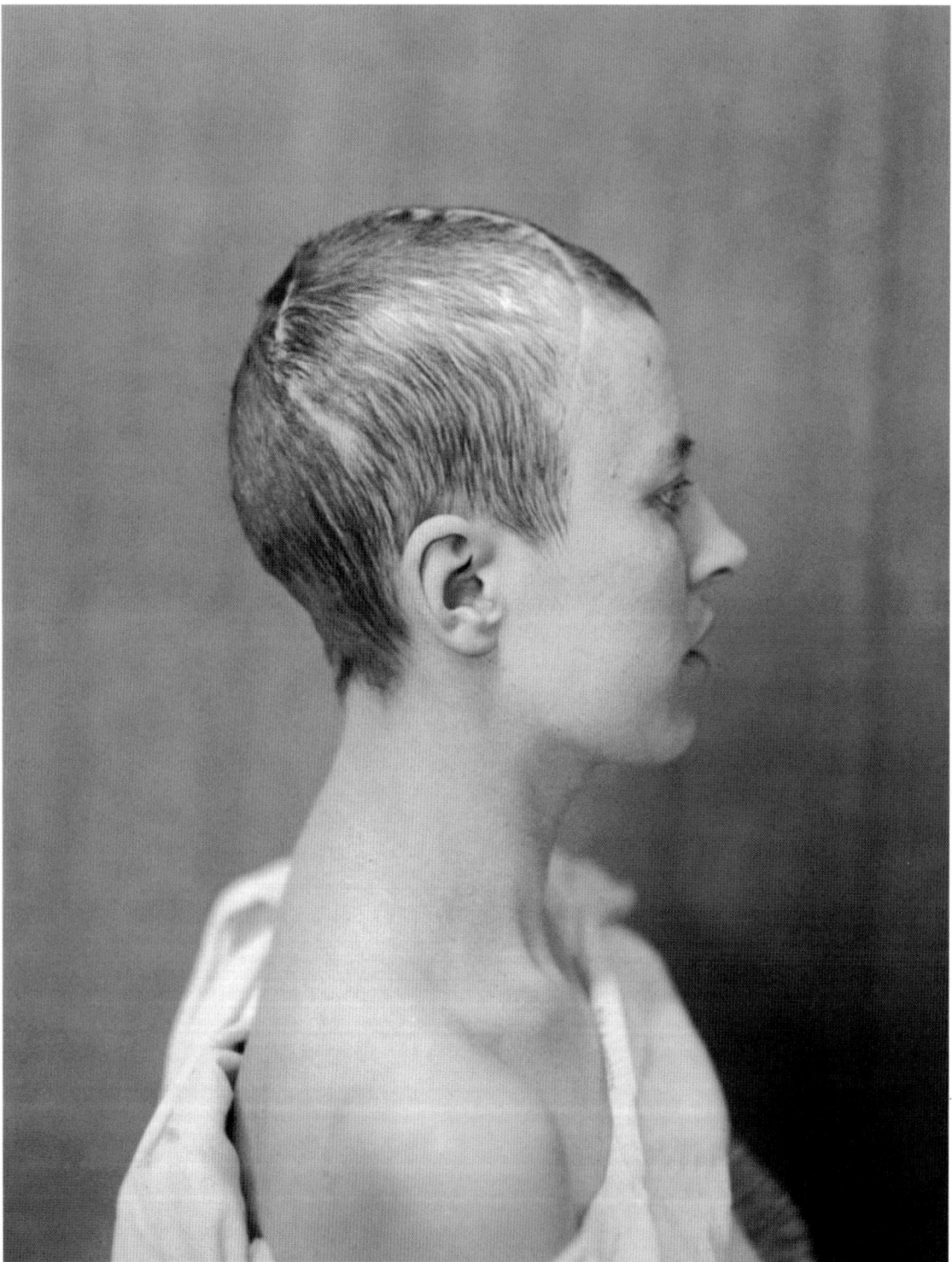

FIG. 6. FOUR WEEKS POSTOPERATIVE.

separation. What undoubtedly should have been done was to have it supported at the time of operation by a collodion dressing and to have left it in position. Yesterday, on her 4th day she had not been feeling well but I did not personally look her over and I presumed that her paralysis must have considerably increased, for after 48 hours she was moving her arm fairly well and this morning she had an arm and leg hemiplegia. The dressing had become slightly stained and was looked at by Dr. McKenzie who found a large fungus cerebri.

The size and the extent of this can be shown by Miss Thing's photograph. The entire upper third of the wound had separated and there was a juicy dripping fungus about 10 cm in length and 5 cm in breadth, such a thing as I have not seen for many years. She was given some salt by rectum which had no appreciable effect on the hernia and some salt intravenously, about 90 cc, which may perhaps have softened the hernia but did not lead to its recession. The major part of it was removed with the blunt end of a scalpel and sutures were placed in the wound while the raw surface was covered with protective.

A lumbar puncture was then performed, a large amount of fluid being secured, about 40 cc being removed. This led to a marked recession of the remaining stump of the fungus, and it is possible that if this procedure had been carried out formerly, a large part of the mass might have been reduced with less excision than I originally made. The layer of buried sutures was reinforced this time with the usual sutures through the scalp, and collodion dressing was applied.

(Dr. Cushing)

February 23, 1923
Dr. Bailey

Sutures removed. Wound well closed, but slightly full under incision.

DISCHARGE NOTE
March 2, 1923

Photograph taken today. Considerable improvement in facial paralysis. Can close left eye. Otherwise conditions same as the chart note.

LETTER TO DR. CUSHING
September 23, 1931

Dear Dr. Cushing

In January 1923, I and my sister (name of patient) from Fostoria, Ohio, visited your hospital and you operated upon (name of patient) for a cerebral tumor. Thinking that you might be interested in her case I am writing to inform you of her death which occurred October 20, 1930. Perhaps Dr. Hale has written to you and if so he has no doubt given the details. In case he has not I will advise that she nearly regained the use of her left hand after the operations which you performed. Her eyesight improved enough for her to be able to write letters but she could not read much. It was too much of a strain on her eyes. She did most of the housework for about a year. Mother passed away in November 1929 and (name of patient) and father kept the home and she did about all the housework. In the winter she had pneumonia and never regained her strength after that. Tuberculosis developed and she gradually slipped away until October 14th when it developed into tubercular meningitis. She was unable to see after that, but talked or whispered and retained her mental faculties until Sunday, October 18.

I have often thought of you and your kind consideration of us while in Boston but knowing how busy you are I never had any occasion to write before. I have not been at home very long at a time since we saw you, so have not been well informed about (name of patient) exact condition, at all times. If you care for any further information which I can give you I will be glad to hear from you.

Yours very sincerely,
Signed

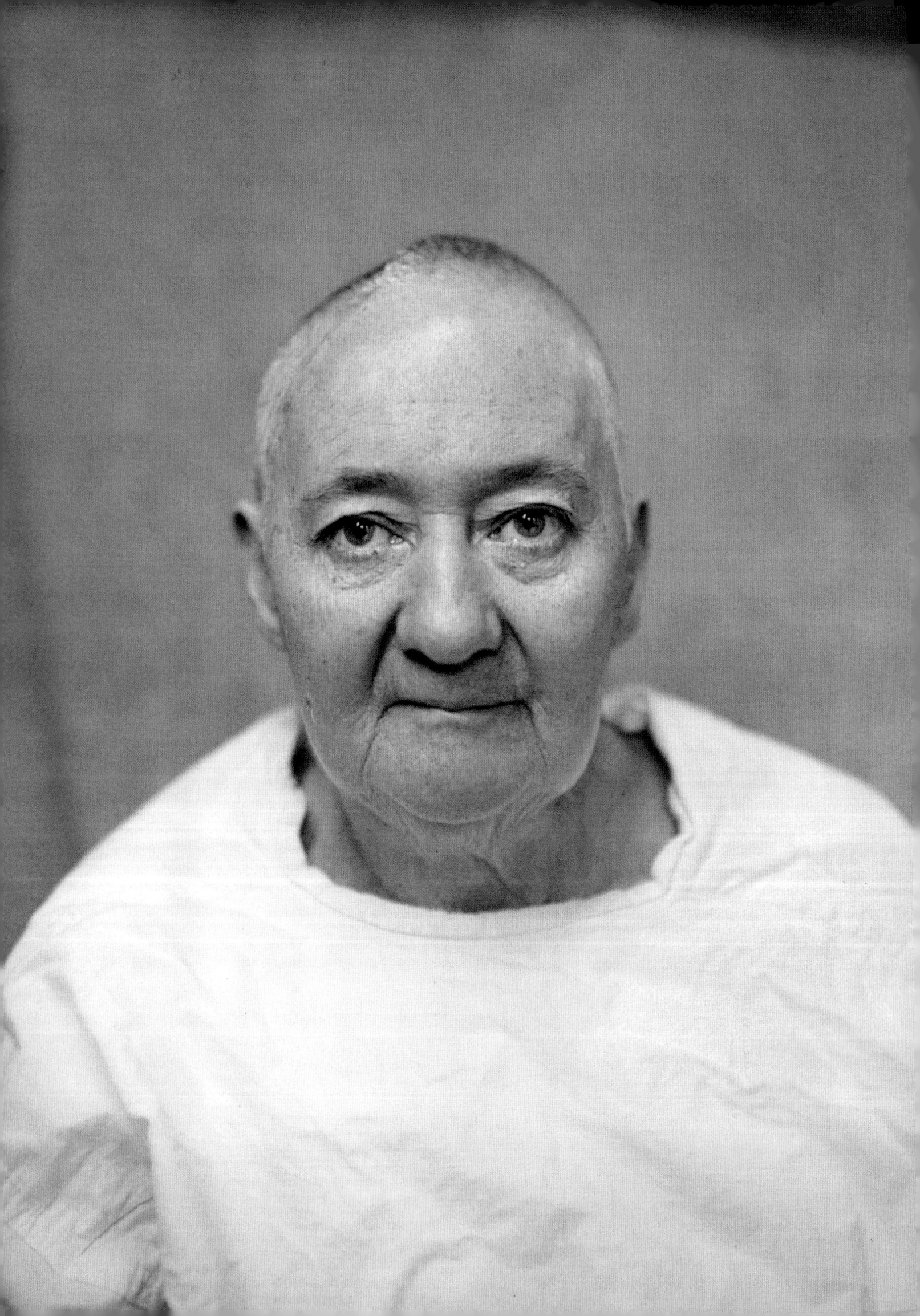

3.7 Parasagittal meningioma

SEX: F; AGE: 62; SURG. NO. 21046; 37882

COMPLAINT

Left-sided convulsions.

SUMMARY OF POSITIVE FINDINGS
March 31, 1924
Dr. Putnam

SUBJECTIVE
1. Left-sided Jacksonian attack beginning with sensory aura, starting in the left foot, and traveling up the left side of the body, and now involving the right foot also for the past 6 years. Extreme pain accompanying the attack.
2. Right craniotomy by Dr. Blair of St. Louis. Nothing was removed and no decompression was done.
3. Hypesthesia, weakness, and soreness of left side of body now very marked.
4. Dyspnea and easy fatigue on exertion.

OBJECTIVE
1. Thick, depressed, adherent scar of old right bone flap.
2. Some tenderness over the upper left parietal region.
3. Hypesthesia of the entire left side of the body, more marked in the foot to light touch. Pin prick and deep palpation felt as more painful on the left side than on the right. Akinesthesia of the left side. Little disturbance of temperature sense.
4. Abdominal reflexes absent on both sides.
5. Deep reflexes much exaggerated on the left as compared to the right. No clonus, however, and ambiguous Babinski.
6. Astereognosis and apraxia on left side.
7. Slight pulmonary emphysema.

IMPRESSION: The gradual onset and progressive character of the attacks beginning in one foot and spreading upwards and now the opposite foot, with little headache and no changes in the discs, seem typical of a meningioma, probably arising from the falx in the parietal region. Of interest is the hyperalgesia of the left side, which would suggest involvement of the left thalamus. Of interest, also, is the definite left anosmia, which is harder to explain. X-ray undoubtedly add further information. A very poor ether risk.

RADIOLOGY REPORT
April 6, 1924
Dr. Sosman

The stereoscopic films of the skull show a large bone flap in the right parietal region with smooth edges, apparently old. There is a small area of decompression at the lower edge where the bone appears somewhat thinned and moth-eaten.

The films show the pineal in the midline and no calcification in the sella.

SPECIAL NOTE
April 7, 1924
Dr. Cushing

This patient has had an earlier operation which did not disclose a definite tumor and since then for the intervening years she has progressively deteriorated until a succession of convulsive attacks accompanied by great muscular cramping and pain and she has also deteriorated mentally. I anticipated finding a large meningioma and was astonished to disclose the small growth which was removed.

OPERATIVE NOTE
April 7, 1924
Anesthesia – Ether – Miss Gerrard

Extirpation of Small Circa, 13 gm, Meningioma from the Right Parasagittal Region. Temporary Muscle Implant. Refusion.

There was no great difficulty in re-elevating the flap though it occasioned a good deal of bleeding, particularly near the midline where we took pains at the time of recutting the flap to remove an extra half inch of bone. This was subsequently increased somewhat until I came actually down to the sinus which required the placement of some bits of muscle which were at hand from another patient before dural bleeding could be well controlled.

Then I made 1–2 punctures without disclosing the tumor and finally excised in a fresh area of dura not exposed at the original operation and in the posterior part of the wound came down upon the mar-

OPPOSITE PAGE. FIG. 1. TWO WEEKS POSTOPERATIVE.

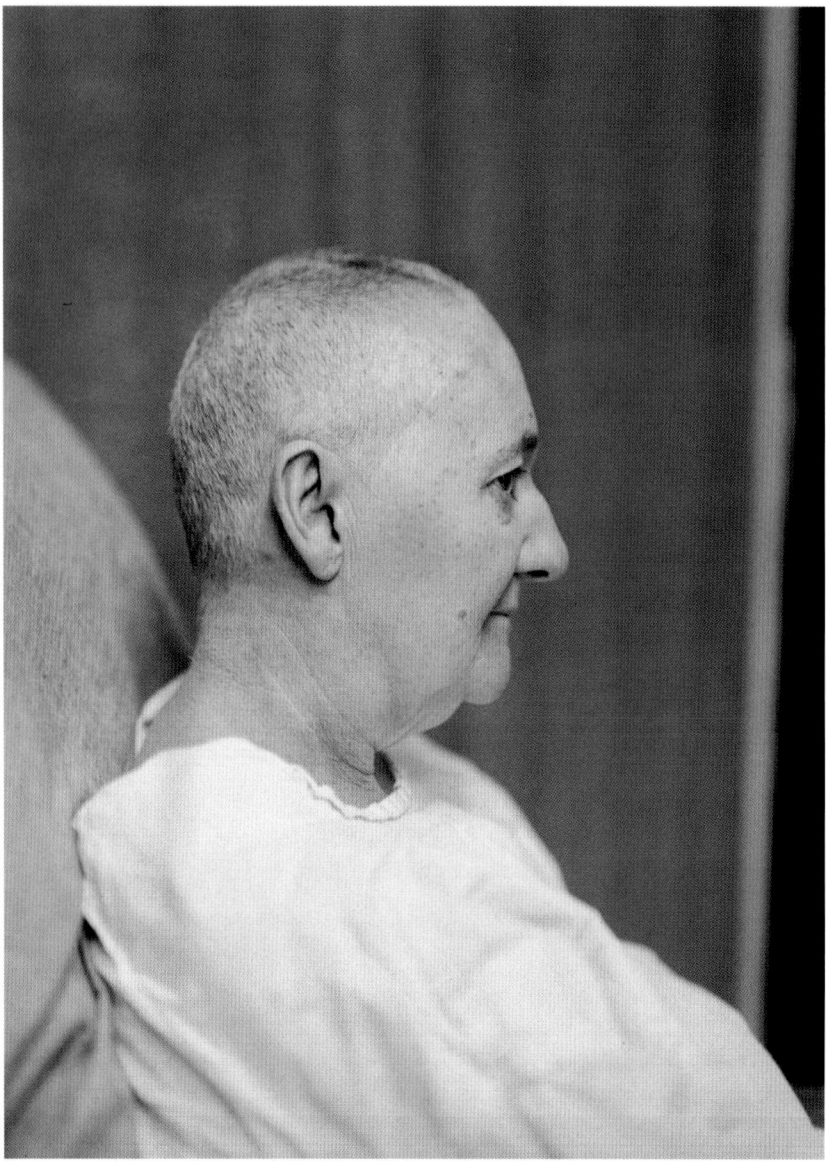

FIG. 2. TWO WEEKS POSTOPERATIVE.

gin of the small meningioma not larger than a pigeon egg. This tumor was adherent to brain and to longitudinal sinus. Fortunately, it was a very fibrous tumor, the capsule of which could easily be caught in clamps and I finally succeeded in tilting it out with only a little loss of blood from the large venous radical coming off from the falx. The margin of dura just at the edge of the sinus was secured with a succession of clamps, finally replaced by clips. Fortunately, there was no great bleeding. **However, she sustained a sharp fall in blood pressure before the bleeding could be fully controlled it was necessary to take muscle from the leg for temporary placement and she was immediately refused by Dr. Davis.** There was a prompt restoration in blood pressure. The flap was replaced and closed as usual in layers securely without a drain.

(Dr. Cushing)

PATHOLOGY REPORT
April 7, 1924

This is a small 13 gram parasagittal meningioma removed from the right rolandic region.

(Dr. Cushing)

DISCHARGE NOTE
April 30, 1924
Dr. Putnam

Patient made an excellent postoperative recovery with remarkable restoration of motor power and was able to walk alone with a cane. The astereognosis persisted and there was still a slight hypaesthesia on the left side. Within a day or two of the operation, however, she had had a slight twitching on the left side.

LETTER TO DR. CUSHING
July 17, 1928
Dear Dr. Cushing:

Mrs. (name of patient) and myself expect to be in Boston about the middle of August, and would like very much to see you for a few minutes. I would appreciate it very much if you would have your Secretary write me a note saying whether or not you will be in Boston at that time. I am glad to say that Mrs. (patient's name) is doing very well and I do not doubt but what you will be pleased to look her over and see for yourself what her condition is.

Hoping that we may have the good fortune to see you next month, I am

Yours very truly,
(Signed) EW

SECOND HOSPITAL ADMISSION

COMPLAINT

The patient had a recurrence of 3 left sided Jacksonian convulsions one week ago and became so apprehensive about having more that she decided to come here immediately.

December 24, 1930
Dr. Henderson

IMPRESSION. Apart from the recent attacks there is no evidence of any recurrence of the tumor and all the physical findings are residual rather than recurrent.

RADIOLOGY REPORT
December 24, 1930
Dr. Sosman

The films of the skull show a right parietal bone flap with smooth edges and with area of bone loss along both upper and lower edges. There are multiple silver clips close to the midline in the posterior half of the operative area, probably along the sagittal sinus. The pineal is in the midline and by measurements is not displaced. There is no evidence of recurrence.

December 26, 1930
Dr. Henderson

No changes since admission. Has not had any attacks.

DISCHARGE NOTE
December 30, 1930
Dr. Henderson

Patient discharged home today. No attacks or other symptoms since admission. Dr. Cushing saw her in OR. She is to take 1½ gr luminal daily and gradually reduce it after 2–3 months.

The last follow up letter from the patient was received on July 31, 1933 (not available in the chart).

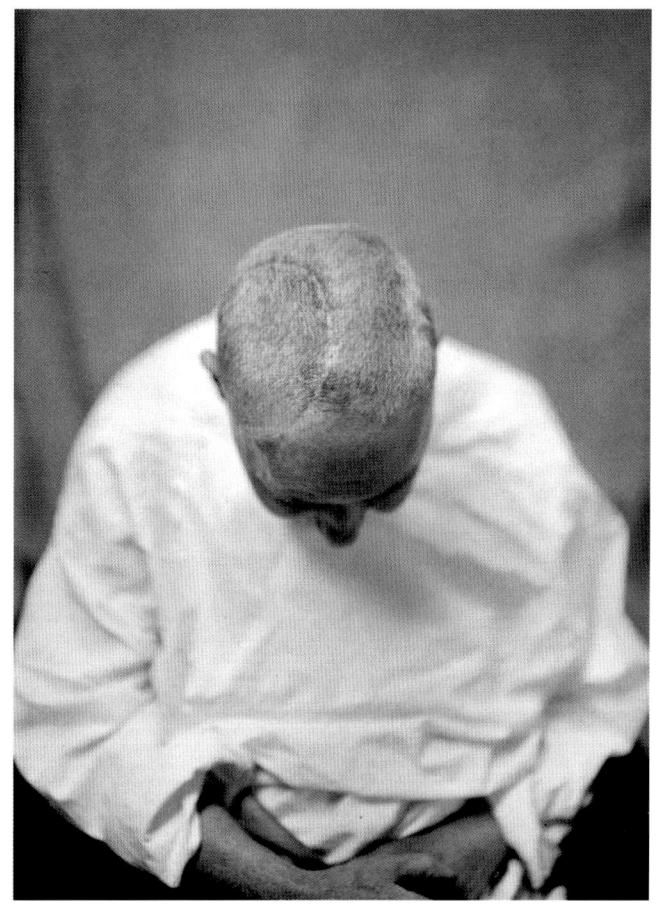

FIG. 3. TWO WEEKS POSTOPERATIVE.

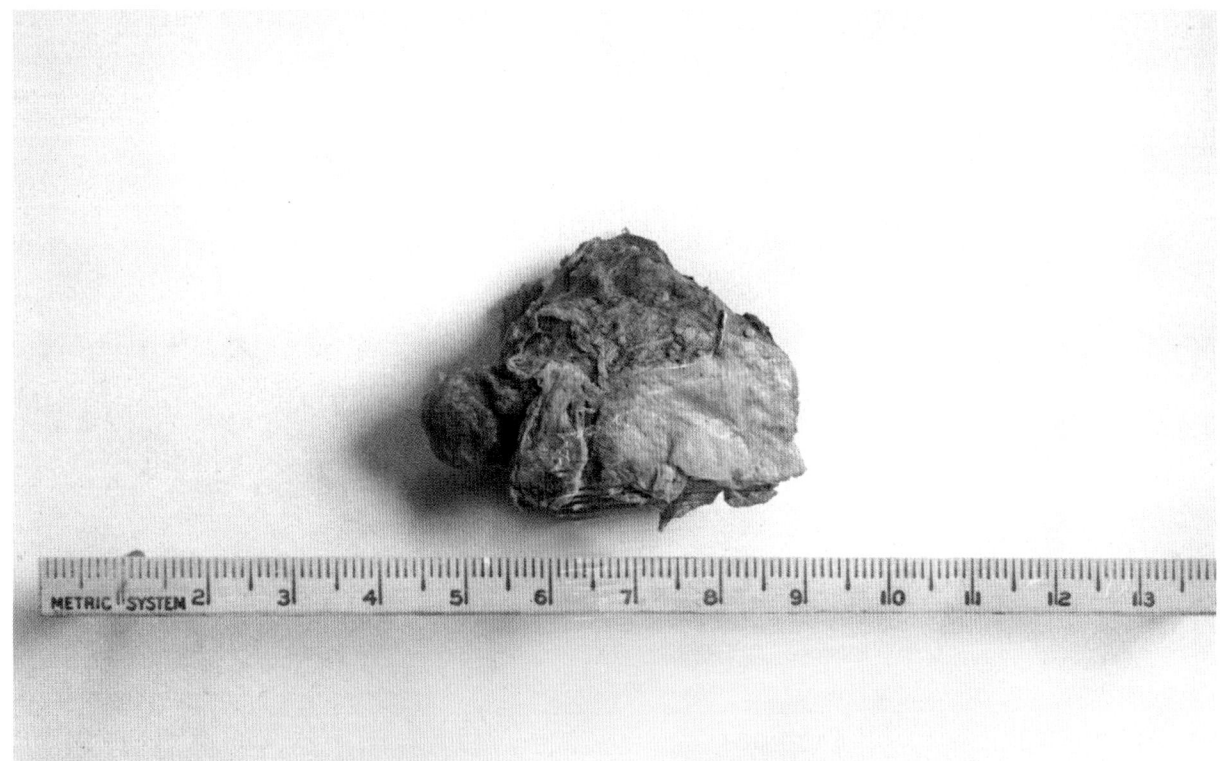

FIG. 4. TUMOR SPECIMEN.

REVIEW OF PATHOLOGY SLIDES
August 28, 1933

Two sections now presented by Dr. Eisenhardt for microscopic description.

The tumor falls into the general group of meningioma and shows only slight cellularity. In a few areas the typical small, oval, perivascular endothelial cells with indistinct borders and one or two tiny, but prominent, nucleoli can be found. Some portions are composed of diffuse cells without perivascular arrangement, but in other fields, slightly elongated cells showing a slight whorled arrangement around a central blood vessel are present. Another type of cell is also seen. These are very large with the same sized nucleoli as those described above, but they have distinct outlines and abundant finely vesicular cytoplasm. In the cellular areas large vacuoles sometimes separate the cells. Hyperchromatic nuclei are uncommon and no mitosis are seen. The tumor is more the psammoma form in which most of the perivascular units have undergone hyalinosis. The tumor is largely composed of hyaline masses of collagen fibrils. The fused whorls of endothelial cells and fibroblasts, which now appear as hyaline spherical bodies showing concentric lamination similar to corpora amylacea, are arranged around a central lumen. These are closed or patent. Some of the lamina contain vessels while many are patent and vacuolated, giving the tumor in places the appearance of a chordoma. On the whole, there are fairly numerous vessels.

Diagnosis – Meningioma.

(Resident pathologist)

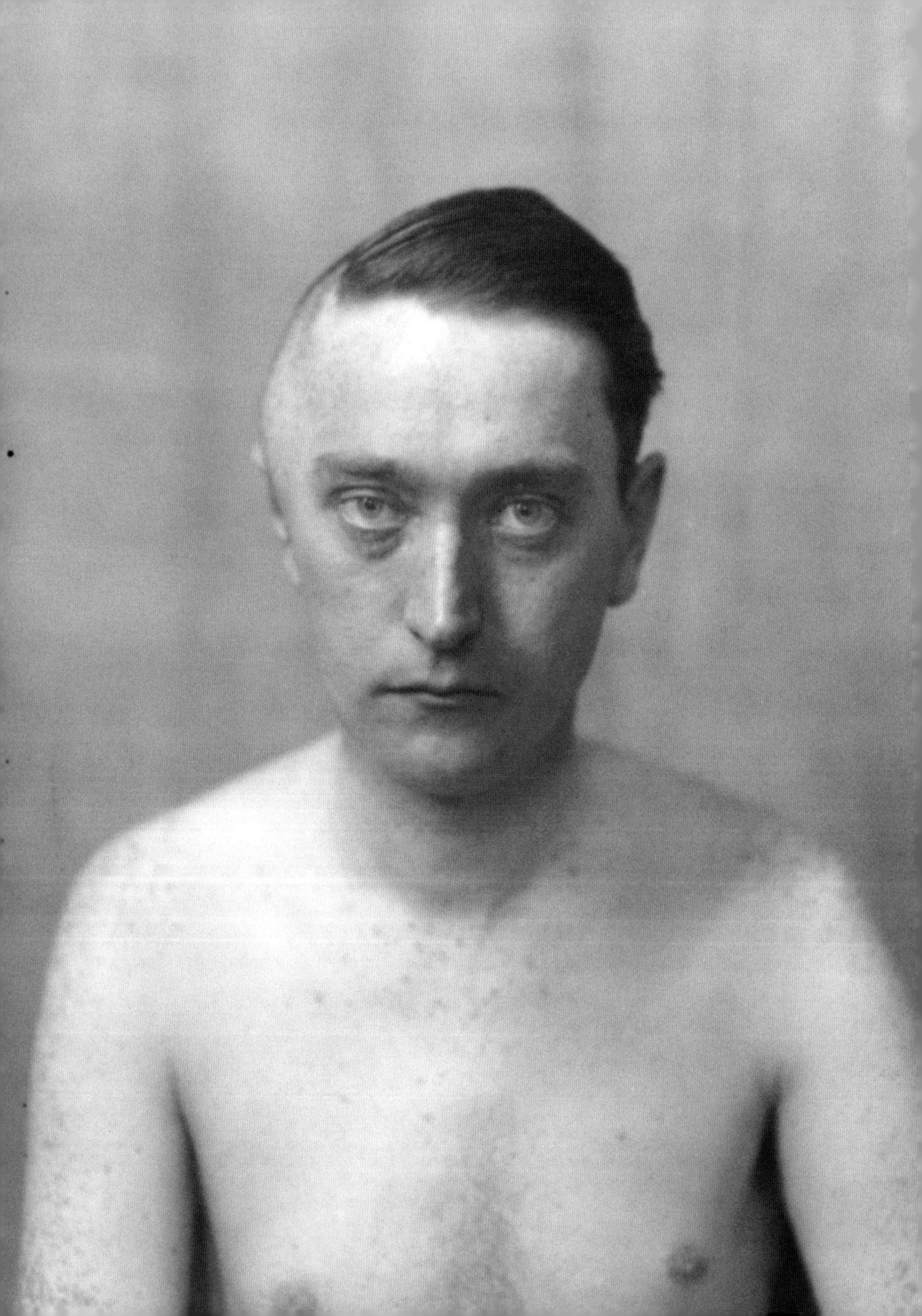

3.8 Frontal meningioma

SEX: M; AGE: 32; SURG. NO. 27038; 30520; 30985; 31682; 32435; 32754

HISTORY

The patient was admitted in the hospital because of "failing vision."

SUMMARY OF POSITIVE FINDINGS
August 23, 1926
Dr. Bailey

SUBJECTIVE
1. Headache over a period of about a year unaccompanied by vomiting.
2. Diminution of vision.

OBJECTIVE
1. Bilateral choked disc 4–5 D.
2. Great diminution in the visual fields without definite hemianopsia.

IMPRESSION: Cerebral tumor without localizing signs.

RADIOLOGY REPORT
August 21, 1926
Dr. Sosman

Right and left stereos, A.P. and P.A. films of skull show the channel for the right middle meningeal artery larger, deeper and more tortuous than the one on the left. It ends about halfway to the vertex in the area of decreased density which appears moth-eaten.

Surrounding this there is a moderate bone reaction. This area involves the posterior edge of the frontal bone and the anterior edge of the parietal bone. There is in addition a large diploetic vein running into this same area across the right parietal bone. The sella turcica appears normal. No other localizing signs of the tumor.

IMPRESSION: The appearance suggests a meningioma.

OPERATIVE NOTE
August 23, 1926
Anaesthesia – Ether – Miss Way

Right Subtemporal Decompression. Evacuation of Only 2–3 cc from Temporal Horn of Ventricle.

The usual procedure was carried out without difficulty until the dura was reached. Here it was noted that there was very great tension and that the supe-

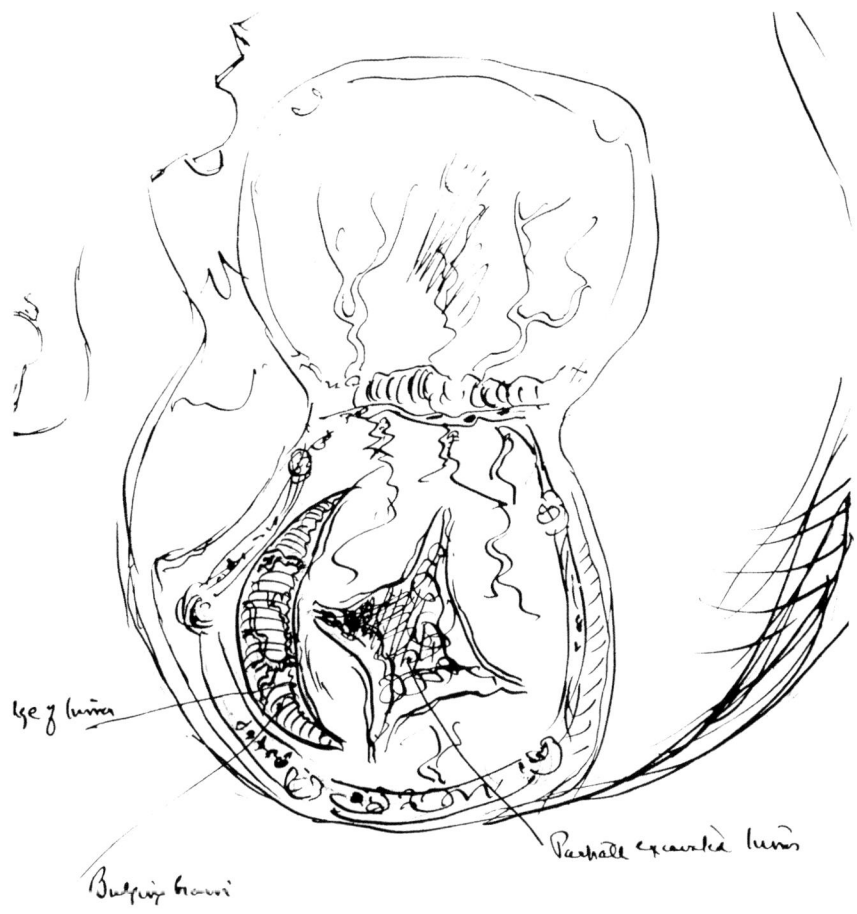

FIG. 2. OPERATIVE SKETCH.

rior branch of the meningeal, which ran along the upper border of the field, was extremely dilated and also extremely tortuous. A nick was made in the lower temporal region and a needle introduced backward and downward reached a few drops of fluid from the temporal horn of the ventricle at a depth of about 4½ cm. There was also a spurt of subdural fluid which came out through the nick, but neither this nor a small amount of fluid contained in the ventricle was sufficient to lower tension to an appreciable degree.

The dura was now opened rapidly by radiating incisions and although the brain bulged quickly and markedly through the opening there was no rupture. There was, however, no time to do any exploring around the edges of the area owing to the danger of rupture of the cortex.

OPPOSITE PAGE. FIG. I. TWO WEEKS POSTOPERATIVE AFTER THE FIRST OPERATION (SUBTEMPORAL DECOMPRESSION).

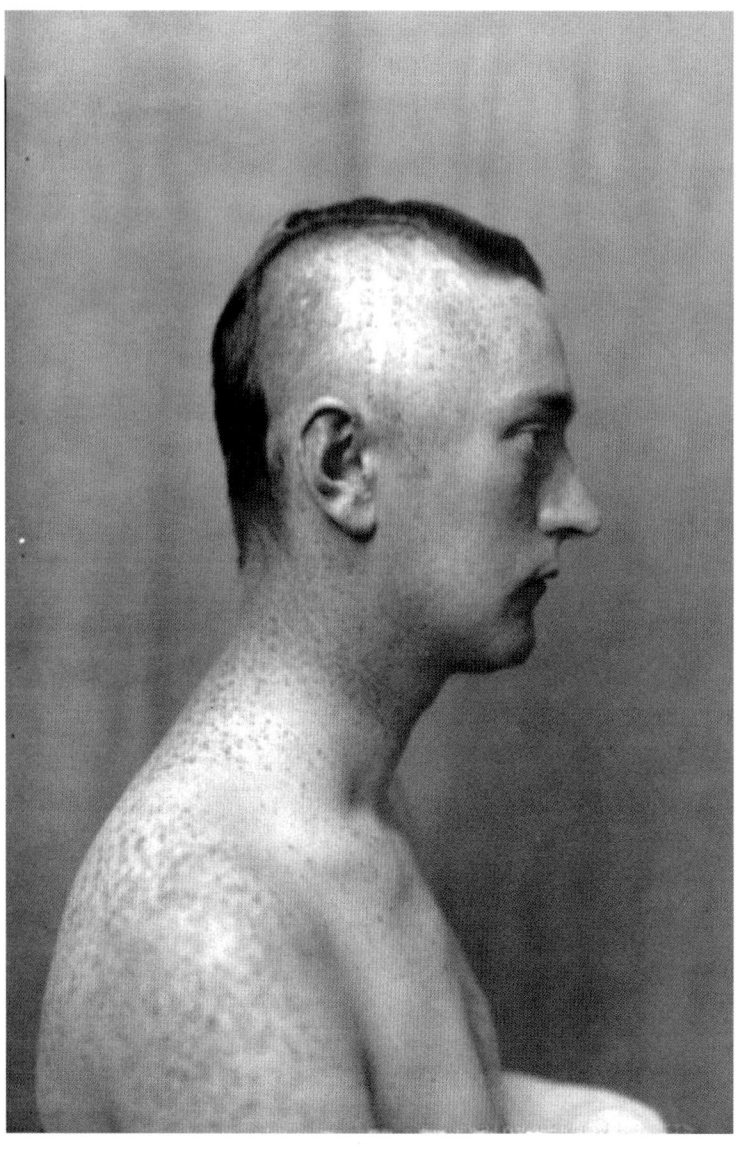

FIG. 3. TWO WEEKS POSTOPERATIVE AFTER THE FIRST OPERATION (SUBTEMPORAL DECOMPRESSION).

The wound was now closed in layers with fine silk without drainage.

(Dr. Horrax)

August 26, 1926
Dr. Horrax

Patient quite comfortable. Marked improvement in vision in left eye, which was the one most affected.

DISCHARGE NOTE
September 9, 1926
Dr. Bailey

Patient relieved of headache. It seems to me there is about 2D swelling in the left eye. No elevation of the right eye, but margins still obscured.

SECOND HOSPITAL ADMISSION

SUMMARY OF POSITIVE FINDINGS
January 24, 1928
Dr. Bagdasar

SUBJECTIVE
1. Subtemporal decompression on August 23, 1926.
2. Rapid failing of vision after operation. Four months later total blindness in left eye and improvement in right one.
3. Pain in left half of head and auditory hallucinations of the left ear when he is sleeping upon that side since the operation.
4. Pain in left face 6–7 months after operation.

OBJECTIVE
1. Bulging of the decompression area on right side.
2. Mydriasis of the left pupil. Does not react to light and accommodation.
3. Secondary optic atrophy with total blindness of left eye.
4. Choked disc – 2D of right eye.
5. Inconstant dorsal flexion of first toe of right foot.

IMPRESSION: The headaches on the left side and pain along the 5th nerve suggest a lesion of the left hemisphere. The auditory hallucinations of the left ear enable me to localize the lesion with some probability, near the auditory center of the left hemisphere. There is no doubt that the lesion is a tumor growing very slowly. He deserves exploration to save the vision of his right eye.

RADIOLOGY REPORT
January 21, 1928
Dr. Sosman

Re-examination of skull shows a smooth-edged decompression in the right temporal region 6.5 cm in diameter. The area of roughening of the bone in the inner table of the skull at the posterior edge of the right frontal lobe, just above and anterior to the decompression remains. There is apparently a slight increase in the amount of bone reaction. The vascularity appears slightly greater than before. This area still suggests a meningioma.

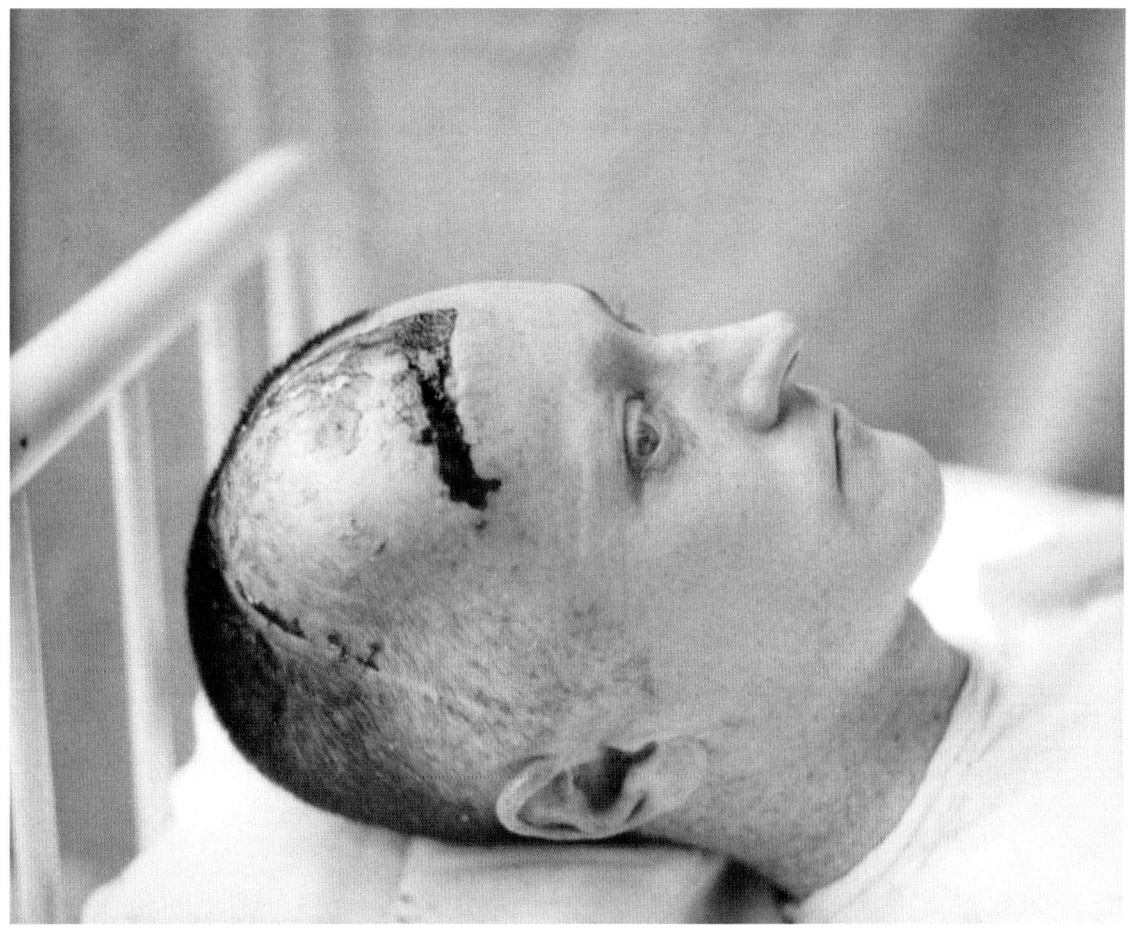

FIG. 4. TWO WEEKS POSTOPERATIVE AFTER THE SECOND SET OF OPERATIONS (RESECTION OPERATIONS).

DISCHARGE NOTE
January 27, 1928
Dr. Bagdasar

Patient to take a holiday and report back later. It is hoped at that time that symptoms will permit of more accurate localization.

THIRD HOSPITAL ADMISSION

SUMMARY OF POSITIVE FINDINGS
March 23, 1928
Dr. Bagdasar

SUBJECTIVE
1. Tinnitus of the left ear since 1918, until 1923, associated with headaches and vomiting. Follows a period of relief of 1 1/2 years.
2. In 1925 recurrence of tinnitus and headache.
3. Flashes before his eyes soon after tinnitus reappeared.
4. Subtemporal decompression on August 23, 1926.

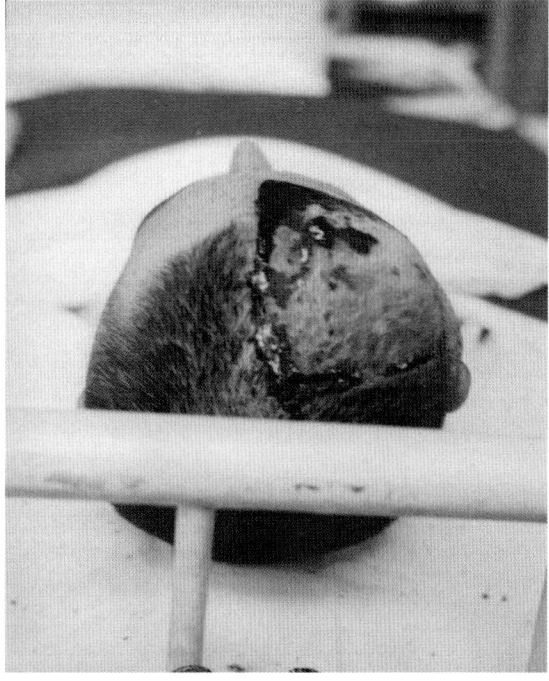

FIG. 5. TWO WEEKS POSTOPERATIVE AFTER THE SECOND SET OF OPERATIONS.

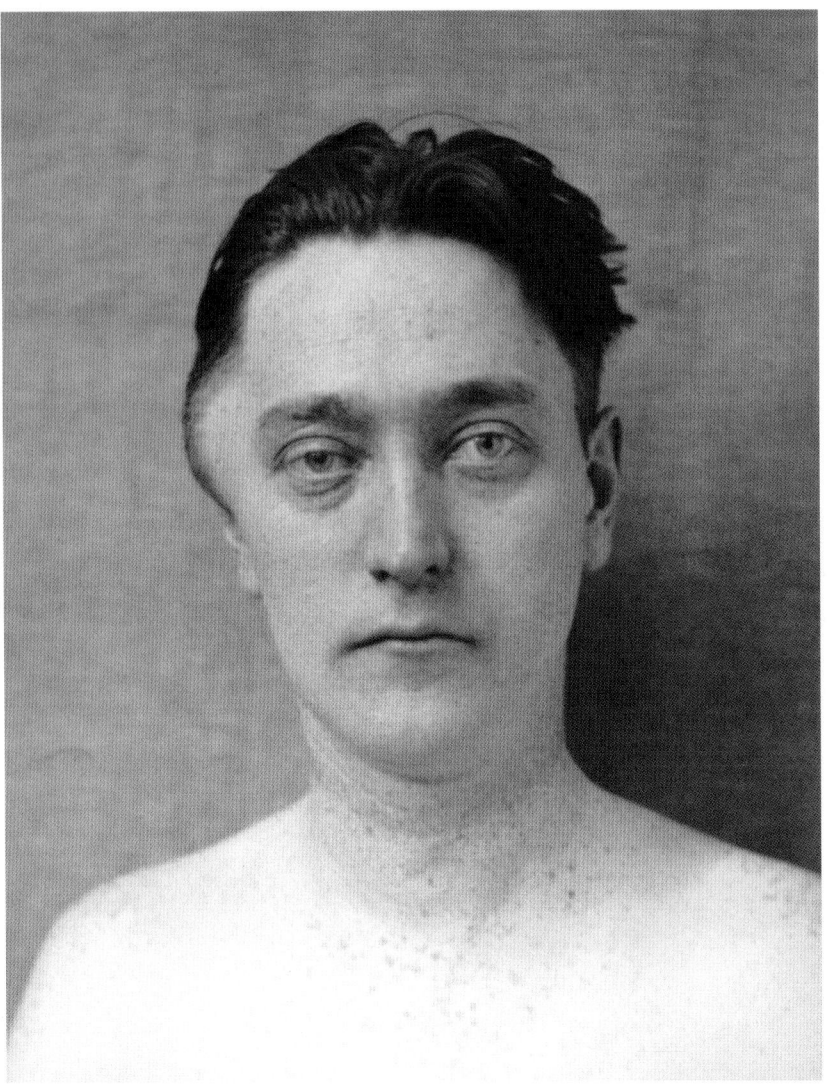

FIG. 6. FOUR MONTHS POSTOPERATIVE AFTER THE SECOND SET OF OPERATIONS.

3. Choked discs, 1D in both eyes and optic atrophy.
4. Slightly increased deep reflexes on the left side and possibly some weakness.
5. Impairment of smell.

IMPRESSION: This is a very embarrassing case. At the last admission he hadn't any objective trouble except total blindness of his left eye and choked disc on the right. So I made a hypothesis of a left temporal tumor on the ground of his only subjective complaint – left auditory hallucinations and pain along the left 5th nerve when he was lying upon the left side. Now with the account of a sudden and transitory attack on the left side, which occurred 2 weeks ago, and slightly increased deep reflexes on this side at the present time with some positive X-ray findings (on the posterior edge of the right frontal lobe) I should rather be in favor of tumor at the base of the right frontal lobe, possibly a ventriculogram could better clear up the localization.

RADIOLOGY REPORT
March 22, 1928
Dr. Sosman

Films show the same irregular, thickened area in the upper posterior portion of the right frontal bone. There is definitive hyperostosis on the external table at this point. This is rather flat and dense. The findings strongly suggest a meningioma.

SPECIAL NOTE
April 5, 1928
Dr. Cushing

5. Rapid failing of vision after operation. Four months later total blindness in left eye and improvement in right one.
6. Pain in left half of head and tinnitus in this ear when he is lying in bed upon this side.
7. Pain in left face 6–7 months after operation, and still lasting.
8. Three weeks ago failing vision of right eye.
9. Two weeks ago sudden and transitory attack of weakness on the left side with falling down.

OBJECTIVE
1. Bulging and tenderness of decompression area.
2. Total blindness of left eye. Left pupil does not react to light. Failing in right. Right visual acuity – 20/40.

We have sadly procrastinated about this man's operation. I never got a very good idea about him and whether had I done the primary decompression I would have been ready to suspect a local meningioma in view of the greatly increased vascularity I do not know. At all events, in view of what I found today, one may assume that the decompression had been exceedingly difficult for there was excessive bleeding from the bone at the lower part of the elevated flap in spite of previous subtemporal defect. At the last time he was in the hospital, there was some suspicion of changes which suggested a meningioma in the frontal region but I for some reason or other let him go out as he seemed in good condition. He has now come back again with his vision poor and the decompression extremely tight.

I chanced to put the case on when there were some Yale applicants for the medical school here and I permitted them to look on but they had certainly enough to discourage them from engaging in my branch of surgery should they ever enter the school.

Though abundant preparations had been made for a possible meningioma, I started out with a very inadequate team and before finishing up had all hands on deck. Even so, it was an extremely difficult case. I do not know when I have encountered worse bleeding from simply turning down a bone flap except possibly in the case of (the name of another patient.)

Good fortune was with me at least in one respect in that I had an abundance of muscle without which I think the man almost certainly would have bled to death.

OPERATIVE NOTE
April 5, 1928
Anesthesia – Novocain
Primary ether – Miss Melanson.

Osteoplastic Resection of Frontally Placed Bone Flap, Excessive Bleeding, Disclosure of Huge, Exceedingly Soft, Stringy Meningioma Occupying Practically the Whole Field. Partial Circumferential Incision of Dura with Bulging Brain, Cross Cut through Dura with Fairly Radical Removal of Core of Tumor by Electro-Surgery and Suction. Sacrifice of Involved Bone Flap, Closure of Scalp Alone.

I was aware almost from the outset that we were going to have great difficulty for there was marked bleeding from the scalp and the surface of the bone was so vascular that it could not be checked even with the abundant use of wax so that there was oozing from the outset.

The lateral incisions were cut with the Gigli saw and when it came to the upper edge this was so vascular and the inner surface so roughened that I did not dare pass the saw through but made a number of perforations and connected them with a Montenovesi forceps.

The flap was then reflected and there was immediate profuse bleeding from 3–4 large dural arteries emerging just below the broken edge of the flap which did not come down quite to the situation of the subtemporal decompression. Before I could get muscle exposed and cut for implantation there had been marked loss of blood but I finally succeeded in getting muscle plastered against the edge and in checking bleeding.

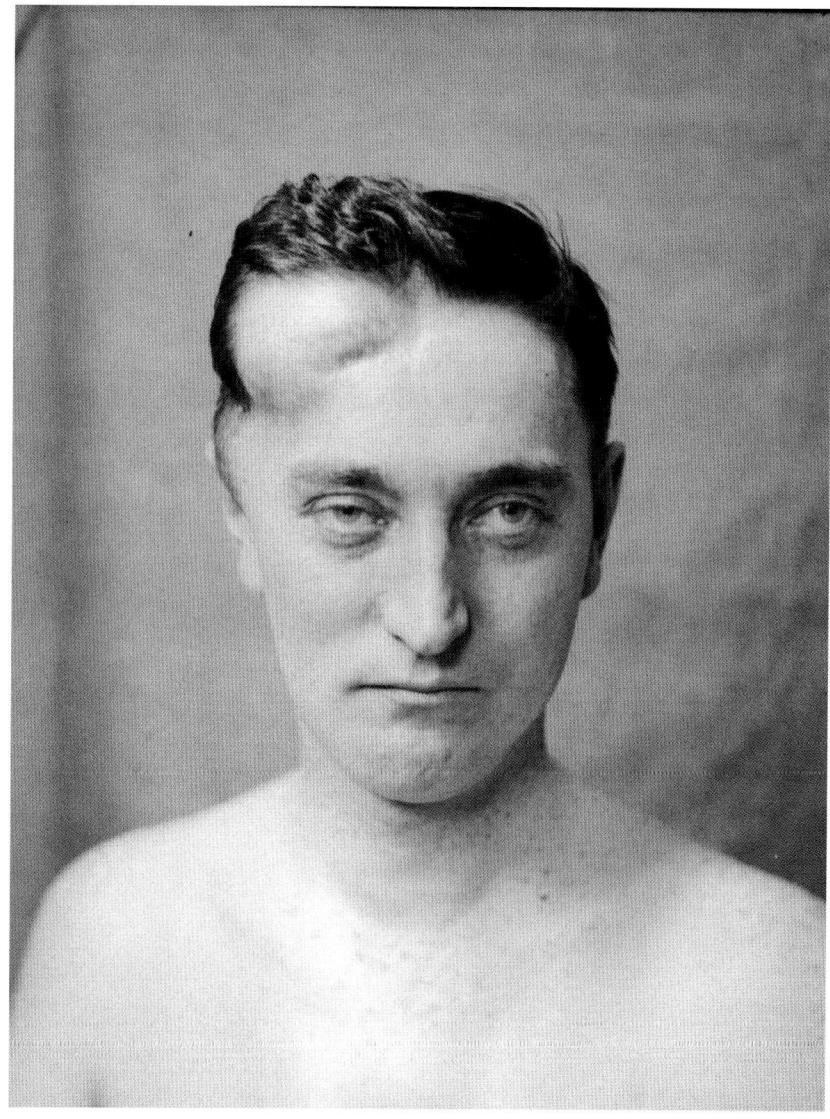

FIG. 7. PREOPERATIVE BEFORE THE LAST RESECTION OPERATION.

It was quite evident that there was a huge meningioma and I was at a loss of knowing what to do, whether to reclose for a second session or to see what could be done at this first session, at least to liberate the growth and perhaps reduce tension.

As shown in the sketch, I made a partial anterior circumferential incision, the brain bulged so markedly that it was promptly evident that I would be unable to replace the flap. I soon came upon the edge of tumor. Thinking that I might perhaps be able to encircle the whole growth by the incision so that the growth would tend to extrude itself, I attempted to make an incision in the posterior part of the field, but immediately came down upon

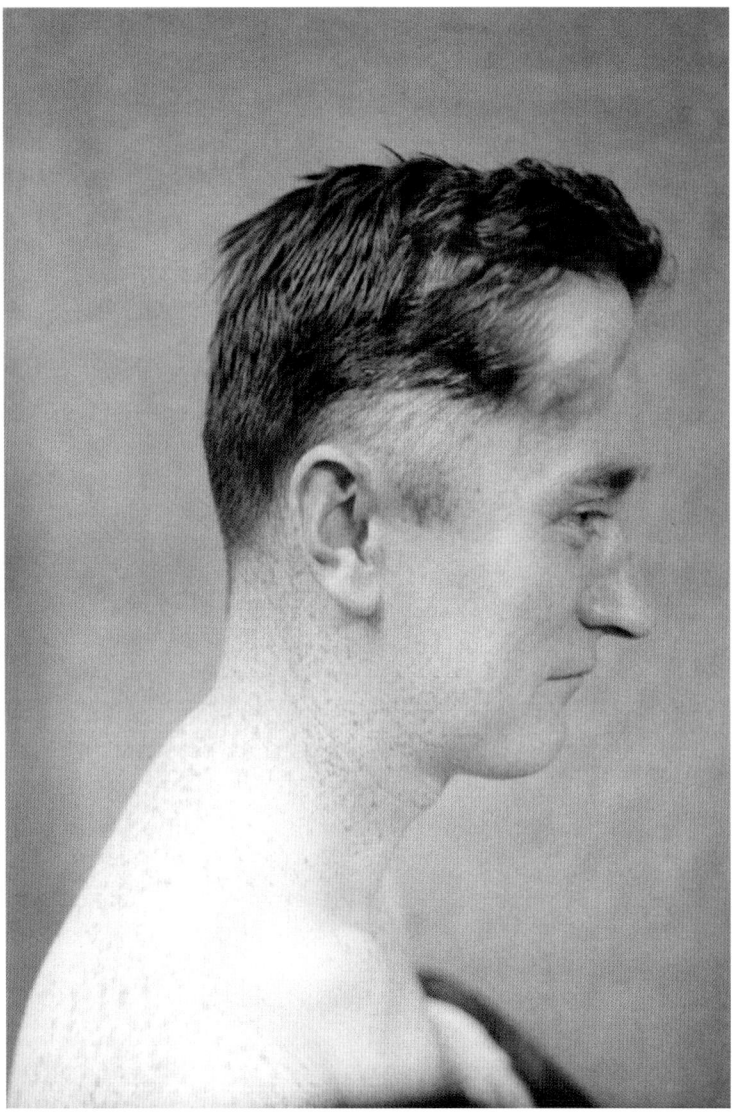

FIG. 8. PREOPERATIVE BEFORE THE LAST RESECTION OPERATION.

tumor so that I anticipate the growth is wider than the exposed field.

I then took a step which I have never before done, making a cross-cut incision through a very vascular dura into the tumor and with the electric loop, I began scooping out great masses of it. The growth was fairly vascular but not excessively so. Its one most striking peculiarity was that it was extremely soft and stringy so that I got fragments for fresh study and masses were pulled out from the depth of the tumor like a lot of stringy seaweed. I excavated the growth as far as I dared and by this time, the patient's pressure was falling off and he was consequently transfused successfully by Dr. Bird.

I might conceivably have gone on from this stage and done more but the operation had already been pretty long and consequently, realizing the bone flap which was evidently involved in the growth had to be sacrificed, I stripped it away and closed the scalp, hoping that the growth would tend to extrude itself and hoping that I might have removed enough from its center to partly relieve tension, though I am not at all convinced of this. Whether at a second session I will have to remove more bone or whether I could coax the growth out of the present field of exposure, I cannot presume to say nor can I tell whether I ought to ligate the external carotid as a preliminary measure. I rather think this ought to be done though it is possible I could work around the lower margin clipping dura as I go without this being necessary.

(Dr. Cushing)

POSTOPERATIVE NOTES
April 5, 1928
Dr. Carlton

Patient's pulse rose embarrassingly during operation (200) and blood pressure dropped to nothing. The tumor had accordingly to be abandoned and a hurried transfusion was carried out as explained in operative note. Patient reacted slowly to the transfusion but toward evening, his blood pressure gradually rose again to 70 and he was returned to the ward at 7:00.

April 6, 1928
Dr. Carlton

Patient vomited frequently during the night, and complained of great discomfort about the head. By morning, pulse was 120, respirations 16, condition objectively good although pulse was slightly weak. Moderate edema of right eye and patient complained of being quite unable to see. Right eye, however, reacted to light. Patient quieter toward evening and though the possibility of a night nurse was considered, it was felt that his condition was sufficiently good to let him stay on ward service. No weakness.

SPECIAL NOTE
April 9, 1928
Dr. Cushing

This poor man's second-stage operation was almost as desperate a business as the first. The scalp had been too tightly closed and the entire edge was involved in a black necrosis which I fear extended the full depth of the flap in some places.

This was probably caused not wholly by too tight closure and perhaps too tight a dressing, but by the fact that the temporal arteries had probably been completely sacrificed in the subtemporal decompression, and also by the fact that there was marked tenderness. On Saturday, I had put a needle into the wound and withdrawn about 30 cc of fluid blood, but the whole region was bulging from the gradual extrusion of the tumor.

If we had had sufficiently good fortune to have had a large enough bony opening, I might have conceivably at the first operation encircled the tumor and allowed it to extrude, and I might then have conceivably removed the whole thing, but as matters turned out, tumor underlay all the lower posterior and upper edge of the flap. It was in other words a huge tumor which I was attempting to remove through an insufficient opening.

OPERATIVE NOTE
April 9, 1928
Anesthesia – Scopolomin – Morphia.

Rough Intracapsular Extirpation of Huge Stringy Meningioma, Partly by Electro-Surgical Methods.

After reflecting the flap, I found it was possible to remove the old muscle implantation without getting bleeding from the lower dura. I attempted to encircle the growth but found that it underlay the bone in the subtemporal region as well as posteriorly and above. Consequently, there was little I could do but to incise the dura with the electric needle and to tear the main portion of the growth out of its capsule. There was a good deal of bleeding following this procedure which was checked with Zenker's and with the electric current.

I used the electric current on the herniated anterior part of the frontal lobe which had been exposed at the previous operation, and did what I could to dissect out the sac of the tumor, leaving raw cerebrum everywhere exposed. However, at the lower posterior and upper part of the field, there was still a large amount of tumor which completely underlay the bony edge. As it was not a growth which evidently was easily stripped away from the brain, I felt I had done as much as circumstances allowed.

A single drain was left into the central portion of the field led out through a new opening. I did the best I could to close in 3 layers with loosely placed sutures around the devascularized margins of the flap.

(Dr. Cushing)

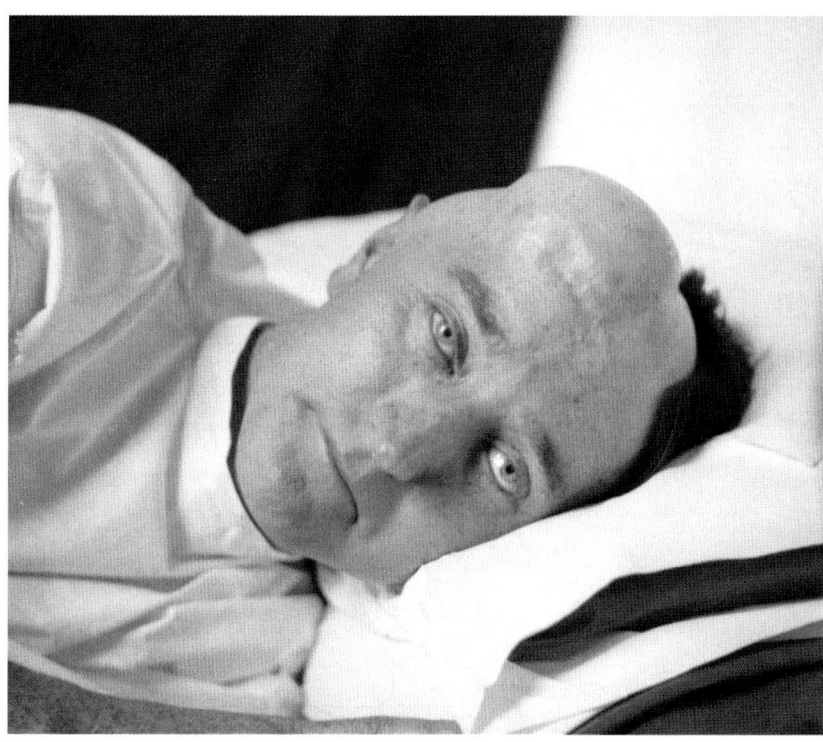

FIGS. 9 AND 10. PREOPERATIVE BEFORE THE LAST RESECTION OPERATION.

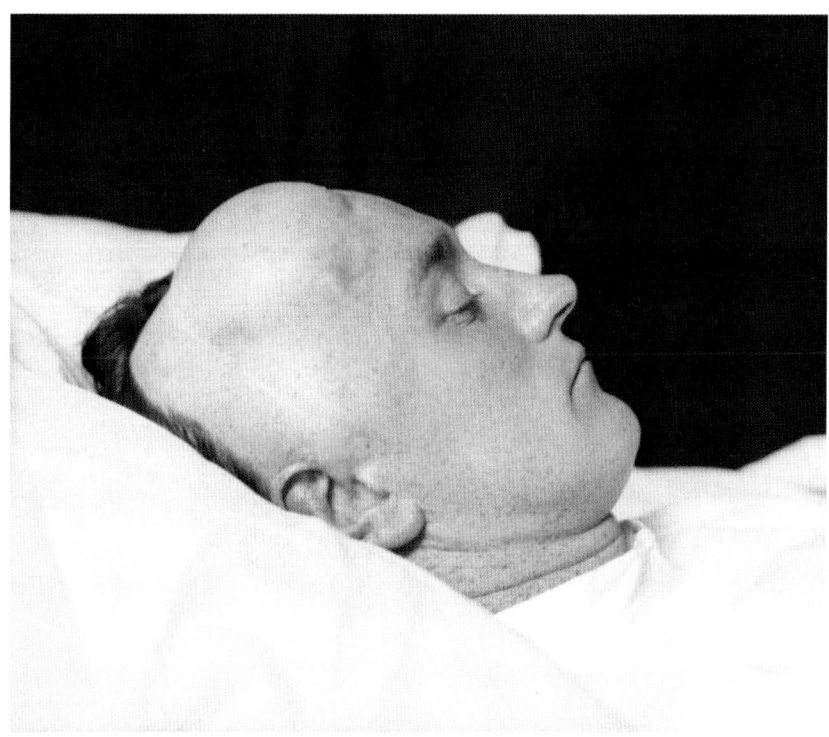

PATHOLOGY REPORT
April 9, 1928

There are two tissues from a case which was operated upon 4 days ago for a meningioma that had a peculiar stringy character. I found that owing to

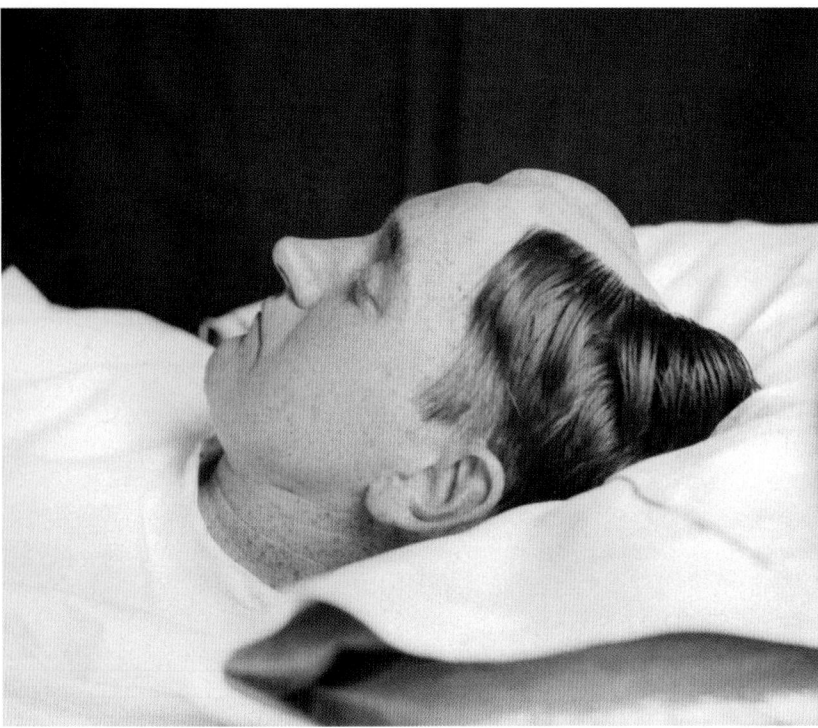

FIG. II. PREOPERATIVE BEFORE THE LAST RESECTION OPERATION.

insufficient room it was impossible to enucleate the tumor as it underlay all bony margins of the flap. Consequently the best I could do was to incise the dura down into tumor and to draw out, scoop and burn out the main portion of the lesion. This chief tumor was put into formalin and there are some perfect pieces for study.

(Dr. Cushing)

Microscopic examination: This is a meningioma with some unusual features as principally large and epithelioid cells forming some of the cell nests and also the finely vacuolated and lipoid laden cells. A great deal of the preparation shows typical meningioma structure so that will be diagnosis adhered to. It is an occasional tumor of this sort which makes me unwilling to accept these meningioma as being of fibroblastic origin.

(Dr. Wolbach)

Postoperative course was uneventful except the concern regarding very tenuous wound edges.

DISCHARGE NOTES
May 20, 1928
Dr. Bagdasar

The patient discharged in a good condition. Visual fields show improvement. He was told to return back for the next resection session as soon as the incision is well healed.

FOURTH HOSPITAL ADMISSION

SUMMARY OF POSITIVE FINDINGS
June 27, 1928
Dr. Farber

SUBJECTIVE
1. Since last operation his sensation of paraesthesia of left arm and leg has gone.
2. His vision has improved. At present he is able to read the fine print of the newspaper with his right eye.
3. No pain in ears since operation.
4. No headaches since operation.
5. Weakness in left leg has improved.
6. About 1 week ago had an attack of vomiting.

OBJECTIVE
1. Bulging, pulsating, subtemporal decompression, right.
2. Optic atrophy, secondary, both fundi, most marked on left. Both discs choked slightly. Pupillary reflexes present, but sluggish in both eyes. Divergent squint of left eye is present.
3. Tendon reflexes hyperactive, a little stronger on left. No clonus.
4. Gait is normal.

IMPRESSION: Patient much improved since operation. In view of this fact diagnosis of meningioma in right frontal lobe is correct. No signs of incomplete removal. No signs of tumor in the left hemisphere.

HOSPITAL COURSE

While in the hospital, the patient's wound, which was completely epithelialized, was dressed with alcohol. There was a noticeable increase in flap protrusion. The tumor had apparently invaded the scar. The patient had a convulsive attack lasting four minutes.

DISCHARGE NOTE
July 3, 1928
Dr. Bagdasar

Dr. Cushing did not want to operate until wound was completely healed, so patient was discharged. Will return 2x weeks for dressing. Will re-enter the hospital. Patient is happy over delay, cooperative.

FIFTH HOSPITAL ADMISSION

SUMMARY OF POSITIVE FINDINGS
October, 1928
Dr. Scarff

SUBJECTIVE
1. High subtemporal decompression, Sept. 1926.
2. Subtotal extirpation of right frontotemporal meningioma, April 1928. Sacrifice of involved bone flap.
3. Return for operation in June 1928: no operation.
4. Since last discharge patient has felt well except the symptoms:
   a) Vomiting: Nausea and vomiting on 2 occasions. Decompression area tight at both times.
   b) Weakness in legs middle of Sept., 1928. No loss of consciousness.
   c) Convulsions, 2 attacks, occurring since Oct. 1928.

OBJECTIVE
1. Fundi – primary optic atrophy slight.
2. Finger to nose test poorly done on right. Heel to shin poorly done on left.
3. Bulging though soft frontal decompression area. Also soft subtemporal decompression.

IMPRESSION: Meningioma, right frontotemporal region, recurrent.

OPERATIVE NOTE
(Unreadable)
October 30, 1928
Anesthesia – Novocain – ether – Miss Melanson.

Reflection of Old Flap With a New Incision Posteriorly – Increase of Bony Opening on All Sides. Gradual Extirpation of Encircling of Meningioma by Electro-Surgical Procedure – Convulsion Produced During Operation – Necessity of Giving Ether.

PATHOLOGY REPORT
October 30, 1928

One section shows a dense connective tissue, presumably dura. The remainder of the section is composed of a fairly vascular meningioma. No mitotic figures are seen.
    Diagnosis – Meningioma
(Dr. Bennett)

HOSPITAL COURSE
The patient had four convulsions the first day after surgery, CSF leakage from the wound was discovered six days later. Dr. Cushing removed some CSF by tapping the flap.

DISCHARGE NOTE
November 21, 1928
Dr. Scarff

General condition excellent. Wound healed and dry, still one small dark scab. Decompression full, soft – not bulging. Vision improved. Taking luminal. To return at once if new symptoms appear.

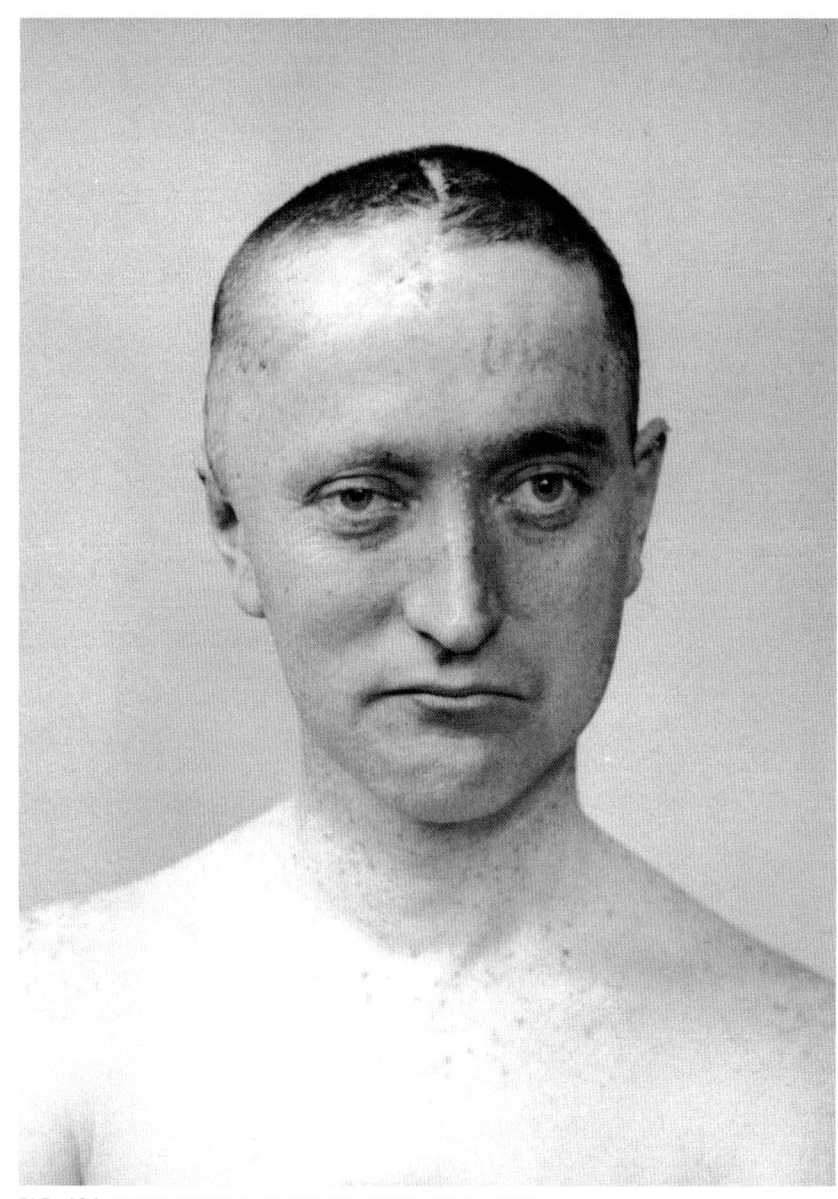

FIG. 12A. TWO WEEKS POSTOPERATIVE AFTER THE LAST OPERATION.

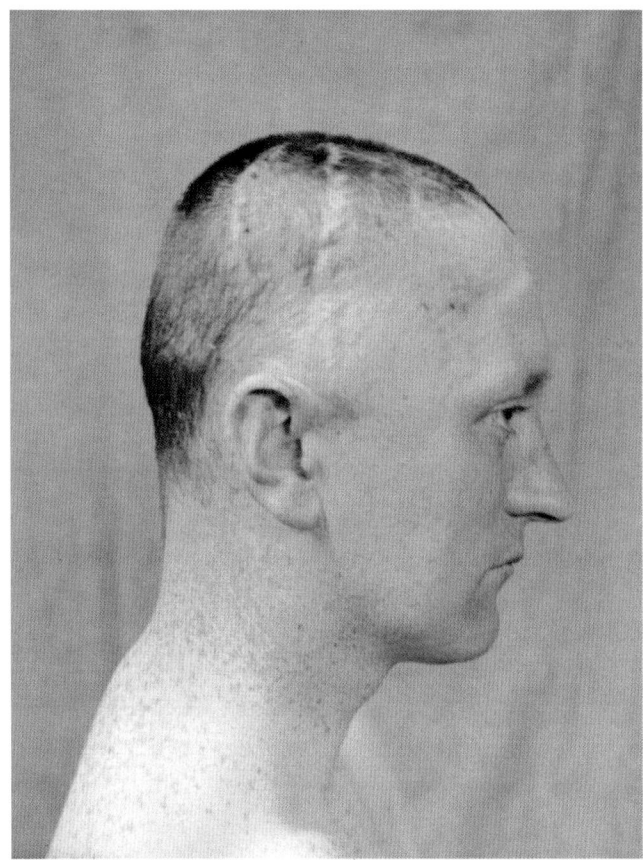

FIG. 12B. TWO WEEKS POSTOPERATIVE AFTER THE LAST OPERATION.

SIXTH HOSPITAL ADMISSION

Patient returned with bulging decompression, headache, fever, and malaise. He was leaking CSF through his incision. Meningitis was suspected. Lumbar taps improved his condition considerably. Staphylococcus was found in the CSF.

November 30, 1928
Dr. Oldberg

Temperature normal. No headache. Still having 2 or 3 dressings daily.

December 5, 1928
Dr. Oldberg

During past 48 hs – slight leakage at night. No leakage in daytime, when patient is up. Dressing 1 or 2 times daily.

December 9, 1928
Dr. Oldberg

Attack of convulsions. About 3 times this morning.
    Today – Tap of the fluctuated area. 50 cc of fluid was removed.

December 17, 1928
Dr. Oldberg

Dry-flap full but not tight up in the walking.

DISCHARGE NOTE
December 19, 1928
Dr. Oldberg

Patient discharged in good conditions. He had one convulsion whole on ward – Jacksonian in type-apparently affected left arm. Discharged with instructions of
1. return at once if trouble occurs;
2. luminal 0.1 mgr qd.

FOLLOW UP NOTES
April 5, 1930
Dr. Henderson

Up till 2 weeks was having a spell once a month – began with clonus in left arm, spreading to leg and face and then with loss of consciousness for few minutes. No aphasia – is left handed.
    During last 2 weeks has had 3 similar attacks, he feels much weaker afterwards. Has been taking 3 luminals (1 mgr each) for 1 mos. – before that taking 2. At night sees colored flashes in right field. Spells are always during the night.

Exam: Decompression soft – not bulging. No tenderness or palpable mass under skin flap.
    Discs: marked secondary atrophy both eyes.
    Nystagmus on looking to right.
    Left lower facial.
    Left hand grip rather weak (is left handed).

Rx: Continue luminal and $MgSO_4$ regime. Report one month.

LAST FOLLOW UP
April 15, 1932
Dr. Kaplan

Continues convulsions.
    Decompression soft.
    Bilateral optic atrophy. Fundi flat.
    Nystagmus to right.
    Weakness of left arm
    Hyperreflexive on left. Hoffman on left.

Seen by Dr. Cushing. Still continues to have old focal dark area (around the incision.) Aborted re-entry for re-exploration.

3.9 Large parasagittal meningioma

SEX: M; AGE: 36; SURG. NO. 27692; 29818; 30376

HISTORY

This patient's illness began in May 1925, when he first noticed a small lump in the mid-parietal region of his head. The lump was not painful, but gradually enlarged and was removed in August 1925 by Dr. Reinholst of Quincy. A "recurrence" occurred four months later. A biopsy was then performed at the Massachusetts General Hospital by Dr. Mixter and X-ray therapy was given. Patient was then referred to Dr. Cushing.

SUMMARY OF POSITIVE FINDINGS
December 1, 1926
Dr. Cairns

OBJECTIVE
1. Bony lump over the middle portion of the sagittal suture.
2. Bilateral papilledema, right – 4.5–5.0 D., left – 4D.
3. Brisk, possibly exaggerated, tendon jerks in the legs, slight weakness of the left leg.

IMPRESSION: Very large meningioma.

ADDITIONAL NOTE
December 7, 1926
Dr. Cairns

Now that the head is shaved a large artery is felt pulsating in the scalp just behind the center of the projection. There is another at the junction of the anterior and middle thirds of the left margin of the lump. X-ray shows very large channels for the meningeal vessels.

SPECIAL NOTE
December 7, 1926
Dr. Cushing

This man had evidently a large midline meningioma crossing the longitudinal sinus, the case being very similar to some of the older cases in the series such as "two other patients' names." It also was from external appearances very like the recent case of (another patient's name), though the extracranial boss was median here, and in that case a little to the side.

What was unusual was the fact that the man has had no focal epileptiform attacks and has had no discomforts. Nevertheless, he has had a high choked disc whereas in (another patient's name) case there was no choked disc. To make it still more surprising, in this case there was a small subdural lesion whereas in (another patient's name) case there was a large one.

OPERATIVE NOTE
December 7, 1926
Anesthesia: Novocain

Removal of Cranial and Extracranial Involvement of a Bilateral Parasagittal Meningioma

A procedure illustrated in the accompanying sketches was carried out without undue difficulty or loss of blood. A flap of scalp, as shown in sketch #1 (Operative sketch for the first operation: Top middle image,) was turned backward and the huge boss encircled by a series of perforations. In the anterior part of the field these perforations went into greatly thickened vascular and obviously involved bone, even outside of the limits of subsequent rongeuring. It should be stated that on reflecting the scalp I got into tumor in the situation of the old scars and had intended to remove the galea in this region had I been able to take the growth out in its entirety. Inasmuch as I could not do so, the flap was replaced with some of this tumor outside the galea still in position.

To go back to the operative field – after the perforations had been made and many of them connected, I scraped off the cap of tumor between bone and pericranium. This was about 1 cm. thick and fully a 10 cm. in its diameter, about twice the size shown in the accompanying sketch. This left a raw area of cranium densely infiltrated with tumor.

I then proceeded with the rongeur to remove this central area piecemeal. In places it was probably about 2 cm. in thickness, the last piece of it coming away in a large fragment.

This left an area about as shown in fig. #2 (Operative sketch for the first operation: Left lower image,) almost the entire exposed area of dura being heavily infiltrated with tumor. I prepared to incise the dura in crescentic fashion on each side of the area carrying the incision up to the region of the longitudinal sinus. In the posterior

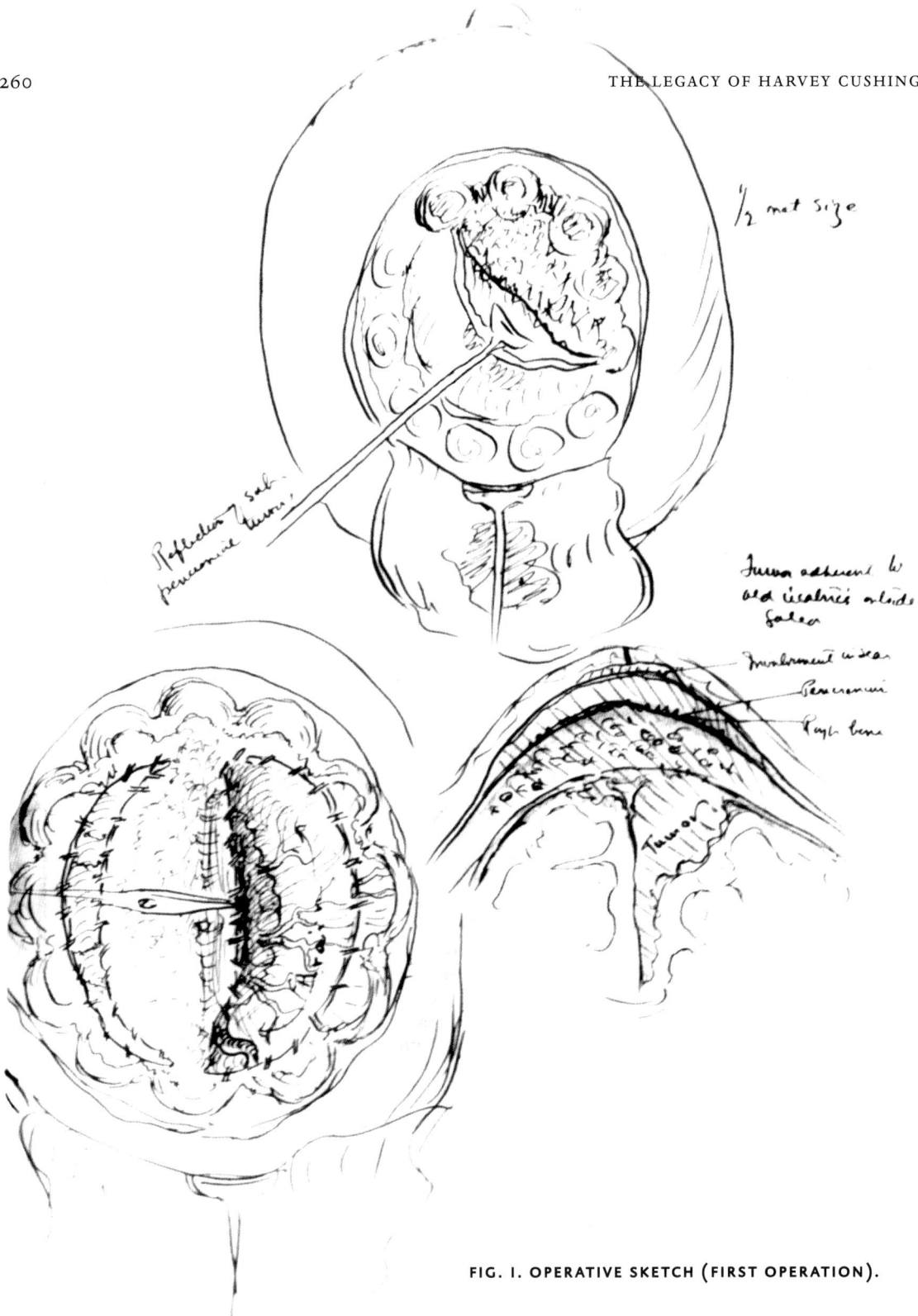

FIG. I. OPERATIVE SKETCH (FIRST OPERATION).

part of the field an enormous vein entering into the sinus was exposed and though I might have divided the sinus and removed the strip in its entirety, it seemed to me unjustifiable, in view of the fact that the tumor was a flat type of tumor and unquestionably spread down the whole length of the falx so that a complete clean extirpation was evidently out of the question.

The interesting and unusual features of the case were a most extensive spread of the growth through the calvarium, far beyond the region of the tumor, the cap between bone and pericranium, and also the involvement outside of the galea. The situation is shown as I understand it in Fig. #3 (Operative sketch for the first operation: Right lower image).

After complete hemostasis the flap was replaced, a single punctured drain being left in at the posterior part of the field as there was still considerable continued oozing.

In view of the fact that this man had never had discomforts and had no epileptiform convulsions I trust that this measure may give him long time at least a complete quiescence from all symptoms, or at least his choked disc should subside. As a matter of fact, there was so little evidence of pressure that I am at a loss to explain why he should have had choked disc at all, unless it may be that the bony tumor was pressing down upon the brain and as soon as it had been removed, the tension was completely relieved.

It should have been mentioned that on reflecting the dura on the left side of the sinus one could see projecting between the cortical meningeal vessels tags of meningioma so that the lesion has actually crossed and in all probability obliterated the sinus.

(Dr. Cushing)

PATHOLOGY REPORT
December 7, 1926

There are tissues from a fragmentary removed meningioma of a longitudinal sinus in its neighborhood.

In Zenker's fluid is a jar of fragments of involved bone. I would be glad to have one or two pieces decalcified and cut to study the character of the bony invasion.

There is also in formalin a large slab of an intracranial portion of the tumor. None of the underlying tumor was removed. This was a typical meningioma of the soft type with tags of seaweed like tumor spreading out over the hemisphere.

(Dr. Cushing)

Microscopic report – Sections representing five blocks show bone which is being invaded by a spindle cell tumor. The spindle cells ... in bundles which run in various directions, and often form small, but very striking whorls. There is a rather large amount of connective tissue mixed with the tumor in many areas. No mitotic figures are noted.
Diagnosis – Meningioma

(Dr. Pinkerton)

Patient had an unremarkable postoperative period.

DISCHARGE NOTE
Dr. Cairns
December 21, 1926

Doing very well. Has had a tranquil convalescence. No headaches. No weakness of legs. Visual acuity improved. Fundi – Right 0.5 D, left to 1.5 D. The wound healed clearly and rapidly, leaving practically no lump behind.

FOLLOW UP NOTE
August 27, 1927

This patient presented to Dr. Cushing on August 27, 1927 with left-sided hemiparesis and Jacksonian attacks starting three days prior to presentation. He was found to have a small hard mass palpable in his previous craniotomy/decompression area. Papilledema was noted. Dr. Cushing was apprehensive to proceed with another surgery.

Patient was readmitted into the hospital on October 7, 1927.

SECOND HOSPITAL ADMISSION

SPECIAL NOTE
Dr. Cushing
October 27, 1927

This man has been waiting about for sometime for me to screw up my courage to attack his case once more. Evidently the tumor has grown thru or continued to grow into the region of the original incision where biopsy was made and I was aware that I would be unable to remove the growth including the central area in toto. Nevertheless, he has been gradually becoming hemiparetic on the left side and there is a firm hard protrusion just to the right of the midline which made me assume that under the butterfly elevation of the dura which had been incised at the first operation, there was a fairly extensive growth.

There are two particularly notable things about this case. One concerns the possibility of removing a block of the longitudinal sinus in the mid-region without getting a spastic hemiplegia – the longitudinal sinus syndrome. The other concerns the possible transformation of a soft meningioma into a stony hard fibroma. We are beginning to feel from the cultural studies of these cases that perhaps meningeal cells may be transformed into fibroblast. There is one case in the series (the name of another patient) in which an occipital lobe tumor was removed and was finally replaced by a dense stony hard fibroma involving the scalp.

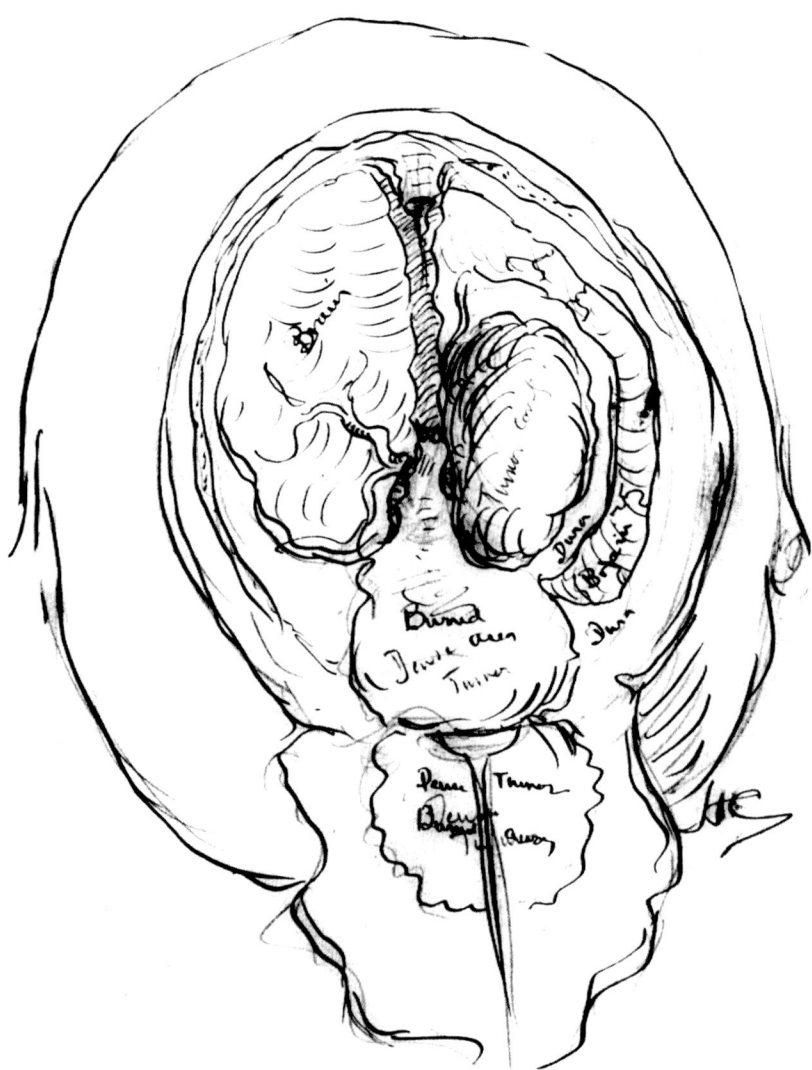

FIG. 2. OPERATIVE SKETCH (SECOND OPERATION).

OPERATIVE NOTE
October 27, 1927
Anesthesia: Novocain

Reflection of Old Flap Disclosing Dense Extensive Continuation of Tumor Growth Completely Involving the Falx with Much Soft Tumor Extension into Mesial Portion of Right Hemisphere – Attempted Removal of Tumor Mass in Toto Abandoned Owing to Fear of Producing Spastic Paraplegia and Owing to the Conclusion that a Total Extirpation at Best Would be Impossible – Fairly Thorough Eradication of Tumor Mass from Cavity in Upper Portion of Right Hemisphere by Electrosurgical Methods – Removal of Block of Longitudinal Sinus Together with Upper Portion of Falx from Long Strip Shown in Sketch.

This long story may be briefly summarized as follows. In the line of the old incision the flap was reflected, to my great surprise, there being no evidence of tumor in the edge of the disclosed bone. It was thin and smooth and looked a little atrophic. I very soon came upon a dense solid extremely stony hard tumor mass which I had to cut thru with the electric current, leaving a disc of it on the reflected flap.

Not knowing as yet what actually lay before us I proceeded to reopen the dura in the anterior part of the field and finally divided through the longitudinal sinus which at its anterior portion I think was not occluded. I then began to lift the tumor involved sinus out of its cavity, dividing it as I proceeded with the electric current and in this process I finally came down to a huge bundle of vessels over the intact left hemisphere which passed into the sinus – or which appeared to me to pass into the sinus. I think I was half hearted perhaps in not immediately dividing these vessels and in proceeding to burn out the areas of the involved sinus but after all it was evident by this time that a total extirpation was going to be impossible but I thought I could benefit the man even though I may not be able to do much more than palliate his lesion.

It was at this juncture uncertain what I had in the right hemisphere and after removing a portion of the growth as far back as shown in the sketch (Operative sketch for the second operation) which involved the sinus, about the best that I could do was with the electric loop to begin to burn off great masses of extensive fibrous stony hard tumor from the inner side of the reflected scalp and from the outer side of the exposed posterior part of the dural field.

It was in the process of this procedure that I finally realized that the reason that I had had difficulty in reflecting the dura as well on the right side as on the left lay in the fact that there was a large soft tumor growing into the hemisphere in this region. This I proceeded to scoop out radically with the electric loop, leaving a cavity about the size of a hen's egg, considerably relieving the tense protrusion on this side which had been present before the operation.

At this stage, I decided to close, leaving a very questionable field for I had two hard areas which were to come in contact with each other when the flap was replaced and I had also removed a large part of the longitudinal sinus which I feared might cause paralysis. The patient, however, was perfectly cooperative through this whole procedure and was moving both feet on request freely and I may have been half hearted in not attacking the region of the left side more radically than I had done, for I conceivably might have carried the dissection down through greatly scarred area and perhaps have removed more of it but even so I do not believe that I could completely have removed the large tumor that was extending into the right hemisphere.

The scalp was then replaced, a single drain being left thru a puncture opening on the posterior region.

(Dr. Cushing)

PATHOLOGY REPORT
October 27, 1927

There are the fragmentary tissue from a recurrent meningioma involving the longitudinal sinus. The tumor was of the type which causes pronounced hyperostosis, the hyperostosis having been removed at preceding operation. Fragments of tissue were taken for immediate fresh study and for histological study. In addition there is a large stony hard part of the tumor which I assume will show nothing but dense fibrous growth owing as I believe to a transformation of the meningeal type of tumor to a fibroma. As will be seen in a previous case (the name of another patient) there was this same occurrence, namely a meningioma which had involved the scalp just as was true in this case which ultimately became transformed into a stony hard fibroma.

(Dr. Cushing)

Microscopic report: Tissue shows a cellular type of tumor supported by and invading …fibrous connective tissue structure (which is probably not dura). The tumor tissue is moderately vascular, and under lower power, has little to suggest any characteristic structure. Under the high power lens however the cells are seen very frequently to be arranged in small whirls of two to four cells each and occasionally more, giving more typical whorl formation. The cells themselves vary in size and shape but are largely oval or slightly spindle shaped and contain large oval nuclei. A few single cells appear to contain hyaloid like masses in their cytoplasm, and frequently they are seen closely applied to or forming small vascular spaces. No mitotic figures are seen.

Diagnosis – Meningioma rapidly growing.

(Dr. Bennett)

POSTOPERATIVE NOTE
October 28, 1927
Dr. Fulton

During operation patient had several attacks, focal in character, affecting his left shoulder; they were persistent and he was finally given ether to stop them. After operation there was noticeable weakness of his left arm and left leg, but not a complete paralysis. Objectively his condition in regard to blood pressure, temperature, etc. was excellent, and he was rational, cooperative, and interested in what was done for him. He was put into bed at 6:30 and taken back to the ward later in the evening. The left sided paresis improved in the course of evening, and he slept in naps.

DISCHARGE NOTE
November 12, 1927
Dr. Fulton

This patient entered the hospital on Oct. 7, 1927 for a second stage removal of a large parasagittal meningioma. This was carried out by electro-surgical methods on Oct. 27th by Dr. Cushing.

Following the operation patient had noticeable paresis of both lower extremities and of the left upper from which he gradually recovered. Five days ago he began to walk for the first time and since then has walked every day without difficulty. He drags his left leg slightly but this is now scarcely perceptible.

P.E. on discharge showed a well healed scalp incision, with soft decompression at his vertex, the central lump which on entry was tough and indurated, was now small and scarcely perceptible. Fundi still show haziness of nasal borders with ½–1D. elevation in both eyes. Veins full and slightly tortuous but much less so than prior to operation. Deep reflexes much exaggerated, especially on the left side. There is a well sustained ankle clonus on the left and poorly sustained clonus on right. Babinski indeterminate but occasionally toes become slightly elevated on the left side. He is able to flex and extend his ankles weakly but can move toes very little on left. There is no astereognosis on either side, nor loss of muscle sense. No disturbance of cutaneous sensibility. Patient has been told to continue luminal and report in a month.

THIRD HOSPITAL ADMISSION

Patient was admitted into the hospital on December 31, 1927, due to discharge of watery fluid from the surgical incision. A piece of epithelialized tumor tissue protruding through the wound was identified. The wound was cleaned with alcohol/bichloride and dressed, no "infection" was found. Discharged on January 4, 1928.

LETTER TO DR. CUSHING
March 9, 1928

Dear Dr. Cushing

I was very much pleased in receiving your kind letter, and I would be very thankful if I could come in some afternoon, when it would be convenient for the doctor, as I am very worried about (name of the patient), his twistering spells have increased for the last three days. He had on Mar. 7, four attacks, Mar. 8, two attacks and Mar. 9, three, the last two were very hard and long. He has increased the pills and is now taking two a day, but they don't seem to relieve him any. The attacks do not make him sick before or after, but as I am uncertain whether they are supposed to follow after the operation, or not. It worries me,

    Thanking you.

Sincerely,
(Signed) AF

LETTER TO DR. CUSHING
(From Quincy City Hospital)
November 14, 1929

Dear Dr. Cushing:
Re: Mr. CF

Patient was admitted to the ward as a stretcher case on July 5th. The physical examination of the patient showed a middle aged man in good state of nutrition. Sensorium clear.

Locally a large soft mass involving the vault of the skull, irregular in outline and of brain tissue consistency. Pupil reflexes equal but sluggish. Weakness of left arm and leg with exaggeration of reflexes. Right sided muscle weakness but no change in reflexes superficial or deep. Paralysis which was spastic became progressively worse so that two months after admission patient was utterly helpless. Bladder and bowel action involuntary.

Patient became greatly emaciated with trophic disturbances and expired on November 1st. The treatment was mostly symptomatic.

X-ray taken on July 11, 1929: X-ray shows a malignant involvement of the dome of the skull with numerous radium seeds in situ with downward extension from posterior border. Dr. Whelan, Roentgenologist.

Yours very truly,
(Signed)
Superintendent

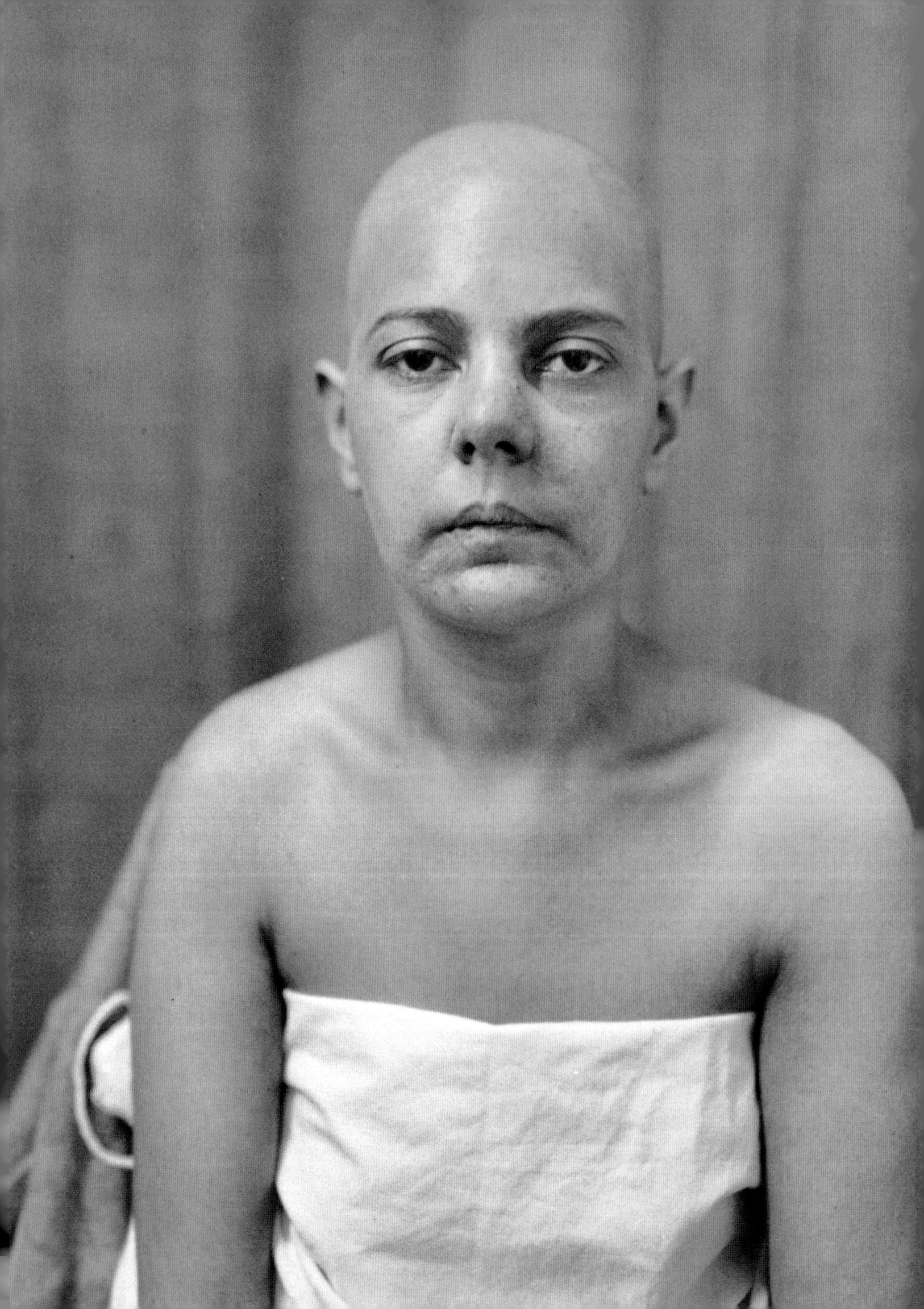

3.10 Occipital meningioma

SEX: F; AGE: 34; SURG. NO. 28752

COMPLAINT

This patient complained of occipital pain of three years duration with blurred vision, and loss of taste/smell more recently.

SUMMARY OF POSITIVE FINDINGS
May 6, 1927
Dr. Putman

SUBJECTIVE
1. Injury to the head at the age of 8, followed by right hemiparesis and astereognosia.
2. Lump of the back of the head first noted 3 years ago which has gradually increased in size.
3. Neuralgia pain in the left side of the occiput and neck beginning 3 years ago and lasting one year.
4. Since then generalized headaches.
5. Failing vision since October 1926.
6. Dizzy spells with tinnitus, relieved by sitting down or lying down, from August to December 1926.
7. Loss of sense of smell for the past 4 months, now gradually returning.
8. Attack of vomiting yesterday, followed by hypaesthesia of the right side of the face.

OBJECTIVE
1. Large diffuse swelling over the back of the skull.
2. Slight relative anosmia on both sides; most of the smells can be recognized.
3. Bilateral choked disc, 2½ and 2-D, with considerable scar tissue.
4. Irregular hemianopsia.
5. Hypaesthesia of the right side of the face.
6. Corneal reflex sluggish. No motor loss.
7. Hemiparesis and slight hemiatrophy of the right arm and leg, with weakness and increased reflexes. No clonus or Babinski. Right astereognosis.

IMPRESSION – Large meningioma of posterior fossa, with increased bone production above it. It is not clear how the 5th nerve on the right is affected. It is conceivable that the growth extends down the side to the skull, to the brain stem, perhaps on both sides to account for the tinnitus which was more marked in the left ear. The field defect is also a most curious and inexplicable one.

RADIOLOGY REPORT

X-ray films showed bony thickening in the occipital region.

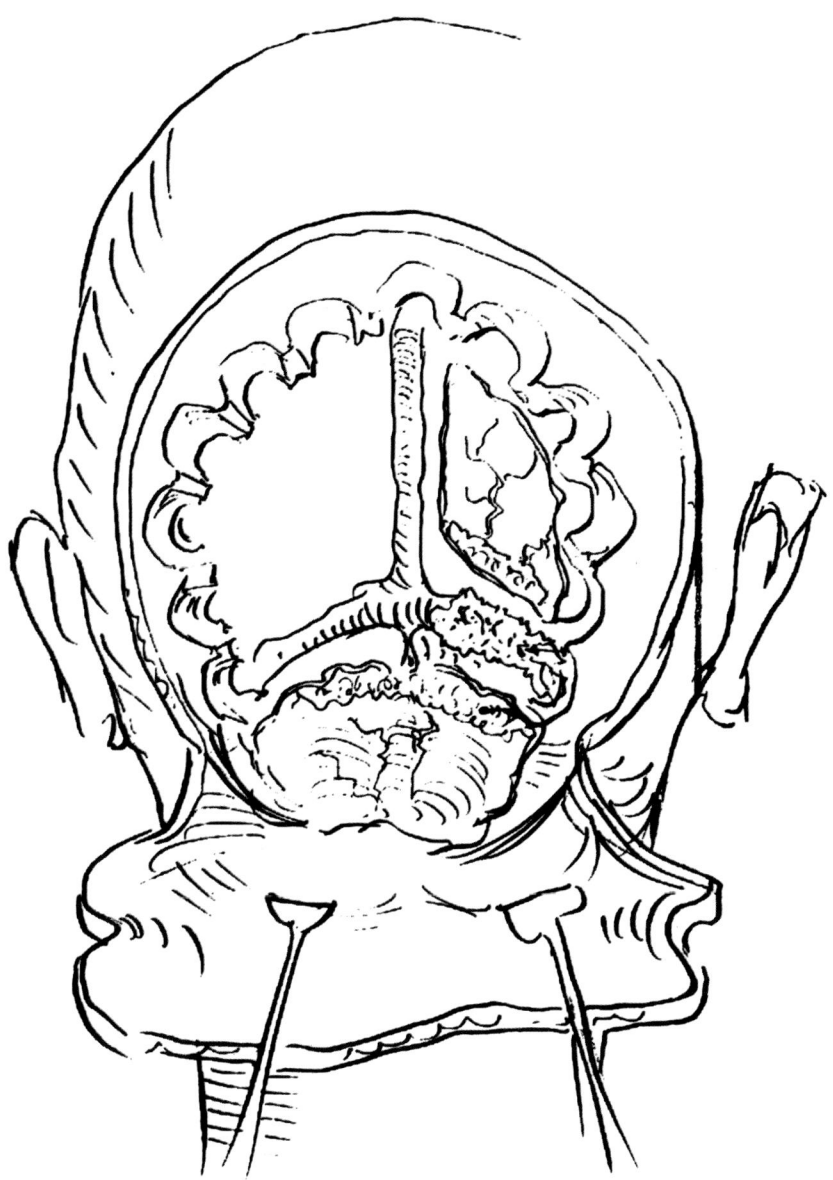

FIG. 2. OPERATIVE SKETCH.

OPPOSITE PAGE. FIG. I. PREOPERATIVE.

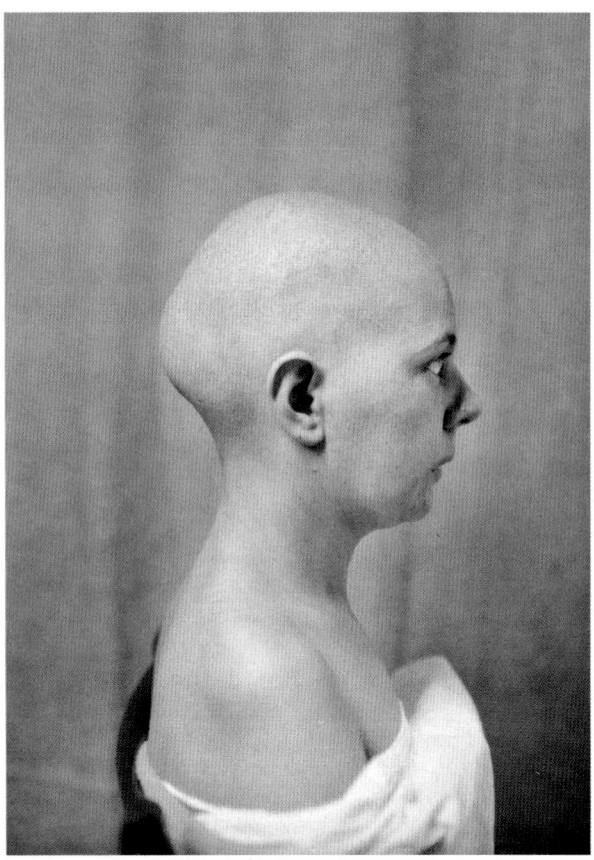

FIGS. 3–4. PREOPERATIVE.

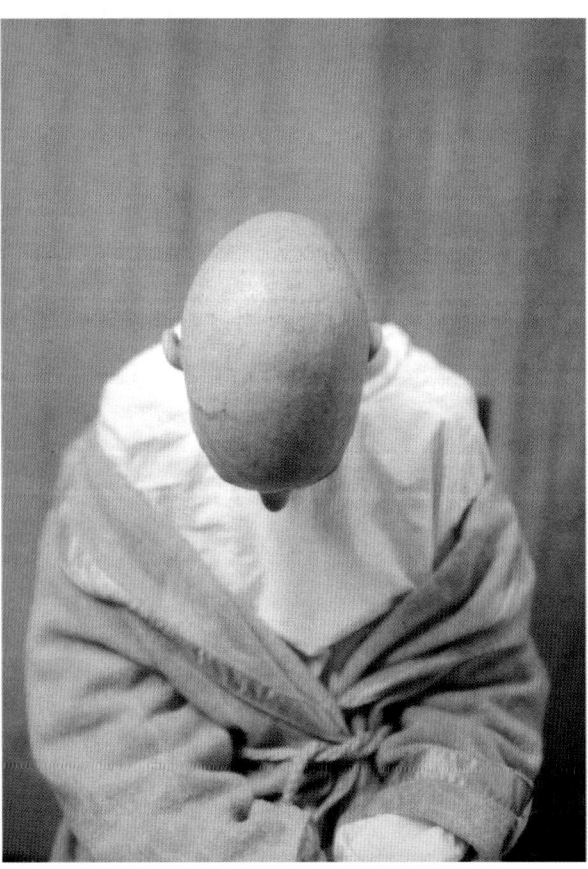

SPECIAL NOTE
May, 14, 1927
Dr. Cushing

This proved to be an enormous hyperosteotic meningioma of the occipital region centering upon the torcula. It would have been scarcely possible to have done more than to have reflected the flap in older day, much less to have removed this extracranial layer of tumor. The perforation of the bone would have required a second stage and I doubt whether we would eventually have been able to open the dura and to give any temporary relief thereby that is without electrosurgical methods.

OPERATIVE NOTE
May, 14, 1927
Anesthesia – Novocain

Reflection of Occipital Flap of Scalp, Disclosing Huge Hyperostotic Tumor Covered by Thin Layer of Tumor Bearing Galea – Scalp Highly Vascular (Cutting Current Used) Superficial Layer of Tumor Dissected Off Also with Cutting Current and Wax used on the Bone. Multitude of Perforations thru the Bone, which was fully 2–3 cm. in Thickness. Piece Meal Removal of Bone. Muscle Implantation over Sinuses – Decompression of Left Occipital Lobe Exposing Parasinusoidal Tumor, Decompression of Cerebellum Exposing Soft Margin of Tumor in Subtentorial Fossa. (5 hour procedure).

We were ready in this case to transfuse and fortunately a breast case had been done so that we had an abundance of muscle. We needed the muscle but got thru without transfusion in one stage.

After novocainizing the large flap circumscribing the tumor I started to turn the flap downward and found it exceedingly bloody. It was necessary to use the coagulating current on innumerable points to control bleeding. The flap was peeled away from the galea but in 2 or 3 places I got into fatty tissue, owing to the fact that there was an extra-cranial tumor which I found difficult to distinguish from galea itself.

The superficial extra-cranial flap was then dissected away with the cutting current comparatively bloodlessly, that is bloodlessly to what it would have been had we endeavored to use a knife for the purpose. This separate piece of tissue was preserved.

Then with the bayonet pointed instruments I made a succession of possibly 12 perforations down thru the tumor to underlying dura. This was followed by the hard burr and in this way as in previous operations of this sort I had the entire tumor pretty well honeycombed. The bone over the region of the lateral sinuses was full, 3 cm. in thickness.

I then proceeded bit by bit to rongeur the bone away and encountered bleeding only over the region of sinuses. Fortunately there was muscle at hand so that the bleeding areas could be controlled. There was very little bleeding over the region of the lateral sinuses, however, which I feared was rather occluded by tumor. Certainly tumor lies both above and below the tentorium.

Lying over the left lateral sinus I left a thin layer of adherent bone as I feared to remove it tho I do not know as it would have made any great difference had I done so. I then, as shown in the sketch, made an opening over the left occipital lobe and allowed the occipital pole to protrude. This opening disclosed soft tumor alongside of and above the lateral sinus. I removed some fragments of it for histological verification.

I then with the cutting current made a transverse incision across the dura of the cerebellum, getting into tumor below the lateral sinuses as indicated in the sketch. I hope in this way that there might be some measure of decompression but I very much feared that the reason for tension was due to the tumor occlusion of the lateral sinuses.

Having completed the hemostasis the flap was replaced and closed securely in two layers, the margin of the galea being sutured to the upper edge of the cerebellar dura so as to shut off the posterior cavity. Patient stood the operation excellently well.

(Dr. Cushing)

PATHOLOGY REPORT
May 14, 1927

Those are tissue from meningioma arising primarily or centering I should say in the region of the torcula. The tumor was present both in the subtentorial (cerebellar) fossa and also in both occipital fossae above the tentorium. The tumor was soft and villous in character, a sort of block endothelioma, not a large nodular tumor, in other words it is the type of tumor which shows hyperostotic changes of the bone overlying it. (1) There are two small bits of tumor proper in separate jars in formalin and Zenker's fluid. (2) There are many fragments of hyperostotic bone, some of which I would like to have cut to verify the presence of tumor. These fragments are all in formalin. (3)

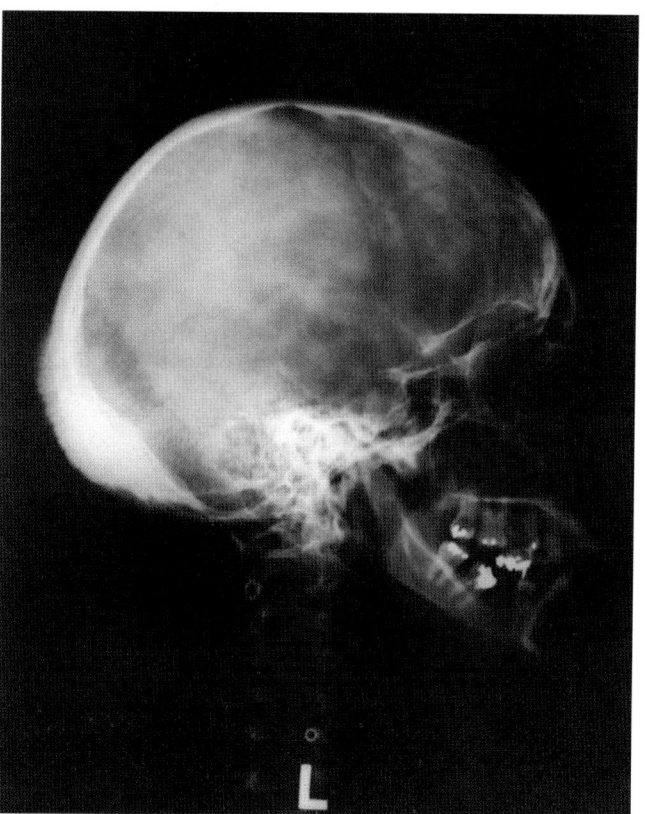

FIG. 5. PREOPERATIVE X-RAY.

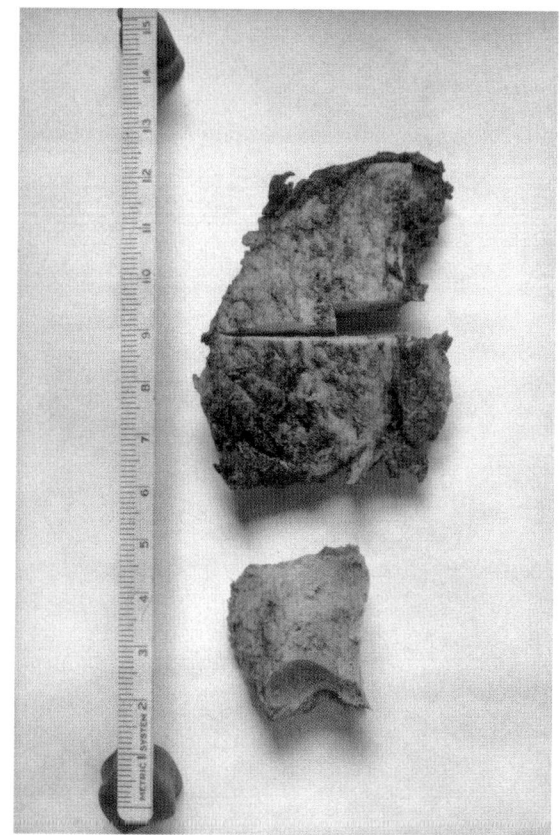

FIG. 6. GROSS TUMOR SPECIMEN WITH BONY INFILTRATION.

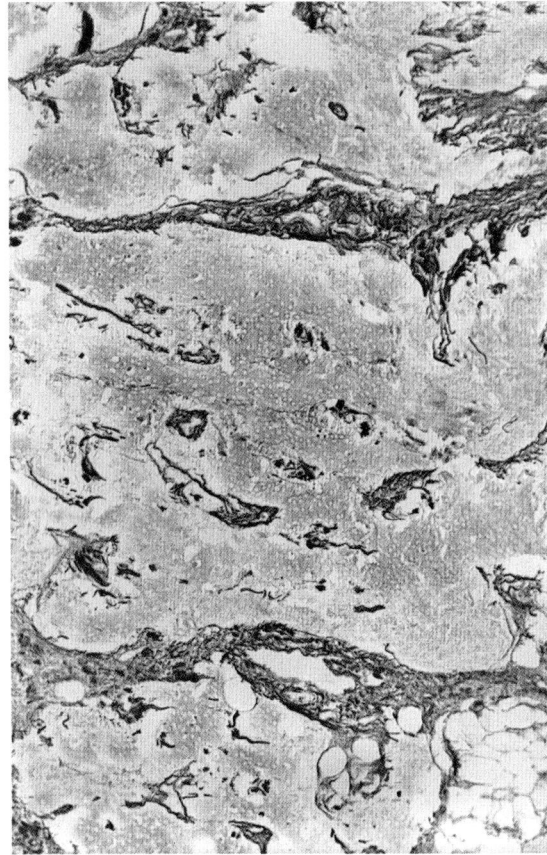

FIG. 7. HISTOLOGY SLIDE.

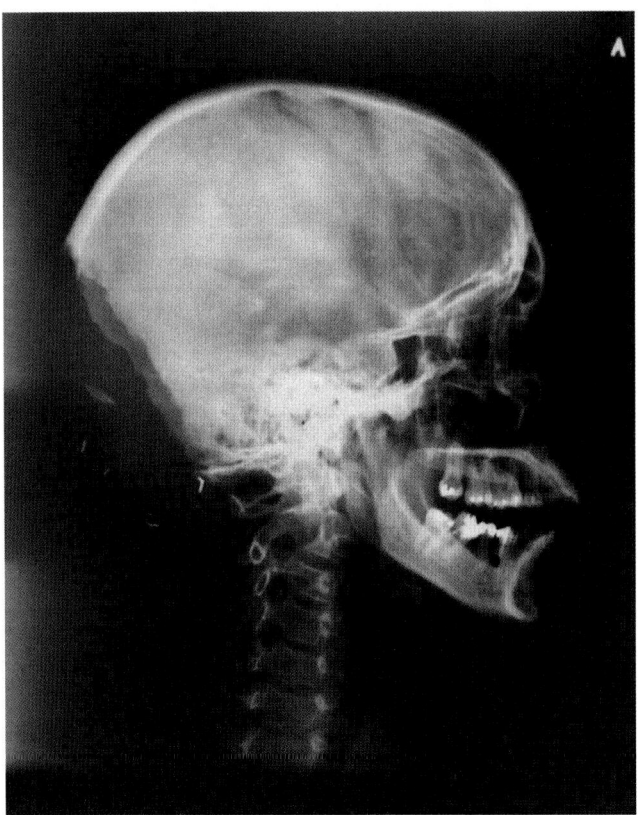

FIG. 8. POSTOPERATIVE X-RAY.

There is a slab of the extracranial thin layer of tumor underlying the galea in formalin in a separate jar, together with all fragments of the whole thickness of the bone which I would like to have photographed and measured.

(Dr. Cushing)

Microscopic report: Sections representing a single block show a small fragment of traumatized hemorrhagic tumor tissue composed of a few islands of rather closely packed spindle shaped cells. No neuroglia fibrils can be seen and no definite mitotic figures are found out. In a few areas, there is definite whorl formation, about blood vessels. Many of the tumor cells are filled with small vacuoles, suggesting fat.

DIAGNOSIS – Meningioma.

(Dr. Pinkerton)

RADIOLOGY REPORT
June 8, 1927
Dr. Sosman

Re-examining of skull shows a large operative defect in the cerebellar and occipital region with a soft tissue mass projecting through the defect. All of the thickened bone previously noted has been removed with the exception of a loose fragment in the soft tissue. Otherwise there is no change.

The postoperative period was complicated by wound dehiscence and infection. On June 16, 1927, Dr. Horrax performed re-opening and drainage of the infected wound. Infected necrotic tissue was found at the base of the wound. Some of the tissue was sent for histological analysis.

PATHOLOGY REPORT
June 16, 1927

Tissue removed at dressing.
   Sections representing a single block show large numbers of polymorphic and large mononuclears supported by a delicate fibrinous network.
   The small parasitic colonies are seen, composed of central cores of coccic organisms, but with definite peripheral club-shaped organisms in each case. The appearance is characteristic of actinomycosis.

DIAGNOSIS – Actinomycosis.

(Dr. Pinkerton)

DISCHARGE NOTE
July, 1, 1927
Dr. Putman

The patient has been having an apparently moribund condition for several weeks. Pockets of pus have been opened in the vicinity of the wound until 5 days ago the last one was opened and drainage appeared to be free and satisfactory. She shows no signs of meningitis or bronchitis although swallowing has been difficult for her and she has had to be fed entirely by nasal tube. Her temperature has gradually subsided but her pulse has remained high and obviously her condition has been extremely poor. I dressed the wound this morning and found it gaping on either side over about 7 cm in length on each side. These large openings led into several cavities, the largest of which underlay the entire skin flap. They were not severely infected but there was a thin, superficial layer of slough overlying a firm, grayish, fibrous feeling tissue which bled whenever it was rubbed, evidently tumor. I do not think the brain or even the dura was exposed anywhere in the pocket. The tissue showed not the least tendency to heal although infection was satisfactorily thrown off. In addition to these pockets the flap was lifted by a large, firm, non-fluctuant mass, evidently tumor. Along the base of the flap was a puffier mass which I suppose represents a hernia of cerebellum.

I have seen a good deal of the patient's husband and have kept constantly in touch with him. He has known for the last 2-3 weeks that there was no hope of the patient's recovery and has expressed his appreciation of what the hospital has done for her. About two weeks ago I first brought up the question of autopsy and explained the situation to him, which he took very well. I felt that I was in as good a position as any members of the staff to make this request of him and pushed the matter as heavily as I could today but without success. He is a very decent fellow but ruled by his feeling and my best efforts were wasted on him. His one definite grievance was that he had brought his wife to the hospital for observation with the distinct understanding that he was to talk to Dr. Cushing before any operation was performed and this was not accomplished. He said he would be glad to pay additional bill that the hospital would send him but could under no circumstances consent to an autopsy and finally I was forced to let the matter drop.

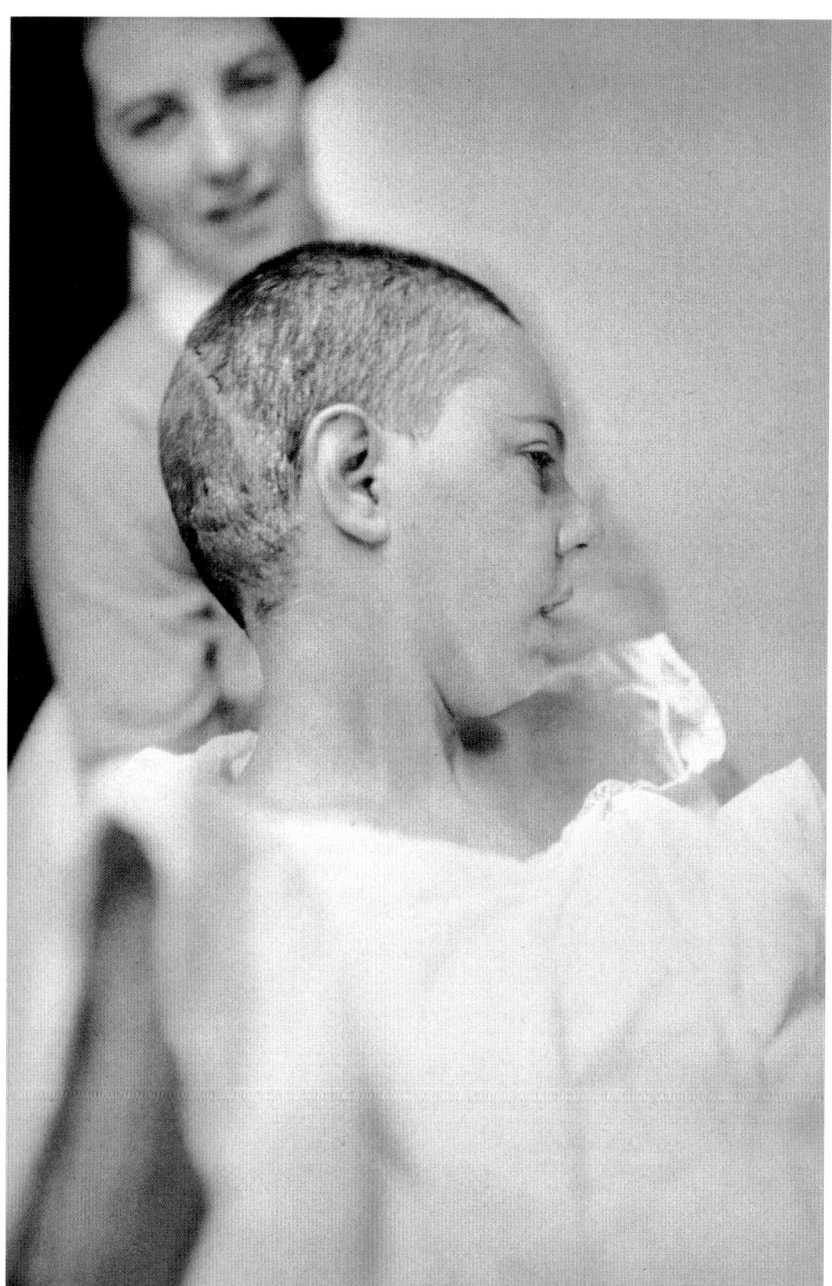

FIG. 9. POSTOPERATIVE – CONDITION OF THE WOUND.

No further hospital notes are available on this patient. Patient expired.

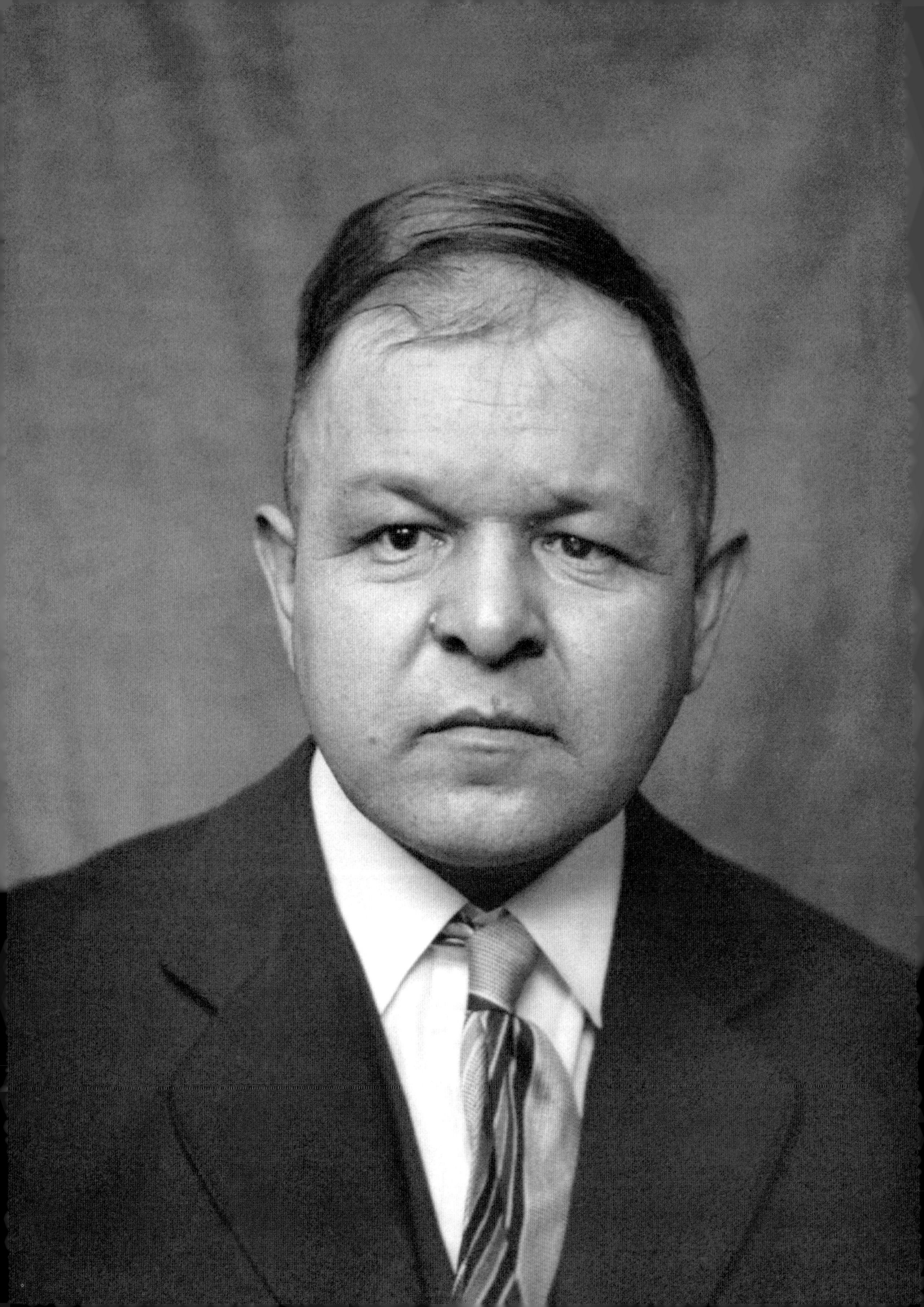

3.11 Parasagittal meningioma

SEX: M; AGE: 42; SURG. NO. 35517; 35670

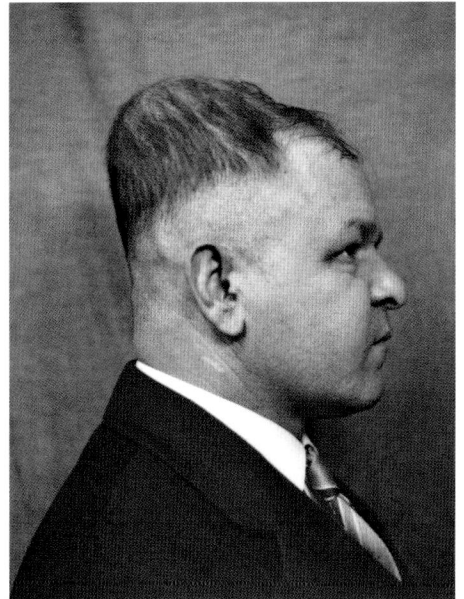
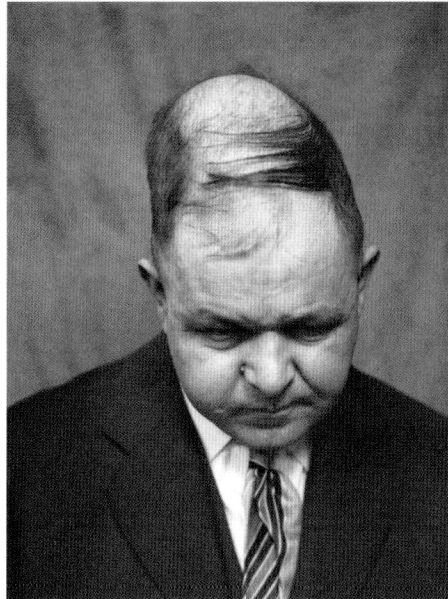
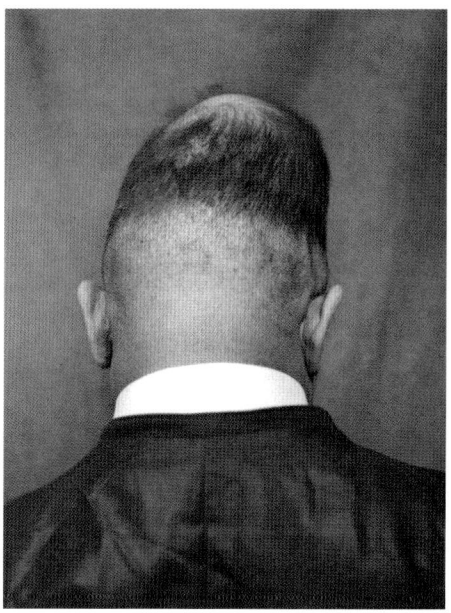

FIGS. 2–4. PREOPERATIVE.

HISTORY

This patient complained of a swelling "on the top of the head" of 10 years duration. Dr. Elliot Cutler of Cleveland made a diagnosis of brain tumor. "In view of the extreme vascularity of the tumor and its great size and knowing Dr. Cushing's interest in this, the patient was sent to this hospital."

SUMMARY OF POSITIVE FINDINGS
December 27, 1929
Dr. Oldberg

SUBJECTIVE
1. History of gradually increasing tumor of the skull of 10 years duration.
2. History of gradual diminution of visual acuity on right eye 7 months of duration. No vision on the left since childhood.
3. History of clumsiness of the left arm and leg with peculiar numb sensation of the left arm of 6–7 weeks duration.

OBJECTIVE
1. Enormous, bilateral, parietal mass, the larger bulk of the mass being on the right.
2. Chronic choked disc of 1D. superimposed on secondary atrophy on the right.
3. Slight left lower facial paresis of central type.
4. Astereognosis on the left.

IMPRESSION: Enormous parasagittal meningioma, invading bone and soft tissue of the scalp, more on right.

RADIOLOGY REPORT
December 27, 1929
Dr. Sosman

Films of skull show a large area of markedly porous bone about 15 cm in A.P. diameter involving both parietal bones, slightly more on the right. The cortex over this area has been destroyed and there is a new cortex laid down about 3 cm beyond the line of the old cortex. This new bone shows a marked spongy appearance and perpendicular spicules, characteristic of meningioma. External to this bony area, there is a fairly large soft tissue mass. The whole process is fairly symmetrical and regular in appearance. There are only slight signs of increased intracranial pressure. The sella is normal, and the mastoid are clean.

Impression – Large parasagittal meningioma.

OPPOSITE PAGE. FIG. 1. PREOPERATIVE.

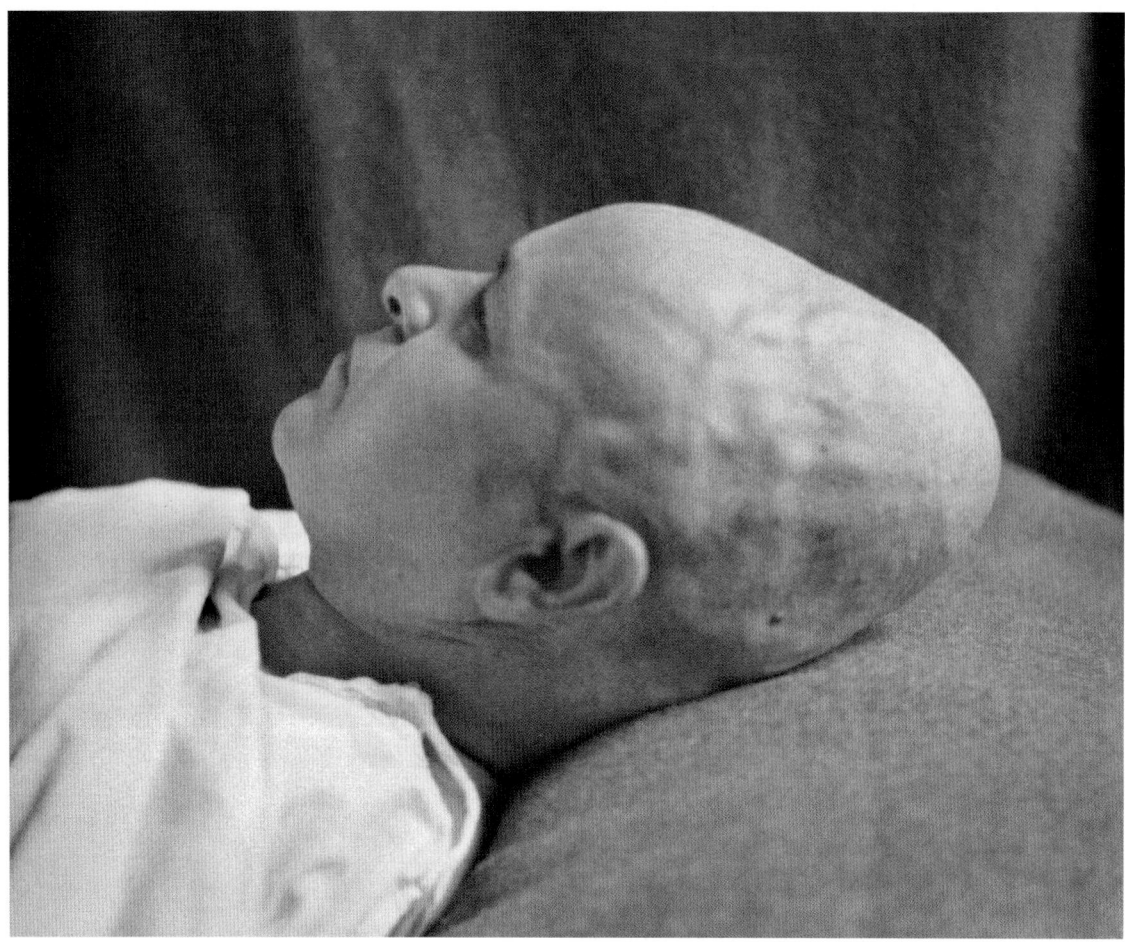

FIG. 5. PHOTOGRAPH TAKEN ON THE OPERATING TABLE BEFORE SURGERY.

DISCHARGE NOTE
December 28, 1929
Dr. Oldberg

Discharged, not willing to consider operation for this time.

SECOND HOSPITAL ADMISSION

Patient presented with failing vision and left lower extremity weakness.

SUMMARY OF POSITIVE FINDINGS
January 20, 1930
Dr. Oldberg

SUBJECTIVE

1. History of previous admission to this hospital on Dec. 27, 1929 with history of gradually increasing tumor of the skull of 10 years duration associated with diminution in visual acuity of 1.5 years duration and paresis and paraesthesia of the left arm and leg of 6 weeks duration.

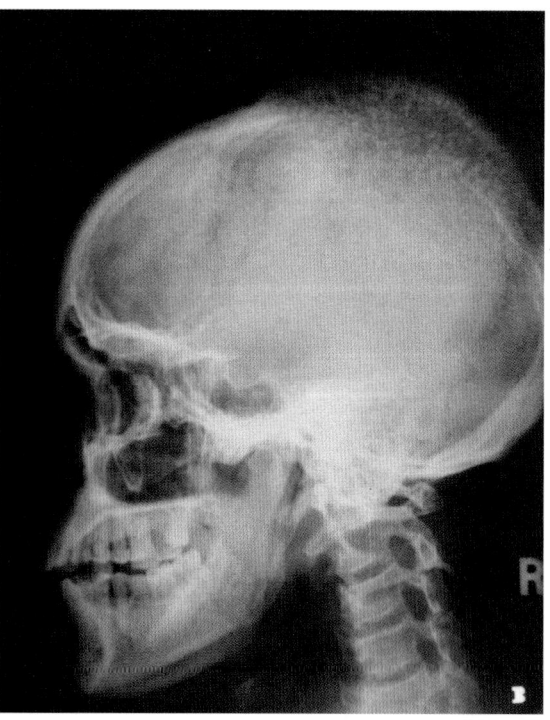

FIG. 6. PREOPERATIVE LATERAL X-RAY.

2. Slight increase in the above described left hemiparesis at that time, the patient not having been treated at his previous admission.

OBJECTIVE
1. Enormous bilateral parietal mass, the larger bulk of the mass being on the right.
2. Chronic choked disc of 3D. superimposed on moderate secondary atrophy on the right.
3. Left internal strabismus.
4. Slight left lower facial weakness of central type.
5. Astereognosis and loss of position sense on the left.

IMPRESSION: Enormous parasagittal meningioma, invading bone and soft tissue of the scalp, more on right.

SPECIAL NOTE
February 10, 1930
Dr. Cushing

I anticipated a far more desperate session with this man than we actually had. Without the electrosurgical device we would have been quite helpless as will be shown I hope by the photograph taken after shaving. There were enormous superficial vessels as big as the little finger coursing over the whole scalp. The tumor itself was evidently soft and apparently pulsating but it had no bruit. The great protuberance spreading over the back of the skull, larger than a hand, was in an awkward position. I first attempted to see if I could get the proper exposure of it in the face down position but it was evident that I would have to take the anterior part of the flap so low that I thought it best to transfer the patient to his back propped up with sand bags, even though in this position I could not get wholly back to the posterior part of the tumor.

OPERATIVE NOTE
February 10, 1930
Anesthesia – Novocain

Reflection Backward of Large Oval Shaped Flap from Over Surface of Tumor – Bleeding in Areas Coagulated in the Process – Electro-Surgical Removal of Extracranial Portion of Tumor – Exposure of a Soft Pulsating Mass, Virtually Communicating Directly with Intra-Cranial Portion of Growth – Replacement of Flap without Drainage.

At about the position shown in the accompanying sketch a large oval flap was turned backward as far as I could possibly go with the patient having a crutch in the back of his occiput. Even so I have left a fringe of extracranial tumor in its posterior position. Making use of digital compression I finally succeeded in getting the flap outlined without undue loss of blood. There was a good deal of bleeding from surface of bone and tumor which I controlled readily by coagulation. I then began peeling off the tumor by the electrical loop and a high cutting current and found that there was much less bleeding in this than I had anticipated. The only difficulty lay in the fact that the current was not working particularly well, the leads being crossed, and it was not until these were adjusted that I could continue well with the procedure. Even so as I peeled off this shell of tumor I kept getting into portions of the fluffy bone and in some areas got into quite soft tumor. The extracranial shell of the growth was finally removed and I cleaned out a great deal more of the tissue by scalloping. The scalloping procedure worked admirably, great slabs full of the soft tumor being removed.

The patient behaved admirably throughout this long five-hour procedure and I might have continued to do more but it was evident that we could not complete the operation at one session. Consequently the operation was abandoned and closure

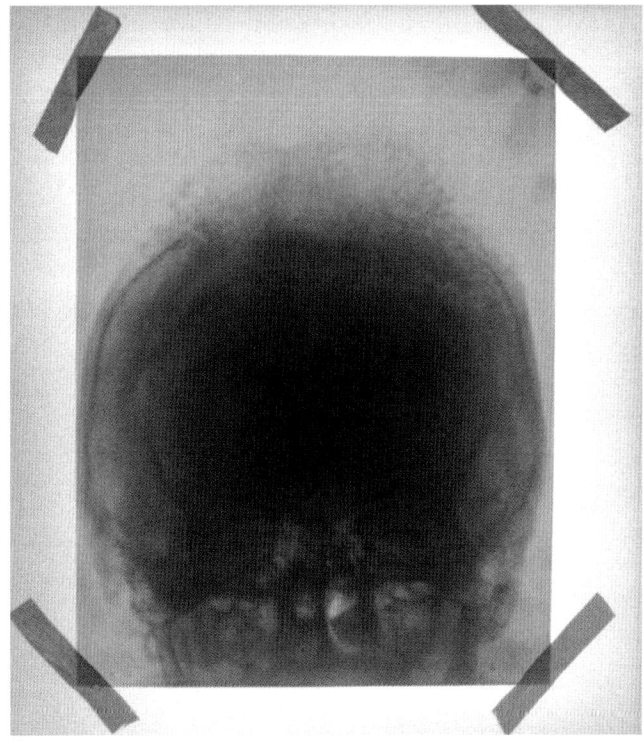

FIG. 7. PREOPERATIVE ANTERO-POSTERIOR X-RAY.

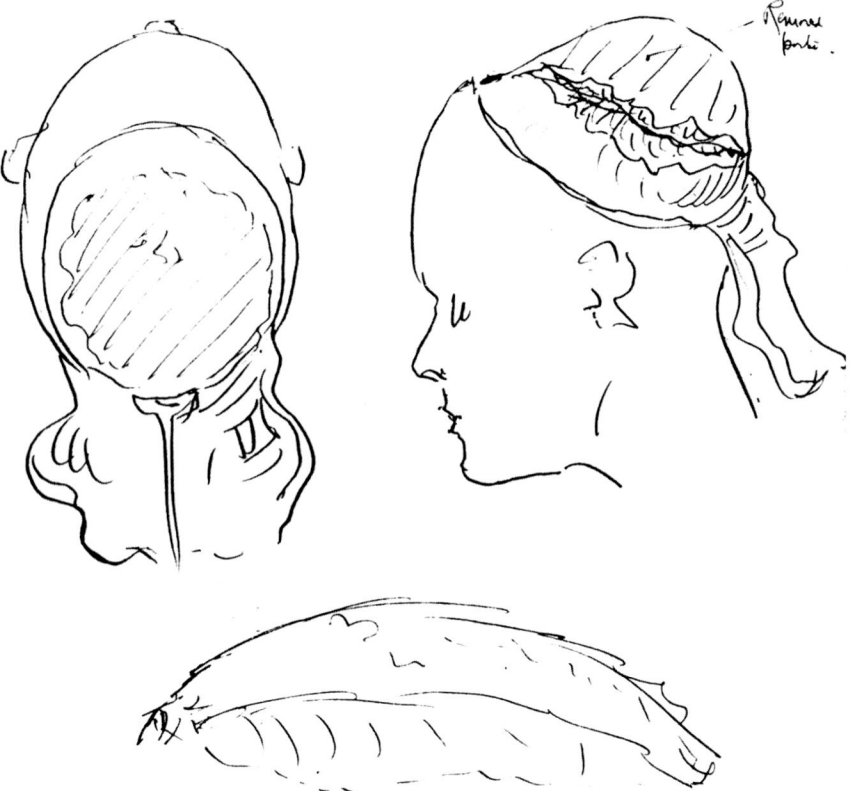

FIG. 8. OPERATIVE SKETCH.

made in the usual way, pressure being exerted against the raw bone to prevent bleeding so far as possible.

I think that in the posterior part of the exposed field there was nothing but soft tissue that probably goes right through to the brain. Of course, the longitudinal sinus was wholly occluded. I shall hope in the next session to clean off the remaining fringes of tumor along the lower parietotemporal and parieto-occipital region and perhaps with the rongeur to take off the bulk of the hyperosteotic bone which is very soft and highly infiltrated with tumor.

I used the electrical current so freely throughout this whole procedure that I doubt whether I have secured tissue worthy of examination, though some of the pieces that were removed with the rongeur at the last stage of the operation from portions adjacent to the soft area that I have mentioned may perhaps not have been affected by the current.

The flap was replaced without a drain.

(Dr. Cushing)

PATHOLOGY REPORT
February 10, 1930
Dr. Eisenhardt

This tissue was of course very hard to cut apart and spread, though a preparation was obtained which by supravital technique shows very definitely the structure of the tumor.

There were numerous whorls (a) in which the nuclei were conspicuously shown, oval in shape, with one or more nucleoli, and then latter were sometimes perfectly enormous (b). There was much collagen present in the form of many strands. The cytoplasm of some cell was nicely defined (d).

Impression–Meningioma.

The weight of resected tumor–230 grams.

SPECIAL NOTE
February 14, 1930
Dr. Cushing

This man since his first operation four days ago has had a most curious tendency of the flap to fill up with highly bloody fluid. Each day I removed over 200 cc of fluid, on one occasion 275 cc of fluid by suction through a lumbar puncture needle introduced into the pocket of blood. This blood counted on one occasion contained 3 million red cells. This has caused me a good deal of mental uncertainty as to what might be going on and I feared that if we let things go with this amount of blood lost every day he might have a secondary anemia. Another very curious thing has been the paralysis of the left arm, which two days ago when I dressed him he was unable to move at all. The leg also was very helpless. I could not explain this unless it might be due to hemorrhage in the tumor within the dura.

The operation today was far less desperate than I had anticipated, although it was bad enough, and required four hours for its completion. This time I had the man face down with his head bent back so I could more easily sew up the flap without getting a pocket of bleeding within it.

OPERATIVE NOTE
February 14, 1930
Anesthesia–Novocain

Reflection of Old Flap. Secondary Removal of a Layer of Tumor and Involved Bone Possibly an Additional 4 cm in Thickness. Bleeding Controlled by Electric Coagulation. Replacement of Flap with Drainage.

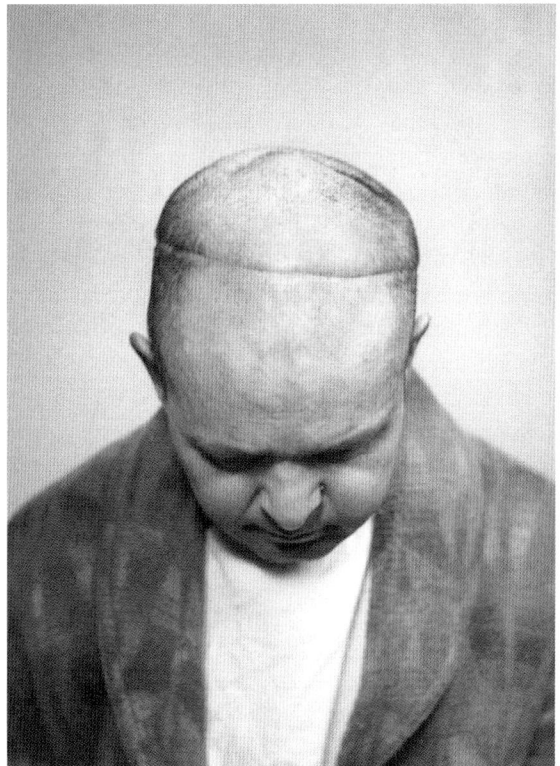
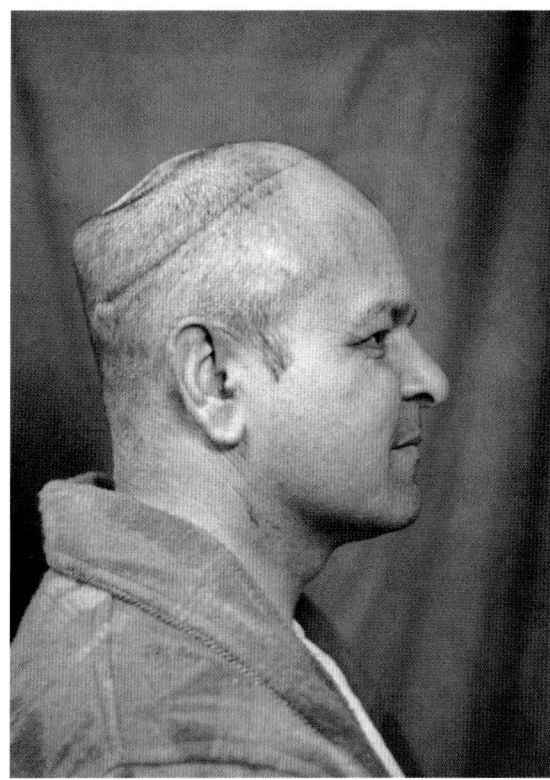

FIGS. 9–11. PHOTOGRAPHS TAKEN AFTER THE SECOND OPERATION.

With the patient in the face-down position and his head bent back somewhat so I could get at the anterior margin of the loop of incision, the scalp was shaved and again novocainized.

In order to remove the posterior crescent of extra-cranial tumor which I had difficulty in exposing at the last session I carried the posterior edge of the incision downward about an inch and then reflected the flap. There was no special bleeding, and I began electrically to take off this remaining posterior extracranial crescentic mass from the region of one ear across the occiput to the other ear.

This accomplished I began scalloping the soft portion of tumor which I referred to in describing the other operation, and I soon found I was down to a depth of a couple of cm and that most of the bone spicules of the growth lay superficial to the soft mass. Indeed as the rongeuring and looping of tissues proceeded I finally had tilted out of the field a mass possibly 4 x 5 inches in diameter which projected above the surface of the remaining part of tumor, and which was elastic, that is, it could be easily depressed and I would again elevate itself. I finally cut off this mass of tumor and it was put in formalin for study.

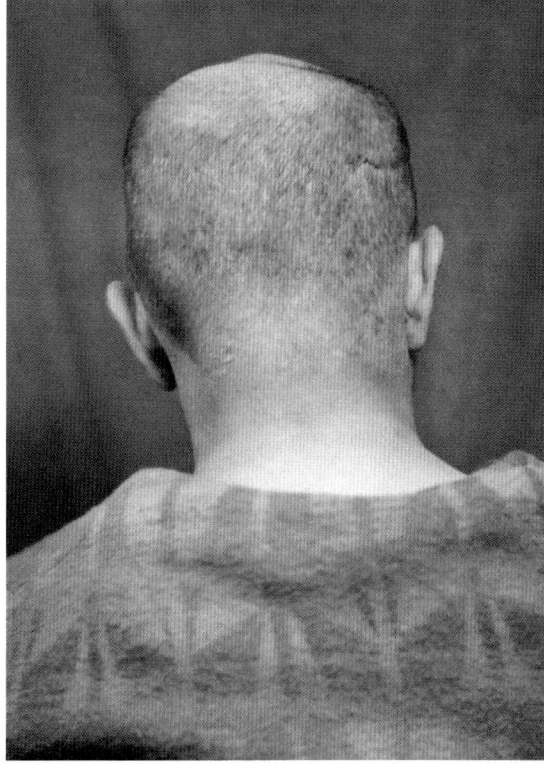

With the Horsley rongeurs I chewed off great masses of tumor well down toward the temporal region, but although there was continued bleeding

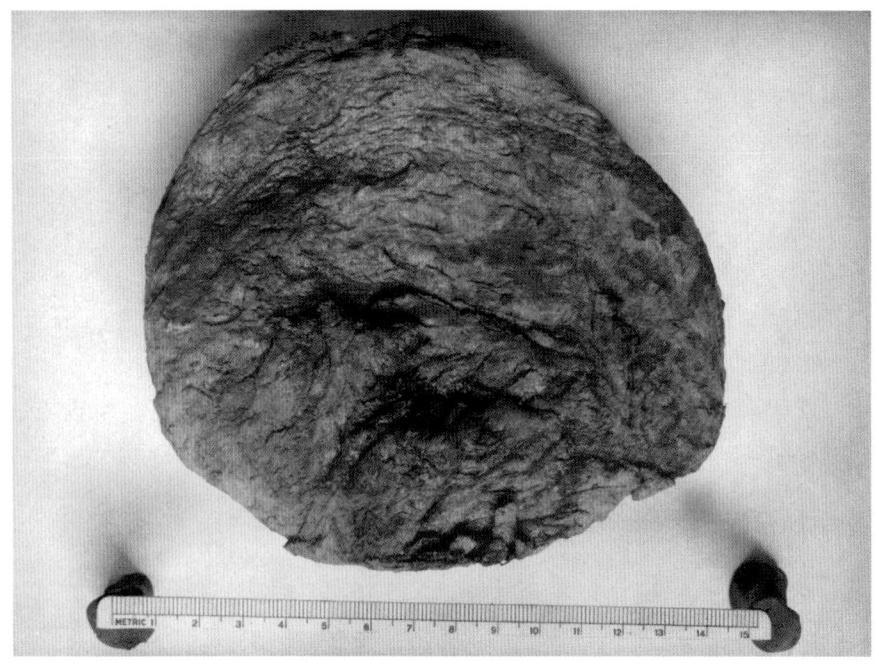

FIG. 12 AND 13. RESECTION SPECIMENS.

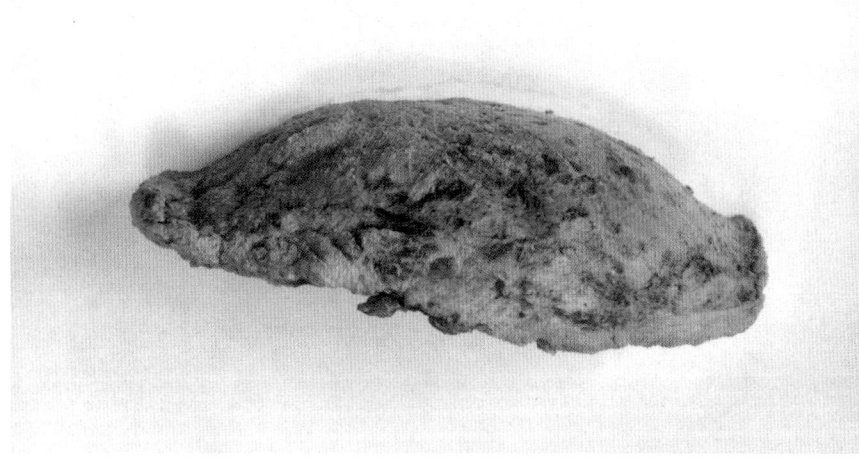

from these zones I managed to keep reasonable control of the loss of blood by coagulation, by Zenker pledgets, and by styptic gauze. As a matter of fact, the bleeding at no time got seriously away from us though as the ether chart will show he had a marked fall of blood pressure after one of these perhaps more radical stages of chewing off great areas of the involved skull. The piece of tissue that was removed at the former operation that was purely extracranial in addition to this morning's session I should say represented a disc of tissue certainly 8 inches in diameter running from one side of the head to the other, and 8 inches in its anteroposterior diameter, and I suppose at its central portion, it was probably about 3 inches in thickness.

I have, of course, only touched the surface of this huge tumor, but in view of the fact that the central portion of it now is quite soft and depressible, I trust that what has been done may serve to let his choked disc subside and to permit his paralyzed right side to recover. This, of course, will largely depend on whether the dura over the chief intracranial mass in the right side has been largely destroyed or whether it is still reasonably intact.

Whether I shall have the courage if we have not gained anything or indeed if we should gain a good deal, to attack this case once more I am at a loss to say. From my present feeling we might leave well enough alone at present, having removed the chief deformity, and I am inclined to feel that we had better see if this growth may not be susceptible to radiation.

(Dr. Cushing)

PATHOLOGY REPORT
February 14, 1930

Gross description: There are further tissue on the case of (the name of patient), who had a wide spread meningioma associated with an enormous hyperostosis. Much better pieces of tissue have been submitted this time than at last and there will be an abundance of well-preserved fragments which can be utilized for study if the earlier tissues are unsatisfactory.

Indeed I think some of the mass in Zenker I should like to have decalcified and examined. I assume that it is an extremely active growing meningioma, bone destruction having been far greater than bone formation.

(Dr. Cushing)

Microscopic diagnosis – Meningioma.

March 1, 1930
Dr. Oldberg

Patient's fundus examined and found flat. There has been a partial reaccumulation of fluid. Tap and X-ray treatment.

March 10, 1930
Dr. Oldberg

Patient has been able to walk without help. Dr. Cushing tapped the fluid on his tumor. 120 cc of yellowish fluid without macroscopic evidence of blood. After the tap, the tumor left in situ seemed to be more elevated than it was before, it might well have been pulled out by the internal pressure. A photograph was taken to be compared with the photos on February 25, 1930.

SPECIAL NOTE
March 22, 1930
Dr. Cushing

I have delayed the 3rd stage of this man partly because of his secondary anemia, partly because I wished to see what radiation would do to the tumor but largely because of the fact that we have had our hands full with other urgent cases during the past two weeks. I put the case on this morning with the expectation of being able to reflect the flap, of taking off some of the remaining rim of involved bone which I was obliged to leave at the other operation and of also attacking the central tumor which has been getting increasingly promi-

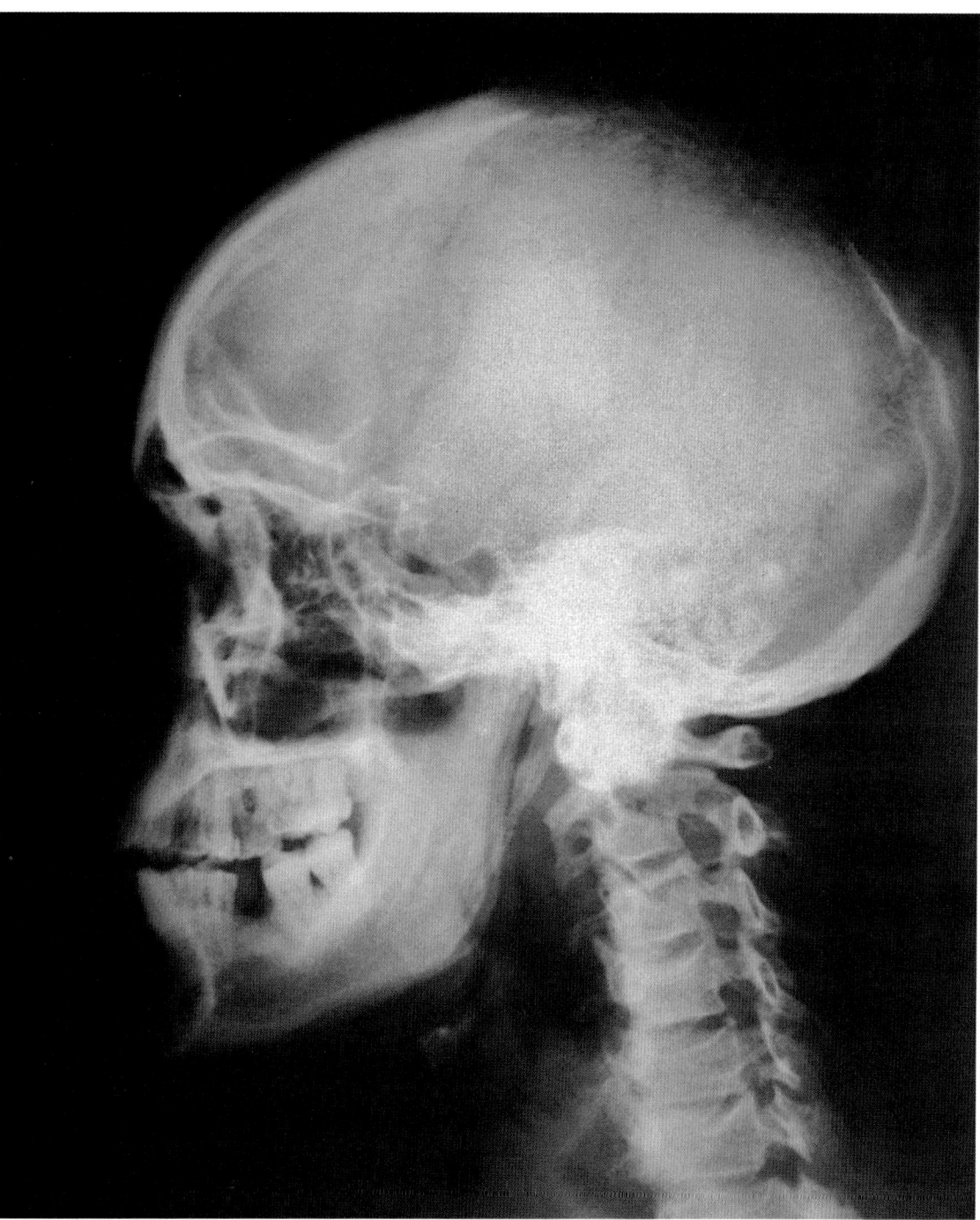

FIG. 14. POSTOPERATIVE LATERAL X RAY.

nent as the man has regained the use of his arm and leg. He was in excellent condition for the operation but I had little warning of the difficulties that we were going to encounter from bleeding so soon as an attempt was made to reflect the flap. Whether these difficulties were due to the marked reaction around the tumor or to the radiation or to our delay until the stage when the wound was wholly granulating I cannot say.

OPERATIVE NOTE
March 22, 1930
Anesthesia – Novocain

Attempted Reflection of Flap – Profuse Venous Bleeding – Procedure Abandoned.

We started in bravely with this operation, and although was aware that we had waited too long to separate the wound by blunt dissection, I had no idea what we would encounter. I made a scratch through the original scar through its whole extent and began at the upper edge to go through to the bone and reflect the scalp but the bleeding was simply overwhelming. As we found that we could not control it by pressure with gauze and as a good deal of blood had been lost there was nothing to do but to take some cutting needles and close the wound.

I then tapped the sac, this having been the first time it had been tapped in possibly two weeks. It contained a slightly mucinoid yellowish fluid, I should think possibly 100 cc. having been secured. With this fluid removed it was evident that the central tumor was much more prominent than at the last tapping. I should like to have this man have a series of deep radiation before his discharge. I am greatly disappointed that I did not have the opportunity to examine this tissue to see what its histological appearance might be after radiation.

In view of what happened, I might add that I could have made a direct median incision the length of the large flap and come down upon the cyst and have attacked the tumor in that way, but if the tumor caused as much bleeding as the scar did, we would have been able to accomplish nothing.

(Dr. Cushing)

March 26, 1930
Dr. Oldberg

Patient was taken down to operating room and tapped by H.C. 50 cc of yellowish fluid. The tumor seems to have grown rapidly – showing the outlines thru the scalp. Dr. Cushing ordered an X-ray treatment. No clinical evidence due to the recurrence of the growth to be found.

March 28, 1930
Dr. Oldberg

Patient was seen by Dr. Sosman, who also not thinks a new X-ray treatment possible until April 10.

DISCHARGE NOTE
April 2, 1930
Dr. Cotton

Wound healed p.p. Patient is referred to Dr. Cutler of Cleveland to get his next X-ray treatment.

FOLLOW UP NOTE
August 5, 1932

The patient subsequently presented with left-sided neurological deficits and was seen by Dr. E.C. Cutler of Cleveland. Dr. Cutler ligated bilateral external carotid arteries and performed a partial extirpation of the tumor.

He was last noted to be in a fair condition in November of 1932. He suffered from Jacksonian seizures, an increased degree of distention and bulging of the scalp flap overlying the area where the skull had been removed, and left-sided hemiparesis.

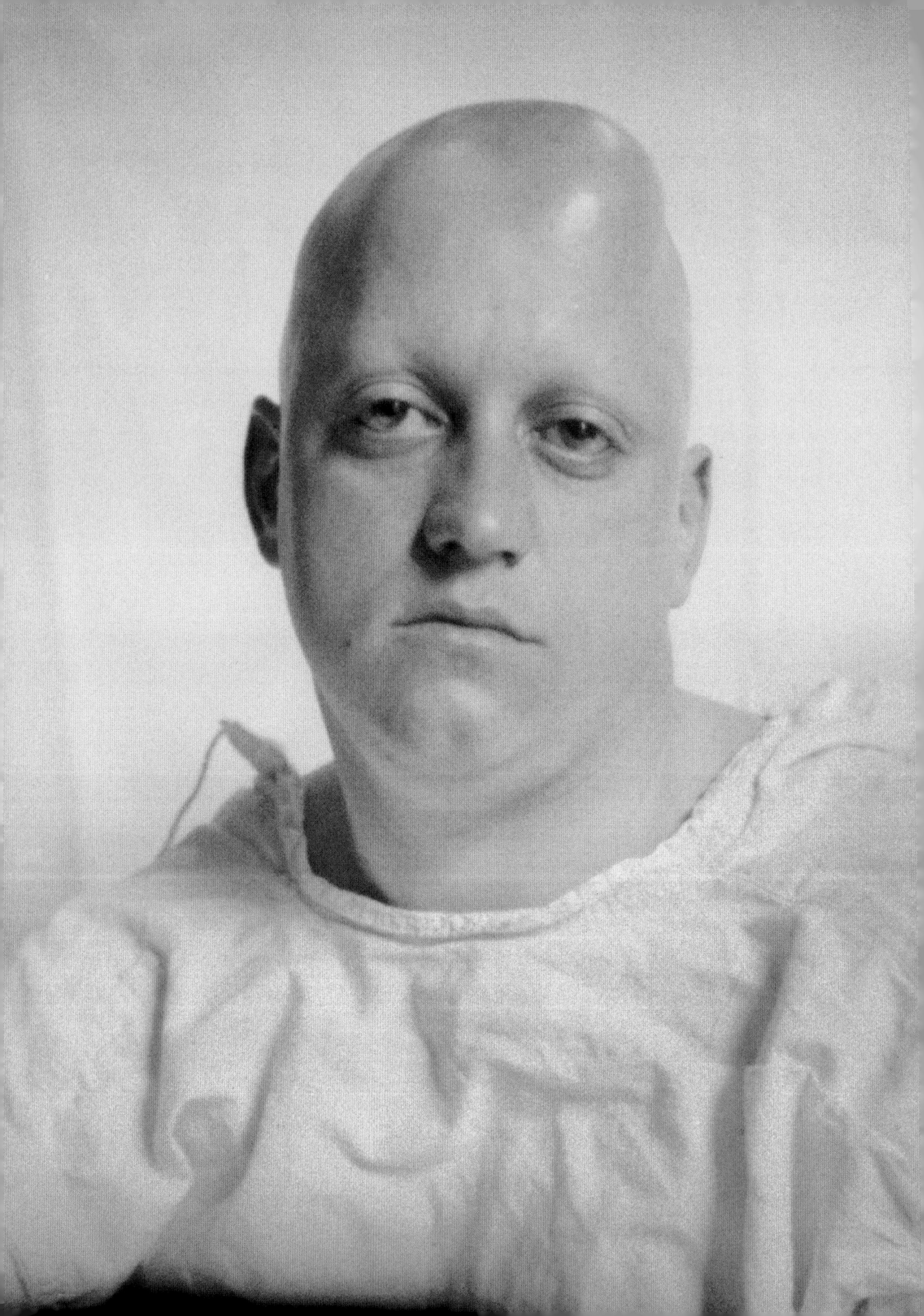

3.12 Parasagittal meningioma

SEX: M; AGE: 32; SURG. NO. 36124

HISTORY

This patient reported swelling in the left frontal region during the last five years.

SUMMARY OF POSITIVE FINDINGS
March 31, 1930
Dr. Oldberg

SUBJECTIVE
1. History of lump in the skull in the left frontal region close to the midline first noticed in 1925, not having consciously increased in size since that time, and having been totally unassociated with any untoward symptoms.

OBJECTIVE
1. Lump in the skull, measuring approximately 5 x 7 cm in area and 2–3 cm in thickness, in the left frontal region close to the midline, with slight increased vascularity in the scalp, particularly in the frontal region in association with this lump.
2. Very slight possible questionable early papilledema in the left eye.

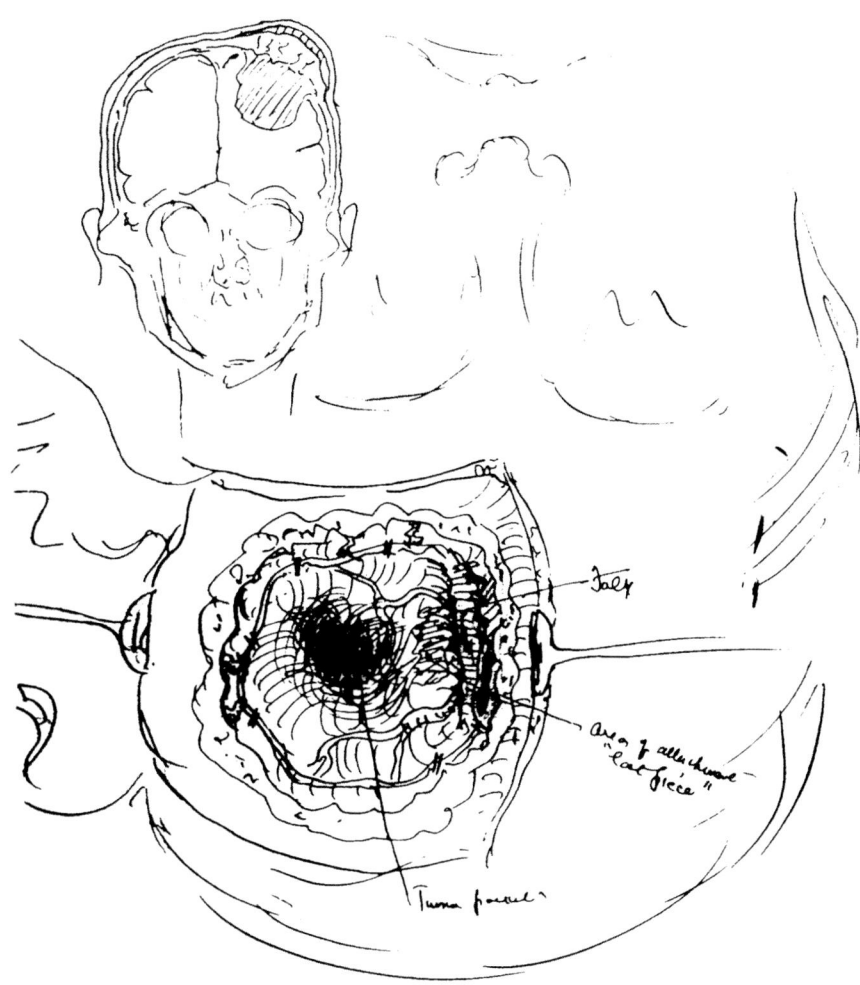

FIG. 3. OPERATIVE SKETCH.

IMPRESSION: Left frontal parasagittal meningioma.

RADIOLOGY REPORT
March 30, 1930
Dr. Sosman

Stereoscopic film of skull show a thin vault, with a fairly large but localized area of increased porosity in the left frontal bone, outer posterior portion, covering an area about 7 cm in diameter. There is fairly marked new bone formation projecting both externally and internally from the bone at this point. The left middle meningeal channel is enlarged and tortuous. There are no general signs of increased pressure. The sella is normal and the mastoids are clear.

Impression – Left frontal meningioma.

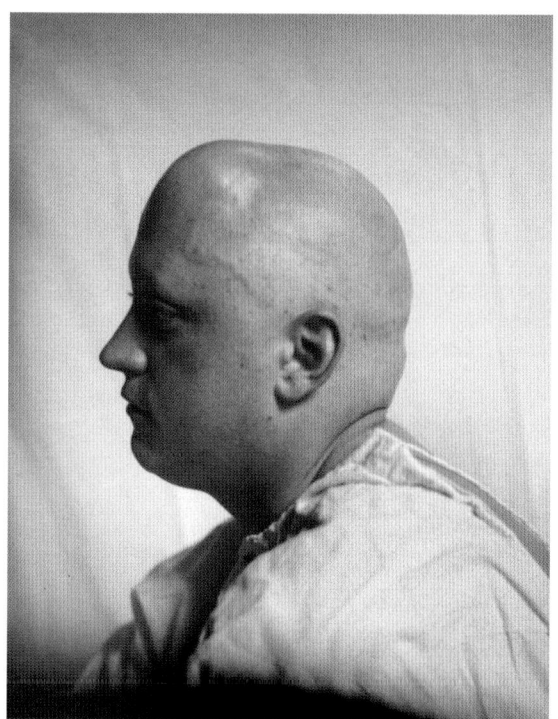

FIG. 2. PREOPERATIVE.

OPPOSITE PAGE. FIG. 1. PREOPERATIVE.

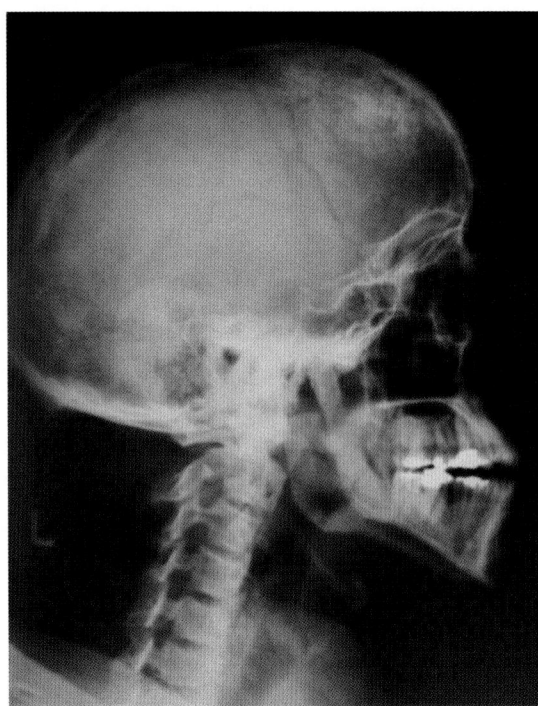

FIG. 4. PREOPERATIVE LATERAL X-RAY.

SPECIAL NOTE
April 7, 1930
Dr. Cushing

This man had an obvious left parasagittal meningioma with a prominent bony hyperostosis and marked vascularity of the scalp. I knew that we might be in for a difficult session and perhaps multiple sessions but as things turned out, the procedure went much more simply than I had anticipated.

OPERATIVE NOTE
(The corresponding operative
note was only partially readable.)
April 7, 1930
Anesthesia – Novocain

Extirpation of Left Fronto–Parasagittal Meningioma in the Separated Episodes –

1. *Layer of extra-cranial tumor.*
2. *Bony tumor itself.*
3. *Intracranial tumor.*

Unavoidable Opening of Longitudinal Sinus – Implantation of Muscle. Coagulation of Suspicious Areas – Closure without Drain.

… with pericranium down to the bone I soon found that I was in a thin extra-cranial shell of tumor. I consequently retraced by steps thru the galea and left a layer which consisted of pericranium and perhaps some inner galea on the surface of the tumor.

Then with electro-surgical needle this thin outer layer of extracranial tumor was removed and I proceed with the burr to encircle boss with

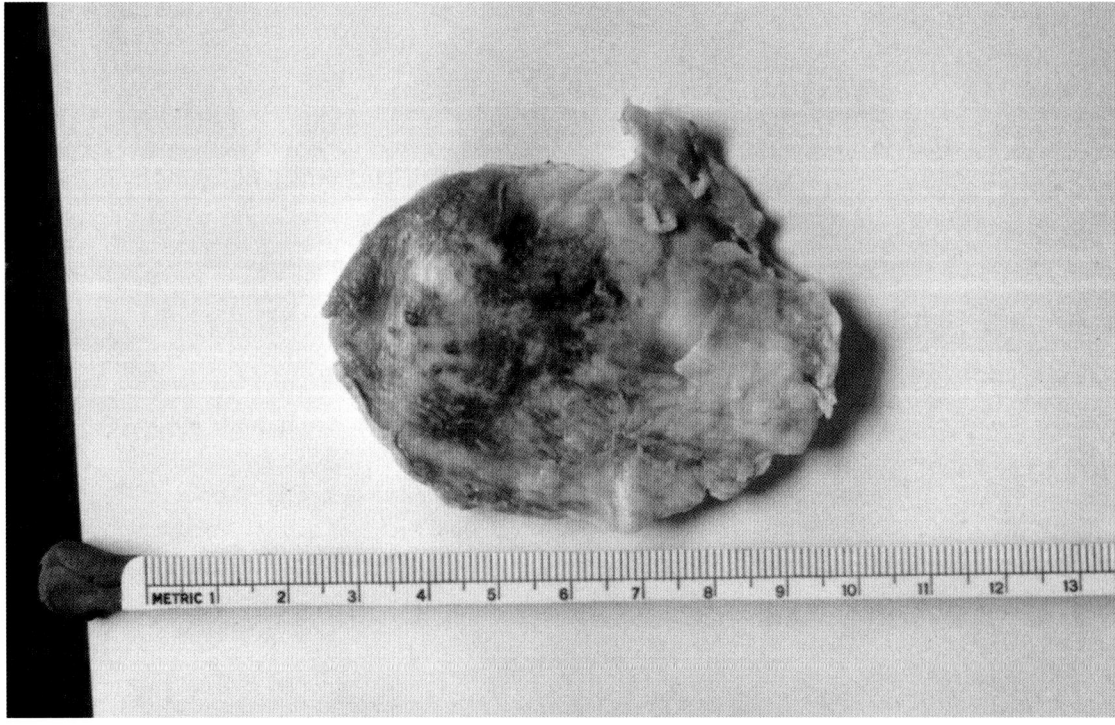

FIG. 5. RESECTED SPECIMEN (TUMOR INFILTRATED BONE FLAP).

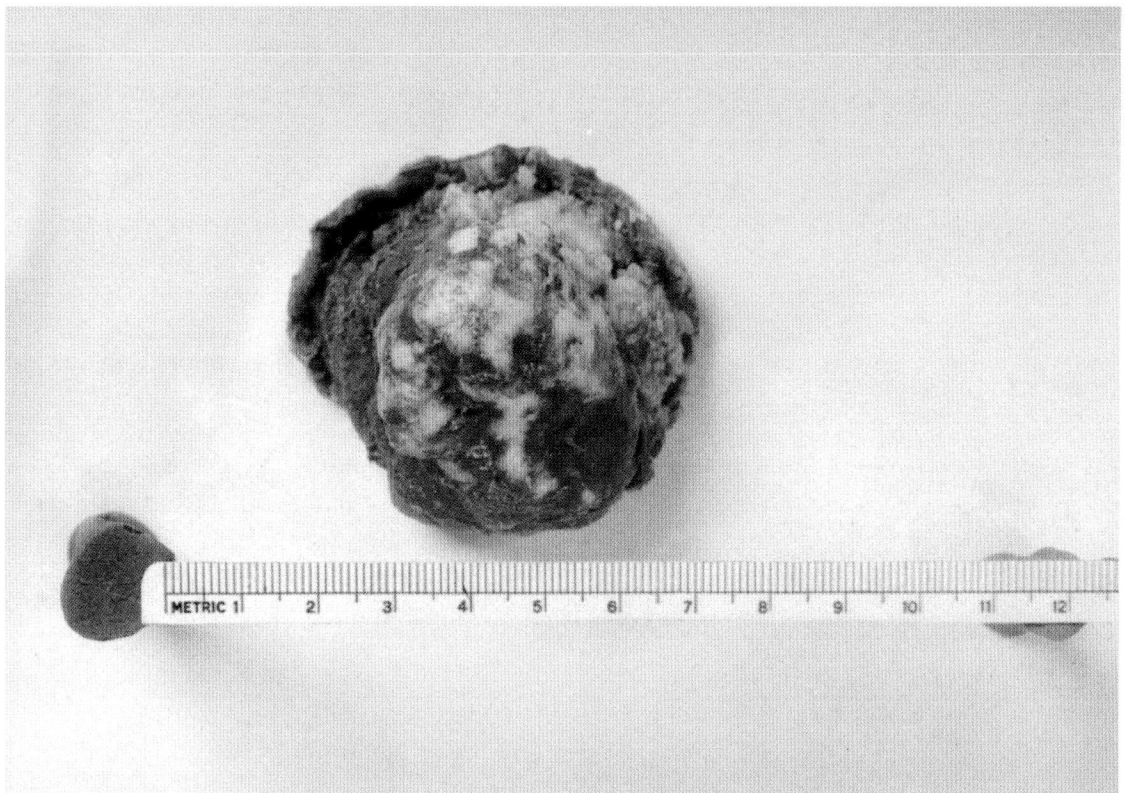

FIG. 6. RESECTED SPECIMEN (INTRADURAL PORTION).

perforations. The bone was very soft but not particularly vascular. I finally connected up between a good many of these perforations and got a gutter around most of the hyperostoses and could not make up my mind whether there was actually underlying tumor of any size or not. I had anticipated if possible taking out the bony tumor together with the extracranial tumor inward often as we have done on other occasions by incising dura thru the gutter. I might conceivably have done so in this case. However, had I attempted it I almost certainly would have gotten trouble from bleeding at the margin of the sinus or I may say at least more trouble from this region than I actually did have.

Altho the field was beginning to be fairly wet I stuck some styptic gauze under the edges of the central boss and in this way secured the more important encountering vessels, notably the huge meningeal vessel, bigger than the radial which entered the tumor from below and which I caught without making lateral incisions in the exposed gutter with the electrical needle.

The bony portion of tumor was then pried off and with it there came out a small piece of the cup of the tumor. There was some bleeding from this area but it was not excessive and was soon checked by pressure with styptic gauze and by cauterizing some of the points.

I then began to encircle the involved field as best I could in dura outside of the area of the central tumor. On the side of the tumor toward the brow I found that I have to remove a little more bone, for a film of the growth was extending down in this region.

The tumor proved to be rather conical shaped, its central portion sticking into the brain a distance I should say about 4 cm. The brain all around there was thickened and it was not until I began to tilt out this central tumor did I find its entering vessels from the cortex. Many of these were clipped and finally I could turn the growth out in the usual old time fashion, so that it was possible to clear along the edge of the longitudinal sinus and to remove the growth, tilting it from left to right across the sinus. I got bleeding here and might have had difficulty with this but a strip of muscle was implanted on this open region without further bleeding.

The margin of the sinus then ... coagulated to destroy any cells which may have been left in the

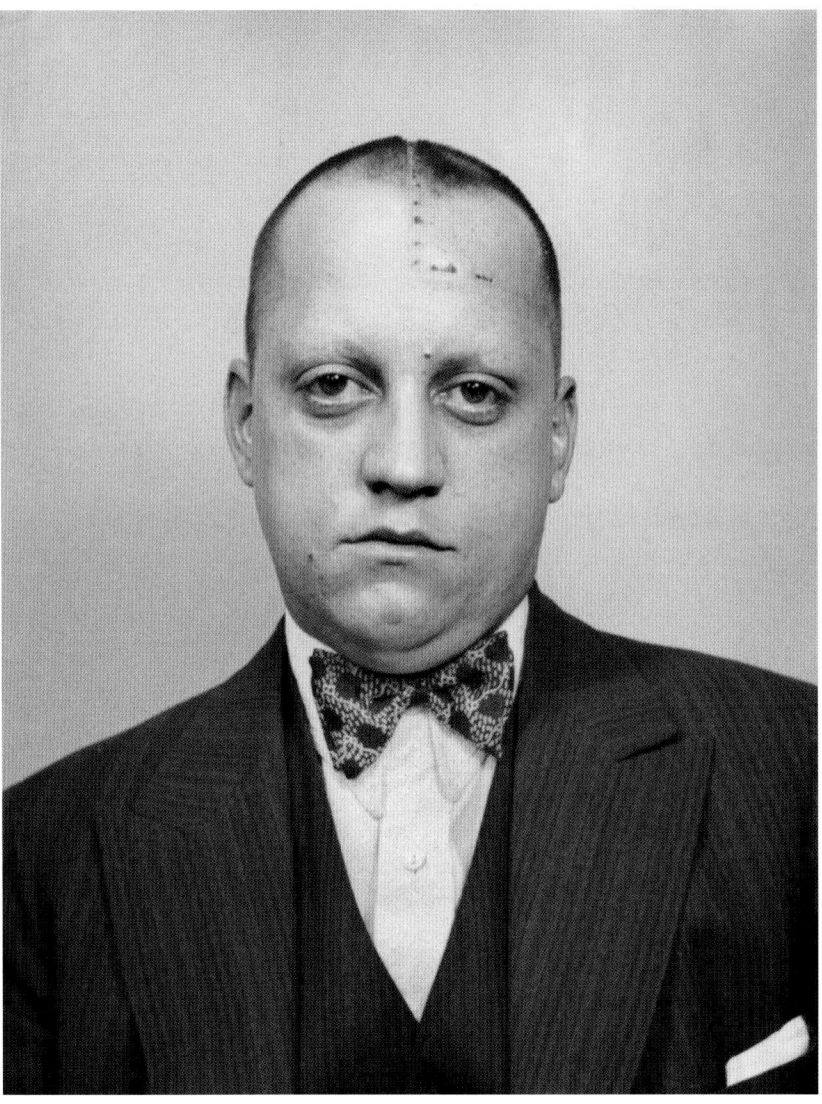

FIG. 7. THREE WEEKS POSTOPERATIVE.

pachyonial edge of the hemispheres which has been … from longitudinal sinus. A considerable part of the falx was exposed which was also coagulated.

(Dr. Cushing)

PATHOLOGY REPORT
April 7, 1930
Dr. Eisenhardt

Supravital Examination
  I. Extracranial portion of tumor. Tissue scraped from inner surface of slab showed meningioma cells, some of them in typical whorl formation. The outer surface did not disclose meningioma cells, one scraping being made.
  II. Small nodule of tumor from just below the bone flap. This looked soft, but actually was so gritty that it was almost as difficult to spread out as bone is. Examination under low power showed huge psammoma bodies, closely packed together, and in some the nuclei around a calcified center of a whorl may be seen even under low power.
  III. Oil immersion. The nuclei in the midst of calcium may be made out quite distinctly in some of the calcified whorls and in between these concentric concretions typical meningioma cells are present.

POSTOPERATIVE NOTE
April 8, 1930
Dr. Oldberg

Dr. Cushing tapped the patient and 75 cc of fluid was removed.

POSTOPERATIVE RADIOLOGY REPORT
April 15, 1930
Dr. Sosman

Re-examination of the skull shows a large operative defect in the upper posterior portion of the left frontal bone, with multiple clips, partially along the edge of the bone defect. The area of operation crosses the channel of the middle meningeal artery. There is no abnormal bone formation or calcification remaining. There is a very small amount of air just beneath the soft tissue opposite the center of the defect.

DISCHARGE NOTE
April 21, 1930
Dr. Oldberg

Patient is perfectly well in every way and has developed no post-op symptoms of any kind.

The last follow-up letter from the patient dated April 2, 1934 was not available in the chart.

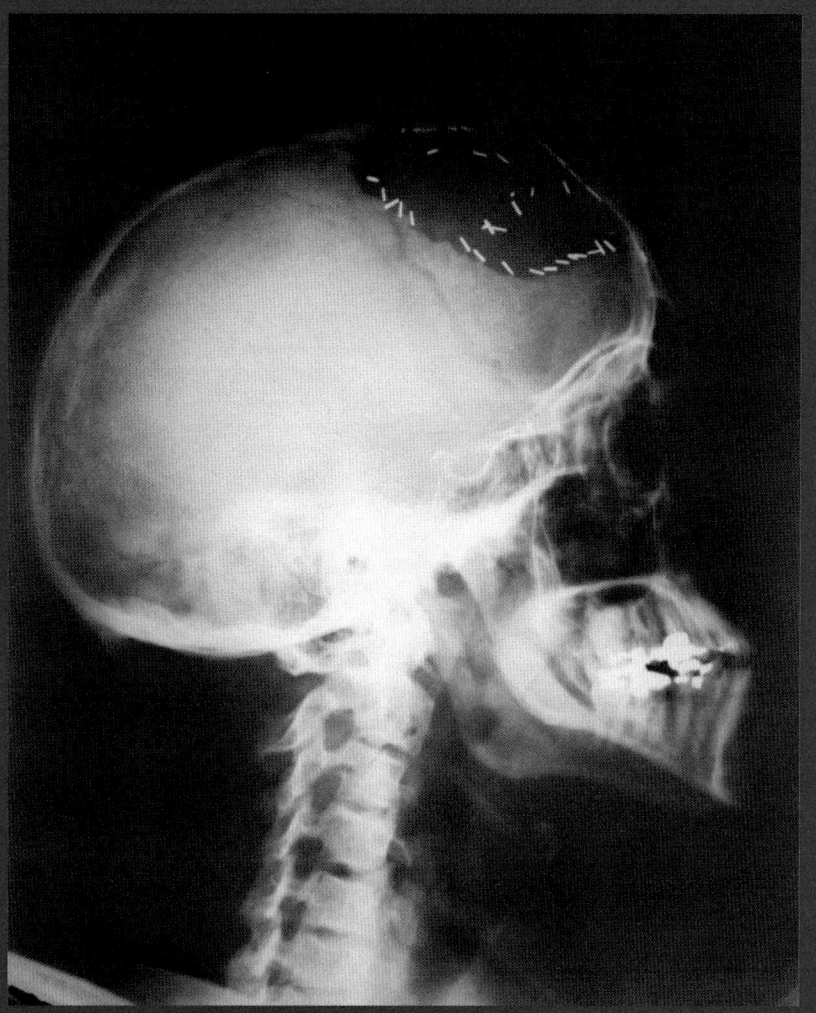
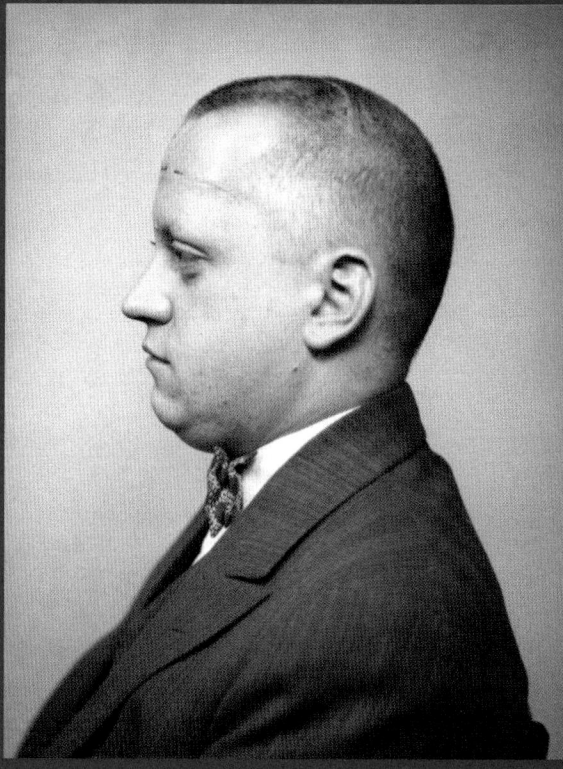
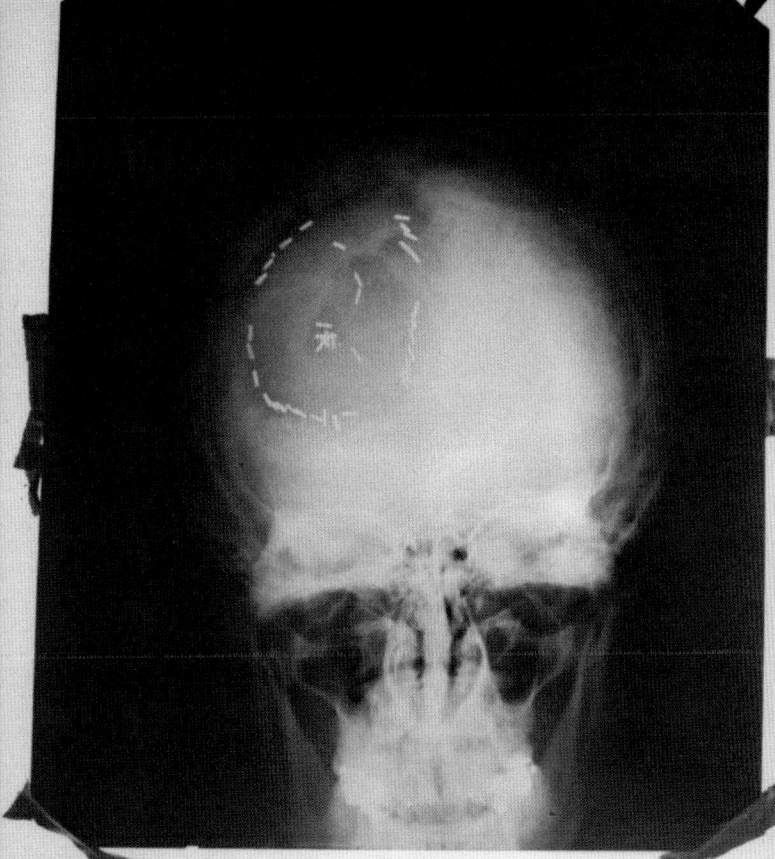

LEFT: FIGS. 8 AND 9. POSTOPERATIVE X-RAYS.
ABOVE: FIG. 10. THREE WEEKS POSTOPERATIVE.

3.13 Meningioma of the Sylvian fissure
SEX: F; AGE: 30; SURG. NO. 36213

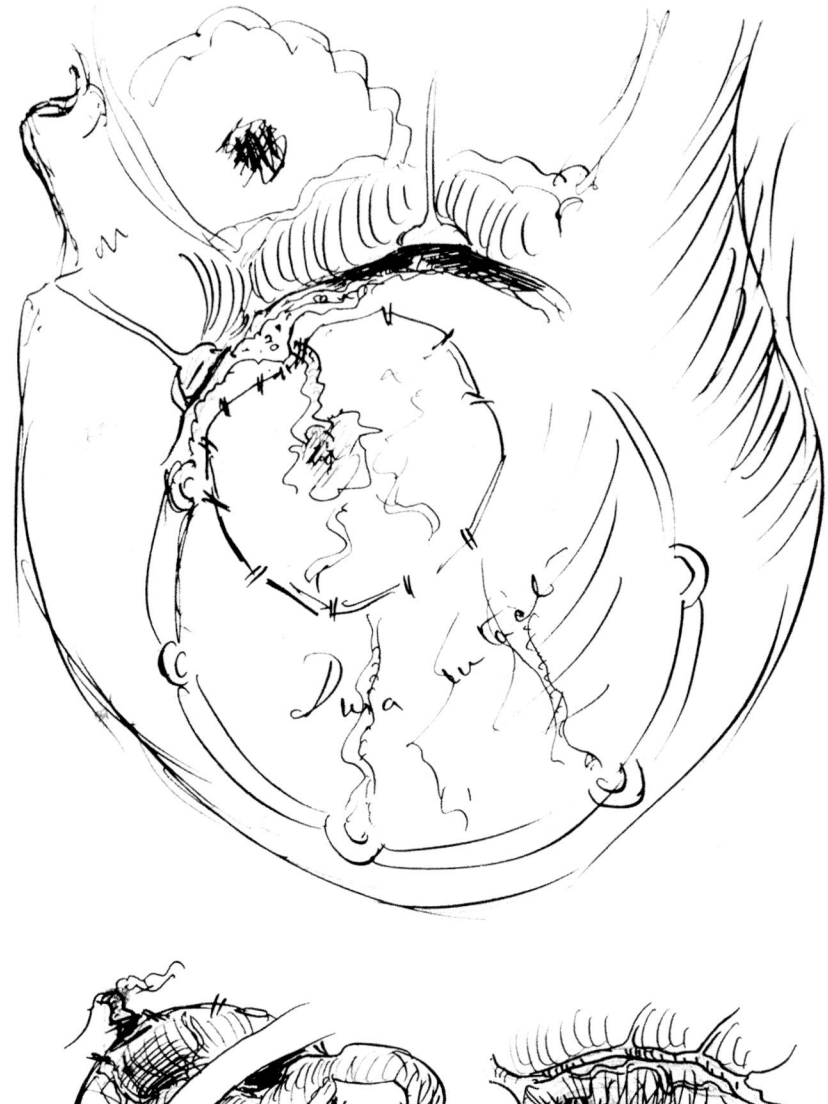

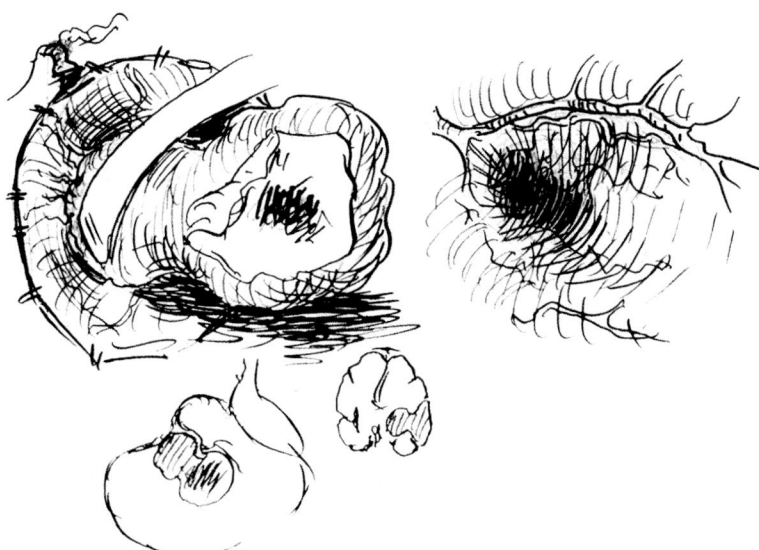

FIG. I. OPERATIVE SKETCH.

HISTORY

About two years before admission, the patient noticed dark spots before her eyes. Three months before admission, her vision began to fail.

SUMMARY OF POSITIVE FINDINGS
April 11, 1930
Dr. Oldberg

SUBJECTIVE
1. History of slight transient difficulty with vision, occurring 2 years ago and reappearing 3 ms ago with rapid diminishing in vision since that time.
2. History of lassitude of 3 months duration.
3. History of occasional pain in the back of the neck on lifting the head upward, of 3 months duration.

OBJECTIVE
1. Bilateral choked disc, 2 D, superimposed upon marked secondary optic atrophy.

IMPRESSION: Ventriculograms indicated, unless X-ray reveals something specific. Not sufficient localizing signs to make a localizing diagnosis.

RADIOLOGY REPORT
April 10, 1930
Dr. Sosman

Right stereo, A.P. and P.A. of skull show a thin vault with moderate signs of increased pressure. There are multiple areas of calcification over the surface of the brain, particularly in the frontal regions, probably in the dura. There is a localized irregular endostosis in the right temporal bone, with slight increase in vascularity around it. This is 5.5 cm above the right external auditory meatus, and slightly in front of it. The sella is atrophic, otherwise apparently normal.

Impression – Right temporal meningioma.

SPECIAL NOTE
April 11, 1930
Dr. Cushing

This woman came in the hospital yesterday with a high grade of choked disc, approaching blindness and nothing else neurologically to show for her trouble until the x-rays came to be taken when they revealed an unmistakable lesion about in the right Sylvian region, representing the stalk of a meningioma. There was no exceptional vascularity around it. We happened to have nothing on today but a ventriculogram and consequently I suggested that this woman be scheduled on the chance that we might be able to put her case thru, a donor and muscle have been provided. Operation relayed with Dr. Horrax.

OPERATIVE NOTE
April 11, 1930
Anesthesia – Novocain

Reflection of Flap, Including Stalk of Tumor – Removal of Involved Area of Bone – Control of Bleeding – Rongeuring of Bone Well Down into the Base of the Sylvian Fissure after Disclosure that Tumor Spread Down in that Region and Lay within the Fissure – Complete Circumscription of Formal Dura – Painstaking Dislodgement of Rather Hour-Glass Shaped Elongated Tumor – Closure without Drainage.

Dr. Horrax had outlined the bone flap when I took over the procedure and reflected the flap. It came away as shown in the sketch with a core of tumor. There was some sharp bleeding from the surface of the dura, but I fortunately caught a large spurting hemangioma with a clamp. There was also considerable bleeding from enlarged dural vessels running up toward the vertex.

While the bleeding from the surface of the dura was being held, I proceeded to make an incision in the lower anterior part of the field and very soon came down upon soft margin of spreading meningioma which made it necessary to remove bone as far down and forward as I could in the Sylvian region. It was somewhat difficult and awkward but I finally managed by clipping and cutting to get across the deep furrow of dura in the Sylvian region and to get just toward the edge of tumor. Circumscription of the growth around the upper and outer margins was then comparatively easy. I should say that in the process of circumscription, I got marked bleeding and it was not until the latter part of the operation that a clamp was placed to secure the vessels.

I then by slow process with dissection began to brush the brain away from the tumor, which appeared at first to be as large as the butt end of a good sized hen's egg. I should say that the Sylvian vessels ran around the lower part of the tumor; in other words pushed downward. I had the good fortune to get the vein and artery away from the tumor without so far as I could see injuring them.

As the enucleation of the tumor began to be more and more completed, I finally found that there was a neck of the growth which led way down into the beginning of the Sylvian region. I was afraid that the middle cerebral artery might run into the tumor in this region, but I finally succeeded in getting it free and coagulated such vessels as I could that passed from cortex into capsule of growth. The capsule of the growth was in places partly stripped away from it, and it is, of course, conceivable that I may have left some fragments of capsule with viable cells, but so far as I could see, the pia arachnoid was intact everywhere. There was very little continued bleeding which was finally checked by a bit of muscle.

After a very careful hemostasis and implantation of muscle, the flap was finally replaced and closed, the major portion of it by Dr. Horrax. Patient behaved admirably throughout this procedure.

(Dr. Cushing)

PATHOLOGY REPORT
April 11, 1930
Dr. Eisenhardt

Tissue is spread without difficulty, although considerable pressure is necessary. Examination by supravital technique show the typical architecture of a meningioma, with masses of cells and numerous whorls. Many of the whorls have central calcium deposit to greater or less degree, as shown above. Some of the whorls are quite large and containing many nuclei.

Diagnosis – Meningioma.

SPECIAL NOTE
April 13, 1930
Dr. Cushing

I was told yesterday afternoon that this girl since the morning of the day before surgery had been having a series of Jacksonian attacks in her left face and that they were becoming more frequent. She came down for a dressing and as at the previous dressing, I found that the flap was a little elevated although it is not mentioned in Dr. Meagher's note of April 12th. I put in a needle and withdrew about

60 cc of highly blood-stained fluid. Patient's condition, however, was such that one would scarcely have considered the likelihood of a clot. Between the attacks, she was perfectly conscious, she had good grip of her left hand.

The attacks evidently originated from the field of operation and began with a twitching of the lip, drawing of the face to the side, contracture of the opposite sterno-mastoid with turning of the head. There were unquestionably also lingual, palatal and laryngeal symptoms in view of the sucking and crowing noises which she made though I did not trouble to open her mouth at the time. She was given a large amount of luminal bromide and finally a hypodermic of morphia but late in the afternoon, I saw that the attacks were getting more frequent and more severe and I did not dare let her go overnight. I thought that we at least ought to look in to see if there might be a clot.

OPERATIVE NOTE
April 13, 1930
Anesthesia – Novocain – Ether

Reflection of Flap; Disclosure of Large Clot

Under novocain-ether, the flap was hurriedly elevated and a large, extradural clot was disclosed. This was cleaned away and there was very little subsequent bleeding. I carefully investigated the region of the operation which was protruding through a hole in the dura and found that there was no evidence of bleeding there. I separated the temporal from the supra-Sylvian convolutions so that I could see the large vessels which had been exposed. The whole area, I may say, was bulging instead of filled with fluid.

The flap was then replaced and closed with a single drain.

(Dr. Cushing)

POSTOPERATIVE NOTE
April 15, 1930
Dr. Cushing

The patient has had no further attacks of any sort, and at the dressing today, the wicks were withdrawn as there had been no discharge of blood or fluid. There was some fullness of the subtemporal region and I did a lumbar puncture and a large amount of clear fluid escaped under tension, as noted by Dr. Meagher above.

DISCHARGE NOTE
May 8, 1930
Dr. Thompson

Patient discharged in a good condition. Vision, however, was markedly reduced.

FOLLOW UP NOTE
August 19, 1933
Dr. Branch

Patient's general condition is quite satisfactory. P.E. has not changed since previous examination. Visual acuity of left eye practically null. Right eye 4/200. Vision has not improved since last visit. Discs show secondary atrophy. Reflexes present and equal. Sensation normal. Cranial nerves normal except for optic. Decompression is soft but somewhat full. No history or signs of increased pressure. Return in 6 months.

FOLLOW UP NOTE
September 13, 1934
Dr. Robertson

No change in general condition. See attached sheet for eye fields and vision. Fundi as above. Reflexes equal and active throughout. No cranial nerve changes except optic. Skull plates taken today show possible recurrence.

X-ray report – re-examination of the skull, right stereo and A.P. show a right parietal bone flap, apparently old with smooth edges. There is a subtemporal decompression 7 x 8 cm in size. There is new a dense mass just to the left of the sella about 2 x 2.2 cm in size.

This may be a new meningioma, parasellar in origin.

Recommend that patient return each month. Clinical course and frequent x-rays to serve as a guide for further therapy.

FOLLOW UP NOTE
July 11, 1935
Dr. Wigley

Patient has no symptoms. The decompression is soft and bulges very slightly. The patient's vision has neither improved nor grown worse. She is able to see fingers at 2 ft. She has not yet learned Braille. Again advised to master Braille.

Color images

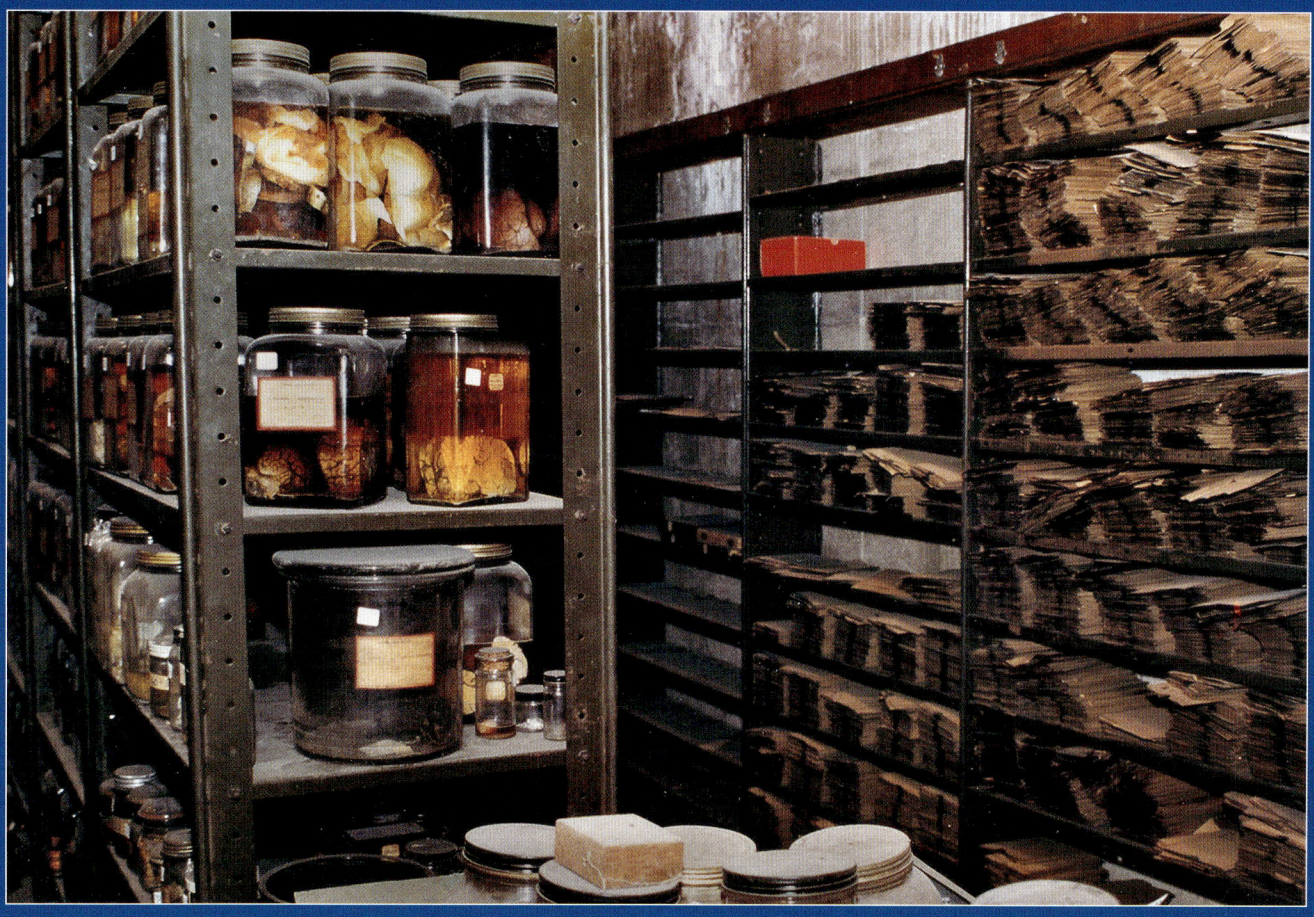

FIG. CS–1A. BRAIN TUMOR REGISTRY. PLEASE SEE PAGE XIX.

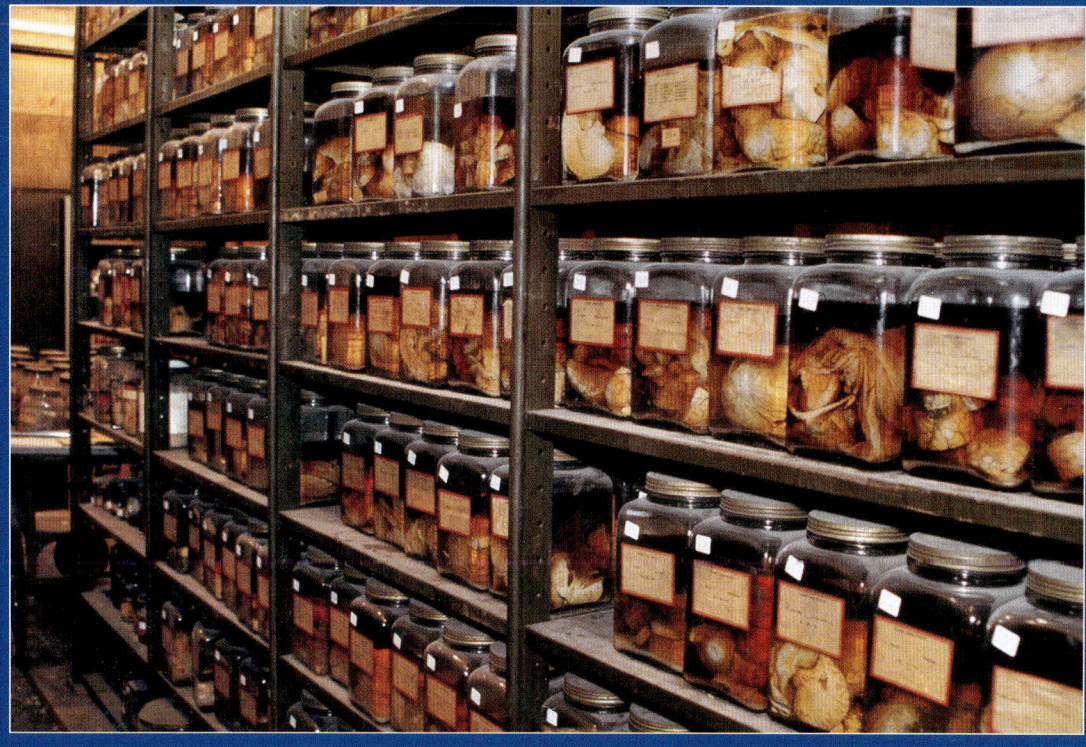

FIG. CS–1B. BRAIN TUMOR REGISTRY. PLEASE SEE PAGE XIX.

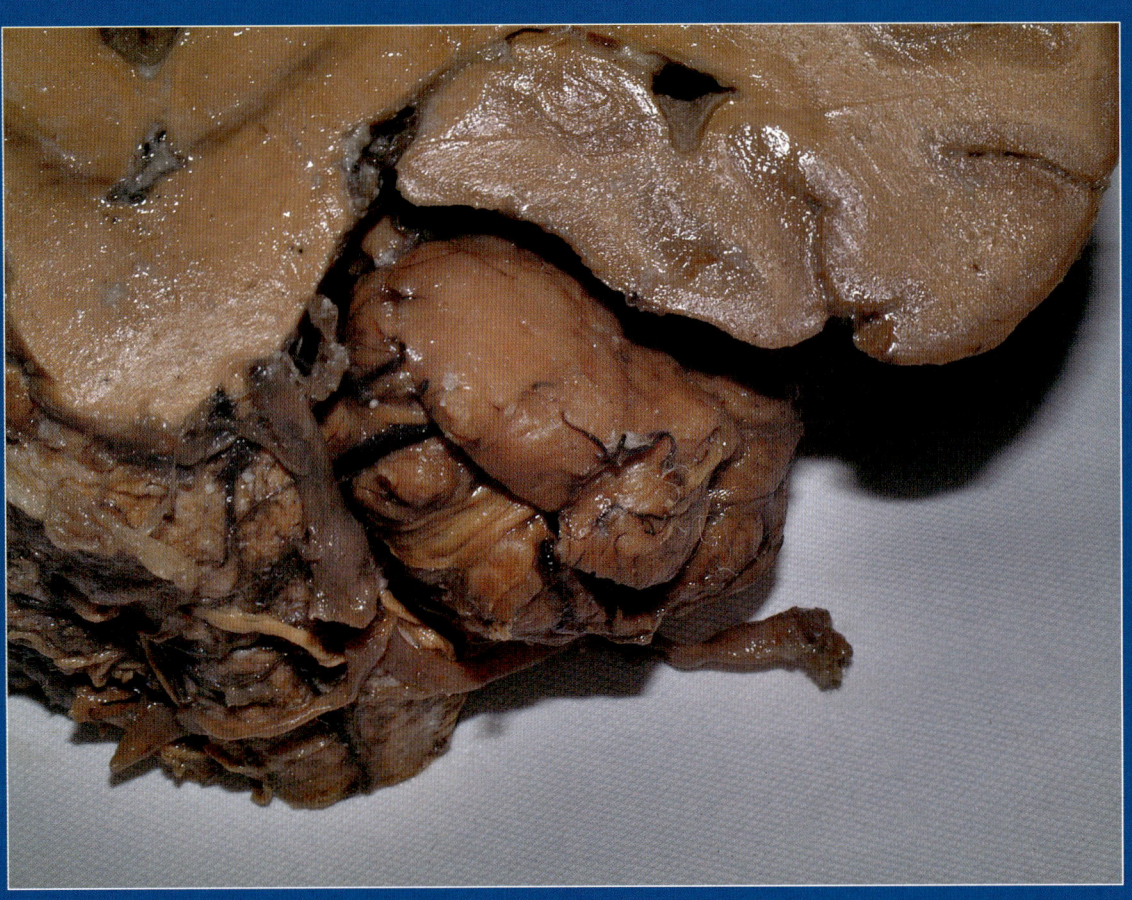

FIG. CS–2. ACOUSTIC NEUROMA.

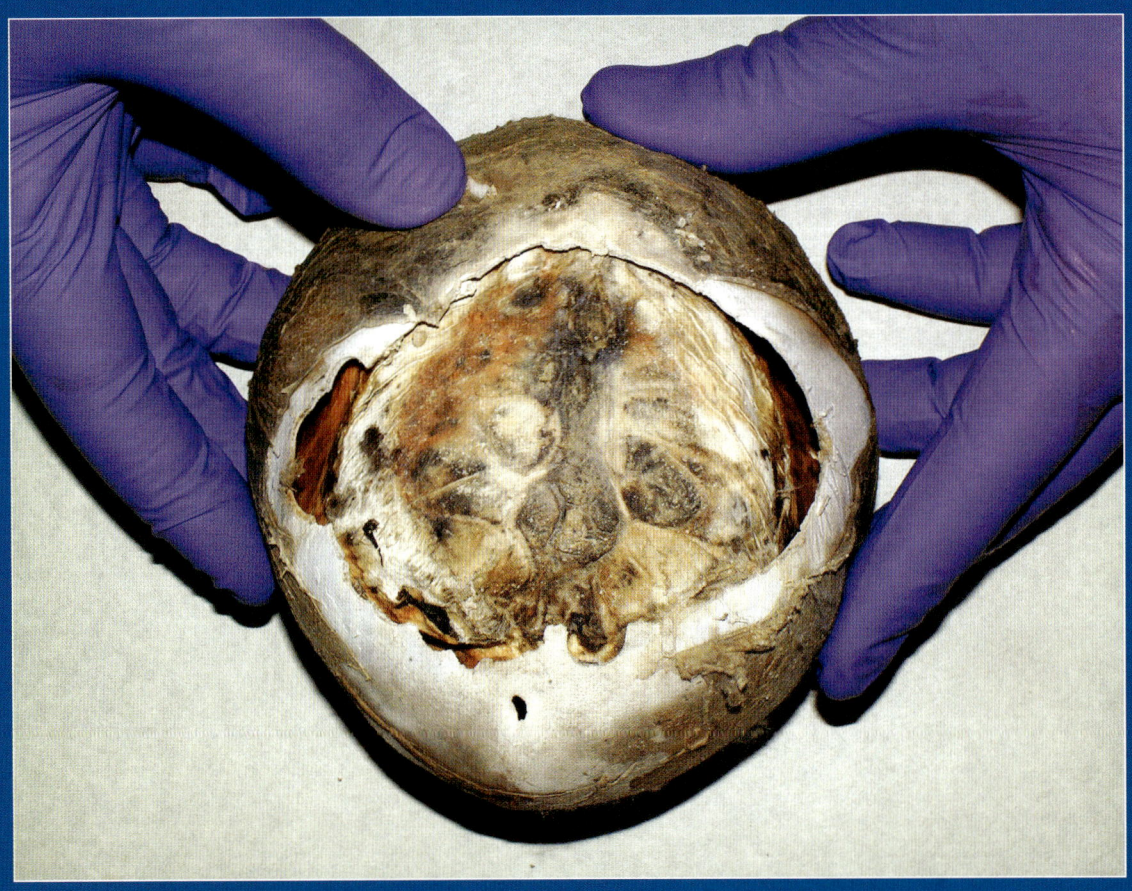

FIG. CS–3. THE HEAD OF PATIENT 6.15 AVAILABLE IN THE COLLECTION TODAY, DEMONSTRATING THE SITE OF CRANIOTOMY. SEE ALSO CHAPTER 6.

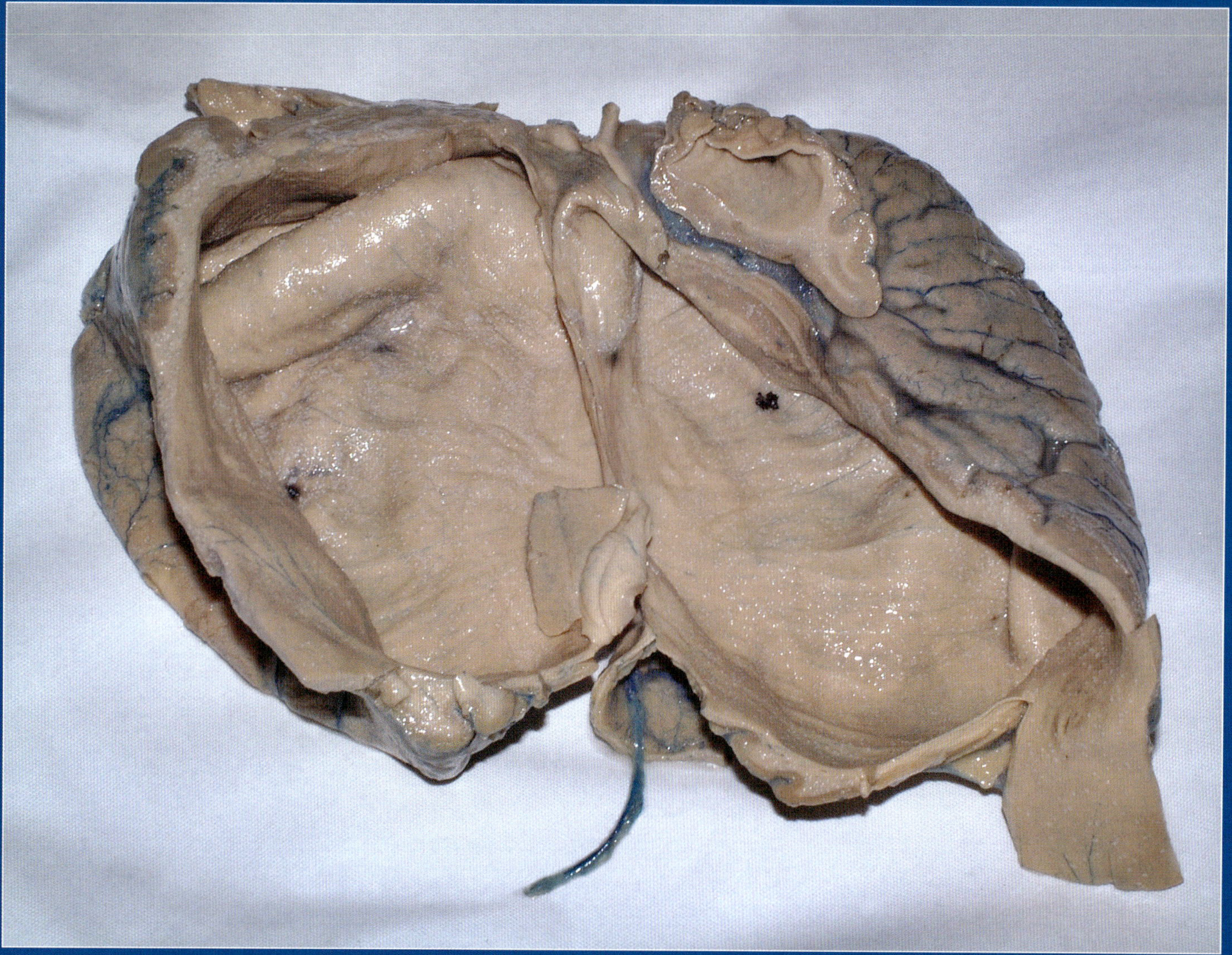

FIG. CS—4. HYDROCEPHALUS.

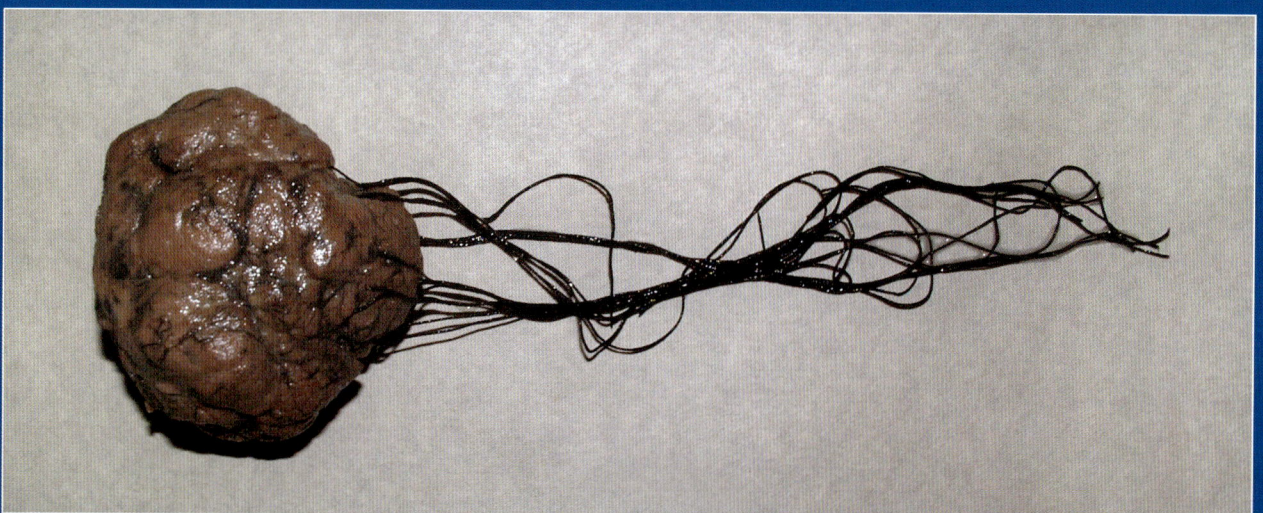

FIG. CS—5. MENINGIOMA SPECIMEN ATTACHED TO SUTURES USED TO ASSIST IN DISLODGING THE TUMOR DURING SURGERY.

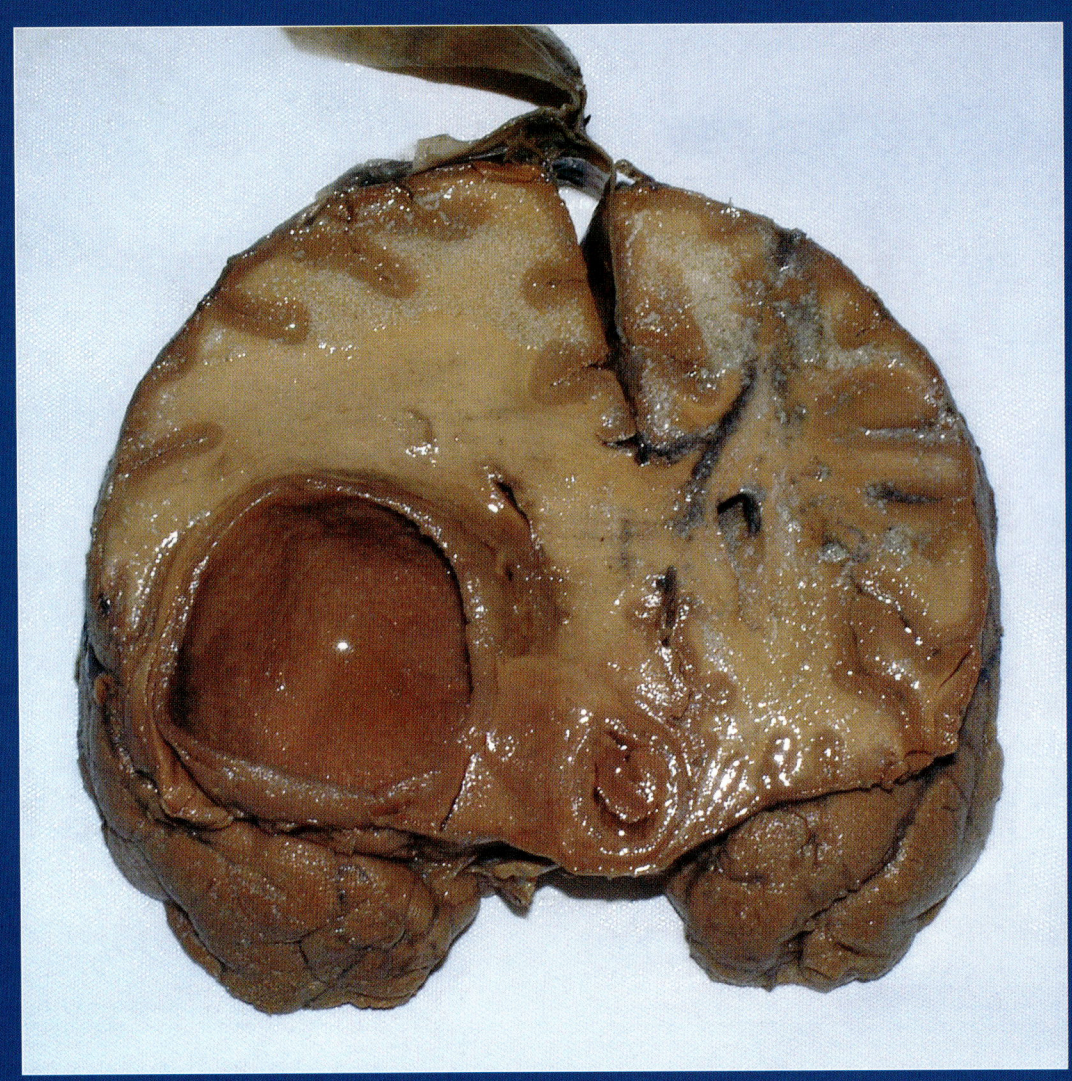

FIG. CS–6. RIGHT FRONTAL ABCESS FROM A PATIENT TREATED AT JOHNS HOPKINS HOSPITAL – 1903.

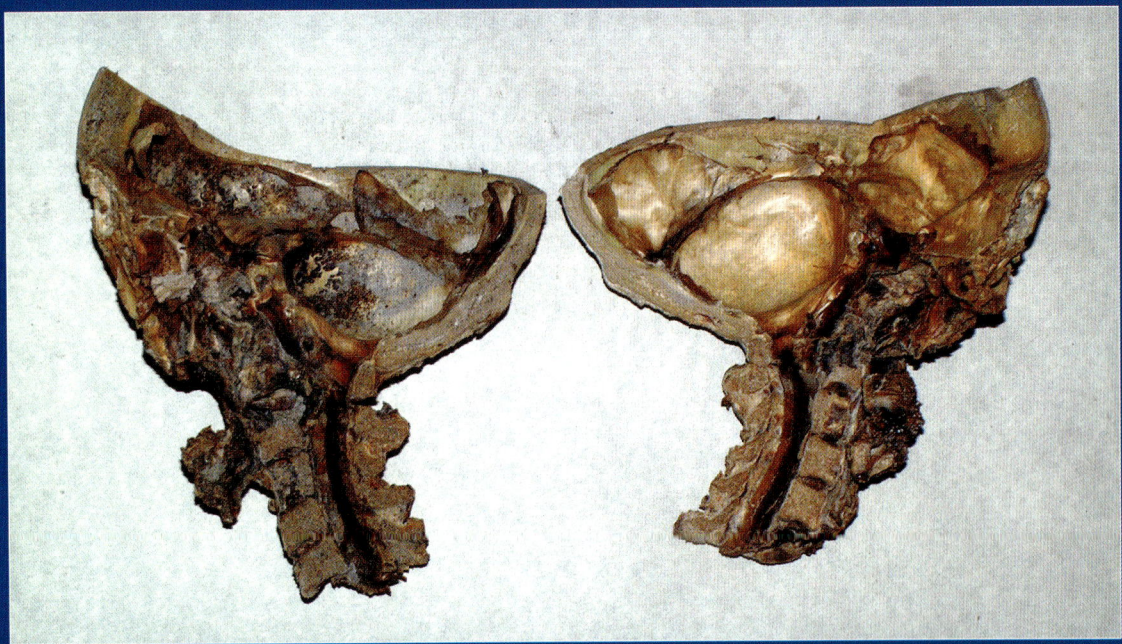

FIG. CS-7. THE AUTOPSY SPECIMENS OF PATIENT 2.5 (ADENOCARCINOMA OF SKULL BASE) CURRENTLY HOUSED AT THE CUSHING TUMOR REGISTRY.

Chapter 4

Cerebral aneurysms and arteriovenous malformations

Introduction

Aneurysms

"Obviously the neuro-surgeon is not likely unexpectedly to encounter one of these aneurysms, for they rarely produce symptoms until there has been leakage, and the aneurysmal sac itself rarely reaches a sufficient size before rupture ... to give symptomatic evidences of its presence. When rupture occurs and the true condition is recognized, whether there are surgical indications such as ligation of the internal carotid, further experience alone can tell."[3]

Harvey Cushing

The first description of an arterial aneurysm was discovered in a paragraph of the Ebers Papyrus.[14] While Galen (129-210 AD) defined an aneurysm, no surgical treatment for this entity was explored until Cooper in 1805 performed the first ligation of the common carotid artery for an aneurysm involving the cervical carotid artery.[1] This patient subsequently developed a hemiplegia eight days later and died. In 1885, Horsley was the first to ligate the carotid artery for an intracranial aneurysm. He incidentally exposed a giant aneurysm in the middle fossa and proceeded to ligate bilateral carotid arteries in the neck and the patient survived.[10] Keen reported that this patient was in a good health five years later.[12]

Despite his focus on brain tumors, Cushing's contributions to the discipline of neurovascular surgery are of great importance. In 1923, Cushing and Sir Charles Symonds[3,18,19] wrote the article titled "Contributions to the clinical study of intracranial aneurysms" in which they described the clinical manifestations of subarachnoid hemorrhage:

"Intracranial aneurysms even those which arise from the internal carotid or Willisian circle, are apt to be comparatively silent lesions until they happen to rupture. Most of them are small, pea-sized lesions, and they may occur in the young or old. Rupture usually causes a characteristic syndrome of sudden extreme cephalgia often followed by unconsciousness, bloody cerebrospinal fluid being disclosed by a lumbar puncture. Should the patient recover, a unilateral palsy of the oculomotorius with numbness in the upper trigeminal skin field is a common sequel of the accident."[2]

In this article, Cushing expressed his lack of enthusiasm for the surgical management of these lesions: "How it is that a surgeon comes to write a note upon a lesion having such remote surgical bearings may be told."[3] He like other surgeons of his time was pessimistic about the surgical treatment of intracranial aneurysms due to the high rate of hemiplegia associated with carotid ligation. He wrote:

"Ligation of internal carotid in the neck for an aneurysm in the region of circle of Willis is futile, inasmuch as the lesion is equally well fed from both sides. Should such a ligation chance to affect the aneurysm favorably, it would be at the same time and for the same reasons in an elderly person be almost certain to cut off the circulation from the hemisphere and cause a contralateral hemiplegia."[2]

Cushing accidentally exposed intracranial aneurysms during his exploratory craniotomies in the search for tumors. Even though he detailed his extensive familiarity with the resection of

---

The following material has been partially excerpted with permission from Cohen-Gadol AA, Spencer DD. Harvey W. Cushing and cerebrovascular surgery: Part I: Aneurysms. *J Neurosurg* 101:547-552, 2004 and Cohen-Gadol AA, Spencer DD. Harvey W. Cushing and cerebrovascular surgery: Part II: Vascular malformations. *J Neurosurg* 101:553-559, 2004.

brain tumors in his various publications, he did not report his experience with the surgical management of cerebral aneurysms.

The early descriptions of the circle of Willis allowed an understanding of the normal cerebral vascular anatomy. The definition of the syndrome of subarachnoid hemorrhage facilitated an earlier recognition of aneurysms in patients before they died. The last step was elucidation of the anatomical details of cerebral aneurysms to permit the development of direct techniques to deal with these lesions. Cushing arrived in history prior to the last stage. The only reliable diagnostic tool available to Cushing to confirm the presence of an aneurysm may have been tapping the aneurysm after its exposure. There was no means of providing an awareness of aneurysmal anatomy relative to the parent artery. For Cushing, the treatment of intracranial aneurysms through a Hunterian carotid ligation was risky and nonselective. Pilz reported a 43% average rate of surgical mortality from carotid ligation in 1868.[17]

Unlike tumors, the surgical treatment of the cerebral vascular disorders highly depends on detailed vascular anatomy and had to wait for the introduction and application of cerebral angiography. For this reason, Cushing was unable to design a safe surgical approach to cerebral aneurysms and believed "whether there are surgical indications such as ligation of the internal carotid, further experience alone can tell."

Cushing consistently used fragments of muscle to control bleeding. Though he first reported this technique, he admitted in a footnote of his paper titled "The Control of Bleeding in Operations for Brain Tumors" that Horsley had previously demonstrated the "hemostatic action of a fragment of muscle on the exposed brain during the progress of a laboratory experiment."[4] Nevertheless, Cushing most likely was the first surgeon to pack and wrap an intracranial aneurysm using muscle pledgets. He passed on this technique to his residents including Norman McComish Dott (Cushing's resident 1923-24). Dott has been recognized as an innovator in cerebrovascular surgery. He performed the first planned direct intracranial operation for an aneurysm in 1931. In this instance, he wrapped an internal carotid artery bifurcation aneurysm with pieces of muscle.[9] He was also the first surgeon to operate on a cerebral aneurysm identified through carotid angiography in 1933.

The most important contribution of Cushing to aneurysm surgery may remain the development of silver clips in 1911.[4] Cushing designed this clip for "placement on inaccessible vessels, which, though within reach of a clamp, are either too delicate or in a position too awkward for safe ligation."[4] The silver clip revolutionized Cushing's ability to maintain homeostasis in tumor operations but Cushing did not employ the clip for obliteration of intracranial aneurysms. Dandy performed the first aneurysm clipping in 1937 using a Cushing silver clip modified by McKenzie, six years after the intracranial operation by Dott.[8] The clip allowed definitive selective exclusion of the aneurysm from cerebral vasculature, therefore pioneering the modern era of aneurysm surgery. Even though the original "silver clip" has undergone significant modifications, its conception and development by Cushing remains a landmark contribution to all subspecialties of neurological surgery. Cushing summarized his surgical approach to aneurysms:

"When a supposed intracerebral cyst was tapped with a large-sized needle and found to be an aneurysm, fine strips of fresh muscle, fortunately at hand for purposes of hemostasis, were fed in through the puncture opening until it became occluded from the inside. It is quite possible that the sac might have been safely filled in this way and have subsequently become solidified with clot."

We reviewed Cushing's "Little Black Book" which has listed all his surgical cases by patients' name and their corresponding pathological diagnosis. These patients were cared for at the Peter Bent Brigham Hospital between 1922-1933. Louise Eisenhardt managed the "Little Black Book" meticulously, keeping records of all the patients who underwent surgery for a "verified" tumor or a tumor "suspect." A review of the tumor "suspect" category revealed nine patients with the diagnosis of an intracranial aneurysm who underwent an operation by Cushing. The clinical details of seven patients have been summarized in Table 1.

In Patient 4.1, Cushing exposed an aneurysm incidentally. He included a note regarding the poor outcome in the patients with aneurysms who were left untreated previously. Incidentally, this patient's brother, a physician, was present at the operation and encouraged Cushing to proceed further to obliterate the aneurysm. Cushing

Pt #	Date of surgery	Presenting symptoms	Physical examination	Imaging findings	Surgical approach	Finding	Intervention	Immediate outcome	Long-term outcome	Last date of f/u
1	12/4/1924 (Patient 4.1)	Facial sensory changes, diplopia, decreased visual acuity	Dec. B visual acuity, R eye proptosis, R trigeminal nerve sensory changes, R temporalis and masseter muscle weakness, R lateral rectus weakness	Skull x-rays; sellar enlargement	R fronto-temporal craniotomy	R internal carotid artery aneurysm	R ICA ligated and aneurysm opened, clot evacuated, muscle strip insertion, aneurysm closed	L hemiplegia, improving	"Sudden death"	9/17/1925
2	7/17/1926 (Patient 4.2)	Loss of vision in the R eye, L vision deteriorating; B UE tingling	B optic nerve atrophy; B temporal hemianopsia	Skull x-rays; unremarkable	R frontal craniotomy	R internal carotid artery aneurysm	Puncture, verified, muscle strip placed over the aneurysm	L eye's vision improved	"Sudden death"	6/15/1929
3	3/5, 14/1927 (Patient 4.3)	L sided weakness (suddenly occurred 2 years ago), vomiting for five days	L homonymous hemianopsia, L hemiparesis, L hemianesthesia	Ventriculogram: L midline shift, compression of R lateral ventricle	R temporal craniotomy	R "temporal" aneurysm from "Willisian branches"	Insertion of muscle strips in the aneurysm after puncture of the dome with a brain needle	No changes, second operation: ligation of the R ICA with worsening of the bruit over the subtemporal decompression	"Stable"	9/16/1932
4	7/9/1929	Bilateral failing vision	L eye with light perception; R vision 10/20; L homonymous hemianopsia; bilateral optic atrophy	Skull x-rays; unremarkable	R frontal craniotomy	Aneurysm in the sella elevating the chiasm	R optic nerve (extremely thin) sectioned to release the L optic nerve	Vision improving	"Sudden death"	12/6/1929
5	9/18/1929	Progressive bilateral visual loss, HA	B optic atrophy, R eye almost blind	Skull x-rays; unremarkable	R frontal craniotomy	Aneurysm under the chiasm	Aneurysm punctured to verify, R optic nerve sectioned to release the L optic nerve	Found dead in bed on the first postoperative night	N/A	N/A
6	4/16/1930 (Patient 4.4)	L sided episodic severe HA's, seizures	B optic nerve atrophy, R lower facial weakness	Ventriculogram: ventriculomegaly and filling defect in frontal horn of lateral ventricle	R frontal craniotomy	Most likely an a-comm artery aneurysm	Aneurysm opened with a needle and packed with muscle	No improvement	Died in an outside hospital, no records	8/10/1939
7	7/7/1930	Epilepsy	Bilateral papilledema	Skull x-rays: R calcified temporal lesion, Ventriculogram: filling defect in the R temporal horn	R temporal craniotomy	Large R "temporal" aneurysm	Verification of aneurysm by puncture, wrapped in muscle	No change	"Sudden death"	8/10/1932

TABLE I. PATIENTS' CLINICAL FEATURES, OPERATIVE FINDINGS, AND OUTCOMES (PATIENTS HARBORING ANEURYSMS).

MEANING OF ABBREVIATIONS: DEC: DECREASED, HA: HEADACHES, B: BILATERAL, R: RIGHT, L: LEFT, ICA: INTERNAL CAROTID ARTERY, UE: UPPER EXTREMITY.

therefore asked Percival Bailey, his assistant during this operation, to expose the ipsilateral carotid artery in the neck and ligate the artery. Cushing apprehensively continues:

"While Dr. Bailey held these ligatures it was evident that pulsation in the tumor was greatly lessened, tho not entirely checked by a ligation of the internal carotid. I felt at last that this was sufficiently diminished pulsation to justify making the step I had proposed to make.

Cushing opened the aneurysm sac and removed its thrombus as illustrated in his operative sketch. He also wrapped the aneurysm in muscle fragments. After the operation was completed, patient awoke from ether with a left hemiplegia. Her weakness much improved upon discharge. She was found dead at home eight months later.

In the case of Patient 4.3 with "congenital aneurysm of the right temporal lobe," Cushing punctured and inserted strands of muscle into the aneurysm with the hope of delayed endosaccular thrombosis. This procedure may remind one of present day endovascular coiling.

The patient did well postoperatively, however, Cairns (one of Cushing's residents at that time) recorded a loud systolic murmur over the patient's head, especially over the parieto-occipital region. These intense surface pulsations prompted Cushing to ligate the patient's right common carotid artery eight days later. Upon ligating the common carotid artery, Cushing noted:

"To my dismay, Dr. Cairns who was listening during this procedure to the subtemporal decompression stated that the bruit which had been for the last day or two somewhat indistinct was increased in its intensity. This I could not account for nor can I now account for it, and perhaps it was foolish to have persisted with the operation and have completed the occlusion of the vessel."

Since the topography of cerebral aneurysms was not appreciated, Cushing may have incorrectly considered the origin of the aneurysm in this patient from the anterior circulation, therefore justifying a carotid ligation. However, the resultant increased aneurysmal pulsations following carotid ligation may highlight the posterior circulation origin of this patient's aneurysm.

Dott and Dandy marked the beginning of the modern era of aneurysm surgery and facilitated subsequent successes in the treatment of aneurysms. Intracranial aneurysms were first detected on imaging in 1933 following the introduction of cerebral angiography by Antonio Caetano de Egas Moniz in 1927.[16] With the application of cerebral angiography, the diagnosis and treatment of intracranial aneurysms entered a new stage.

Arteriovenous malformations

"What is to be done surgically with an angioma venosum when it is exposed? It would be nothing less than foolhardy to attack one of the deep-seated racemose lesions which we have, at some pains, endeavoured to distinguish from the more superficial and serpentine variety. But even with this latter and surgically speaking more favourable type, there is little encouragement to be had on the side of radical treatment from our single experience in which attempted [cortical vein] ligation led to calamitous results. Nor would the cases in the literature serve other than to make a surgeon hold his hand, should he happen to be familiar with the bibliography of the subject. ..."[6]

Harvey Cushing

The first recognition of a cerebral vascular malformation is unknown. An early reference may have been made in the Old Testament. The experience of the Shuanmmite's son is reminiscent of an apoplexy: "And when the child was grown, it fell on a day, that he went out to his father to the reapers: And he said unto his father, 'My head, my head' ... And when he had taken him, and brought him to his mother, he sat on her knees till noon, and then died. ..." (II Kings 4:18-20) The exact cause of his apoplexy is not clear. Considering the reference to a child, we suspect the cause of the apoplexy may be more likely related to the rupture of an intracranial arteriovenous malformation (AVM) rather than an aneurysm.[10]

Gaupp reported one of the earlier cases of cerebral AVM in 1888; the lesion was described as "hemorrhoid of the pia mater."[11] Prior to Cushing, a handful of surgeons unexpectedly exposed vascular malformations during exploratory craniotomies, however; their attempts at resection led to disastrous results due to uncontrollable hemorrhage. Among these, Fedor Krause (1908)[13] and Sir Charles Ballance (1921)[20] disclosed AVM's during intracranial explorations for epilepsy. They ligated the large cortical veins, however; excessive bleeding required temporary tamponade of the brain and packing of the wound with gauze. They returned a week later to remove the gauze but it was thoroughly embedded and a portion of the gauze was left in the brain. They reported an eventual significant recovery in the patient's deficits caused by the operation.

Though scattered reports of cerebral vascular malformations were present before 1928, Cushing's personal account with these lesions, which appeared in his 1928 book titled, *Tumors Arising from the Blood-Vessels of the Brain: Angiomatous Malformations and Hemangioblastomas,* was a significant contribution. As in the case of cerebral aneurysms, the lack of adequate surgical methods (microsurgical techniques) and imaging to reveal surgical angioarchitecture (angiography) dissuaded Cushing from an aggressive resection of vascular malformations. Nonetheless, Cushing should be credited with the first successful removal of an AVM in 1927 as described in the Patient Case 4.5. This malformation was radiated three years before the resective operation. He considered the excision of these lesions in their non-radiated "active state" "unthinkable." Even though Walter Dandy around the same time period reported the radical resection of an AVM, this patient expired from an intraventicular hemorrhage on the seventh postoperative day.[7]

Cushing categorized these malformations into three groups: (a) telangiectases, (b) venous angiomas, and (c) arterial or arteriovenous angiomas. Anatomical varieties of venous angiomas included the simple varices, serpentine varices, and racemose or circoid types.[6] While telangiectases correspond to the contemporary capillary telangiectasias, Cushing considered venous angiomas as "hugely dilated, thin-walled, non-pulsating veins in a circumscribed area of the cerebral cortex" with no involvement of the arteries. He defined the angioma arteriale as dilated vessels "through which the arterial blood passes from enlarged entering arteries directly into one or more greatly dilated veins of exit usually with the production of an audible bruit." Though Cushing advocated that venous angiomas are purely venous structures, Walter Dandy in his paper published within the same year corrected Cushing by claiming that all vascular malformations have an arterial connection from the outset.[7]

Based on his favorable experience with radiotherapy for vascular malformations, Cushing became especially interested in their preoperative diagnosis to avoid the risks of an exploratory craniotomy. In his time, the vast majority of these lesions were diagnosed inadvertently during an operation or postmortem examination since angiography was not available. Cushing believed that "the crux of the pathological diagnosis lay in the presence or absence of an audible bruit."[6] He proposed that the increased scalp vascularity, increased size of the carotid artery, and cardiac hypertrophy observed in some of the patients with AVM's is related to the increase in blood volume as a consequence of the high flow through the arteriovenous fistula.[6] The relatively high epileptogenic propensity of vascular malformations was thought to be related to the relationship of these lesions to the paracentral lobule.

Monopolar electrocautery offered Cushing minimal efficacy in resection of vascular malformations. This mode of electrocoagulation failed to provide homeostasis especially for the small feeding arteries present at the depth of the AVM; therefore, the removal of non-radiated malformations was considered technically unfeasible. Earlier catastrophic attempts of Cushing by ligating large cortical veins in venous angiomas (Table 2, Case III) diverted his attention to using his silver clips to obliterate large cortical feeding arteries in arterial angiomas. The disappointing results in Case III (Table 2) as evident by massive brain swelling tapered his enthusiasm for pursuing cortical vein ligations in venous angiomas and he employed a more "cautious attitude" towards similar lesions.[6] This adjustment may have reflected Cushing's improved understanding of flow dynamics through AVMs.

Radiation treatment for cerebral angiomas was used based on the favorable experience of this therapy on cutaneous angiomas. Wilhelm Magnus of Oslo may have been the first to treat a cerebral vascular malformation with radiotherapy in 1914.[15] In his patient, a venous angioma of the left central lobule region was exposed unexpectedly during an exploratory craniotomy for epilepsy. Following a decompressive procedure, the patient received "radium therapy." Subsequently, his seizures gradually disappeared. Cushing clearly verified the efficacy of radiotherapy for the treatment of inoperable vascular malformations in a relatively large group of patients. After resection of the radiated lesion (Case VI, Table 2), Cushing for the first time demonstrated the radiation-induced occlusion of the vessels in the AVM by intimal proliferation.[6] The dimension of the AVM during radiation treatments was followed by assessing the reduction in the bruit auscultated over the craniotomy defect. If the bruit disappeared after the last radiation treatment, the lesion was considered obliterated.

The review of the medical records of 1870 consecutive tumor registry patients indexed by demographic data revealed the records of 11 patients with the diagnosis of an intracranial vascular malformation who underwent surgery between 1913-1932 (Table 2). Dr. Cushing previously reported 14 patients harboring vascular malformations in his publications mentioned above;[6] however, the records of four of these 14 patients could not be found in our database, two of these were managed non-operatively and another one underwent a surgical exploration at the Johns Hopkins Hospital by Cushing. One patient who was not included in his published series was among our 11 patients collected from the database (Patient XI, Table 2); he was treated after Cushing published his series. Patient 4.5 (Case VI, Table 2) is the first report of a

Pt #	Lesion	Date of surgery	Presenting symptoms	Physical examination	Imaging and other studies	Surgical approach	Finding	Intervention	Immediate outcome	Long-term outcome	Last date of f/u
I	Angioma venosum	9/4/1920	R temporal swelling, R exophthalmos	R exophthalmos	Skull x-rays: R temporal bone erosion	R temporo-parietal craniotomy	Dilated veins	Two venous trunks ligated	Exophthalmos slightly improved	Unchanged neurologically, no bruit	10/27/27
II	Angioma venosum	3/18/1921	Epilepsy, recent R leg weakness	Unremarkable	Skull x-rays: increased prominence of L frontal meningeal channels	L fronto-parietal craniotomy	Angiomatous vessels	Ligation of a cortical vein; significant bleeding/ Post-op radiotherapy	R arm and facial weakness, slight dysphasia	Free of seizures, no neuro deficits	10/19/26
III	Angioma venosum	4/25/1921	Epilepsy, severe HA	Haziness of L optic disk	Skull x-rays: L large meningeal vessel channels	L fronto-parietal craniotomy	Large cortical veins	Ligation of veins, brain swelling, implantation of muscle fragments; bone flap was not replaced	R sided hemiplegia, aphasia	Free of seizures, only slight R arm weakness	1/8/27
IV	Angioma venosum	12/28/1922	Epilepsy, HA's	"Choked" optic disks, right hemihypesthesia	None noted	L parietal craniotomy	A tangle of large tortuous thin-walled veins	Radiotherapy	No change	Occasional focal seizures	6/21/26
V	Angioma arteriole	7/19/1922	HA, failing vision, staggering gait	B optic atrophy, B exophthalmos, systolic bruit over the R mastoid region	Skull x-rays: increased prominence of R meningeal channels	R temporal craniotomy	Angioma	Subtemporal decompression/ Radiotherapy	Unchanged	Sudden death	2/22/24
VI	Angioma arteriole	1/17/1924, 3/7/1927 (Patient 4.5)	Epilepsy, memory difficulties	Slight dysphasia, R foot "clumsy"	Skull x-rays: L enlarged meningeal channels; calcified lesion	L fronto-parietal craniotomy	Significant bleeding during elevation of the bone flap, large cortical veins and tangle of vessels exposed	Radiotherapy/ Radical resection of the lesion during a second operation	R hemiplegia, unable to speak	Much improved	7/18/28
VII	Angioma arteriole	5/16/1924, 2/2/1927	Blurred vision, epilepsy	R lower quadrantanopsia, slight dysphasia; "unusual carotid bruit over the L neck"	Skull x-rays: unremarkable	L fronto-parietal	Tangled mass of small pulsating arterioles, several large pulsating veins	Subtemporal decompression, second operation: ligation of the L external/internal carotid and superior thyroid arteries/ Radiotherapy	Unchanged, bruit continues	Died after a severe HA	5/15/28
VIII	Angioma arteriole	9/26/1925	Failing vision, gait unsteadiness	"Cracked pot sound" on percussion of the head, B "choked" optic disks, cerebellar signs	Skull x-rays: Erosion of the dorsum sella, Ventriculography: ventriculomegaly	Suboccipital craniectomy	A tangle of large pulsating vessels	Suboccipital decompression/ Post-op radiotherapy	Subsidence of "choked" optic disks	A faint systolic bruit audible over the decompression	10/5/27
IX	Angioma arteriole	4/23/1926	Failing vision, L ear sounds	L exophthalmos; L optic atrophy, loud bruit over the L occipital region, R homonymous hemianopsia	Skull x-rays: thinning of L occipital bone and increased vascularity	L neck exposure and L occipital craniotomy	Racemose aneurysmal varix	Bilateral ligation of external carotid arteries/ Post-op radiotherapy	Bruit much less audible	No auscultable bruit	2/28/28
X	Angioma arteriole	3/30/1927, 4/9/1927	Epilepsy	L abducens palsy, L quadrantal hemianopsia	Ventriculogram: R occipital filling defect	R occipital craniotomy	A large tangle of vessels	Radiotherapy/Second operation after a dose of radiation: attempted coagulation halted by bleeding, implantation of muscle	Improved	Occasional seizures	2/1/33
XI	Angioma arteriole	1/23/1932	Epilepsy	Unremarkable	Skull x-ray: R temporal calcifications, ventriculogram: filling defect of the L lateral ventricle	L fronto-parietal craniotomy	Tangle of vessels, venous varix	An arterial feeder clipped, surface vessels coagulated, post-op radiotherapy	Unchanged	No bruit	3/3/34

TABLE 2: PATIENT'S CLINICAL FEATURES, OPERATIVE FINDINGS, ADJUVANT THERAPY, AND OUTCOME (PATIENTS HARBORING ARTERIOVENOUS MALFORMATIONS).

successful resection of an intracranial vascular malformation and therefore will be elaborated upon. Cushing's operative note during this first operation reveals his desperation and unfamiliarity in dealing with intracranial hemostasis and arteriovenous malformations, respectively.

During the first operation (Patient 4.5), Cushing found further manipulation of this mass risky and a subtemporal decompression was performed. This patient awoke from the anesthetic hemiplegic, aphasic, and underwent a series of "X-ray" treatments. His neurological deficits significantly improved on discharge. He returned to Cushing three years later due to the worsening of his preoperative symptoms. With the introduction of Bovie's electrosurgical instrument in 1926,[5] Cushing was encouraged to attempt a removal of the lesion during a second operation.

Cushing's treatment armamentarium for AVMs mainly comprised of external carotid ligation, decompressive craniectomy, and radiotherapy. He realized the limitations of his surgical techniques: "… half-hearted ligations of a few errant arteries … are probably futile when one realizes, … that one or more large arterial trunks may enter the growth from the depth." Ligations of the external carotids may have reduced flow from the external circulation and decreased blood loss during a decompressive procedure. Craniectomy was believed to facilitate the penetration of radiation as the roentgenologists "were under the impression that the skull might serve as a partially effective filter for the therapeutic rays."[6] The following summarizes Cushing's experience in resection of vascular malformations:

"From our personal experience it is evident: that surgery at its present state of development offers little as a means of controlling one of these lesions in the brain by direct intervention; …"[6]

Aaron A. Cohen-Gadol, M.D., M.Sc.
Indianapolis, IN

Dennis D. Spencer, M.D.
New Haven, CT

Fredric B. Meyer, M.D.
Rochester, MN

References

1. Cooper A: A case of aneurysm of the carotid artery. *Med Chir Trans* 1:1-12, 1809
2. Cushing H: The chiasmal syndrome. *Arch Ophthal Chicago* 3:505-551, 1930
3. Cushing H: Contributions to the clinical study of intracranial aneurysms. *Guy's Hosp Rep* 73:159-163, 1923
4. Cushing H: The control of bleeding in operations for brain tumors. With the description of silver "clips" for the occlusion of vessels inaccessible to the ligature. *Ann Surg* 54:1-19, 1911
5. Cushing H: Electro-surgery as an aid to the removal of intracranial tumors. with a preliminary note on a new surgical-current generator by WT Bovie, PhD, Chicago. *Surg Gynecol Obstet* 47:751-784, 1928
6. Cushing H, Bailey P: *Tumors arising from the blood vessels of the brain.* Springfield, IL: Charles C. Thomas, 1928
7. Dandy W: Arteriovenous aneurysm of the brain. *Arch Surg* 17:190-243, 1928
8. Dandy W: Intracranial aneurysm of the internal carotid artery. *Ann Surg* :654-659, 1938
9. Dott N: Intracranial aneurysms: Cerebral arterio-radiography: surgical treatment. *Edind Med J*: 219-234, 1933
10. Drake CG: Earlier times in aneurysm surgery. *Clin Neurol* 32:41-50, 1985
11. Gaupp J: Casuistische Beitrage zur pathologischen anatomie des ruckenmarks und seiner haute. II. Hemorrhoiden der pia-mater spinalis in gebiete des lendenmarks. *Ziegler's Beitr z. Path Anat u. z. allg Path* 2:515-524, 1888
12. Keen W: Intracranial lesions. *Med News* 57:439-449, 1890
13. Krause F: Krankenvorstellung aus der hirnchrurgie. *Zentralbl fur Chir* 35:61-67, 1908
14. Lippi D: An aneurysm in the Papyrus of Ebers. (108, 3-9). *Med Secoli* 2:1-4, 1990
15. Magnus V: Bidrag til hjernechirurgiens klinik og resultater. Kristiania, 1921. *Trykt i Merkur*: 138, 1921
16. Moniz E: Arterial encephalography, its importance in the localization of cerebral tumors. *Rev Neurol*: 72-89, 1927
17. Pilz C: Zur ligatur de arteria carotis communis, nebst einer statistik dieser operation. *Archiv fur Klinische Chirurgie* 9:257-445, 1868
18. Symonds C: Contributions to the clinical study of intracranial aneurysms. *Guy's Hosp Rep* 72:139-158, 1923
19. Symonds C: Spontaneous subarachnoid hemorrhage. *Q J Med* 18:93-122, 1924
20. Worster-Drought C, Ballance C: Venous angioma of the cerebral cortex. *The Lancet* (London) 203:125-127, 1922

4.1 Aneurysm of the right internal carotid artery

SEX: F; AGE: 58; SURG. NO. 22647

HISTORY

This patient had two episodes of severe right facial pain, sensory loss and weakness associated with diplopia. Seven years prior to admission, the patient had a right neck abscess treated by surgical drainage.

SUMMARY OF POSITIVE FINDINGS
November 21, 1924
Dr. Van Wagenen

OBJECTIVE

1. Paralysis of the right temporal and masseter muscles.
2. Hypesthesia of the right half of tongue.
3. Corneal reflex absent on right with increased lacrimation.
4. Weber's test lateralized more to the left than the right.
5. Paresis of right external rectus with a slight right internal squint.
6. Numerous small, raised, brownish pigmented areas and subcutaneous nodules over lower thorax, both sides, similar to those seen in Von Recklinghausen's disease, duration less than 1 year.
7. BP 150/90.

IMPRESSION: This is quite apparently a tumor involving the 5th, 6th, and 7th nerves, most likely in region of Gasserian ganglion. The pigmented areas in the chest suggest Von Recklinghausen's disease, making one consider this as being the basis of whole complaint and there are palpable nodules on peripheral nerves to be made out over the surface of the chest where the pigmented spots exist.

RADIOLOGY REPORT
November 22, 1924
Dr. Sosman

Right stereoscopic films of the skull show marked

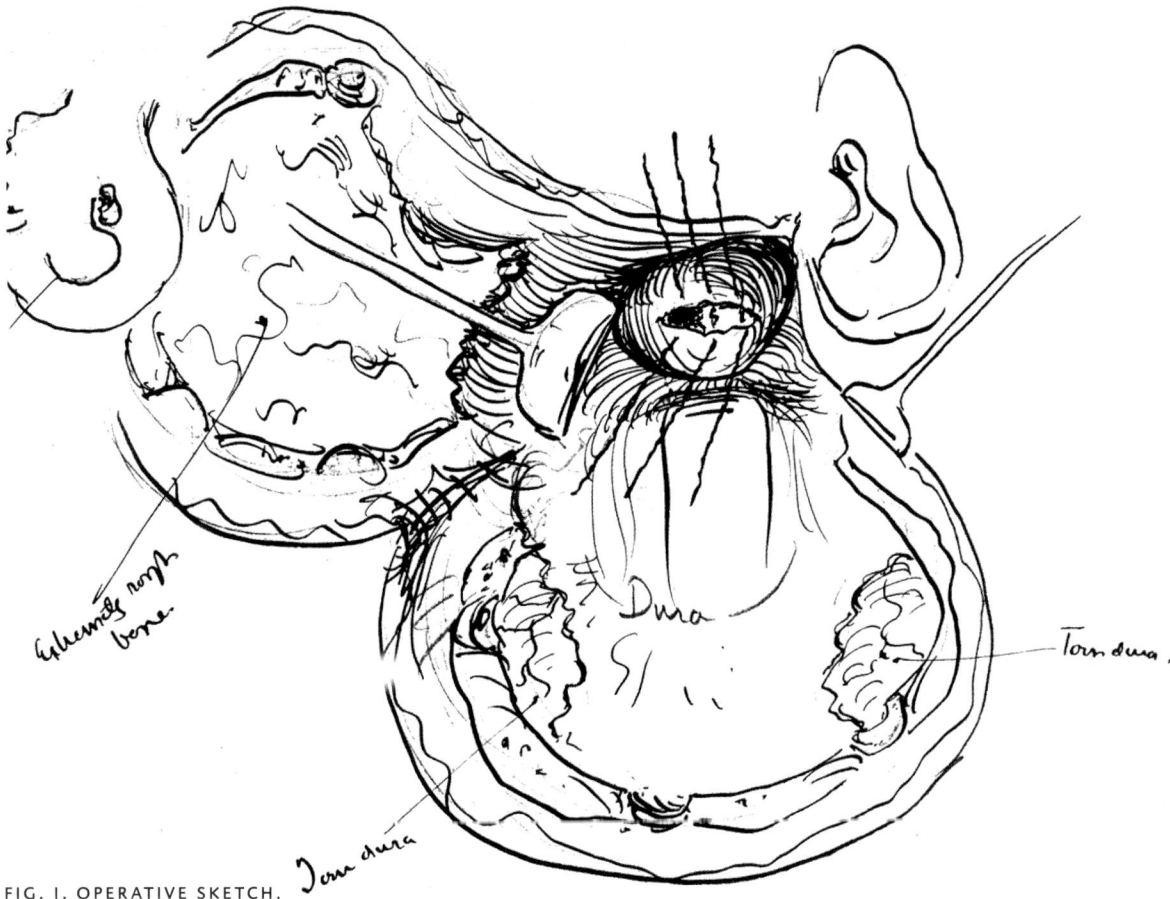

FIG. 1. OPERATIVE SKETCH.

calcification over the frontal region, probably in the meninges and bilateral. The sella is slightly larger than usual and the posterior clinoids are quite irregular and indistinct. The pineal is in the midline. No localizing signs of tumor.

SPECIAL NOTE
December 4, 1924
Dr. Cushing

We had great difficulty in making certain of a diagnosis in this woman's case. I don't know how accurate the history may be in view of the findings, but all that we could learn was that she had had two periods of pain in her right face with gradual loss of sensation in the trigeminal area. So far as I could make out this was slowly progressing lesion and not an acute, sudden one. At this admission she was clearing up from her last attack of pain and there was almost complete loss of sensation in the trigeminal area. Otherwise nothing – no choked discs, no arterio-vascular disorder, no evidence of any intracranial lesion whatever, except a probable involvement of the Gasserian ganglion from some process, that she had a benign tumor, probably a meningioma arising from the trigeminal sheath.

I had no very definite inspiration as to just how I should go about this operation. There were two possible things to do. One, to satisfy myself with the avulsion of the sensory root so as to spare her any further pain in case the tumor was one beyond removal. The other was to make a large exploration and to expose a larger part of the hemisphere so as to prepare the field for tumor extirpation. I rather fell between the two possibilities.

OPERATIVE NOTE
December 4, 1924
Anesthesia – Ether – Miss Way

1. *Exposure of Trigeminal Area by Usual Gasserian Incision.*

2. *Subsequent Osteoplastic Flap with Disclosure of Lesion.*

3. *Ligation of Right Internal Carotid with Treatment of Lesion.*

A large flap was outlined in the right temporal region much larger... that we might have to turn down a bone flap. The lower part of the field alone was incised except for a small opening in the bone over the temporal region. There was great difficulty in separating the dura from the bone. The dura was torn in one place so that I was fearful of causing some damage to the temporal lobe. It was impossible not to cause a good deal of bleeding to get down to the neighborhood of the trigeminus and I only succeeded in exposing the meningeal artery and dividing it between clips and then exposing the third division of the nerve. I was unable to elevate the temporal lobe owing to resistant mass which I thought unquestionably must be meningioma.

Stage 2. In view of the finding it seemed best, in as much as the patient's condition was good, to turn down the flap corresponding with the size of the outlined skin incision. Here I encountered extraordinary difficulty which we perhaps should have foretold by the extraordinary irregularities of the undersurface made plain in the X-ray plates. It was impossible to separate dura without several tears, and finally on elevating the flap and turning it forward as shown in the accompanying sketch, the dura was torn in several places, luckily not injuring the underlying cortex.

With the flap turned forward it was then possible to go down under the temporal lobe and to elevate the dura, getting a wider view than we had in the first stage of the operation. The margin of the flap adherent to the dura was divided and there came into view a rounded, smooth tumor about the size of a pigeon's egg which I thought to be almost certainly meningioma. In further preparing the field and in elevating the dura away from it I found that the tumor was actually extradural, and that what we were peeling away was the dura itself, so that I was aware that we must be confronted with some unusual situation. On further study of this tense tumor it was obvious from the first that it was pulsating and we evidently had exposed the large part of an unusual big aneurysm of the internal carotid, which, as is unusual, did not show in the X-ray plates for there were no lime salts in its capsule.

It possibly would have been best to have withdrawn at this stage, but, having in mind the last of these patients who had come into the hospital with the diagnosis of tumor in this situation which could be seen upon the X-ray plates and after debating the advisability of ligating the internal carotid in the hope that she might escape from any further successive episodes connected with periodical rupture of

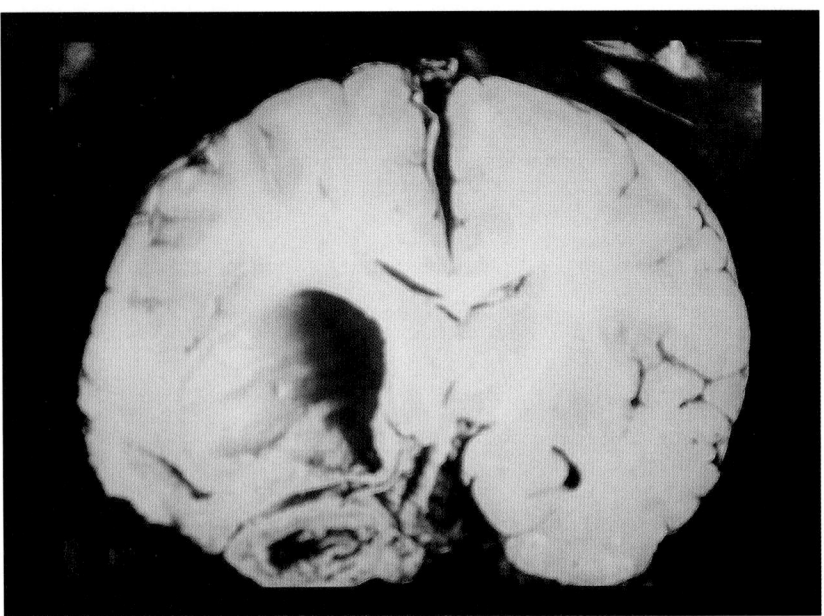

FIG. 2. AUTOPSY SLICE DEMONSTRATING THE SIZE OF THE ANEURYSM.

the aneurysm – I say that in view of this case which we did not treat and which ended in sudden fatality in two to three weeks after leaving the hospital, I thought that I ought to go ahead with this woman and was encouraged to do this by her brother, a doctor who was present at the operation.

Consequently the internal carotid was then exposed and a double ligature thrown around it. While Dr. Bailey held these ligatures it was evident that pulsation in the tumor was greatly lessened, tho not entirely checked by a ligation of the internal carotid. I felt at last that there was sufficiently diminished pulsation to justify making the step I had proposed to make.

It should be stated that before I had been absolutely certain that this was an aneurysm rather than possibly a pulsating vascular meningioma I had made an incision in the cortex and had come down upon the characteristic layers of old blood clots within the capsule of the sac. This incision was possibly 2 cm. in length and before going ahead with the clearing out of the sac I placed a lot of sutures and took a mass of muscle from the sternomastoid muscle in the neck, if by chance we should get into unexpected bleeding difficult to control.

Thus prepared, with a pituitary spoon the contents of the sac were scooped out in great masses and I thought that in the entire sac we were going to find nothing but these layers of coagulated blood which was peeled out like the layers of an onion.

However, after the sac was completely emptied there was a sudden and uncontrollable gush of blood from the lower portion and consequently I inserted the mass of muscle in through the incision and by some pressure wet pledgets implanted on the collapsed sac, and to my great relief the bleeding was thus secured. At this junction the internal carotid was tied and I closed the capsule of the sac to over the muscle implantation. I think it was perhaps a foolish step for in all possibilities it would have been possible to remove the muscle and then to have enfolded the sac as one would do in a aneurysmorrhaphy.

I could not be sure whether the circulation in the hemisphere had been interrupted by this procedure from the appearances of the hemisphere thru the tears in the dura, tho I felt a little dubious about it. It should have been stated that although the patient had shown no elevation in blood pressure before the operation and we did not for a moment suspect that she had any arterio-vascular disease, she showed an enormous high blood pressure as soon as she took the ether, the pressure running about 260 all thru the operation with a pulse of well over 100. So soon as the operation was completed and ether was withdrawn an extraordinary fall in this pressure level took place as shown by the ether chart.

The flap was replaced and closed carefully in layers. The patient made a slow recovery from her anaesthetic which was perhaps natural as the operation was a long one – 4-5 hour procedure. There was a left hemiplegia, and I am told at this writing (24 hours later) that this is very evident, tho she has had some movement in her left arm.

(Dr. Cushing)

DISCHARGE NOTE
January 29, 1925

The patient was in the hospital for 69 days. She was discharged with a left-sided hemiparesis. Her preoperative symptoms were unchanged.

FOLLOW-UP NOTE

The patient died on June 17, 1925 (Phone call.)

4.2 Aneurysm of the internal carotid artery

SEX: F; AGE: 52; SURG. NO. 26733

HISTORY

This patient came to Boston from Buffalo after a year and half of unsuccessful treatment for her gradual diminution of vision.

SUMMARY OF POSITIVE FINDINGS
July 10, 1926
Dr. Morelle

SUBJECTIVE
1. Gradual loss of vision in the right eye for 1½ years.
2. Impairment of vision in the left eye for 4 months.
3. Impossibility of reading for the past 3 months.
4. Appearance of tingling sensation in both arms for last 2 months.

OBJECTIVE
1. Bilateral primary atrophy, more pronounced in the right eye.
2. Bitemporal hemianopsia.

IMPRESSION: Suprasellar tumor.

RADIOLOGY REPORT
July 12, 1926

Right stereo and P.A. films show a porous cranial vault without localized changes. The pituitary fossa is not enlarged but it appears atrophic, and the anterior clinoids appear eroded. The pineal is close to the mid-line and is not measurably displaced. Impression-appearance is compatible with a supra-sellar meningioma.

SPECIAL NOTE
July 17, 1926
Dr. Cushing

This is the first time that I have ever exposed at operation a parasellar aneurysm of the internal carotid tho I have long expected to do so as in this case, with a syndrome such as this woman presented. The essentials of the case are a middle aged patient becoming blind from primary atrophy, showing field defects evidently due to a tumor of some sort in the chiasmal region and a normal or approximately normal sella.

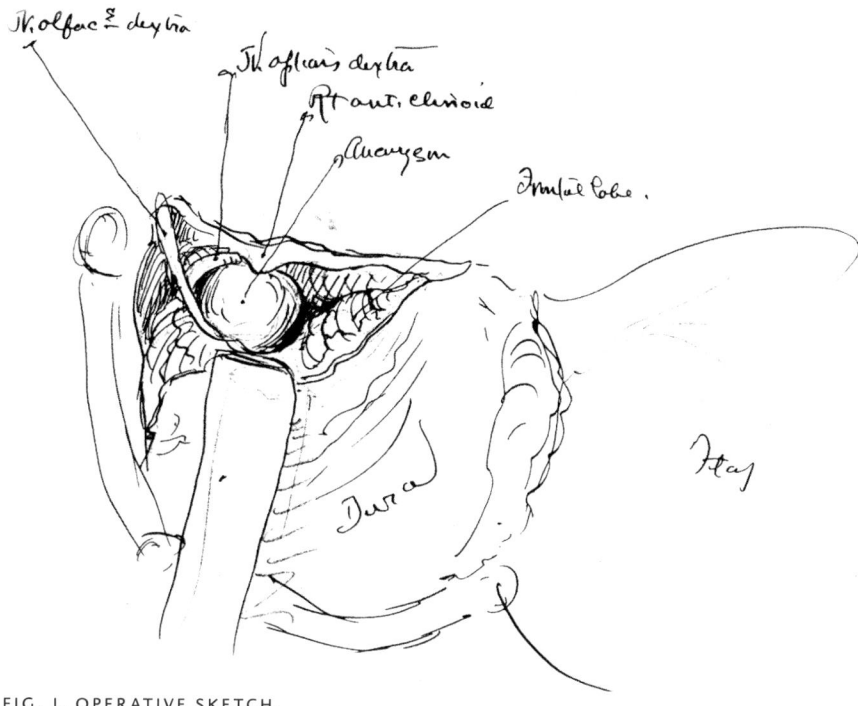

FIG. I. OPERATIVE SKETCH.

In this case the anterior clinoid showed a good deal of pressure absorption and we were led to favor a suprasellar meningioma which after all is the most common lesion giving this syndrome in patients past middle life.

In view of the disclosure of a tumor to the right side of the chiasm pushing the right optic nerve far off to the left as I had never before seen it pushed by a tumor in this region, I should feel that she almost certainly must have had a left homonymous hemianopsia and regret that someone with a little more experience with the perimetry had not taken her fields before the operation. However, two independent observers had agreed on there being evidence of bitemporal hemianopsia and on these observations the case must rest unless this can be corroborated by subsequent fields.

OPERATIVE NOTE
July 17, 1926
Anesthesia – Ether – Miss Mellanson

Right Transfrontal Exploration for Presumed Suprasellar Meningioma – Disclosure of Saccular Aneurysm – Puncture of Aneurysm for Verification – Closure.

This was a fairly easy transfrontal operation in spite of a rather thick bone and rather adherent dura. Fortunately the flap was elevated without a tear in the mucous membrane which was found free from tension.

The dura was elevated as usual from the orbit and an incision made along the sphenoidal ridge as usual. I elevated the frontal lobe and condition of things shown in the accompanying sketch was found. The right optic nerve was pushed far to the left ... On exposing its surface there was nothing to indicate anything other than it might have been a pharyngeal pouch cyst and had I not had a perfectly good view of it and been unfamiliar with the pharyngeal pouch cyst in this situation I might well I think have punctured it with a large needle in the expectation of emptying it.

However pressure with a blunt instrument against the structure showed that it had a very definite heave and I wish that I might have listened to it with the stethoscope but I can hardly believe that there is a bruit. Even so I did not feel absolutely certain that we might not have a sort of pulsating kind of tumor or that the pulsation which I detected might not have been transmitted.

Consequently a fine Gentile needle was inserted into the tumor and pure blood came from its lumen. On withdrawing the needle there was a spurt of blood well out into the wound and I feared for a moment that we might have difficulty in checking it. Fortunately I had taken a snip of muscle from the temporal region in anticipation of bleeding and this was planted on the bleeding point so far as I could place it and then held in position by cotton pledgets for 10 or 15 minutes. Bleeding was checked and there had fortunately been no soiling or extravasation of blood thru the meninges.

I finally removed with great care individual pledgets and the muscle floated off afterward, leaving the aneurismal wall perfectly dry and without further bleeding. **Nevertheless I attempted to permanently implant a piece of muscle over what may be a weakened spot and after filling the cavity with salt solution replaced the bone flap and withdrew in the usual fashion.**

A large part of the closure was done by Dr. Horrax.
(Dr. Cushing)

POSTOPERATIVE NOTES

July 18, 1926
Dr. Morelle

Patient stood the operation very well and is in good condition.

July 19, 1926
Dr. Morelle

Edema of eyelids on both sides. Patient feels comfortable.

Sutures cut but left in place. Wound in good condition. No elevation of the flap. Crinoline dressing re-applied.

July 31, 1926
Dr. Schaltenbrand

Visual fields did not change very much since July 16 and 12.

DISCHARGE NOTE

August 6, 1926
Dr. Schaltenbrand

Patient feels comfortable. Discharged in good condition.

FOLLOW-UP NOTE

The last letter from this patient was from June 15, 1929. The letter was not available in the chart.

4.3 Congenital aneurysm of the right temporal lobe

SEX: F; AGE: 10; SURG. NO. 28235

HISTORY

This child had a history of progressive weakness of left upper and lower extremities and visual changes for approximately two years prior to admission.

SUMMARY OF POSITIVE FINDINGS
February 17, 1927
Dr. Cairns

SUBJECTIVE
1. Left hemiparesis coming on quite suddenly in Jan. 1925; that is two years ago. It has persisted ever since; according to Dr. Schwab it has progressed but the parent does not confirm this.
2. Left hemi-hypaesthesia, probably for a similar period.
3. Left hemianopsia noticed first 9-10 months ago, apparently has gradually progressed.
4. Headaches. Slight right frontal headaches for the last 3 weeks occasionally.
5. Vomiting once 5 days ago.
6. The child is said to be very nervous.

OBJECTIVE
1. Left homonymous hemianopsia with splitting of macula.
2. Left hemiparesis, flaccid in type. The weakness concerns particularly the fine movements rather than the coarse movements.

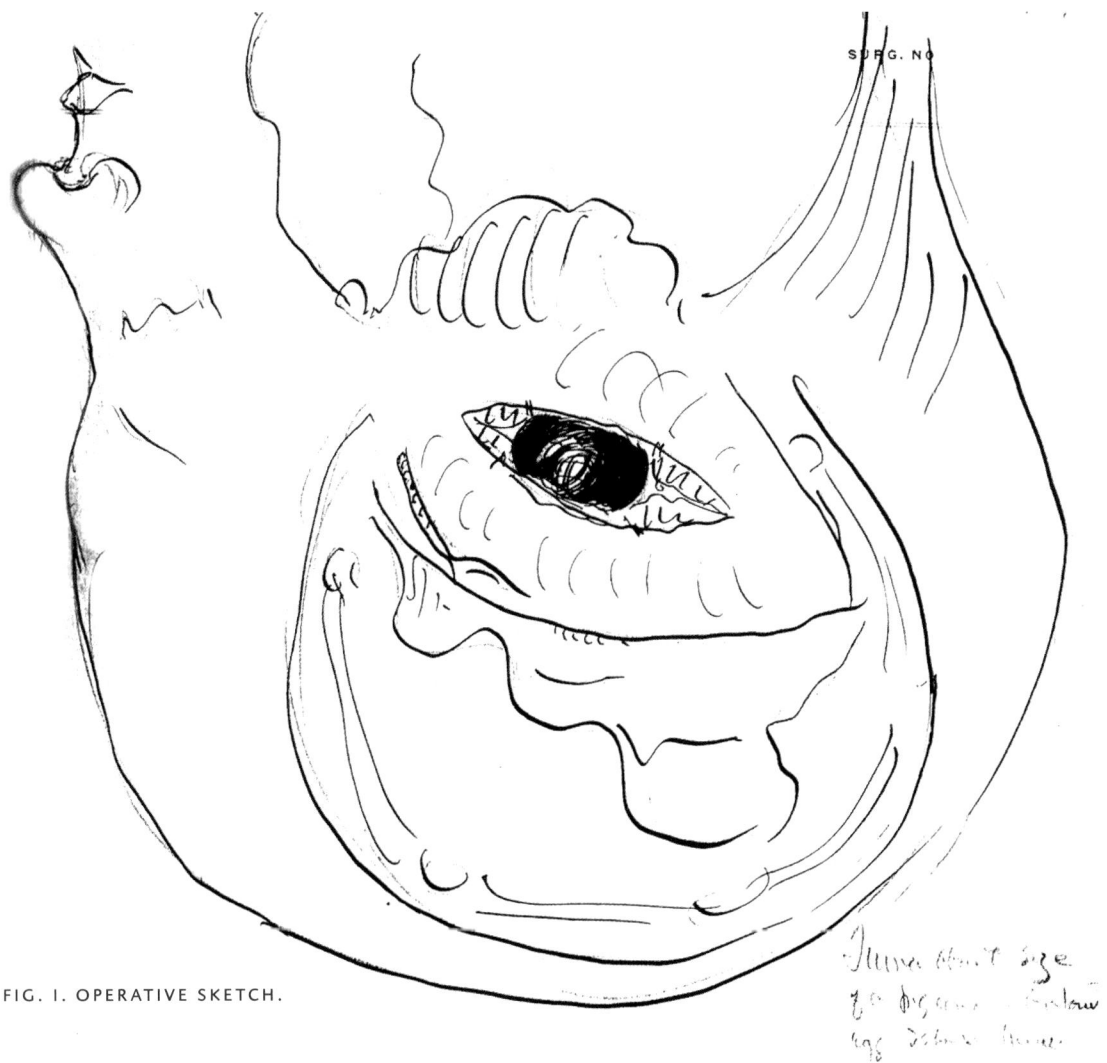

FIG. I. OPERATIVE SKETCH.

With it there is diminution of the abdominal reflexes on the left side, and a left Babinski. Also slight increase of the tendon jerks.

3. Diminished sensation of pin prick on the left side.
4. Very doubtful primary optic atrophy in the left eye. The left pupil reacts sluggishly to light and is larger than the right.
5. Nystagmus on lateral movements of the eye.

IMPRESSION: This is a progressive lesion of the right hemisphere and evidently therefore tumor. From the suddenness with which it produced left hemiparesis it is almost certainly deep seated. Deep seated glioma. Right parieto-temporal region.

SPECIAL NOTE
March 5, 1927
Dr. Cushing

This little girl was a great puzzle to us until ventriculograms disclosed what was unmistakably a tumor of some sort in the right temporal lobe. I felt that this tumor must certainly be very deep to have given the pyramidal tract symptoms, but still in certain examples particularly of large neuroblastomas the tumor has extended deeply into the brain and actually caused pressure against the brain stem.

Thinking from the X-ray that the case must be tumor I inquired more fully into the antecedent part of the history and the child remembered distinctly having been troubled by headaches before the onset of the hemiplegia, they being severe enough to have caused her mother to take her to an ophthalmologist who prescribed glasses.

I do not believe any of us had the slightest intimation that this might be aneurysm, nor do I believe that the skull was ausculted. The child certainly never complained of whizzing sounds in her head and this has better be inquired into should she recover.

We were impelled to discount the aortic lesion and whether it has any bearing upon the production of the aneurysm which might conceivably be a congenital aneurysm, it is difficult to tell. I understood Dr. Levine's note to imply that this was a congenital lesion of the aortic orifice without significance. The temporal lesion was undoubtedly thin to palpation. Cranial tabes might easily enough have been observed as the operation disclosed. There was tenderness all over the right temporal fossa and there was, I thought, some little bulging there.

OPERATIVE NOTE
March 5, 1927
Anesthesia – Novocain; Ether - Miss Melanson

Right Osteoplastic Exploration with Subtemporal Decompression. Disclosure of Bulging Temporal Lobe. Needle Introduced into Lobe Met a Resistance at a Depth of about 2 cm. Fortunately it was not Pushed Farther to see Whether It Was Cyst. Incision of Temporal Lobe Disclosing Aneurysm; Verified by Puncture. **Several Strands of Muscle from Another Case were Pushed into the Sac Hoping to Encourage Coagulation. Muscle Stamp. Closure of Wound.**

I have not encountered an aneurysm since the case of Mrs. (the name of another patient) operated upon with the expectation of finding a suprasellar meningioma. In that case I succeeded in stopping bleeding after puncture of the aneurysm, and the case according to subsequent symptoms may possibly have coagulated. In this case we went further as will be told.

Flap was turned down without difficulty, the bone being very thin particularly in the temporal region where it was so rubbery that it nearly bent over without fracture. Anticipating a large glioma I made a generous subtemporal decompression. The dura was incised and reflected upward as shown in the accompanying sketch and to my great surprise I found a fairly wet brain but an unmistakably bulging temporal lobe, the convolutions of which were somewhat flattened. The sylvian vessels and fissure were markedly dislocated upward.

Palpation of the lobe showed it to be distinctly firm.

I then punctured in two directions and posteriorly came down upon a resistant mass at about a depth of 4 cm. Anteriorly, I struck the same resistant mass at a depth of about 2 cm. I thought that possibly we were going to find a solid tumor, perhaps a congenital tumor.

An incision was then made down through the cortex and for a time I thought that I might be in a glioma owing to the passing in the procedure in the incision through a broad strip of gray cortex. However I proceeded through this, and finally came down upon a perfectly smooth surface of a dark colored tumor, the surface resembling very closely that of a thin dura.

I could not make out that this was definitely pulsating apart from the pulsations of the brain and consequently I made a small nick in the membrane which did not bleed and then inserted a needle through what must evidently have been a thin layer of lamellated clot, and found that I was in the center of aneurysm. Blood spurted from the end of the needle. The needle was then withdrawn and holding the sucker in the neighborhood of the opening which was bleeding profusely I made use of a but of muscle which fortunately was at hand to plant it over the opening. Bleeding promptly stopped and I found I could remove the muscle.

I was then at a loss to know what further to do. I of course did not know where the aneurysm originated but presumed it must be from one of the Willisian branches. The circulation of the temporal lobe and the sylvian veins I should add were perfectly normal although to be sure I had not exposed the motor area and it is conceivable that there may have been some degeneration there, but I doubt this.

Having used the ordinary brain needle for the puncture I thought I might possibly take some strips of the muscle which I had at hand and insert them through the opening with the aid of Mayo plunger of the needle. This I found was an extremely simple procedure, and I put in several strands of muscle into the cavity amounting all told I should think to a strip 4–5 cm in length and possibly 3–4 mm in diameter.

I then put over the opening a small bit of muscle to check bleeding. The wound was then closed in layers without a drain.

(Dr. Cushing)

SPECIAL NOTE
March 13, 1927
Dr. Cushing

This child has done surprisingly well from her operation but we have observed since the aneurysm was disclosed that she has a systolic bruit, heard pretty well over the whole left side of the head perhaps particularly marked just above the mastoid and also over the site of the decompression on the right side. The decompression seems somewhat full and is pulsating as though the aneurysm was almost under the surface.

The child was interested in listening with a stethoscope not only to her heart but also to this bruit and she was then conscious of the fact that this was the sound she had been hearing for no-one knows how long, and that she regarded it as nothing abnormal. **Dr. Cairns adds that the child says she used to count herself to sleep by it.**

Evidently the insertion of the muscle has not served to cause, at least as yet, clotting in the aneurysm, and it has not been possible by compression of the jugular against the carotid tubercle to put a complete stop to the bruit largely because the vessel tends to slide off the tubercle and cannot easily hold, and partly because the child objects to the pressure.

Inspite of this fact I felt that occlusion of the vessel would be a timely procedure and regretted not having occluded it at the time of her operation since the aneurysm was disclosed.

OPERATIVE NOTE
March 13, 1927
Anesthesia – Novocain

Banding of Right Common Carotid.

This was a somewhat awkwardly done procedure. I hoped I might avoid a scar by making a transverse incision in a fold of one of the creases in the neck. Consequently I did not get a very easy exposure of the artery. When it was exposed it proved to be of unexpectedly large size so that the primary band which was put upon it was not broad enough to hold the vessel.

What is more, somewhat to my dismay, Dr. Cairns who was listening during this procedure to the subtemporal decompression stated that the bruit which had been for the last day or two somewhat indistinct was increased in its intensity. This I could not account for nor can I now account for it, and perhaps it was foolish to have persisted with the operation and have completed the occlusion of the vessel.

Vessel was then slipped out of the primarily placed band and a broader one put upon the vessel (and I am speaking of the Matas aluminum band) and was closed down, cut, and infolded and dropped in place. So far as could be told at the time, and so far as subsequent events show, this procedure had no influence whatever on the bruit or pulsation of the aneurysm.

During the preceding week and subsequently, the child insisted that she had much better use of her arm and hand than previously but whether this was purely a subjective impression on the child's part I could not be quite sure. Her father, however, seemed to think that she used her hand much better.

(Dr. Cushing)

RADIOLOGY REPORT
March 25, 1927
Dr. Sosman

Fluoroscopy showed the aorta smooth in outline as far as seen, with no narrowing at the isthmus. No evidence of any congenital lesion of heart or aorta.

DISCHARGE NOTE
March 26, 1927
Dr. Cairns

The patient has done very well. Her wounds in the neck and in the head have healed perfectly. The bone flap is absolutely flush with the rest of her skull. The decompression, though slightly firm, is not bulging.

The bruit is still the same as it was after ligation of the common carotid. It is heard all over the skull and is conducted down onto the neck and onto the face. It is heard best immediately behind the posterior leg of the craniotomy. The child herself now says that she has heard this noise in her head for as long as she can remember. She said that she used to count herself to sleep with them at night, but she never thought this was anything out of the ordinary so she did not tell her father.

Eyes – Vision is unchanged being still slightly diminished in the left eye. The fields show no change nor do the fundi in which the temporal half of the left disc still shows a rather abnormal pallor suggestive of a slight degree of optic atrophy.

Hemiparesis – The child states that there is a definite improvement in the movements of the left hand. She says that she can make believe at playing the piano much better than she used to do. Her nurse who was with her for some time before the operation states that she thinks there is an improvement. The patient does much more with her left hand than she did before operation. This improvement if such it be, is too slight for me to pronounce upon, objectively. One point of significance which was perhaps rather under emphasized hitherto is the fact that the left arm is definitely shorter than the right and the left hand definitely smaller than the right. This suggests that the hemiparesis was of long standing and points as does the child's statement about the constancy of the bruit to a congenital origin of the aneurysm.

She still has fine nystagmus on looking to the right or left. The left pupil is slightly larger than the right and reacts a little sluggishly to light.

Photographs have been taken.

FOLLOW-UP NOTE

The last letter received from the patient was dated September 16, 1932. The letter was not included in the chart.

4.4 Anterior cerebral artery aneurysm

SEX: M; AGE: 32; SURG. NO. 36214

HISTORY

There was a history of headaches since December of 1929 possibly related to frontal sinusitis, treated by an operation in January of 1930. The patient complained of dizziness and blurred vision for the last 2-3 months.

SUMMARY OF POSITIVE FINDINGS
April 11, 1930
Dr. Oldberg

SUBJECTIVE

1. History of frequent, rather severe frontal headache, located just to the left side, beginning 3½ months ago and being unassociated with nausea or vomiting.
2. Mental aberration beginning immediately after operation, supposed on the patient's sinuses, being most intense at that time and having gradually disappeared.
3. History of generalized weakness of 3 months' duration.

OBJECTIVE

1. Mental aberration, manifesting itself chiefly in lack of memory and unreliability of statements.
2. Bilateral early choked disc without measurable elevation.
3. Right lower facial weakness of central type.
4. Diminished deep reflexes.

IMPRESSION: Ventriculograms indicated. Possibly a deep left fronto-temporal tumor.

RADIOLOGY REPORT
April 11, 1930
Dr. Sosman

Left stereo, A.P. and P.A. of skull show a thin vault without localized changes or signs of pressure. The sella is normal. The mastoids are clear. The pineal shadow is not visible on the A.P. view. By measurements, the pineal is at the upper limits of normal, not displaced in the antero-posterior diameter.

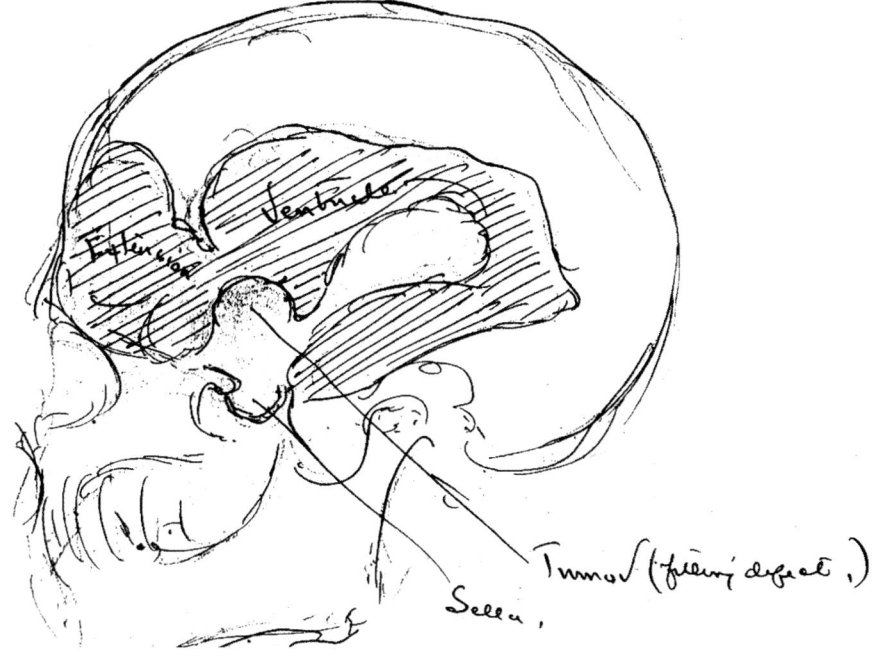

FIG. 1. OPERATIVE SKETCH 1.

OPERATIVE NOTE
April 16, 1930
Anesthesia – Novocain – Miss Geizer

Right Ventriculogram

Patient was placed upon the table, prepared in the usual fashion and an area in the right posterior parietal region which had been infiltrated with Novocain, was incised. Skull of average thickness, was burred without encountering undue vascularity, and dura split. A thickened, bluish-arachnoid bulged somewhat into the burr opening and in order to get a somewhat better exposure, a small amount of bone was rongeured away from the medial edge of the burr hole for a distance of possibly half a cm. The thickened, tough arachnoid was than pricked, and a ventricular needle was inserted in the usual direction. At a depth of about 4 cm., needle plunged into ventricle and clear, colorless spinal fluid began to escape under moderately increased initial pressure. Fluid air interchange was then begun until 150 cc. of perfectly clear, colorless spinal fluid had been withdrawn and had been replaced by approximately 130 cc of air. Rotation of the head during this procedure gave one the impression of there being a free passage of air from one ventricle to the other. Wound was closed in the usual fashion with fine silk and was silvered and collodion dressed. Patient, who stood the operation well, except for one or two emotional outbursts, was then taken to X-ray.

(Dr. Oldberg)

RADIOLOGY REPORT
April 16, 1930
Dr. Sosman

Ventriculograms show marked dilation of the ventricles, including the third ventricle. They are not displaced or deformed by external pressure. There is a large irregular collection of air in the right frontal region communicating with the anterior horn of the ventricle thru a wide opening, and apparently reaching the skull wall anteriorly and inferiorly. There is no evidence of osteoma or of tumor in frontal or ethmoid sinuses. The left anterior horn appears normal except for their dilatation.

SPECIAL NOTE
April 16, 1930
Dr. Cushing

We had looked over this man yesterday afternoon and he had very little to show for what this morning's ventriculogram and exploration disclosed. There was a low grade of choked disc with no field defect. He had an apparent weakness of his lower right face and it was stated that he had once had some aphasia. He spoke Italian but Dr. DeCoppet could not make out that he had any defective speech nor from such English that he spoke could I make out that there was any anomia. Nevertheless I suspected that there might possibly be a left temporal tumor and to make certain of our ground it seemed advisable to make ventricular studies.

OPERATIVE NOTE
April 16, 1930
Ventriculography

A tap was made as usual in the right ventricle. Both ventricles were found to be widely dilated but on the right side there was a most extraordinary exclusion of the right ventricle into the anterior pole of the right frontal lobe. On examining the wet plates, as in Sketch I (Please see the operative sketch I), there is a rough indication of what the left lateral stereogram showed. Bulging up above the sella was what I took to be an evident filling defect and that probably this represented the lesion and that it was perhaps to be a 3rd ventricle lesion. I did not suspect for a moment an aneurysm. There was no bruit, blood pressure was low and the patient had no evidence of artero-sclerosis. I assume that his Wassermann was negative.

(Dr. Cushing)

OPERATIVE NOTE
April 16, 1930
Anesthesia-Novocain

Right Fronto-Central Flap of (the name of another patient)'s Type-Subtemporal Decompression—Exceedingly Vascular Dura-Markedly Bulging Hemisphere with Thickened Arachnoid—Puncture of Ventricle, Releasing Air—Transcortical Frontal Incision, Disclosing Huge Cavity Lined by Normal Appearing White Matter- Reddish Tumor, the Size of a Plum in the Base—Puncture of Tumor, Supposedly Aneurysm without Bleeding—Foramen of Monro Adjacent and Tumor had Communication Between Frontal Cavity and Right Lateral Ventricle. Muscle Inserted into Cavity of Aneurysm. (Muscle taken from patient's leg). Closure with Drain.

The patient had become so uncooperative and so unruly after the ventriculogram that ether was necessary at the outset. Dr. Horrax had turned down a generous flap on reflection of which there was profuse bleeding from the dura. It was at this juncture that I took over the operation and made an incision thru the dura along the lower frontal margin of the exposed field. The brain bulged markedly thru this opening. I finally put a needle into it and released a great deal of air, but nevertheless continued full.

It was evident that we were going to meet tension and I then proceeded to make a fairly generous subtemporal decompression and the dural incision was carried down into the temporal region, disclosing a large bundle of about 6 sylvian vessels, as shown in Sketch II (Please see the operative sketch II.)

During all of this time there was continued troublesome bleeding from the surface of the dura and consequently it was reflected upward, as shown in Sketch II and I managed to get some of the large bleeding dural veins by sutures. It was evident that there was going to be troublesome bleed-

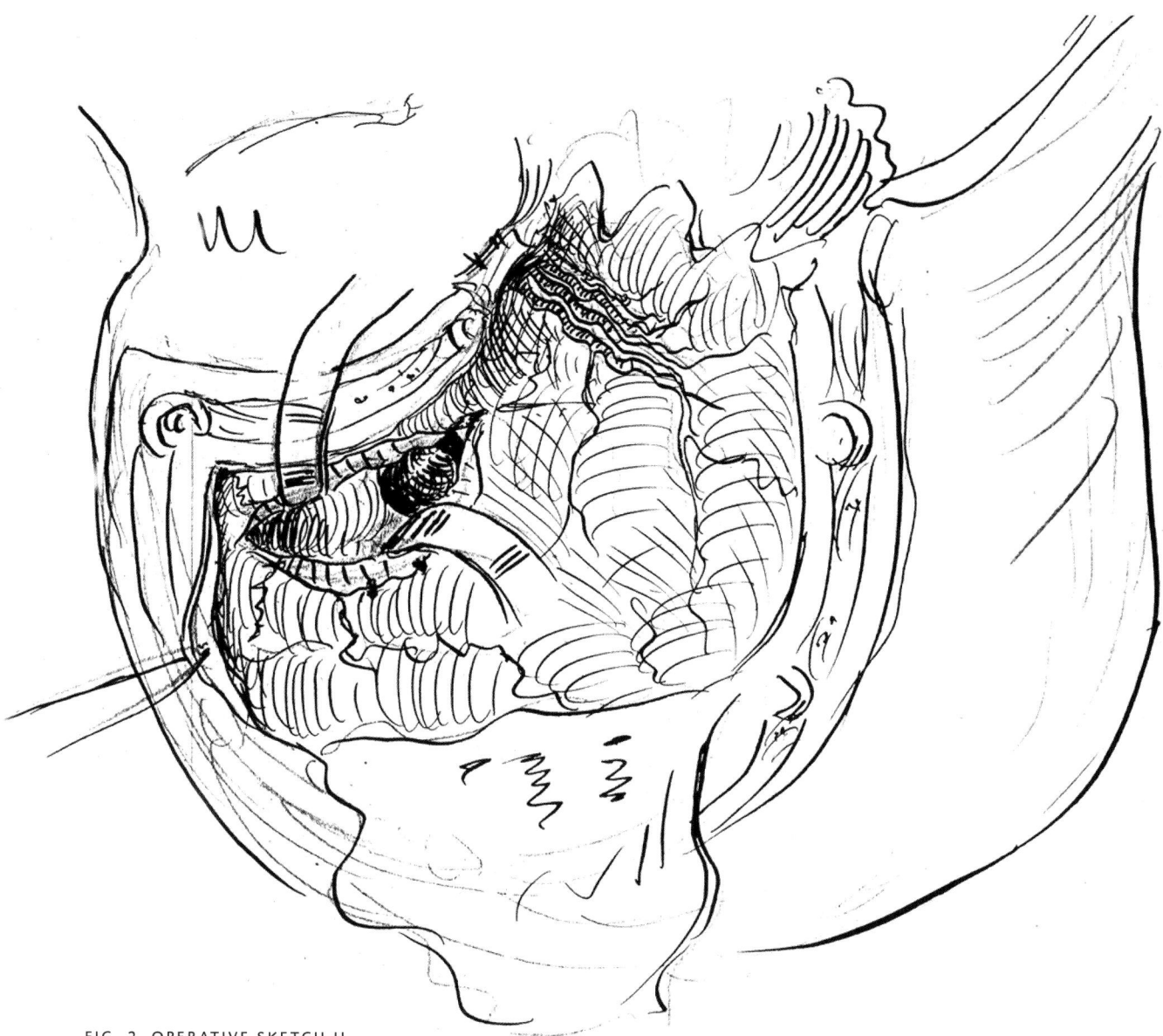

FIG. 2. OPERATIVE SKETCH II.

ing and Dr. Horrax came in and took some muscle from the patient's leg.

I then made an electrical incision thru the cortex, in the position shown in the sketch, and got into a huge cavity, exactly like the aerocele in the case of (the name of another patient). The cavity was not lined much by membrane, merely by smooth white matter with the exact appearance of the tissue on the inside of the ventricle. Whether it was lined by ependyma I should doubt very little.

By holding the walls, as shown in Sketch II, I could see a plum-colored, purplish tumor, projecting into the cavity well down toward the region of the sella turcica. This tumor or whatever it might be was absolutely uncovered by any membrane or by nervous tissue. The appearance was a most extraordinary one. The tumor was visibly pulsating but still the whole brain was slightly pulsating. It moreover was firm on pressure and it had all the appearance of enucleability. I began brushing the brain away from it until it was laid bare well down to its middle circumference.

There was little question but that from its situation and from its appearance the tumor was an aneurysm. Dr. Wolbach was called in and had a good chance to look at it and he thought unmistakably it must be an aneurysm.

Being certain of this I prepared to pack around the tumor, to put a lumbar puncture needle into it, and as I was sure of meeting with a sharp gush of

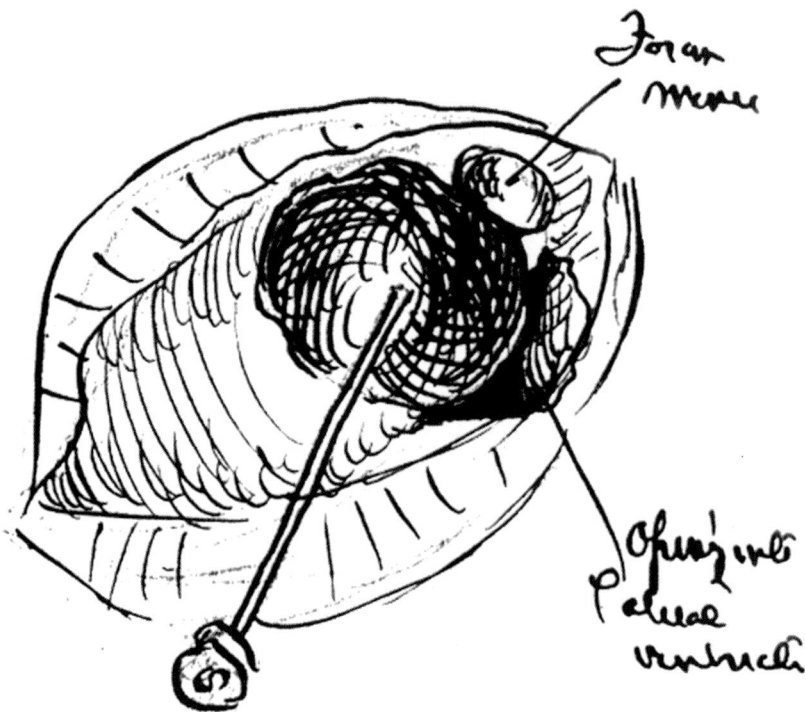

FIG. 3. OPERATIVE SKETCH III.

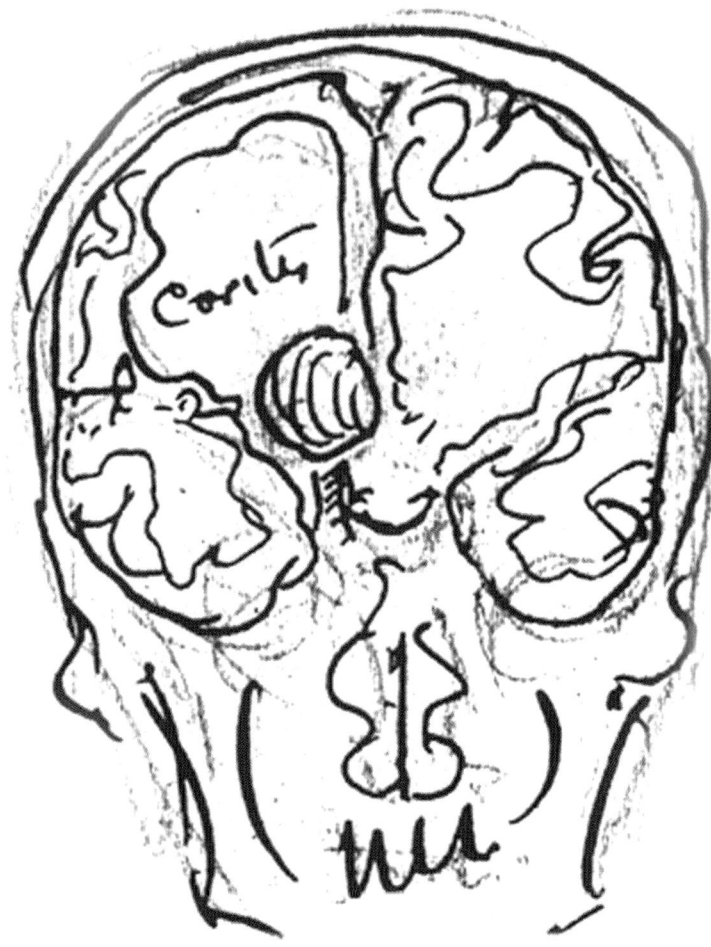

FIG. 3. OPERATIVE SKETCH IV.

blood I was ready with muscle to cover the opening or to insert into the opening. No bleeding, however, was encountered.

Thru the opening made I then inserted a strip of muscle to plug up the hole from the inside.

In order to make sure of the situation of the lesion since the brain was completely collapsed I looked in under the frontal lobe, saw the anterior nerves, exposed the right optic nerve, stripped the tough arachnoid away from it and then had the carotid artery exposed. On then looking into the cavity of the frontal lobe at the tumor with this thin part of cortex between me and the exposed carotid, it was evident that tumor lay just above the carotid artery-unquestionably, I think, tumor of the anterior cerebral branch.

It was quite possible that this growth might have been excavated and that I might have caught the anterior cerebral artery but the chances are that it came off so near the growth that I almost certainly would have gotten into difficulties. I suppose that I might have ligated the carotid itself but this did not seem to me to be really a justifiable procedure as I might very possibly have gotten a hemiplegia.

On turning to the aneurysm itself and investigating it still further I could demonstrate to Dr. Wolbach a widely dilated foramen of Monro to its inner side, as shown in Sketch III (Please see the operative sketch III) and also a large opening into the hugely dilated ventricle to the outer side and above-that is above, in speaking in terms of the top of the patient's head.

After irrigating the walls of the cavity with salt solution, the dura was resutured in place, muscle implants were made over the bleeding dura and the flap was then replaced and closed securely in layers, the last part by Dr. Oldberg.

(Dr. Cushing)

DISCHARGE NOTE
May 5, 1930

The patient was discharged "improved."

FOLLOW-UP NOTE

This patient died on August 10, 1939 at the Westborough State Hospital. "Reported by the pathologist there." No information was attached in the chart.

4.5 Angioma of left hemisphere

SEX: M; AGE: 64; SURG. NO. 20504; 28283

HISTORY

Long-standing history of generalized convulsions.

SUMMARY OF POSITIVE FINDINGS
January 11, 1924
Dr. Putman

SUBJECTIVE

1. Generalized convulsion beginning in right arm, with loss of consciousness beginning at the age 18, possibly following an injury.
2. Disappearance of convulsive attacks with loss of consciousness and instead nocturnal attacks with incontinence of urine from age of about 20 until 2 years ago.
3. During past two years many similar convulsive attacks, sometimes associated with numbness of fingers of the right hand, and epileptic absences, during which he was able to walk about and perform certain attacks without retaining consciousness.
4. Definite loss of memory, euphoria, and inadequate emotional reaction for at least a year.
5. Blood and spinal fluid Wassermann taken in N.Y., negative.

OBJECTIVE

1. Very marked euphoria, expansiveness, and memory defect. Slight speech defect.
2. Tenderness over left fronto-parietal region.
3. Slight fullness of disc and retinal veins.
4. Right foot slightly more clumsy than left.

IMPRESSION: Left fronto-temporal endothelioma.

RADIOLOGY REPORT
January 12, 1924
Dr. Sosman

Findings indicate a good-sized tumor on the left, either a large glioma reaching the surface, or endothelioma dipping rather deeply into brain.

SPECIAL NOTE
January 17, 1924
Dr. Cushing

This proved to be a very desperate operation. Had it not been for the fact that an amputation of the

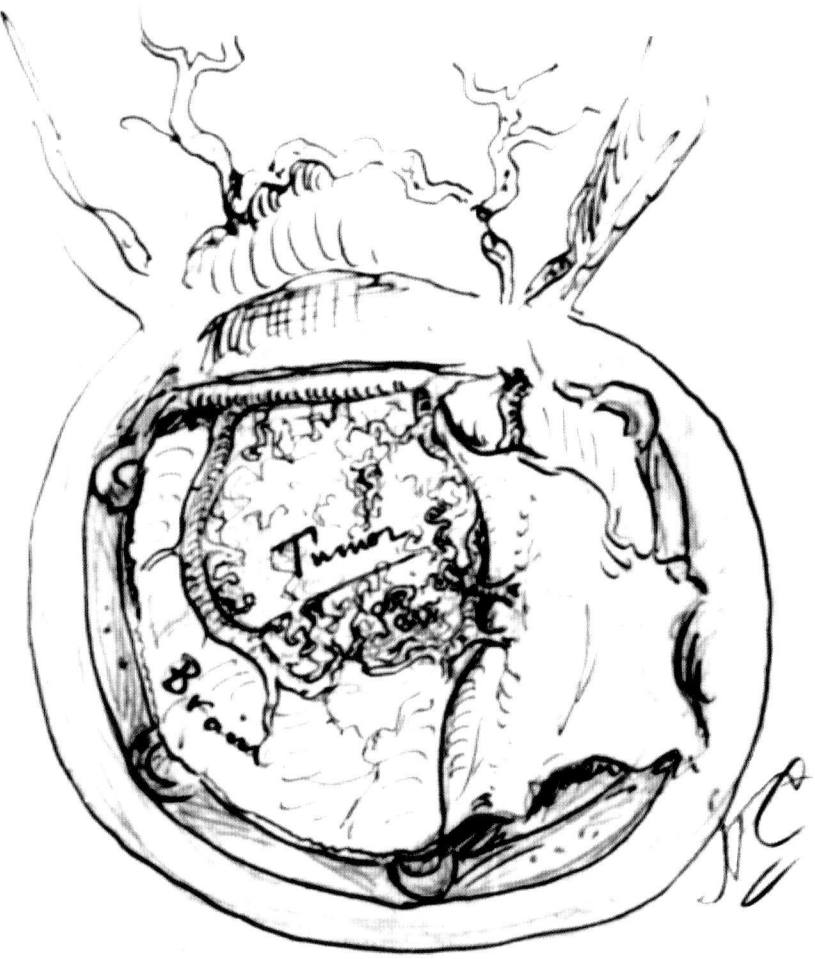

FIG. I. OPERATIVE SKETCH – FIRST OPERATION.

leg had just been done in the other room, so that we had plenty of muscle at hand and had we not been ready for a refusion of blood I am quite sure that this man would never have left the table. Whether we ought to have foretold the nature of this tumor, I do not know, but I assumed from the X-rays that it was in all probability a meningioma in which there was an abundance of psammoma bodies.

OPERATIVE NOTE
January 17, 1924
Anesthesia – Ether – Miss Gerrard

Osteoplastic Flap to Disclose Tumor of Left Hemisphere.

There was a good deal of difficulty encountered from the first owing to bleeding in the bone, some of the burr holes spurting in such a way that they were difficult to control with wax.

In passing a guide for the Gigli saw I was a little dubious in regards to the separation of the dura and on one occasion the guide had evidently passed in between two layers of what was a very thin and easily friable dura. At the upper part of the field indeed I was so doubtful that the saw was used to divide the bone which was then cracked with a blow of the mallet and chisel.

The flap was then elevated and turned back, profuse bleeding following this procedure. The dura had in large part come away with the bone flap. Fortunately, however, not in its entirety for had this been the case we would almost certainly have had a fatal hemorrhage because from the surface of the tumor there were a number of big arterial branches which connected tumor with the dura. A glance at the inner surface of the reflected bone showed the outer layer of dura densely adherent to it had come away with the bone and the dura had been torn in elevating the flap on the side of the posterior part of the wound almost all the way around.

The surface of the remaining portion was bleeding and spurting and finally with the placement of great masses of muscle I succeeded in checking the bleeding points and covered it with masses of cotton.

The blood pressure, as shown in the chart, had dropped down almost to nothing but fortunately a large amount of blood had been gathered in by Dr. Putman during this time and patient was immediately refused by Dr. Davis, the blood pressure picking up so that it was possible finally to remove most of the muscle implantations and to get a good view of the field. By good fortune there had been no damage to the cortex in all this procedure and by still greater good fortune there was no tension due to tumor, otherwise we might have had a very desperate situation. On finally, reflecting the dura which was covered by huge branches of a greatly dilated meningeal it was found that some of these branches passed directly from the dura into the tumor and thinking that it might still be possible to in some way enucleate this bloody growth, one of these vessels was doubly clipped and divided but there proved to be half a dozen of them, some with such short stems that I did not feel justified in pursuing this procedure further. The tumor itself which was hard in consistency and measuring about 5 cm on the surface, lay in the middle of the field, perhaps a little lower than I had expected and just above what must have been the Sylvian fissure. At its lower margin was an enormous artery about the size of a lead pencil which sent off a branch embracing the tumor in the posterior part of its exposed surface. From this large branch countless smaller branches passed on the surface of the tumor which was more tangle of small pulsating arterioles. The tumor felt firm in consistency and doubtless was enucleable but in all certainly had throughout its circumference similar vascular attachments and it would have been foolhardy to attempt its enucleation.

A partial subtemporal decompression was made corresponding about to the situation of the tumor. The dura was replaced and caught at its corners where it was possible to cut out a fragment of dura at the situation of the perforations and it was possible to withdraw leaving the field in very much better shape than would have been thought possible at the moment of elevating the flap.

A description of the transfusion will be given by Dr. Davis.

At the end of the operation the patient's condition was better than could have been expected.

(Dr. Cushing)

The postoperative course was without complications. Before discharge, the patient received two X-ray treatments.

DISCHARGE NOTE
February 18, 1924
Dr. Putman

Patient had done extremely well. He feels much better and is able to walk.

No difference in power between the two hands. He will continue to get X-ray treatments.

FOLLOW UP LETTER
October 31, 1924

Dear Dr. Cushing

We have just returned from Chicago where Mr. (name of patient) has been on business. While there, he was subject to three short mild attacks during the night and one period of aphasia lasting twenty minutes. He had continued to be well from the time I last wrote you, the first of September until this week.

I was anxious to do some thing about it as soon

as possible so talked with Dr. Ross Golden immediately upon arrival yesterday. He seemed to favor a course of perhaps three more X-rays but wishes to consult you and Dr. Sosman before proceeding.

In your last letter you said that further X-rays were a matter of uncertainty in your mind. You were kind in asking me what I think. It seems that in view of the decided improvement which showed up with each X-ray – in speech, energy and general well being, I would like to have a few more treatments – but of course I realize how ignorant I am, of the other side of the question. Would it be disturbing rather than beneficial?

May I have a word of advice from you at your earliest convenience?

Please do not think that I am nervous or over anxious. Everything had been running along so happily and smoothly that we just want to keep it so.

I expect to run home to Boston for a few days next week. I would like to make you a short call, may I?

Sincerely
(signed) FJ (The wife of the patient)

SECOND HOSPITAL ADMISSION

COMPLAINT

Grand mal, petit mal, and Jacksonian epilepsy, periods of disorientation, headaches, failure of speech.

Patient had received 16 X-ray treatments since the first operation. The last X-ray treatment was in February 9, 1927.

SUMMARY OF POSITIVE FINDINGS
February 26, 1927
Dr. Cairns

SUBJECTIVE
1. Epileptic attacks consisting of grand mal, petit mal and Jacksonian seizures in the form of numbness of the right hand and right face beginning first at the age 18.
2. Failing memory.
3. Changes in character, loss of normal inhibitions.
4. Osteoplastic exploration revealing an extremely vascular tumor probably perithelioma in the left parietal lobe on Jan. 17, 1924.
5. Epileptic symptoms and aphasia, partially controlled by X-ray treatment until 4 weeks ago.

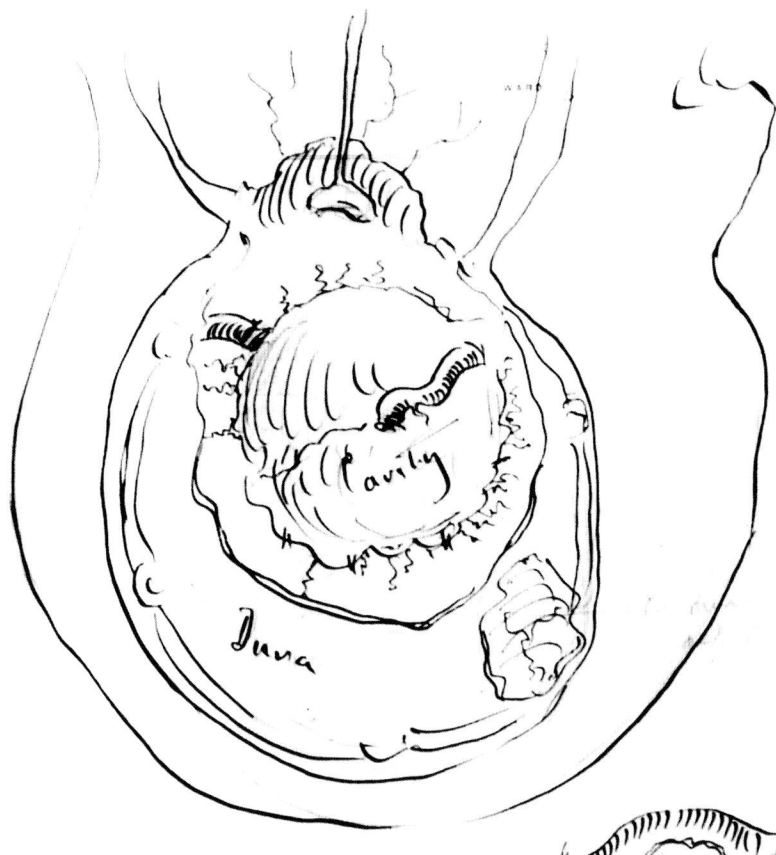

FIG. 2. OPERATIVE SKETCH – SECOND OPERATION.

OBJECTIVE
1. Slight papilledema with slight secondary atrophy. Right not measurable, left 1D.
2. Slight aphasia affecting only spontaneous speech and power of naming objects.
3. Personality changes – loss of inhibitions.
4. Weakness of right lower face.
5. Diminished sensation to pin prick in right face and slightly in right leg.
6. Slight decrease of auditory acuity on left side.

IMPRESSION: Vascular cortical neoplasm of left hemisphere.

RADIOLOGY REPORT
February 26, 1927
Dr. Sosman

Re-examination of the skull, left stereo, A.P. and P.A. shows the irregular mass of calcification in the left hemisphere opposite the lower edge of the bone flap. There are two silver clips on the surface of the brain almost directly over this calcified area. The size and distribution of calcification is practically the same as that previously noted.

SPECIAL NOTE
March 7, 1927
Dr. Cushing

I doubt whether I can adequately describe this operation. I went ahead with great misgivings. At the previous session we exposed a large aneurismal varix in the Sylvian region as big as an orange. We almost lost the patient from exanguination merely in turning back the flap. He has done reasonably well and has had a multitude of X-ray treatments, just how many I do not know, but it would be wise to get a complete chronological list of them with the dosage. Lately he has begun to get somewhat worse as will have been described in the history. I had doubts as to whether we would ever be able to expose the tumor and feared that no attempt at extirpation would be possible. Consequently all preparations were made for transfusion, in getting muscle from the leg and Dr. Bovie was on hand on the chance that we might be able to coagulate the growth. As it turned out I finally exposed the lesion which had largely died out. Whether in extirpating I have taken at the same time the entire arterial supply to his left hemisphere time only can tell.

OPERATIVE NOTE
March 7, 1927
Anesthesia – Novocain – Ether

Extirpation of a "Dead" Circoid Angioma, Super-Sylvian Region of the Left Hemisphere, Including What Appeared to Be All of Greatly Dilated Sylvian Vessels.

The operative note is not available.

PATHOLOGY REPORT
March 7, 1927

Material: This represents a ball of what was once a circoid angioma of the Sylvian region, a tumor which had been exposed some two years or so ago and abandoned as inoperable. The patient has since had an abundance of deep radiations and at the operation practically a dead tumor was found. There were many minute little pearly nodules of calcification encountered during the process of the excision. The huge vessel which lay practically on the anterior side of the tumor will be photographed. The entire tumor was put in formalin.

Microscopic report: The tissue is seen to consist of varying sized blood vessels supported by a moderate amount of stroma chiefly connective tissue. In the stain for elastic tissue only a small amount of elastic tissue is seen to remain and that only in a few vessels. Some of the blood sinuses show old thrombosis with recanalization, others show more recent thrombosis.

DIAGNOSIS – Hemangioma.

(Dr. Bennett)

POSTOPERATIVE NOTES

The patient suffered from aphasia and dense right-sided hemiparesis after surgery. These deficits improved significantly by the time of the discharge on April 10.

FOLLOW UP LETTER
July 18, 1928

My dear Dr. Cushing:

Toward the last of May he was very much better than he had been since his last operation in March 1927. He could speak as many as eight or nine consecutive words and seemed to have a good deal of strength, going up and down stairs by himself two or three times a day. Rather suddenly about June 1 perhaps he overtired himself, plus the confusion of my sister and her husband's arrival here and departure for Europe – Dad had a decided slump from which he has not recovered. He is despondent not complaining but terribly quiet and sad and it is only with the greatest difficulty that he can make one word understood even by the nurses. Certain words, such as "I want, all right, fine, yes and no," he says easily but not always meaning what he says. During the past 3 or 4 days he has had intervals 3 times a day of several minutes duration of acute pain in the left side of his head. He shudders all over and winces away from it in agony. These pains come without any warning and from no apparent cause. On the 4th of July it was necessary to stuff his ears with cotton because the explosions of the fire crackers caused severe shooting pain.

(The patient's daughter)

Chapter 5
Spinal tumors

Introduction

"The device for extricating the customary small thoracic meningioma, which we came to employ in the Brigham Clinic in later years, is to draw upon the attached growth as one may draw a patient to the side of his bed by pulling on the sheet beneath him." [4]

Harvey Cushing

The surgery of intradural spinal tumors emerged as Horsley and Gowers pioneered the operation in 1887.[5] Other surgeons including Putnam, Krauss, Shultze attempted similar operations with success after Horsley.[3] Cushing's resection of a C6-7 intradural fibrosarcoma in 1903 at the Johns Hopkins Hospital may be the 10th reported successful operation for the resection of an intradural spinal neoplasm.[3] The note by Sir William Osler who referred this patient to Cushing reads as:

"When the patient first consulted me I suspected cervical caries or pachymeningitis. It was not until after his admission to the hospital, and a more careful study of the case with Dr. H. M. Thomas, that tumor was suspected. I urged early operation, feeling sure that the condition would not be made worse."[3]

This patient recovered from his preoperative neurological deficits after surgery.

Harvey Cushing's refinement of Halsted's meticulous surgical techniques facilitated safe resection of intradural spinal tumors. Though Cushing focused his attention on the tumors of the brain at the Peter Bent Brigham Hospital, his numerous contributions to the treatment of intradural spine tumors include the description of these tumors' life history and their histological classification. The application of his experienced intracranial surgical techniques to the resection of spinal tumors improved the outcomes from the spinal operations. Cushing believed that a "successful operation for a spinal meningioma represents one of the more gratifying of all operative procedures."[4]

Our review of the 1870 patients' records available at the Cushing's Tumor Registry disclosed 60 patients with spinal tumors. This registry includes patients who underwent an operation between 1912 and 1932. The dominating intradural spinal pathologies verified in this series included meningiomas (23 patients), neurofibromas (4), "sarcomas" (8), ependymomas (3), and astrocytomas (4). Using his initial histopathological experience with these tumors, he later tailored his resection based on different tumor types. Cushing did not believe in lipiodol myelography for tumor localization. He was concerned with the efficacy of this technique in relation to its risks.

Cushing's surgical techniques evolved throughout his career. Cushing's meticulous attention to aseptic techniques and wound closure increased the safety of the intradural spinal procedures. Gentle handing of the spinal cord allowed neurological recovery following decompressive surgery. Tumor classification tailored the resection approach and permitted selection of adjuvant treatment strategies. The application of radiotherapy as an example of such adjuvant treatment modality may have improved outcomes. The absence of adequate imaging methods made localization of spinal tumors dependent on a detailed neurological exam, therefore exploratory laminectomies had to be often extended for proper tumor exposure. Microsurgical techniques were not developed and therefore

---

The following material has been partially excerpted with permission from Cohen-Gadol AA, Spencer DD, Krauss WE. The development of techniques for resection of spinal cord tumors by Harvey W. Cushing. *J Neurosurg-Spine* 2: 92-97, 2005.

the resection of intraparenchymal spinal cord tumors was considered challenging and risky.

Intraoperative hemostasis remained a challenge. Cushing designed his silver clip in 1911 and electrocautery was incorporated into practice in 1926.[2] Despite these developments, Cushing continued to use muscle pledgets to facilitate hemostasis; he adopted this technique from Horsley. Cushing and Bailey completed the classification of tumor histologies by 1926[1] and radiotherapy was implemented in Cushing's practice by 1920. These advances may have been responsible for the reduction of operative mortality and improved outcomes during the latter part of Cushing's career. However, adjuvant spinal stabilization strategies were not well-developed and delayed deformities after extensive exploratory laminectomies were left untreated. Tumor localization was paramount and if he did not find a tumor upon opening the spinal dura, he passed a flexible catheter proximally and caudally parallel to the cord intradurally to search for a block caused by the tumor.

Cushing's practice contained one spinal meningioma for every 16 intracranial meningiomas, reflecting Cushing's interest and his referral patterns for intracranial pathology. Charles A. Elsberg, who practiced neurological surgery in New York at the same time as Cushing, had an especial interest in spinal lesions and contributed substantially to the field. The ratio of surgical cases in Elsberg's series was one spinal to every 2.5 intracranial meningiomas.[4] Cushing emphasized the importance of recognizing meningiomas from neurinomas. The latter are "attached to a nerve root and though they may project into and enlarge the intervertebral foramen, they can be in most instances cleanly dislodged without risk of recurrence, leaving the adjacent meninges intact."[4] Cushing's contributions to the surgery of spinal tumors became a foundation upon which future neurosurgeons refined their techniques and progressively increased the operative safety with the introduction of the microsurgical techniques. In the following chapter, we present a group of patients who underwent resection of their spinal tumors by Dr. Cushing to illustrate some of the techniques used in the early history of spinal surgery.

The first patient (5.1) underwent resection of a spinal meningioma. Based on his intracranial experience in meningioma surgery,[4] Cushing resected the meningioma and involved dura to reduce the risk of recurrence. The picture of the lantern slide is an example of slides used for Cushing's lectures. For Patient 5.2, although we have abbreviated the neurological exam, the portions included demonstrate the depth of detail which was necessary to approximate the spinal location of the lesion preoperatively in the absence of appropriate imaging. In the operative report, Cushing candidly admits to his mistake:

"There was no sign of any damage having been done to the cord by the slipped instrument mentioned in the description of the first step of the operation."

Similarly, in the operative report of Patient 5.8, Cushing criticizes himself for being too aggressive in resecting the tumor:

"I think I would have done very well if I had done nothing more than do this upper laminectomy and dislodge from the canal the lesion I have mentioned since the patient's symptoms corresponded to the line of about the 10th thoracic which was above the level of the visible tumor, namely at about the 1st lumbar and 12th thoracic. If I had contented myself with this measure it is quite conceivable that the child might have been well and have regained some of the lost function."

The series of letters exchanged among different investigators regarding the pathology of the tumor resected in Patient 5.4 is intriguing. In Patient 5.5, as was customary, if Cushing did not find a tumor upon opening the spinal dura, he passed a flexible catheter (searcher or filiform bougie) proximally and caudally parallel to the cord intradurally to search for a block caused by the tumor. In the same patient, Cushing summarizes his technique in resection of spinal meningiomas in his operative sketch.

Exploratory laminectomies spanning many segments exposed Patient 5.9 to delayed development of spinal deformity. This deformity was left untreated causing disabling spinal cord compression.

Finally, in the operative note of Patient 5.10, we can appreciate Cushing's maturation of surgical techniques and application of electrosurgical instrument in the resection of spinal lesions. Based on this operative note, one can witness the progress in resection of spinal cord tumors during Cushing's lifetime.

Aaron A. Cohen-Gadol, M.D., M.Sc.
Indianapolis, IN

William E. Krauss, M.D.
Rochester, MN

Paul C. McCormick, M.D.
New York, NY

References

1. Bailey P, Cushing H: *A classification of the tumors of the glioma group on a histogenetic basis with a correlated study of prognosis.* Philadelphia: JB Lippincott Co, 1926
2. Cushing H: The control of bleeding in operations for brain tumors. With the description of silver "clips" for the occlusion of vessels inaccessible to the ligature. *Ann Surg* 54:1-19, 1911
3. Cushing H: Intradural tumor of the cervical meninges with early restoration of function in the cord after removal of the tumor. *Ann Surg* 39:935-936, 1904
4. Cushing H, Eisenhardt L: *Meningiomas: Their classification, regional behaviour, life history, and surgical end results.* Springfield, IL: Charles C. Thomas, 1938
5. Gowers W, Horsley V: A case of tumor of the spinal cord. *Med Chir Trans* 71:377-428, 1888
6. Laws Jr E: Trainees in Neurological Surgery: The Peter Bent Brigham Hospital., in Black P, Moore MR, Rossitch E, Jr. (eds): *Harvey Cushing at the Brigham.* Park Ridge, IL: AANS, 1993, pp 143-154

5.1 Spinal meningioma

SEX: F; AGE: 53; SURG. NO. 1420

HISTORY

The main complaints included progressive weakness of the left leg for the past two years prior to admission associated with pain in bilateral lower extremities and twitching of both legs for the past 18 months.

SUMMARY OF POSITIVE FINDINGS
July 10, 1914
Dr. Horrax

1. Definite hypoesthesia to pain, touch and temperature below line running from the costal cartilage about to the 11th thoracic spine. Heat and cold not distinguished over the right leg and thigh. Questionable area of hyperesthesia at the level just above the hypoesthesia.
2. Marked spasticity of lower extremities-more left.
3. Left leg and thigh practically helpless.
4. Reflexes
   Abdominal and epigastric not elicited.
   Plantar very active and equal.
   KK and TA extremely lively, greater left.
   Positive ankle clonus both right and left.
   Positive patella clonus left.
   Babinski positive right and left.
   Oppenheim and Cordon suggestive each side.

IMPRESSION: A left sided lesion at 7th and 8th segments which means the 4th and 5th thoracic vertebras.

The Wassermann reaction was double plus on the blood and negative on the spinal fluid. X-rays showed several indistinct shadows of the density of lime salts to the left of the third lumbar vertebra.

OPERATIVE NOTE
July 17, 1914
Anesthesia – Ether – Boothby

Mid Thoracic Laminectomy and Removal of Arachnoidal Endothelioma.

With the patient on the cerebellar table, the spinal canal was exposed about the mid-thoracic region, it having been estimated from the patient's symptoms that the upper level of disturbance of the sensory skin fields was about at the T VII, so that it was estimated that the lesion, if any, was to be found to lie 2 or 3 vertebra higher and it was found about opposite the spine of T V.

The exposure was dry as usual and the laminæ were removed without difficulty. On exposing the dura, the tumor could be seen through the membrane exactly in the middle of the exposed field as shown in the sketch. The dura was opened with some little escape of arachnoid fluid, but it was apparent nevertheless that the arachnoid caudad to the lesion bulged slightly more than did the membrane cephalad to the lesion. Running over the posterior surface of the tumor was a nerve root, apparently the 6th thoracic root, very possi-

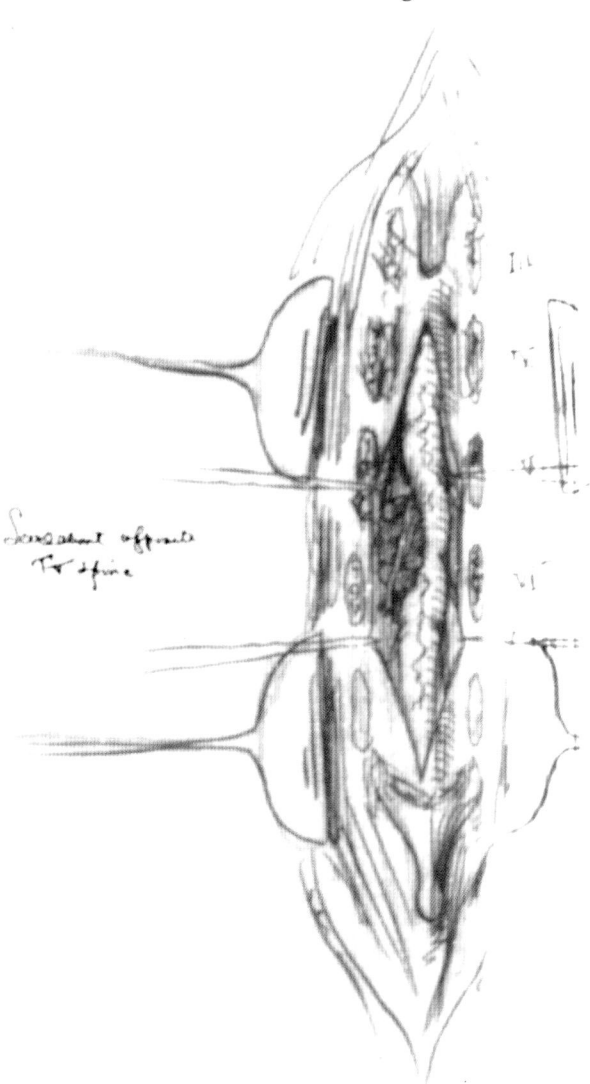

FIG. 1. SURGEON'S DRAWING.

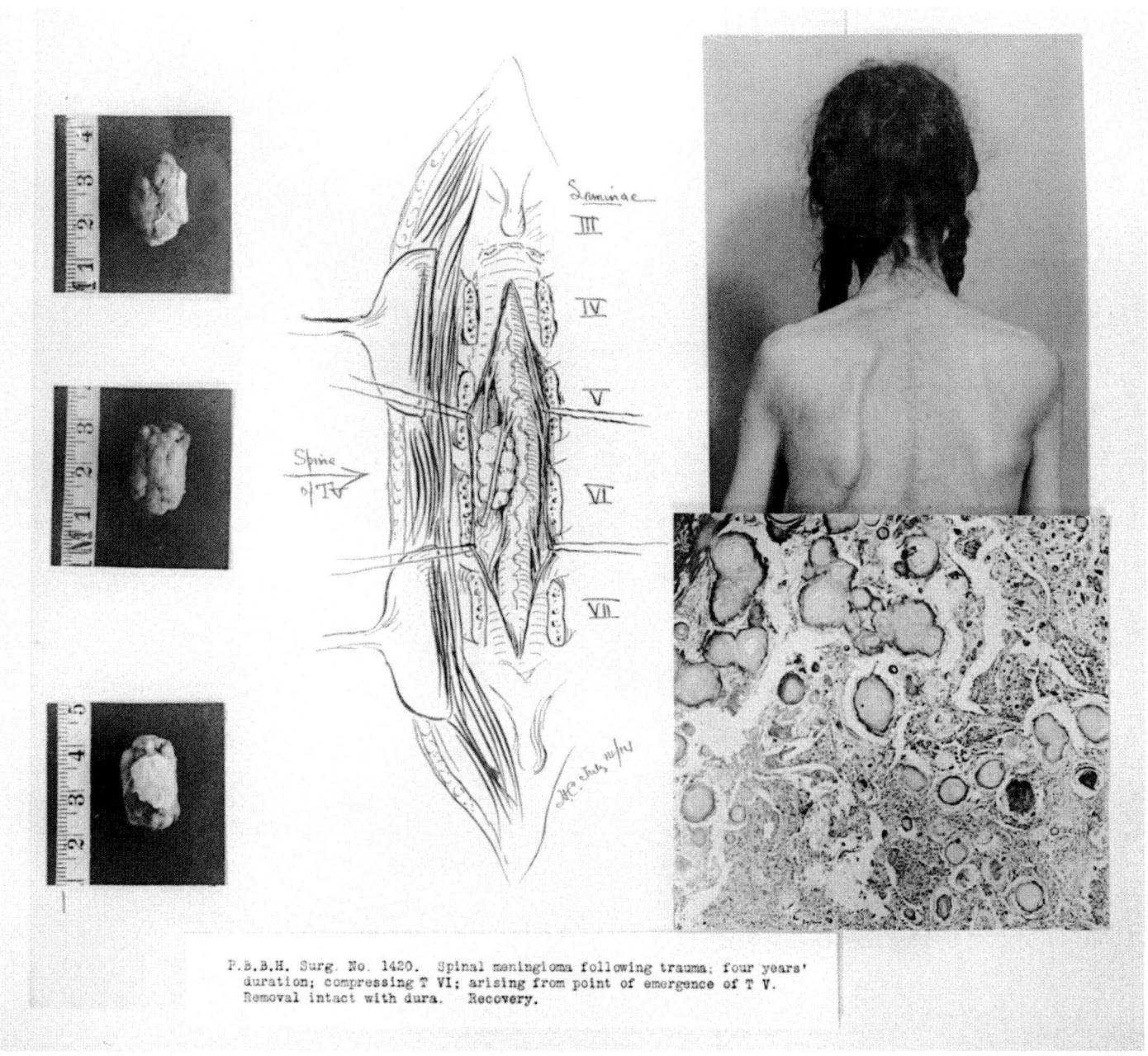

FIG. 2. CUSHING'S LECTURE SLIDE.

bly the 7th. Instead of dividing this root as has been usually done, the root was pulled to the side and preserved. In this manipulation, it became evident that the tumor lay within the arachnoid and probably, as is true of the intracranial lesions, of a similar nature. It had arisen from the arachnoid mesothelium and not from the dura. The growth was unusually nodular, but it was firm and its point of attachment was on the dura to the outer side at the point of emergence of the nerve root above the one which overlay the tumor. The tumor was tilted outward and the small patch of dura about 1 cm. in diameter to which it was adherent was cut away with the growth which was intact.

There was some slight bleeding from the neighborhood of the excision, but this was finally checked with 2 or 3 bits of muscle taken from the raw surface of rector spinæ muscle.

After some delay, the oozing was stilled and the wound was closed as usual in many superimposed layers.

(Dr. Cushing)

PATHOLOGY REPORT
July 17, 1914
Dr. Cushing

Gross description: Tumor received fresh. It weighs 2.3 grams. It consists of oval mass about the size of a small dove's egg. It measures 2.3 cm from pole to pole, averages 1.4 cm in diameter. The ends are rather blunt, the sides somewhat flattened. It has a verucous appearance. On one side the tumor mass is attached to a layer of fibrous tissue 1 cm in length and .9 cm in width, and about 1 to 2 mm thickness. This resembles dura. There is no definite pedicle.
(Dr. Cushing)

MICROSCOPIC REPORT: Tumor not cut, reserved for specimen.
(Resident pathologist)

July 31, 1914
Dr. Rand

The patient's sensations were again gone over for the first time after operation. The patient is feeling much better than before operation. All dressings have been removed, and she is anxious to be up and about the ward.

DISCHARGE NOTE
September 4, 1914
Dr. Rand

Patient's general condition has been improving steadily. She is now able to walk without help and there is practically no difference in the strength of the two sides, some tendency to foot drop on the left. Sensation now practically normal. Has been given KL and HG from time to time. General condition much improved over that on admission. There is no longer any root pain nor has she been troubled with shortness of breath recently. Her cardiac condition at present is good. Discharged.

LETTER TO DR. CUSHING
December 23, 1915

My Dear Doctor,

Many times since my return to Utica I have wished I were able to write you a little note of gratitude. Accept, Doctor Cushing, my most sincere thanks for your kindness to me while I was in the hospital, it was which I shall never forget.

I am now under the care of Doctor Hyland and feel I am recovering nicely.

Again thanking you Doctor Cushing and wishing you every success in life, I remain

Sincerely,
(Signed by patient)

On the previous page is the slide used by Dr. Cushing during his lectures related to this patient.

5.2 Metastatic carcinoma of the spine

SEX: F; AGE: 66; SURG. NO. 4411

HISTORY

Three years prior to her admission, the patient was diagnosed with "neuritis of sciatic nerve." One year prior to admission, in May 1915, she was found to have a small "tumor of left breast" which was removed completely.

One month ago, she noticed that her legs were getting weak. A week or ten days later, she began to have numbness of both feet. The numbness gradually "worked up the legs" as far as the hips, and finally, for the last 10 days, there was a belt of numbness about the waist.

SPINAL EXAM (SUMMARIZED)
March 12, 1916
Dr. Horrax

MOTOR

All muscle groups of both arms are of equal and normal strength.

Lower extremities show a definite weakness on both sides in all muscles groups, but motion in all directions is possible. Flexion of the thigh and dorsal flexion of the foot are perhaps the weakest motions made out.

SENSORY

Sensation is normal on the head, neck, arms and chest. The legs, buttocks and abdomen are hypoesthetic to light touch, pain and temperature, but there is still a considerable degree of sensation retained. The thermal sensation is perhaps the least impaired of the three. The upper line of impaired sensation in front follows the costal border and from here a belt of hypoesthesia which is less marked than that below extends down to about 5 cm, above the umbilicus. Below this second line of hypoesthesia is greater. In back the belt of lessened hypoesthesia extends around in an area between the 8th-12th dorsal spines, below the 12th sensation being still further impaired.

REFLEXES

Superficial

Corneal active and equal both sides.
Epigastric and abdominal not elicited either side.

Deep

Biceps, triceps, periosteo-radials equal and brisk both sides.

KK, patella and achilles greatly exaggerated. Possibly a little more on right than left.

Plantar response active and there is probably a positive Babinski, but response is so great that it is rather hard to determine it exactly.

Oppenheim is suggestive.

There is a bilateral, non persistent ankle clonus.

VASO-MOTOR

No change.

SPHINCTERS

Are practically normal, although there is some difficulty in starting urination during the last few days.

IMPRESSION: Metastatic carcinoma of spinal column. Here is the possibility of a benign growth from the old history of trouble 3 years ago.

RADIOLOGY REPORT
March 13, 1916

The examination of the chest shows a very marked increase of fibrous tissue about the hilus region. There is a diffuse dilatation of the arch of the aorta and moderate enlargement of the heart shadow. There is generalized absorption of lime salts of the bones, especially marked in the lower thoracic and lumbar spine. There are, however, no evidence of any focus of destruction.

OPERATIVE NOTE
March 18, 1916
Anesthesia – Ether – Dr. Boothby

Exploratory Laminectomy – Disclosure of Carcinoma of Right Side of Spinal Cord Involving Bones – Division of Three Nerve Roots Passing off from Distorted Cord.

The usual laminectomy was performed with dissection of muscles away from the spines and laminæ. There was considerably more bleeding than usual, doubtless owing to the growth which was subsequently exposed. At one point the blunt dissector which was being used went unexpectedly directly through the lamina into a growth. The laminæ

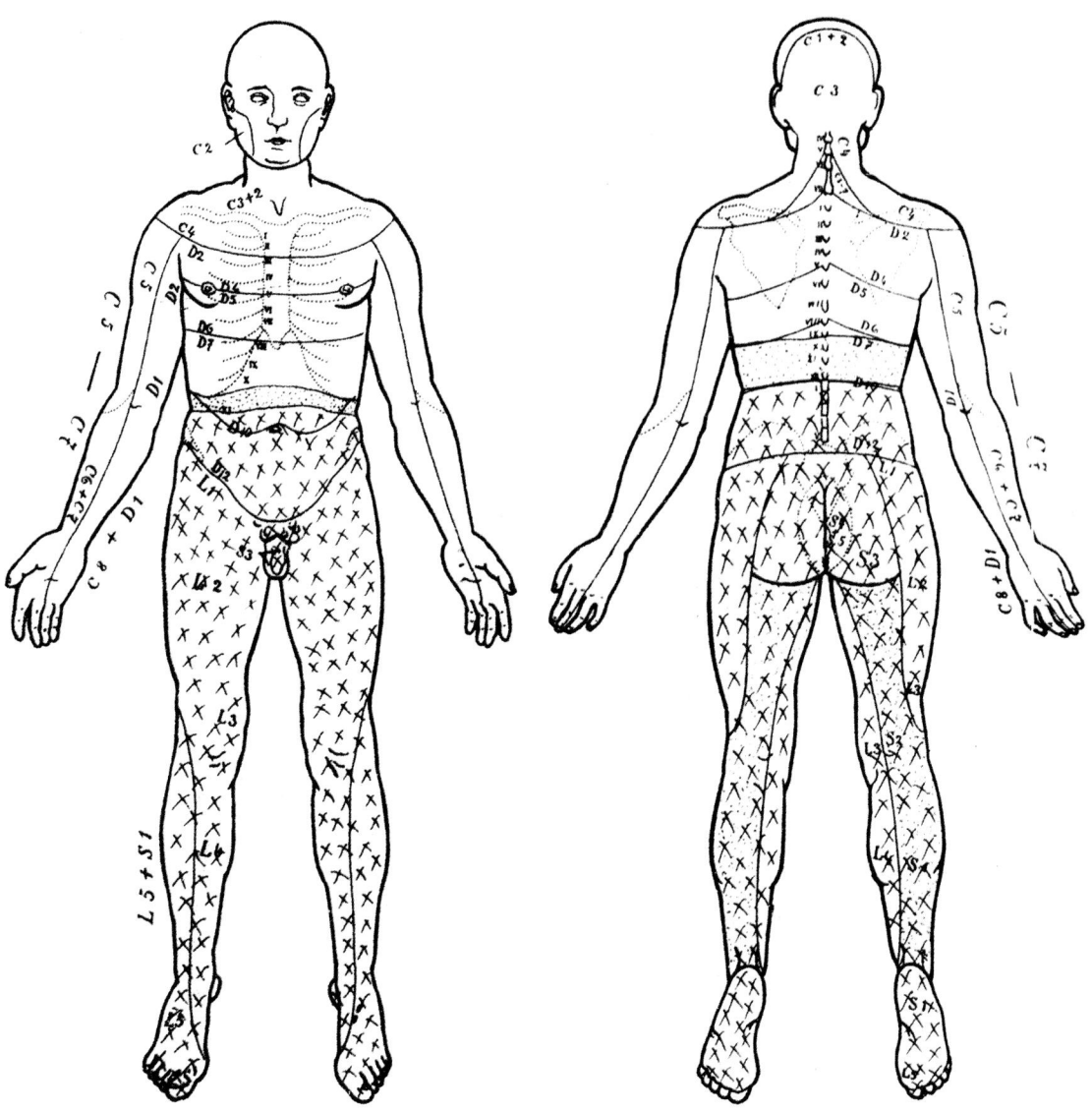

FIG. 1. PREOPERATIVE EXAM. CROSSED AREAS INDICATE REGIONS OF DECREASED SENSATION.

FIG. 2. PREOPERATIVE EXAM. CROSSED AREAS INDICATE REGIONS OF DECREASED SENSATION.

were removed with great difficulty owing to the fact that in the center of the field bone was invaded by tumor. Also on the right side there was a good deal of invasion of muscle by tumor. Finally a fairly good exposure was secured and the tumor was finally cut away to give a good exposure. It had broken through the side of the cord and must have completely involved the transverse process possibly of the 7th and 8th thoracic vertebræ. When the cord was finally exposed a remarkable condition was brought into view, for the cord was so twisted that the nerve roots for the right side actually came off from the left side of the cord as shown in the sketch. Three of these nerve roots were divided, the peripheral stump of each of them being caught with a silver clip. One of them directly entered the tumor.

The first two, namely, the lower cords, were divided without anæsthetizing the nerves, but before dividing the upper one the nerve was novocainized. On the division of the first two roots there was a sudden respiratory irregularity which Dr. Boothby suggested might be due to the intercostals supply to the diaphragm. The tumor was scooped out as thoroughly as possible and the bleeding was checked by the occasional placement of clips and of bits of fibrin leaf, and the wound was finally closed without drainage. It was left apparently dry.

There was no sign of any damage having been done to the cord by the slipped instrument mentioned in the description of the first step of the operation.

(Dr. Cushing)

PATHOLOGY REPORT
March 18, 1916

Gross description: Fragment of spinal tumor fixed in formalin.

Microscopic report: Tumor shows the characteristics of an adenocarcinoma of rather slow growth, mitotic figures being comparatively infrequent.

Diagnosis – Adenocarcinoma.
(Dr. Goodpasture)

April 6, 1916
Dr. Horrax

Her condition improved very slowly, but gradually each day. She is sitting up in bed a little better now and also sits up in a chair a short while during the day. The latter is a considerable effort, however, and she often has more pain in left side after she has been up. She is moving her legs more freely and thinks they are improving in strength.

DISCHARGE NOTE
April 16, 1916
Dr. Horrax

She is now sitting up in a chair for longer periods each day and is considerably less tired by the effort. She still complains, however, of pain in the left side as before, but this is made easier while sitting up by a tight binder.

Inspection reveals the same tendency toward abdominal rather than thoracic breathing as before. The spine shows only the abnormality due to loss of the laminæ at the site of operation. The muscle strength in all groups of the upper extremities is very good and equal on the both sides. The lower extremities show a marked improvement in strength in all groups. Flexion of the thigh and flexion and extension of the foot being quite evidently much better than before operation. She is now also able to walk with assistance a little each day and although she could walk slightly before operation with assistance this has improved and she feels much stronger on her feet. Sensation has also improved on her body and especially on the legs below the knee. There is an area on the right side of the chest, however, which is anesthetic and corresponds to the areas of the sensory root distribution which were cut at the operation. She was discharged today to her home in very fair general health and considerably improved from the operation.

LETTER TO DR. CUSHING
January 9, 1917

Dear Dr. Cushing

I have just returned from seeing my sister, upon whom you operated for spinal tumor (cancer) and I write to ask if treatment now given her is all that can be done to relieve the awful agony of her suffering. Of course, I realize there is no hope of her recovery, as her body is now, by paralysis, more than half dead. Are they doing all that can be done? Would that God could see fit to take her from this death by inches. I enclose the treatment given, written out by the nurse. For an early answer-will be under great obligations.

Yours truly,
(Signed) E.C.

Copy of treatment
Morphine gr ½ (sub cu) during day every three hours. Hyoscine hydrobromide gr 1/150. Morphine sulphate. Atropine gr 1/200.

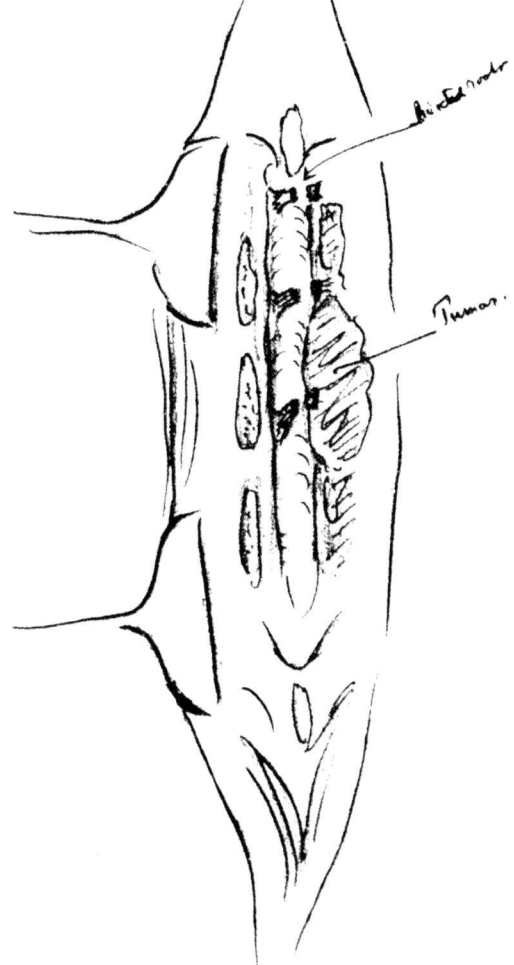

FIG. 2. OPERATIVE SKETCH.

5.3 Cauda equina fibrosarcoma

SEX: F; AGE: 50; SURG. NO. 13231

HISTORY

The patient presented with a 20-year history of back and right lower extremity pain, with first manifestation during labor. She subsequently developed progressive lower extremity weakness. In March 1919, she underwent a "pelvic operation" by Dr. Gullen. Following the operation, she became more "uncomfortable and never could regain her strength."

In 1919, she visited the Mayo Clinic and was evaluated by Dr. Housternan and Dr. Will Mayo. They made a diagnosis of "pressure on spine." She subsequently saw Dr. Barker, Dr. Meyer and Dr. Homas in Baltimore for this pain; their conclusion was that the disorder was functional. Dr. Barker advised pelvic operation and promised that "after this there would be no pain."

In November 1919, she returned back to the Mayo Clinic and saw Dr. Charles Mayo, Dr. Houseman, Dr. Piper and Dr. Shelby. They told her that her trouble was in "nerves and that she would always have it and advised no operative treatment." Their impression was that this disorder was functional. They did not perform a lumbar puncture.

Dr. Milliken from Dallas made a spinal puncture a few weeks ago and first diagnosed a spinal cord tumor. The patient was then referred to Dr. Cushing.

SUMMARY OF POSITIVE FINDINGS
September 28, 1920
Dr. Locke

SUBJECTIVE
1. Since 1920 patient has had a numb tingling sensation of right leg brought on particularly by fatigue.
2. Also about 20 years patient has had attacks of sharp, stabbing pain in the small of her back and down her right leg. This pain is brought on by laughing, straining at stool and coughing.
3. In March 1919, after a pelvic operation, patient started to experience pain in her left lower extremity.
4. In January 1920 legs became flaccid.
5. In July 1920 L.M.D. on lumbar puncture found yellow fluid which solidified soon after being drawn.

OBJECTIVE
1. Gait is unsteady and is one of weakness.
2. There is an unusual lordosis of the lower spine in the lumbar region, and slight scoliosis.
3. There is rather marked weakness of both lower extremities, especially the left. The weakness is particularly marked in the adductor groups.
4. There is general slight atrophy of all muscles and rather marked atrophy of the

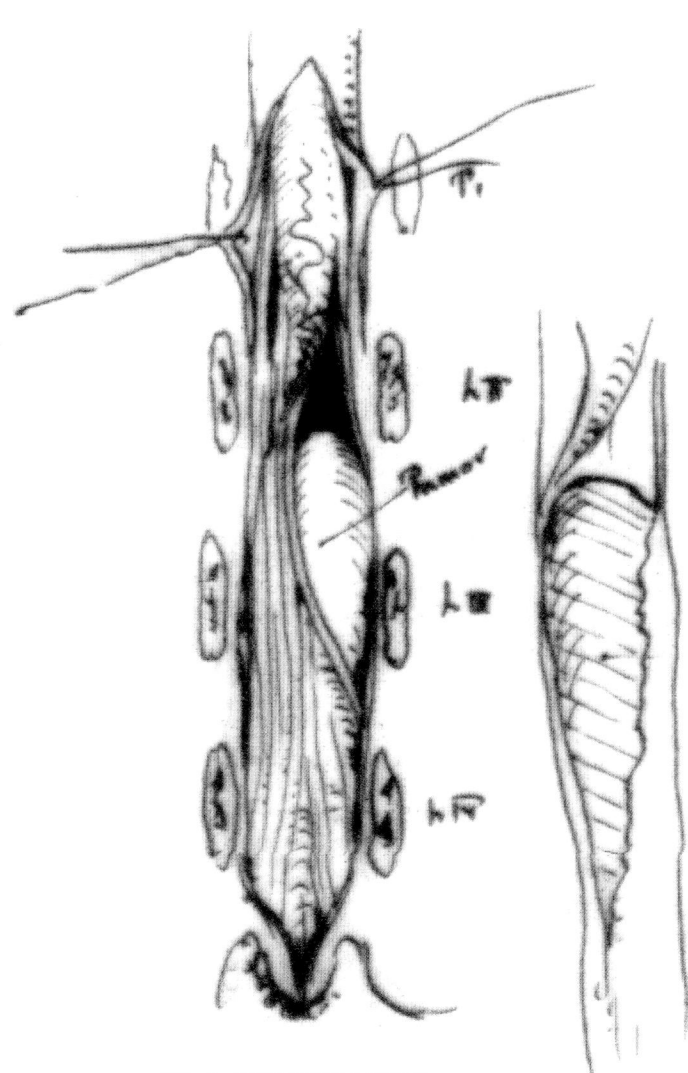

FIG. 1. OPERATIVE SKETCH.

adductor groups on either side, more marked on left.

5. There is rather marked flaccidity of lower extremities.
6. Deep reflexes on the left are absent and on right are present only with reinforcement.
7. There is diminished sensation to touch and pain prick of lower extremities; some hyperæsthesia to cold.
8. There is diminished vibratory sense in the lower extremities on the left and right.
9. Some hypertrophic changes of the spine.

RADIOLOGY REPORT
September 25, 1920

X-ray-lateral spine shows hypertrophic arthritic changes along the dorsal vertebras.

SPECIAL NOTE
September 28, 1920
Dr. Cushing

It has been practically certain in this woman's history that she must have had from the outset, namely for 20 years, a tumor involving the lower cord of possibly cauda equina. The fact that there was so very marked motor involvement with comparatively slight sensory involvement and that the deep reflexes at knee and ankle were abolished, whereas a normal plantar reflex was preserved, made it seem almost certain that the tumor must be a fairly extensive one involving the cauda equina. The presence of tumor moreover was certified almost beyond any doubt by the history of a highly colored fluid which clotted on standing, that had been removed by puncture from the lower cord some weeks ago. The operative findings led me to believe that the growth which in a short time would have largely absorbed the lamina of the 2nd, 3rd, and 4th lumbar vertebra, was of the endothelioma variety. Certainly if it has been present for 20 years it can have no great malignancy, and I assume that if it is fibroblastic it belongs to the fibro-endothelioma group.

OPERATIVE NOTE
September 28, 1920
Anesthesia-Ether-Miss Gerard

Laminectomy was performed exposing the lower part of the cord and lumbar region including the laminæ from the L1 or possibly T12 to L4. Great

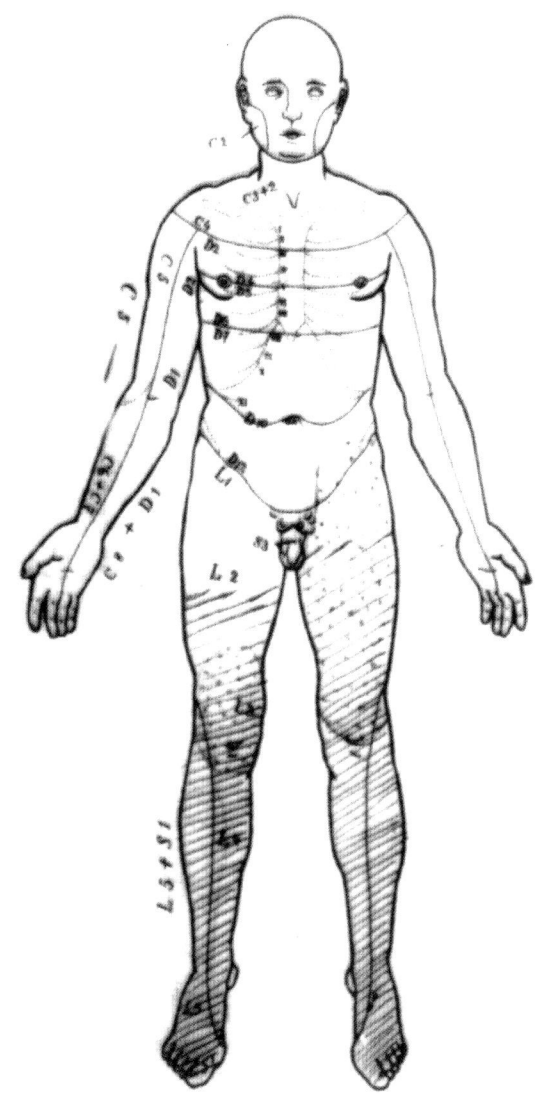

FIG. 2. PREOPERATIVE EXAM. HASHED AREAS DEMONSTRATE THE REGIONS OF DECREASED SENSATION TO PIN PRICK.

care was exercised in stripping muscles from the lamina, particularly as it was found early that the lamina appeared soft and not particularly well developed. Finally after removing the spines and separating the muscles well to the side, a very extraordinary appearance was found. The laminæ were small, evidently undergoing absorption and between them there bulged the contents of the canal; particularly between L3 and L4 there was a separation of the laminæ for about 2 cm and there projected backward a round swelling indicating unquestionably the presence of some growth in the canal. Between the other laminæ there was a similar appearance, though perhaps less marked.

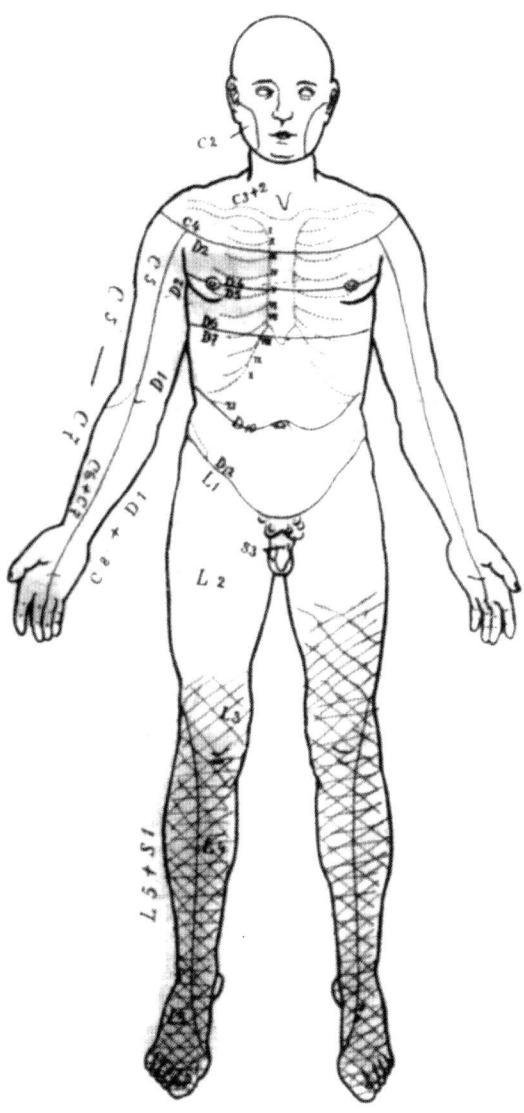

FIG. 3. PREOPERATIVE EXAM. CROSSED AREAS DEMONSTRATE THE REGIONS OF DECREASED SENSATION TO COTTON.

The usual form of removal of the laminæ was therefore precluded and they were nibbled away bit by bit as carefully as possible to avoid damage. When this was done the contents of the canal protruded backward much as after removal of bone in the skull in the presence of tumor the brain protrudes.

On incising the dura throughout the length of the exposure the normal lower portion of the lumbar enlargement was exposed and a mass of the nerve roots of the cauda equine were laid bare. On separating these nerve roots, the operator came down upon a solid smooth tumor evidently attached to the anterior surface of the canal and projecting backward. Its upper pole was easily approached and it was seen that the entire tumor could not be dislodged. In the hope of removing as much of it as possible its capsule was split and it was treated somewhat in the fashion of an acoustic neuroma, and a large mass of the growth being gradually tilted out from above downward. The tumor was fibrous and tended to split in a curious fashion in a longitudinal direction. It was not particularly vascular and it is possible that much more of it with further manipulations might have been removed.

The patient had been reported by Miss Gerard as being in not particularly good condition early in the operation, and therefore I did not feel justified in prolonging the procedure to a great length. A fragment of tissue sent to the laboratory was reported as possibly fibro-sarcoma. The chief mass of the tumor was fixed in formalin for further study. It should be said that during the early stage of the laminectomy tumor was entered along side of the laminæ on the right, where it had evidently squeezed its way through between laminæ, and where it was evidently invading, though not in a malignant sense, the extra-vertebral tissues.

Wound was closed securely in layers without a drain.

(Dr. Cushing)

PATHOLOGY REPORT
September 28, 1920

Microscopic description: There are two sections which show well the structure of the main tumor. That from the tip of the tumor is very cellular, consisting of long spindle cells lying in very collagenous stroma. The cells vary somewhat in size. Nucleus is eliptical, sometimes more or less rounded. The amount of stroma varies in parts. Where the cells are most numerous a moderate number of mitoses are seen. There is moderate number of small, thin walled blood vessels. Section which apparently is very near its attachment to the dura shows an increased amount of collagen stroma and cells are fewer and more matured. There are many small hemorrhages in parts, most recent, a few old. The picture of the tumor at the tip is that of the fibrosarcoma. At its base it suggests a dural origin. Several stains reveal no nerve or glia elements.

Diagnosis: Fibrosarcoma

(Dr. Wolbach)

September 30, 1920
Dr. Locke

Patient still complains of "terrible pain" and says that she does not know what it is to be comfortable. She is very low in spirits and cannot be cheered up although strenuous efforts have been made. The movements of her legs are about the same. Thinks there is a little bit of improvement on the left.

October 13, 1920
Dr. Locke

The day before yesterday the posterior cast was removed, wound found to be well healed and excellently approximated. No evidence of any subcutaneous hemorrhage. Patient is a little bit more bright and slept 5 hours last night.

October 26, 1920
Dr. Locke

In the last two days patient has been up in a wheel chair but there is no real improvement in her subjectively. Dr. Cushing has told her that the course of last resort would be to cut the dorsal root but has also told her that he does not want to do this unless it is absolutely necessary.

DISCHARGE NOTE
November 3, 1920
Dr. Locke

Following operation the patient complained of a great deal of pain and insisted that her condition was not any better, yet nearly every day she showed objective improvement to her general condition. She also had some improvement in the motor function of her legs. Wound healed extremely rapidly. She received two X-ray treatments and is to have some at home.

LETTER TO DR. CUSHING
FROM THE REFERRING PHYSICIAN
(Readable portions)
March 18, 1922

Patient had several applications of radium. No discovered metastasis. She died of starvation and ... use of morphia. I regret that a post mortum could not be obtained, that you might have more complete data for your records. I think it possible however to get the last X-ray picture, showing the softening of the vertebra mentioned above, and if you wish, I will try to furnish it.

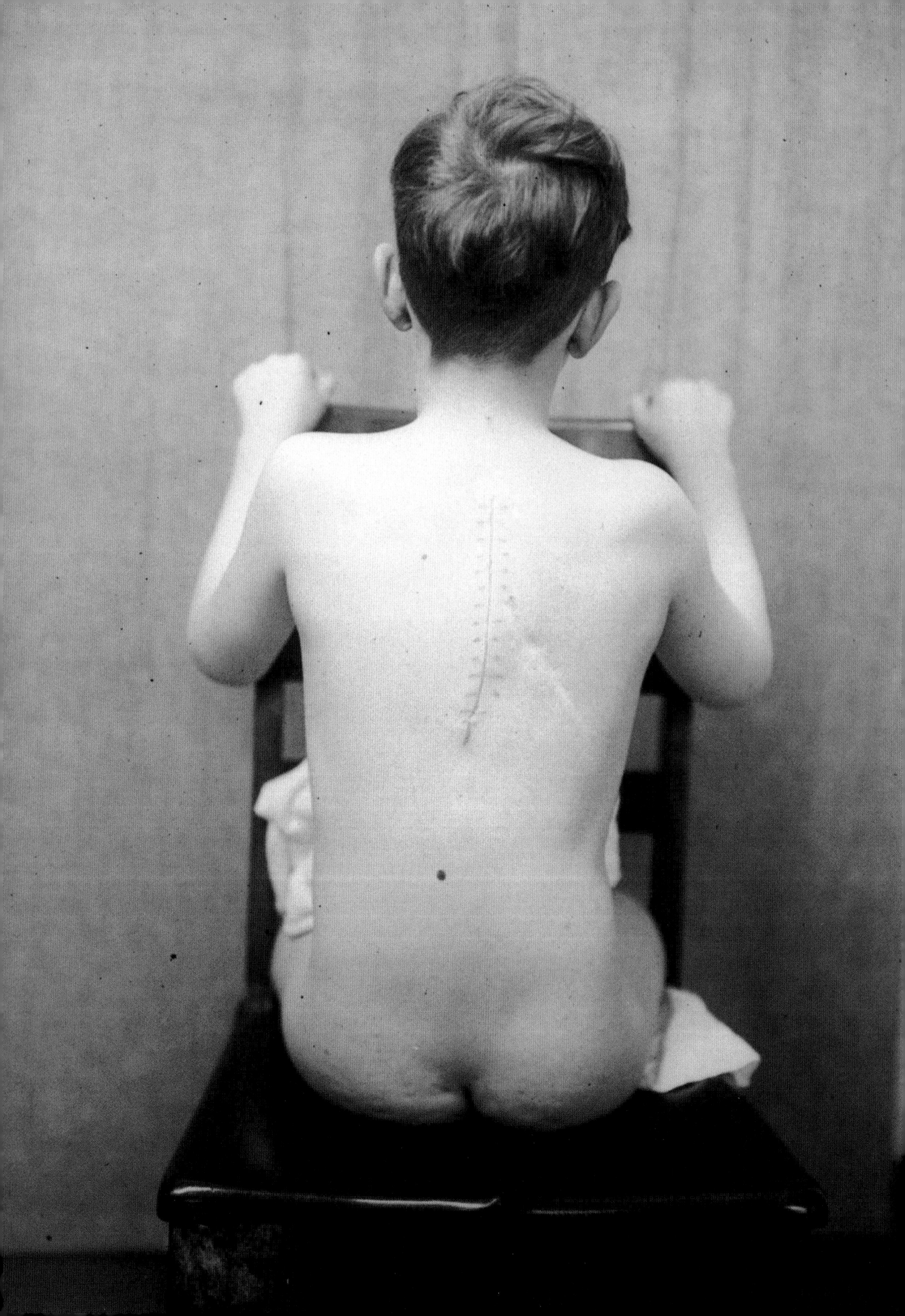

5.4 Ganglioneuroma of spinal cord

SEX: M; AGE: 11; SURG. NO. 14560

HISTORY

When the child was two years old, he was diagnosed with a spinal tumor which was removed by Dr. McGuire. The pathology of the resected lesion was consistent with fibrosarcoma. During the month after surgery, the tumor "increased in size" and was treated by "Coley's serum" with an improvement of symptoms. His condition gradually improved although there was a loss of bowel and bladder function. Of note, the patient's father was a family doctor.

SUMMARY OF POSITIVE FINDINGS
May 19, 1921
Dr. Wheeler

SUBJECTIVE
1. In April 1911 father noted some awkwardness in walking, especially a weakness of the left leg.
2. One week later father noticed that right foot could not be raised over a broom stick
3. At the same time a nodule about the size of butter bean was found on the right side of the vertebrae, at the level of the angle of scapula.
4. May 1, 1911 weakness had spread up the trunk, finally involving the arms and hands.
5. During May 1911 patient had what was diagnosed as T.S. meningitis.
6. About the 1st of June 1911, after illness patient could not move either leg and would only move the hands across the abdomen.
7. At this time there was a loss of rectal and urinary control.
8. June 8, 1911 Dr. McGuire removed a tumor of the back which was diagnosed sarcoma.
9. About July 1, 1911 tumor had definitely increased in size.
10. July 8, 1911 Coley serum treatment began. Tumor gradually disappeared.
11. Since 1914 without treatment patient has regained strength in his arms and hands and since 1919 has been able walk about on crutches.

OBJECTIVE
1. Marked weakness of both lower extremities.
2. Spasticity of both lower extremities with slight contracture of the knee.
3. Exaggerated reflexes, right and left.
4. Patellar and ankle clonus.
5. Positive Babinski and Oppenheim reflexes.
6. Cutaneous sense alteration questionable.
7. Left leg longer than the right, 1 cm.
8. Operative scar of the right side of the back, upper end, at the level of 6th thoracic, lower end at the 12th thoracic, but about 18 cm. to the right.

Examination of the spine – There are no prominences of the vertebrae. No tenderness to percussion. No limitation of motion but there is a scar where a tumor was removed just to the right of the spine at the level of the 6th thoracic extending obliquely out under the angle of the scapula. There is no evidence of new tumor growth in the scar and there is some slight nodule just beneath the edges of the old scar.

X-rays revealed "shadows of increased density" along the 7th cervical vertebrae.

May 19, 1921
Dr. Wheeler

Pressure of the groin gives a marked flexion of the legs on the thighs with erection and marked cremasteric retraction. Pin prick of penis gives adductor spasm. Chief flexor spasm comes from pinching skin of front of the thigh. Please note the image titled "Fig. 2. Preoperative physical examination by Dr. Wheeler."

OPERATIVE NOTE
May 21, 1921
Anesthesia – Ether – Miss Gerrard

Laminectomy with Exposure of Intraspinal Diffuse Extradural Tumor.

With the position of the old scar representing the original seat of the tumor a short laminectomy was performed, three vertebrae only having their spines removed. This proved to be an insufficient exposure and finally two upper vertebrae and one lower were removed before there was sufficient room to expose the bulk of the tumor.

FIG. 1. THREE WEEKS POSTOPERATIVE.

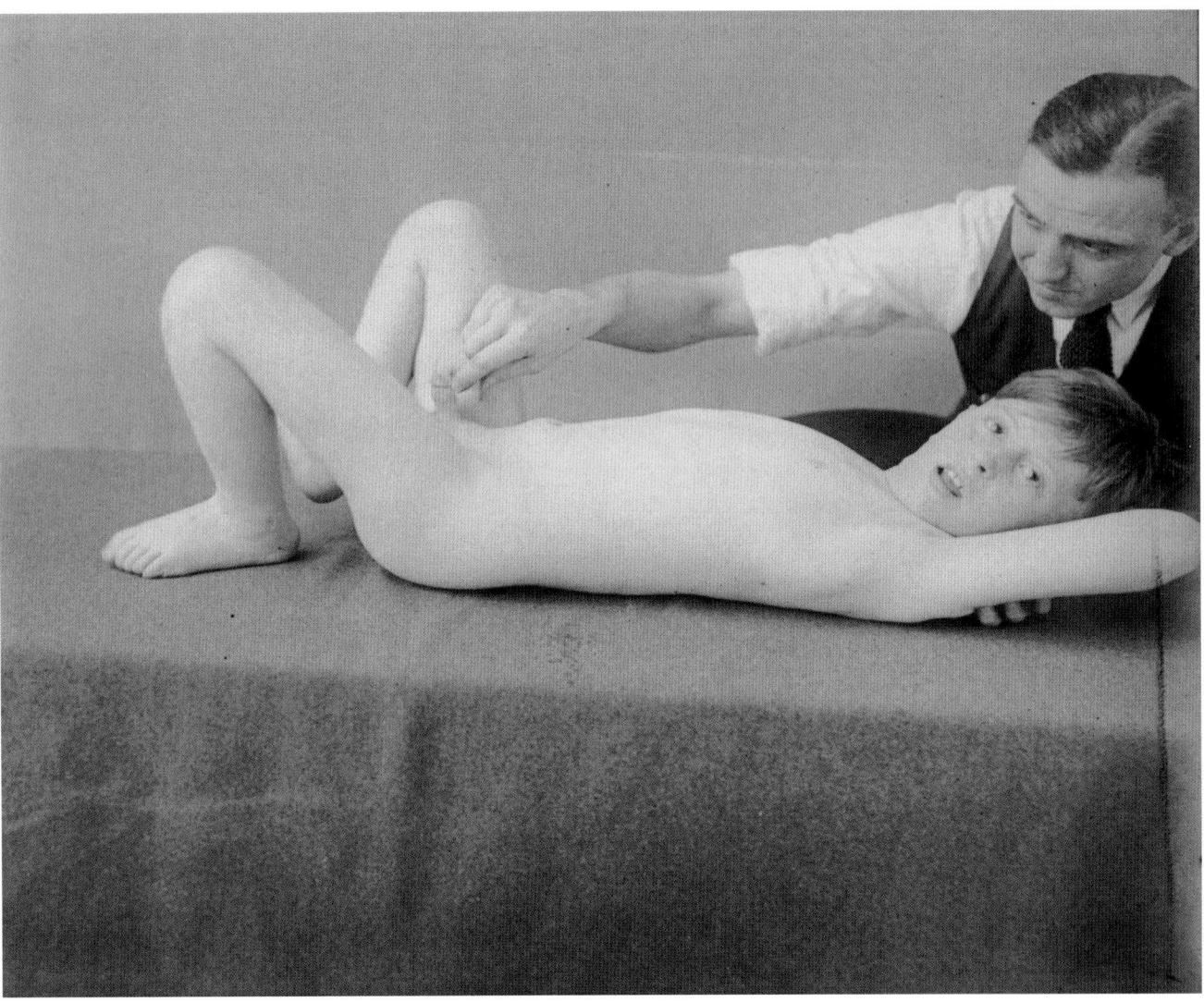

FIG. 2. PREOPERATIVE PHYSICAL EXAMINATION BY DR. WHEELER. PLEASE SEE TEXT.

It may be said that there was no apparent lesion of the bone, and the tumor must have found its way out in some intravertebral spaces. Indeed it may possibly have originated from one of the posterior root ganglia, a source of origin which the histological finding makes still more probable.

After removing the laminae there was a very peculiar appearance to the underlying intraspinal tissues. Instead of the usual fatty tissue filling in the canal there was a fairly dense scar-like tissue which appeared to completely fill the canal. An incision was made down into this scar and it seemed unending, giving the appearance of being carried through the entire canal without disclosing cord. I could not be sure at one time whether I was actually inside or still outside of the dura. The tissue as throughout was exceedingly vascular and there were many spurting arteries, some of which had to be caught with clips or clamps.

It became almost certain that this tissue was tumor tissue and indeed it looked to me on making the separation of bone from overlying muscle on the right side that there was tumor tissue possibly in the muscle.

It was at this juncture that the two preaxial vertebrae were removed, and I got in just above where this thickened envelope surrounded the cord, the dura appearing normal.

From this point downward the tissue was made scraped away from the dura to which it was not adherent – the same dense, grayish, vascular tissue. In order to get below it was necessary as stated to remove another vertebra on the postaxial side of the area of exposure.

A fragment of this tissue taken by Dr. Wolbach gave him the impression of its being a ganglia neuroma, and it is quite possible that this may indicate the seat of origin. Just at one place opposite to the original scar, in other words opposite the original seat of tumor, there was a particularly dense mass which I endeavored to push away with rongeurs and then to remove with the curette unsuccessfully owing to bleeding. I felt almost certain that this represented a space between two vertebrae which led out therefore into the region of a posterior root ganglion, and which communicated outside of the canal with the tumor mass which was there.

Some of the bleeding was checked with pieces of muscle. A fragment of the extra-vertebral area of tissue under suspicion was removed for study and the wound was closed in layers with fine black silk sutures. A cigarette drain being left in position owing to the continued closing.

Note – This is a very extraordinary story, namely of an original large tumor which was diagnosed fibrosarcoma though Dr. Stuart McGuire says the tissues have been lost. The tumor disappeared under Coley's serum. It is now 10 years later and the cord is surrounded by this cuff of tumor, and what is more the X-ray shows a good deal of extravertebral fibrosis or ossification just about in the position corresponding with the tumor and which were found within the canal.

(Dr. Cushing)

PATHOLOGY REPORT
May 21, 1921
Material – Tissue from spinal canal (extra-dural)

It is rather difficult to interpret this material as a tumor consisting as it does of nerve cells and fibrous tissue of the type found to nerve sheaths. Evidence of the growth, however, is present in the irregular extensions into fat and muscle and in the cones of small, deeply staining cells with large nuclei which seem to be precursors of the ganglion cells.

DIAGNOSIS – Giant cell neuro-ganglioma

(Dr. Wolbach)

DISCHARGE NOTE
June 17, 1921
Dr. Wheeler

Deep reflexes of the arms and legs are active, but more marked on the left. Ankle and patellar clonus bilateral. Hypesthesia is definite as before operation. Patient walking is much better but far from normal. Discharged with improvement. Photo taken.

CORRESPONDENCE REGARDING THE PATHOLOGY
December 20, 1921

Dear Dr Cushing:

I have at last been able to find the original slides of the tissue removed from the tumor of the cervical spine by Dr. Steward McGuire, in May 1911, in the case of BW. At that time, the lump was plainly palpable and suggested the presence of a lipoma or collection of broken-down tuberculous tissue. On exposing the growth, it was found to be a well-defined tumor springing from the laminae and transverse processes of the vertebrae. Microscopical examination made by Dr. E. Guy Hopkins of Richmond (Professor of Pathology of the University College of Medicine) proved it to be fibro-sarcoma. Pathological examination made by Dr. James Ewing, March 29, 1912 reads:

"In fact the case of BW, I am unable to offer a positive and exact diagnosis. It is certain that you deal with a malignant tumor which may very well be called sarcoma. I am inclined to think it is either an endothelioma secondary to the cerebral growth, or possibly a neurocytoma derived from misplaced nerve tissue in the cranium."

I would be very glad to send you a slide, if you will be good enough to let me have one of yours, of the tumor removed ten years later. I have already written you twice about it but I imagine it has slipped your mind. The case is of extreme interest and I think you will be pleased to have a slide of the original tumor. Ewing was certain that it was a malignant tumor at the time. If so, it must have been modified by the treatment. If not, we have a rapidly-growing tumor occurring in a child who had been perfectly well until Feb. 1911, when he was thrown from a wagon, and developing one month after the injury.

The case greatly interests me and I would like very much to get your full, authoritative opinion on it.

With best wishes for Christmas and the New Year believe me Sincerely yours, Dr. Coley

January 6, 1922

Dear Harvey,

I have been over the two slides from the first operation on the boy BW which were sent by Coley.

At first glance, it appears to be essentially a spindle cell tumor but peculiar in that it is broken up into positions by connective tissue bands. With the stain employed it is impossible to see the cell outlines and the impression of spindle shaped cells is given wholly by the oval nuclei. The nature of the tumor, however, is made apparently by third type of intercellular substance, namely large bands composed of extremely delicate fibrils which with the hematoxilin-eosin stain take a very faint bluish color. The grouping, size and general arrangement of these fibrils agree perfectly with those in neuroblastoma in general.

I should not hesitate to make a diagnosis of neuroblastoma here. This tumor is very much cellular than the one you removed and does not show any differentiation into ganglion cells. I am going to have drawings and photomicrographs made because the case must be published.

Sincerely yours,

February 12, 1924

Dear Harvey:

Thanks for the abstract of the BW case. That is just what we want. The primary reason for registering it is that Coley believes it to be a case of bone sarcoma, although you and your pathologist call it a Neurocytoma, Coley may be right. Although I agree with you that is unwise to call such tumors bone sarcomas, still there was undoubtedly a clinical confusion and your record states that the X-ray showed bone production. I should appreciate very much a print of this X-ray and will send a copy of this letter to Doctor Howland to see if he can obtain one for us from the X-ray department.

Furthermore, I am very glad to register this case because the slides will be of great interest and probably somewhat instructive to the laboratories who are helping to study these bone tumors.

Unless I keep the laboratories interested they are likely to get tired of the problem and such a case is indeed very interesting.

You yourself may be interested in the following copy of Ewing's report on this same tumor made in Match 1912, (copied from Dr. Coley's Brussells Paper, 1914):

In the case of Baby W, I am unable to offer a positive and exact diagnosis. It is certain that you deal with a malignant tumor which may very well be called sarcoma. I am inclined to think it is either an endothelioma secondary to the cerebral growth, or possibly a neurocytoma derived from misplaced nerve tissue in the cranium.

This showed that Ewing suspected the origin of the tumor at that time and the slide which Coley has forwarded to me shows the same histology as that from the specimen which you took.

May I call your attention to the fact that your instructive case of Cavernous angioma of the skull, (the name of another patient) lacks a slide and the laboratories of the country are therefore not having benefit of having this case passed around to them.

I regard this much as another case which would create interest and wake up the slumbering. It would be particularly interesting as a pair with Bevans' case of a huge tumor of the pelvis which he has considered sarcoma and was apparently cured by X-ray.

Sincerely,

FOLLOW UP NOTE

August 2, 1926

Abstracted from the letter of the patient's father (Dr. Wilkinson) to Dr. Cushing:

He has fair control of his bladder. His cutaneous sensation seems to be good. He gets up, dresses himself, and walking around most of the time with one crutch, he can walk across the floor without a crutch. He has helped me right much in the drug store this summer, and he goes to the barn hitches his pony himself and drives around town any where he wants.

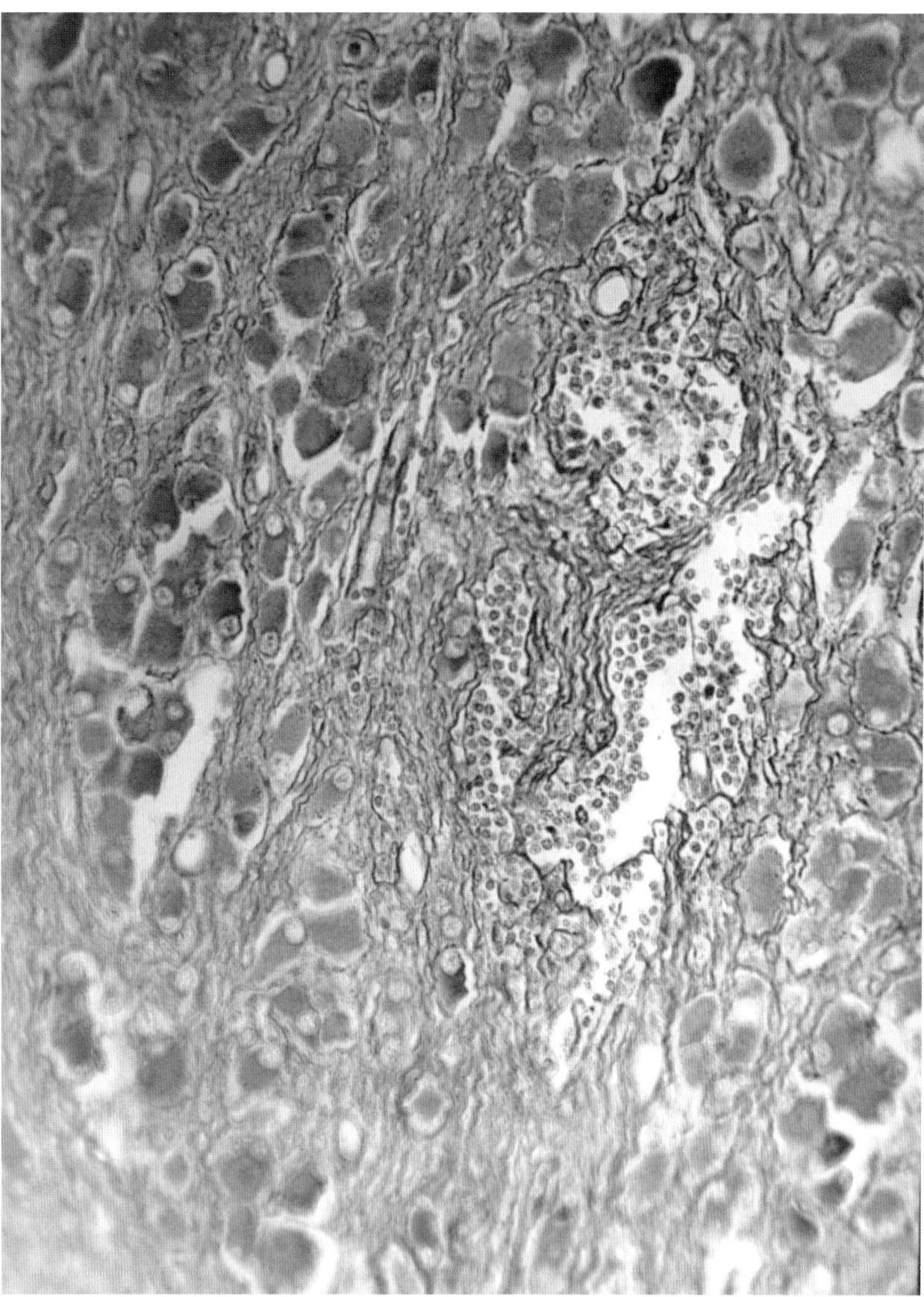

FIG. 3. HISTOLOGY SLIDE.

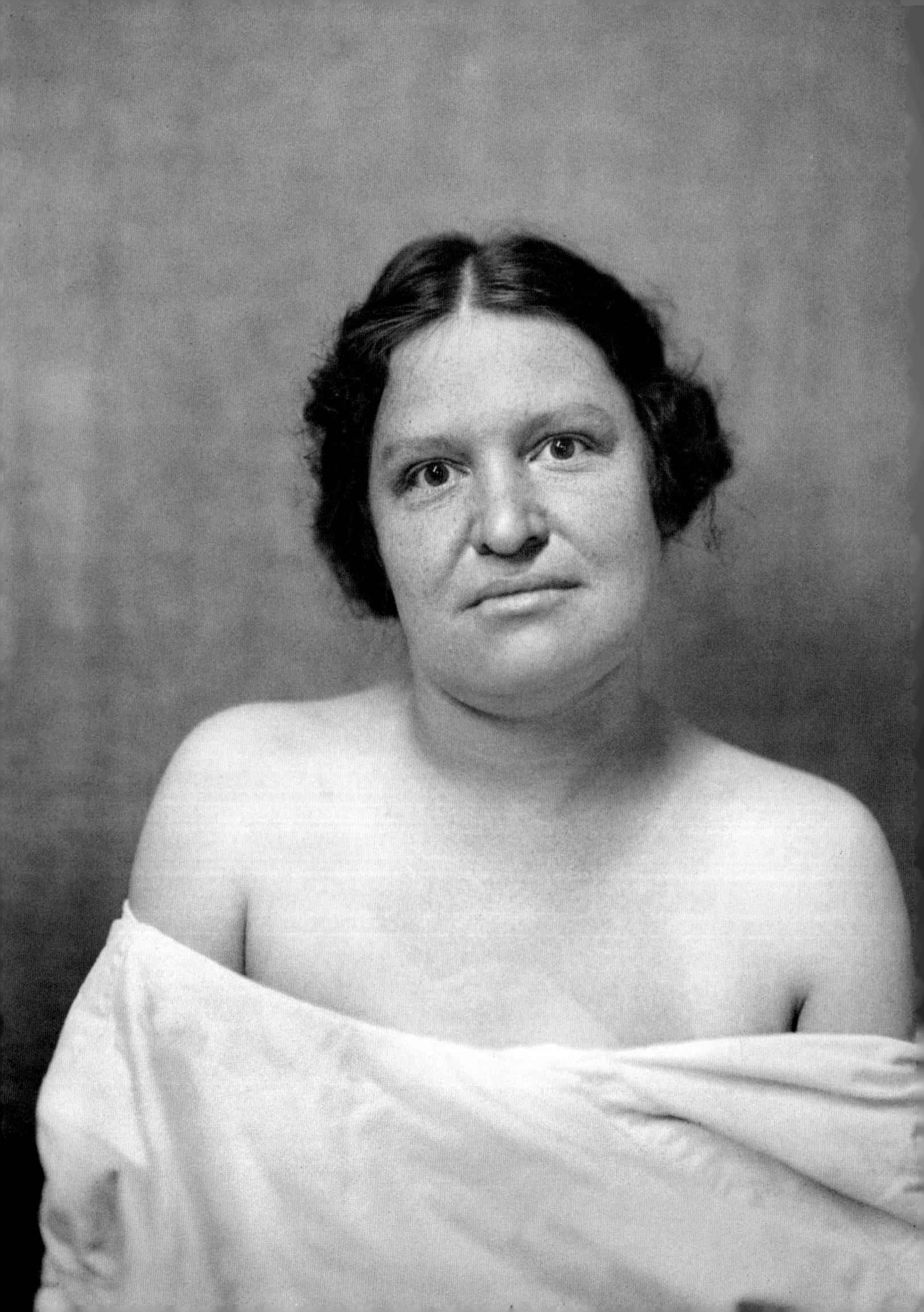

5.5 Spinal meningioma

SEX: F; AGE: 34; SURG. NO. 24039

HISTORY

This patient complained of five-month history of bilateral leg numbness. Following her pregnancy in January of 1925, she noticed right leg weakness and inability to move the right foot. Both feet and right leg felt cold. Her right leg became progressively weaker more recently.

SUMMARY OF POSITIVE FINDINGS
June 10, 1925
Dr. Van Dessel

OBJECTIVE

1. Bilateral increased reflexes of the upper extremities.
2. Absence of abdominal reflexes.
3. Weakness of the right leg, quadriceps and hamstrings of the knee.
4. Patellar jerks increased more to the right, bilateral clonus.
5. Bilateral ankle clonus, more marked to the right.
6. Slight Babinski on the right; indifferent on the left.
7. Definite hypæsthesia to pain over the 1st, 2nd, 3rd, 4th and 5th lumbar skin distribution on the right, over the 2nd, 3rd, 4th on the left.
   Light touch is hypæsthetic on the right over lumbars 3 and 4.
   Pain, light touch and pressure normal over sacral 2, 3, 4, and 5.
8. Vibratory sensation is abnormal in lower extremities.
9. Sensation of position is normal.

IMPRESSION: Cord tumor at the level of the first sacral nerve at the height of the 12th dorsal vertebra.

SPECIAL NOTE
June 24, 1925
Dr. Cushing

It was difficult to tell whether this woman actually had tumor or spinal sclerosis. Opinions differed in this respect and one could have been persuaded either way. She had practically no pain though to be sure that pain was produced by coughing and sneezing. There was no evidence of spinal block which is curious in view of the operative findings. The sensory symptoms on the two sides were much more marked than I would have expected until I saw how far anterior the tumor lay, contrary to its usual position. There was no spinal tenderness or pressure anywhere that I could detect. There was no loss of common sensation, merely a relative loss to pain and temperature. The level of anesthesia pointed toward the upper level at the 11th thoracic. I estimated, therefore, that the tumor would be about at the 9th thoracic and

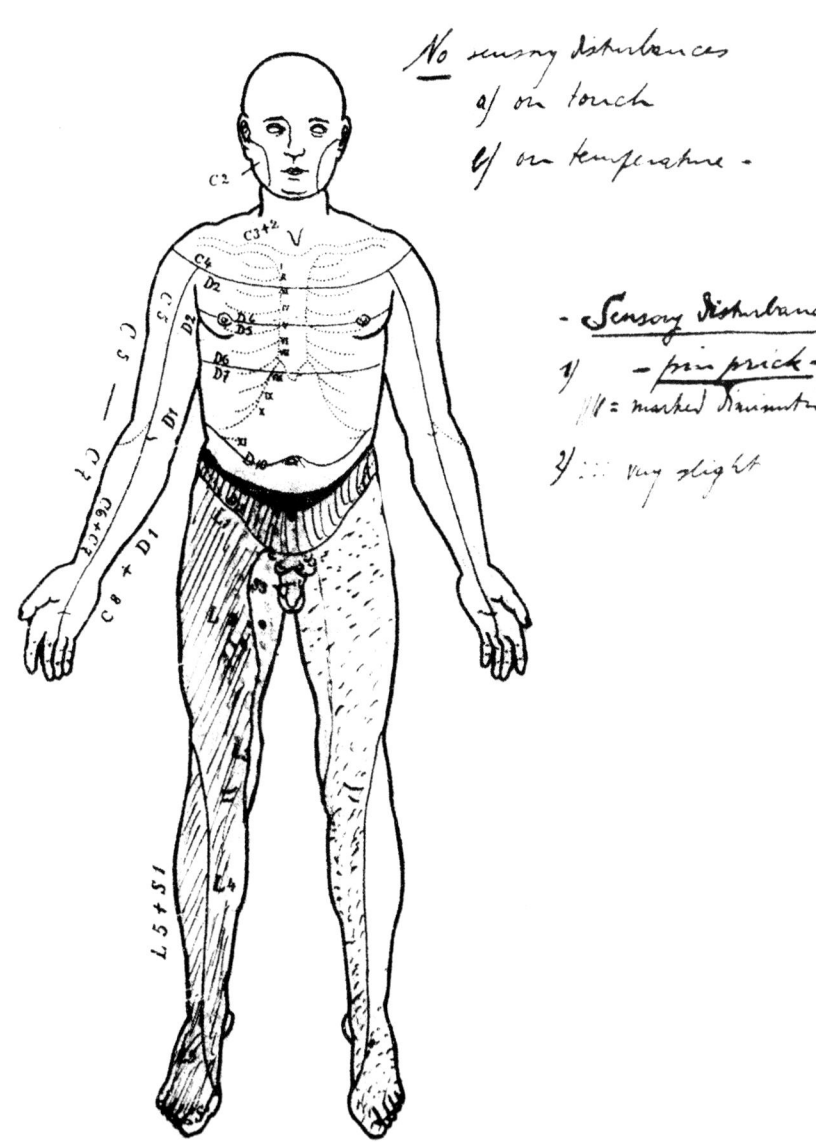

FIG. 1. PREOPERATIVE NEUROLOGICAL EXAMINATION. SENSORY CHANGES.

OPPOSITE PAGE: FIG. 2. POSTOPERATIVE.

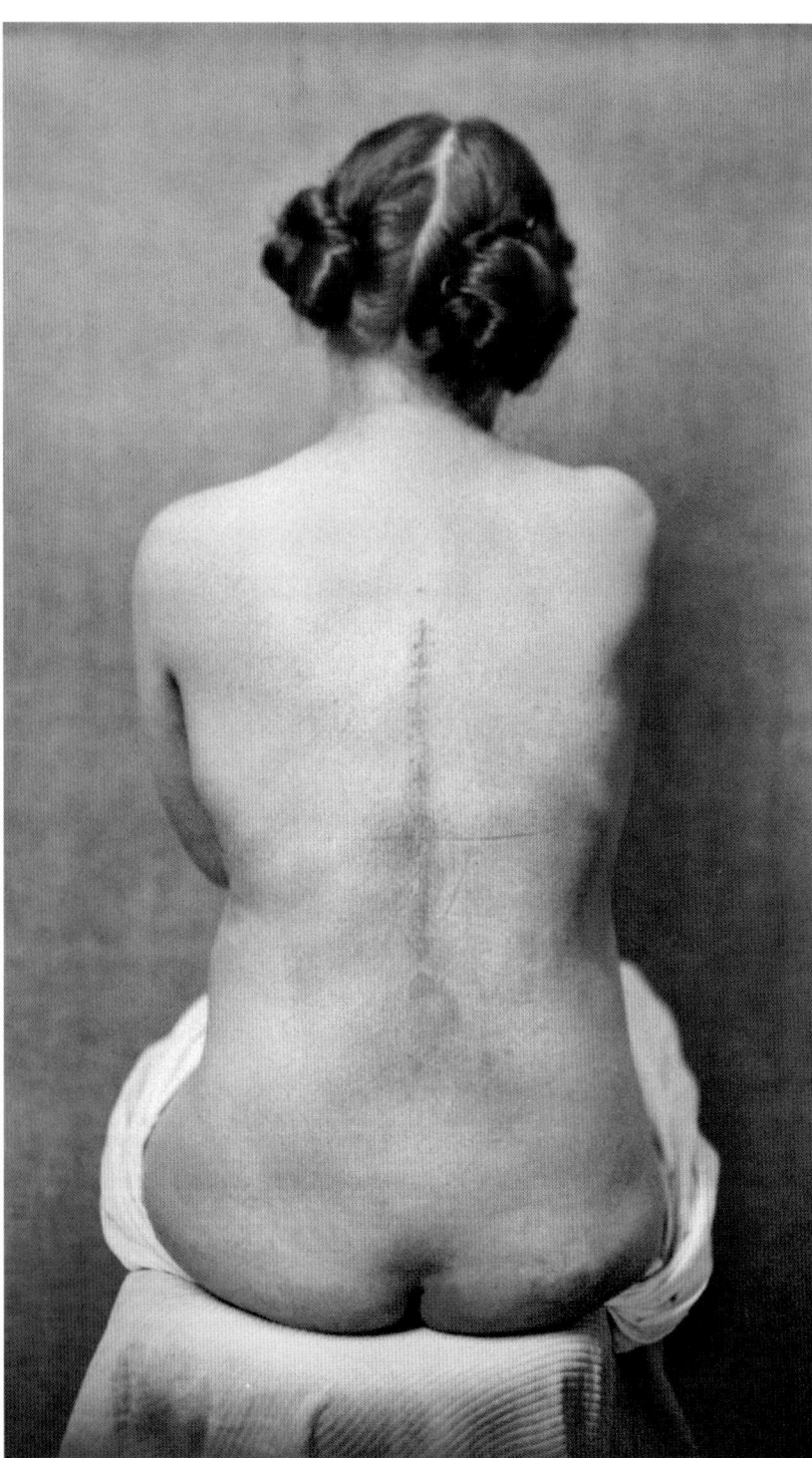

FIG. 3. THREE WEEKS POSTOPERATIVE, SHOWING WOUND.

ject have pointed out why it is that these people have pain. This, I think, is due to the fact that the tumor arises from an arachnoid tumor at the point of emergence of one of the nerve roots so that any change in position causes pain which might not be caused by a tumor otherwise situated. This, too, is a very important matter in regard to the treatment. That is, if one does not wish to face the possibility of recurrence, the tumor must be taken out in its entirety with its attached dura. This was done in the present case and indeed the tumor could not have been possibly dislodged without fragmenting it unless it had been drawn down as shown in the sketches by the dura as dura was incised around the tumor after division of the main nerve root. There is another very interesting matter in connection with these cases, namely, identification of the situation of the tumor by the venous stasis shown on the posterior part of the cord. I do not know that I have ever had this so clearly brought to my attention. The searcher, or filiform bougie, passed readily up the cord between the dura and arachnoid without meeting any resistance. I would not have removed the two upper vertebræ, thereby exposing the tumor, had it not been for this evidence of stasis.

Lipoidal, as in the last one of these cases, certainly would have gravitated promptly to the lower spinal region. There is one other factor to be mentioned, namely the method of getting into the canal without trauma. This I think is preferably done by a succession of burrs. I believe that Miss Warner has already made some sketches of this procedure.

OPERATIVE NOTE
June 24, 1925
Anesthesia – Ether – Miss Way

Laminectomy of Possibly 8th to 12th Thoracic Spines with Negative Findings. Additional Removal of Two Further Dorsal Spines Disclosing Tumor on the Anterior part of the Canal. Total Enucleation with Dura of Arachnoid Tumor.

found it, I think, about at the 7th. I would like to have an x-ray taken after the operation to see just what spines are missing. I take it that one spine higher than the site of the lesion will be absent.

The whole subject of these spinal meningiomas is an interesting one. I do not know that Elsberg and others who have written on the sub-

This operation was entered into half-heartedly for I was a little doubtful of the diagnosis. With the presumed seat of tumor at about the 9th thoracic spine at the center of the incision, the spines were exposed as usual with removal of perhaps the lower five thoracic spines and laminæ. The wound was held open as usual by strippers.

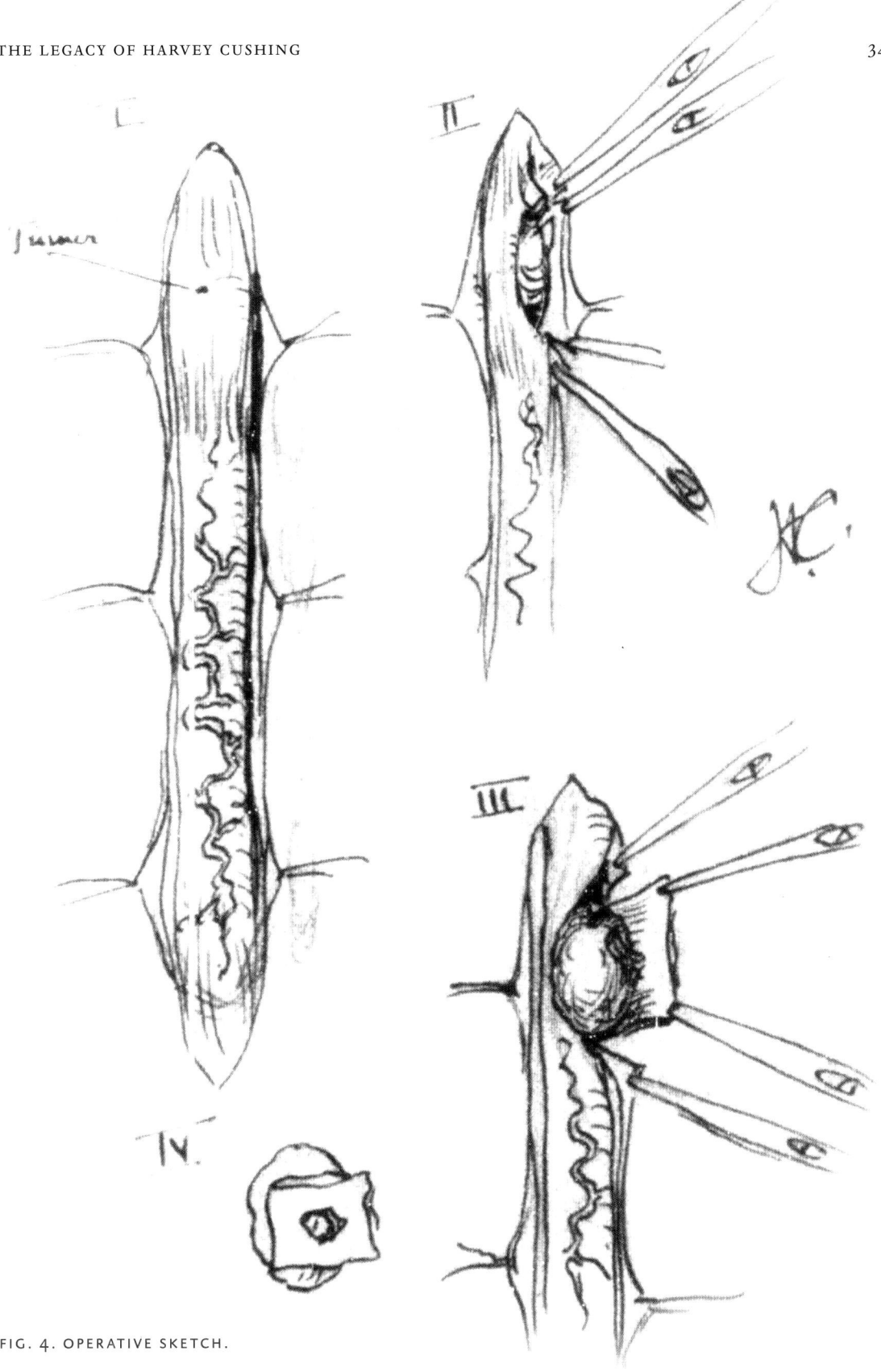

FIG. 4. OPERATIVE SKETCH.

There was no unusual bleeding. The dura was opened without injuring the arachnoid, disclosing a normal but somewhat vascular cord as could be seen through the glistening arachnoid. A searcher in the shape of the usual soft bougie was passed up between dura and arachnoid without detecting a lesion. On further inspecting the cord, I was struck by the markedly dilated vessels an appearance which I could not account for unless there was some stasis above.

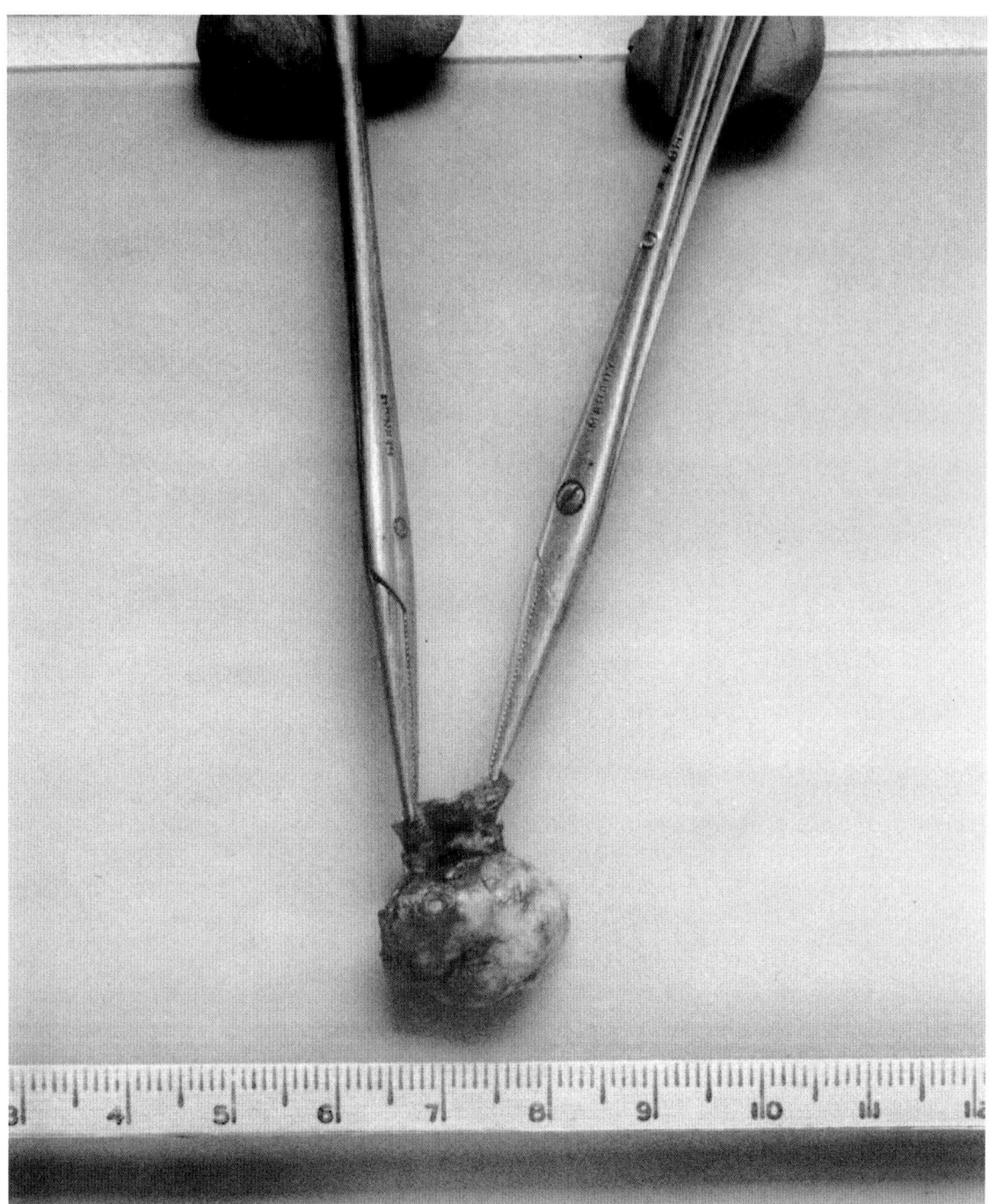

FIG. 5. TUMOR SPECIMEN.

I had a hunch that the tumor would be found higher up and so removed the laminæ of the next two higher vertebræ with the spine of the third vertebra still farther up. On opening the canal and dividing the dura, I came down upon a condition represented in sketch I (Left upper sketch, please see the operative sketch), namely a protrusion of the cord with neovascular appearance, evidently due to tumor within the cord itself or anterior to it.

I had never seen this appearance in a case of spinal meningioma, for almost invariably the tumor is visible. I searched on the right side where the tumor was supposed to lie; opened a little arachnoid space along side the nerve root which I could see and came down upon the smooth, reddish surface of what evidently was going to be an enucleable tumor.

The nerve root was then divided as shown in

sketch II (Right upper sketch), and the tumor began to be apparent. The cord, much flattened, being gradually pushed to the left side with just as little trauma as possible.

I then saw that I was going to have a large, roundish meningioma which could not be withdrawn without breaking it and without causing damage to the cord unless some device could be hit upon.

I consequently, as in fig. III (Right lower sketch), split the dura down on each side of the tumor and began to draw the tumor out and it finally popped from its position in the canal as shown in sketch III. The dura was then divided beneath it, the spinal root being divided in this process and causing a little temporal bleeding. This was controlled by placement of a bit of muscle.

After careful blood-stilling, the dura was reclosed all except for a square portion of it which was withdrawn with the tumor. The wound was closed as usual in layers carefully without a drain.

(Dr. Cushing)

PATHOLOGY NOTE
June 24, 1925
Dr. Bailey

Material consists of a small meningioma removed from the anterior aspect of the spinal canal. The nature of the tumor is obvious and I am not sure that Dr. Cushing wishes to submit any for histological examination.

DISCHARGE NOTE
July 17, 1925
Dr. Bailey

Patient walks with support. Babinski phenomenon is not so easily elicited on the right. Ankle clonus persists on both sides. Right foot is still weak. No hypæsthesia, on the contrary increased hyperesthesia below the 11th level.

LETTER TO DR. CUSHING FROM THE REFERRING PHYSICIAN, 7 YEARS LATER
September 9, 1932

Dear Dr. Cushing:

The patient has no nerve symptoms at present except a numbness in first and second toes of right foot. She has a considerable pain in her back if she exerts herself especially in stooping. She has had two children born since the operation, making now six children living. Her days are of course full of many activities. She wishes me to again express her thanks for what you did for her.

Very respectfully yours,
David E. Dolloff, M.D.

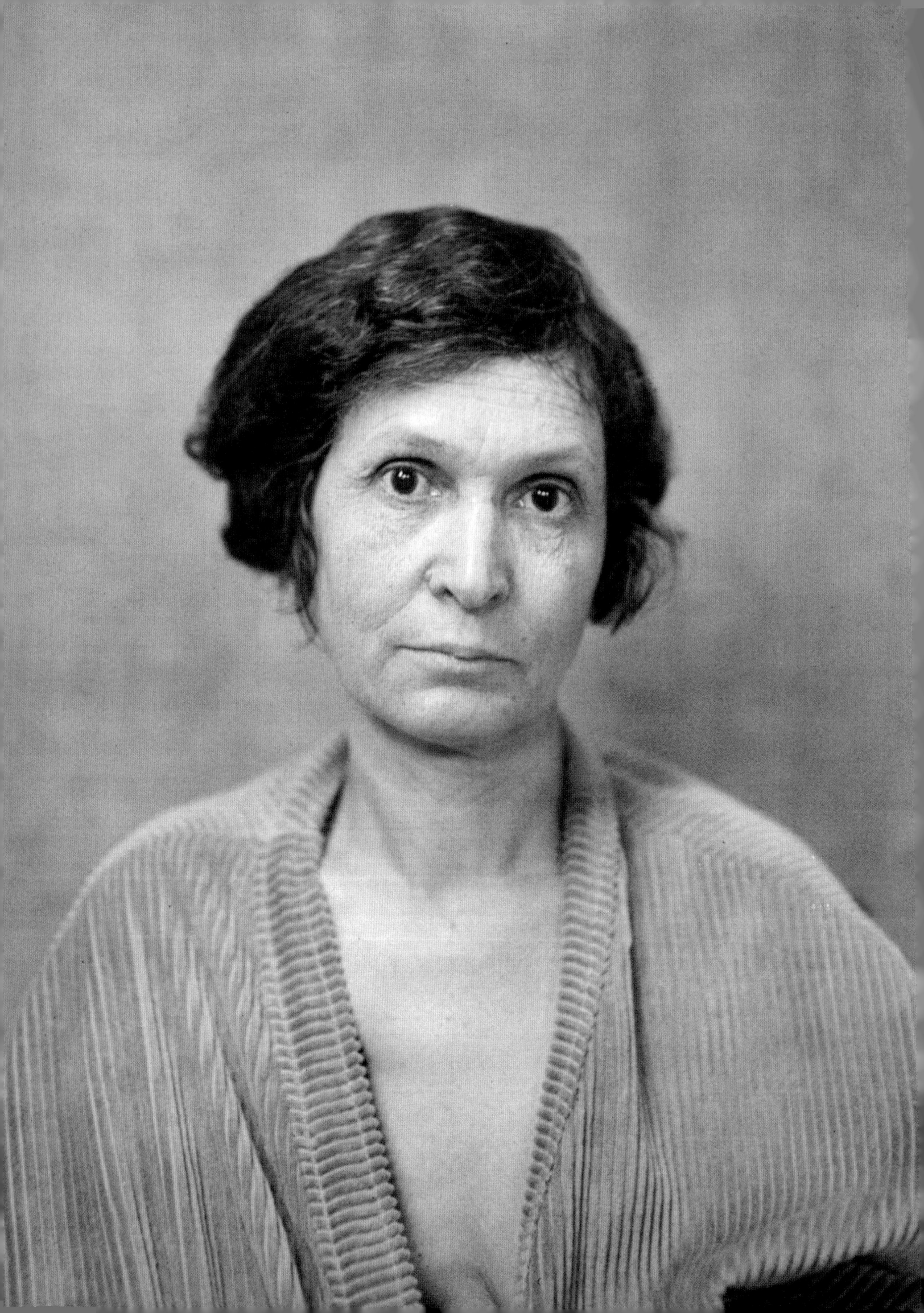

5.6 Spinal meningioma

SEX: F; AGE: 51; SURG. NO. 25237

HISTORY

The letter of referral to Dr. Cushing from Dr. G.H. Walker (Lincoln, Nebraska.)

Dear Doctor:

I will not attempt to give you a thorough history of this case, as you will procure a much more complete one than I could furnish.

However, we suspect cancer, (spinal) especially on account of a breast tumor which had removed in 1915. She also had a uterine fibroid removed about that time.

I first saw Mrs. (name of the patient) in 1922, when she was complaining of occipital pain and insomnia. Examination at that time was negative, with the exception of some slight stomach and abdominal disturbances, which readily responded to treatment.

In April, 1925, she had considerable pain over the liver region, which improved under treatment. In June, she first complained of pain in her feet, arches and legs, which later developed into a motor disturbance, especially of the right leg. We first suspected a sacroiliac synchondrosis, as the Roentgen-ray examination disclosed a slight separation of the sacroiliac joint. However, this was speedily disproved by other symptoms.

The blood examination was negative. The Wasserman was made August 10, 1925.

The spinal examination was made October 15th, with the following results: Normal pressure. Cell count, 136 per cc.—mostly mononuclear. Globulin reaction–trace. Spinal Wasserman–negative. Colloidial gold test, (Lange's), negative.

Following the spinal puncture, she suffered considerably with a severe pain at the base of skull. This was aggravated on attempting an upright position.

Pardon this narrative history, but we think that there is a spinal cord lesion, with a big possibility of it being cancerous.

We are very anxious for Mrs (name of the patient) to see you. She is a lovely woman, very sensible and willing to cooperate in every way.

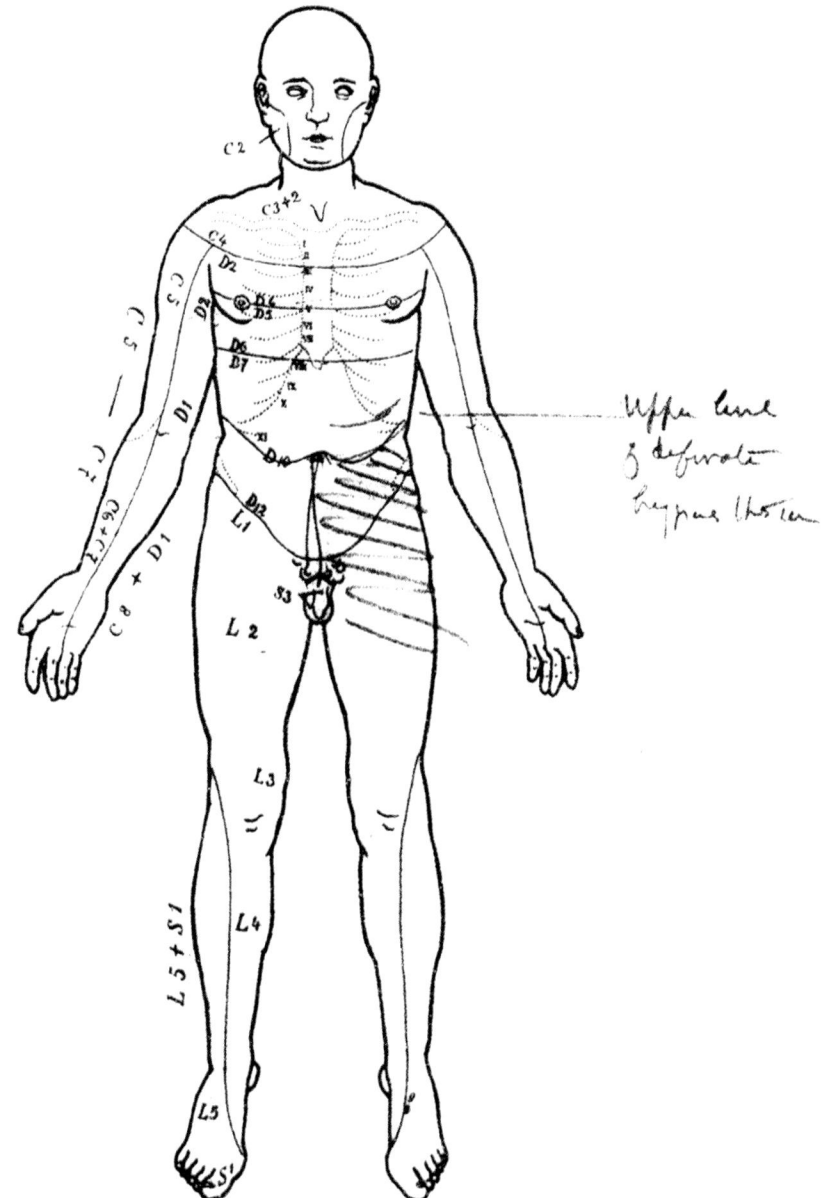

FIG. 2. PREOPERATIVE SENSORY CHART.

My consultants have been Drs H.H. Everett, of Lincoln, and LeRoy Crummer of Omaha, both of whom have the honor to know you personally.

We will all appreciate anything you can do for us in this case.

Yours truly
George H. Walker

OPPOSITE PAGE: FIG. I. TWO WEEKS POSTOPERATIVE.

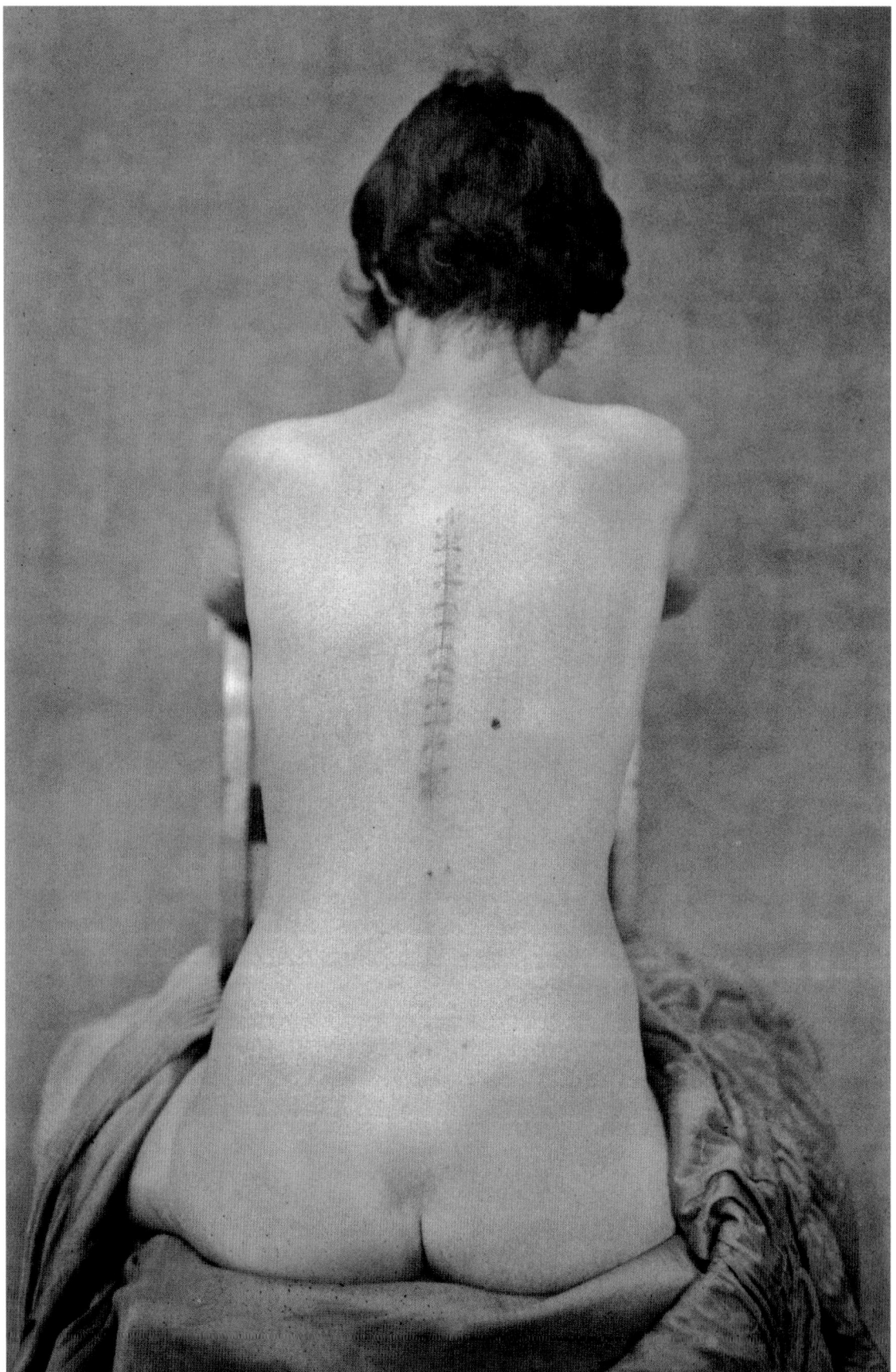

FIG. 3. TWO WEEKS POSTOPERATIVE.

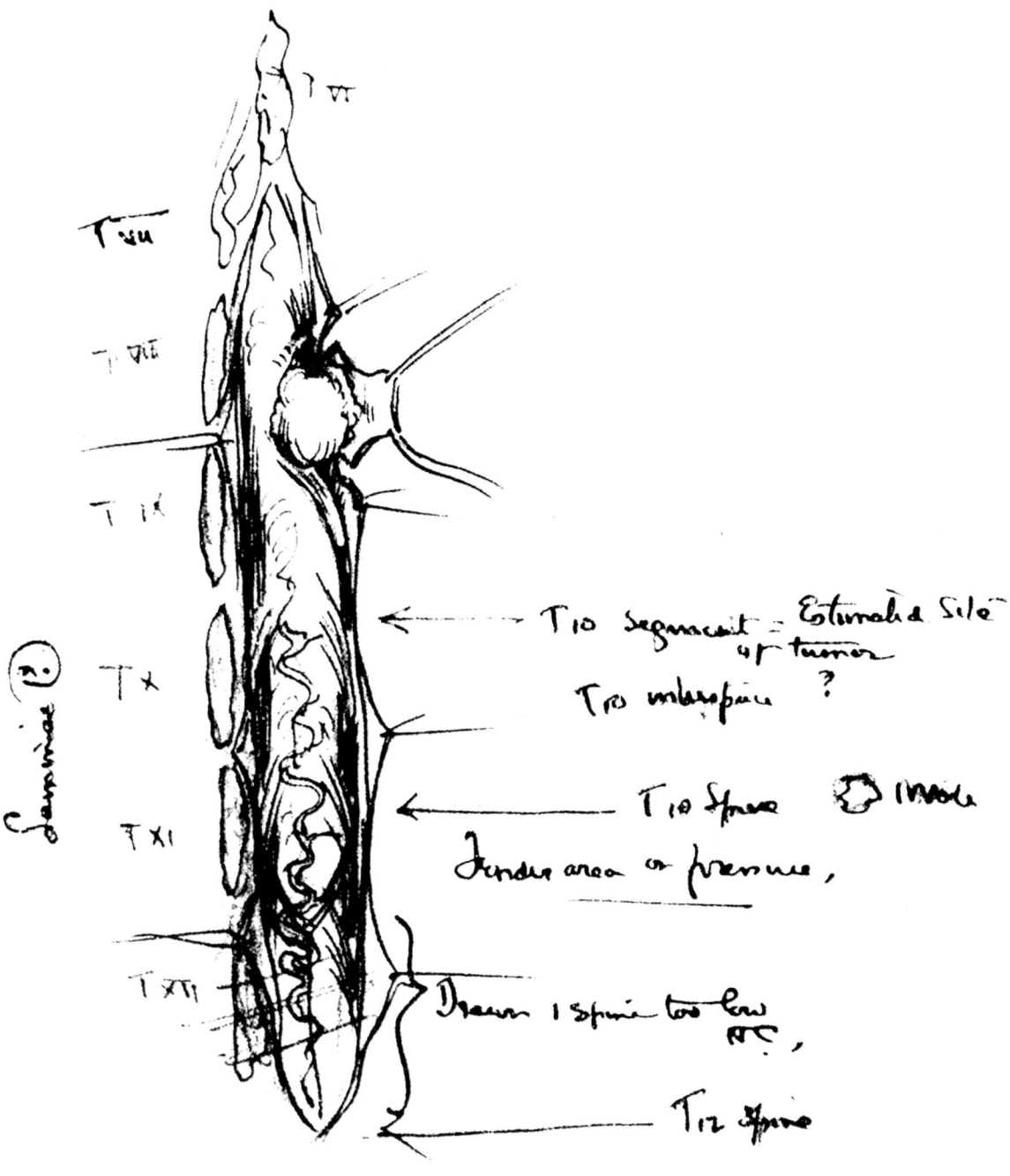

FIG. 4. OPERATIVE SKETCH.

SUMMARY OF POSITIVE FINDINGS
November 22, 1925
Dr. Davidoff

SUBJECTIVE:
1. Sensation of pain in toes and arches and legs, 6 months ago.
2. Feeling of numbness in the toes of both feet, especially on the right, gradually creeping up to the pelvis.
3. Sensation of girdle-like constriction in the region of the pelvis, for two weeks.
4. Difficulty with walking for 5 weeks, especially with weakness of the right leg.
5. Constipation and slight delay in starting urinary stream, for the past few weeks.
6. Sensation of tightness and drawing up of the right lower extremity for the past two or three days.
7. History of amputation of right breast 12 years ago, for "incipient malignancy."

OBJECTIVE:
1. Sensory disturbances of left lower extremity

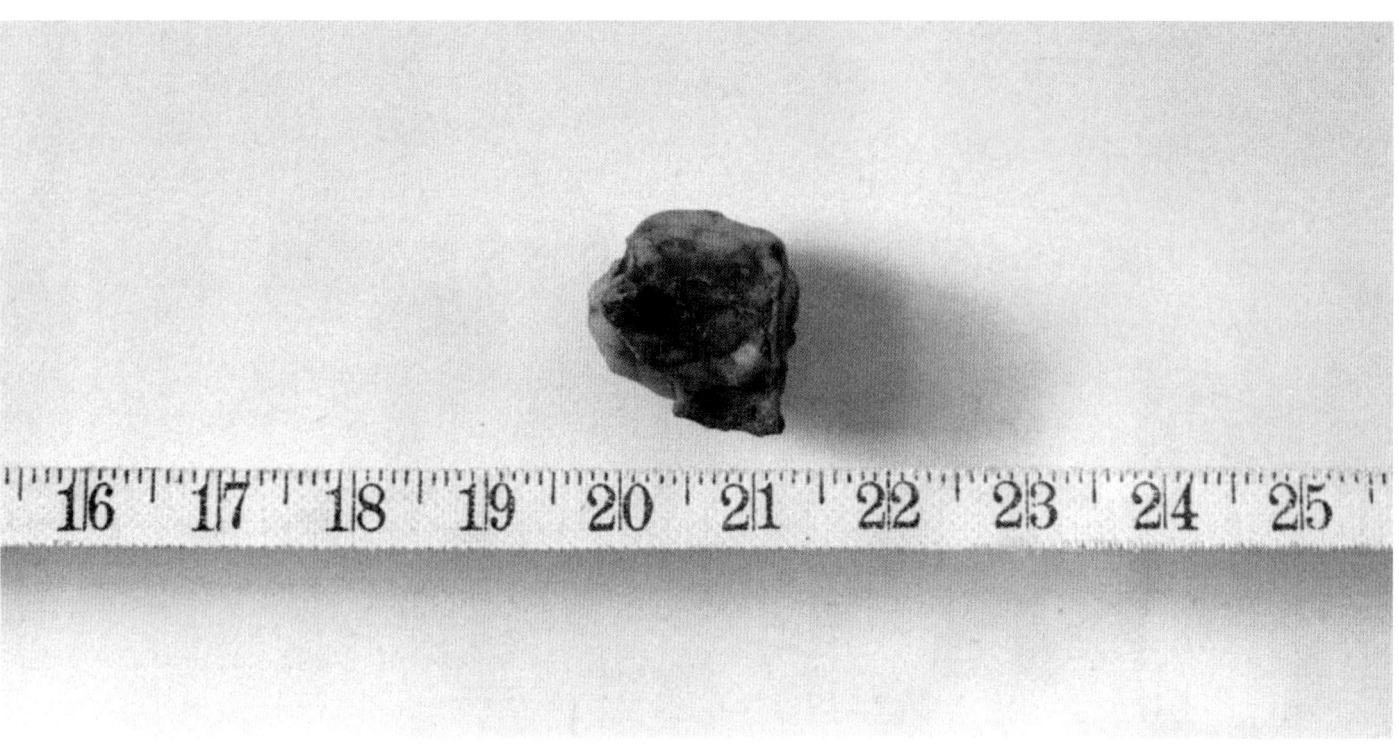

FIG. 5. RESECTION SPECIMEN.

from region of the pelvis down (See chart).
2. Slight spasticity and motor weakness of right lower extremity.
3. Positive Babinski and Oppenheim on the right.
4. Slight ankle clonus on the right.
5. Loss of deep sensation of the right lower extremity.
6. Positive Romberg. Slight dragging of the right foot when walking.

IMPRESSION: In view of the relatively short history and the fairly well-marked Brown-Sequard syndrome, it seems to me that the most likely diagnosis would be an extramedullary tumor of the spinal cord, located in the region of the lower two thoracic and the lumbar spinal cord segment on the right. The history of breast amputation twelve years ago is so remote that it seems hardly likely that a supposed malignancy will have been quiescent until this time, and begin showing signs of metastases now.

SPECIAL NOTE
December 3, 1925
Dr. Cushing

We would gather by the note given yesterday, when we examined this patient, that I had no very definite expectation of finding a tumor, even should she actually have one. Moreover, some objective symptoms she could detect, namely an upper level of sensory disturbance at the 10th skin field, and tenderness to pressure along the 10th, 11th, and 12th spines, particularly about the 12th spine. On the other hand, her old history of pain in the gallbladder region was at least an objective indication of the fact that this symptom, as actually due to tumor, must be caused by one higher in the spinal region.

I do not know that the general history brings out the fact that the patient, at the present time, is having practically no discomfort and only on solicitations does she confess to some little occasional gallbladder discomfort, on straining or coughing.

OPERATIVE NOTE
December 3, 1925
Anesthesia-Ether-Miss Way

Laminectomy of T VII – T XI. Exposure of Right-Sided Meningioma after Removing One of the Extra Spines. Though Tumor Was Exposed in the Upper Part of the First Field.

This was an uncomplicated procedure with bleeding fairly well controlled. The laminectomy was performed in the usual fashion with removal of the spines. And as much of the laminæ as possible, with the flat giant rongeur, followed by serial perforation so that there remained little to be removed, except the intervertebral bridges of tissue.

In the upper part of the exposed field, which I imagine took in T XI to T VII, I could palpate a tumor and could see pulsating dura above, whereas below the dura remained full and was non-pulsating.

I consequently removed the other spine and the corresponding lamina, which I take to have been T VII. I would be glad to have this patient's spine x-rayed, so as to be sure as to the exact number of laminæ removed.

This gave me about three to four cm headway to the tumor. The dura was then excised, leaving the arachnoid intact, and on reflecting it, it showed, as in the sketch, a nodule of tumor about the size shown, laid bare. Into this tumor a nerve root extended, and below it another nerve root passed down into the next intervertebral foramen.

This last nerve was separated from the tumor, and the upper nerve divided between clasps, as shown. The segment of dura corresponding to the tumor was drawn out, and as in the last several extirpations of tumors of this kind, the growth was removed together with the section of dura.

It was adherent and also the point of perforation of the nerve toward the intervertebral foramen.

After complete blood stilling, the dura was resutured, except for this large defect, which was left, and it corresponded to a marked indentation in the cord, though so far as I could tell, the cord was not damaged. It may be said in passing, that the tumor was a little more adherent to the cord than I have ordinarily seen. Apparently, in other words, it was adherent to the pia and had to be gently brought away from almost a pia-like actual substance. However, there is no doubt that the growth was removed in its entirety.

The wound was closed securely and carefully in the usual six to eight layers, without drain. It was left reasonably dry before the final suture could take.

(Dr. Cushing)

PATHOLOGY REPORT
December 3, 1925

Specimen consists of what appears to be an intact meningioma removed from the right spinal cord above apposite the VIIth thoracic segment.

The patient had fairly typical symptoms of a spinal tumor in this region which had been long misdiagnosed as gallstone.

Measurement of specimen 1 x 1.5 x 2 cm in its three dimensions. It is somewhat nodular.

Diagnosis: Meningioma.

(Resident pathologist)

SPECIAL NOTE
January 3, 1926
Dr. Davidoff

No objective signs of disturbance of either motor or sensory functions on either lower extremity. When walking, however, patient still is a little tottery without any characteristic disturbance of gait.

DISCHARGE NOTE
January 5, 1926
Dr. Davidoff

Patient still a little easily fatigued when walking, otherwise perfectly well. Discharged home today.

LETTER TO DR. CUSHING
September 10, 1932

Dear Dr. Cushing:

I am sorry Dr. Walker has neglected to report on my case. Had I known that, I would have reported myself. I am very glad to be able to tell that I am in good health and have been most of the time since I was in Boston. I weigh 118 lbs. and have kept the gain I made following the operation. I have Dr. Walker check on my condition every few months and he says he finds no symptoms of my former trouble.

Our papers carried a notice of your retirement from the university and Peter Bent Brigham. I hope this doesn't mean you are giving up your practice permanently. We need your skill.

Sincerely yours,
Mrs. JS

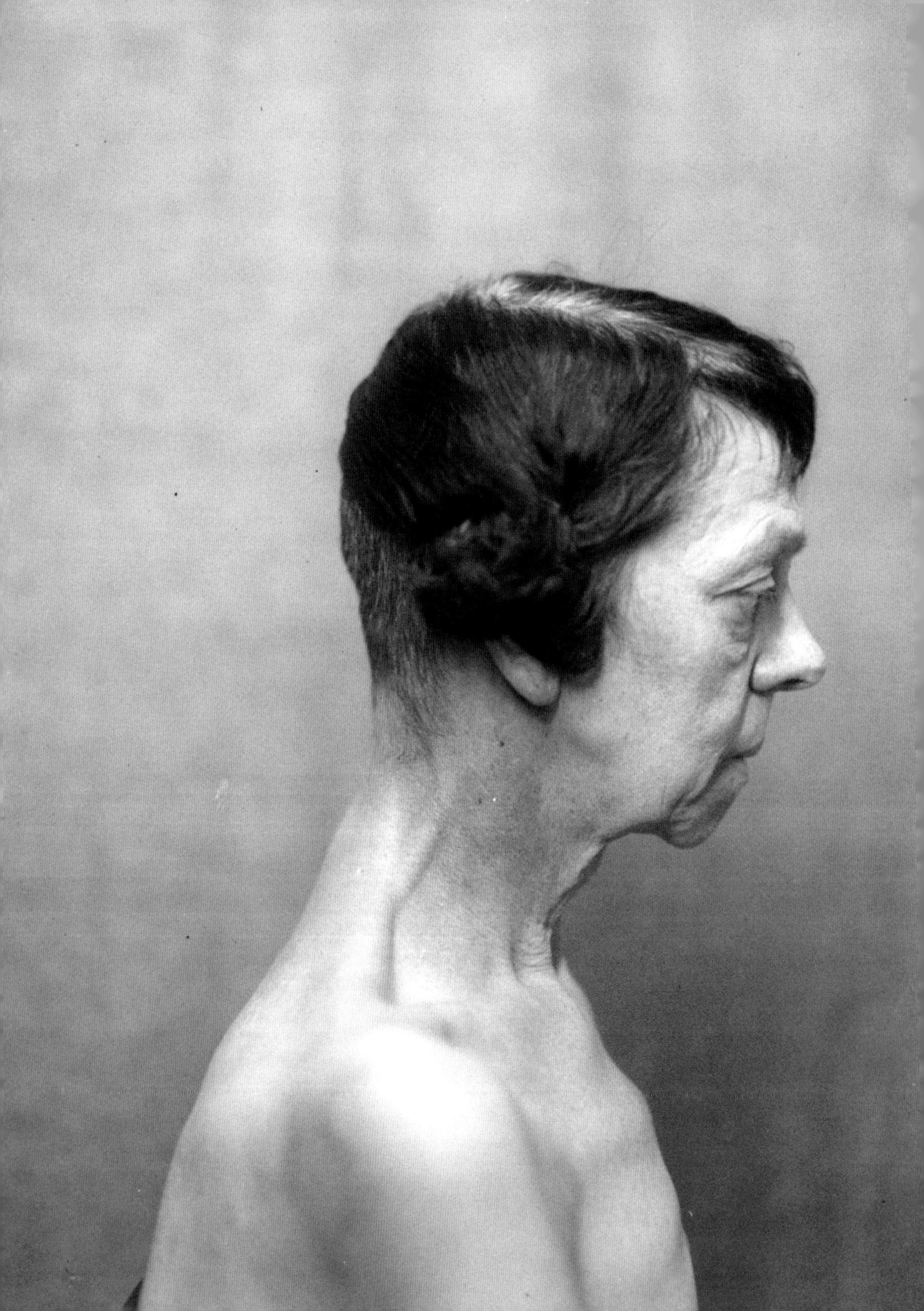

5.7 Spinal meningioma

SEX: F; AGE: 47; SURG. NO. UNKNOWN

HISTORY

The patient complained of progressive pain in the upper neck/occipital region and weakness of the left arm and leg.

January 6, 1926
Dr. Horrax

Examination revealed weakness of the left hand, arm, leg, with some muscular atrophy in the left hand. Exaggerated reflexes and positive Babinski were present on the left. Sensory level was determined at the 1st thoracic spine posteriorly.

IMPRESSION: Spinal cord tumor at the 5th-6th cervical segments.

Dr. Cushing's hand-written "Special Note" was not readable.

OPERATIVE NOTE
January 11, 1926
Anesthesia – Ether – Miss Way

Laminectomy.

This woman as told in the special note of yesterday evidently has high tumor, I thought probably of a tumor involving the root of suboccipital nerve owing to the pain in her suboccipital region. The tumor could hardly have done this although the fact of her atrophic hand would have suggested tumor of the lower cervical region. The accompanying sketch shows fairly well the situation which was found.

The laminectomy was performed easy and the spines and laminae removed by the large rongeurs without difficulty. The occipito-atlantal ligament seemed full… Nevertheless, suspecting a tumor in the upper region I removed a portion of the suboccipital bone, including the posterior rim of the foramen magnum. The tumor as a matter of fact, proved to have projected upward for possibly a cm. of this rim. The dura was then opened without injuring the arachnoid at the upper part of the field …

A surprisingly large tumor was then disclosed and only the lower part of the cord could be seen. I began, as I have done in recent cases to incise the dura down to the attachment of the tumor but as a matter of fact found to my dismay that the attach-

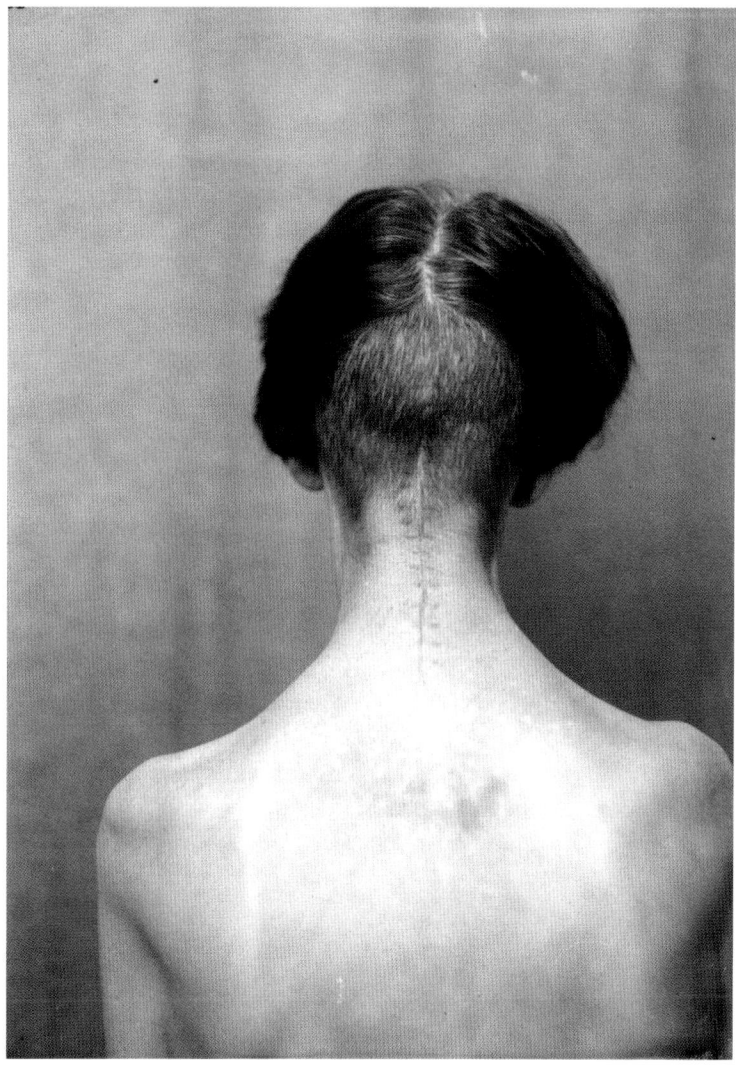

FIG. 2. THREE WEEKS POSTOPERATIVE.

ment was apparently from the anterior portion of the dura, as in the case of (the name of another patient) of years ago. I feared that it may be impossible to dislodge the growth without contusion of the cord. Consequently made, as shown in the sketch a median incision in the tumor and scooped possibly the third of the contents within the capsule. Then, I drew together the edges with 4-5 silk stitches, used as stays, I could tilt the growth slightly outward and began to deliver it … Last step being taken by elevating it with the periosteal element … To my gratification there seemed to be no rupture of the tumor capsule. Cf. photograph.

OPPOSITE PAGE: FIG. 1. THREE WEEKS POSTOPERATIVE.

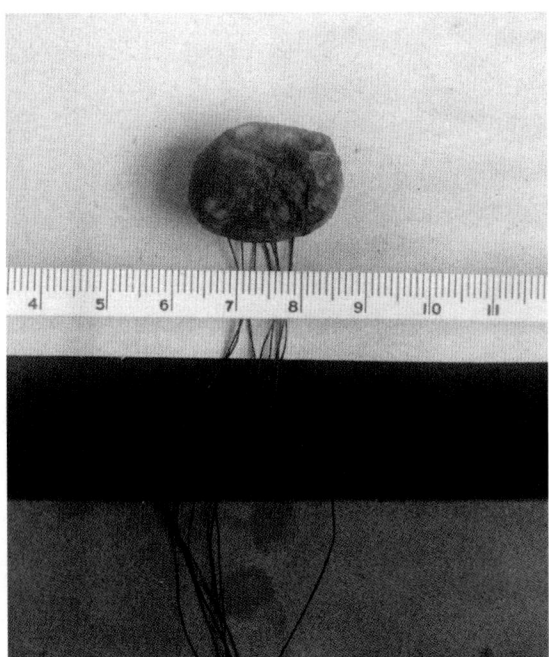

FIG. 3. RESECTED TUMOR ON SUTURES.

There was a little bleeding from the cavity which was checked and filled. The dura was then resutured not as perfectly as I might have otherwise done had it not been for the lateral incision in the membrane on the left side.

Patient stood the operation perfectly, the wound was closed in layers with a few silver sutures but otherwise by fine silk. Weight of the tumor removed was 4.65 gms.

(Dr. Cushing)

PATHOLOGY REPORT
January 11, 1926

Material – Tissue consists of a few fragments of a meningioma (dural endothelioma) exposed at operation at about the region of the foramen magnum. The tumor was incised and a partial intracapsular decompression performed before it was dislodged. The tumor itself is preserved for Dr. Cushing's collection and for subsequent study.

Microscopic description – The slides made up of elongate cells arranged in whorls or rings, some forming spaces, others forming rounded, concentric masses filling endothelial spaces. There is a small amount of fibrous tissue stroma.

Diagnosis – Dural endothelioma.

("Resident pathologist")

Postoperative course was without complications.

DISCHARGE NOTE
February 9, 1926
Dr. Davidoff

Sensory function is normal. Patient still has some interosseous and "hyperthernar" atrophies. Discharged with improvement.

FOLLOW UP NOTES
August 19, 1926
Dr. Davidoff

Patient reports here on her way through Boston. She is very happy with her newly acquired health and very grateful to the operator. She has complete use of her arm and leg, walks perfectly, and boasts that she even dances. All the interosseous and hyperthernar atrophies present before the operation and to some extent at the time of discharge have entirely disappeared. The region of the operation is almost invisible, movements of her neck are quite free and unassociated with pain or discomfort. No examinations were made of sensory functions but the presumption is that they continue to be normal as they were at the time of discharge.

October 9, 1926
Dr. Horrax

Patient has no pain or discomfort. Nor conscious of any weakness of left arm or leg. Could scarcely lift her left leg before and now well, dances, etc. No objective weakness of left arm or leg. No sensory disparity of two sides except that the left occipital area is still anesthetic. Deep reflexes slightly diminished on left.

LETTER FROM THE PATIENT
January 20, 1928
Dear Dr. Cushing:

Thank you very much for your greetings and interest in me. I think of the condition I was in two years ago, it doesn't seem like that this can be me. I am so much better, and I don't believe people will ever cease talking about what was done for me. I hope when I go to Boston, that both you and Dr. Homans will have one free moment to look at me.

Very gratefully,
(Signed)

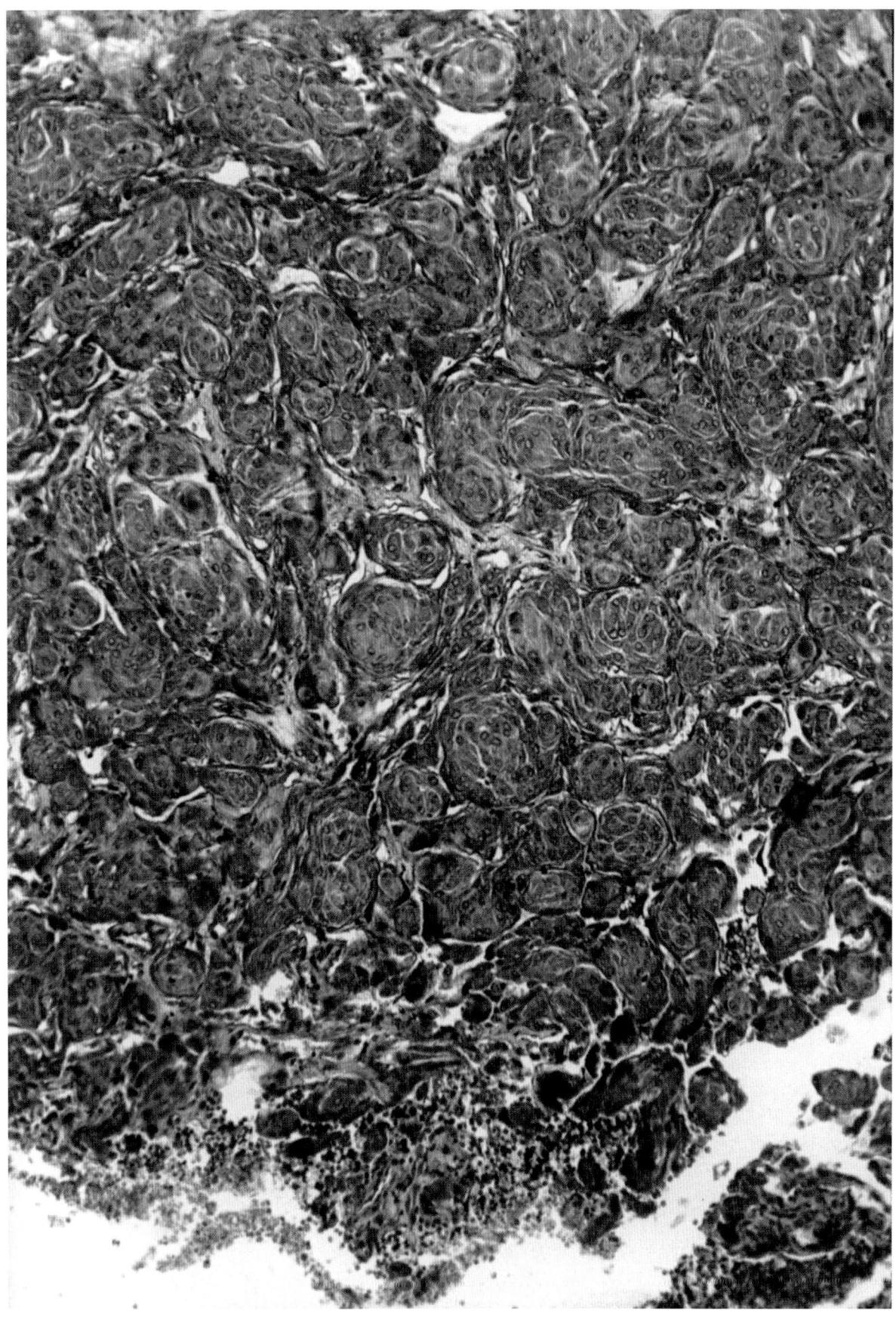

FIG. 4. HISTOLOGY SLIDE.

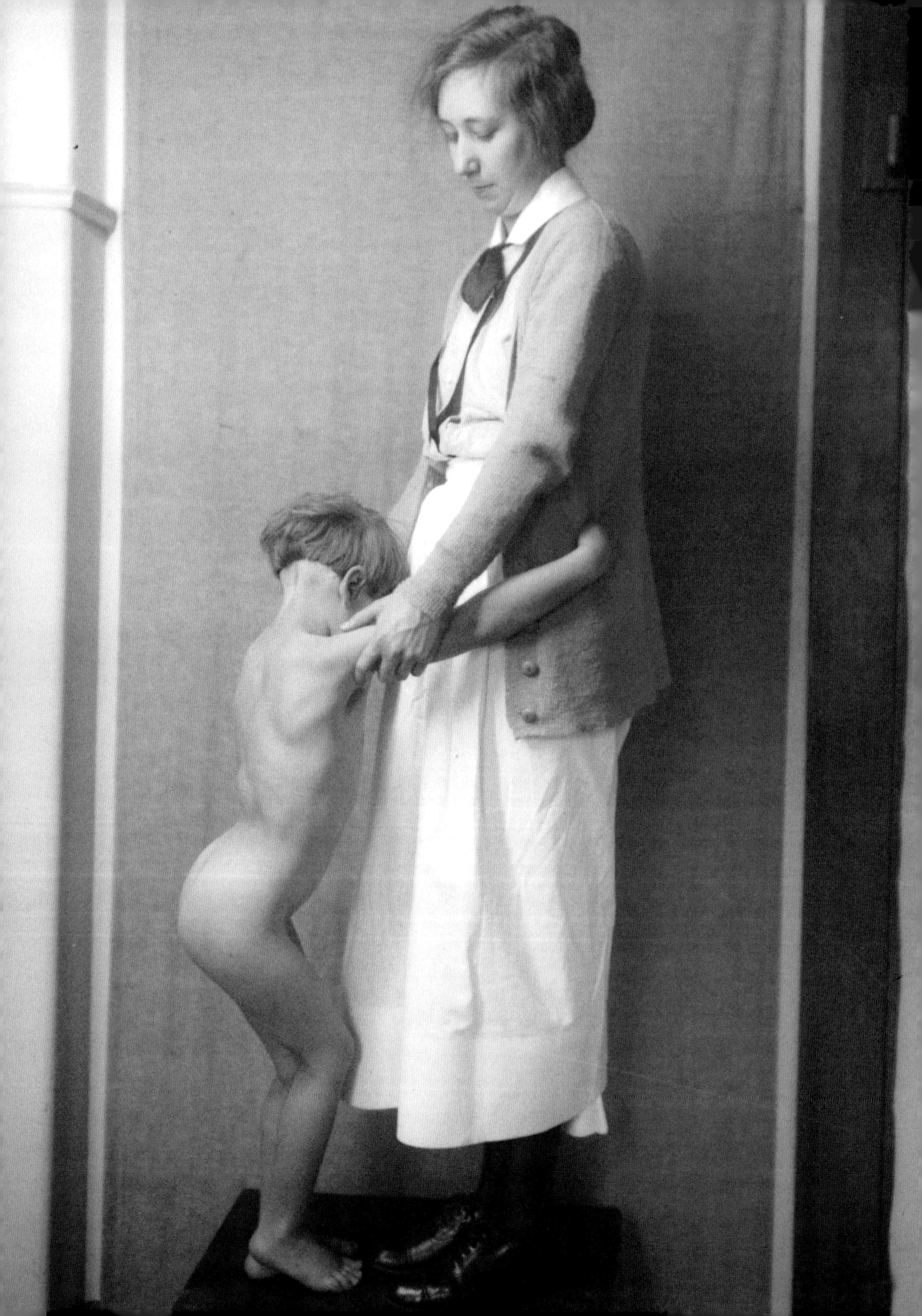

5.8 Spina bifida: Intraspinal lipoma

SEX: F; AGE: 7; SURG. NO. 26384

HISTORY

The child was born with "spina bifida." On the 11th day of age, a "dermoid cyst" was removed from the region of the lumbar spine. At age 5, due to spinal deformity, she was taken to the Children's Hospital and was placed in a "posterior shell" and was then taken to the Peabody Home where she continued her rehabilitation for her lower extremity weakness. The shell was removed several weeks later and she continued to wear a plaster jacket most of the time. She was recently seen by Dr. Cushing who advised her admission to undergo surgery.

SUMMARY OF POSITIVE FINDINGS
May 15, 1926
Dr. Schaltenbrand

SUBJECTIVE
1. Spina bifida first noticed at birth.
2. Eleven days after birth a dermoid cyst over the spina bifida was removed by Dr. Cutler in the Children's Hospital.
3. When the patient began to walk at one year, the parents noticed dragging of the right foot.

OBJECTIVE
1. Kyphosis and scoliosis of the dorsal spine. Lordosis of the lumbar spine.
2. Spina bifida in the height of the last thoracic and first two lumbar vertebrae.
3. Abdominal reflexes absent on both sides.
4. Legs atrophic, especially the right one.
5. Spasticity of the right leg.
6. Paresis of adduction and abduction of the thighs. Paresis of flexion of the knees and of dorsal flexion of the feet.
7. Exaggerated knee and ankle jerks on right side.
8. Absent knee reflex on left side.
9. Positive Babinski on both sides.
10. Sphincters not contracted.

IMPRESSION: *Bilateral paresis of the leg due to spina bifida.*

SPECIAL NOTE
May 17, 1926
Dr. Fallon

The following is a copy of the C.H. operative note obtained over the telephone: May 17, 1919

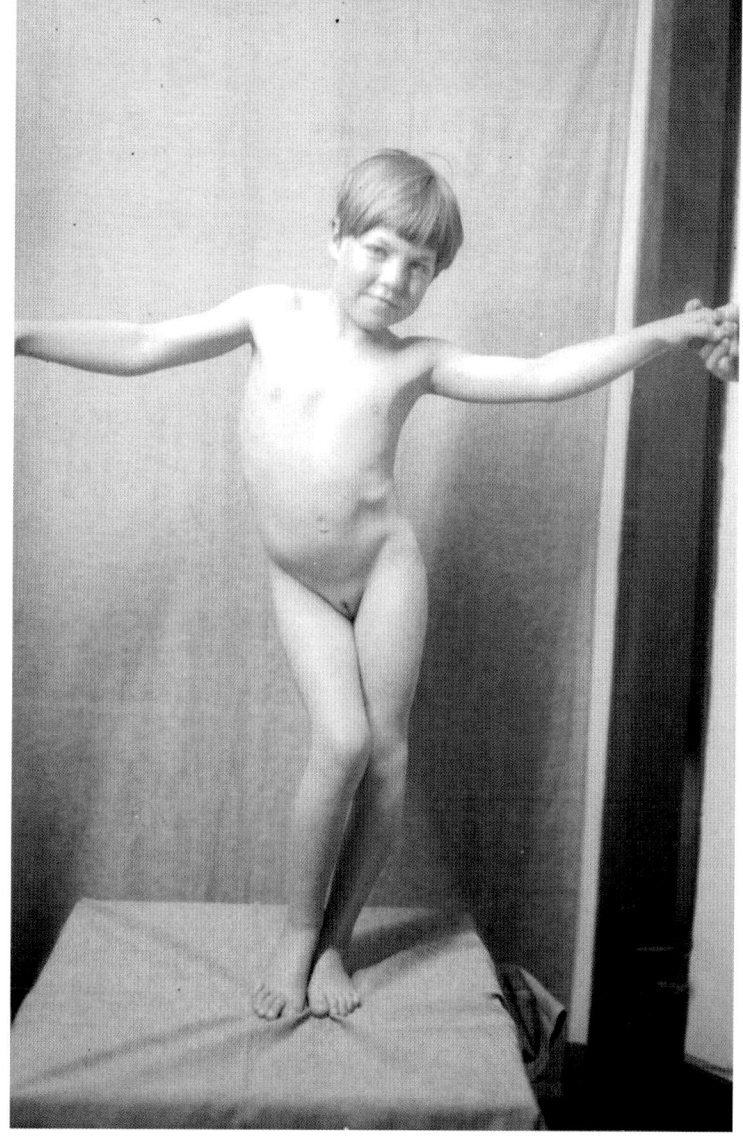

FIG. 2. PREOPERATIVE.

Operator: Dr. C. Mixter
Anaesthesia: ether
Dermoid of the back.

Transverse elliptical incision excising the sinus carried down to process of bone. Periosteum incised along left side of base of process. Process lifted up and venous plexus closed beneath suggesting veins over membranes cord. Projecting portion of process excised and base left to cover in defect. Periosteum and lumbar fascia closed with interrupted chromic catgut. Skin closed with S.W.G.

OPPOSITE PAGE: FIG. 1. PREOPERATIVE.

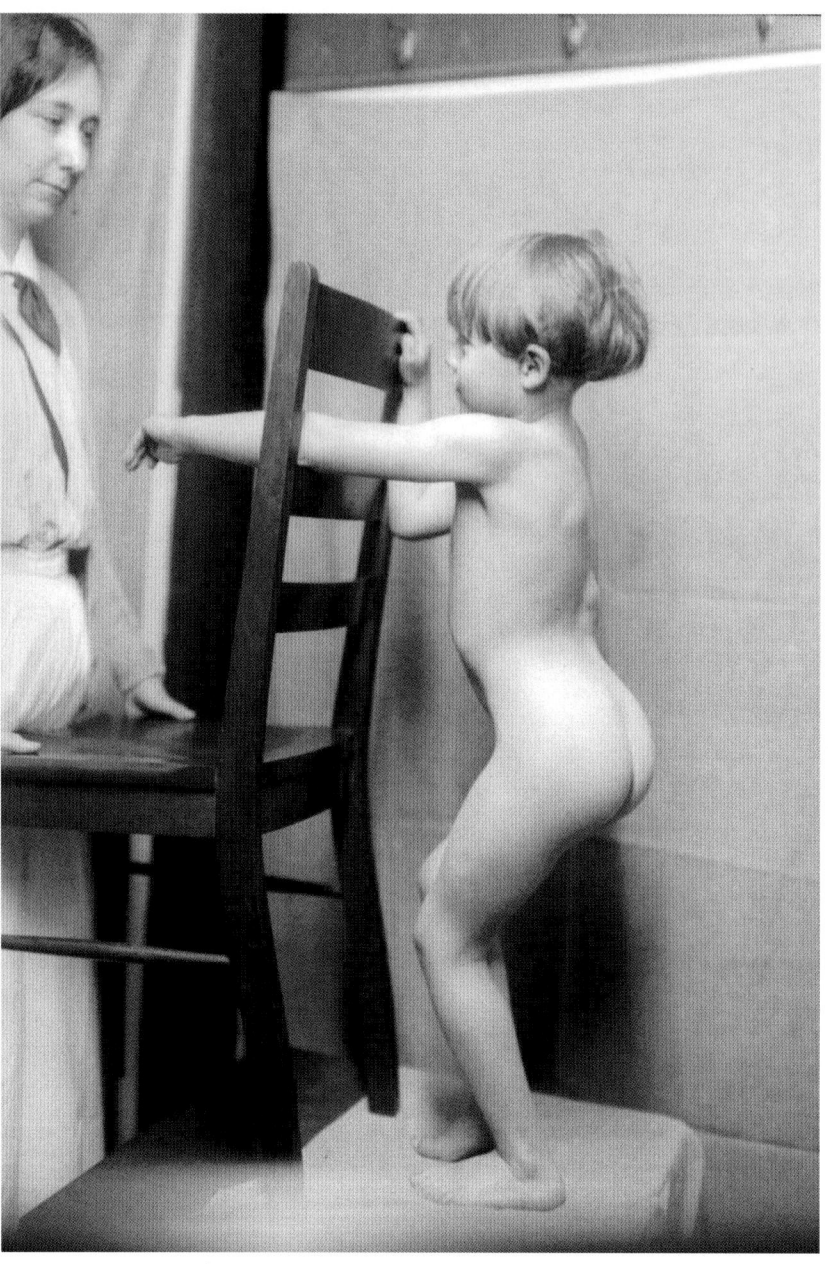

FIG. 3. PREOPERATIVE.

and horsehair. Local examination, preoperative: A circular tumor over lower dorsal region: firm and apparently bony with sloughing of skin for an area of half an inch at apex. Diameter of tumor nearly 2 cm.

The record room at the C.H. says that they have no pathology report.

RADIOLOGY REPORT
May 17, 1926
Dr. Sosman

A.P. and lateral films of the spine and pelvis show there is apparently a congenital anomaly. There is a spina bifida involving the 11th and 12th dorsal vertebrae and the 1st, 2nd and 3rd lumbar vertebrae. The 1st and 2nd lumbar vertebrae are fused and are much narrowed on the left then on the right... Lateral view shows collapse of the body of the 11th dorsal vertebra.

SPECIAL NOTE
May, 17, 1926
Dr. Cushing

This child has a history of having been operated upon a few days after birth for a presumed spina bifida. There is now a transverse scar 10 cm in length about over the 1st lumbar vertebra. Corresponding to this scar is a somewhat fluctuant swelling which is not tender and it is obviously associated even without the X-ray with an anomalous condition of the spine. One can palpate spinal processes down to the 9th thoracic and then they become obscured until one comes possibly to the 2nd lumbar. There are several irregular bony prominences, one of which lies directly under the scar of the old operation and appears to be almost a transverse bony prominence. There is a tendency to excessive growth of hair over the protrusion. The child sits erect without difficulty. She is well pigmented from sun exposure. When erect the swelling is much more prominent. There is a marked dorsal scoliosis to the right or dorsal curve to the right which I should think was due rather to defect rather than to an actual scoliotic twist.

There is a slight patch of pale skin in the midline, about at the level of the posterior spine of the ilium. I do not see any especial evidence of change in the skin in the cutaneous fields below the level of the lesion. The child is well developed and nourished and is a normal baby apparently above this lesion. The patient is able with help to take a few steps, the left leg being much better than the right but she is evidently very spastic on both sides. The deep reflexes are exaggerated with clonus easily elicited on the right and a pretty constant extension of the great toe. On the left no clonus was elicited and the spasticity is distinctly less.

Sensory test – The sensation is a little difficult to test but the child is very cooperative. There is evidently on the left leg up to the level of the crest of the ilium a relative hypoesthesia which is perhaps present on the right leg but less markedly so. In other ... there is a suggestion of a Brown-Sequard type of lesion. This is what one might expect in view of the fact that the swelling in the back is more marked on the right side and I assume just here the foramen with the communication thru the spinal canal occurs on the right side

Visceral reflexes are impaired with incontinence. There is very definite thermic disparity to the two sides, the left feet being colder than the right as it should be.

The x-ray show a very interesting condition with what appears to me to be a defect in spine from the 9th thoracic down to and indicating the 1st lumbar. The 12th thoracic and the 1st lumbar are fused, representing a single vertebra on the left and double on the right. There is a marked lateral curve with an acute angulation at this level.

The anomalies are not particularly clear. There is evidently a sacralized 5th lumbar vertebra.

SPECIAL NOTE
May 18, 1926
Dr. Cushing

I was sadly misled in my interpretation of this child's case by a report that there had been found at operation when the child was a few weeks old a dermoid which was of the collar-button type, portion of which projecting into the spinal canal probably not having been removed and that there had been a recurrence of the tumor with increasing spasticity and incapacitation during the past year or so. I could not conceive of a congenital defect of the nervous system behaving in this way.

Knowing that I might have difficulty in untangling the lesion from the very anomalous vertebrae I nevertheless went into the operation with no expectation of the difficulties we were to encounter.

OPERATIVE NOTE
May 18, 1926
Anesthesia – Ether – Miss Way

Laminectomy of Old Spinal Defect with a Tangled Spina Bifida Surmounted by Fatty Tumor which Projected up into the Spinal Canal. Fragmentary Removal of the Lesion.

A very careful and painstaking laminectomy was performed from about the 8th or 9th dorsal spine down across the lesion to the lower lumbar region. The upper part of the laminectomy was easily performed and covering the middle of the field was a tumor mass which looked very much like a fatty tumor. I did not realize at the time that it might not be the dermoid.

The spines and laminae of the supposed normal lower thoracic vertebrae were removed and the canal opened, disclosing an intraspinal extension of the fatty tumor mass. Fortunately this mass could be pulled out of the canal and I then, for the first time, saw normal cord. It looked very much at this juncture as though it were going to be a very easy matter to peel the fatty tumor away from the outer surface of the dura. I soon, however, came down upon a dense attachment and finally had to open the dura and I then saw that the lesion above

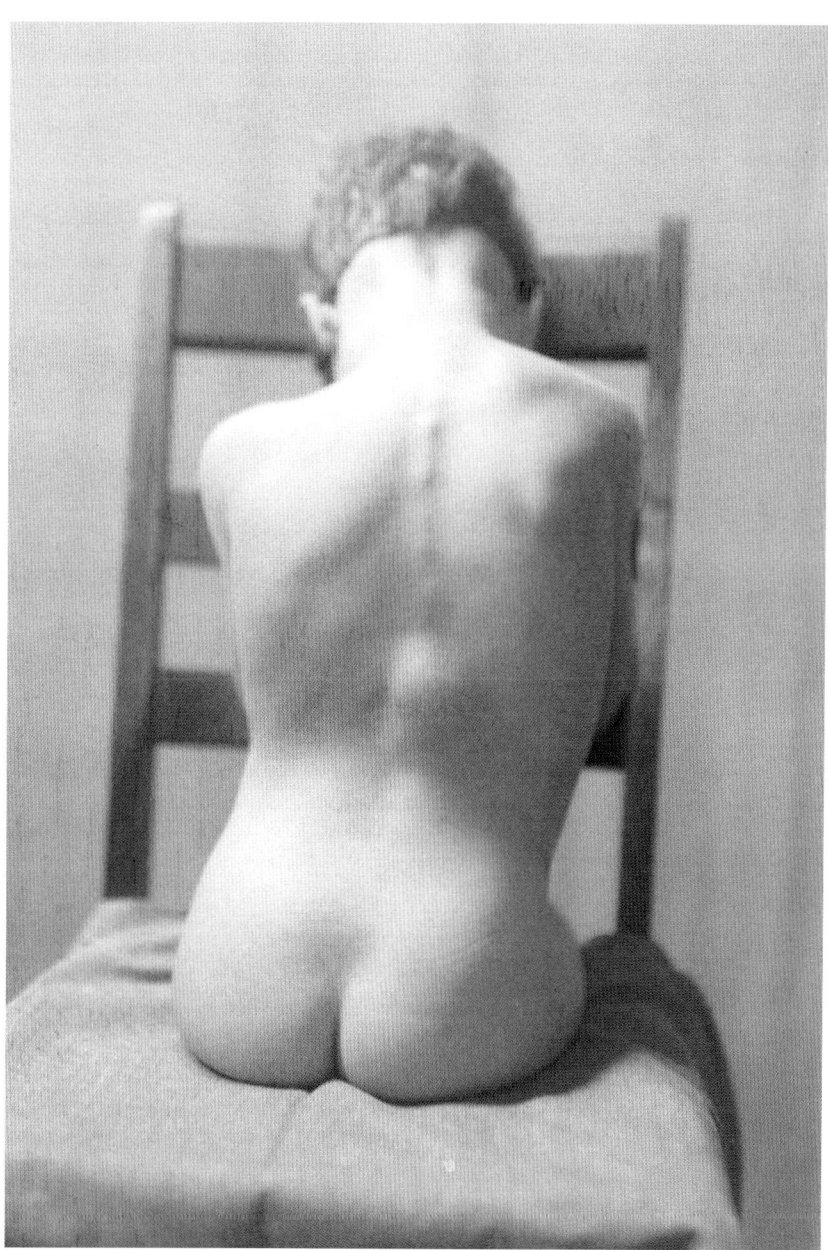

FIG. 4. PREOPERATIVE.

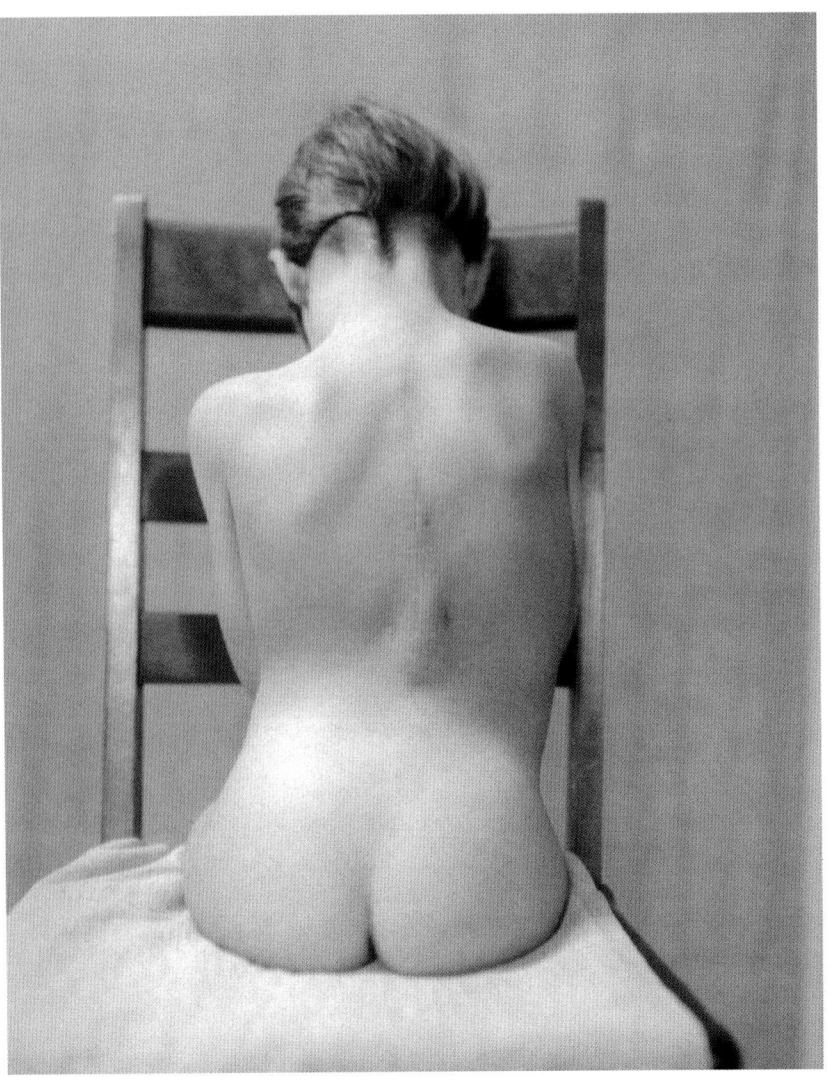

FIG. 5. THREE WEEKS POSTOPERATIVE.

1st lumbar and 12th thoracic. **If I had contented myself with this measure it is quite conceivable that the child might have been well and have regained some of the lost function.**

However, I was in for it and had partly excised the major tumor. I finally in desperation cut longitudinally through the tumor hoping that I might come down to dermoid but nothing was exposed but dense, cicatricial fibrous tissue, in which I thought I could see nerve fibers. It appeared to me that what was left of the spinal cord was being pulled out of the wound by traction on the tumor. I finally cut across the lesion at its base, leaving a considerable portion of it behind.

I should have stated that in freeing the central tumor mass from the cord, I found many curious anomalous fragments of the old laminae and then a great cup where there was a defect in the canal certainly 2 cm in width. The neck of this defect was filled with the fibrous tumor which I have been describing.

I had opened the spinal meninges headward to the lesion and almost on each side, getting into a large arachnoid space which I thought was probably anterior to cord.

Closure was then begun in the usual fashion but it was difficult because of this wide defect and I had to make lateral incision in the muscles of the back so as to free tissue sufficiently to bring margins together in the midline over the lesion. There was some leakage of cerebrospinal fluid and whether I succeeded in getting a dry closure which will not leak I am not sure of.

The child took the anaesthetic well and seemed in good condition at the close.

(Dr. Cushing)

PATHOLOGY REPORT
May 18, 1926

Material – There are fragmentary tissue removed from over a lumbo-thoracic spinal defect in a child of 7 who had been operated upon when 11 days old at the Children's Hospital, that is, 7 years ago. The diagnosis at the time was dermoid cyst and I had supposed that this present lesion was merely a recurrent cyst with an intraspinal projection which had not been removed.

The tissues were hard and fibrous, sapped by a fibroid tumor mass, a portion of which projected into the canal. The tissues were fully incorporated with spinal cord and dura and were only removed

it was intradural and adherent to the anomalous cord. I hoped that I might be able to dissect this away from the scar but it was so vascular and adherent that about the best I could do was to cut off the external tumor mass which I think contained nervous tissue as well as a lipomatous and very fibrous mass.

At the upper part of the exposed lesion underneath the aforementioned fatty mass which was dislodged from the canal, there was disclosed a cyst which I for some time assumed must be the intraspinal dermoid portion of the lesion. I think I would have done very well if I had done nothing more than do this upper laminectomy and dislodge from the canal the lesion I have mentioned since the patient's symptoms corresponded to the line of about the 10th thoracic which was above the level of the visible tumor, namely at about the

in fragmentary fashion. There is one small part of the tumor which was slightly cystic and which may prove to be epidermal in character but it contained fluid and not atheromatous material. The entire block is in formalin for study in the pathological laboratory.

(Dr. Cushing)

Microscopic exam – The sections all contain an old mixture of fibrous tissue, neuroglia and the sheaths of degenerated nerve fibers. In one section a few spicules of bone are seen. There is nothing in the nature of a tumor present except the nerve fibers. An interpretation of the findings is difficult, but the condition might be regarded as in the nature of an amputation neuroma, with proliferation of nerves following operation, and with great fibrosis and gliosis due to its location.

Diagnosis – Proliferation of nerves with gliosis and fibrosis.

POSTOPERATIVE NOTES
May 20, 1926
Dr. Davidoff

Patient recovered promptly from anaesthesia and seemed immediately quite comfortable. In the two days that have passed, no improvement can be noted in use of extremities but ever since return of consciousness she has been conscious of bladder distention when it occurs, and has been quite continent.

May 26, 1926
Dr. Schaltenbrand

Movements of the legs have improved, bending of the knees is better, the spasticity has diminished.

May 27, 1926
Dr. Davidoff

Cast removed. Dressing done. Wound is beautifully healed. Suture removed. Left leg seems almost normal in tone and movements. Right one still quite spastic but less than before operation. Bends knee even on this side fairly well. Very little movement at ankle.

DISCHARGE NOTE
June 9, 1926
Dr. Davidoff

Considerable motor function improvement since operation. No changes in hypoesthetic area. Still positive Babinski, right and left. Present epigas-

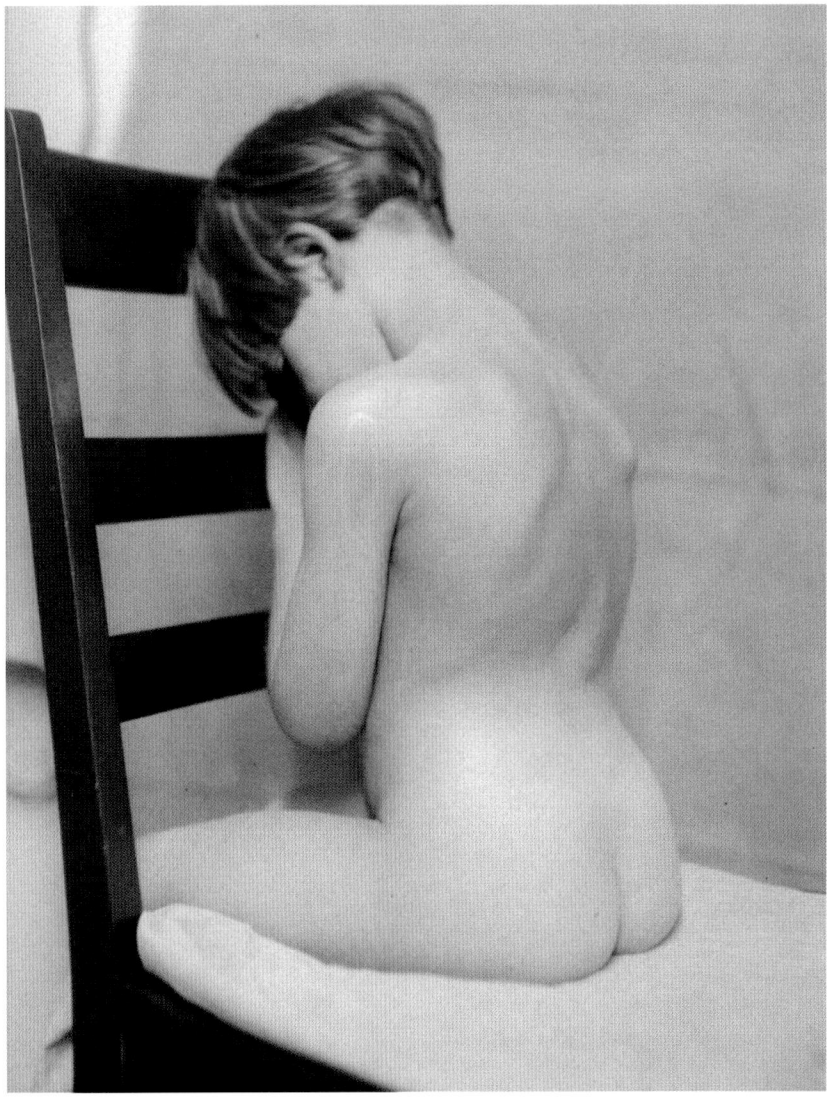

FIG. 6. THREE WEEKS POSTOPERATIVE.

tric and absent gastric reflexes. Discharged to Peabody Home.

FOLLOW UP NOTE
May 25, 1928
Dear Dr. Cushing

Your letter received asking about my daughter Margaret, she is getting along very good. The cord of her right leg is somewhat stiff but better then it was. I take her in the Childrens Hospital every Wednesday morning for massage and exercise and that is helping her.

If you would like to see her I could bring her in to the Out Patient Department any time if you let me know when.

Very sincerely yours,
(Signed) Mrs. W

5.9 Spinal cord ependyoma

SEX: F; AGE: 8; SURG. NO. 27176; 36444; 37305

HISTORY

This patient was transferred to the Peter Bent Brigham Hospital from the Children's Hospital complaining of a stiff neck for 2 years. After a fall in October 1924, the child complained of stiff neck. She was unable to voluntarily correct a right torticollis. She was treated in bed for 8 weeks by her local medical doctor. X-rays were negative. She made a gradual recovery. About two months before admission, there appeared a muscular weakness of both arms.

SUMMARY OF POSITIVE FINDINGS
September 13, 1926
Dr. Bailey

SUBJECTIVE
1. Stiffness and pain in the neck and down the back.
2. Weakness of the arms.

OBJECTIVE
1. Rigidity of the neck in anterior flexion.
2. Atrophy and weakness of all the muscles of the upper extremities predominating in the muscles of the proximal extremities and the small muscles of the left hand.
3. Absent triceps and radial reflexes in both arms.
4. Scoliosis.
5. Abdominal reflexes not obtained. Exaggeration of tendon reflexes in lower extremities with clonus at each ankle.
6. Sensory loss, especially to heat, over both upper extremities.

IMPRESSION: The two most likely possibilities are: (1) Pott's disease. Against this diagnosis it may be urged that the X-ray findings are negative. This is not sufficient to rule it out as Pott's disease, especially in children, they show nothing in the X-ray. (2) Is that of an intramedullary tumor.

SPECIAL NOTE
September 17, 1926
Dr. Cushing

This was an extraordinarily interesting case in a little girl who showed very few symptoms except a flexed head with stiff, rigid cervical vertebræ and a

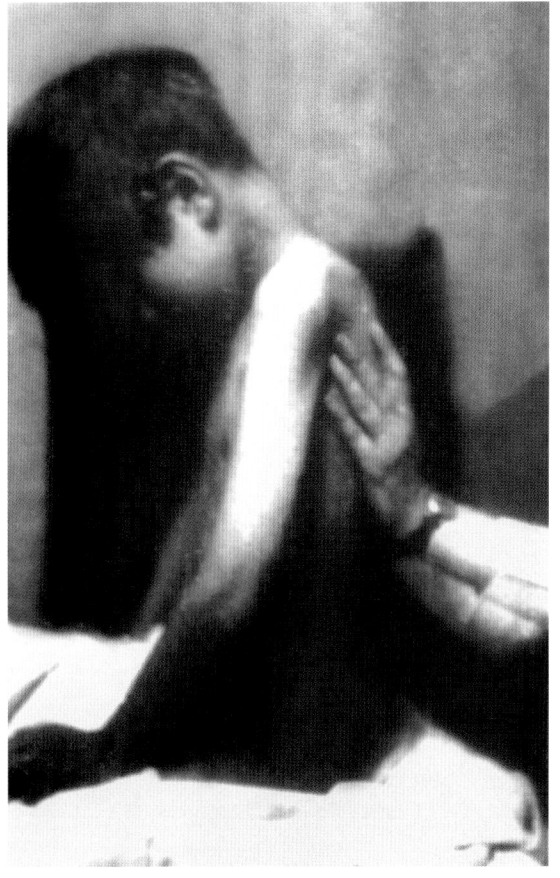

FIG. 1. PREOPERATIVE.

spasm of the cervical muscles which made the condition closely resemble cervical T.B.

The child also had a little fever but the x-rays showed no demonstrable lesion in the vertebræ.

She had some slight spasticity of the lower extremities with increased reflexes but nevertheless was able to walk. There was no definite sensory loss except for some vague hyperæsthesia difficult to plot. She had some evident weakness of the muscles of the upper extremities with atrophy, particularly well shown in the intrinsic muscles of the hand on the left, tho there was also some atrophy of the shoulder girdle muscles.

There had not been any Von Pirquet's test made. The child had not had a lumbar puncture nor had there been any lipiodol studies made.

I was under the impression that whatever the lesion might be, it certainly must be within the

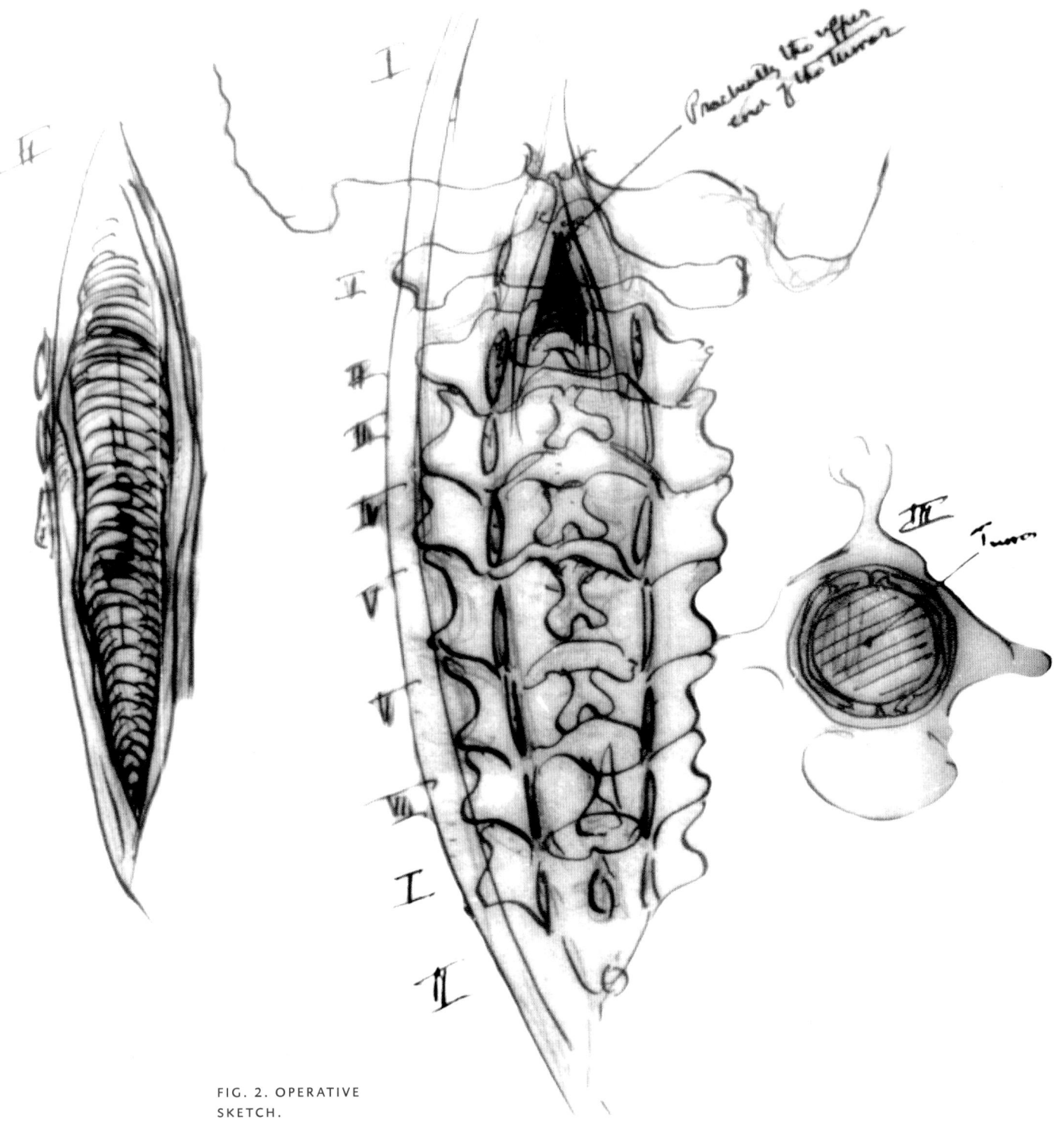

FIG. 2. OPERATIVE SKETCH.

spinal canal and that we would do little more than to upset the child by making dynamic studies of the cerebrospinal fluid.

When after the child had been anesthetized and attempted to do a lumbar puncture to get fluid, I was particularly glad that we had not punctured the child before operation, particularly so that we had not attempted a cisternal puncture.

OPERATIVE NOTE
Sept. 17, 1926
Anesthesia – Ether – Miss Way

Lumbar Puncture. Negative Tap. Cervicodorsal Laminectomy of 8 Vertebrae, Disclosing Greatly Dilated Spinal Canal with Medullar Gliomatous Tumor Extending the Full Length of the Exposed Wound and at least the Full Length of the Spinal Cord. Incision of Posterior

Columns–Removal by Suction of Soft Tumor from the Center of an Enormously Dilated Spinal Cord–Closure.

A photograph was taken before operating to determine the position of the head. The child was then etherized and a lumbar puncture performed. This procedure I carried out more for the matter of satisfying my curiosities as to whether there would be xanthochromic fluid. As a matter of fact, I made two punctures between the 4th and 5th and the 3rd and 4th vertebræ without getting fluid. The needle indeed entered to a surprising depth without encountering any resistance, so that I was absolutely lost in a large space. On a 3rd tap directly in the midline, I got a few drops of yellowish bloody fluid. There was no question but that I must have encountered tumor.

This experience was that we were probably dealing with an intraspinal tumor but since the symptoms referable to the cervical cord were the most serious symptoms I thought that we had better continue with the operation as planned.

Laminectomy consequently was performed and it proved to be extremely easy, the laminæ being so spread out, thinned and widened in their vertical dimensions that they were extremely easy to remove, leaving a broad space fully an inch wide as shown in the accompanying sketch #1 (The middle image in the operative sketch).

Directly under the laminæ was the tense dura without any intervening fat. It seemed to be quite evident that the position of the child's head was largely due to the distention of the spinal canal and widening of these laminæ for the muscular spasm which completely relaxed under the anæsthetic nevertheless left the neck arched up there, much in the position the child held it while on the ward.

An incision was then made in the dura, no fluid being secured, but I came down upon what I took to be a fibro-fatty tumor which as a matter of fact was nothing more than the greatly distended spinal cord which bulged thru the dural opening as I enlarged it upward and downward.

This early laminectomy covered only about the 2nd to the 6th vertebræ and seeing that we had a tumor which extended a much greater length than this the Atlas was laminectomized and then the last cervical and first 2nd thoracic vertebra.

I think I got above the tumor so soon as the dural incision was carried upwards as far as the foramen magnum but in the lower part of the field

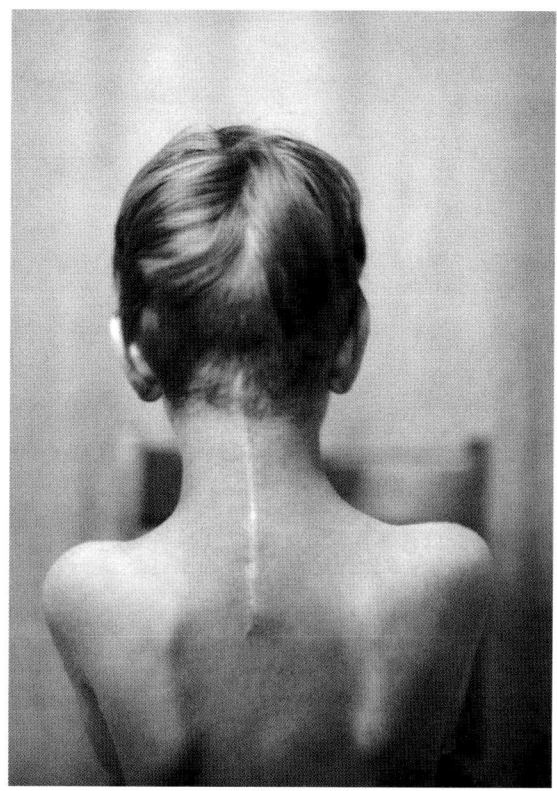

FIG. 3. ONE MONTH POSTOPERATIVE.

we were still dealing with tumor, tho the incision in the dura was made down to the 2nd thoracic, if I mistake not.

It soon became perfectly evident that we had an inter-spinal tumor causing the cord to bulge in an extremely peculiar fashion. There was one place that looked thin and dark, strongly suggesting a cyst. With the assumption that it might be syringomyelia, a needle was inserted without getting fluid.

I then deliberately split the thin, stretched out posterior columns the full length of the incision, that is from about the foramen magnum down to the 2nd thoracic segment. An elongated and dark tumor mass began to extrude about as shown in figure #2 (The left image in the operative sketch).

With the spoon two or three large fragments of this soft tumor were removed and put in Zenker's and saline and then with the sucker this whole tumor of tissue was totally removed. There was practically no connective tissue and it was relatively non-vascular, such little bleeding as was occasioned being easily controlled by irrigation and temporary placement of some muscle from another case.

I was somewhat at a loss to know whether to proceed with the exposure of the entire spinal cord

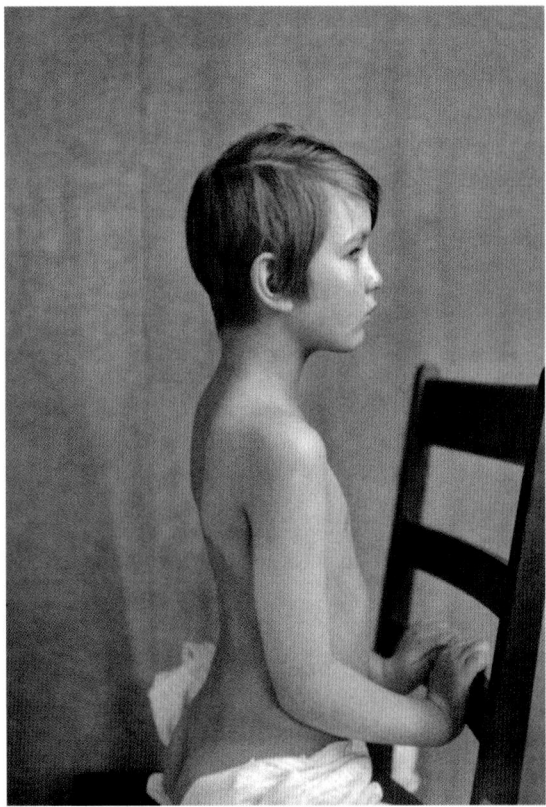 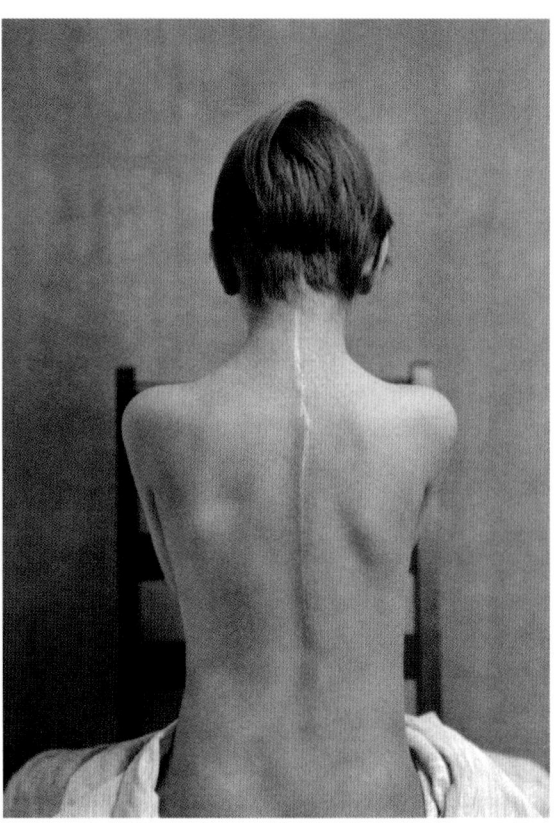

FIGS. 4 AND 5. TWO MONTHS POSTOPERATIVE.

or to let things go with the repair simply of this cervical region. It seemed to me that this was best, and I assume that a second operation with laminectomy of the remaining vertebræ and upper lumbar vertebræ will undoubtedly be called for. It is quite possible that the child may do extremely well after such an operation but I at least cannot say how well she will react to this cervical procedure.

The wound then closed securely in successive layers with fine silk sutures. It should be stated that the original wound was novocainized so that the anæsthetic was withdrawn early in the operation about the time closure was begun.

(Dr. Cushing)

POSTOPERATIVE NOTE
September 17, 1926
Dr. Davidoff

The patient made a very quick recovery from anæsthesia and was able to move all four extremities as well as before operation. She complained of "prickles" in both hands which disappeared after three to four hours.

SPECIAL NOTE
October 7, 1926
Dr. Bailey

Much more comfortable. Definite improvement in arms. Muscles of the shoulder girdles especially. Can abduct both arms at shoulder. Extension of fingers of left hand much better. Still cannot spread out fingers of left hand. Abdominal reflex present on either side. Dorsi-flexion of both feet very weak. Both legs very spastic with exaggerated reflexes and clonus at both knee and ankle. Bilateral Babinski response today. Has ceased to be incontinent. No sensory disturbance could be discovered to pin prick, touch or temperature. Wound well healed. Movements of neck somewhat restricted but not painful.

SPECIAL NOTE
November 2, 1926
Dr. Cushing

This child has made an astonishingly good recovery from her former operation with better movement in her claw-like hand, with freedom of movement in the neck and she is now up and walking

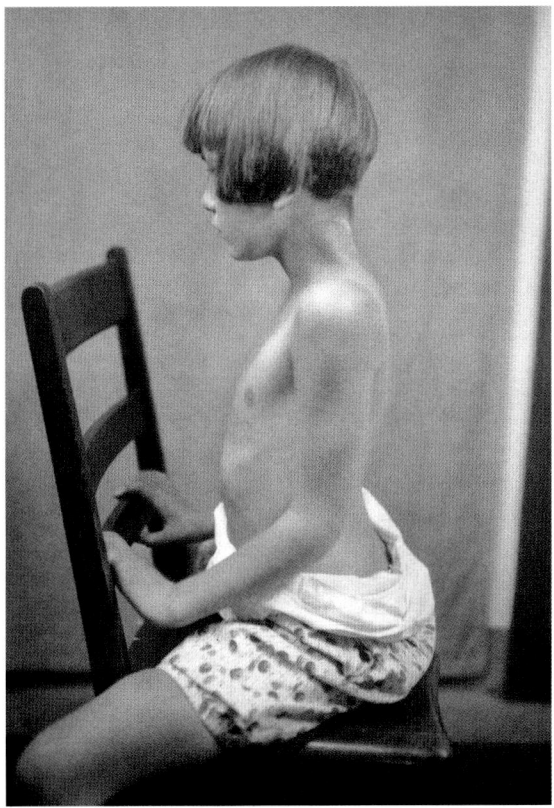 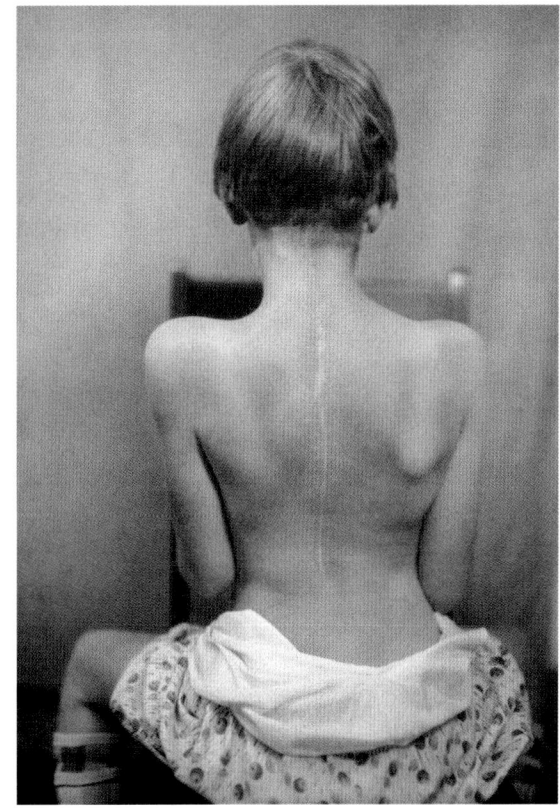

FIGS. 6 AND 7. TWO YEARS POSTOPERATIVE.

though with some unsteadiness and with exaggerated reflexes. I anticipated fully finding an extension of the tumor down to the lumbar region but now that the operation is over I cannot explain how it was that I got a negative spinal tap. It is, of course, entirely inconceivable that the growth should have disappeared under the x-ray and I can only assume that the chief tumor mass ended at about the upper thoracic cord which was the lowest portion exposed at the first operation. I set out to do an extensive laminectomy from the second thoracic through to the mid-lumbar region.

OPERATIVE NOTE
November 2, 1926
Anesthesia – Ether – Miss Melanson

Laminectomy for Supposed Tumor. Disclosure of Merely Dilated Central Canal after Incision of Exposed Cord.

This operation was conducted without difficulty. A long laminectomy was performed, the spines and laminæ were removed by rongeurs without difficulty and with very little bleeding, some thinned laminæ being exposed first in the upper operative field.

The x-ray had misled us in regard to the apparent absorption of some of the laminæ and spines in the mid-thoracic region. The laminæ were all well formed though as I felt flattened and broadened. I secured a wide exposure of dura and on incising dura came down upon what looked like an extremely wide and somewhat pale spinal cord, which was soft on pressure. At the upper part of the field just below the old laminectomy one could see that the cord was collapsed so that I assume this was the lowest end of the tumor.

Being somewhat taken back by its appearance, I made an incision at about the mid-thoracic region down thru the cord expecting to come upon tumor. A little bleb of brownish tissue looking like the original tumor finally presented itself and on going through this I came into a greatly dilated spinal canal about the size of a lead pencil, no tumor being present.

The dura was slit the full length of the exposed field, the wound was closed securely in layers, the last part by Dr. Bailey, without a drain. The child stood the operation well.

This, then, is a case of a cervical ependymoma with dilated spinal canal below, surrounded possibly by a thin film of ependymoma. I regret that I did not take a snip of this tissue for histological

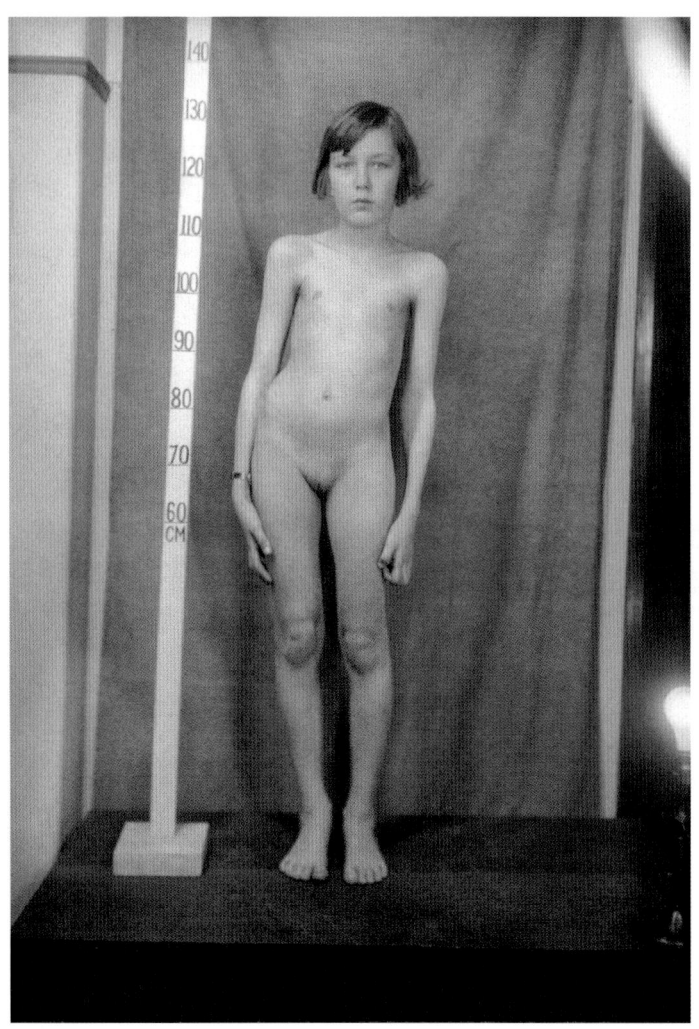
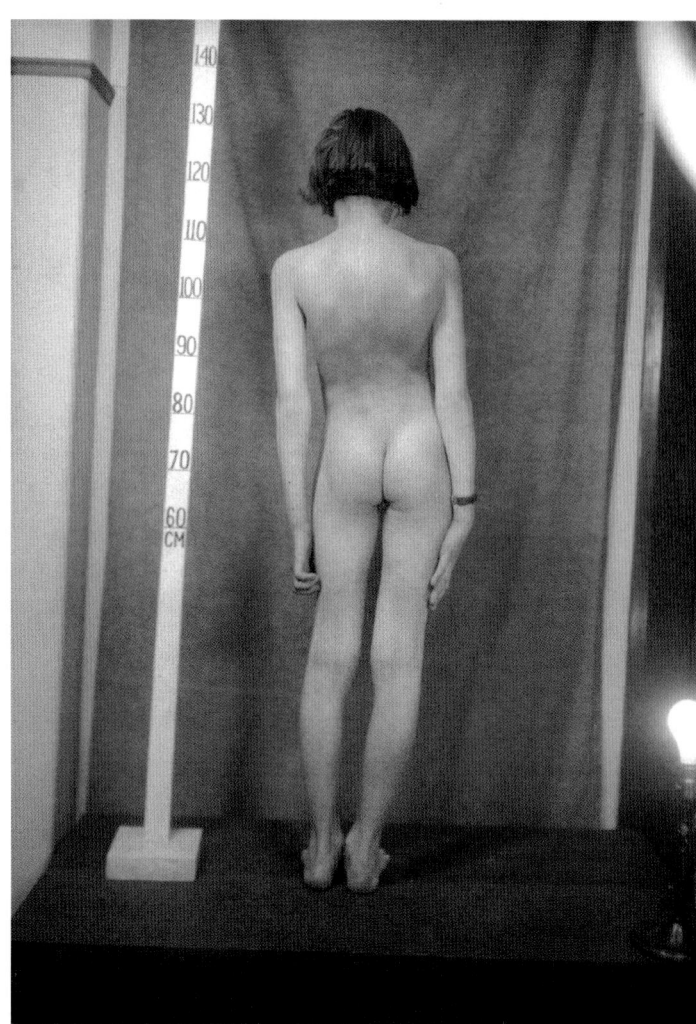

FIGS. 8, 9, 10, 11, 12. TWO AND A HALF YEARS POSTOPERATIVE.

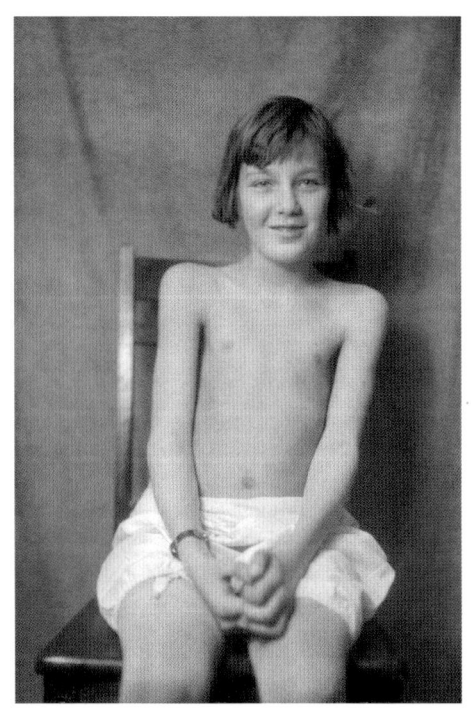
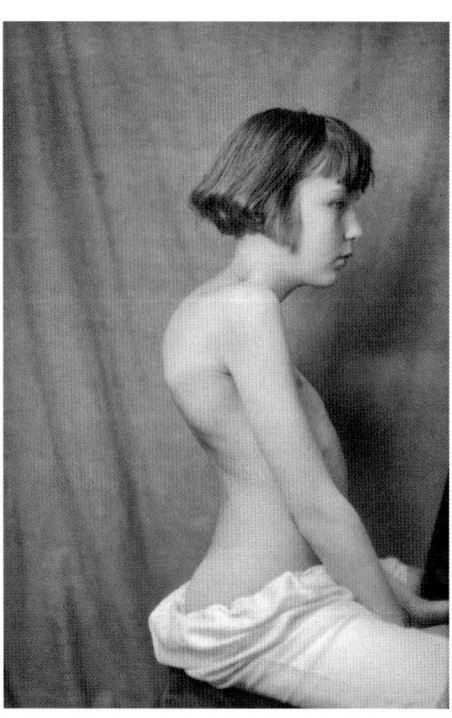
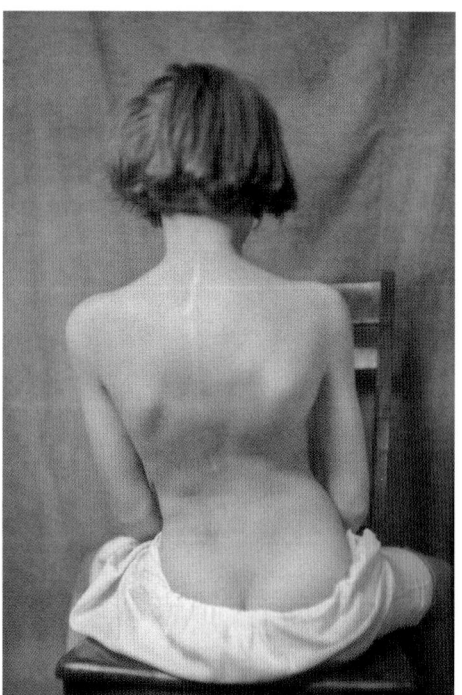

examination. I assume that the condition is one which had the tumor absorbed spontaneously would have left what would be regarded as a syringomyelia.

(Dr. Cushing)

POSTOPERATIVE NOTE
November 3, 1926
Dr. Bailey

Temperature elevated. After last operation also went to 101.2. Pulse rapid but strong. Cast is wet with urine but will not allow it to be changed. Probably wiser to leave her alone.

SPECIAL NOTE
November 23, 1926
Dr. Cairns

Is making rapid strides with her walking. Already can walk by herself and she thinks that her walking is, even so soon as this, better than it was before the first operation.

DISCHARGE NOTE
November 27, 1926
Dr. Cairns

Patient walking very well now though her steps are short and she seems to be hobbling along. There is rapid daily improvement. Head position is much improved. On admission her head was flexed. Now she is able to hyperextend it about 15 degrees beyond the ventral. There is very great subjective improvement of hand movement. Sphincters are fully controlled.

FOLLOWUP NOTE
December, 18, 1926
Dr. Horrax

Child seems perfectly well except tendency to hold head a little forward. No sensory changes made out. Deep reflexes +++ R and L, greater on the left with clonus at left ankle.

SECOND HOSPITAL ADMISSION

Patient was admitted in hospital with complaint of momentary spasmodic contractions of the abdomen with pain for 10 days.

DIAGNOSIS: Intraspinal tumor, recurrent with spinal lordosis, kyphosis and scoliosis.

PLAN: Patient received a course of X-ray therapy to

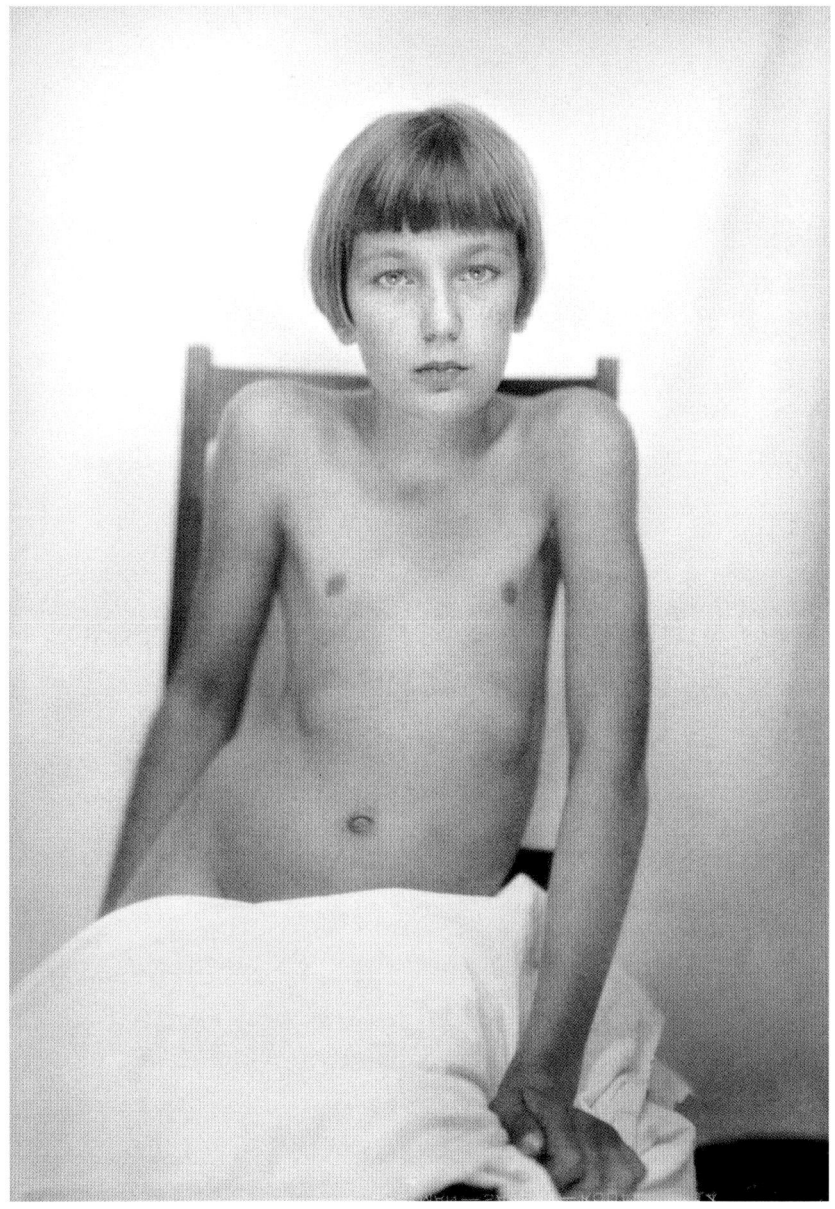

FIG. 13. THREE YEARS POSTOPERATIVE.

spinal region. She was discharged with slight subjective improvement of symptoms.

THIRD HOSPITAL ADMISSION

HISTORY

This 12-year-old girl enters the hospital for the 3rd time because of inability to walk.

September 20, 1930
Dr. Hoen

The patient after first admission improved to such an extent that 2 months after her discharge she was

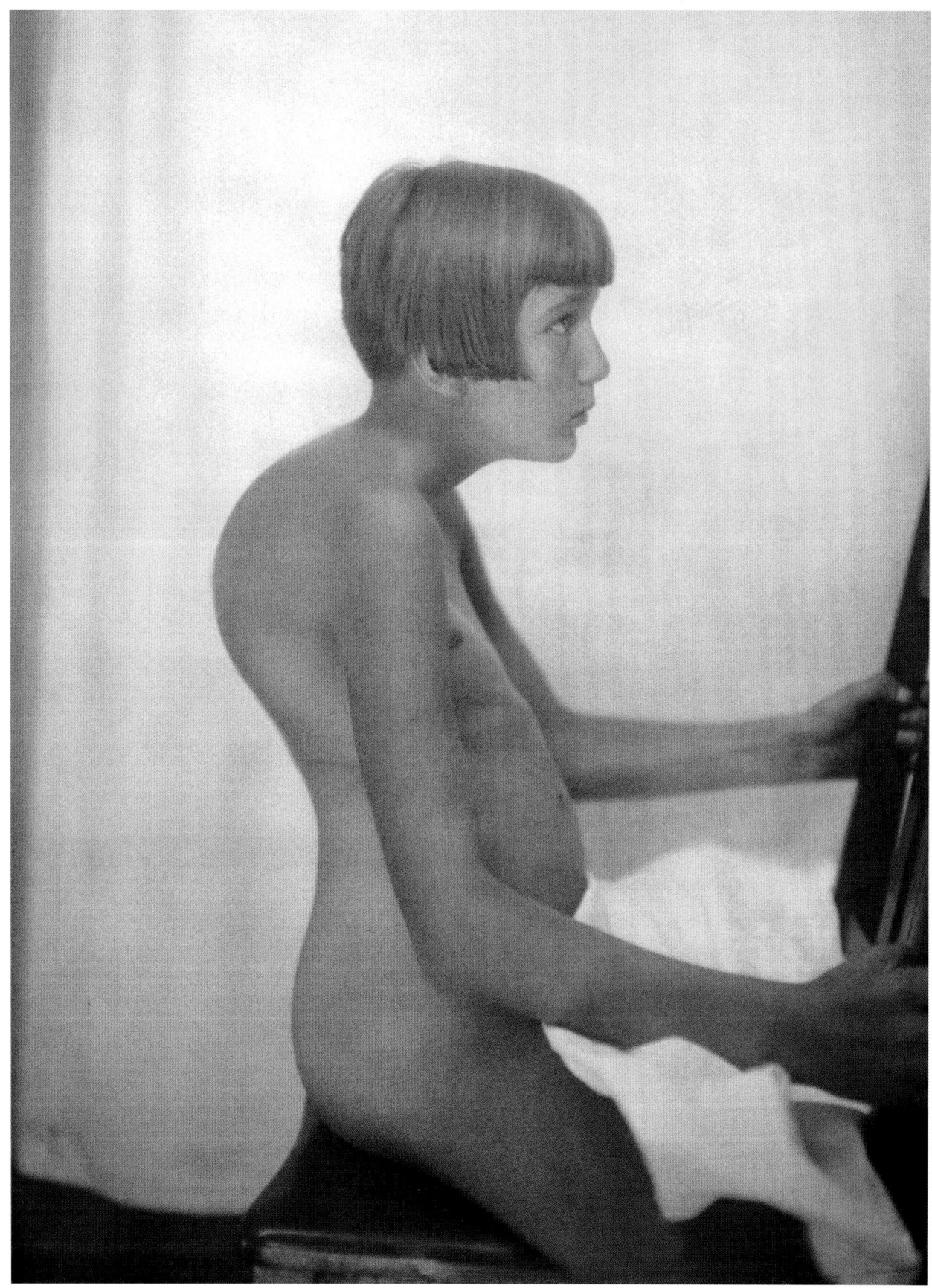

FIG. 14. THREE YEARS POSTOPERATIVE.

able to take part in a dancing performance without any noticeable deformity. There was no return of neurological symptoms until April 1929, when her parents noticed some weakness of the left leg. During the following summer she had a course of X-ray treatments followed by some improvement. In December 1929 it was noted that the child's posture was not good but she had no complaints until May, 1930, when she complained of severe cramplike pains in her abdomen as well as considerable stiffness in her legs and some difficulty in walking. She also had less sphincter control than she had before. She was readmitted to the hospital in May 1930. During her stay in the hospital the patient was kept at complete rest and given a course of X-ray therapy. After 2.5 weeks of this regime the patient was slightly improved and was discharged home. There was possibly some improvement during few months following her discharge. She was able to walk around, to go in swimming and enjoy herself. She has no pain or discomfort and she had good control of her sphincters. About the first of September, she got up to walk and discovered suddenly that her legs would not support her. Since this time she has made no attempt to walk and has remained in bed almost the entire time. During this time also she has had almost no control of bowels or urine.

Readmitted in hospital with diagnosis: Tumor of the spinal cord, recurrent, probable level of last cervical or 1st thoracic vertebra.

This girl is certainly very much worse since her last admission. There is now slight weakness of the right arm, progressively increasing spinal deformity, together with very marked weakness of the right leg as well as the left.

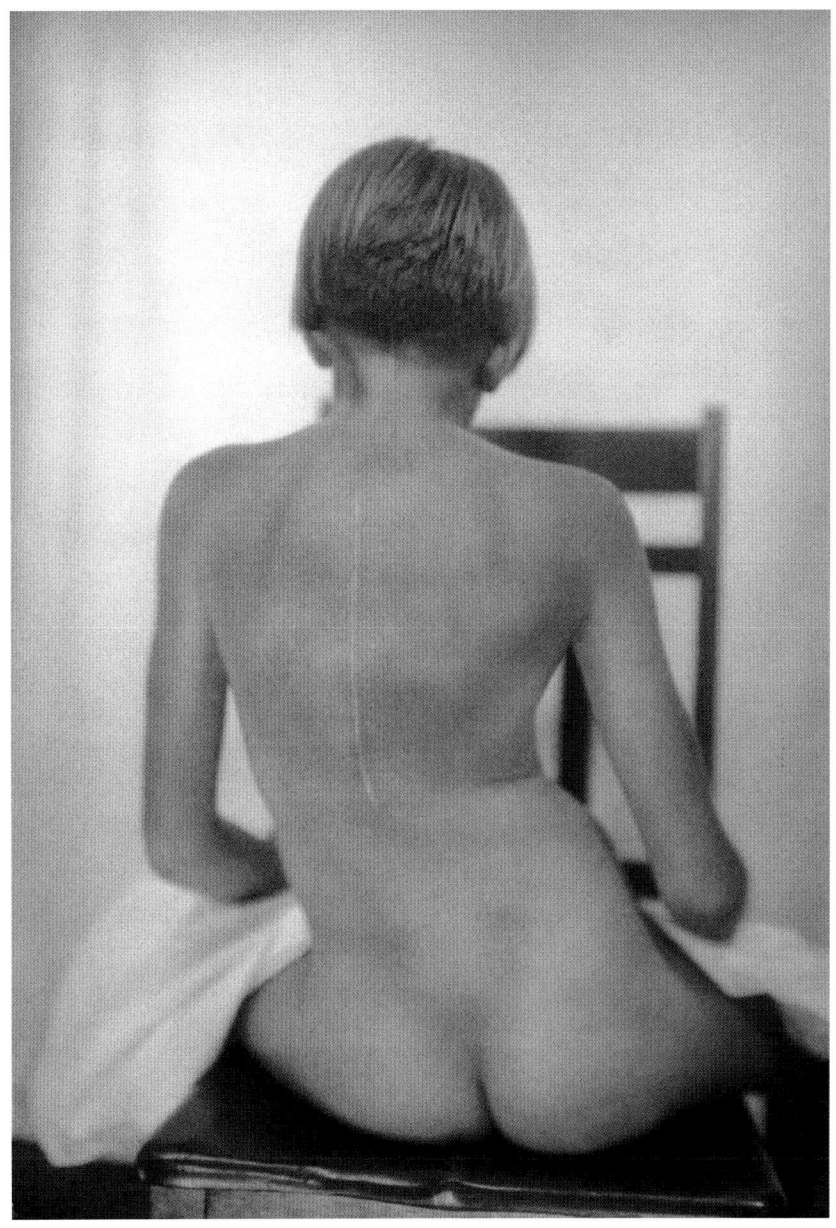

FIG. 15. THREE YEARS POSTOPERATIVE.

DISCHARGE NOTE
October 1, 1930
Dr. Hoen

Discharged today without treatment.

March 11, 1931

Patient died at home.

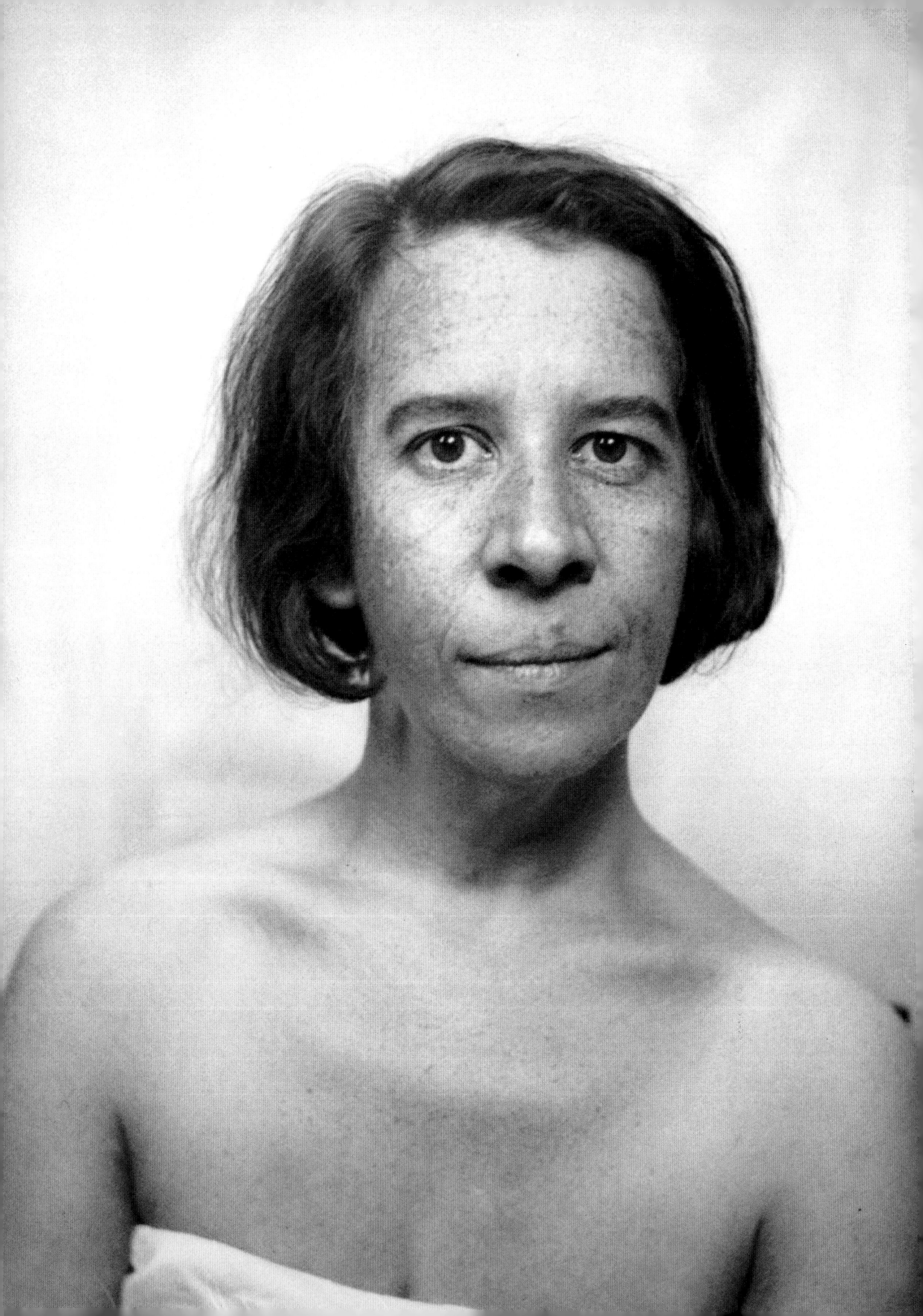

5.10 Spinal neurinoma

SEX: F; AGE: 40; SURG. NO. 39890

HISTORY

This patient presented with bilateral lower extremity weakness.

SUMMARY OF POSITIVE FINDINGS
October 25, 1931
Dr. Mahoney

SUBJECTIVE
1. Pain in the dorso-lumbar region of the back radiating around to the groin, 2 years.
2. Beginning difficulty in walking 2 years ago with gradual dragging of the right leg for 10 months, extending to the left leg in the last 2 months, since which time she has been unable to walk at all.
3. Sphincteric disturbances, 4 months.
4. Edema of legs, 2 months.
5. Paræsthesia in legs, 6 months with disturbed position sense for 2 months.

OBJECTIVE
1. Markedly edematous legs from knees down.
2. Inability to move legs.
3. Spasticity of legs with marked hyperactive reflexes and pathological Babinski.
4. Sensibility changes below last lumbar region bilaterally to pin-prick, touch and temperature.

IMPRESSION: Spinal cord tumor, extra-medullary below dorsal.

RADIOLOGY REPORT

X-ray – No apparent variation from the normal.

SPECIAL NOTE
October 31, 1931
Dr. Horrax

This woman had unmistakable signs and symptoms of a pretty complete cord lesion at the level of the 11th dorsal segment. Her troubles started some two years ago with beginning weakness of the right leg and also pain down the legs. Gradually, the left leg also became weak, but the sensory changes on the left side were apparently always more advanced than on the right and this was true to our examinations at the present time, there

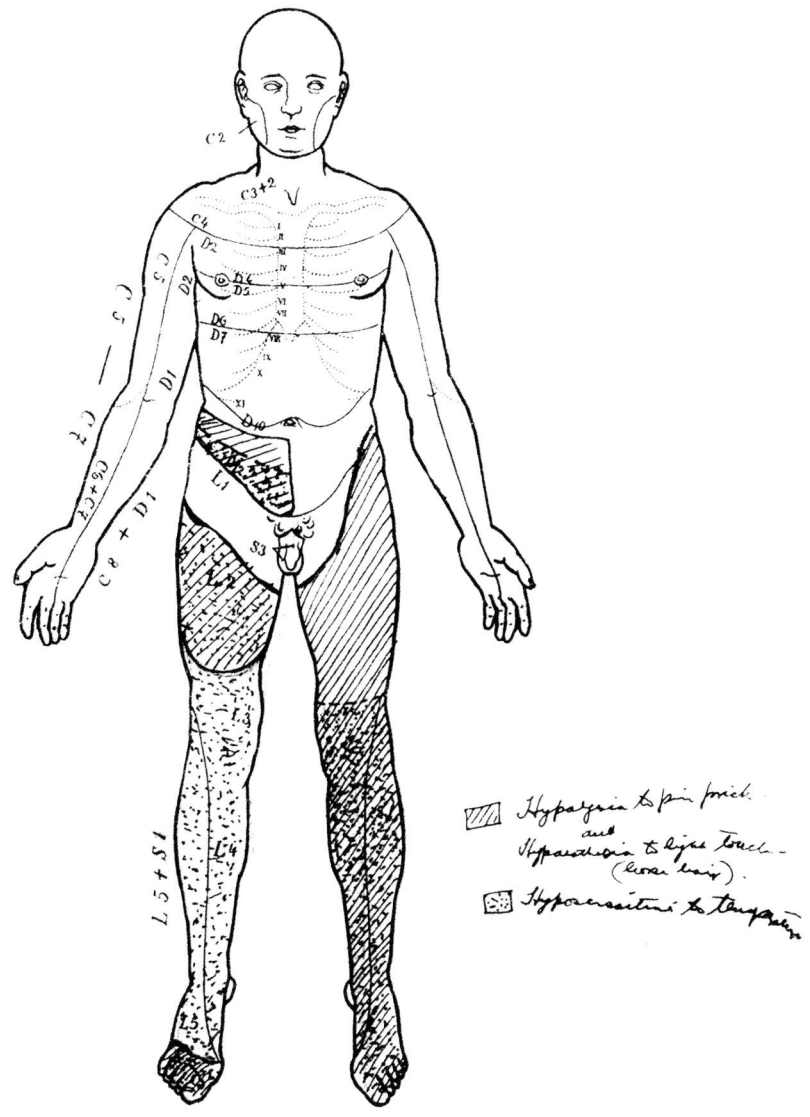

FIG. 2. PREOPERATIVE EXAM.

being much more complete loss of sensation to all forms on the left than on the right, this being especially true below the knees. This, therefore, represented a definite Brown-Sequard syndrome. Lumbar puncture elsewhere had revealed what was taken to be a partial block with clear fluid but in view of the findings at operation there must certainly have been a complete block and also the fluid below the level of the tumor was distinctly yellow at the time of operation. It did not seem necessary to repeat the lumbar puncture here

OPPOSITE PAGE: FIG. 1. THREE WEEKS POSTOPERATIVE.

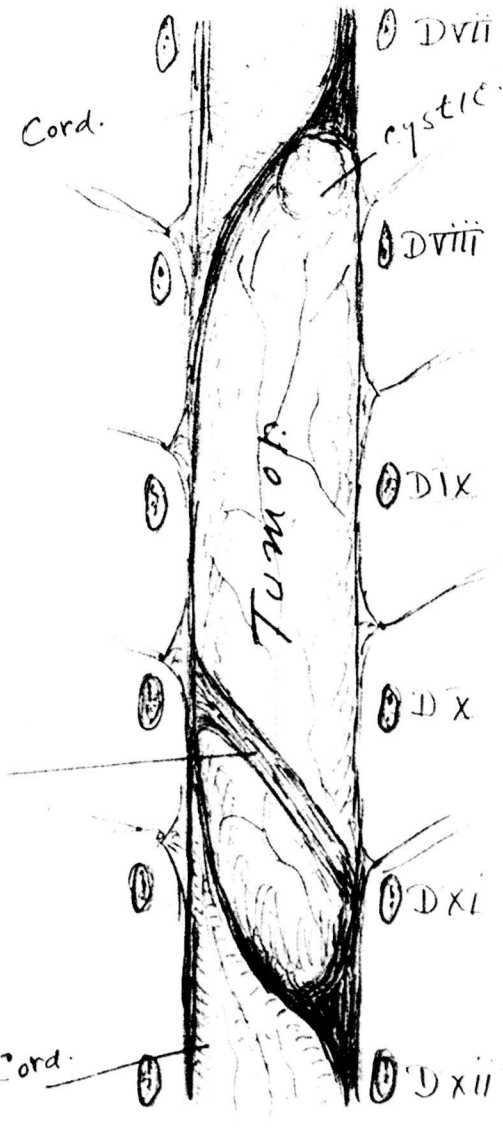
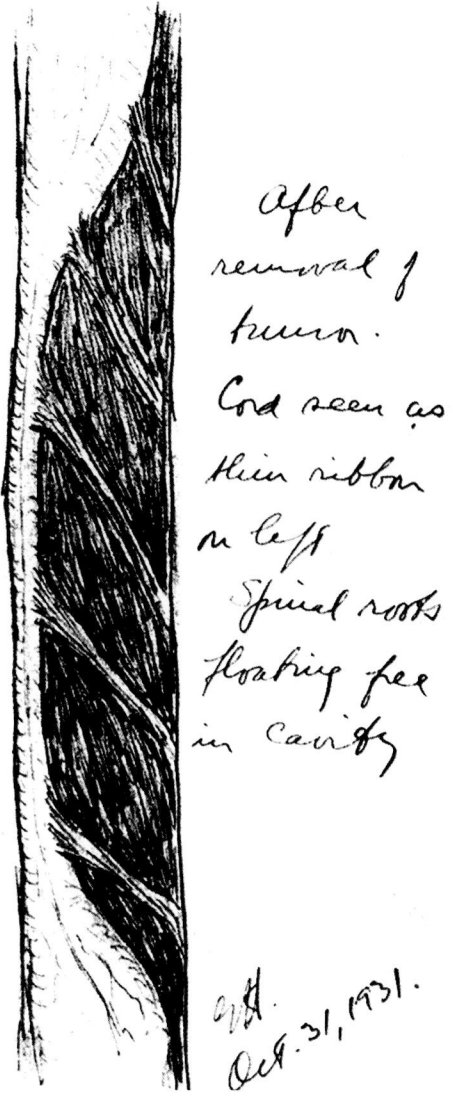

FIG. 3. OPERATIVE SKETCH.

because of the very definite neurological findings. The patient also had very marked swelling and edema of both legs which I see no reason to account for on the basis of her spinal cord tumor. The operation was a long, difficulty one, lasting possibly five hours.

OPERATIVE NOTE
October 31, 1931
Anesthesia: Novocain–Avertin–Ether, Miss Geizer

Lower Dorsal Laminectomy with Removal, Piecemeal, of Long, Solid, Encapsulated Tumor, Measuring Approximately 5 Inches in Length and Compressing the Cord to a Ribbon along the Left Side of the Canal.

The usual straight incision was made over the spines of the 7th to 12th dorsal and first lumbar vertebræ, and the spines and laminæ of the six lower dorsal vertebra removed. This exposed dura was also darkly discolored and felt very firm so that there was an unmistakable tumor lying underneath. The dura was now opened over the entire length of the field and held apart with silk sutures. The tumor occupied approximately the whole length of the incision, normal cord being visible above for a distance of perhaps half a cm and for the same distance below. It could be seen also that the cord was compressed over to the left side of the canal although this region of cord was at first hidden by growth.

An attempt was now made to dislodge first the upper pole of the tumor and then the lower pole, but it was very adherent at both ends and there were numerous tangles of blood vessels between it and the cord so that this separation of tumor from cord could not be accomplished for the time being. Also the tumor was so large that there was no room at all to work around on either side of it and in any case this would have been inadvisable on the left side because in so doing, cord would have been badly contused. At the upper end of the growth there was a small cystic area but this was finally punctured and the room thus obtained gave me a chance to work at the growth from its end. When it finally became evident that the long tumor could not be tilted out as can usually be done with the ordinary managements of the cord, my one resource was to scoop out growth from within its capsule which I now proceeded to do from one end to the other, partly by pituitary scoop and partly by suction. It proved to be moderately but not excessively vascular and the electrosurgical needle was used in 1-2 places to control bleeding. It was necessary to sacrifice one sensory root running over the lower pole of growth and after this area had been excavated it was then possible to tilt out the lower end, freeing it from the cord and anterior roots in so doing and in this way peel it outward and upward away from the thinned out cord on the left side. In this way practically all of the remaining growth and capsule was removed. There was, however, a small bit at the upper end which had to be freed and teased out in the same way. When the tumor had finally been removed, there was a large cavity with a clean bed of dura and nerve roots below and along the right side and on the left side the greatly attenuated but not contused cord. It is probable, however, that at the upper pole of the tumor there still remained some cells which could not be entirely removed from the tangle of vessels between them and the cord. It was, however, a practically complete extirpation and will in all probability give the patient a good many years of freedom from symptoms.

After all bleeding points were carefully secured, one especially at the lower end of the field where some small bits of muscle were necessary, the dura was closed by interrupted sutures of silk, the muscles with several silver wire sutures and the upper tissues and layers with fine silk as usual. The patient was in good condition at the end of the operation although her blood pressure had gradually fallen off to 80 mm. This, however, began to improve toward the end.

(Dr. Horrax)

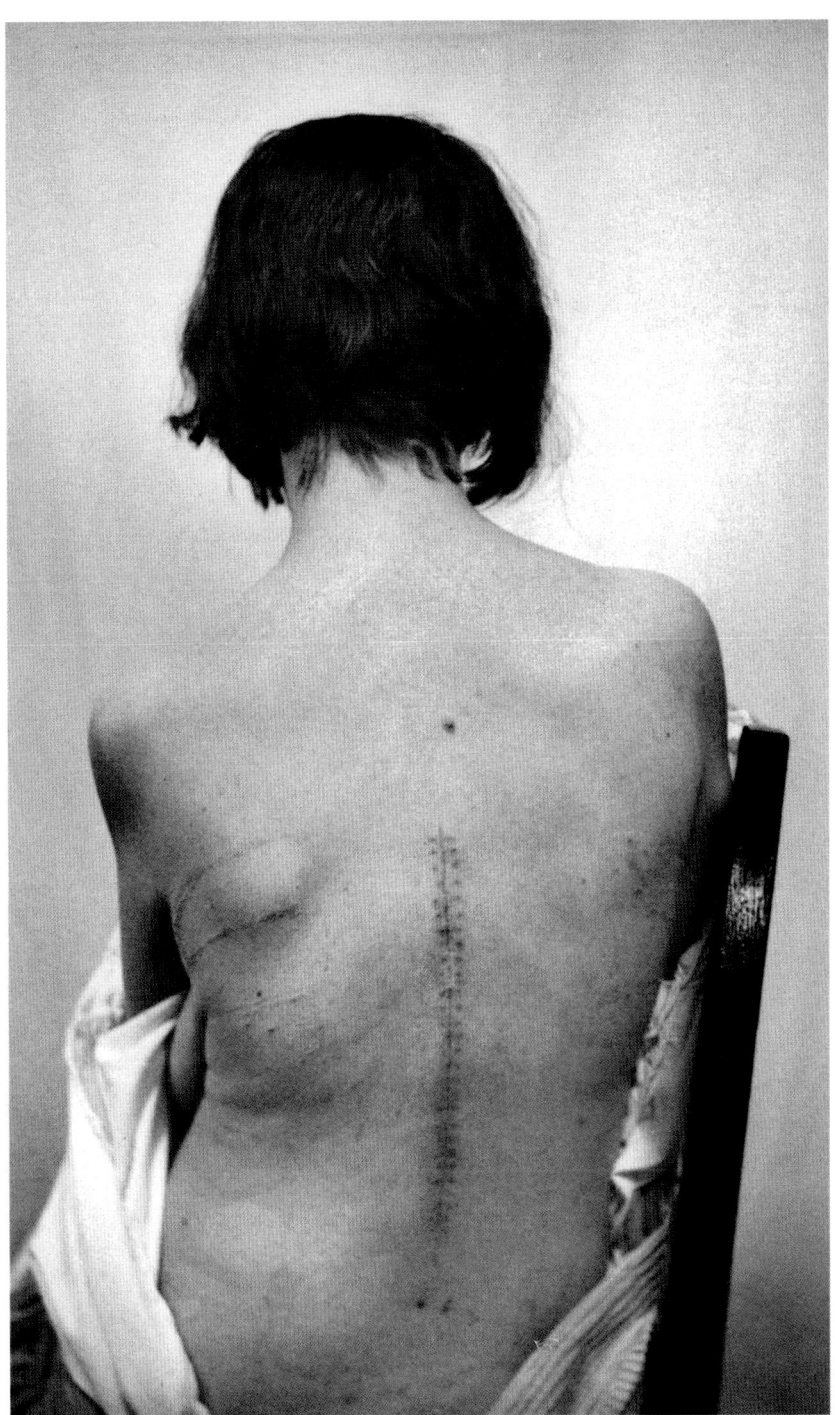

FIG. 4. THREE WEEKS POSTOPERATIVE — WOUND.

PATHOLOGY NOTE
October 31, 1931
Dr. Eisenhardt

Examination by supravital technique shows an exceedingly vascular fragment of tissue. There are some patches of fusiform cells such as one sees in a neurinoma and this is the most likely diagnosis. However I would like to see another piece of tissue

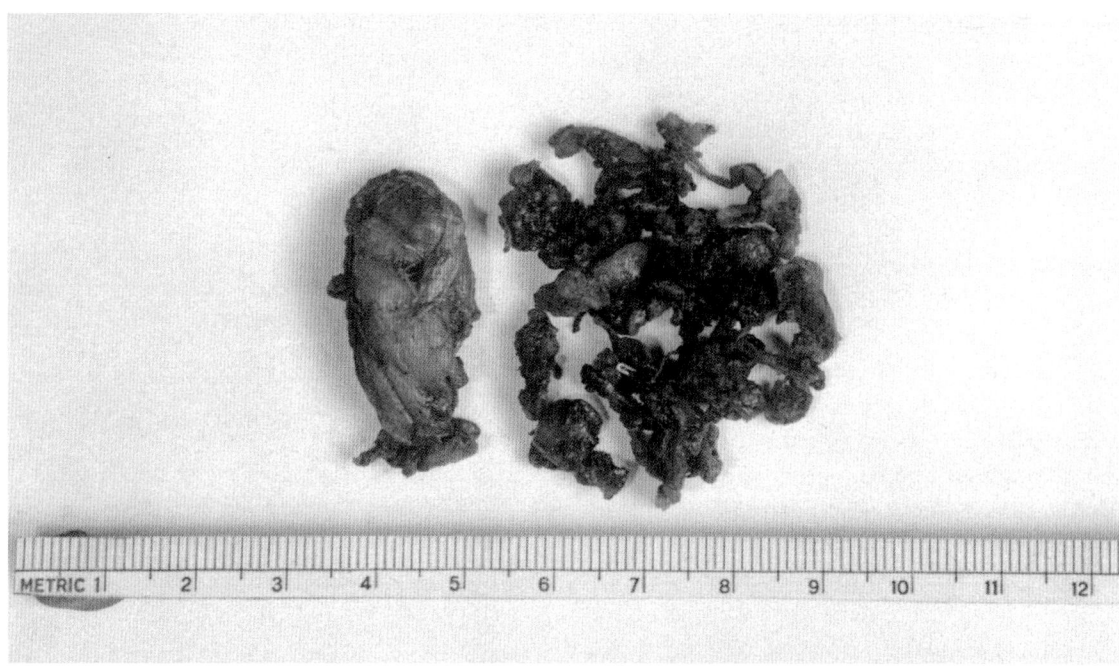

FIG. 5. GROSS TUMOR SPECIMEN.

to be sure that this is only a tangle of capillaries rather than part of a vessel lumen. The structure is not typical of a meningioma.

DISCHARGE NOTE
November 21, 1931
Dr. Mahoney

Discharged improved to patient's home.
Motor: can move both legs and left better than right.
Sensory: slightly hypoesthetic to pinprick and temperature.
Sphincters: not wholly constrict, but doing better.
Reflexes: KJ AJ equally hypoactive.
Bilateral ankle clonus
Bilateral Babinski
Wound well healed.

LETTER TO DR. CUSHING
November 17, 1932

Dear Dr. Cushing:

I have your communication of Nov. 8. Even though I did not, as your note indicates, sever my connection with the Peter Bent Brigham Hospital completely when I left it a year ago, I am very happy to give you a report of my condition. I began to walk with a great deal of assistance about six weeks after the operation; in about ten weeks I managed to get about with the help of one person and a cane, and seemed to improve gradually until February. At that time I was greatly bothered with the painful and involuntary drawing up of the right leg. I also became even more bent over than before. That condition continued until June when I began to feel very much better. On my return to Pittsburgh Sept. 1st, I resumed my household duties gradually, and am now doing all my work with the exception of that which requires kneeling or climbing. I still tire more easily than normally, and with too much exertion my right hip and lower back ache a little and my right leg draws up. But, I note improvement in all these things from week to week and feel that I have reason to hope to be practically normal in the course of time.

If there are other points of my condition that you would like information about, I shall be very glad to tell you anything that might help your work in any way or that might relieve any patient's distress of body or mind in the slightest degree. All my friends feel that Dr. Horrax performed a miracle on me. I cannot say too much in praise of the Peter Bent Brigham Hospital in general and of your neurosurgical department in particular.

Very sincerely yours,
DC

The last letter from patient was received on October 31, 1935 (not available in the chart).

Chapter 6

Posterior fossa tumors and other pathologies

Introduction

"When an experience such as this is now looked back upon, it seems that only stupidity could have so long delayed our better understanding of these lesions."[7]

Harvey Cushing

Development of posterior fossa surgery remains one of the hallmark contributions of Dr. Harvey Cushing to neurological surgery. During the pre-Cushing era, posterior fossa lesions were mostly considered "gliomas" and inoperable and merely bony decompressive surgery was offered. Surgical and anesthetic techniques were in their infancy and manipulation of the delicate nervous tissues required technical refinement. The lack of adequate hemostatic agents and transfusion strategies offered special challenges.

Cushing realized early in his career that early diagnosis would improve surgical outcomes. He therefore attempted to increase the awareness of the medical community regarding the diagnosis of cerebellar tumors through his lectures. In 1927, he wrote:

"… that a median tumor of the cerebellum is so common a lesion in preadolescence that when a child has unexplained vomiting, shows a possible enlargement of its head, and gives a story of periodical unsteadiness, it is well to be on guard and to have a look at the eye grounds every week or two."[9]

In 1905, Cushing described a decompressive suboccipital procedure for posterior fossa lesions through a crossbow incision.[6] Resective surgery for such lesions became a reality as he developed various surgical maneuvers during his career. The development of techniques such as lateral ventricular puncture to decrease cerebellar herniation after dural opening, transvermian approach to midline tumors (especially in pediatric patients), and electrocoagulation were the key factors in his triumph to pioneer posterior fossa surgery. His recognition of the importance of the tumor mural nodule in cyst recurrence and elucidation of the histogenesis of posterior fossa tumors to tailor treatment including radiotherapy facilitated improved outcomes. These techniques are reviewed in the following paragraphs.

Lateral ventricular puncture

The technique of lateral ventricular puncture was first noted in his record in 1909.[7] The release of CSF reduced "extracranial" bleeding from the bone and dura and prevented life-threatening cerebellar herniation upon opening of the dura. Such complications previously prevented operations in the infratentorial space. Reduction of the intracranial pressure in the posterior fossa allowed detailed examination of the cerebellar topography to localize the underlying mass lesion. Cushing subsequently routinely used ventricular puncture throughout his career to decrease blood loss especially in children.

Resection of tumor mural nodule

Initial surgical treatment of cerebellar tumors involved a subtemporal or suboccipital bony decompression to relieve mass effect from hydrocephalus or a posterior fossa mass lesion, respectively. Cushing conducted such procedures at the Johns Hopkins Hospital because his attempts at resection were associated with a high rate of postoperative fatality. When he arrived at the Peter Bent Brigham Hospital, he began aspiration of cerebellar cysts using a lumbar needle, followed

---

The following material has been partially excerpted with permission from Cohen-Gadol AA, Spencer DD. Inauguration of pediatric neurosurgery by Harvey W. Cushing: his contributions to the surgery of posterior fossa tumors in children. *Historical Vignette J Neurosurg: Peds* 100(2 Suppl):225-31, 2004

by destruction of the cyst wall by excision or formalin/Zenker solution fixation. During this time, since all cerebellar tumors were considered malignant and unresectable based on the classification by Virchow, cyst aspiration was considered the reasonable palliative option.

When Cushing reflected upon his initial experience, he noted in a 1915 operative report that cyst aspiration was associated with a high rate of symptomatic recurrence. As he removed part of or all the mural nodule solely for the purpose of histological studies, he discovered that the patients who had the whole nodule removed benefited from a decreased rate of cyst recurrence. Consequently, sometime in 1922, the significance of mural nodule secretion in maintenance of cyst fluid was definitively appreciated and removal of the nodule became his standard practice during the subsequent posterior fossa operations.

Introduction of 'electro-surgical' methods

Dr. Cushing's "electro-surgical method" was a landmark in his quest for radical resection of posterior fossa tumors. The terms "intracapsular tumor enucleation" and "adequate hemostasis" began to regularly appear in Cushing's operative notes in 1927 when he employed Bovie's electrocautery machine.[4,5] Around the same time, Cushing began to consider wound re-exploration for possible clot evacuation or staged gross total tumor removal; we did not find such considerations in his postoperative notes prior to this time.

Cushing recognized the importance of adequate hemostasis in the limited posterior fossa space as seven early postoperative autopsy cases disclosed a clot associated with brain stem compression. Vascular tumors were more effectively dealt with in the latter part of Cushing's career. Availability of electrocoagulation allowed Cushing to consider earlier operations and reoperations despite the risks. To attain hemostasis, he used pledgets of gauze, cotton, or muscle (initially described by Horsley). Ultimately, Cushing's introduction of silver clips and electrocautery may be considered the two most important success factors in improving the safety of posterior fossa operations.

Electrosurgical methods transformed Cushing's surgical technique from palliative decompressive surgery to curative resective surgery. Electrocautery allowed safe vermian sectioning, facilitating exposure of the tumor and its resection. Such technical advances were instrumental in Cushing's success at achieving gross total tumor resections during 1928-32.

Ventriculograms

Cushing did not advocate vetriculograms for children with posterior fossa mass lesions. There are multiple underlying reasons for such practice.[10] In his clinical experience, one of the three patients in the present series who underwent a ventriculogram became significantly restless with worsening of her admission symptoms requiring an increase in the amount of ether anesthesia used to keep her at rest during surgery. The other two patients became comatose with respiratory irregularities a day after their ventriculograms, requiring an immediate ventricular puncture.

He believed all cerebellar tumors could be localized based on a detailed neurological examination. Should any confusion occur regarding tumor localization, Cushing preferred to complete the transverse leg of his cross-bow incision under local anesthesia and punctured both lateral ventricles. If the ventricles were punctured in the usual fashion without piercing a mass and the CSF was under pressure, he would proceed with an exploratory suboccipital craniectomy. If not, further work-up was needed. Our review of the nine autopsy reports for the patients who had no findings during their posterior fossa operations supports his claim that no supratentorial mass lesion had gone undetected in these patients.

Cushing's series of posterior fossa tumors represents the earliest attempts to tackle lesions in the posterior fossa in children. The application of Halstedian meticulous surgical techniques by Harvey Cushing, who was encouraged by Sir William Osler, provided the substance upon which surgery in the subtentorial space was established. Subsequent refinement and further development of these surgical techniques and the application of electrocautery by Cushing defined the safety of such operations.[1,2,15,16]

Surgical considerations for posterior fossa lesions

Magnesium sulfate enema was used to reduce intracranial hypertension while patients were awaiting surgery.

The patient was placed on a "cerebellar headholder." Anesthesia consisted of a local injection of Novocain, and was supplemented by inhalation of ether only if the patient was restless. Cushing avoided ether since he believed it might cause respiratory difficulties especially in patients with brain stem compression. Patients undergoing surgery from 1929-1932 received Avertine (tribromoethanol) per rectum combined with ether – this cocktail was considered a safer and faster anesthetic. Cushing's idea of monitoring etherized patients by recording their respiration and pulse was a critical contribution especially during surgery of posterior fossa tumors.[14]

A crossbow incision was Cushing's distinctive trademark to expose both sides of the suboccipital area to allow complete bony removal down to the foramen magnum and up to both transverse sinuses. This incision consisted of a transverse leg nearly from ear to ear, joint by a vertical midline incision. Such exposure allowed exploratory decompression of both cerebellar hemispheres. Evidence of excessive "extracranial bleeding" from the dura and bone required puncture of the lateral ventricle using a ventricular needle; such technique was performed in almost every case. Upon puncturing the lateral ventricle, he routinely documented in his note the distance the brisk flow of the CSF traveled from the operating table to illustrate the amount of "tension."

A piece of dura and the occipital sinus were cut and removed, both cerebellar hemispheres were exposed for visual and tactile inspection. Sinus bleeding was controlled using Cushing's silver clips.[4,11,13] If tactile and visual inspection of the surface anatomy did not reveal any suspicious abnormality, the cerebellopontine angle was explored. If this exploration was not revealing, a lumbar needle was then passed into both cerebellar hemispheres to the depth of approximately 5 cm to find the wall of a cyst or tumor. If a mass was noted deeper, it was considered too deep and resection was not contemplated.

He used pituitary and "Horsley" rongeurs to biopsy a piece of the tumor for histological analysis. Introduction and refinement of the suction apparatus and "electrosurgical needle" by William T. Bovie in 1927 allowed radical resection of these tumors.[5,17] He used pieces of cotton gauze to "brush the tumor away." The surgical cavity was filled with the salt solution. The skin was closed using fine silk sutures and an elaborate cerebellar dressing was applied. Blood transfusion was arranged by the direct transfer of blood from a donor to the patient.

Postoperatively, prior to application of the dressing, some patients were left in the prone position on the operating room table up to 24 hours after surgery to recover from ether anesthesia. The surgical instruments remained available during this time. Cushing believed that such arrangement would allow timely wound re-exploration if a compressive clot was suspected. Furthermore, it was a safer position for patients at risk of vomiting following infratentorial surgery.

Postoperative high fever in the absence of an infectious source was thought to be due to blood in the CSF space and Cushing advised his residents to perform a series of lumbar punctures until the blood tinged CSF cleared. If a patient's status continued to deteriorate postoperatively, Cushing often tapped the lateral ventricle and surgical cavity using a ventricular needle through the skin to drain fluid and provide decompression.

Cushing's contributions in the area of basic science research for brain tumors is evident in his attempts to implant xenografts of tumor cells in the spinal canals of rhesus monkeys, attempting to recapitulate the seeding of the spinal canal so commonly seen in the patients with posterior fossa malignancies. He noted that the absence of tumor growth in the monkeys was more than likely due to experimental technique, since the cells could grow in "hanging-drop preparations made synchronously with the injections."[8] Further, Bailey and Cushing attempted to elucidate the differentiation pathway of the "primitive cells of the medulloblastomas" via histological analyses and cell culture.[12]

The following patients' records may illustrate the details of Cushing's attempts at the lesions of posterior fossa. Other pathologies which could not be classified in the other chapters have been included here.

The picture of Patient 6.1 suffering from trigeminal neuralgia (holding the right side of his right face with his hand) may represent the first available picture of a patient with this disease treated surgically (1913). The letter sent to Cushing by this patient 20 year after his surgery demonstrates the sincere appreciation of the patient. Patient 6.2 underwent a delayed repair of her myelomeningocele at the age of seven months. During the early part of Cushing's career, closure of myelomeningoceles may have been done in a delayed fashion due to a lack of recognition of this disease as amenable to surgery. In addition, the children may have tolerated surgical conditions of the time more safely if the child had matured more physically. The operative sketch and report describe the application of Bayer myocutaneous flap for sac closure.[3]

Based on the available record, Cushing may have not been involved in the care of Patient 6.3. Charles Bagley, Cushing's first resident at Brigham, performed the cyst aspiration. The details of preoperative work-up are scarce in this case. Patient 6.4 underwent subtotal resection of his acoustic neuroma (Cushing firmly believed radical resection of acoustic tumors was risky and advocated intracapsular enucleation.) In 1916, prior to further classification of brain tumors, this tumor was initially thought to be a "glioma." In 1923, this pathological diagnosis was corrected to be "acoustic neuroma." Upon the return of symptoms, the patient underwent radiation treatment.

The hospital records of Patients 6.6, 6.7, 6.9-11, 6.14–16, and 6.20 are not available in the Brain Tumor Registry. The images have been included to illustrate the diversity of Cushing's surgical practice.

In Patient 6.8, Cushing attempted facial nerve rhizotomy using alcohol around the styloid process. Although this procedure was unsuccessful, it verified "neuralgia of facial nerve origin." Before performing further heroic measures, Cushing documented the details of patient's symptoms in his usual "special note." He then resected a portion of facial nerve through drilling the mastoid bone. During this procedure, the two ends of the facial nerve were left "in near approximation."

Patients 6.9 and 6.15 underwent craniectomy procedures for craniosynostosis. The autopsy head specimen of Patient 6.15 in the Registry demonstrates the site of craniectomy. Patient 6.11 most likely suffered from progeria and may have been evaluated by Cushing for pituitary disease. Patient 6.12 underwent intradural rhizotomy of spinal accessory nerve and upper cervical roots with an acceptable result. Patient 6.14 underwent a similar operation but including bilateral sternocleidomastoid rhizotomies. He suffered from a temporary right-sided shoulder weakness postoperatively.

Patient 6.13 is of special significance because he is one of the early patients who underwent a total resection of an acoustic neuroma by Cushing. Dandy reported his experience with total extirpation of an acoustic neuroma in 1922. Cushing performed his total extirpation of an acoustic tumor earlier in September 1921 (This patient is mentioned in the operative report of Patient 6.7).

Cushing's experience with the surgical treatment of peripheral nerve disease is illustrated in the patient record of 6.17. The details of operative report of Patient 6.18 for removal of a petroclival epidermoid illustrate Cushing's mastery and evolution of neurosurgical techniques. The tumor was first approached through a subtemporal approach and later in another session through the suboccipital corridor. In the "special note" of the first operation, Cushing describes an alternative route to the Gasserian ganglion. Patient 6.20 most likely underwent resection of a carotid body tumor.

Cushing's most important pediatric neurosurgery contribution is his personal account with cerebellar tumor resections which appeared in *Surgery, Gynecology and Obstetrics* in 1931 titled "Experiences with Cerebellar Astrocytomas: A Critical Review of 76 Cases."[7] The evolution of Cushing's surgical expertise from performance of suboccipital decompressions to total extirpation of vascular fourth ventricular tumors combined with a dramatic decrease in his operative mortality rate reflects the maturation of modern neurosurgical techniques.

Aaron A. Cohen-Gadol, M.D, M.Sc.
Indianapolis, IN

Amandip S. Gill, B.S.
Irvine, CA

Devin Binder, M.D., Ph.D.
Irvine, CA

References

1. Black PM: Harvey Cushing at the Peter Bent Brigham Hospital. *Neurosurgery* 45:990-1001, 1999
2. Black PM: Peter Bent Brigham Hospital. *J Neurosurg* 75:987-988, 1991
3. Cohen-Gadol AA, Nahed BV, Voorhees JR, Maher CO, Spencer DD: Cushing's experience with the surgical treatment of spinal dysraphism. *J Neurosurg* 102:441-444, 2005
4. Cushing H: The control of bleeding in operations for brain tumors. with the description of silver "clips" for the occlusion of vessels inaccessible to the ligature. *Ann Surg* 54:1-19, 1911
5. Cushing H: Electro-surgery as an aid to the removal of intracranial tumors. with a preliminary note on a new surgical-current generator by WT Bovie, PhD, Chicago. *Surg Gynecol Obstet* 47:751-784, 1928
6. Cushing H: The establishment of cerebral hernia as a decompressive measure for inaccessible brain tumors; with the description of intramuscular methods of making the bone defect in temporal and occipital regions. *Surg Gynecol Obstet* 1:297-314, 1905
7. Cushing H: Experiences with the cerebellar astrocytomas: a critical review of seventy-six cases. *Surg Gynecol Obstet* 52:129-204, 1931
8. Cushing H: Experiences with the cerebellar medulloblastomas: a critical review. *Acta Pathologica et Microbiologica Scandinavica* 7:1-86, 1930
9. Cushing H: The intracranial tumors of preadolescence. *Am J Dis Child* 4:551-584, 1927
10. Fox W: The Cushing-Dandy controversy. *Surg Neurol* 3:661-666, 1975
11. Horrax G: Some of Harvey Cushing's contributions to neurological surgery. *J Neurosurg* 54:436-447, 1981
12. Kunschner LJ: Harvey Cushing and medulloblastoma. Arch Neurol 59:642-645, 2002
13. Light RU: The contributions of Harvey Cushing to the techniques of neurosurgery. *Surg Neurol* 35:69-73, 1991
14. Long DM: Harvey Cushing at Johns Hopkins. *Neurosurgery* 45:983-989, 1999
15. Moore MR, Rossitch E, Jr., Black PM: The development of neurosurgical techniques: the postoperative notes and sketches of Dr. Harvey Cushing. *Acta Neurochir (Wien)* 101:93-99, 1989
16. Moore MR, Rossitch E, Jr., Shillito J, Jr.: Cushing and epilepsy surgery: two successfully treated cases with long-term follow-up. *Surg Neurol* 32:241-245, 1989
17. O'Connor JL, Bloom DA: William T. Bovie and electrosurgery. *Surgery* 119:390-396, 1996

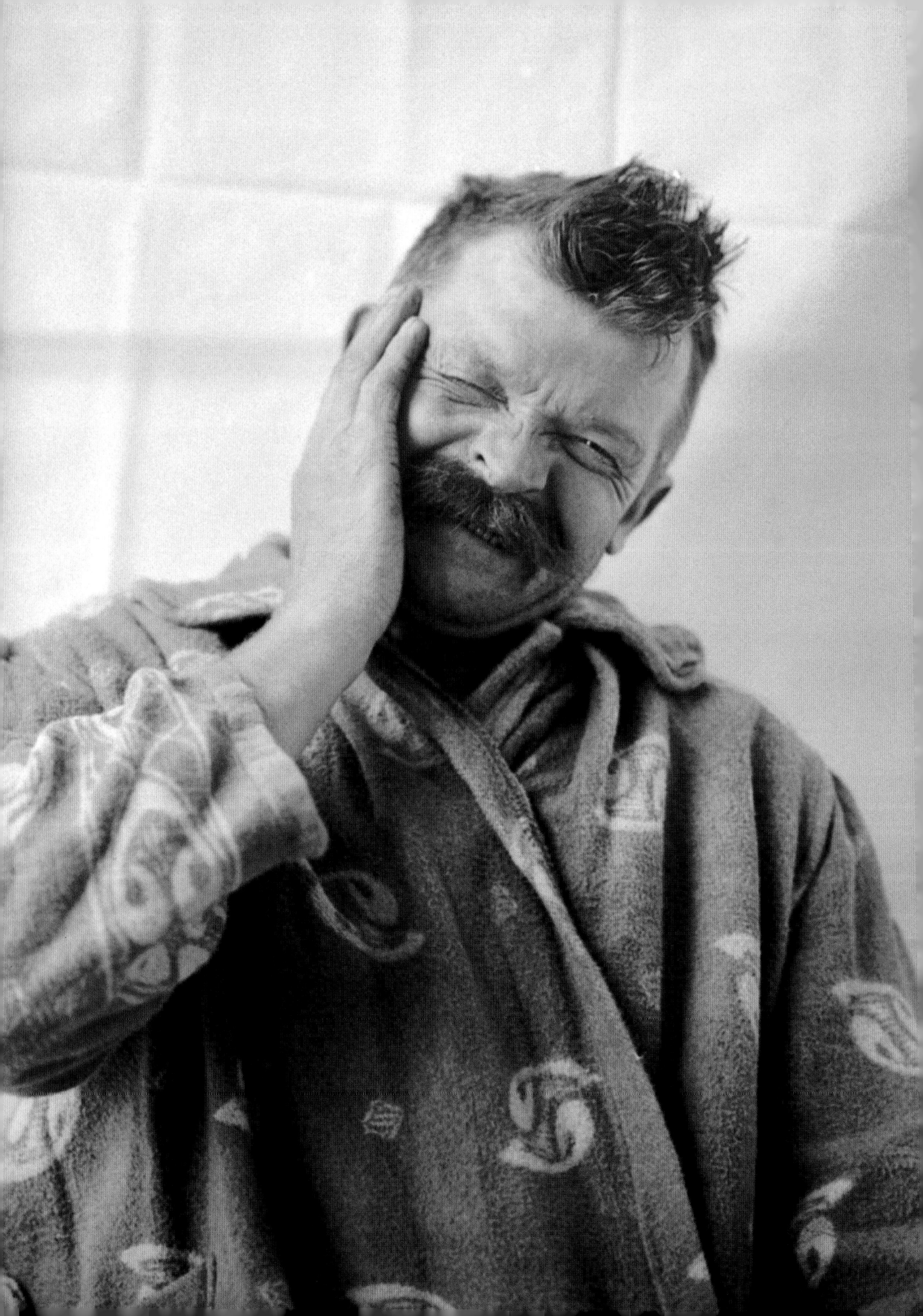

6.1 Trigeminal neuralgia

SEX: M; AGE: 45; SURG. NO. 206

HISTORY

This patient suffered from right-sided facial neuralgia for 25 years. He was first treated by teeth extraction, "medication," "electricity," and "injection." Eighteen years ago he had "the nerve cut under the right eye," with some pain relief, however; after a year and a half the pain returned. During the last five weeks prior to admission, he had four alcohol injections. He continued to have pain in the "upper and lower" part of the right side of his face.

EXAMINATION

June 29, 1913
Dr. Cobb

III – Left pupil dilated considerably – more so than right – both react actively. Quick nystagmoid movements to left, fine in character.

V – Trigeminus

SUBJECTIVE

Pain over area of distribution of 1st, 2nd and 3rd division of right side for past 20–25 years.

OBJECTIVE

Beneath right eye is a scar running across the face horizontally over distribution of 2nd division of nerve.

Pain–touch–temperature sense, seem equally acute on both sides except in region directly under right eye which is less acute. No disturbance of taste.

Muscle of mastication equally firm on both sides. Pain is excited by these tests and patient stops them by smacking his tongue against the roof of his mouth and pressure on the right side of his neck.

VII – Facial

Slight paralysis of facial muscles below the right eye. Naso-labial folds not so prominent on this side. Face has somewhat placid expression.

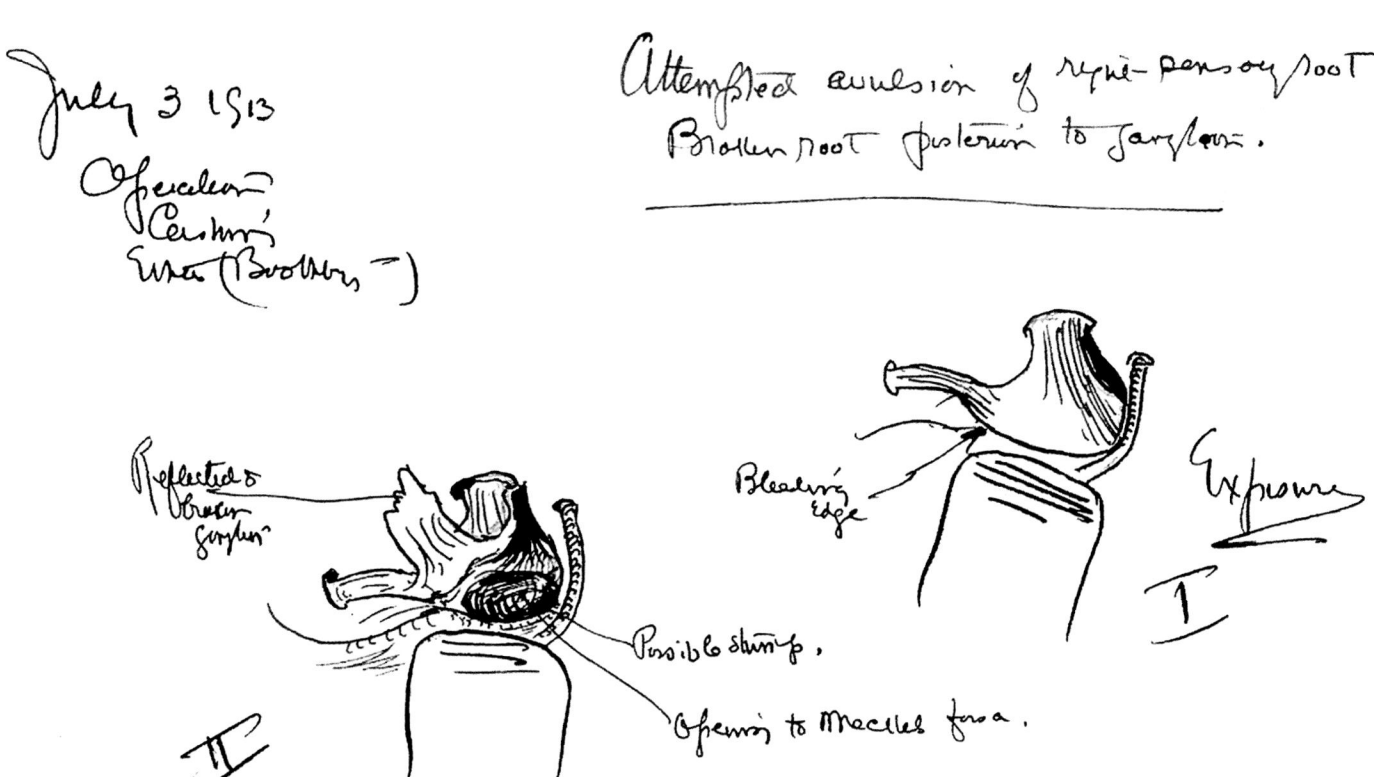

FIG. 2. OPERATIVE SKETCH.

OPPOSITE PAGE: FIG. I. PREOPERATIVE.

OPERATIVE NOTE
July 3, 1913
Dr. Cushing
Anesthesia – Ether – Dr. Boothby

Attempted Avulsion of Right Sensory Root. Broken Root Posterior to Ganglion.

The usual approach was made and no especial difficulty met with in the exposure of the ganglion. The ganglion was lifted away from the base of the skull. Unfortunately there was some bleeding from underneath the structure. However, this difficulty was overcome and finally the upper surface of the ganglion was exposed. It was much larger than usual and as the meningeal artery entered the foramen spinosum at a considerable distance it was possible to lift the dura well up and to expose the larger part of the ganglion as shown in the sketch.

Bleeding had been met with along the reflected margin of the dura and there was one or two points of attachment between the ganglion and this reflected edge of dura which could not be separated without causing trouble from hemorrhage.

The first division was then freed and the attempt made to lift out the sensory root. There was a considerable escape of cerebro-spinal fluid and the latter stage of the operation was conducted without difficulty and with a good exposure. On lifting out the sensory root, however, the root did not come as clearly as expected and there seemed to be some adhesion between the root and the reflected dura. It is quite probable, in other words that the upper portion of the dissection liberating the very posterior margin of the ganglion itself from the dura had not been fully accomplished.

The portion of the ganglion as shown in Fig. II (Please see the operative sketch,) which was reflected left the opening in the dura passing into the sub-arachnoid space well exposed and no trace of further nervous or ganglionic structure could be found. It is possible, therefore, that the avulsion may have been more definitely and completely carried out than seemed to be the case at the time. This cannot be determined, however, until it is possible after the operation to test for sensation.

Wound was closed as usual in layers without drainage. *(Dr. Cushing)*

POSTOPERATIVE NOTES
July 5, 1913
Dr. Bagley

First dressing. All sutures removed – wound completely healed. Eye in excellent condition – some mucus discharge, but no conjunctival congestion. Anaesthesia over area of 1st division, apparently complete. Foil, gauze and crinoline reapplied.

July 18, 1913
Dr. Bagley

Condition excellent, eye in good condition, anaesthesia complete over 1st division.

DISCHARGE NOTE
July 19, 1913
Dr. Bagley

Discharged today in good condition.

LETTER TO DR. CUSHING
(20 years later)
June 26, 1933

Dear Professor Cushing,

I have not written to you in many years, because I feel that your time is too valuable. Also, the condition of my health has been perfect.

Twenty years ago Dr. Davidson of Seattle, Wash. sent me to you with Tic Douloureux, from which I had suffered for twenty-five years. July 3, 1913 was the day you successfully performed the operation.

For this reason, I am writing to you, to thank you, after twenty years of good health for your interest and kindness.

Today I am in very fine health and life has been a great pleasure and success, made possible for me by your skill, kindness and interest.

I am enclosing a picture of myself, in which you can see the scars below the right eye caused by former unsuccessful operation performed in the Netherlands in 1895. (The picture was not included due to its poor quality.)

Wishing to thank you again for my very fine condition of health, I remain,

Sincerely yours,
(Signed) WJ

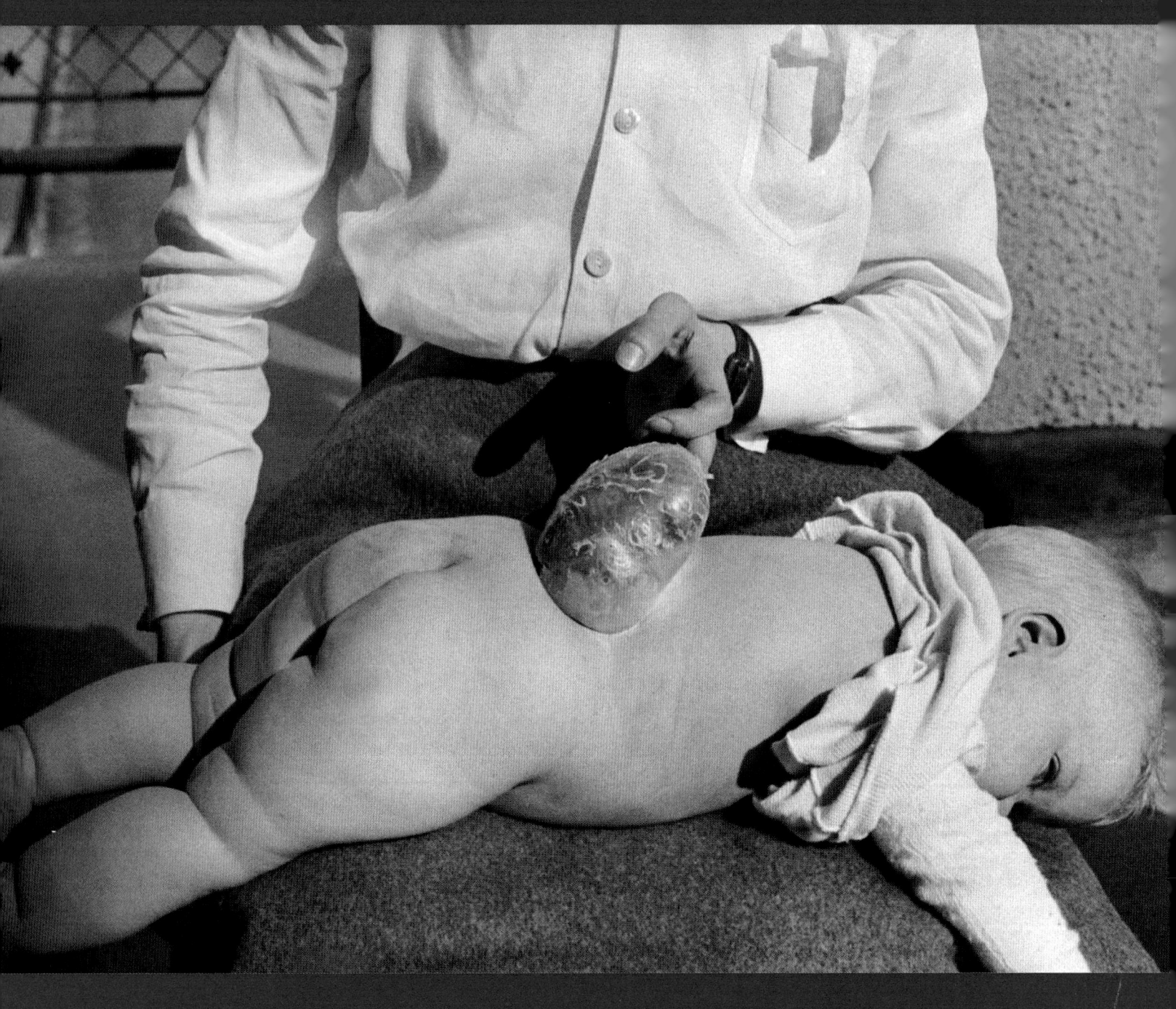

6.2 Myelomeningocele

SEX: F; AGE: 7 MONTHS; SURG. NO. 5456

HISTORY

The parents noted a mass at the lumbar region at the time of the child's birth. The mass has increased in size with the growth of the child. The right lower extremity has been immobile for the last two months.

SUMMARY OF POSITIVE FINDINGS
July 1, 1913
Dr. Cobb

SUBJECTIVE

Since birth – gradually increasing in size of spina-bifida sack – apparently no increase of intracranial pressure.

OBJECTIVE

1. Spina-bifida sack.
2. Posterior fontanelle closed.
3. Anterior fontanelle 6 cm. in antero-posterior and lateral diameter.
4. Loss of muscle power of right lower extremity – first noticed two months ago.
5. Complete loss of sensation of right lower extremity – first noticed two months ago.
6. Apparently no disturbance of left lower extremity.

IMPRESSION: Myelomeningocele.

OPERATIVE NOTE
July 7, 1913

Anesthesia – Ether – Boothby

Exploration of Sac of Myelomeningocele with Reduction of Cord and Closure by Plastic.

An incision was made around the stalk of the large sac saving as much of the cutaneous normal tissue as possible for subsequent closure. On carrying this incision down towards the stalk, the usual juicy succulent tissue was encountered. This was dissected back by blunt dissection until the defect

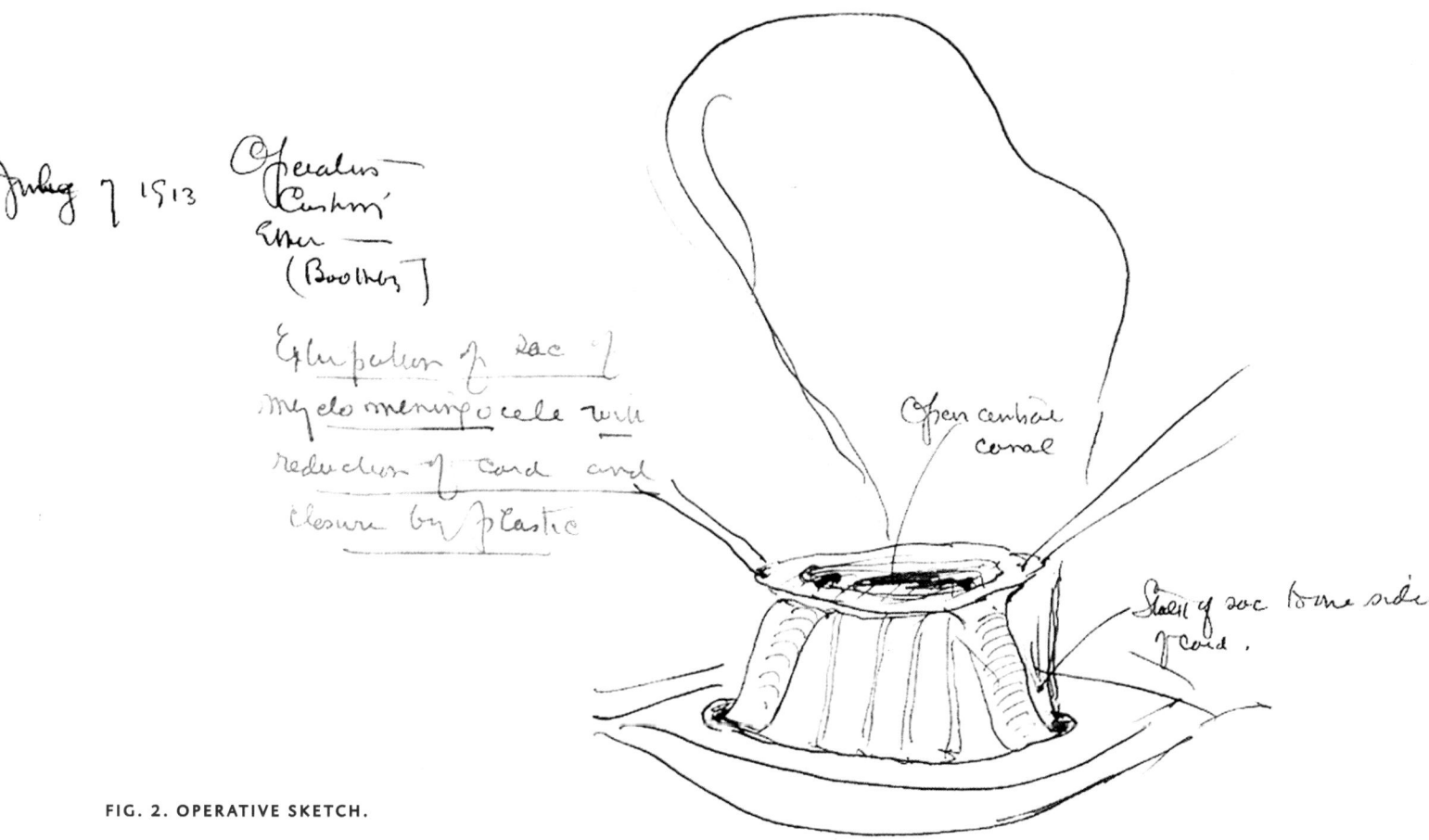

FIG. 2. OPERATIVE SKETCH.

OPPOSITE PAGE: FIG. I. PREOPERATIVE.

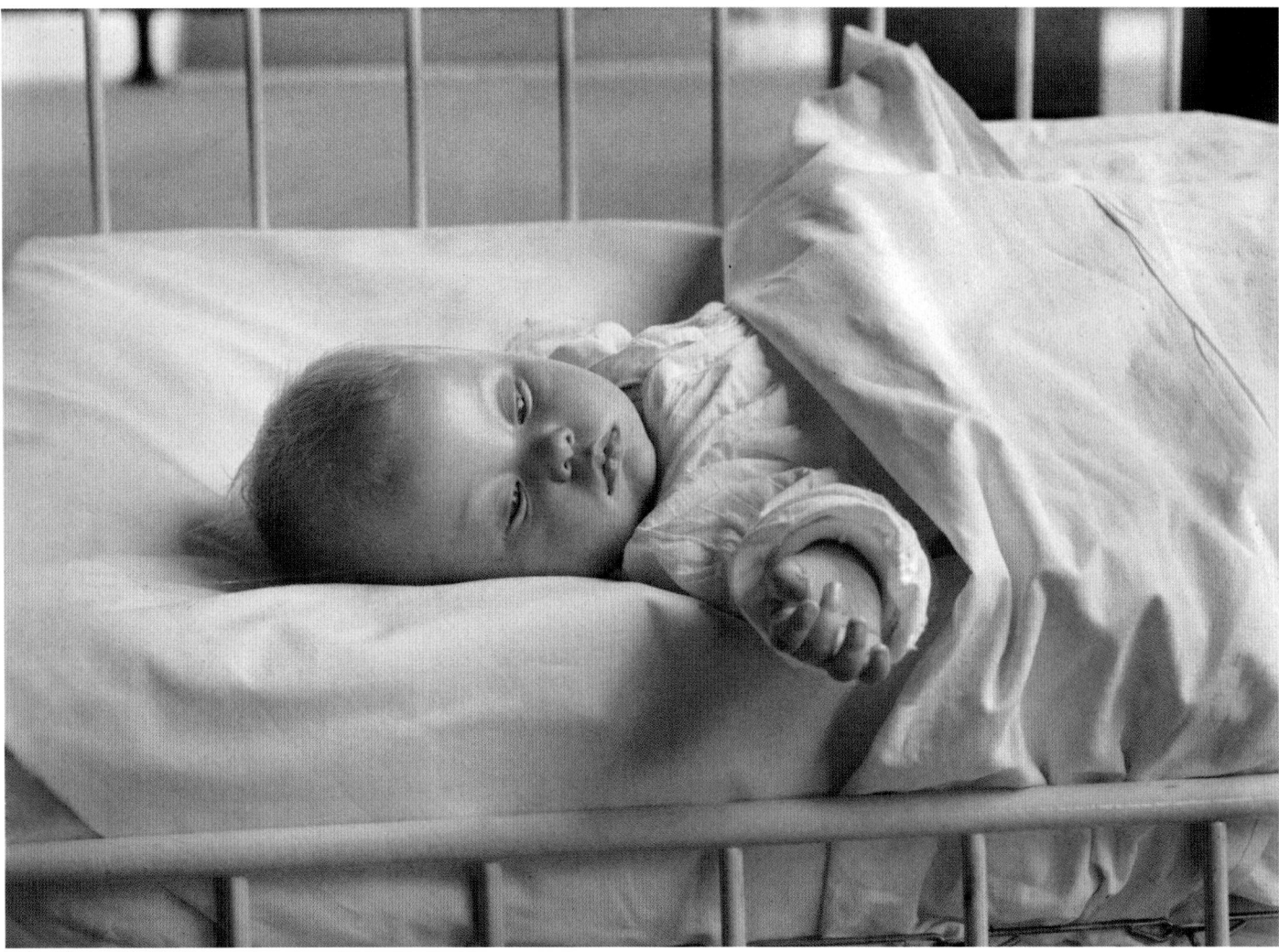

FIG. 3. POSTOPERATIVE.

in the spine was brought into view. It was evident that the cord and nerve protruded as was expected into the sac, though not in the way expected, for the sac itself lay to one side and it was possible to separate the sac from the proximal end of the cord to divide it and to close it by sutures.

With the cord both at its proximal and distal ends in view it was possible by careful and close dissection to remove the herniated portion of the cord from the sac itself, showing clearly as in the sketch of the open canal. Though there was not a great deal of room in the cavity which was left by freeing the tissues at the side the cord could be reduced and the tissues in a primary layer closed over the cord. Subsequently three additional layers were made—the last one drawing over the loosened spinal muscles on each side so that a very firm closure was finally obtained. The skin was then sutured as usual in one or two layers and the wound thus closed without drainage.

(Dr. Cushing)

DISCHARGE NOTE
August 3, 1913
Dr. Bagley

Head—Anterior fontanelles tight and bulging. Entire frontal bone beginning to seem elevated. Veins over fronto-temporal region markedly distended, also over bridge of nose. Circumference— 48.4 cm. A rather sudden increase of ½ cm. since note of July 29. Elevation of outer canthus still well marked. There is apparently but very little headache recently.

Child has been very comfortable and bright, mother much encouraged.

The incision in the lumbar region is quite firm

and still somewhat ridged. Photographs made 48 hrs. ago.

There is evidently slight movement of toes — right lower extremity. This, however, is very slight and though left lower extremity is moved actively right is always in more or less flaccid position.

Apparently no return of sensation.

Child discharged today to return in Sept. for relief of internal hydrocephalus.

LAST FOLLOW UP
December 15, 1915
Dr. Cushing

Wonderfully well. No Hydrocephalus! Very bright. 3 years old. Right foot is better. Has not walked yet. Is at Children's Hospital, getting braces. Head = 53 cm. Has control of bowel and bladder. No diaper necessary.

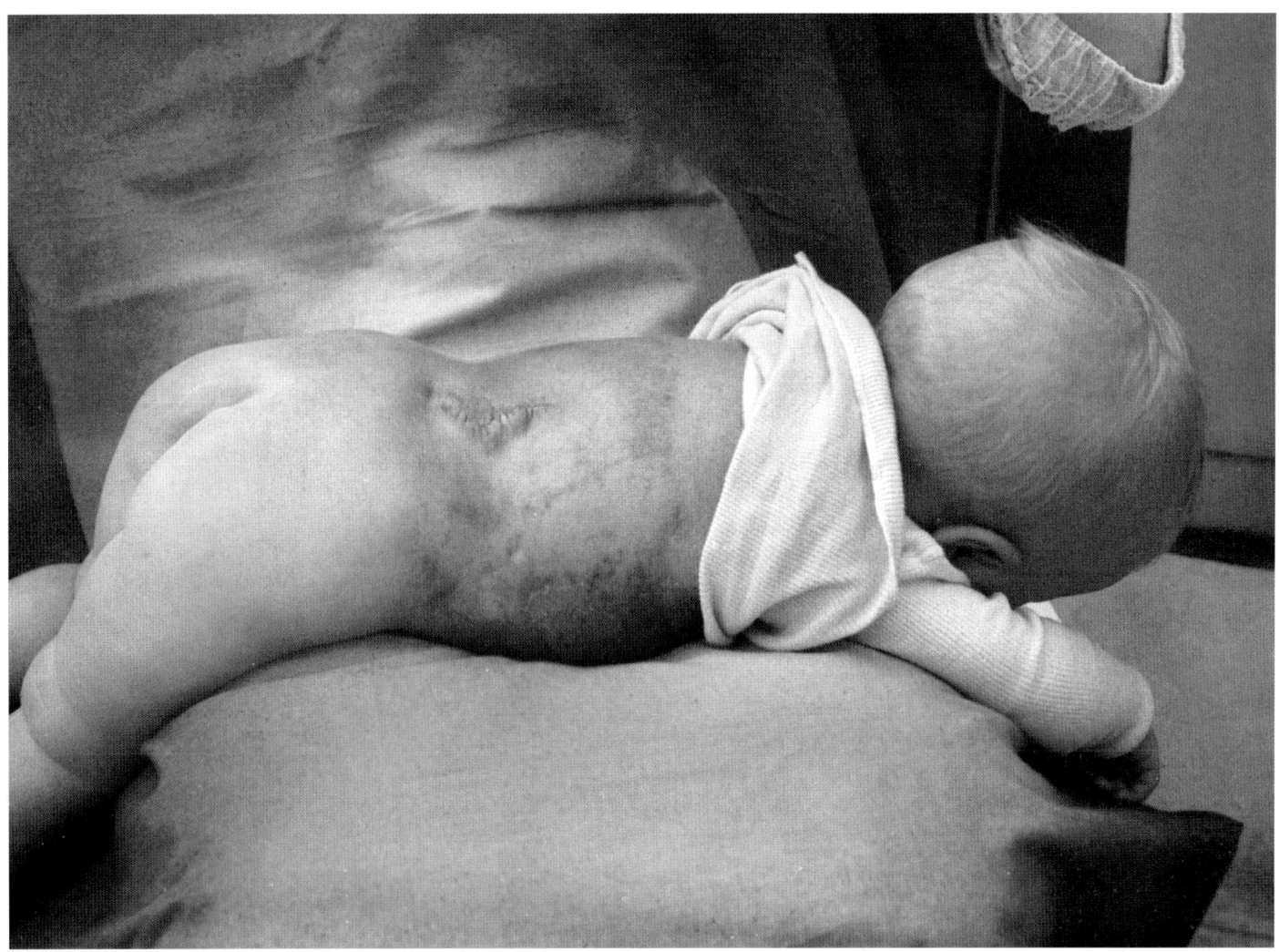

FIG. 4. POSTOPERATIVE.

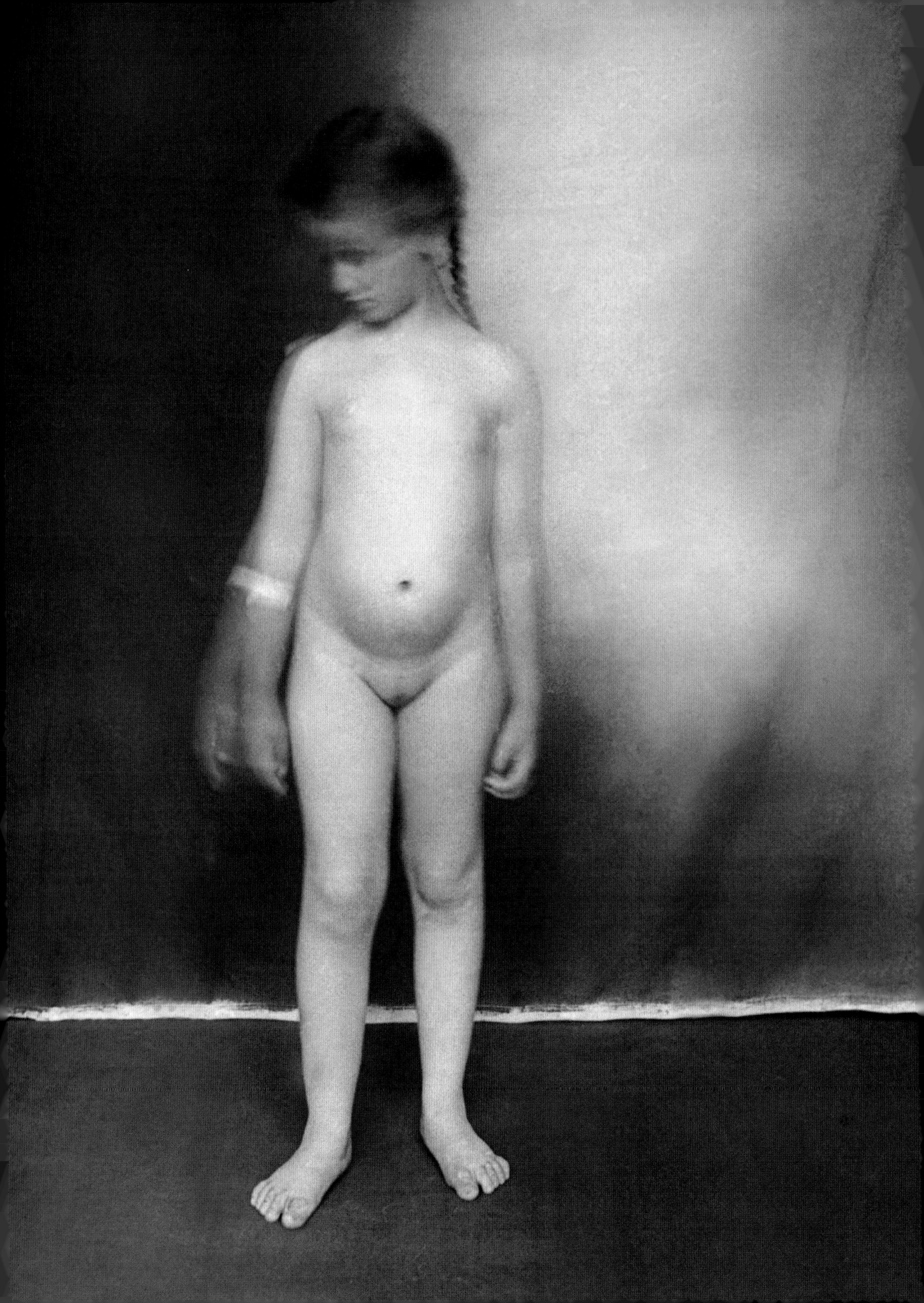

6.3 Porencephalic cyst

SEX: F; AGE: 6; SURG. NO. 345; 429

This six-year-old child was born with "water on the brain" and was suffering from seizure "spells" at irregular intervals since 3½ years of age. She underwent a rapid growth spurt until the second year of life. She was mentally underdeveloped since birth. Her past medical history was remarkable for her premature birth.

SUMMARY OF POSITIVE FINDINGS
August 27, 1913
Dr. Bagley

SUBJECTIVE
1. Condition present since birth. Difficult labor – duration 33 hours – forceps delivered with great difficulty. Small child weight 3 lbs. Head grew rapidly until 2 yrs of age.
2. Convulsive seizures: Since 3 years of age. Still present though less frequently.
3. Muscle weakness: Right upper and lower extremities and left side of face noticed since birth.
4. Skin: Always dry
5. Development: Walked and talked late. Mental development has been poor and entirely out of proportion with physical development. Mammary glands enlarged during last 6 months.
6. Adiposity: First noticed 6 months ago – gradually increasing.
7. Pubic hair: First noticed several months ago – increasing since.

OBJECTIVE
1. Marked over-growth.
   Child seemingly 13 or 15 yrs of age.
   Weight – 34.6 kilo.
   Height – 133 cm.
2. Distinct asymmetry of face.
   Left side less well developed.
   Prognathism – fairly well marked.
3. Skin
   Dry, though not scaly.
4. Adiposity
   Fairly well marked.
5. Mammary glands
   Markedly over-growth.
6. Optic

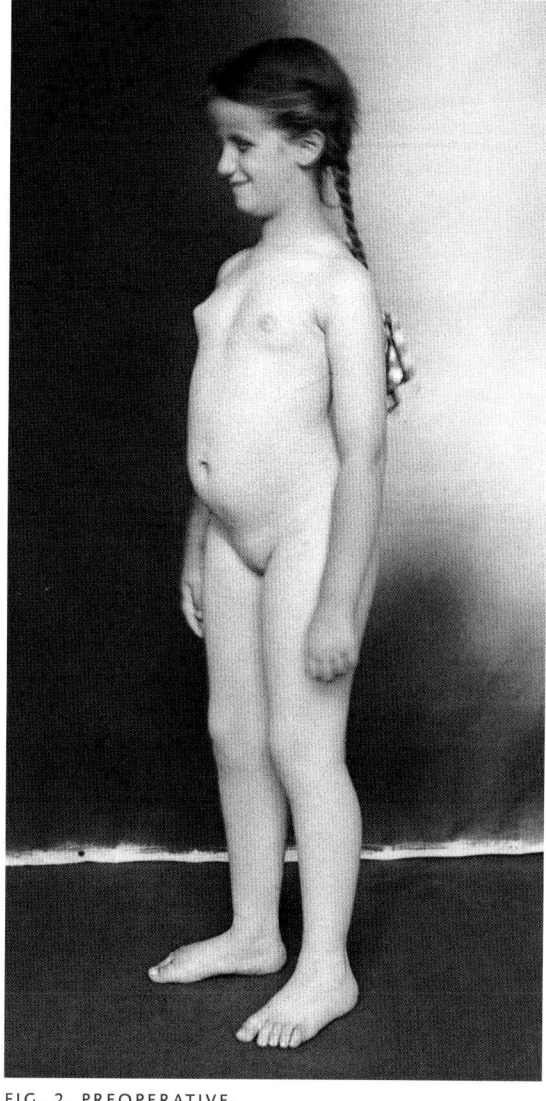

FIG. 2. PREOPERATIVE.

No chocked disc. Quite active nystagmus looking forward and to left side. Atypical nystagmus looking upward.
7. Definite voice changes. Voice is much heavier than other children of her age.
8. Mental development has been poor.
9. Gait
   Disturbed, perhaps due to weakness of right side.
10. Reflexes
    K.J. diminished on left-slightly exaggerated on right. No clonus.
11. Sphincter reflex O.K.

OPPOSITE PAGE: FIG. I. PREOPERATIVE.

DISCHARGE NOTE
August 27, 1913
Dr. Bagley

Not treated. Discharged for consultation with Dr. Cushing and Dr. Bagley in September.

SECOND HOSPITAL ADMISSION
September 30, 1913
Dr. Bagley

Child readmitted for further examination. Since leaving hospital there has been no change in condition with the exception of improvement in nervous excitement which father believes is due to the fact that child was separated from companion, a young woman of 17 yrs. with whom she has been sleeping as noted at time of previous examination.

No further studies available in chart.

OPERATIVE NOTE
October 9, 1913
Dr. Bagley
Anesthesia – Ether – Dr. Boothby

Puncture of Porencephalic Cyst. Left Hemisphere.

After shaving of hairs in region of anterior fontanel a slight bulging about 5 cm across base was found extending from midline down on the left. An incision of 4 cm. in length was made over the apex of this area, burr opening made, dura incised about ½ cm. Through the incision a membrane protruded entirely different in appearance from the normal cortex. It was evident the membrane was quite thin as it presented with a bluish reflex. A small incision was made in the protruding membrane – where clear fluid was evacuated under great pressure. This flow under pressure continued and about 100–150 cc of fluid was evacuated and the opening was plugged with moist cotton and further escape prevented. The fluid was clear, resembling cerebrospinal fluid. No suggestion of yellow tinged cyst fluid. The flow was also influenced by respiratory movement suggesting communication with ventricle. A blunt ventricular puncture needle was then passed through the small aperture downward to the depth of the brain a distance of 10 cm, but did not come in contact with cortex. Further measurements not made as too large a quantity of fluid was being evacuated. Cavity was filled with normal salt and wound was closed in usual manner.

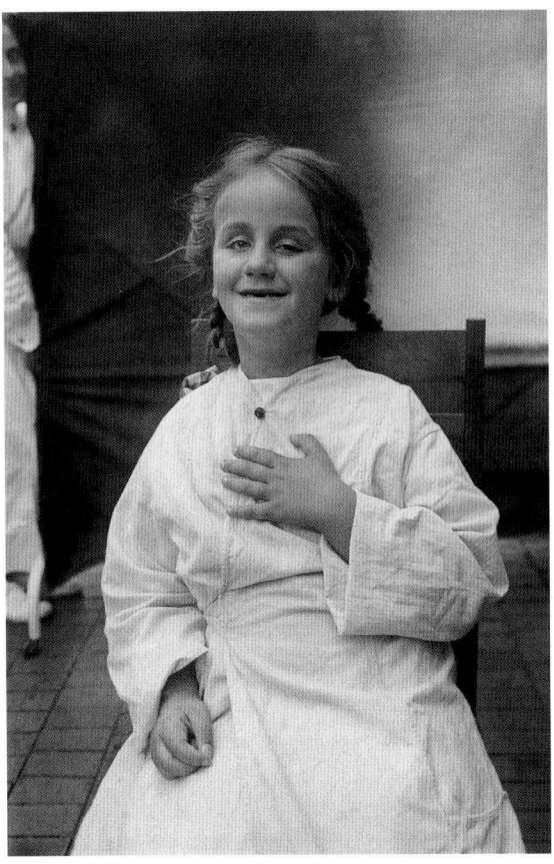

FIGS. 3 AND 4. PREOPERATIVE.

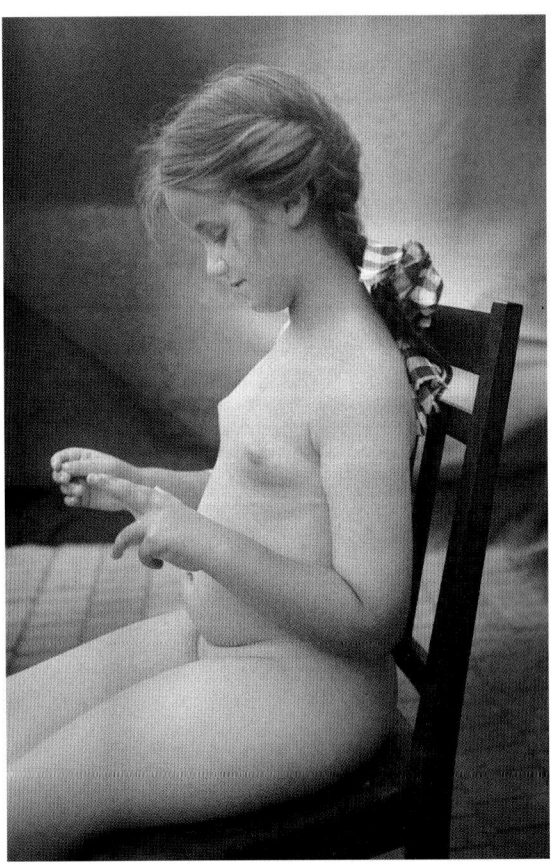

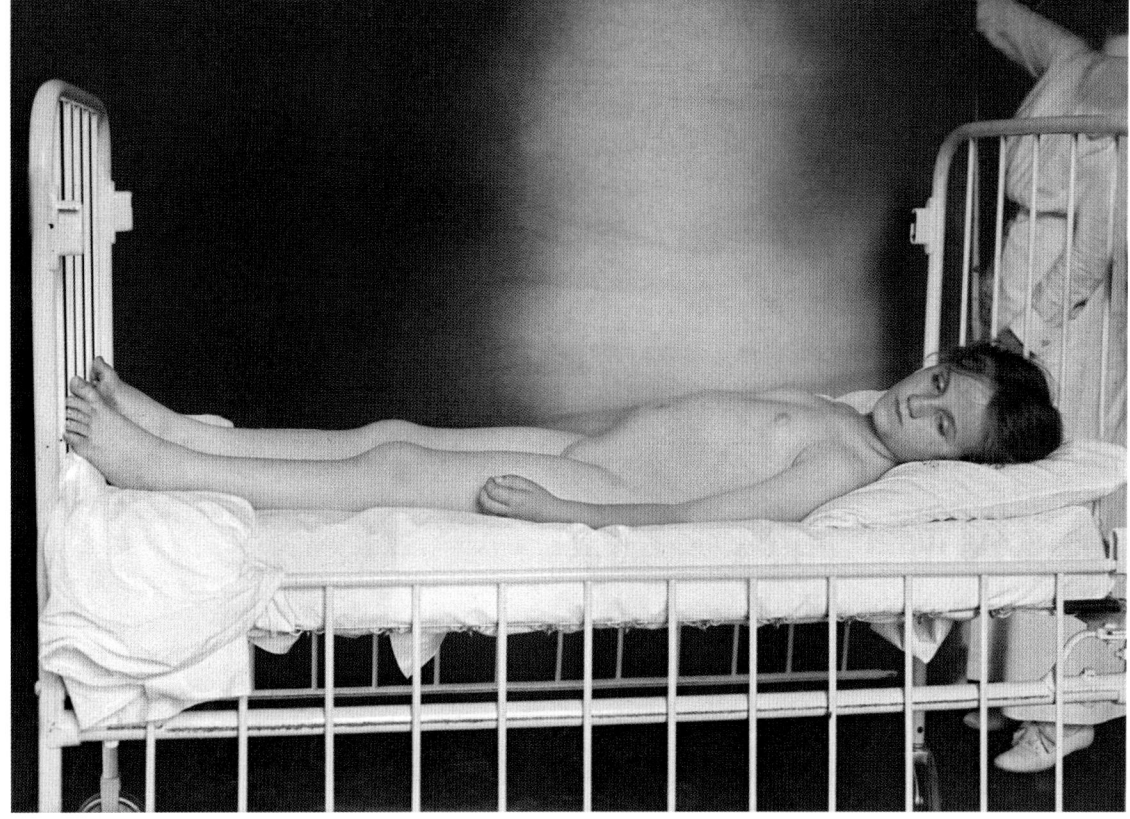

FIG. 5. PREOPERATIVE.

Anaesthetic well borne – condition quite satisfactory.

(Dr. Bagley)

POSTOPERATIVE NOTES
October 11, 1913
Dr. Bagley

Very good recovery. Wound healed. Sutures removed. There is some air in tissues for a distance of about 4 cm. from wound on all sides.

October 14, 1913
Dr. Rand

Following puncture of cyst by Dr. Bagley, patient's temperature rose to about 102°, where it remained constantly until October 11. Patient apparently perfectly comfortable, appetite good, slept well. Since Oct. 11, temperature has varied between 100 and 102°, q.d. gradually, however, becoming more nearly normal. Dressing changed by Dr. Bagley on Oct. 11, as noted above.

October 21, 1913
Dr. Bagley

Second dressing.

Since the operation child has been quite fretful, appetite poor, muscle membranes pale, expression suggestive of discomfort. Quite nervous, sings frequently. Dressing removed today – wound firmly healed though there is evidently free communication between the scalp and cyst cavity as the scar is elevated and tense during crying, etc. Crinolin dressings reapplied.

DISCHARGE NOTE
November 4, 1913
Dr. Rand

Since last note child's condition has been much the same – better. There is marked bulging over the operative field. This marks the point where the ventricular puncture was made. This bulging is tense when child cries or coughs – possibly elevated about 1 ½ cm and 3–4 cm in diameter. Mental condition unchanged. Discharged.

LAST FOLLOW UP NOTE
January 27, 1916

Mother reports that child's foot is bad.

6.4 Acoustic neuroma

SEX: M; AGE: 30; SURG. NO. 4139; 10811; 13072; 13469; 18709; 22295; 25560

Diagnosis: Surg. No 4139 – Cerebellopontine angle tumor, endothelioma.

Surg. No 10811; 13072; 13469; 18709; 22295; 25560 – Acoustic tumor.

Extracerebellar group. Neurinoma.

HISTORY

This patient was admitted complaining of left facial twitching, headaches, gastric distress, dysphagia, speech difficulty, inability to walk, failing vision, and "uncinate gyrus attacks."

SUMMARY OF POSITIVE FINDINGS
January 18, 1916
Dr. Jones

SUBJECTIVE
1. Headache – 1½ years
2. Gastric distress – nausea and vomiting – 1 year.
3. Twitching of left side of face – 9–10 years.
4. Twitching of hand and leg – about 1 year.
5. Dysphagia – 1 year.
6. Inability to walk – 4 months.
7. Failing vision – especially during last year.
8. Difficulty in speech – 5–6 months.

OBJECTIVE
1. Tenderness over right parietal region.
2. Left facial twitching.
3. Bilateral choked disc – 5D.
4. Weakness of left side of body.
5. Reflexes hyperactive – upper extremities.
6. Ankle clonus on left.
7. Hyperaesthesia on whole left side.
8. Deaf in left ear.
9. Ataxia.
10. Nystagmus – lateral and upper.

RADIOLOGY REPORT
January 19, 1916

Thickness of the skull is 5 mm. The sutures are slightly distended. There is a rarefaction in the skull in the region of the upper coronal suture. The venous channels are enlarged. The arterial

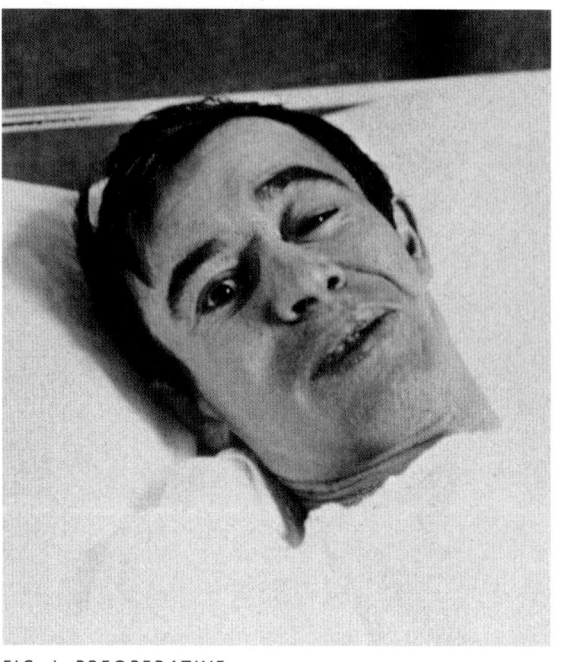

FIG. I. PREOPERATIVE.

grooves are not seen. The antero-posterior diameter of the sella is 12 mm. It is 10 mm deep. The anterior clinoid processes are distinct. The dorsum is plainly seen. There is a slight, but definite pressure atrophy of the posterior clinoid processes.

SPECIAL NOTE
January 24, 1916
Dr. Cushing

Though the case clearly suggests left cerebellopontine growth, the periodic left facial spasm with the hemi-hypesthesia, the increased reflexes and positive Babinski, naturally suggest a right-sided lesion.

However, the dysarthria, nystagmus, and extracerebellar (nerve) symptoms, more than counter-balance the above possibility.

OPERATIVE NOTE
January 24, 1916
Anesthesia – Ether – Dr. Boothby

Occipital Exploration with Partial Removal of Left Cerebello-Pontine Tumor (Endothelioma or Glioma) – Puncture of Left Lateral Ventricle.

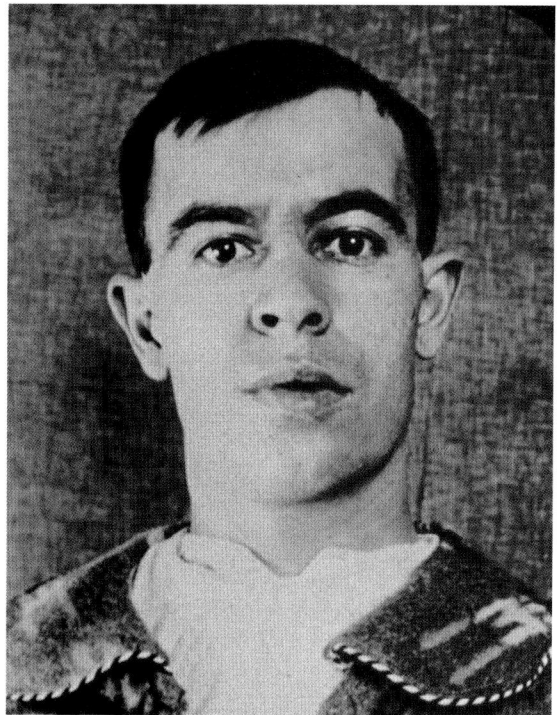

FIGS. 2–3. POSTOPERATIVE.

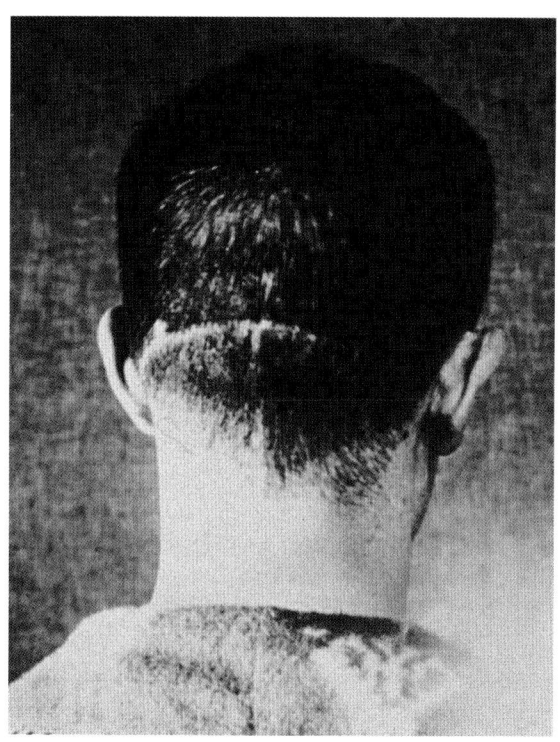

The usual cross-bow incision with much less bleeding than usual. The bone was very thick with no evidence of pressure thinning whatsoever. A generous opening was finally made including the foramen, but the dural tension was so great as to render a primary dural opening injudicious.

The left ventricle was then punctured and a large amount of fluid secured. (Specimen sent to Dr. Harvey). This lowered the tension so greatly that the dura was opened. There were no adhesions and no median sinus. Indeed, the appearances would hardly have made one believe that there was a subtentorial tumor. On exploring towards the left recess the margin of a large bluish cyst was brought into view. This cyst was low down and very near the bony opening. It was capped by a margin of cerebellum. On retracting this margin the cyst was very largely exposed, but it finally ruptured and a considerable amount of fluid escaped. This rupture showed that a tumor, lying in the left side of the fossa and doubtless coming from the recess was really capped by a cyst. The tumor was covered by large vessels, one bundle in particular having to be secured with clips. The surface of the tumor was soft and bleeding. It was much less tense and yellowish than in the usual type of recess tumor of the endothelioma variety. A considerable portion of the tumor was scooped out and this maneuver opened another cyst further in from which much fluid was evacuated. The tension was thus entirely relieved and the retracted hemisphere stayed well away from the cavity.

The cavity was then filled with fluid, and the wound closed in layers without a drain.

This was a very simple operative case in spite of the spasms aroused by the deglutory difficulties from which the patient was suffering. It is the only case, moreover, in which I have seen these facial spasms of distinctly epileptiform nature, though it may be said that the spasms appeared to come on under emotion or excitement, and at the time of taking the photographs this morning after a 5–10 minute rest, speaking to the patient or attracting his attention would be apt to produce a spasm.

(Dr. Cushing)

PATHOLOGY REPORT
January 24, 1916

A frozen section shows spindle nuclei in relation with fine fibers and running irregularly. Probably fibrous. A peculiarity in the presence of large masses of hyaline in connection with vessels. The masses containing numerous nuclei.

There are numerous hyalinised blood vessels and masses of cicatricial tissue. The general mass of tumor is fibrous, syncytial in character with enormous masses of fibrils between the cells

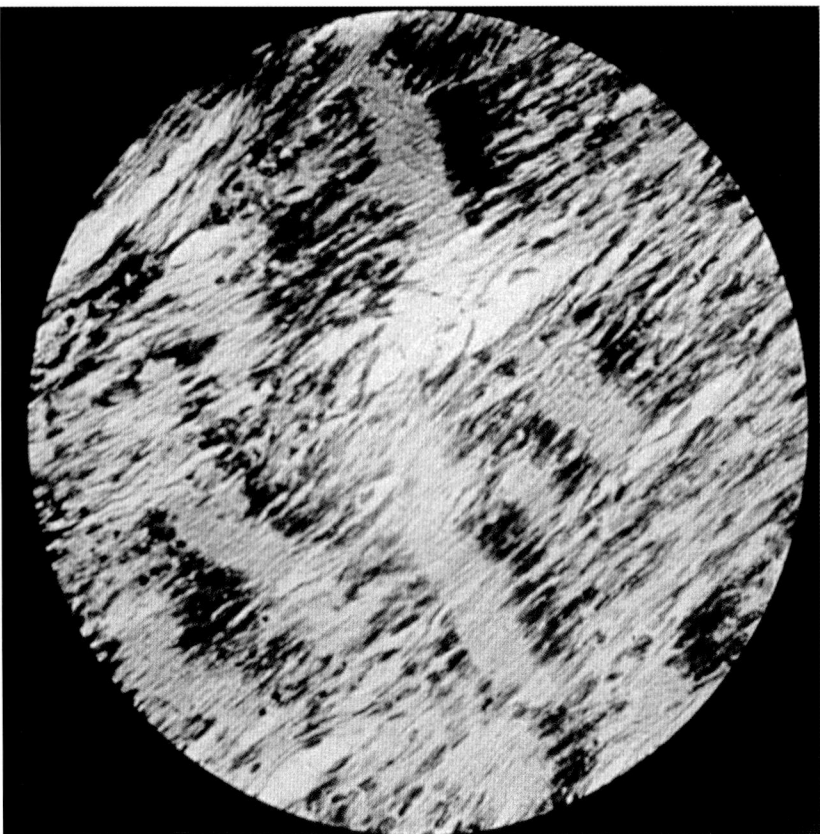

FIG. 4. HISTOLOGY SLIDE.

which also contains a considerable amount of hyaline fibroid. Among the tumor cells there are a number of large multinuclear cells probably resulting in direct division.

Diagnosis – Glioma.

(Dr. Councilman)

Patient had an uncomplicated postoperative course.

DISCHARGE NOTE
March 3, 1916
Dr. Grey

The patient shows a very marked improvement since operation. He has put on about 25 lbs. in weight and is able to be up and about the ward in comparative comfort. There have been no appreciable headaches since operation and no nausea or vomiting for some time. Speech has improved and there is very slight dysphagia. The wound has healed perfectly. It is soft and shows no abnormal fullness. The left side of the body is still a trifle weak and there is practically the same subjective disturbance in sensation at present as noted by the patient before operation. Ataxia is definitely less – very slight on left. Nystagmus is absent on looking forward, but continues fairly marked on looking to either side and upward. Jerks show no difference in character on either side. There is no definite impairment of conjugate deviation to either side. Facial spasm is not present now and there is only a trace of weakness on this side. The discs have greatly receded, measuring at the present time about 1 D on either side. Hearing has definitely improved on the left side.

FOLLOW UP NOTE
August 19, 1916
Dr. Gray

Patient returns for observation in response to a letter recently mailed to him. He walked into the clinic, appearing like any average normal adult. His gait subjectively is a very trifle unsteady, more marked especially after fatigue. Objectively, however, it is good. In the Romberg position there is no swaying with the eyes open but still considerable instability with the eyes closed. There is practically no ataxia on the right side but with the left arm, though no definite ataxic movement, there is noticeable a moderate amount of dysmetria. He only has occasional mild headaches – bifrontal. No nausea or vomiting. The wound is firm throughout and there is no fullness of either side. Nothing characteristics in the attitudes of the head. The eyelids are still a trifle puffy. Vision (corrected perhaps with glasses) is quite good. He reads the ordinary print. There is practically no nystagmus on looking forward and to the left – a few slow jerks; – looking to the right there are fairly marked, rather rapid oscillations. He still has occasional spasms of the left face, but these only occur at infrequent intervals, though he states that the last one was more severe than any for the past 7–8 weeks. The face is symmetrical now and moves well on either side. No tinnitus. He can distinctly hear a soft watch tick with the left ear, the right ear being firmly plugged. In view of this latter finding a caloric test seemed superfluous. Careful X-ray examination of the porus acousticus on either side was made by Dr. Carr, and rapid examination discloses no material difference in the size of the shadows on either side.

The late onset of the acoustic nerve phenomena coupled with the lack of any enlargement of the left porus acousticus seems to argue against the lesion being a true acoustic nerve tumor.

SECOND HOSPITAL ADMISSION
(Summary from Dr. Locke's Note)

The patient was readmitted in the hospital on July 12, 1919. He complained of facial twitching, staggering gait and slight dizziness.

Dr. Cushing found no suboccipital fullness. It was decided not to operate unless "general pressure symptoms appeared."

THIRD HOSPITAL ADMISSION
August 31, 1920

The patient complained of frontal and suboccipital headaches, vomiting, unsteady gait, and difficulty in speech. Dr. Cushing advised X-ray treatment. One X-ray treatment was given. By the time of his discharge, the patient reported improvement of equilibrium and clearing of nausea and vomiting.

FOURTH HOSPITAL ADMISSION
November 5, 1920

This admission was merely for radiotherapy. There was considerable improvement in symptoms since last entry. He had received 3 X-ray treatments. He was walking fairly well. He had slight headaches and nausea. He was still unable to work.

FOLLOW UP NOTE
November 15, 1922

X-ray treatments during past year have numbered about 15. All signs seem better than at last note.

FIFTH HOSPITAL ADMISSION
(Summary from Dr. Rioch's Note)
April 26, 1923

SUBJECTIVE: Readmitted for weakness "all down left side." Also complains of slight dysphagia, unsteadiness of gait, vomiting with nausea and epigastric discomforts. Uncinate attacks.

OBJECTIVE: Nystagmus, lateral (marked) and vertical (slight); contraction of left side of face; hypotonia of left arm and leg; hypermetria of left arm and leg; dysdiadochocinesia, left; Romberg positive; "cerebellar gait"; abnormal plantar response and slightly increased deep reflexes on left.

IMPRESSION. Recurrence of cerebellopontine tumor.

SPECIAL NOTE
May 9, 1923

Dr. Cushing confirms the alteration in diagnosis and states that there is no doubt that this was an Acoustic Neuroma.

DISCHARGE NOTE
May 16, 1923

During stay in hospital his main complaint has been gastric discomfort and constipation, flatulence. He never vomits or does not suffer acute pain. G.I. series negative. Cerebellar symptomatology remains the same as on admission.

SIXTH HOSPITAL ADMISSION
October 3, 1924
Dr. Cox

Patient complains of headaches and dizziness; gastric discomfort with nausea and vomiting especially in morning; weakness, especially left arm and leg; dysphagia and dysarthria; inability to walk without support; failing vision and occasional black spots before eyes; failure of memory; history of urinary retention 4 weeks ago; catheterization.

This patient 8 years ago had operation for left cerebello-pontine tumor with relief of symptoms. In the interval since this time there has been a gradual return of symptoms, progressive in form.

IMPRESSION: Tumor of left cerebello-pontine angle, no signs of pressure. Probable X-ray damage.

DISCHARGE NOTE
October 8, 1924

Dr. Cushing believes that too intensive X-ray treatment may account for present condition. Recommended that no further treatment be given for some time at least.

SEVENTH HOSPITAL ADMISSION
January 11, 1926
Dr. Rioca

Patient exam shows partial left facial paralysis, suboccipital tenderness (left) an old scar (suboccipital); partial closure of left eye; nystagmus to right and left; – also vertical nystagmus on looking up; slight inequality on pupils (left smaller); hyperesthesia of left side of face; tongue protruded to right; "husky" voice; a few moist rales with slightly prolonged expiration; marked emaciation; wasting of extremities on left more pronounced than on right; exaggerated and equal reflexes in upper and lower extremities; ankle clonus on left; deafness in left ear.

IMPRESSION: Acoustic neuroma. Pyorrhoea alveolaris. Left inguinal hernia.

DISCHARGE NOTE
January 27, 1926

Patient in a deplorable state requiring daily catheterization, feeding by nasal tube. Seen by Dr. Cushing who feels, that further operation not justified. Discharged.

LETTER TO DR. CUSHING
December 15, 1927

Dear Sir:

JC (name of patient) died June 7, 1926 at 7:30 p.m. and was conscious up to about 4:30 in the afternoon. Hoping this is all the information desired. I am,

Sincerely yours,
(Signed) VC

Attached you can find Dr. Cushing's teaching slide related to this patient.

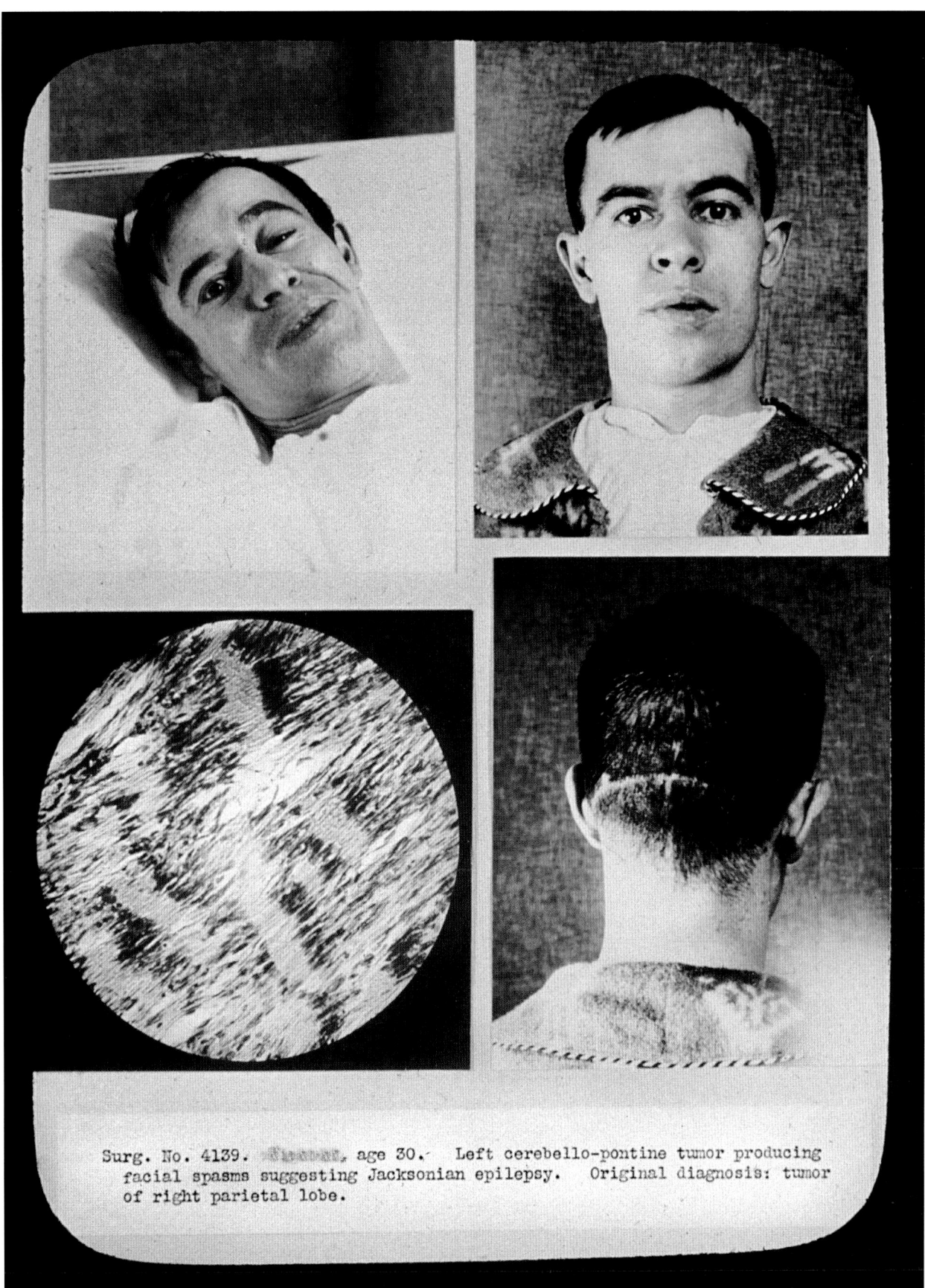

FIG. 5. TEACHING SLIDE.

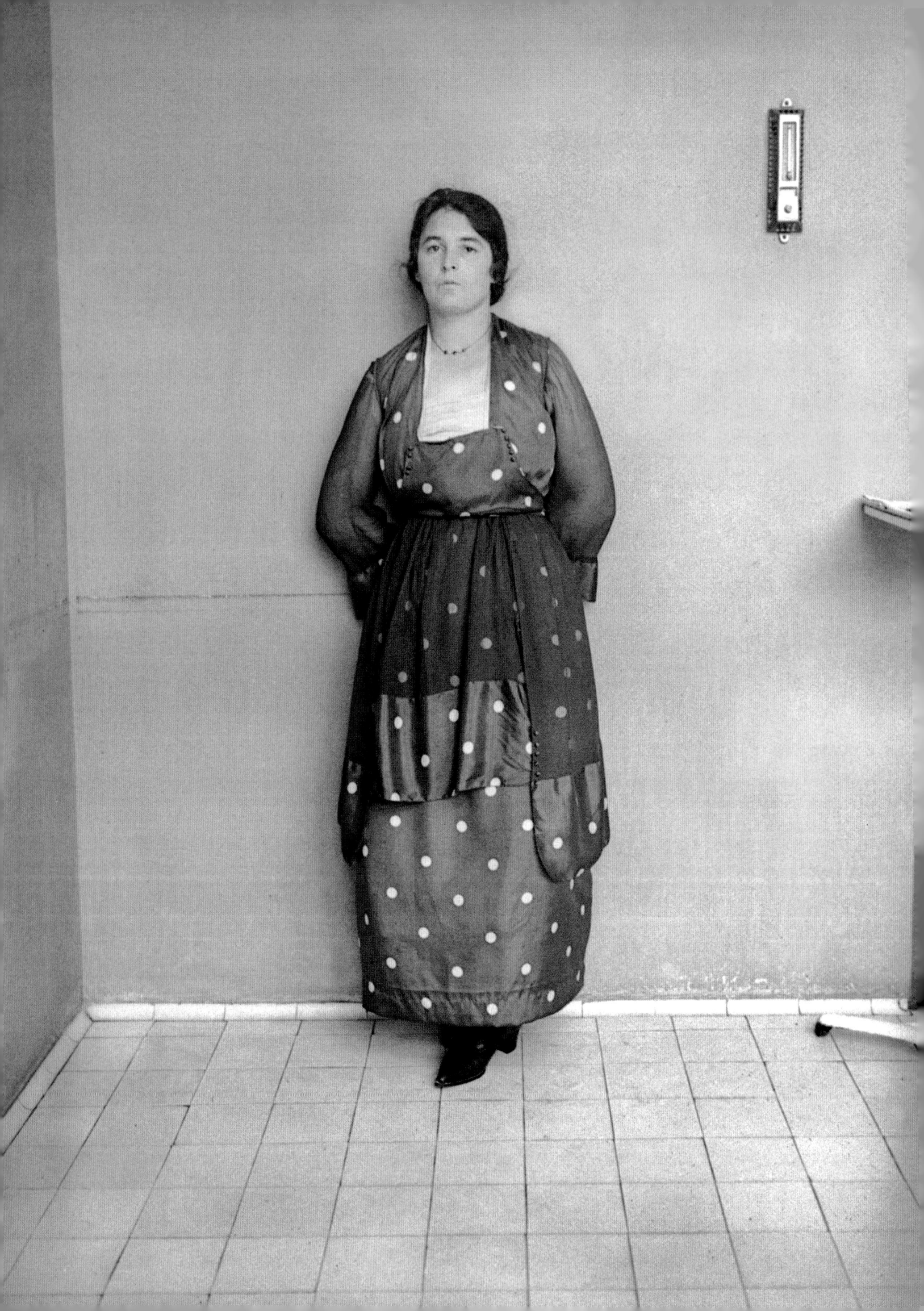

6.5 Epidermoid of the fourth ventricle

SEX: F; AGE: 28; SURG. NO. 10302

HISTORY

This 28-year-old right-handed female developed a severe headache with vomiting five and a half years ago during her first pregnancy. The headaches and vomiting persisted and were primarily during the mornings. Nine months before admission she noticed "a singing noise" in her left ear and her vision began to fail. The noise grew louder until she began to stagger and "her friends commented that she walked as though drunk."

In November 1918, her evaluation at the Bay State Hospital included a lumbar puncture. She had an immediate relief of her headaches and her physician gave her an injection of Novarsenobensol. Three weeks prior to her admission to the Peter Bent Brigham Hospital, her vision worsened and she began to fall to the left and backwards. She developed left hand weakness and her personality began to change; she stopped working, sewing, and playing with her son. She changed from "happy go lucky to irritable and emotionally unstable."

SUMMARY OF POSITIVE FINDINGS
April 14, 1919
Dr. Bailey

SUBJECTIVE
1. Tinnitus.
2. Slight nausea.
3. Headaches, mainly temporal, sometimes occipital.
4. Failing vision.
5. Twitching in the eyes.

OBJECTIVE
1. There is nystagmus on looking to the left and right, more marked on looking to the left, with quick component to left.
2. Hearing less acute in left ear.
3. Defective memory.
4. Emotional instability.
5. Ataxia in left upper and lower extremities.
6. Positive Romberg and tendency to go always to the left in walking.
7. Epigastric and abdominal reflexes not elicited.

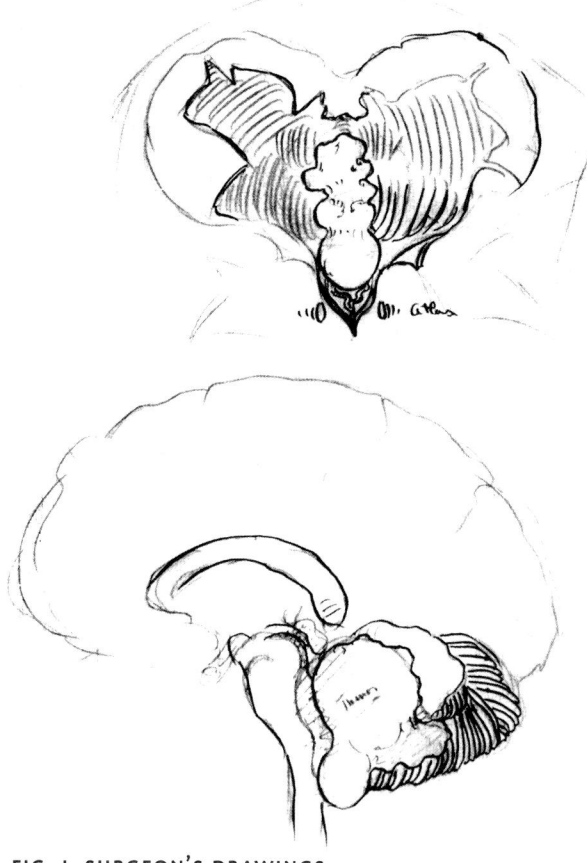

FIG. 1. SURGEON'S DRAWINGS.

Dr. Cushing believed that the skull x-rays did not reveal any abnormalities.

OPERATIVE NOTE
April 21, 1919
Anaesthesia – Ether – Miss Hunt

Extirpation of Cholesteatoma from Roof of Fourth Ventricle – Removal of Atlas Piece-Meal – Enucleation of Tumor the Size of Golf Ball, Extending Well into Region of the Aqueduct of Sylvius, and Laying Over the Entire Roof of the Fourth Ventricle.

With the patient on the cerebellar table the usual cross-bow incision with lateral flaps was made. An extensive bone defect including the margin of the foramen magnum was made without difficulty. The dura was not excessively tense. On opening the dura near the foramen a very, very large posterior cistern was disclosed and through the fluid in this cistern a glistening white, smooth

OPPOSITE PAGE: FIG. 2. POSTOPERATIVE.

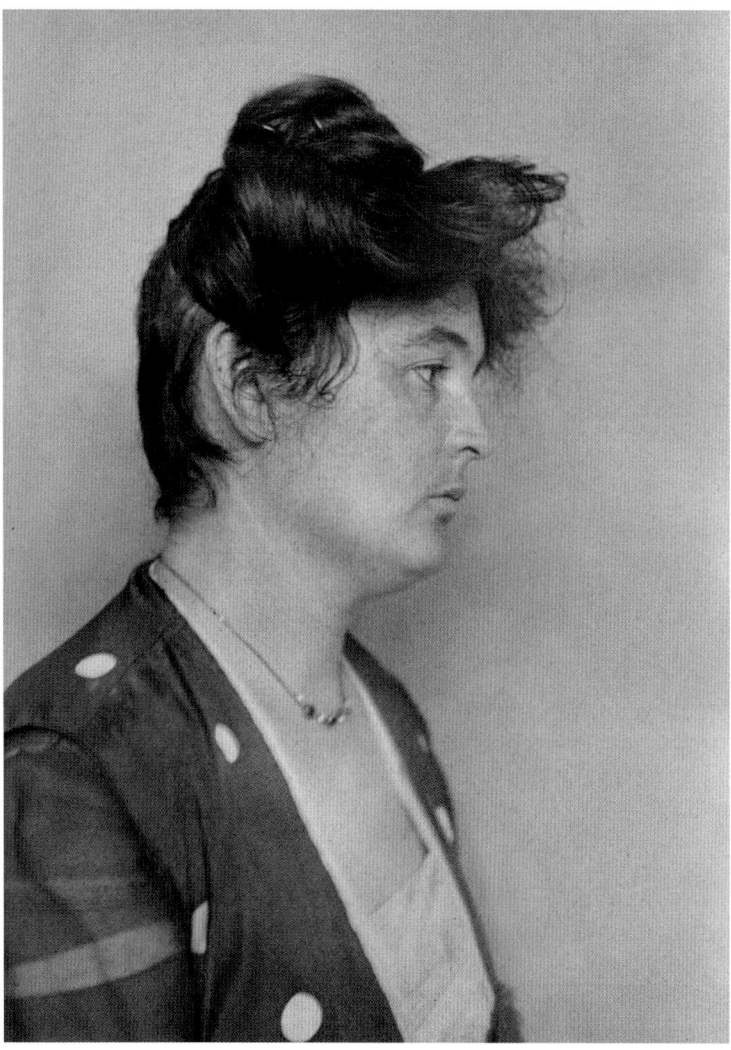

FIG. 3. POSTOPERATIVE.

nodule could be seen looking as though a pledget of white cotton underlay the somewhat thickened arachnoid membrane. The wall of the cistern was opened and a most extraordinary appearance came into view, a typical pearly, nodular, glistening, smooth growth. It was found that this growth extended down into the spinal canal so that it was necessary to remove the posterior half of the atlas and to incise the dura down to the axis. This brought into view a large nodule passing down into the spinal canal lying directly upon the fourth ventricle. **The appearance of the growth was exactly that of mother-of-pearl, with a brilliant glistening surface.** The tumor, however, was of about the consistency of a somewhat hard marshmallow, so that it crushed easily, but nevertheless it was possible to free it from the overlying and but slightly adherent brain. This dissection was carried down for a long period until finally it became evident that the growth was extremely deep. A larger part of the lesion was removed, the scaly contents of the growth being spooned out of the cavity with a blunt spoon.

It was finally possible to remove the glistening capsule of the growth from the depths, leaving a perfectly clean, smooth-walled cavity of the fourth ventricle, a most extraordinary appearance, with a dilated fourth ventricle at the bottom of the deep hole and the distended Iter through which fluid was pulsating as shown above. One could look almost into the third ventricle. There was extraordinarily little upset to the patient during this long delayed procedure and no bleeding whatsoever. The great cavity was filled with salt solution and the wound closed in layers without drainage.

The operation lasted fully four hours and the anaesthetic was very smoothly taken without the slightest upset.

(Dr. Cushing)

PATHOLOGY REPORT
April 21, 1919

Gross description – Tumor as it lay in the tissue presented a characteristic Mother of Pearl appearance. The outside capsule is a very tough membrane. The tumor was so extensive as to be unable to be removed entirely. The interior of the tumor consists of a putty-like, white material which was dug cut with a pituitary spoon. The tumor extended from below the medulla oblongata to the aqueduct of Sylvius, and it caused considerable atrophy of both hemispheres.

The specimen removed consists of a number of fragments of capsule, highly lustrous, pearly

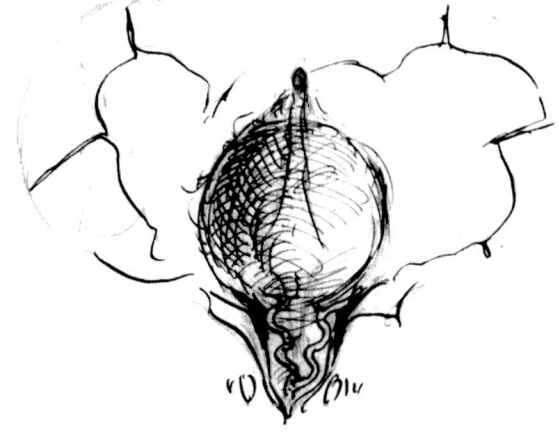

FIG. 4. SURGEON'S DRAWING.

membrane and many masses of white, cheeky material which was dug out with a spoon. Tumor is avascular.

(Dr. Cushing)

Microscopic reports – Three sections consist of lamellated keratinized epithelial remains. No epithelial cells can be seen but the outlines of cells are present in places, also a small amount of fresh blood.

Diagnosis – Cholesteatoma.

(Dr. Wolbach)

POSTOPERATIVE NOTE
April 22, 1919
Dr. Bailey

Good recovery from anesthetic. In excellent general condition, but has a paresis of right external rectus muscle.

SPECIAL NOTE
May 3, 1919
Dr. Cushing

Patient has made a perfect recovery. Photograph taken today.

DISCHARGE NOTE
May 24, 1919
Dr. Stone

Thirty-four days ago the patient had a cholesteatoma removed from the roof of the 4th ventricle. The patient made a good ether recovery but developed a paresis of the right external rectus muscle which has persisted. She now has no subjective disturbance but has nystagmus, and coarse static and intentional tremor. Slight ataxia of both upper extremities, mild emotional disturbance, positive Romberg and distinctly cerebellar walk. Discharged today.

FOLLOW UP NOTE
August 6, 1919

The patient was seen in clinic with only slight dis-diadokinesis and slight nystagmus bilaterally.

The patient was seen on two other occasions postoperatively, once following a trolley accident in 1922 and her final visit with Dr. Cushing in 1925 when he thought she had a cold. She was apparently very concerned about her head on both occasions but continued to demonstrate the exam noted in August of 1919.

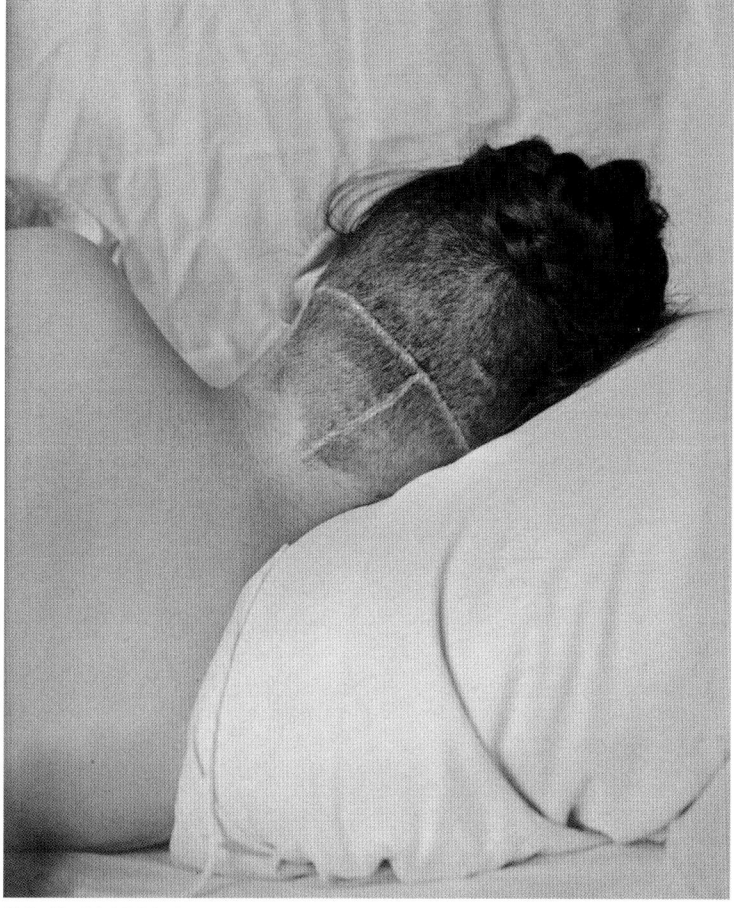

FIG. 5. POSTOPERATIVE.

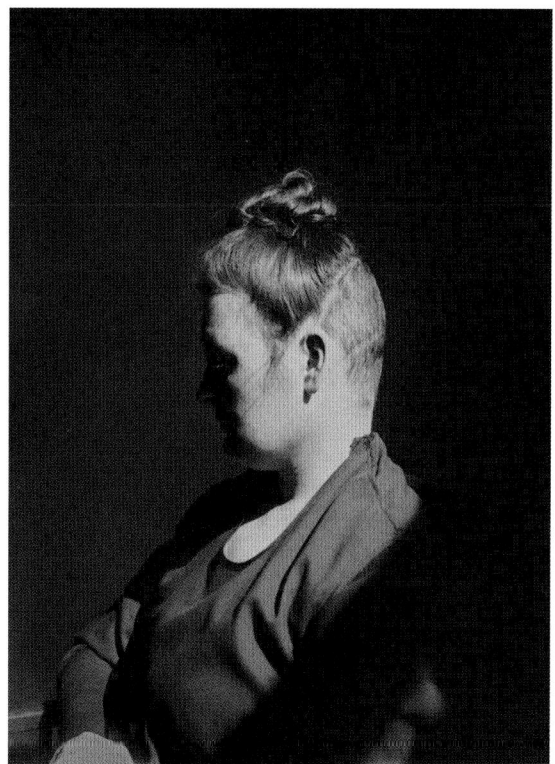

FIG. 6. POSTOPERATIVE.

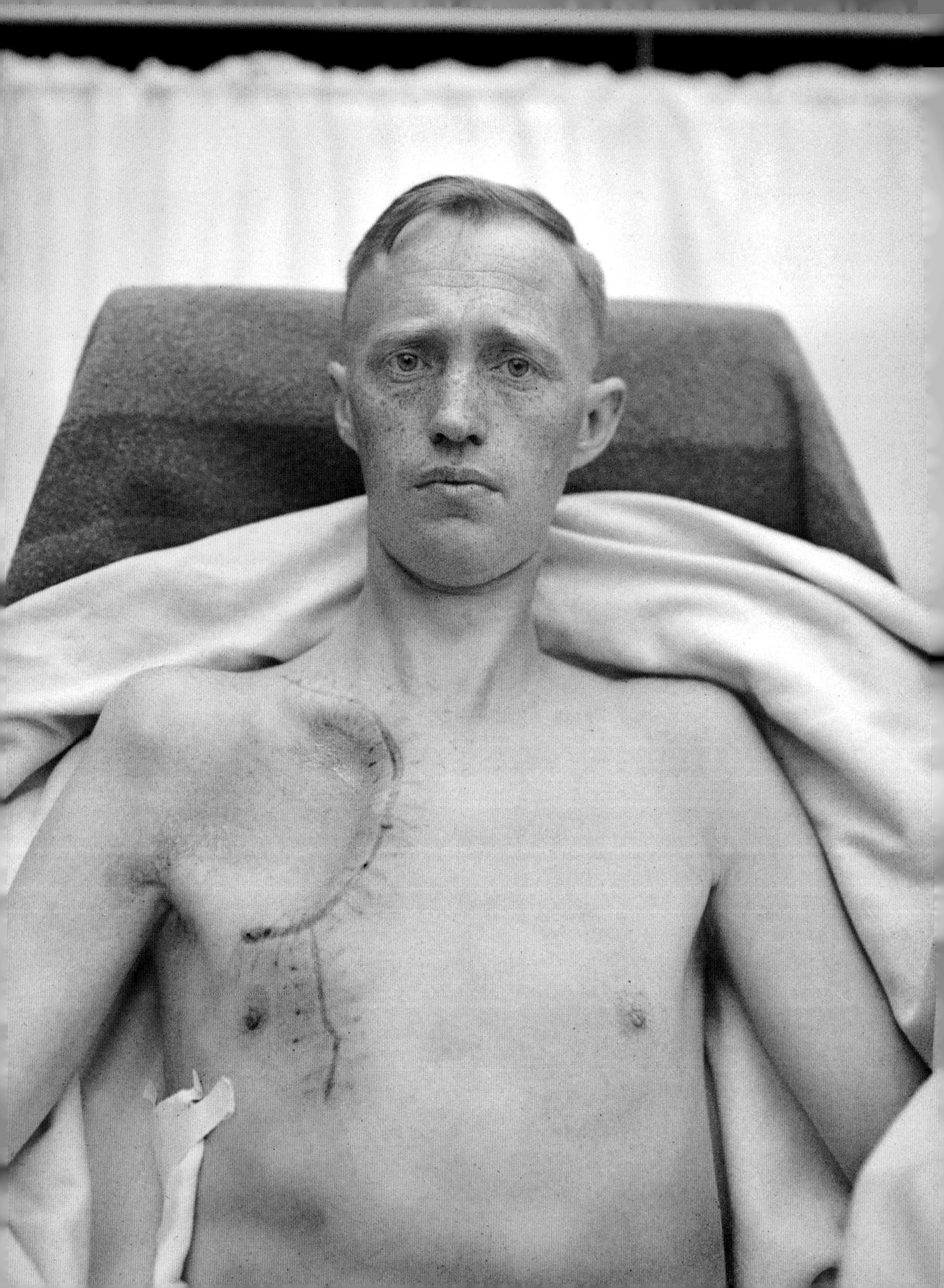

6.6 Brachial plexus tumor

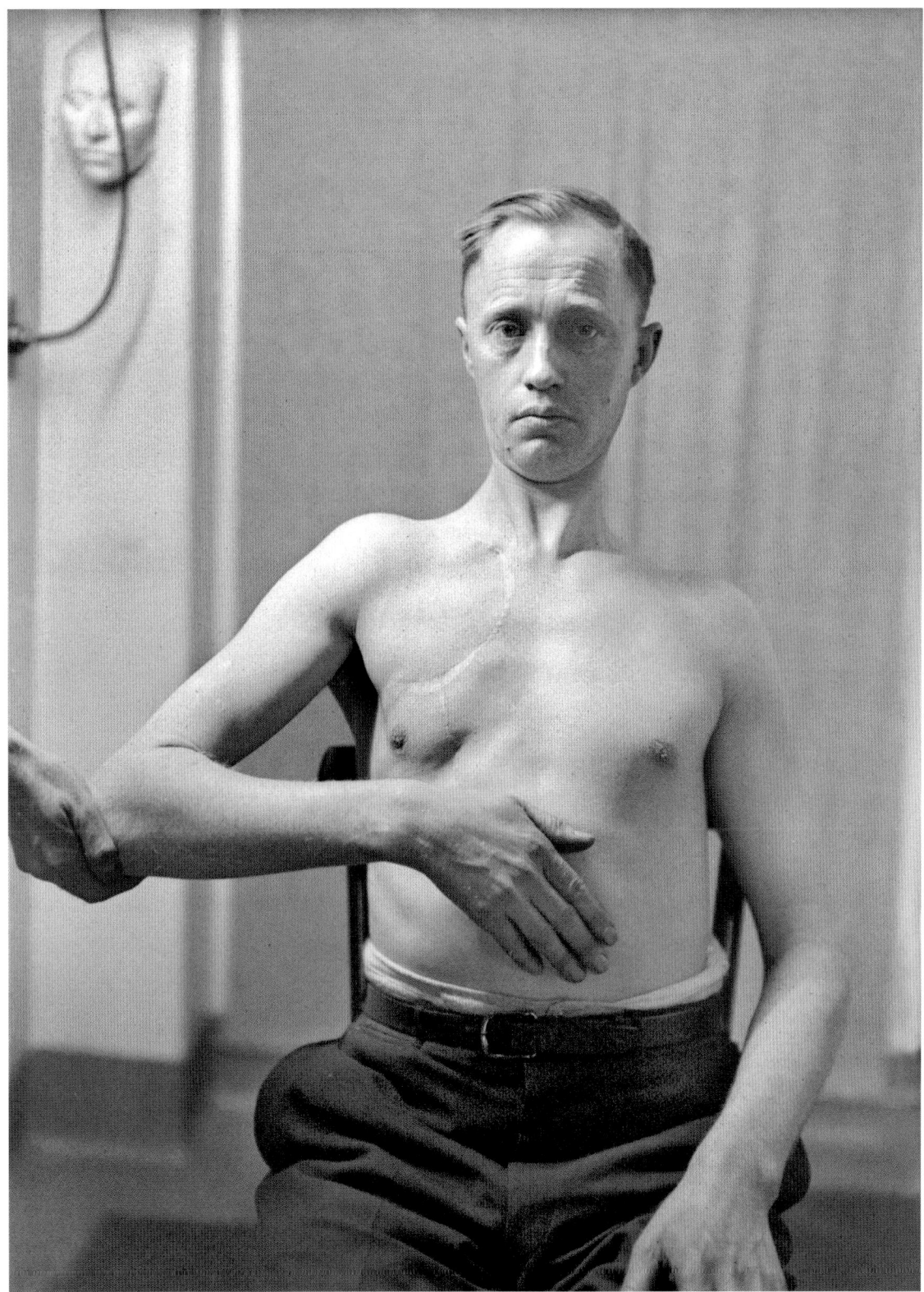

FIG. 2. THREE MONTHS POSTOPERATIVE — DELTOID WEAKNESS.

OPPOSITE PAGE: FIG.I. THREE WEEKS POSTOPERATIVE.

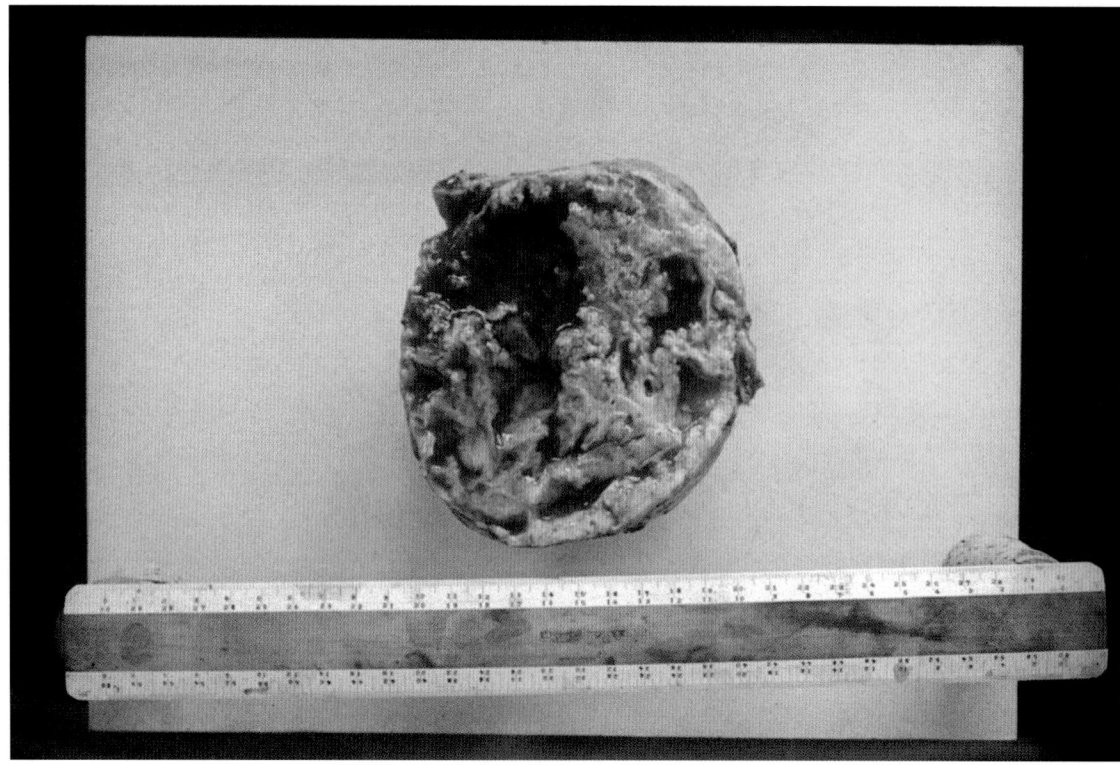

ABOVE: FIG. 3. RESECTED TUMOR.
BELOW: FIG. 4. THREE MONTHS POST-OPERATIVE.

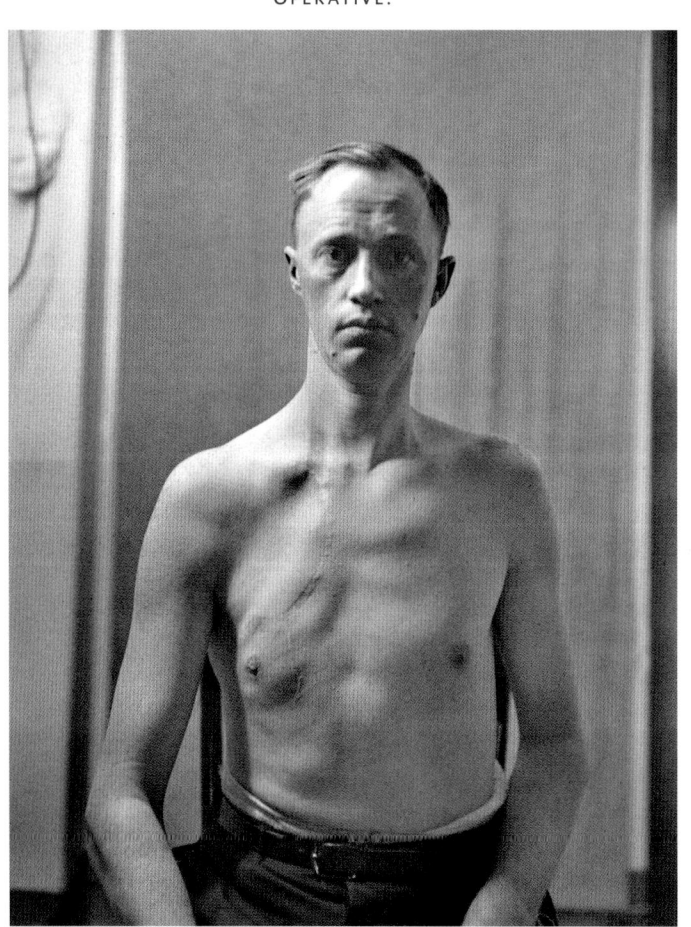

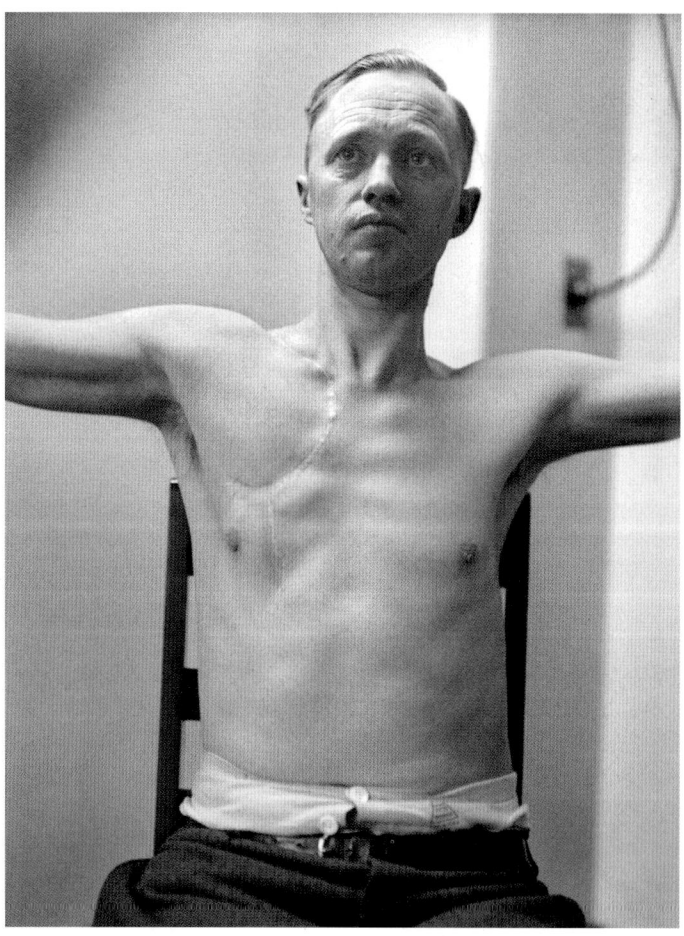

FIG. 5. SIXTEEN MONTHS POSTOPERATIVE — RESOLUTION OF DELTOID WEAKNESS.

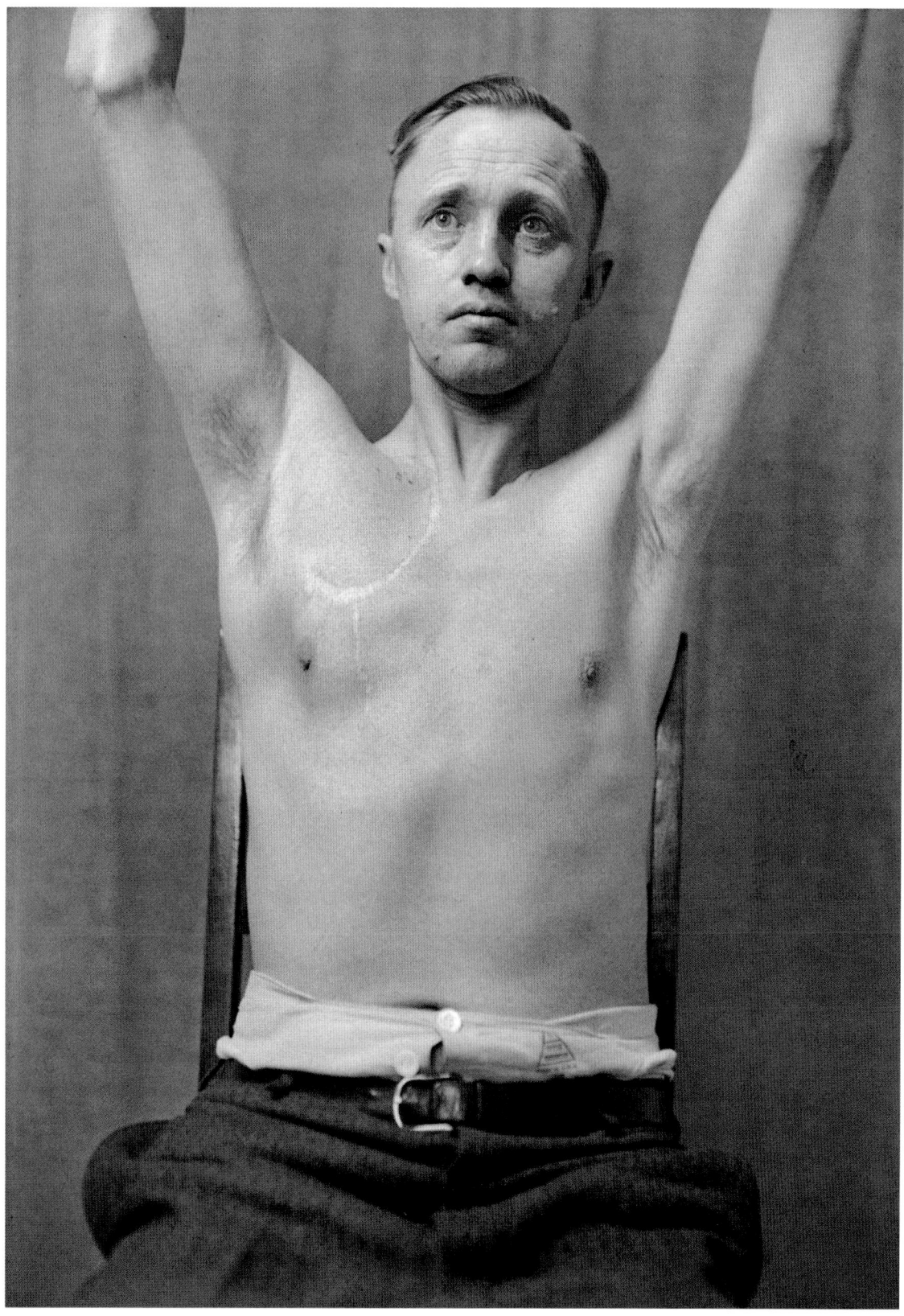

FIG. 6. SIXTEEN MONTHS POSTOPERATIVE.

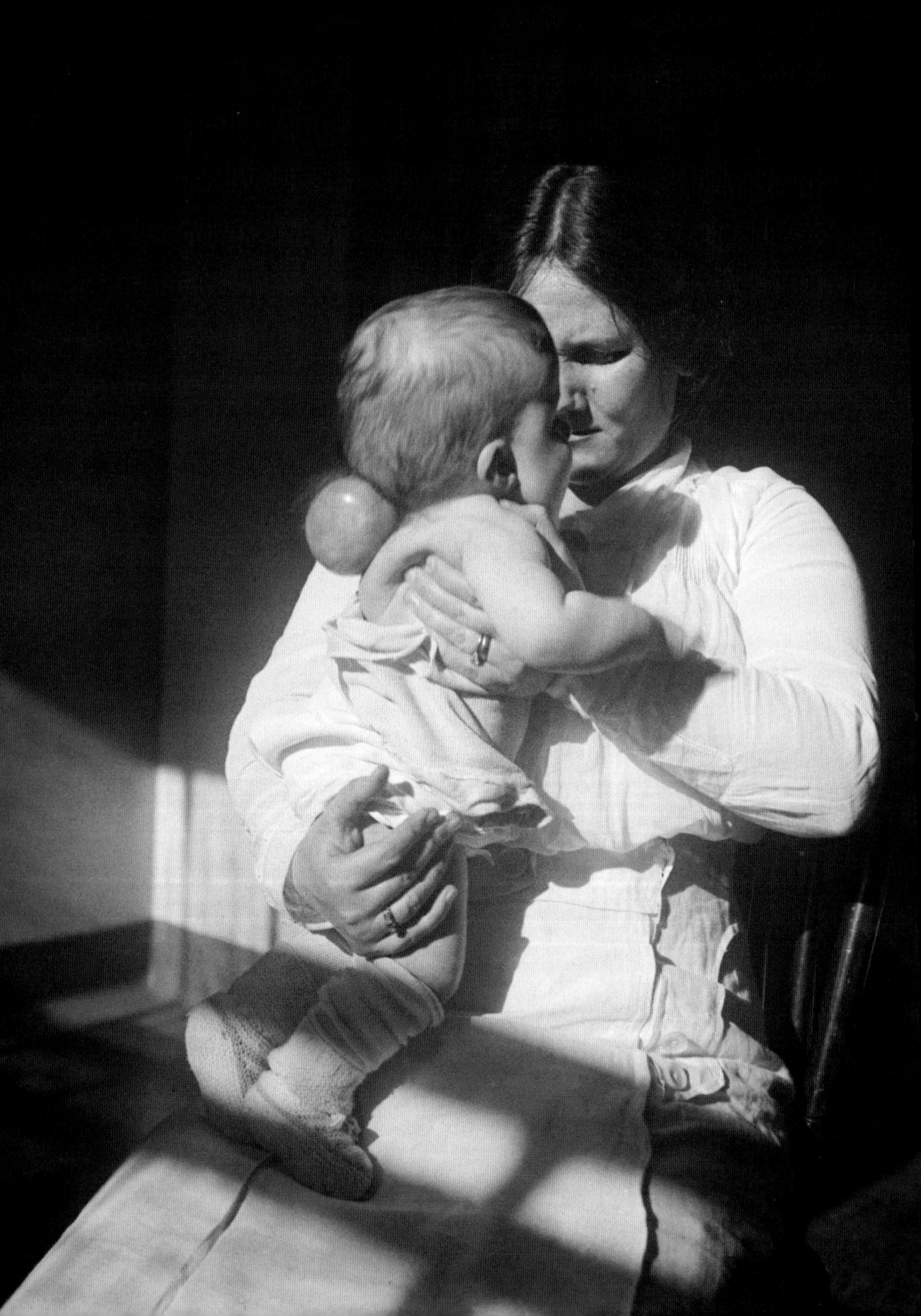

6.7 Cervical meningocele (three different patients)

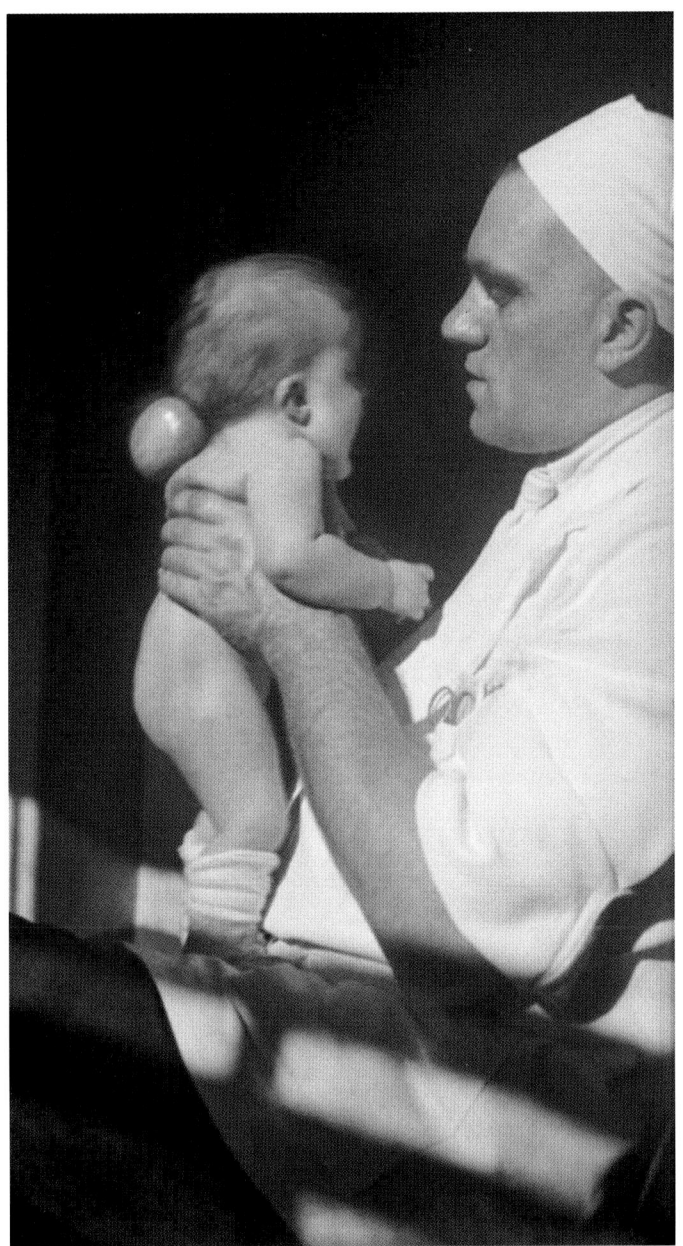

FIG. 2. PATIENT I. ADOLPH WATZKA, CUSHING'S ORDERLY, HOLDING THE CHILD.

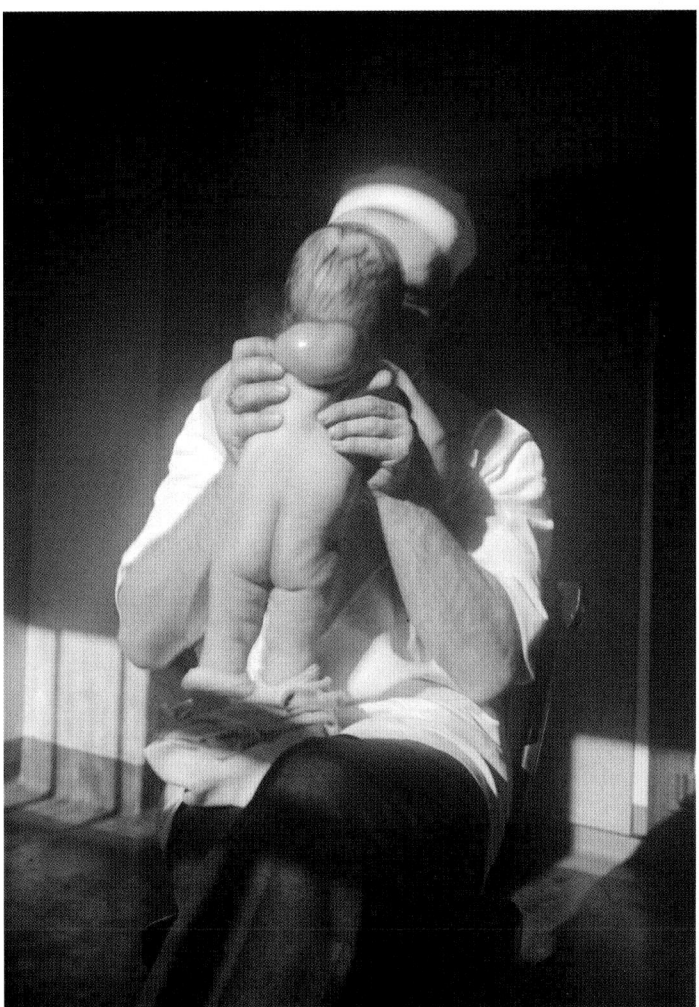

FIG. 3. PATIENT I. ADOLPH WATZKA, CUSHING'S ORDERLY, HOLDING THE CHILD.

OPPOSITE PAGE: FIG.I. PATIENT I. MOTHER HOLDING THE CHILD.

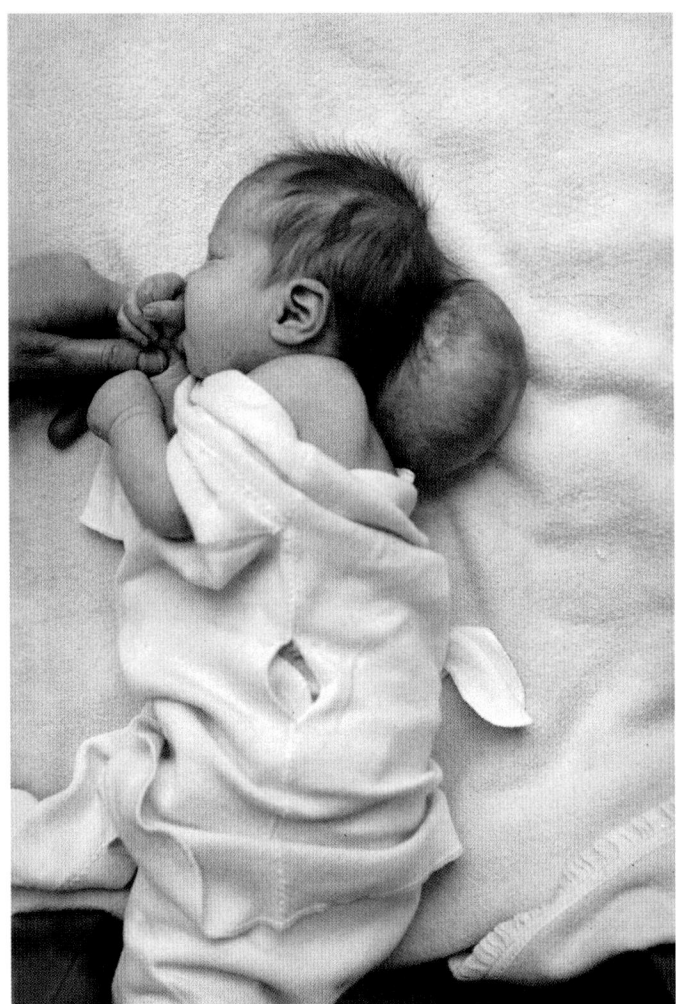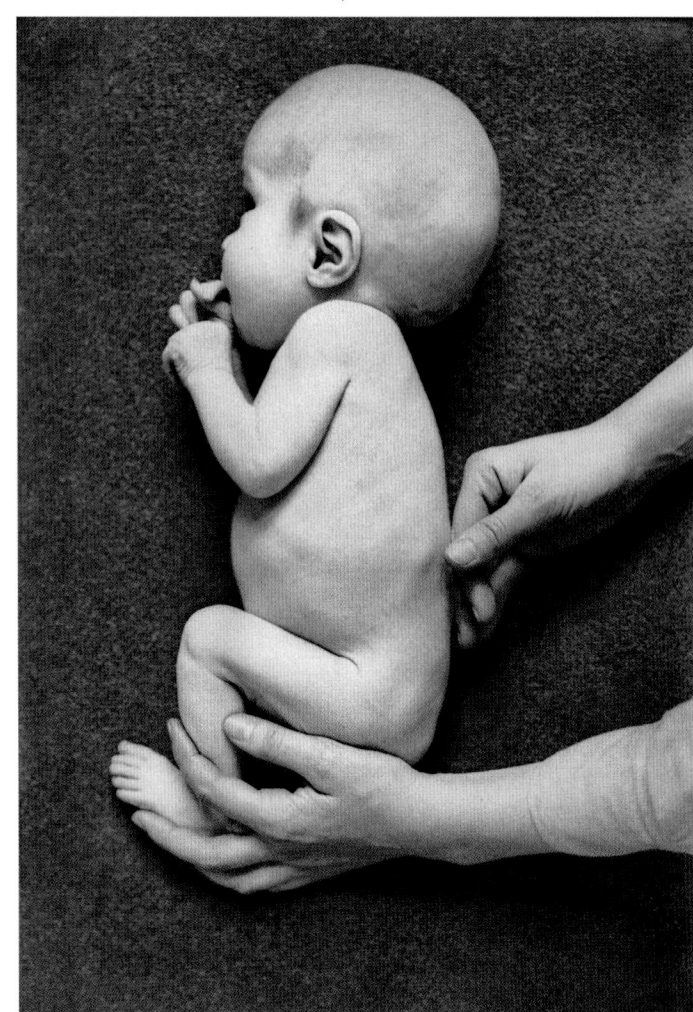

FIGS. 4 AND 5. PATIENT II. PREOPERATIVE (LEFT) AND POSTOPERATIVE.

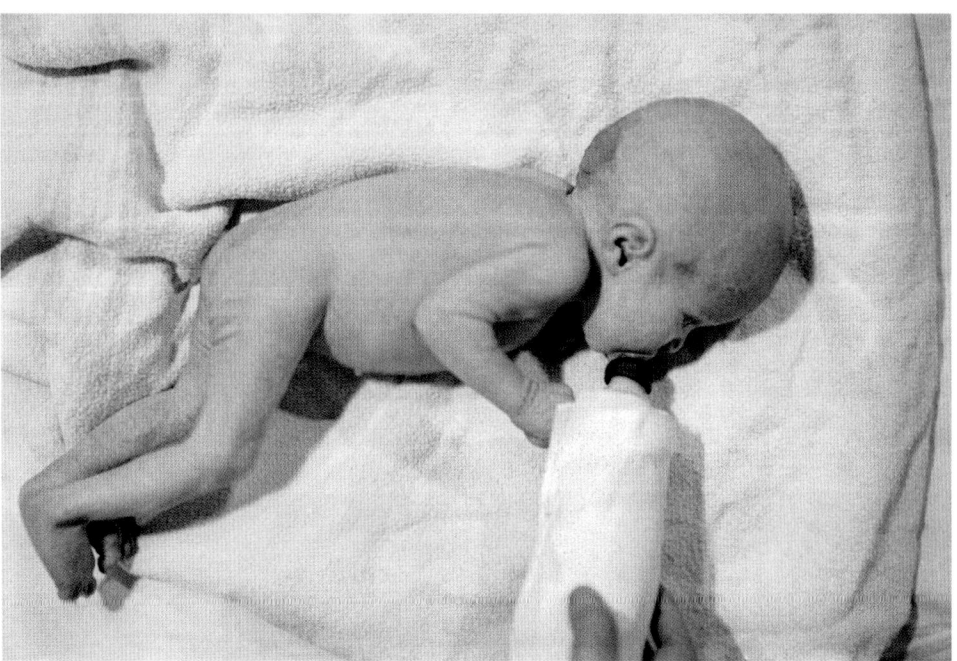

FIG. 6. PATIENT II. POSTOPERATIVE.

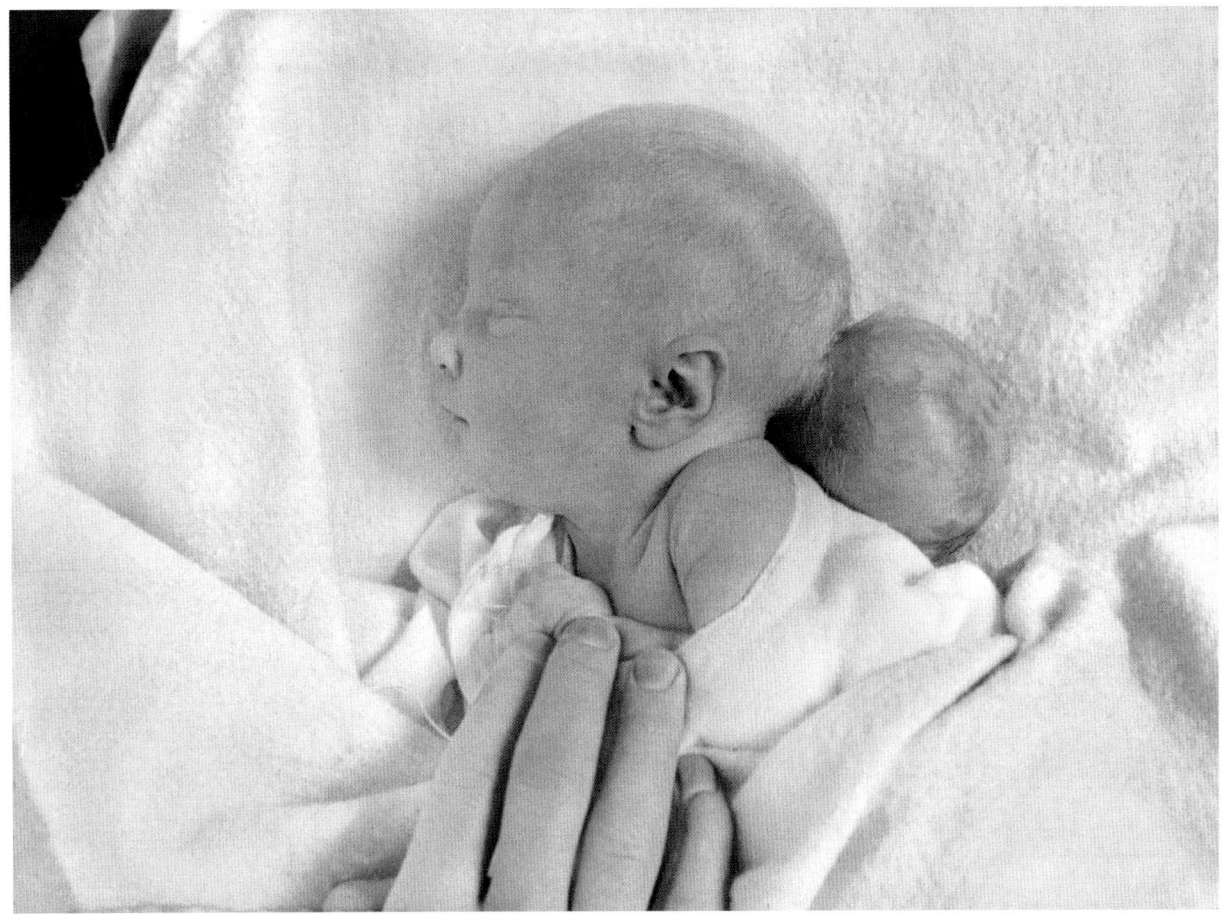

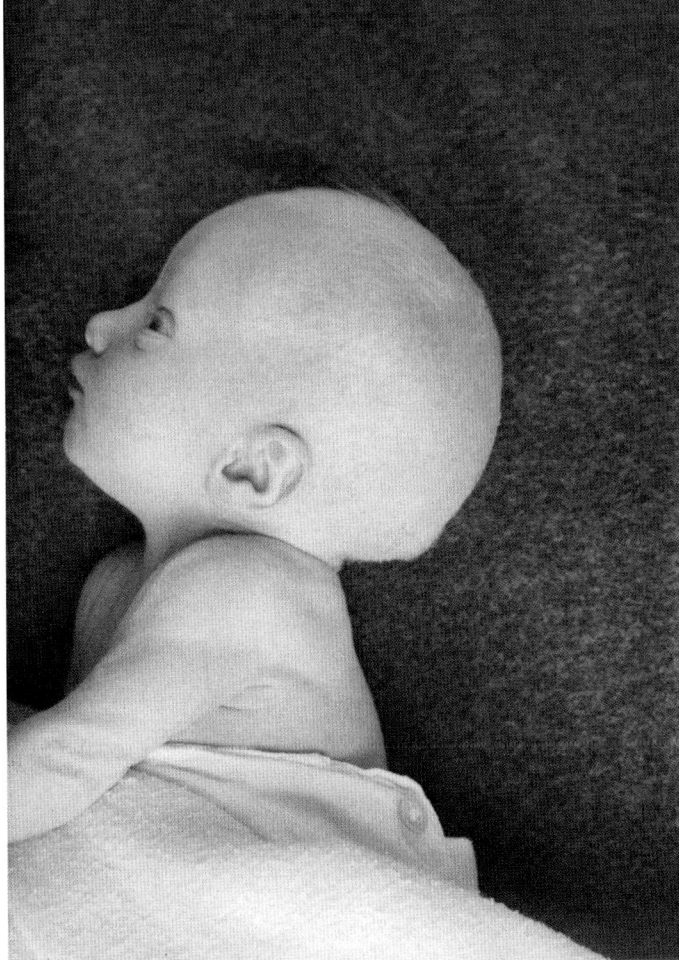

FIGS. 7 AND 8. PATIENT III. PREOPERATIVE (ABOVE) AND POSTOPERATIVE (LEFT).

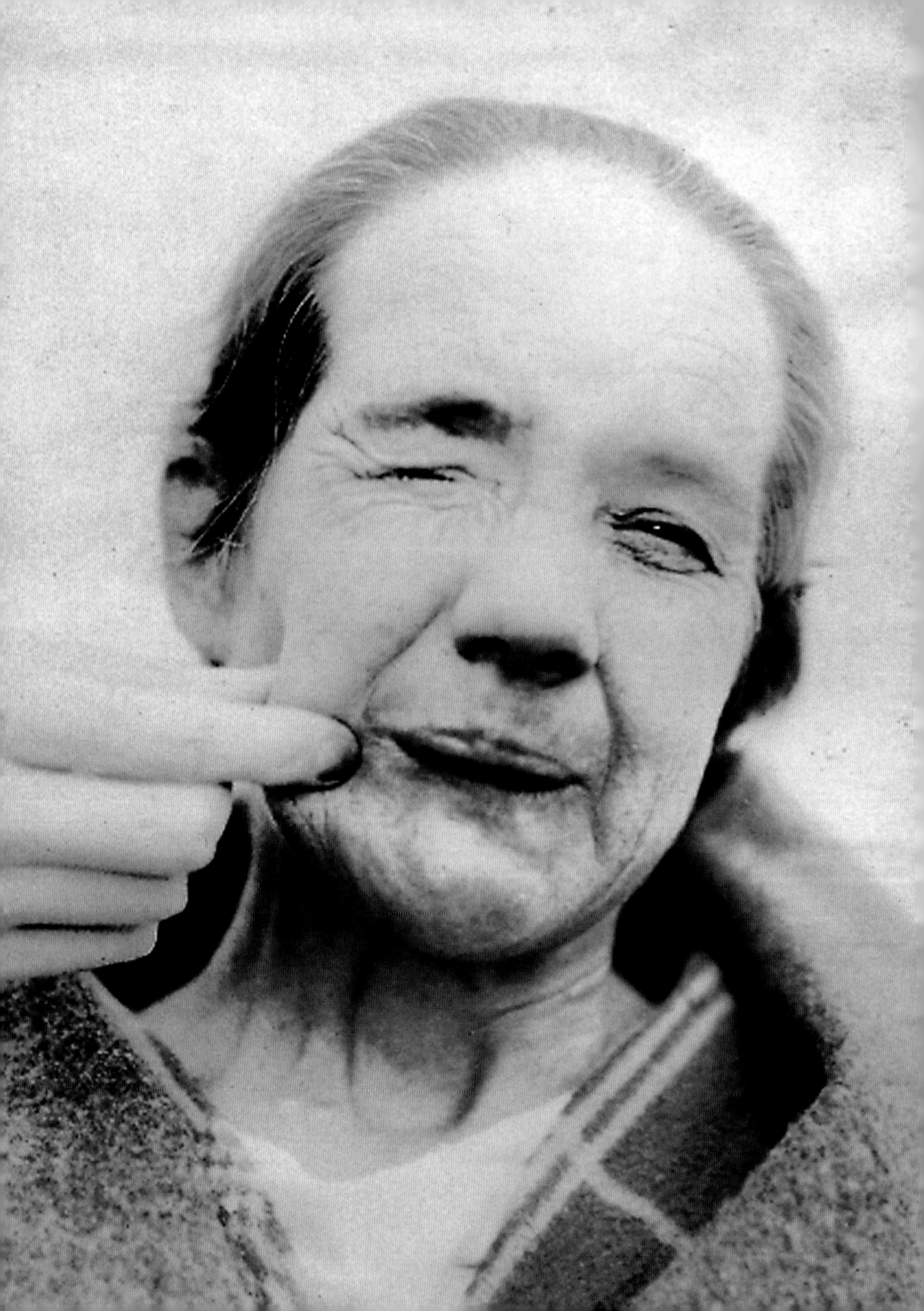

6.8 Hemifacial spasm (trigeminal neuralgia)

SEX: F; AGE: 54; SURG. NO. 13482

HISTORY

This patient suffered from a four-year history of right "trigeminal neuralgia" involving the 2nd and 3rd divisions. She underwent nine operations on her nose and throat for relief of her symptoms and a number of her teeth were removed without relief. She also underwent right Gasserian ganglion sensory root avulsion by Dr. Jacobson, made a good recovery following the operation but still complained of pain. She came to Peter Bent Brigham Hospital for observation under Dr. Cushing's service.

SUMMARY OF POSITIVE FINDINGS
November 16, 1920
Dr. Locke

SUBJECTIVE

1. Rather remarkable history of numerous types and all kinds of operations.
2. In 1918 Dr. Jacobson performed an avulsion of sensory root of the right trigeminal nerve for painful neuralgia associated with much twitching.
3. Operation failed to relive condition and patient has had continuation with twitching of her facial musculature associated with pain.

OBJECTIVE

1. Almost constant voluntary ptosis of OD associated with little twitching of orbicularis orbitus.
2. Twitching of right corner of mouth, both of these being associated with pain as demonstrated by patient's actions.
3. Complete anaesthesia over all 3 divisions of the right trigeminal nerve.
4. Loss of taste on anterior 2/3rd of tongue on the right.
5. Slight inequality of pupils.
6. Dysarthria probably due to false teeth and facial spasm.
7. Asymmetry of face with much more wrinkling on the right side probably due to over action of that side with the twitching.

November 17, 1920
Dr. Locke

Since patient's entry into the hospital she has continued to have the pain which she described in the right side of her face, associated with drawing movements of her whole facial musculature. She also often speaks of an "engine" in her head which seems to "wind up."

OPERATIVE NOTE
November 18, 1920
Dr. Cushing
Anesthesia – None

Attempted Puncture of the Facial Nerve.

A needle was inserted at the tip of the mastoid and carried inward and upward in the direction of the styloid process and facial canal. Curiously enough this puncture gave the patient just the same kind of discomfort in the nose and forehead which she complains of during her bad paroxysms, an observation strongly suggestive of the fact that she may actually be having neuralgia of the facial nerve. About 1 cc of alcohol was injected without, however, securing a paralysis. This measure will probably have to be repeated.

(Dr. Cushing)

POSTOPERATIVE NOTES
November 19, 1920
Dr. Locke

Yesterday Dr. Cushing had an unsuccessful attempt at injecting the facial nerve. Patient complained of a good deal of pain during the injection which was similar to the pain she complains of ordinarily. Today she has no evidence of any facial paralysis but the injected area is merely tender.

November 21, 1920
Dr. Locke

Patient continues about the same with the same complaint of her "engine." Dr. Cushing has seen her recently and it has been noted that the sensation of her face is quite anaesthetic to superficial stimulation such as pin prick or pinching the skin with a fine pair of forceps. However grasping the deeper tissues of the face between the thumb and forefinger, causing pressure gives patient a good deal of pain (Please note the preoperative image.) She complains of this not only in her face but all over that side of her body, over arms and trunk, and the opposite side of her body gives her no pain on this pressure between the thumb and forefinger.

There is definitely a neurotic element in the patient's condition and she is not altogether balanced mentally.

November 25, 1920
Dr. Locke

Condition remains about the same. Patient is doing a good deal of work about the ward such as carrying trays and says she feels better when she has something to do.

December 5, 1920
Dr. Locke

No particular change in patient's condition. She continues to have painful spasmodic tic with marked drawing up of the face. It seems to be worse at night and she says when things are quiet her pain is worse. When she can be doing things it is less severe.

SPECIAL NOTE
December 9, 1920
Dr. Cushing

Patient describes her pain as starting in the temporal region, passing down into the region of the 2nd division of the face and ending up with sharp stabs in the side of nose. It does not go across the median line. The pain which she says she had before the operation was largely over the temporal region up into the frontal but never crossing the midline. There has also been pain down into the lower jaw and lip, and in describing it she gives exactly the same description and designation of the usual trigeminal victim. She insists upon the fact that the twitching was all over the facial area before the operation, but that pain was in the frontal region thru temporal, in and around the ear. What she describes as an engine is directly in the ear. It is quite possible that this might be regarded as a true otalgia of the Ramsey Hunt type. Just 6 years ago this January she began having this pain behind the ear shooting thru the eye. No blisters or herpes. She has been deaf in the right ear for a long period.

2 weeks before she had what she calls a shock with extravasation in the eye she went to a doctor for pain in and around the ear. Evidently she was given an insufflation.

Several years before, the exact time is uncertain, she became deaf in the right ear. She never had any facial paralysis, certainly no Bell's palsy. At present there is a spasmodic tic which at times goes into a more or less tonic spasm, involving the whole musculature on the right side, including the platysma; face draws and the eye closes. Gasserian operation has left a total 5th anaesthetic seeing field. The jaw opens in the midline. The masseter can be felt to contract and I judge the motor root has been preserved.

She has no nystagmus or unsteadiness. It is difficult to believe that this could be due to an acoustic tumor. Among her complaints she says that protrusion of the tongue or putting the tongue on the right side starts the "engine" going or starts the pain. On deep pressure everywhere on the right side of the face and particularly on pinching the lips or cheek or orbicularis region or platysma pain is produced. She also complains greatly of soreness in the back of the mouth. There is great soreness on pressure against the posterior third of tongue.

Tuning fork lateralized to left ear; hears the fork slightly in right ear; by air conduction: bone conduction apparently less on right than left but not in abeyance. There is also great tenderness in the region of the facial nerve and pressure there brings on bad facial spasm. The patient says that after the Gasserian operation the twitching stopped from December to May. She says that the "engine" in her ear and pain was there just the same. Twitching began again after 6 months.

December 10, 1920
Dr. Locke

Yesterday Dr. Cushing made an unsuccessful attempt to inject the 7th nerve. During this process pressure behind the ear and pressure in the region of the 7th nerve gave patient pain similar to that which she calls her "engine." No facial paralysis or weakness has followed this injection.

OPERATIVE NOTE
December 17, 1920
Dr. Cushing
Anesthesia – Local

Resection of 3 mm Fragment of the Right Facial Nerve in its Course through the Mastoid.

I had intended in this case to find the facial at its point of emergence but at the last moment it seemed that it would be much more simple to burr through the mastoid and to expose the nerve at the aqueduct of Fallopius. It may be added that this procedure served to show why we had such difficulty in paralyzing the nerve with alcohol, for it did not lie in the canal but lay along side of inner side of the mastoid without penetrating the bone, at least up to a distance of 2 cm., above where it ordinarily should have emerged from the stylo-mastoid foramen. In short this foramen was missing.

The interesting feature of the procedure lay in the fact that as soon as the operator got down near the nerve, whenever the region was touched she had her characteristic great pain referred to the nose, eye, cheek, and later on when the nerve was really exposed, to the ear. I had to remove a surprising amount of the bone with the burr before I was able to identify a nerve, for I kept expecting to come down into the canal, whereas the nerve lay entirely outside of the bone, and about a cm., and a half of it was exposed before it was actually identified. It lay, as a matter of fact, in a slight groove but not in a canal. It was necessary during the latter part of the exposure to give some chloroform as she complained so greatly whenever the region was touched. Very slight touch of the nerve with an instrument caused this great pain in eye, nose and ear.

The nerve was finally exposed and divided, and a small fragment as stated was excised, the two ends being left in near approximation. Wound was perfectly dry and closed in layers over the cavity. A complete facial paralysis resulted from the procedure. I immediately tried pinching the face and am not really sure whether she has some sensation in it, but certainly pinching of the lip does not give pain as heretofore.

(Dr. Cushing)

POSTOPERATIVE NOTE
December 21, 1920
Dr. Locke

Dressing today showed wound in good condition. Stitches were removed and silver foil dressing applied.

Since operation there has been a complete facial paralysis. There has been no more spasmodic twitching. Punching of the cheek is not so tender as it was before but still gives some discomfort. Patient says that the engine still goes. She says there is burning sensation of her face and eye which is very distressing. However, she is much relieved in not having the painful twitching.

RADIOLOGY REPORT
January 24, 1921

Plates of the skull in a right and left lateral position show an operative defect in the right temporal region. There is no evidence of increased intracranial pressure, and no change in the sella turcica itself.

DISCHARGE NOTE
February 12, 1921
Dr. Locke

The mental depression is still well marked and she complains of the engine that keeps her awake at night. The roof of the mouth seems to be a trigger point and anything touching this causes severe pain over right side of nose and forehead.

The complete sensory loss as well as complete motor paralysis of the right face is present. The painful twitching of the right face is no longer present yet this other pain has taken its place.

The eye is in remarkably good condition and patient taking good care of it. She seemed to have a great dread of leaving the hospital. Discharged.

FOLLOW UP NOTE
July 20, 1921
Dr. Cushing

The facial nerve is evidently undergoing spontaneous regeneration. The whole right face draws up well. She has no longer any facial spasmodic tic, but complains of the "engine." She has evidently gained weight, and looks to me in much better condition. She says that she is still having pain in her face, and that she cannot take anything hot or cold or hard in her mouth without a return of the pain. She will report again in a few months.

On December 3, 1923, this patient was admitted in the hospital with the diagnosis of facial neuralgia (unknown origin). She underwent cervical sympathectomy. There is no medical record available for this admission.

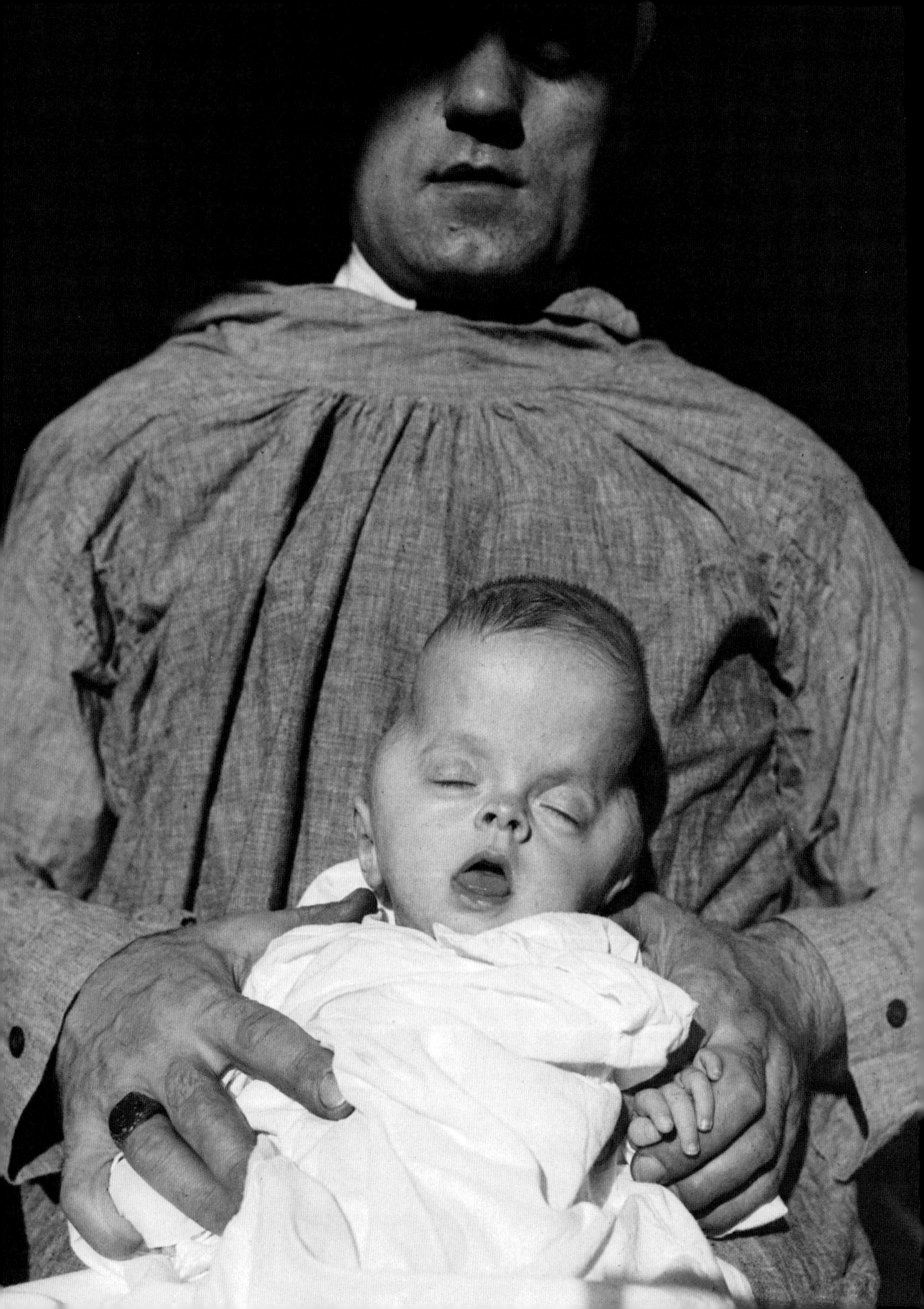

6.9 Craniosynostosis

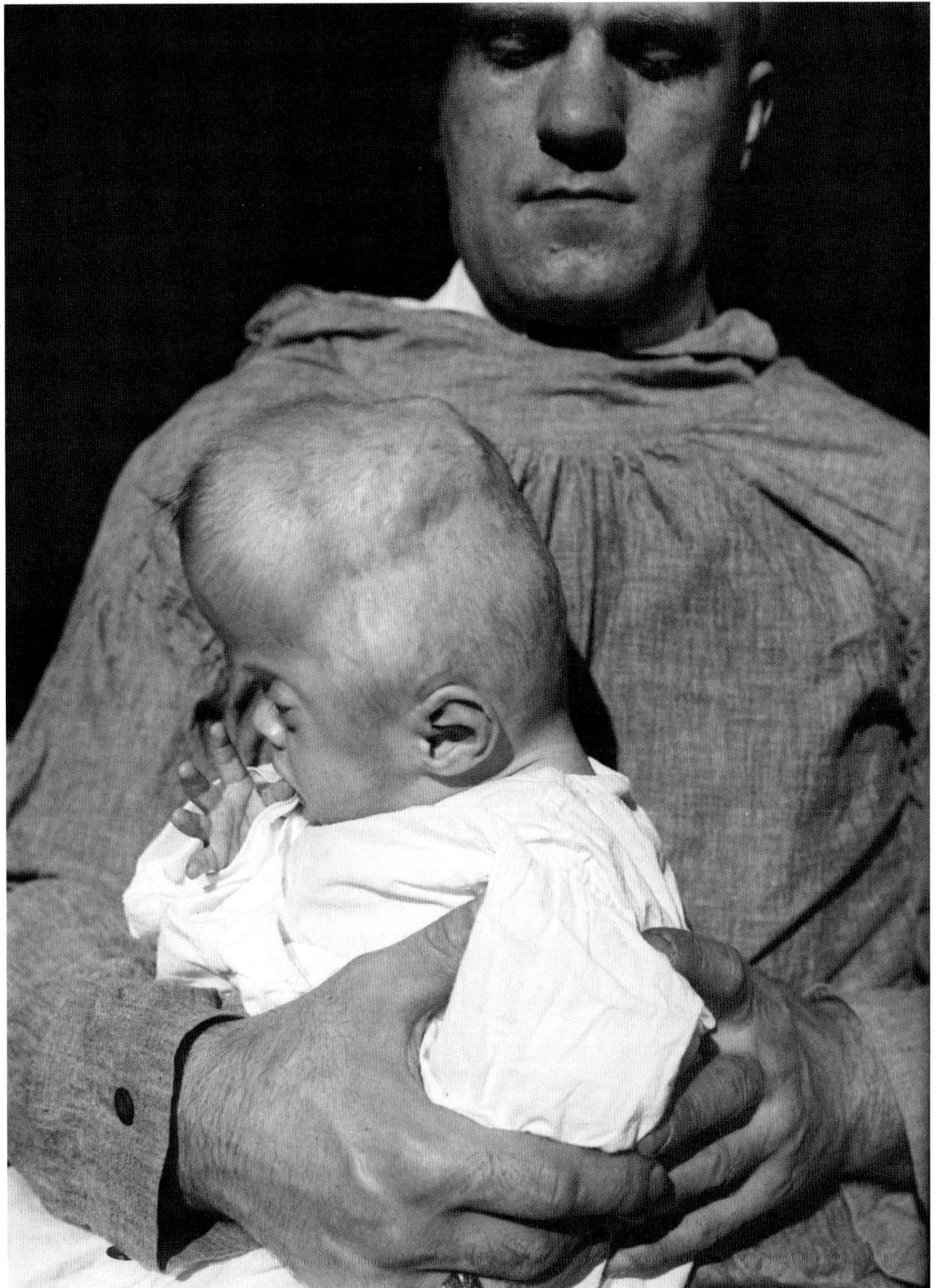

FIG. 2. PREOPERATIVE.

OPPOSITE PAGE. FIG. 1. PREOPERATIVE.

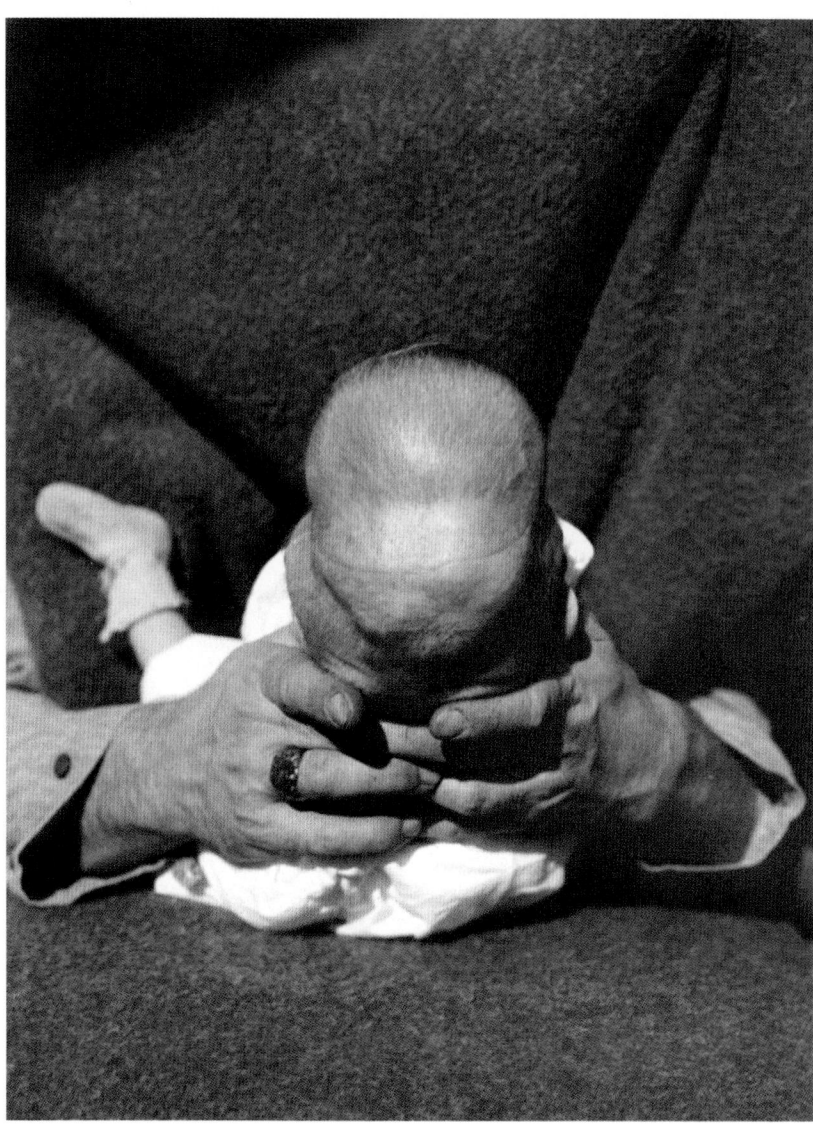

FIG. 3. PREOPERATIVE.

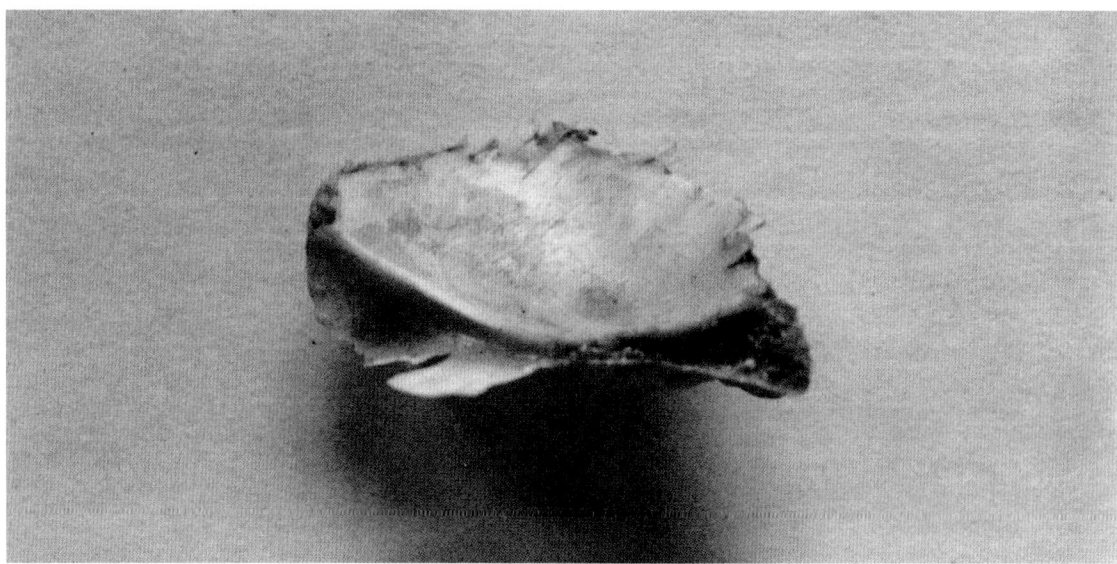

FIG. 4. RESECTED BONE FRAGMENT.

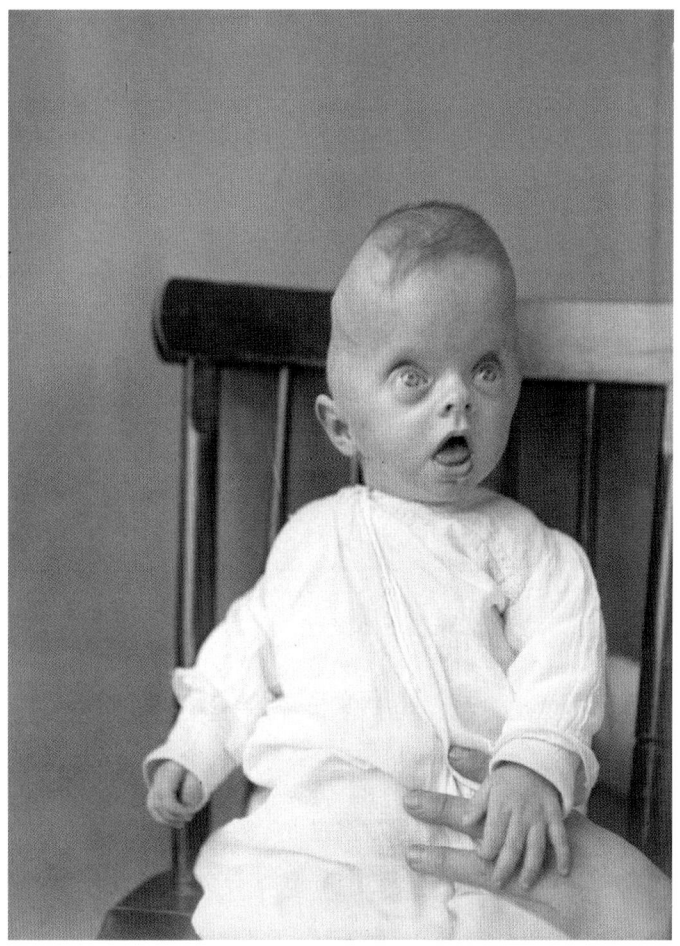
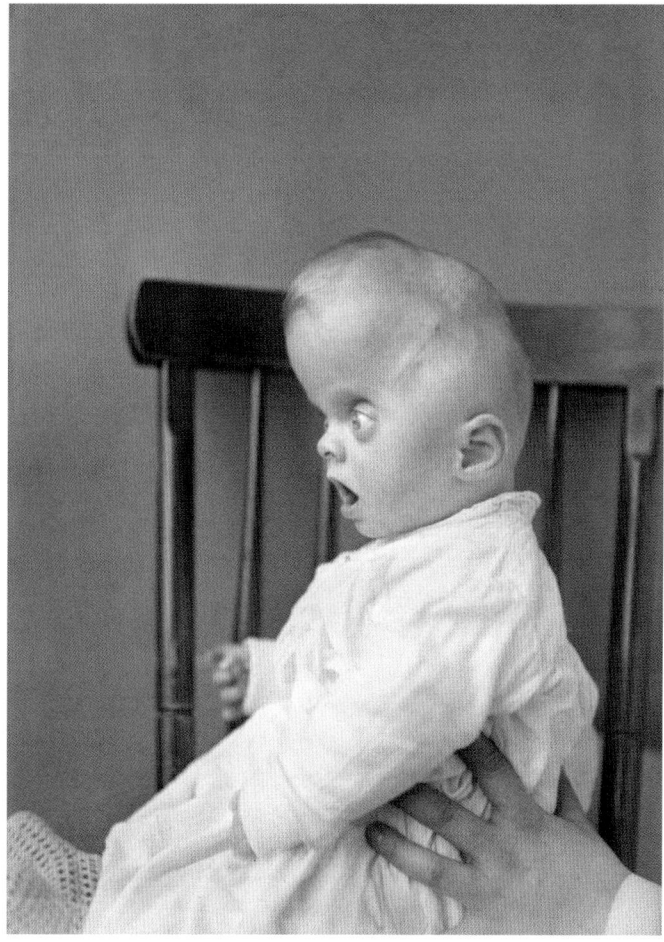

FIG. 5, 6, 7. THREE WEEKS POSTOPERATIVE.

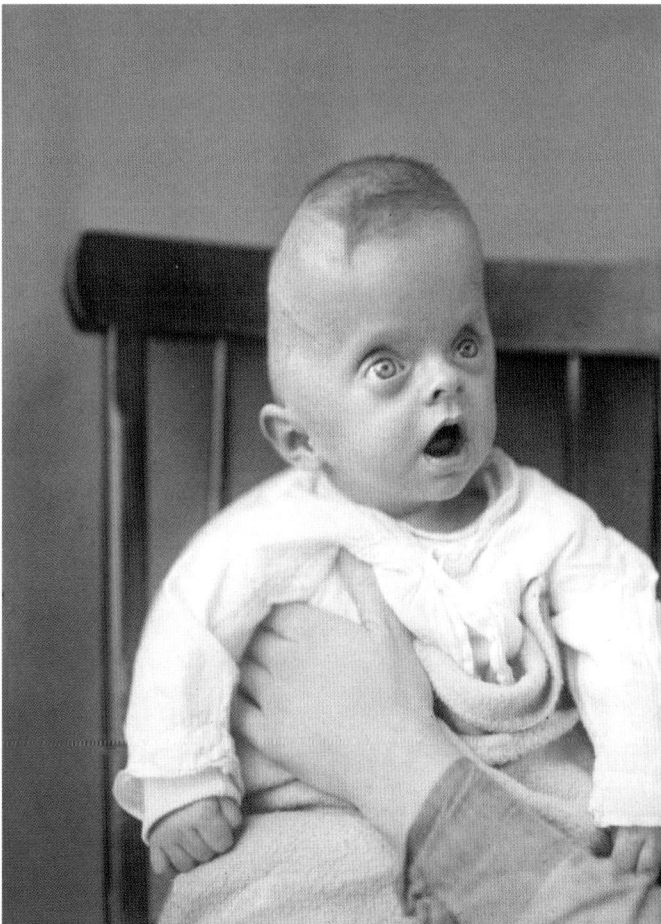

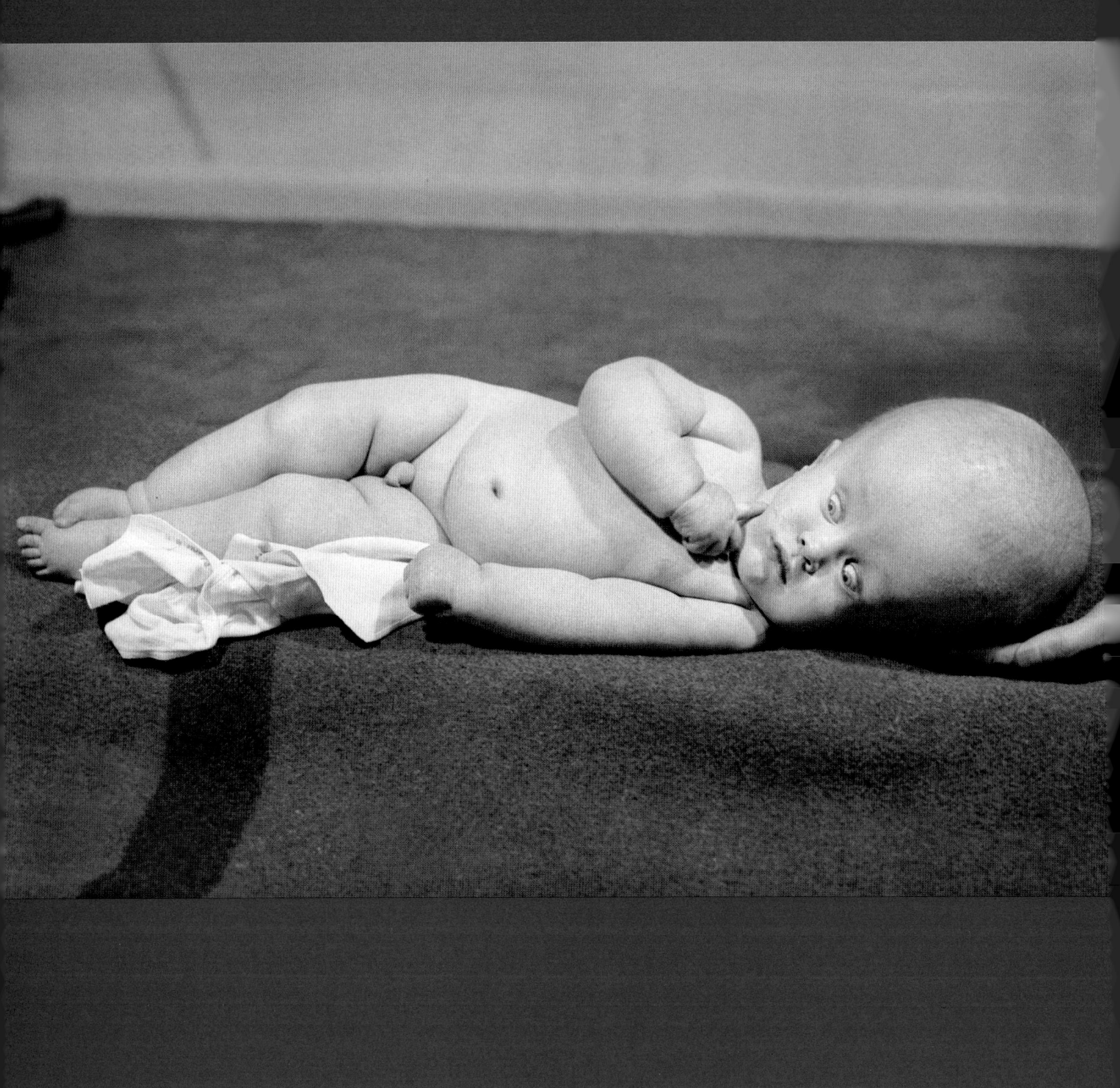

5.10 Hydrocephalus

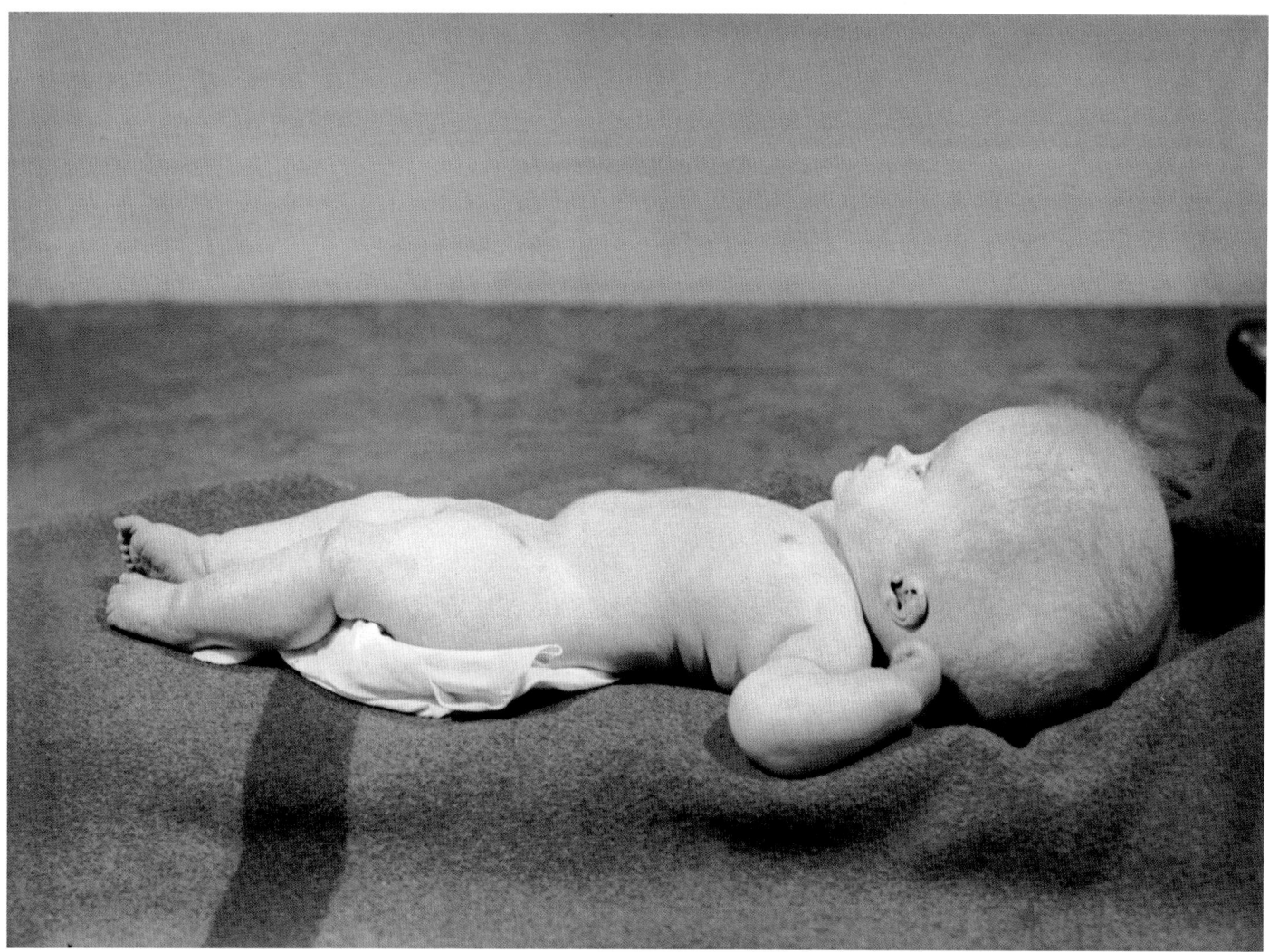

FIG. 2. HYDROCEPHALUS.

OPPOSITE PAGE. FIG. 1. HYDROCEPHALUS.

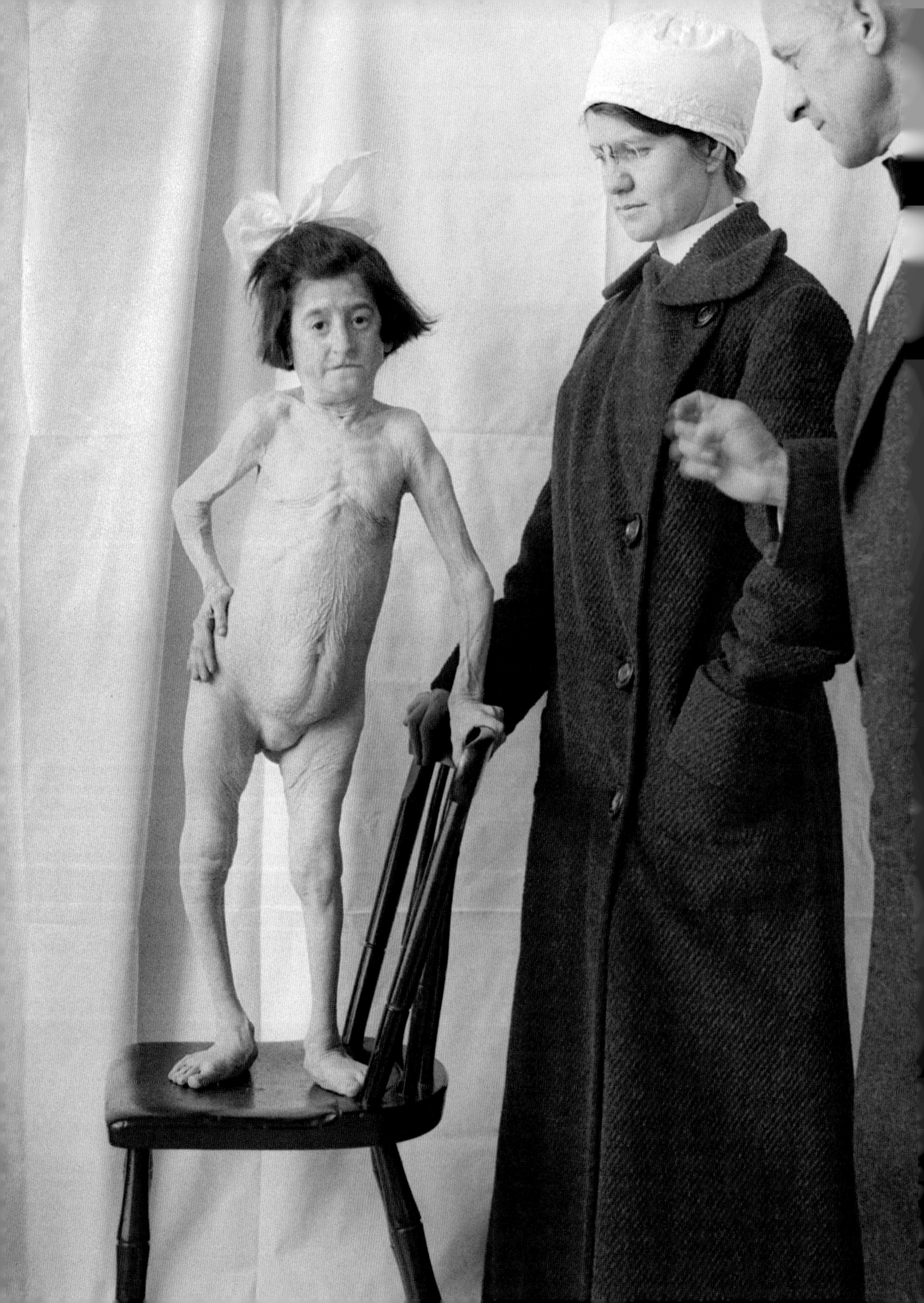

6.11 Progeria

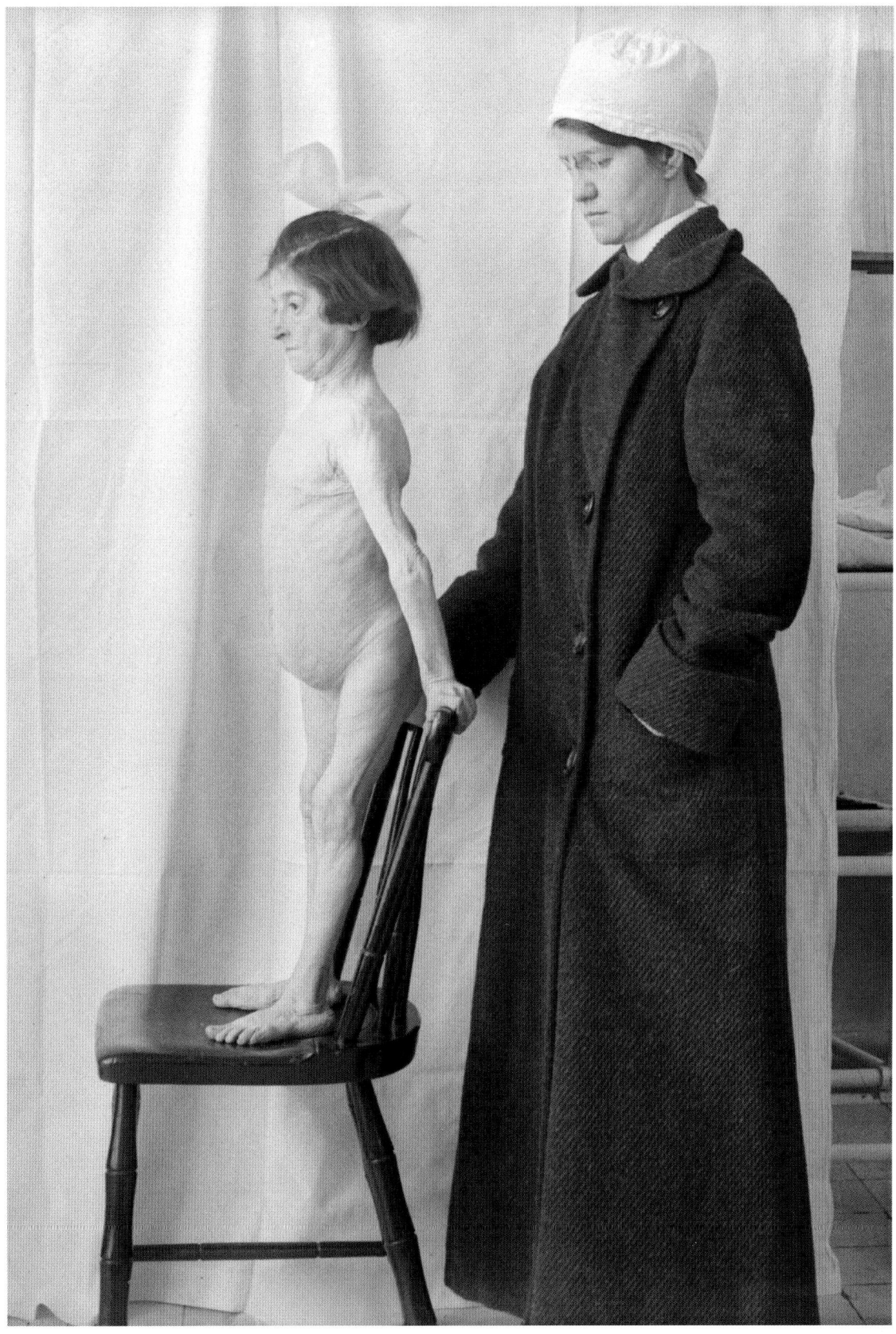

OPPOSITE PAGE. FIG. I. ABOVE: FIG. 2.

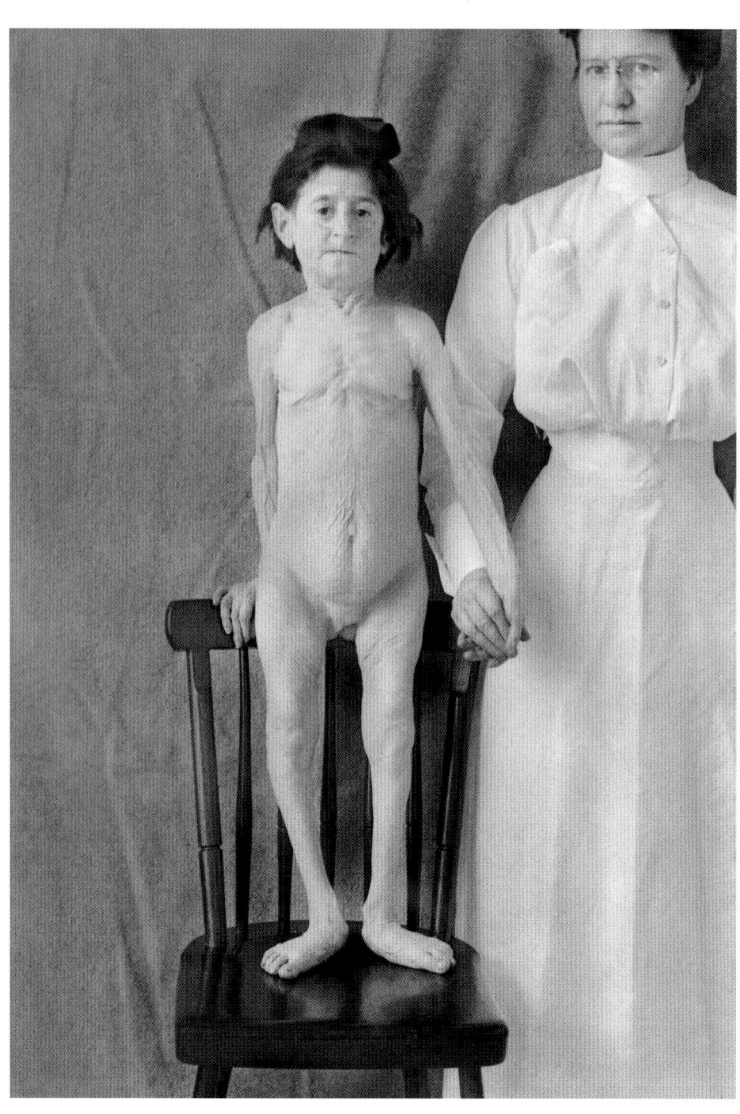
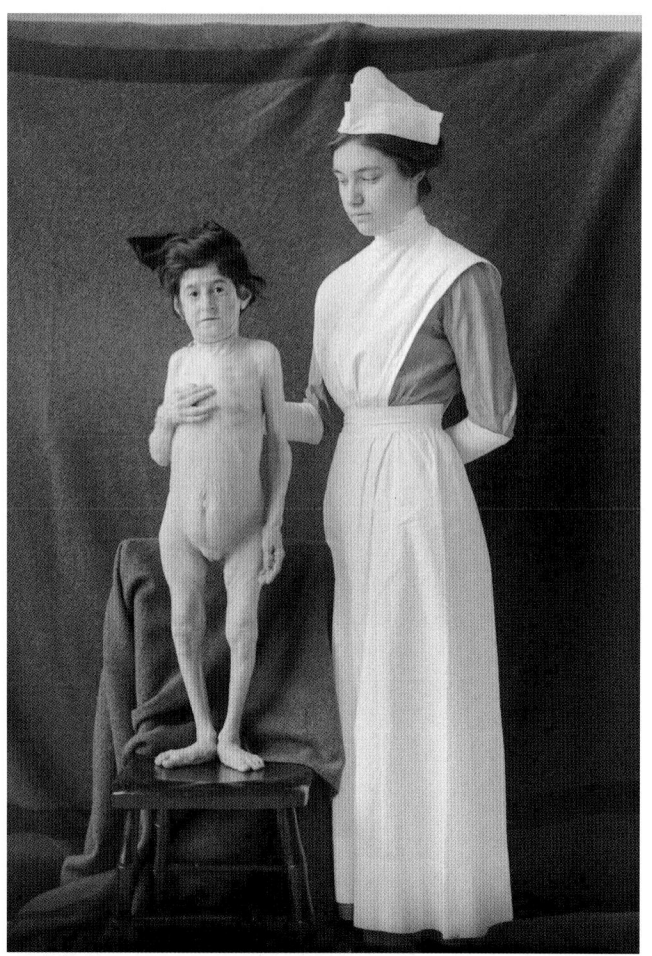
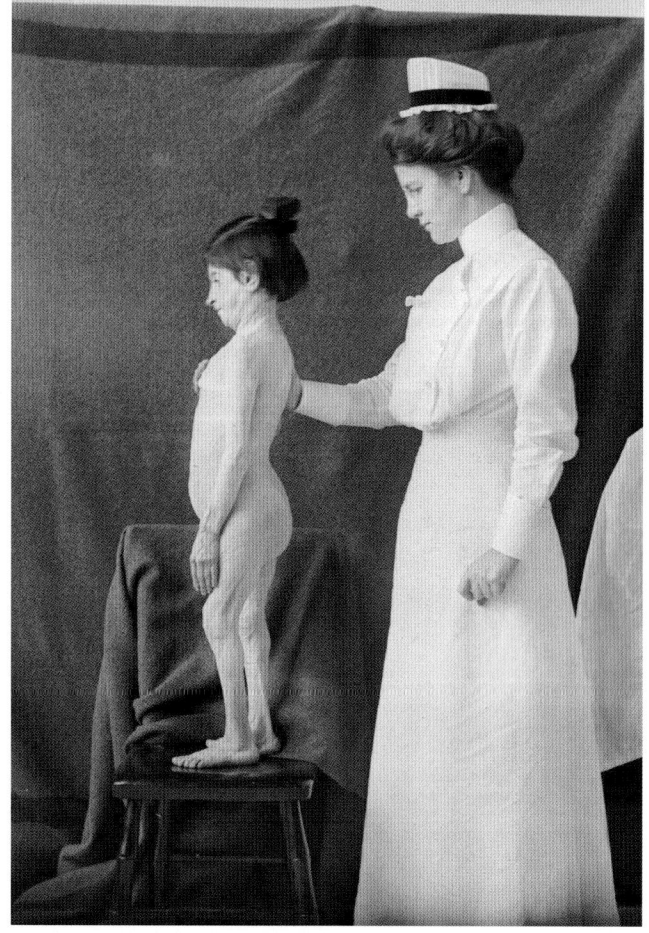

FIGS. 3, 4, 5.

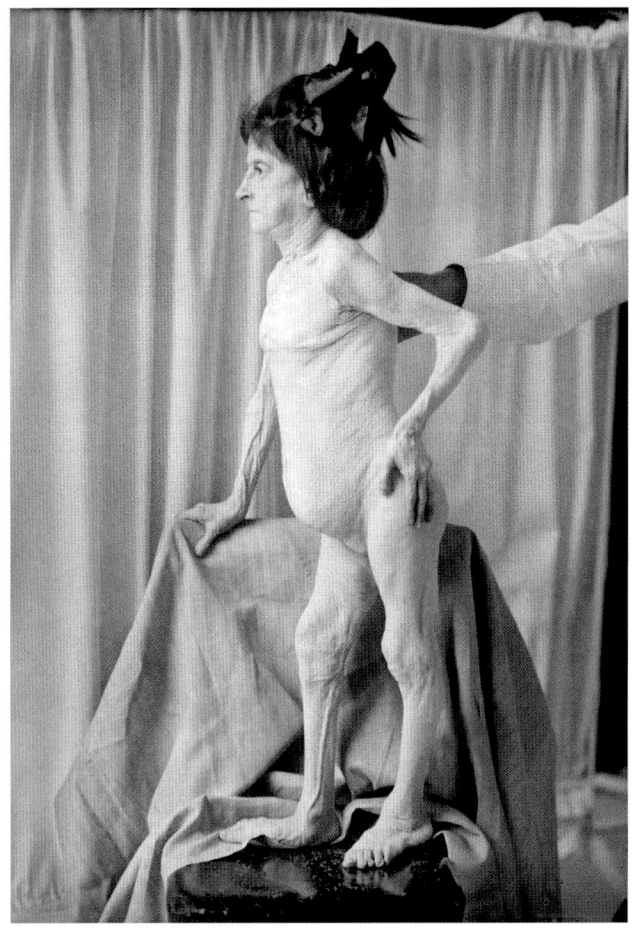

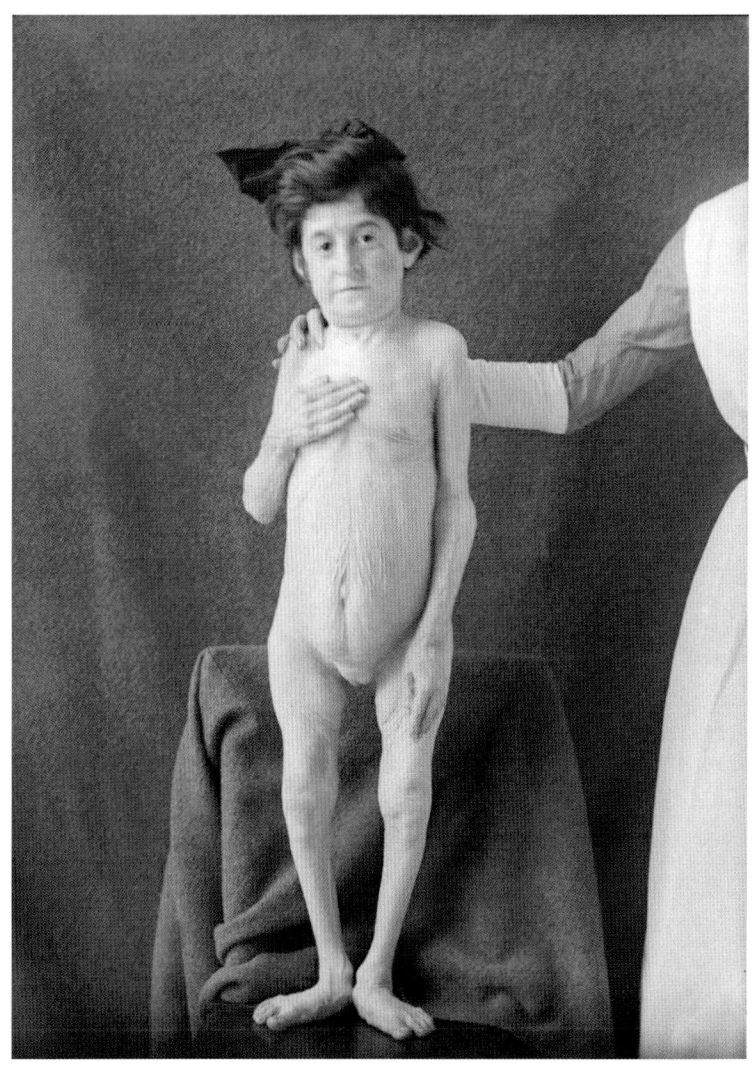

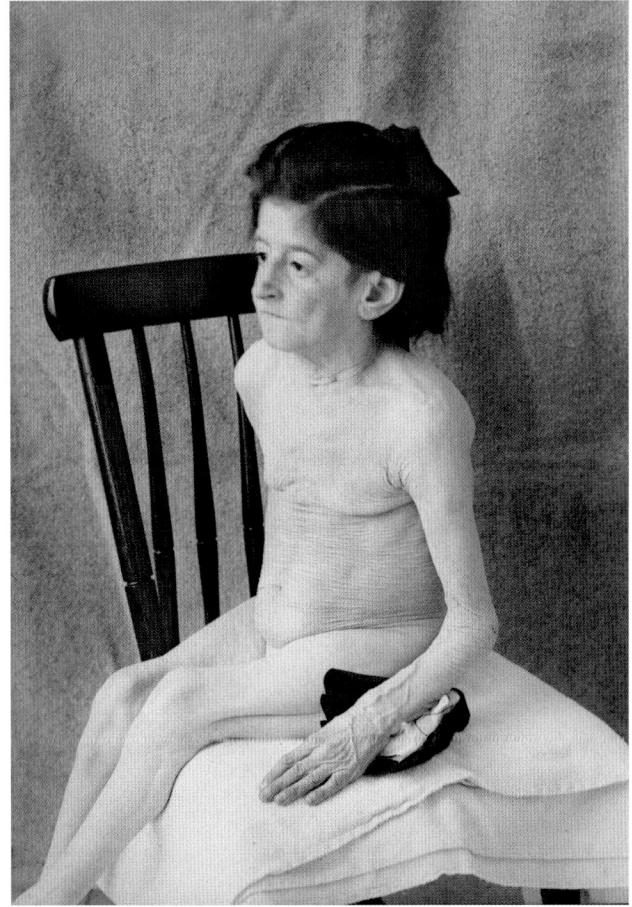

FIGS. 6, 7, 8.

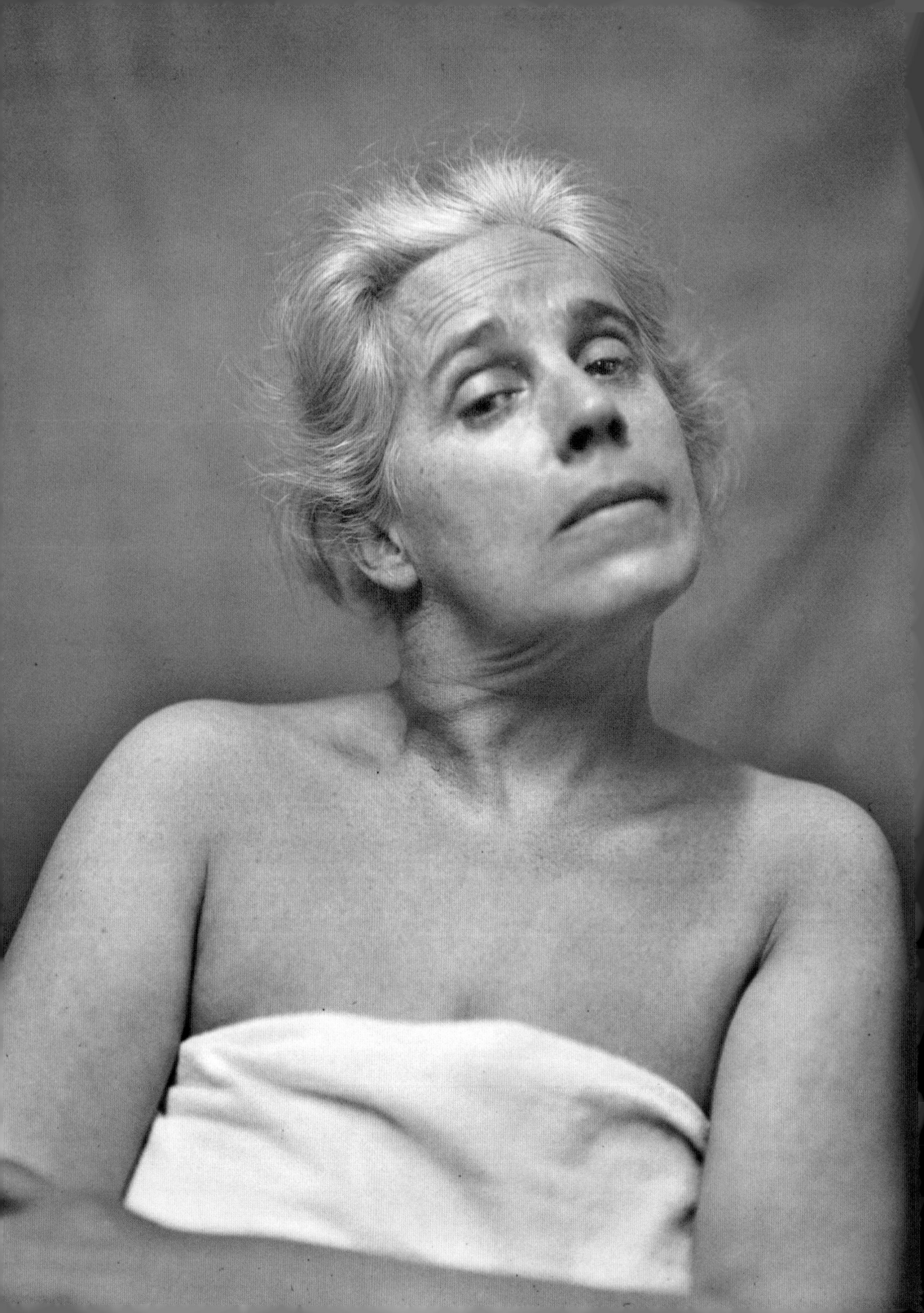

6.12 Left rotational torticollis

SEX: F; AGE: 51; SURG. NO. 18028

HISTORY

This patient has been suffering from left rotational torticollis with phasic component.

SUMMARY OF POSITIVE FINDINGS
January 3, 1923
Dr. McKenzie

SUBJECTIVE
1. History of almost constant side to side shaking of the head for the last 3 years.
2. History of right sided suboccipital pain associated with a tilting of the head to the right and the pulling of the skin to the left for the last year.

OBJECTIVE
1. Side to side motion of the head, especially noted when the patient is up out of bed. This is associated with a tilting of the head to the right and a pulling of the skin to the left, and a spasm of the right sternomastoid muscle.
2. Limitation of rotation of the head to the right to one-half normal, accounted for by the spasm of the right sternomastoid muscle.

IMPRESSION: Torticollis with involvement chiefly of the right sternomastoid muscle.

SPECIAL NOTE
January 13, 1923
Dr. Cushing

This woman has a motor grade of torticollis with painful spasm involving the right sternomastoid, trapezius and all the deep group of cervical rotatories on the right side of the upper neck. So far as I am aware there was no diaphragmatic spasm observed. It seemed to me to be a case in which the nerve supply to this group of muscles might be divided intracranially and intraspinally though so far as I am aware such a performance heretofore has not been undertaken anywhere. I at first contemplated making merely a vertical incision but in view of her short neck and tendency of the head to hyperextend I thought that I would have insufficient room and so made a reflection of the deep muscles on one side as would bilaterally be done in the usual cerebellar operation.

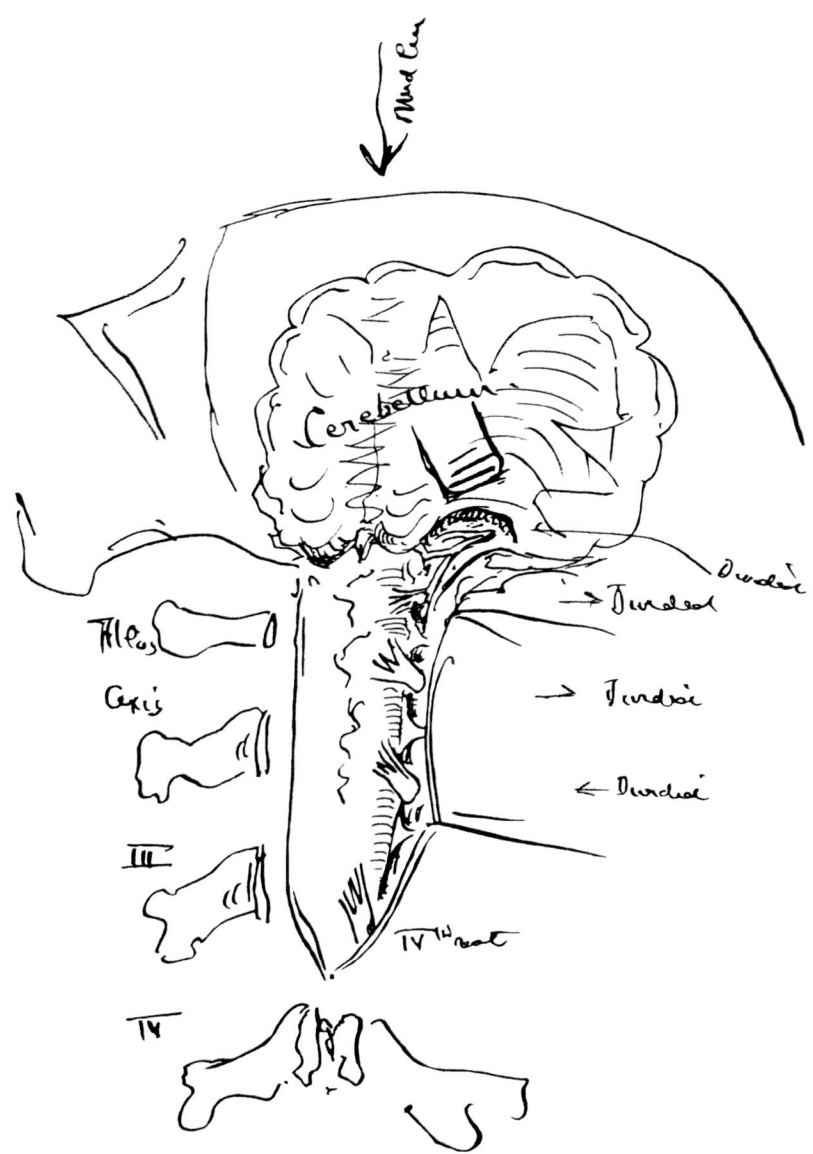

FIG. 2. SURGEON'S DRAWING.

OPERATIVE NOTE
January 13, 1923
Anesthesia – Ether – Miss Gerrard

Combined Cerebellar and Upper Cord Exposure with Laminectomy of Three Upper Cervical Vertebrae.

The flap was reflected on the right as usual care being taken to keep in the median line. The spines of the upper vertebrae were identified, the 2nd and 3rd being bifid as usual. The spines were removed and also the laminae without difficulty. About as

OPPOSITE PAGE. FIG. 1. PREOPERATIVE.

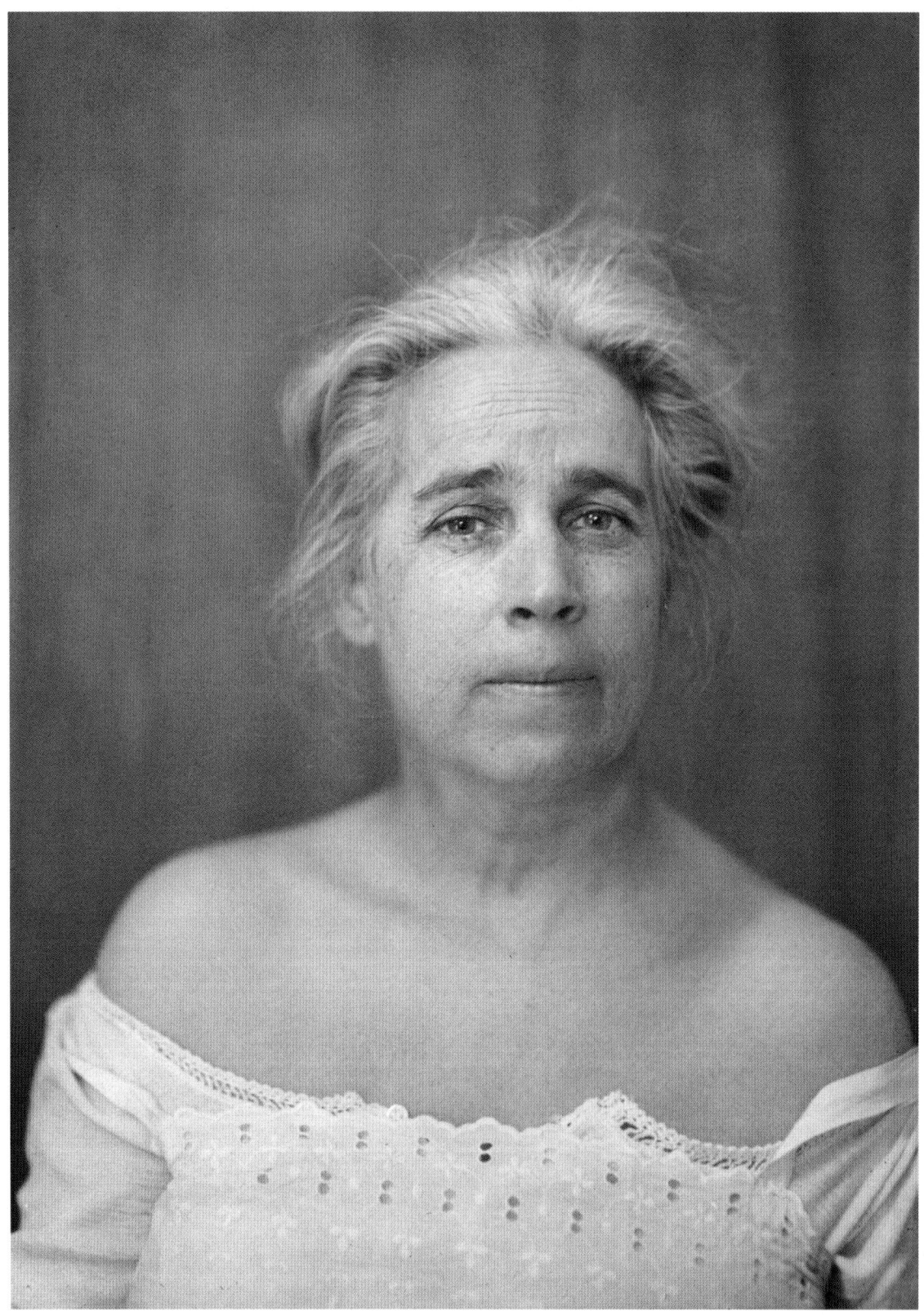

FIG. 3. POSTOPERATIVE.

much of the occipital region was removed as is shown in the sketch. The dura was opened and the incision carried down the length of the laminectomy to the spine of the 4th cervical. There was a very large posterior cistern with thin transparent arachnoid through which it was possible to see all of the nerve roots and the spinal accessory before the arachnoid was opened and the fluid evacuated. This was finally done and the spinal accessory was followed up to its point of emergence from the skull. The fibres of the glossopharynges were easily seen and it is of interest that on touching the various fibres going into the spinal accessory from the upper cord there was no twitching of muscles nor when the long direct cord was touched did the shoulder muscles jerk. I assume therefore that these upper fibres are not motor. The nerve was divided just about at its point of entry into the jugular foremen though I am not sure that it was necessary to divide it this high.

The first, 2nd and 3rd nerves were then divided with fine scissors at their point of emergence outside the arachnoid. It was far easier to expose them from above than to expose them by peeling the arachnoid away for there seemed to me to be an unusual number of arachnoid adhesions though I am not sufficiently familiar with this region to be sure of this. The dentate ligament was also divided and the cord rolled to the side so that I am sure that the divisions were complete. It was perfectly easy to identify the 4th root passing down to emerge below the 3rd lamina.

I had some difficulty from bleeding at the time of dividing the 2nd cervical which was the largest of these roots. I must have cut a minute artery and it was necessary to implant a bit of muscle and to delay for some time before I could proceed with the other divisions. The 3rd was then divided and it was some little time before I could make sure of the 1st which after all was the most difficult of all to divide for it lay in a tangle of small vessels and spinal accessory branches. It was very easy to determine the situation of the fibres, however, and to identify them because on touching them with the instrument the deep cervical muscles all twitched just as the shoul-

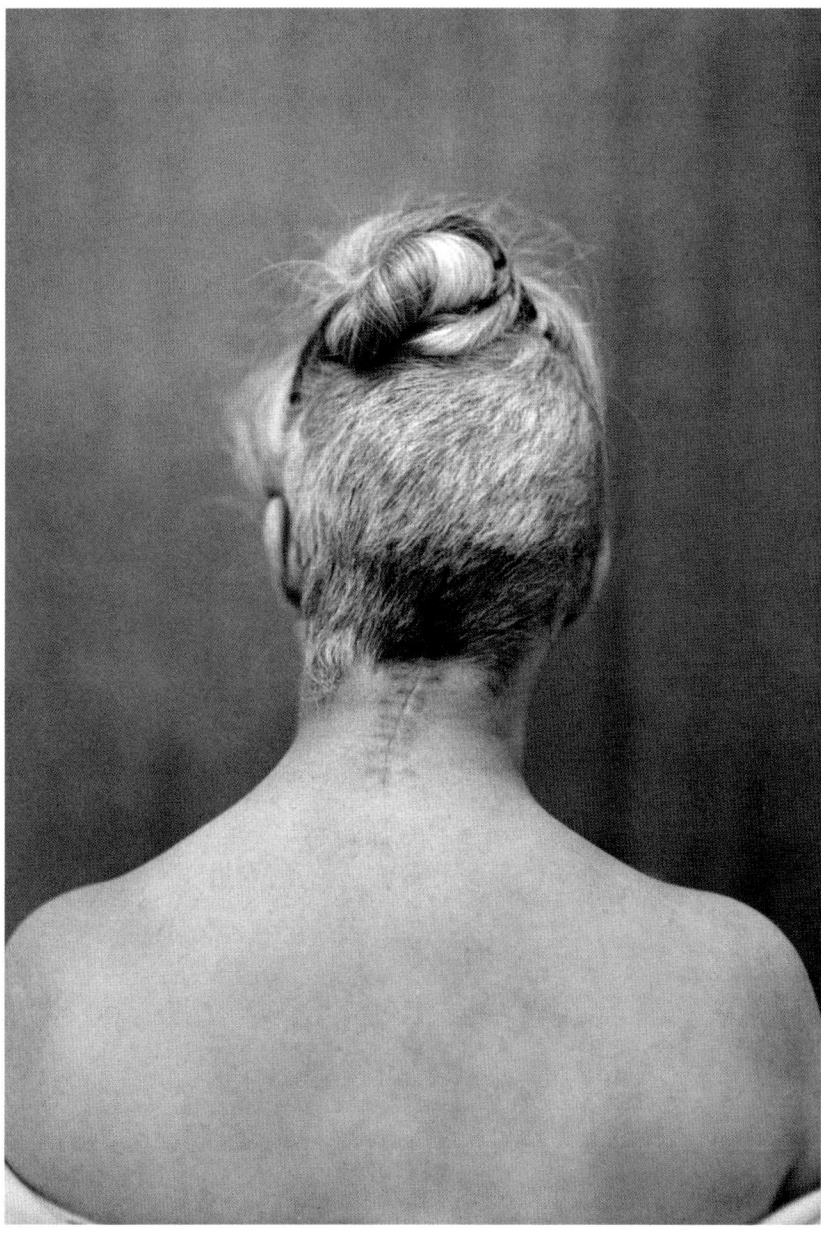

FIG. 4. POSTOPERATIVE.

der muscle twitched when the spinal accessory was divided. I regret that I did not make this test before dividing the 2nd and 3rd bundles.

The patient stood the operation well and wound was left dry and closed as usual in layers.

(Dr. Cushing)

This patient was discharged in an "improved" condition.

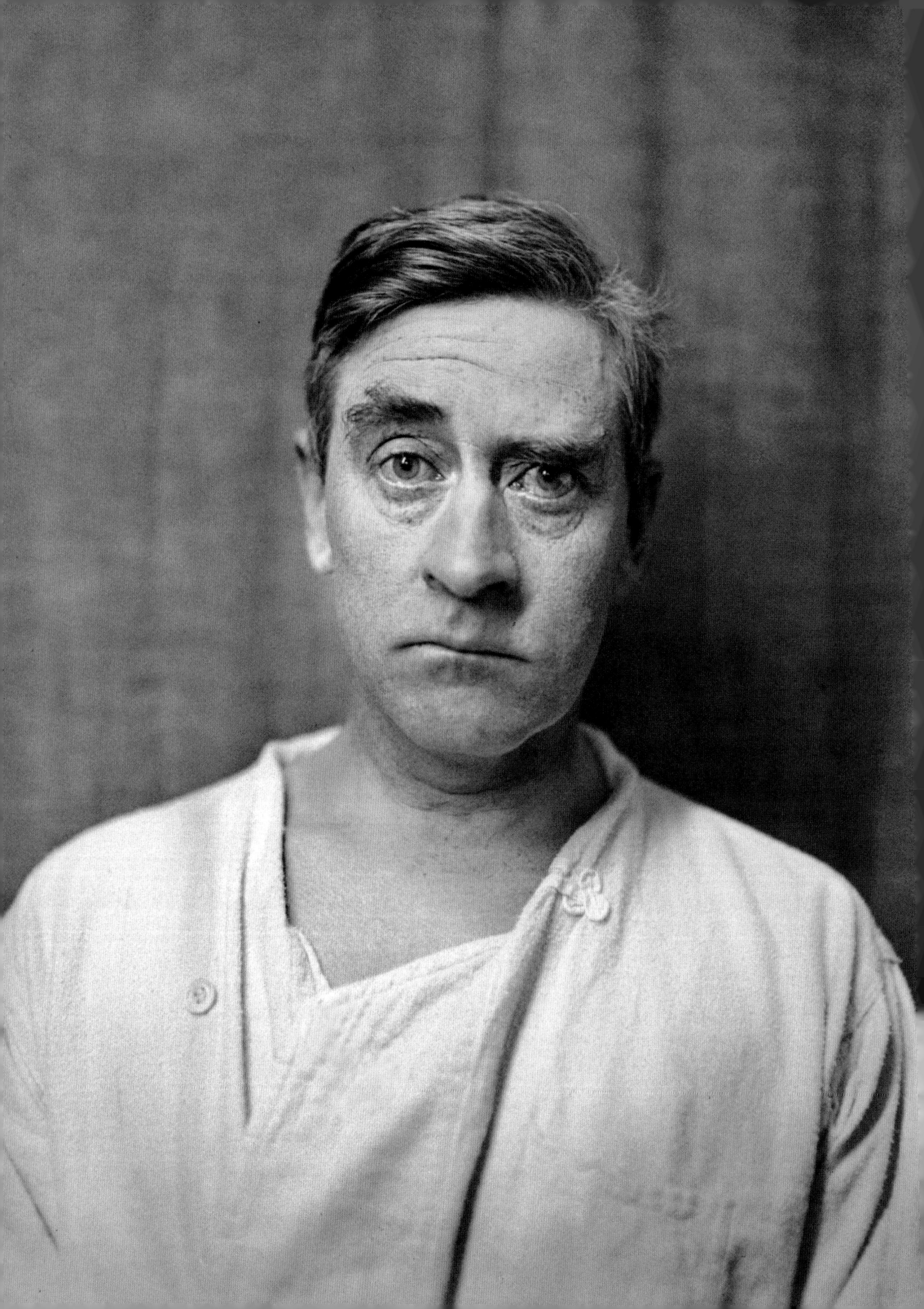

6.13 Acoustic neuroma

SEX: M; AGE: 44; SURG. NO. 19796

HISTORY

The patient suffered from several months of headaches, hearing loss, numbness of the face and blurry vision. After ophthalmological evaluation, he was referred to Dr. Cushing.

SUMMARY OF POSITIVE FINDINGS
October 1, 1923
Dr. Stimson

SUBJECTIVE

1. "Bursting" severe parietal headaches for 7 months, progressively more frequent. "Dull, heavy feeling" in head constantly.
2. Difficult walking, uncertain gait, falling toward left.
3. Tinnitus, left, of rushing type, for 7 months.
4. Dyspnea, partial deafness, left, of sudden onset, 8½ months ago.
5. Blurring of vision for 6 months. Occasional diplopia during past 2 weeks.
6. Numbness of left side of face for 6 months.
7. Vomiting, non-projectile, 3 times in past month.
8. Vertigo on standing or walking, for 7 months.

OBJECTIVE

1. Coarse nystagmus, lateral, more to left.
2. Left pupil larger than right, both dilated; left corneal reflex absent.
3. Partial deafness, left.
4. Hypesthesia to pinprick, left face.
5. Gait uncertain, veers to left, leans to left in Romberg position, walks with wide base.
6. K.J. and A.J. hyperactive, equal. Tendency to ankle clonus.
7. Bilateral choked disc, with beginning secondary atrophy, one or two small retinal hemorrhages.

IMPRESSION – Acoustic neuroma, left.

ADDITIONAL FINDINGS ON EXAM
October 1, 1923
Dr. McKenzie

CRANIAL NERVES

II. Optic

SUBJECTIVE: There has been intermittent dimness of vision for the past 7 months. During the past month dimness of vision has been constant and gradually increasing.

OBJECTIVE: Both discs have obliterated margins, small petechial hemorrhages in the left disc with large blotching hemorrhages. There is considerable burying of the vessels and pallor of the disc showing thru, 6D elevation on both sides. Vessels are quite tortuous. VOS 20/100 corrected; VOD 20/50 corrected.

V. Trigeminus

SUBJECTIVE: Numbness of the left face has been noticed for the past few weeks.

OBJECTIVE: Left corneal reflex is absent. There is marked diminution in sensation over the left face to pin prick and light touch. Also there is very slight motor weakness.

VII. Facial

There is no facial weakness to be noted. Both platysma stand out very prominently.

VIII. Acoustic

SUBJECTIVE: 12 months ago diminution in hearing was noted in the left ear and this has been gradually getting worse. Careful questioning does not elicit the fact that there were any noises noted in this ear before the deafness.

OBJECTIVE: Both eardrums appear normal. Watch heard 3 feet in the right ear, not heard when placed against the head, left. Ao greater than Bo on both sides, markedly diminished on the left. However, tuning fork is heard. Also he states that he can hear loud clock ticking with left ear. Weber not tried.

OPPOSITE PAGE. FIG. 1. THREE WEEKS POSTOPERATIVE.

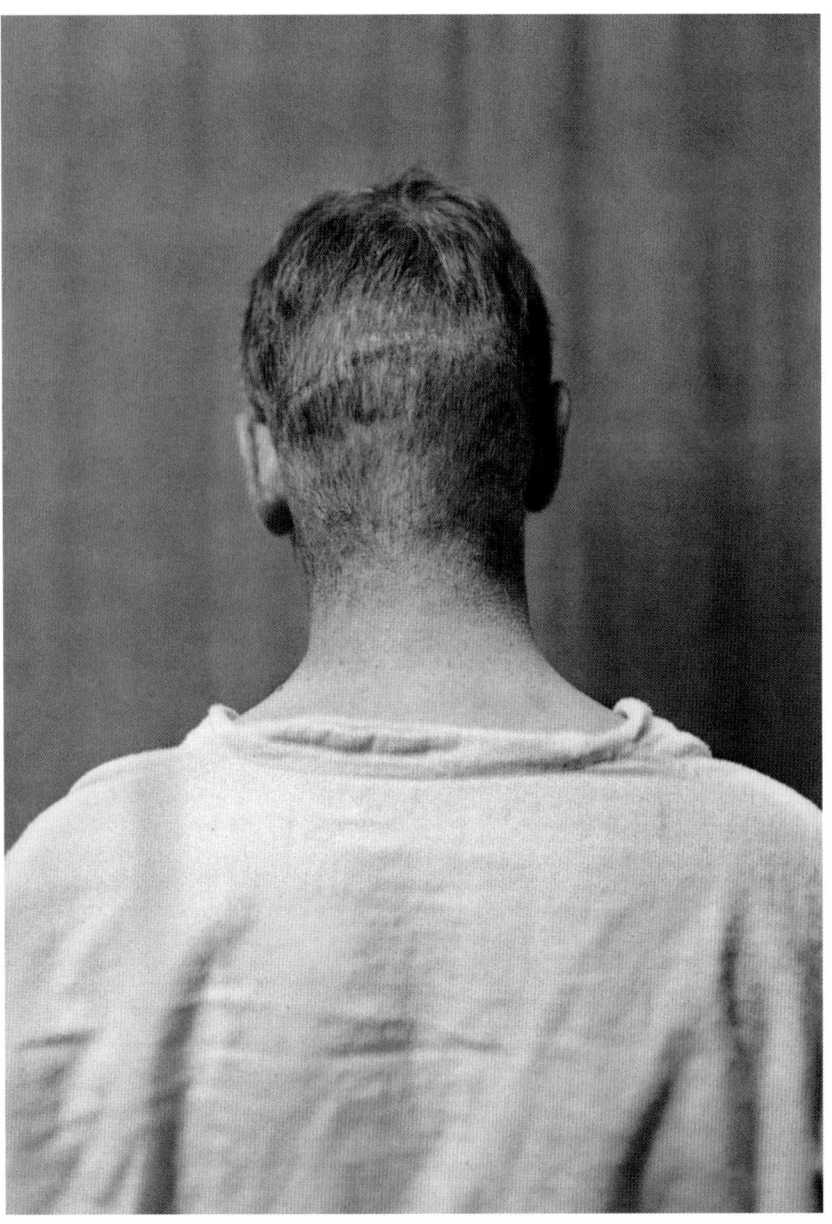

FIG. 2. THREE WEEKS POSTOPERATIVE.

Vestibular

Subjective – There has been unsteadiness but no dizziness.

CEREBELLUM

Slow horizontal nystagmus to the right and left, more marked on the left. With eyes closed and heels and toes together the patient falls to the left. On walking he staggers to the left. Unable to stand on either foot alone, especially the left. Unable to stand in tandem position.

IMPRESSION: Acoustic neuroma, left.

RADIOLOGY REPORT
October 2, 1923
Dr. Sosman

No localizing signs of tumor.

SPECIAL NOTE
Oct. 5, 1923
Dr. Cushing

This man unfortunately has had such advanced pressure symptoms that he has largely lost vision. There seemed to me very little doubt but that he had an acoustic tumor which possibly was of longer duration than his history indicated. His loss of hearing was discovered on the chance observation one day when testing his watch which he thought had stopped until he tried it in both ears. I expected to find a large acoustic neuroma which, however, had probably not undergone marked fatty degeneration if it was as recent as the history indicated.

OPERATIVE NOTE
October 5, 1923
Anesthesia – Ether – Miss Gerrard

Suboccipital Exploration. Total Enucleation of Cystic Left Acoustic Neurinoma.

This was an extremely simple, straightforward, uncomplicated operation which from beginning to end lasted only 2 ½ hours. A fairly good suboccipital exposure was secured and the bone removed. The dura was tense and a ventricular puncture withdrew a large amount of fluid but did not greatly lessen tension. This was not relieved until after the dura had been opened, the cerebellum exposed, and an attempt made to get into the left lateral recess when there was an escape of a large amount of cerebrospinal fluid from the spaces around the 9th, 10th, and 11th nerves – fluid which largely came from the spinal canal.

There was at first no sign of tumor and it was not until the cerebellum was widely disclosed that the surface of a smooth tumor covered by strands of arachnoid was seen. It was elastic and had the appearance of a meningioma.

I decided that I would split the tumor and treat it like an acoustic neuroma getting a fragment meanwhile to identify its histological character, but on splitting it I got into a cyst which must have held 4–5 cc of fluid and the walls partly collapsed.

I was able with the pituitary rongeurs to grasp the walls and by slow and careful brushing and dissection to deliver the entire cyst. There were 1–2 tags of nerve which were adherent and which may possibly be the 7th and 8th nerves.

A little bleeding followed the final delivery of the tumor, but this was controlled by muscle which I had previously secured, from the patient's leg. One fairly good muscle mass was left on the lateral recess on the raw surface in the region from which the tumor was delivered until late in the closure when it was removed without apparent bleeding.

At the time of the dislodgement of the tumor there was some little disturbance of pulse and respiration, which however, appeared to quiet down, and as a matter of fact the other chart shows a very regular pulse rate.

Only on one other occasion have I succeeded in this way in drawing out an acoustic tumor in its totality, a woman who had a cystic acoustic tumor of very much this same kind, though in her case there was much less tissue in the tumor wall than in the present case.

It may be said that the tumor wall in both of these instances was surprisingly tough and thick, and it may be that we are dealing with quite a different tumor, for I have never known of an acoustic tumor wall being as resistant as this and as unlikely to tear, for in the manipulations to deliver this tumor the wall held without tearing even though it was being torn out by the sharp-billed pituitary rongeurs.

The wound was closed securely in layers without a drain.

(Dr. Cushing)

PATHOLOGY REPORT
October 5, 1923

Specimen consists of a tumor of the acoustic nerve. 3½ x 2½ x 2½ cm and weighing 14.5 gms. It was deleted out intact. This is very rare for acoustic neuromas which are usually dug out with a pituitary spoon. There was apparently a cystic cavity in the interior of the tumor. The tumor was fixed immediately in 10% formalin and was retained in the Surgical Laboratory, no material being submitted for microscopic examination.

(Dr. Cushing)

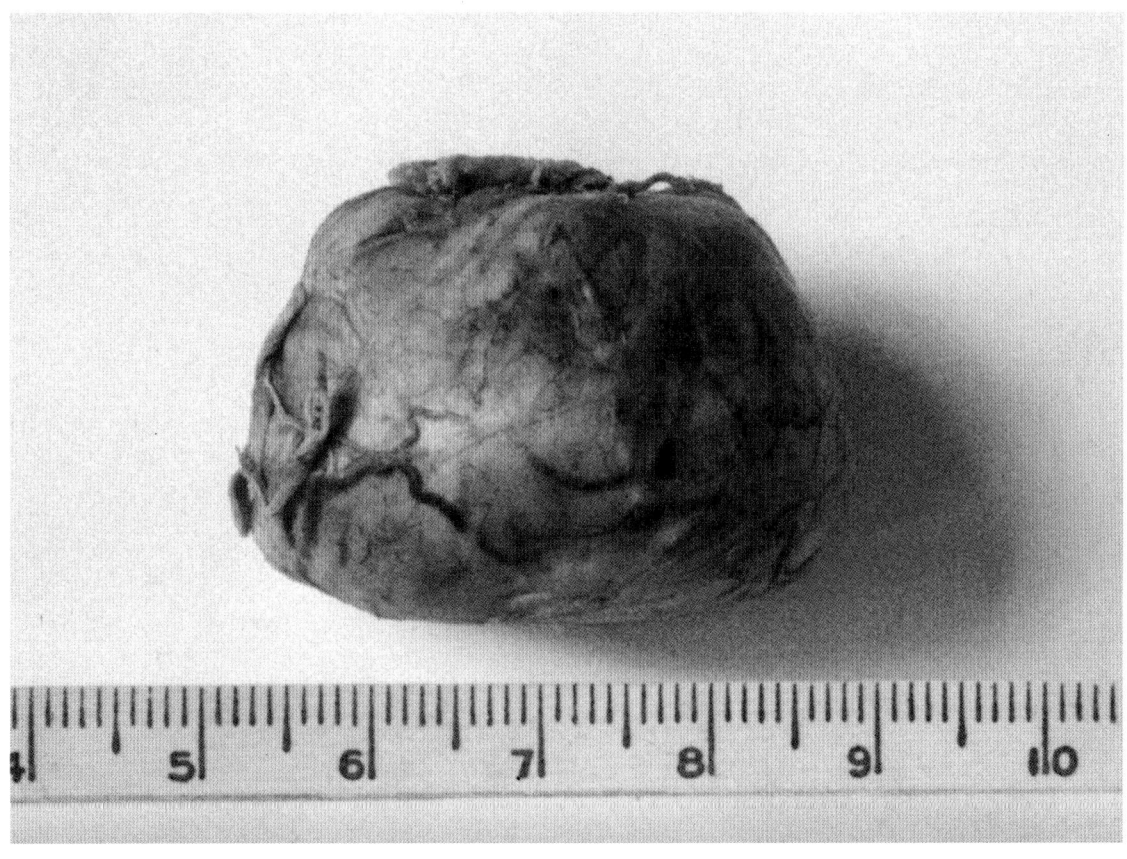

FIG. 3. TUMOR SPECIMEN.

MICROSCOPIC REPORT: Two sections—one, E 7 B stain, one, PTAH. These sections consist of a very small portion of the periphery of the tumor. Here the tissue is composed of dense tissue arranged in interlacing bands. The cells are spindle shaped with long nuclei and a small amount of cytoplasm stringing from one or either end. Nuclei are sometimes found in palisades. Centrally, some of the tumor cells assume a different appearance. The tissue is less dense and there are more blood vessels. Here cells have round, granular nuclei and an abundant vacuolated cytoplasm. The tissue in this region shows retrograde changes and necrosis.

IMPRESSION: Neurofibroma of acoustic nerve with necrosis.

(Dr. Wolbach)

POSTOPERATIVE NOTES
October 6, 1923
Dr. McKenzie

Complete left facial was noted when patient was taken off the table. He rallied quickly from his anaesthetic. His general condition this morning is quite satisfactory.

October 9, 1923
Dr. McKenzie

Patient has been progressing favorably. Complete facial persists. Both discs still 4–5 D. 5th nerve remains as before operation, that is a dulling sensation only.

DISCHARGE NOTE
October 26, 1923
Dr. McKenzie

Both discs are flat. Vision is practically as before operation. Has reading vision in the right eye. Up and about, feeling well. Cerebellar incoordination is only moderately marked and is well lateralized to the left side. This incoordination is improving every day and he feels that he will be able to return to work before long.

LETTER TO DR. CUSHING
March 5, 1926

Dear Dr. Cushing

(Name of the patient) enjoys excellent health. Is working every day. He has probably a permanent facial paralysis.

Very truly,
(signed) L.P.Crawford, M.D.

LETTER TO DR. CUSHING
September, 1931

Dear Dr. Cushing

I have not seen (name of the patient) for about a year. He had a facial paralysis at that time no disturbed vision. He was in good health.

Yours truly,
(signed) L.P. Crawford, M.D.

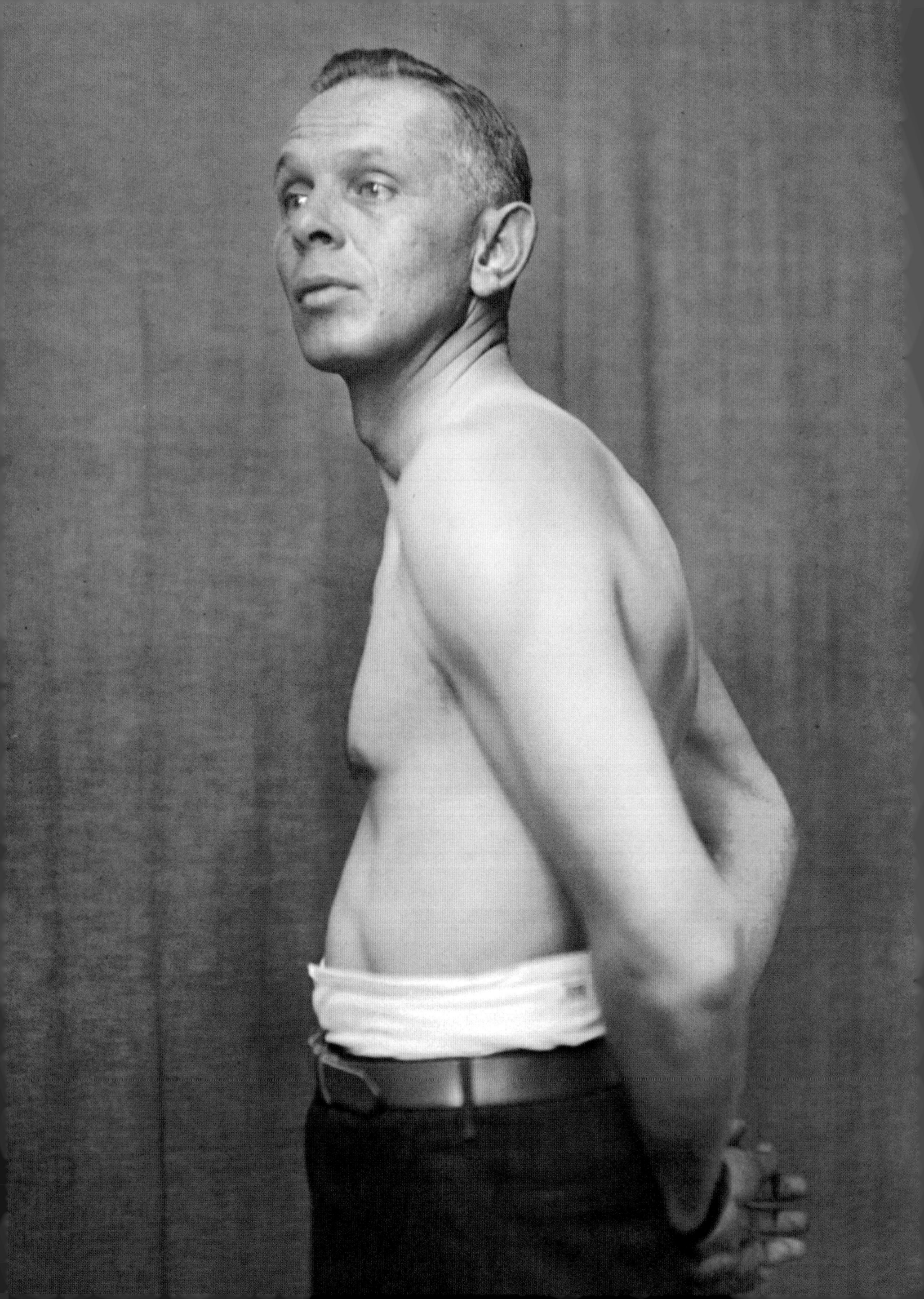

THE LEGACY OF HARVEY CUSHING

6.14 Left rotational torticollis

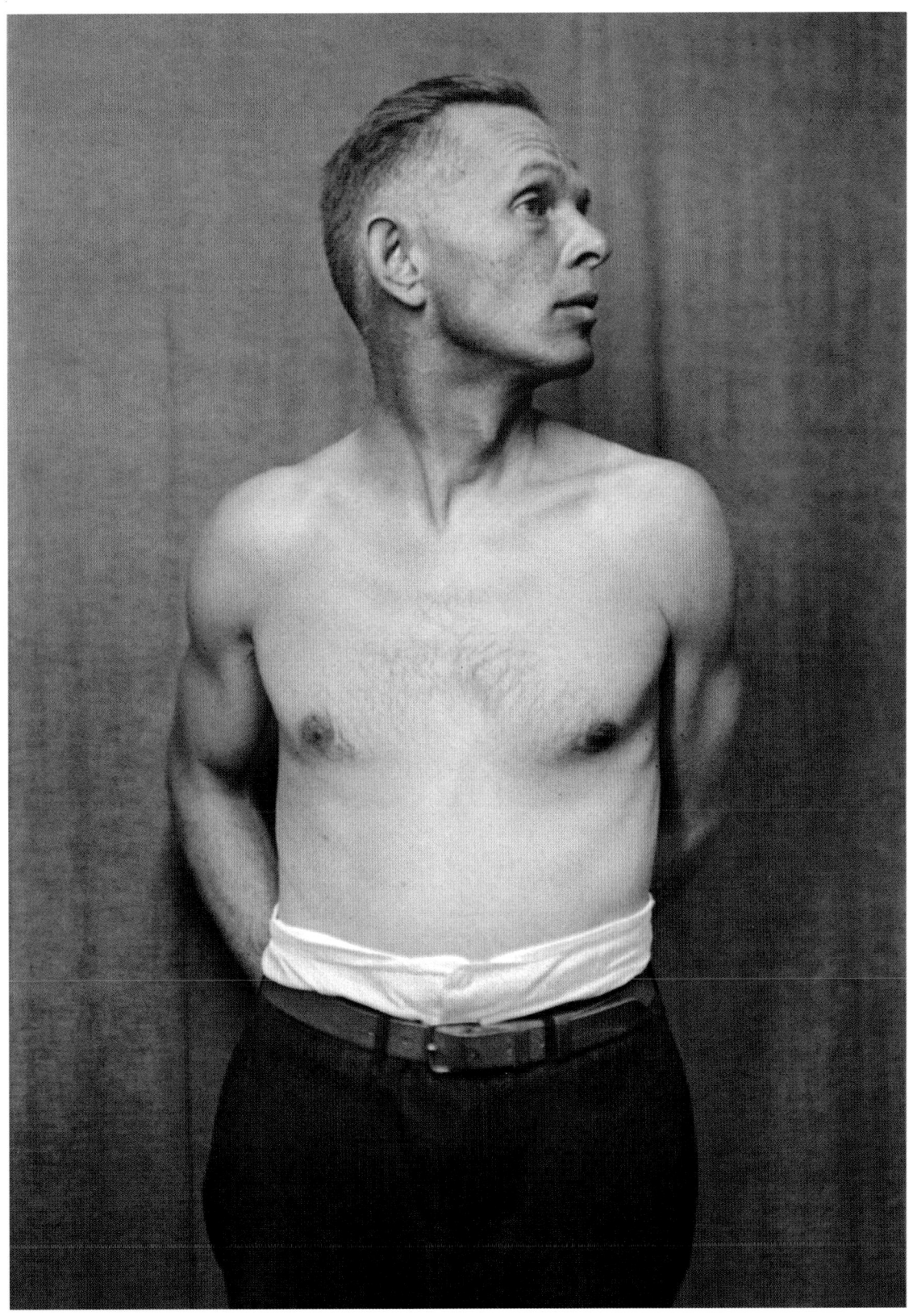

OPPOSITE PAGE. FIG. 1. PREOPERATIVE. ABOVE: FIG. 2. PREOPERATIVE.

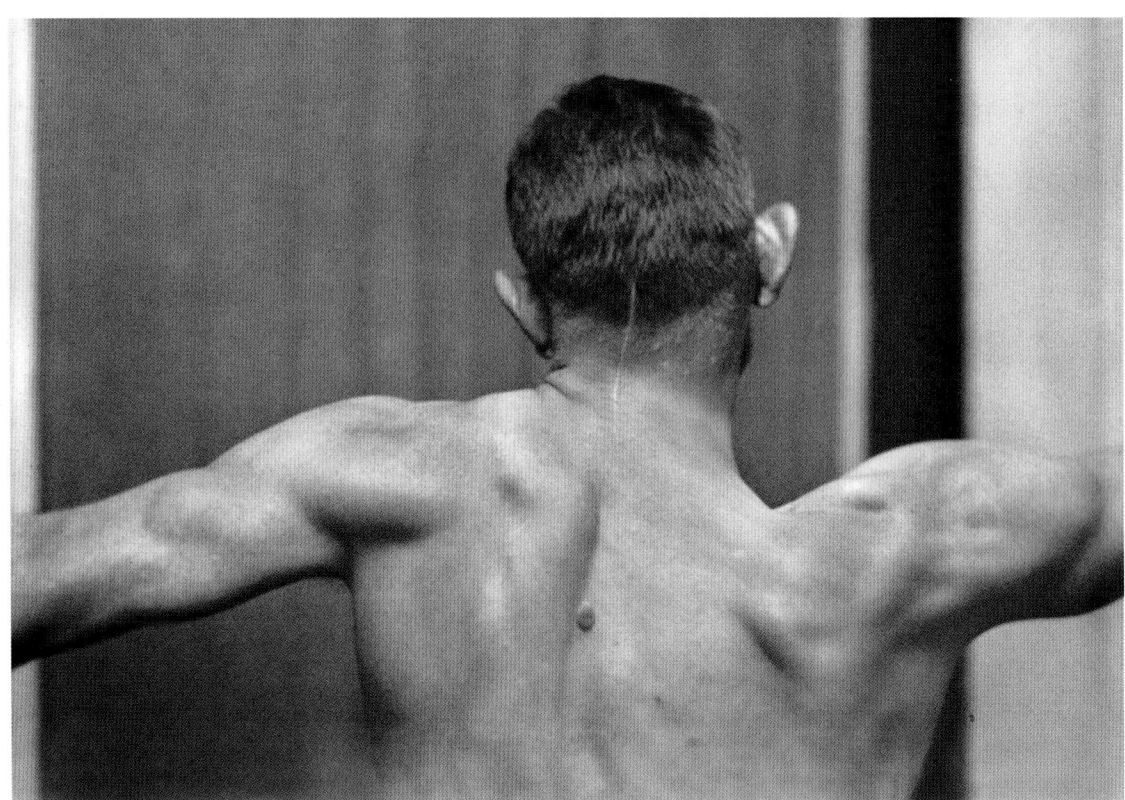

FIG. 3. FOUR MONTHS POSTOPERATIVE — RIGHT SHOULDER WEAKNESS.

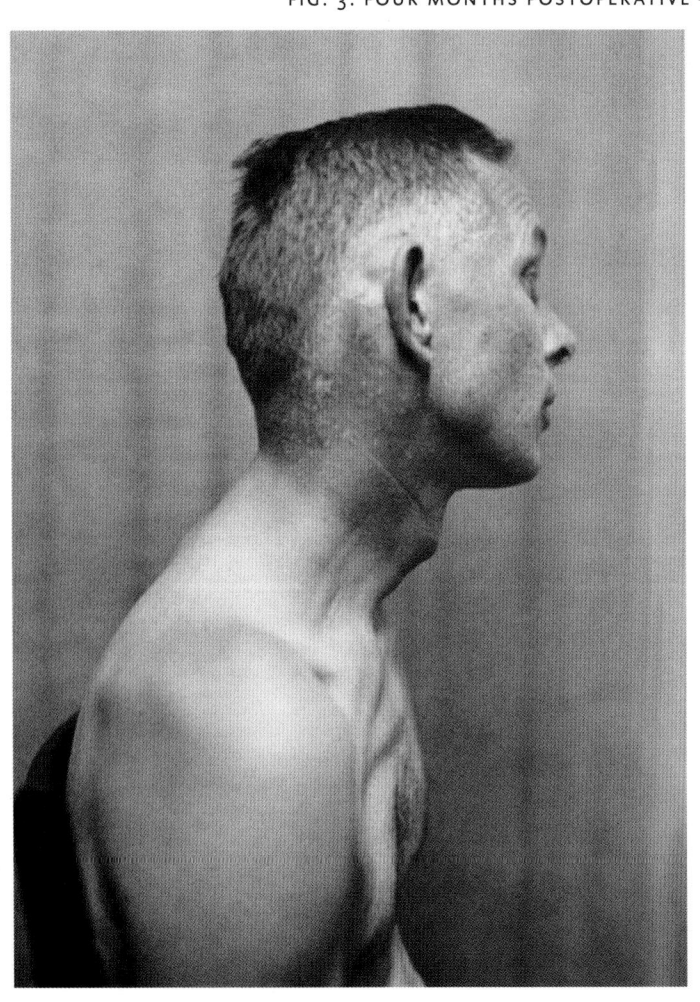

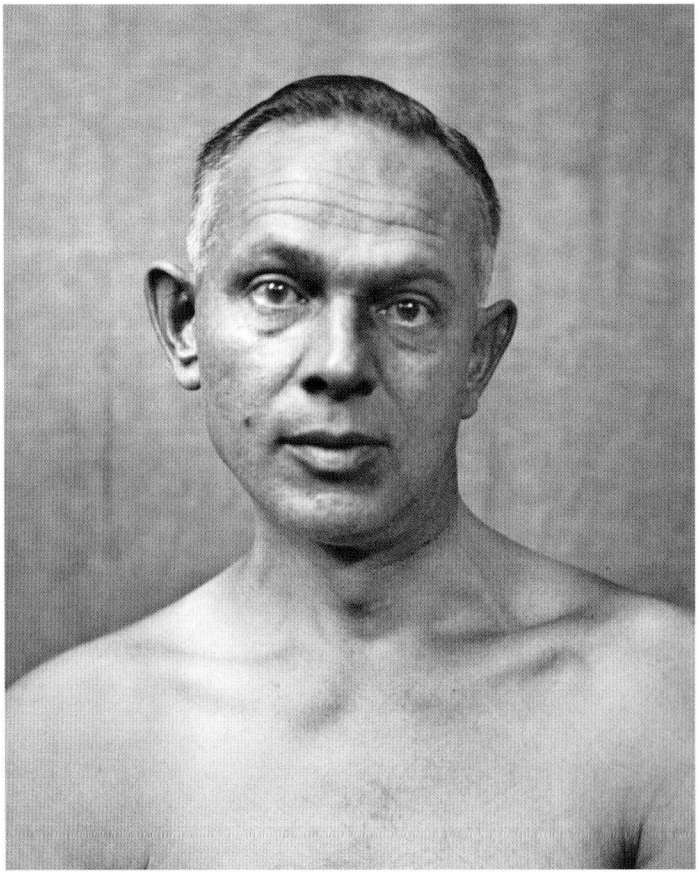

FIG. 4 (LEFT). FOUR MONTHS POSTOPERATIVE. FIG. 5 (ABOVE). FOUR YEARS POSTOPERATIVE — CORRECTION OF NECK POSTURE.

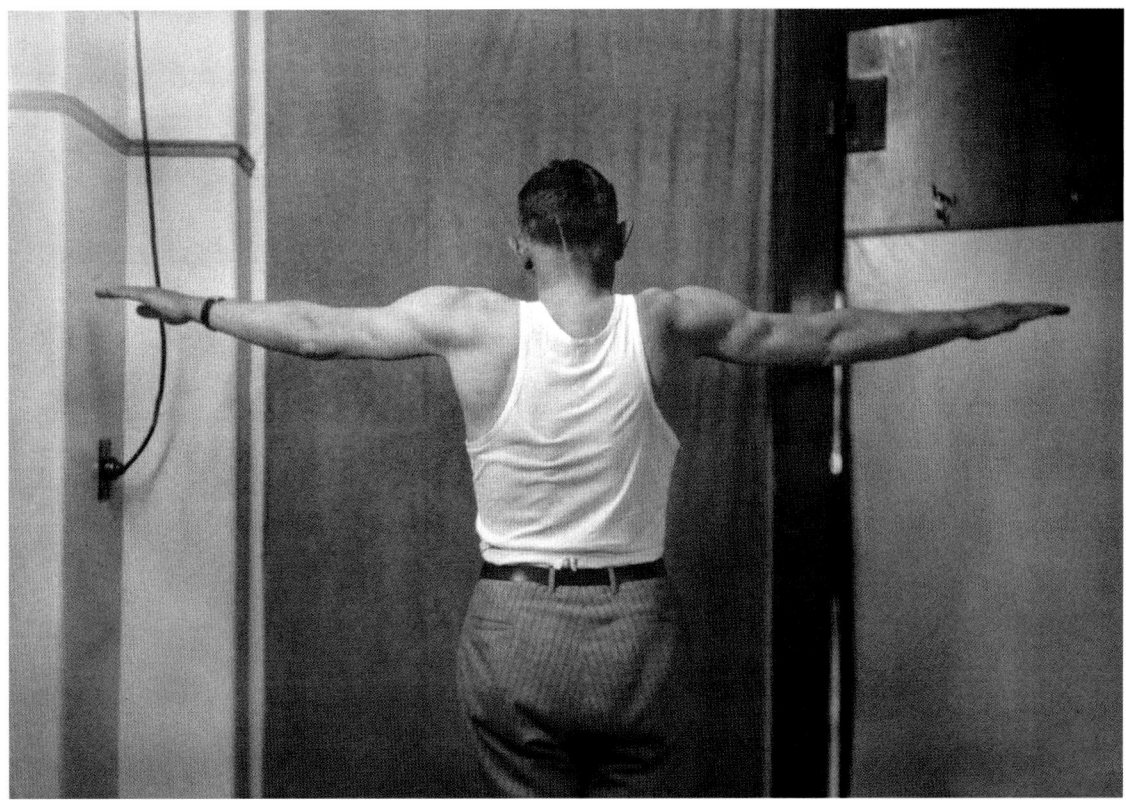

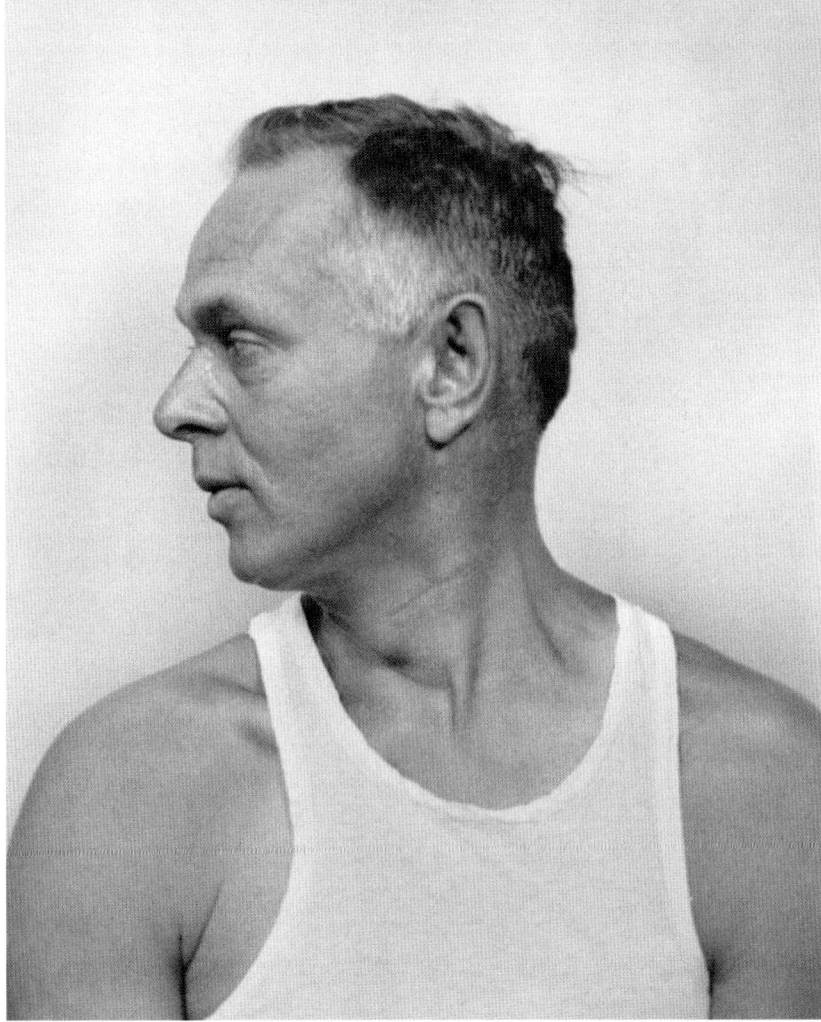

FIG. 6 (ABOVE). FOUR YEARS POSTOPERATIVE – RESOLUTION OF SHOULDER WEAKNESS.

FIG. 7 (LEFT). FOUR YEARS POSTOPERATIVE.

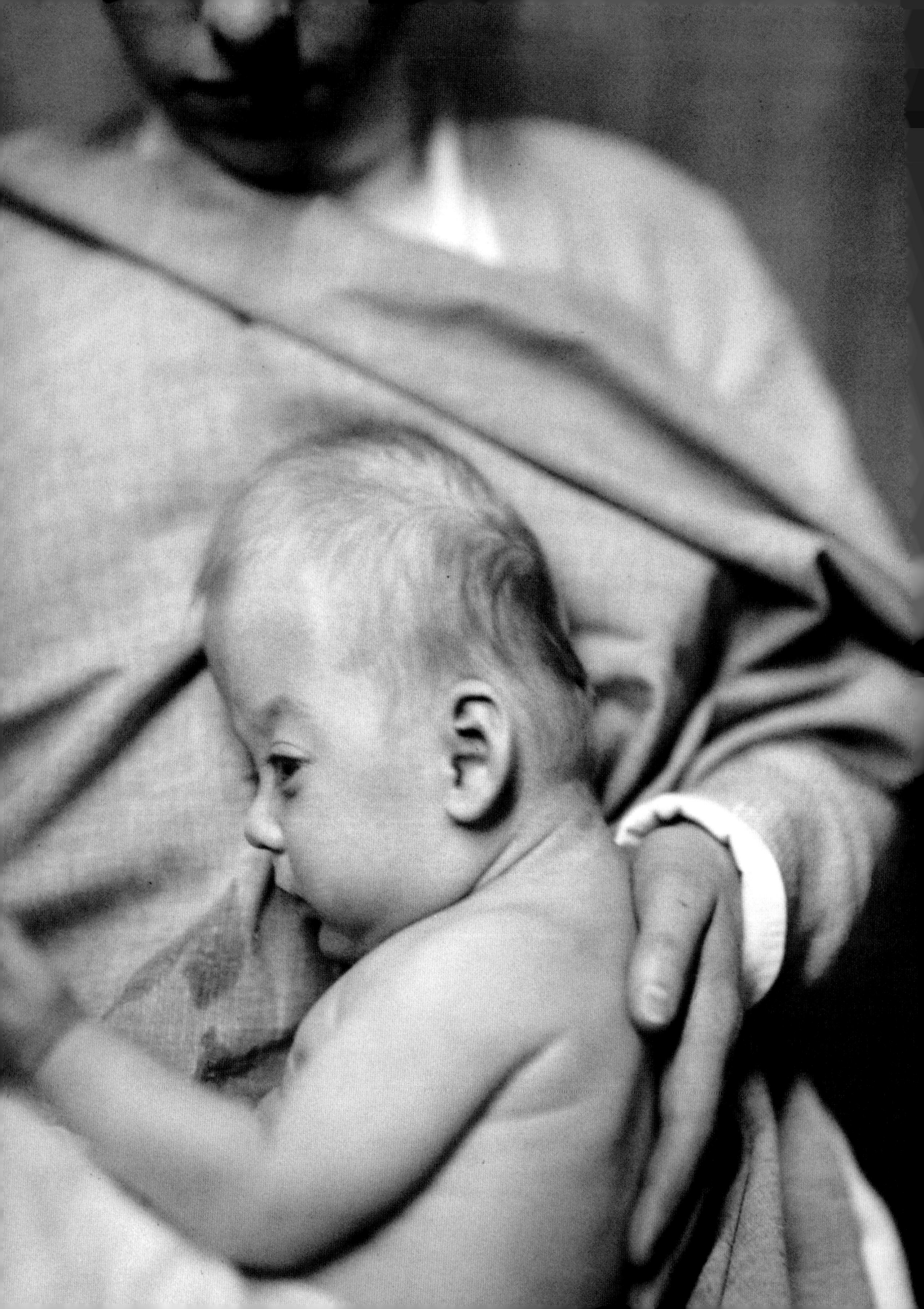

6.15 Craniosynostosis

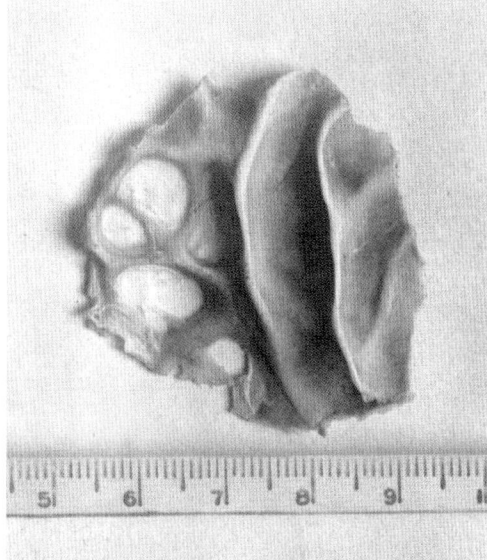

FIG. 4. CRANIECTOMY FLAP.

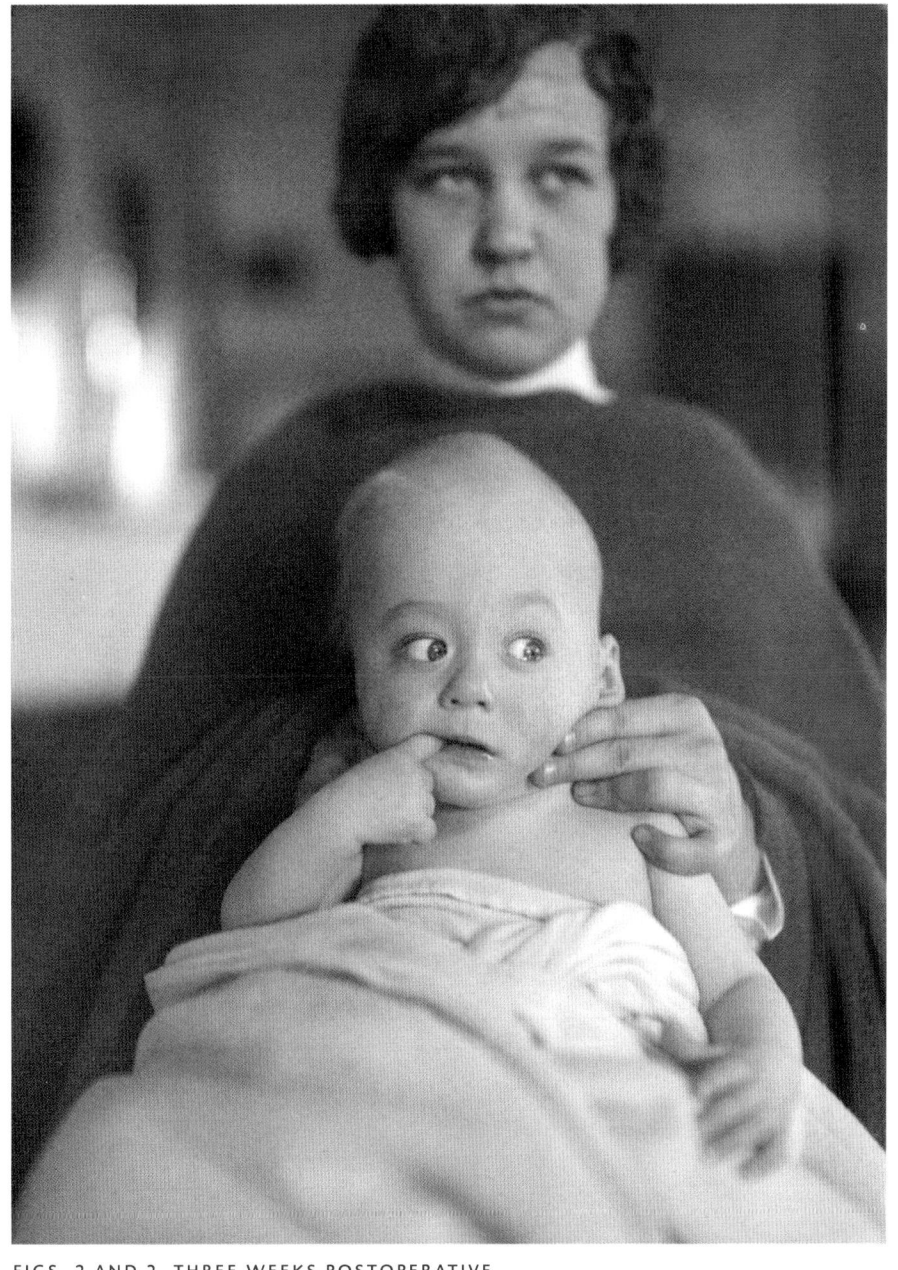

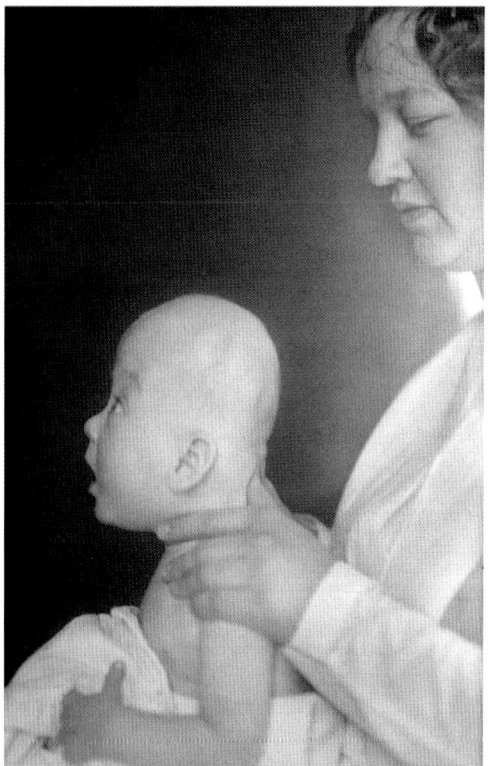

FIGS. 2 AND 3. THREE WEEKS POSTOPERATIVE.

OPPOSITE PAGE. FIG. 1. PREOPERATIVE.

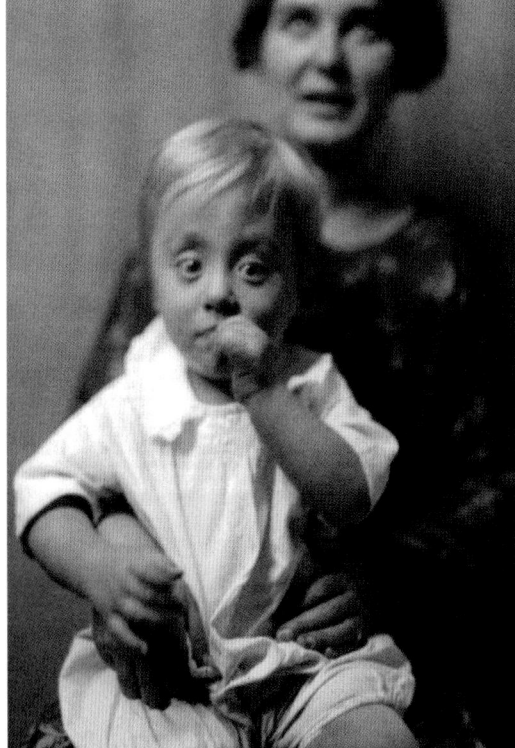
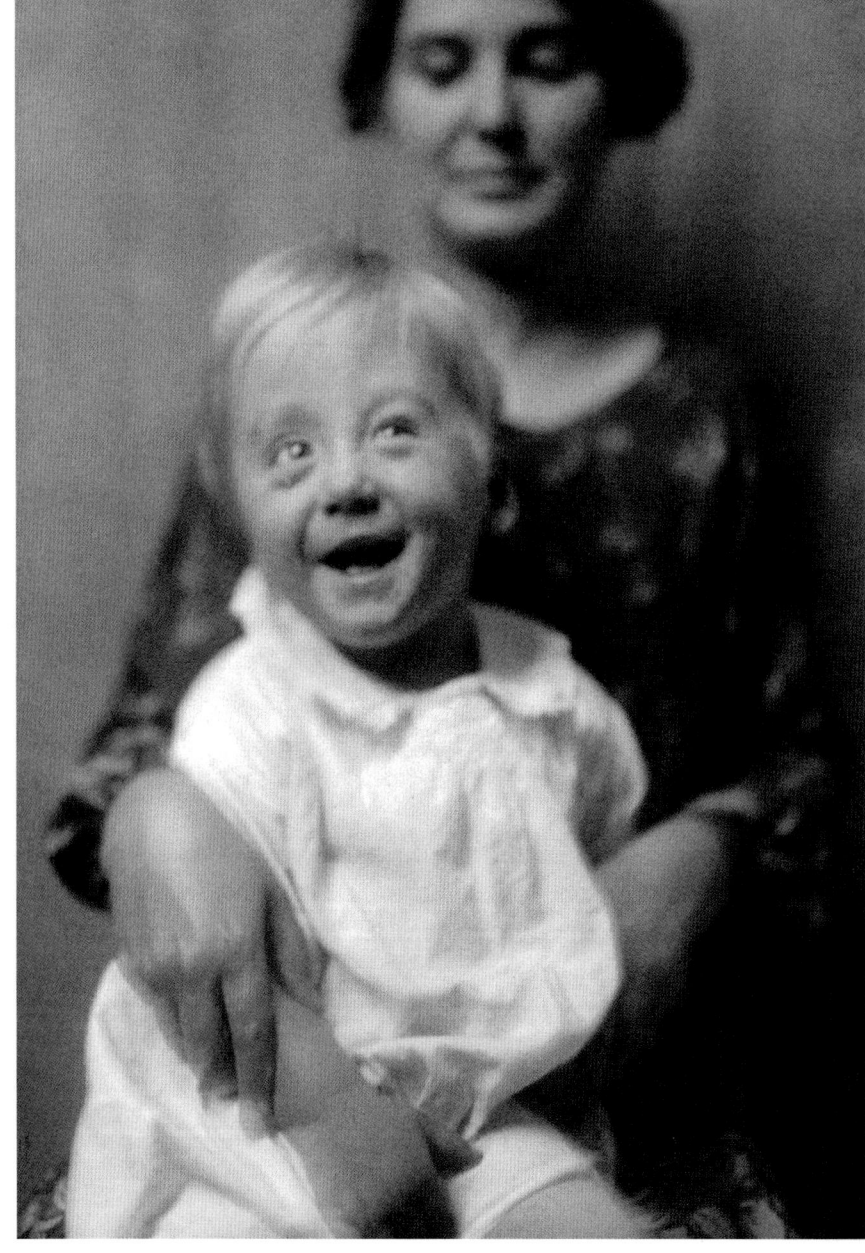

FIGS. 5 AND 6. ONE YEAR FOLLOW UP.

6.16 Fungus cerebri

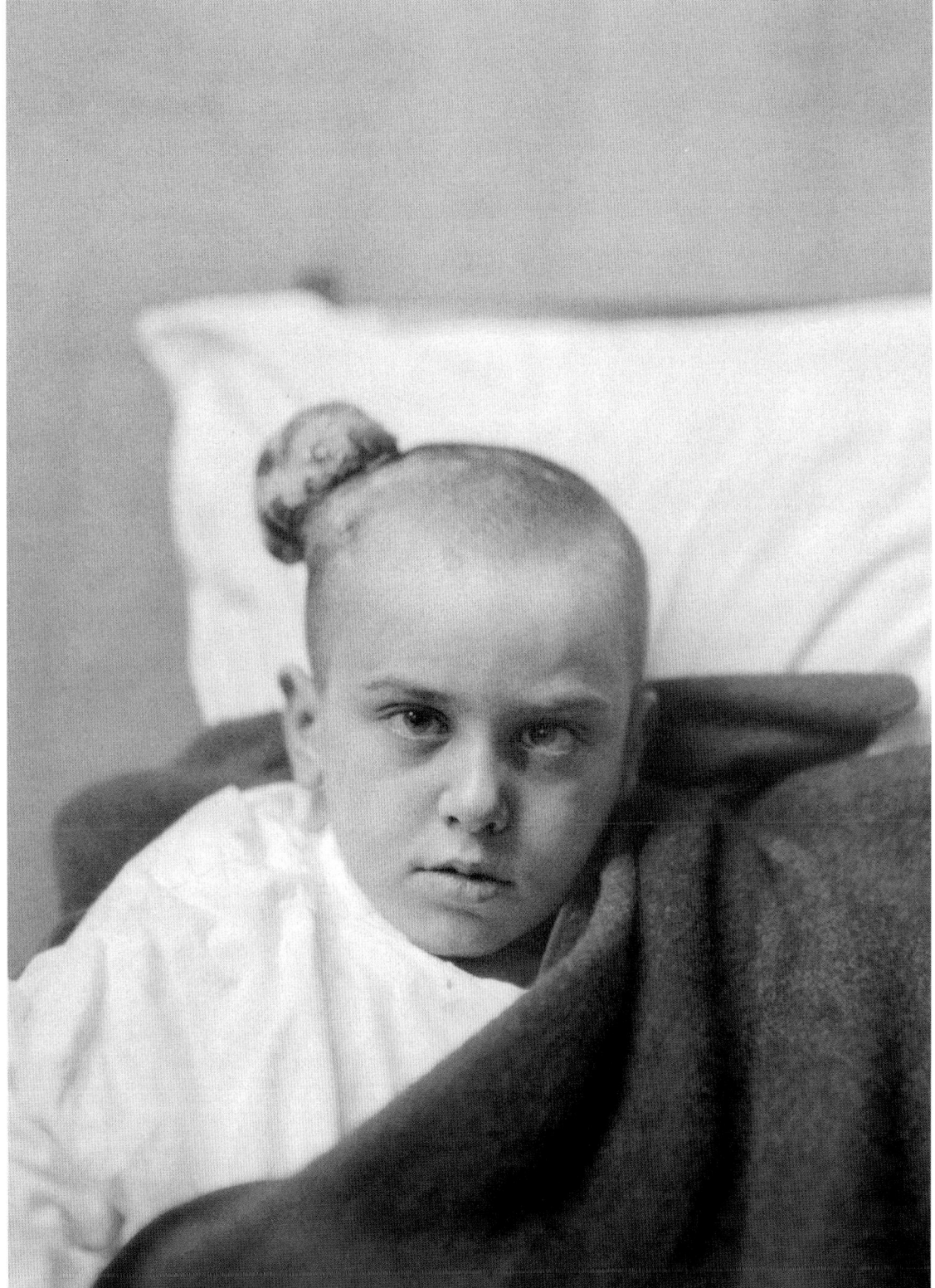

FIG. 2. FIVE DAYS POSTOPERATIVE.

OPPOSITE PAGE. FIG. 1. FIVE DAYS POSTOPERATIVE.

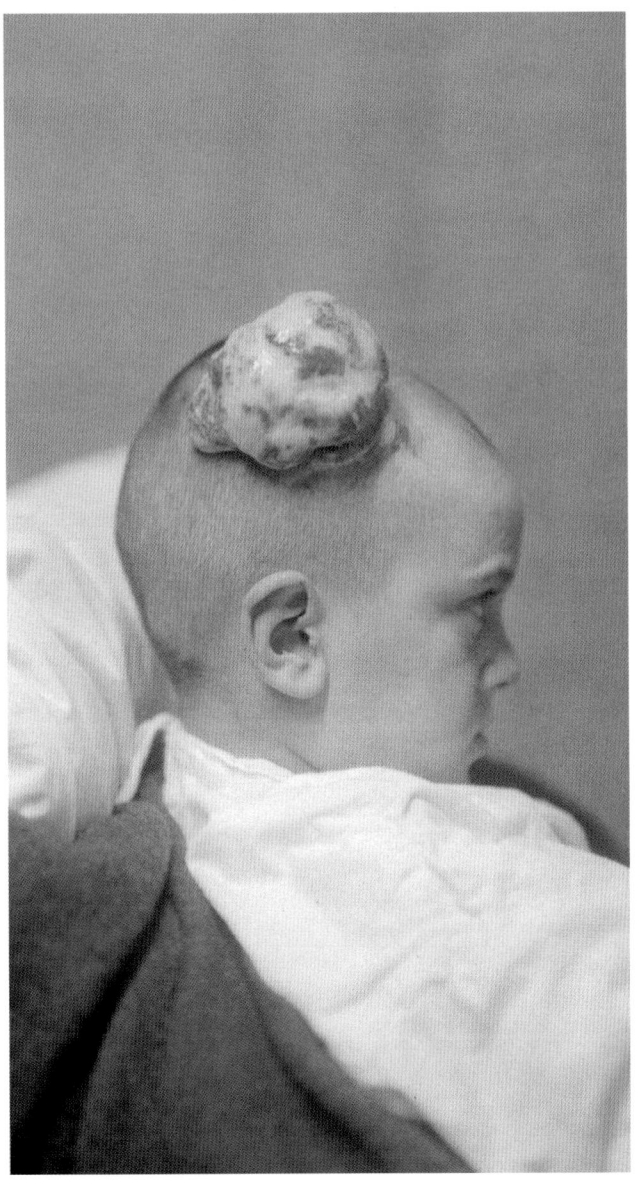

FIG. 3. FIVE DAYS POSTOPERATIVE.

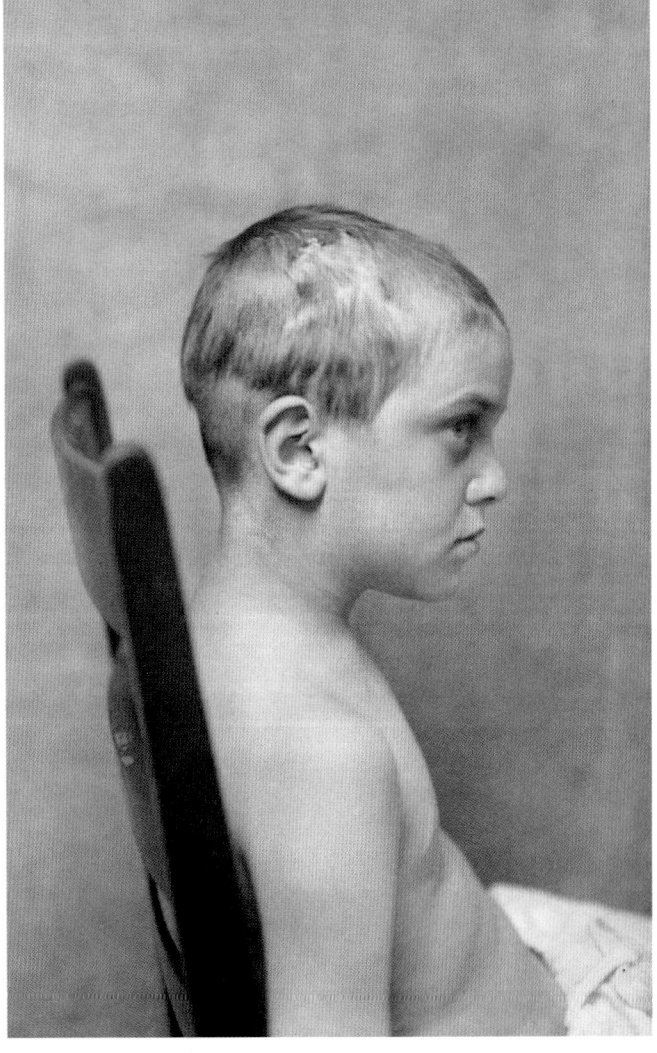

FIG. 4. TWO MONTHS POSTOPERATIVE.

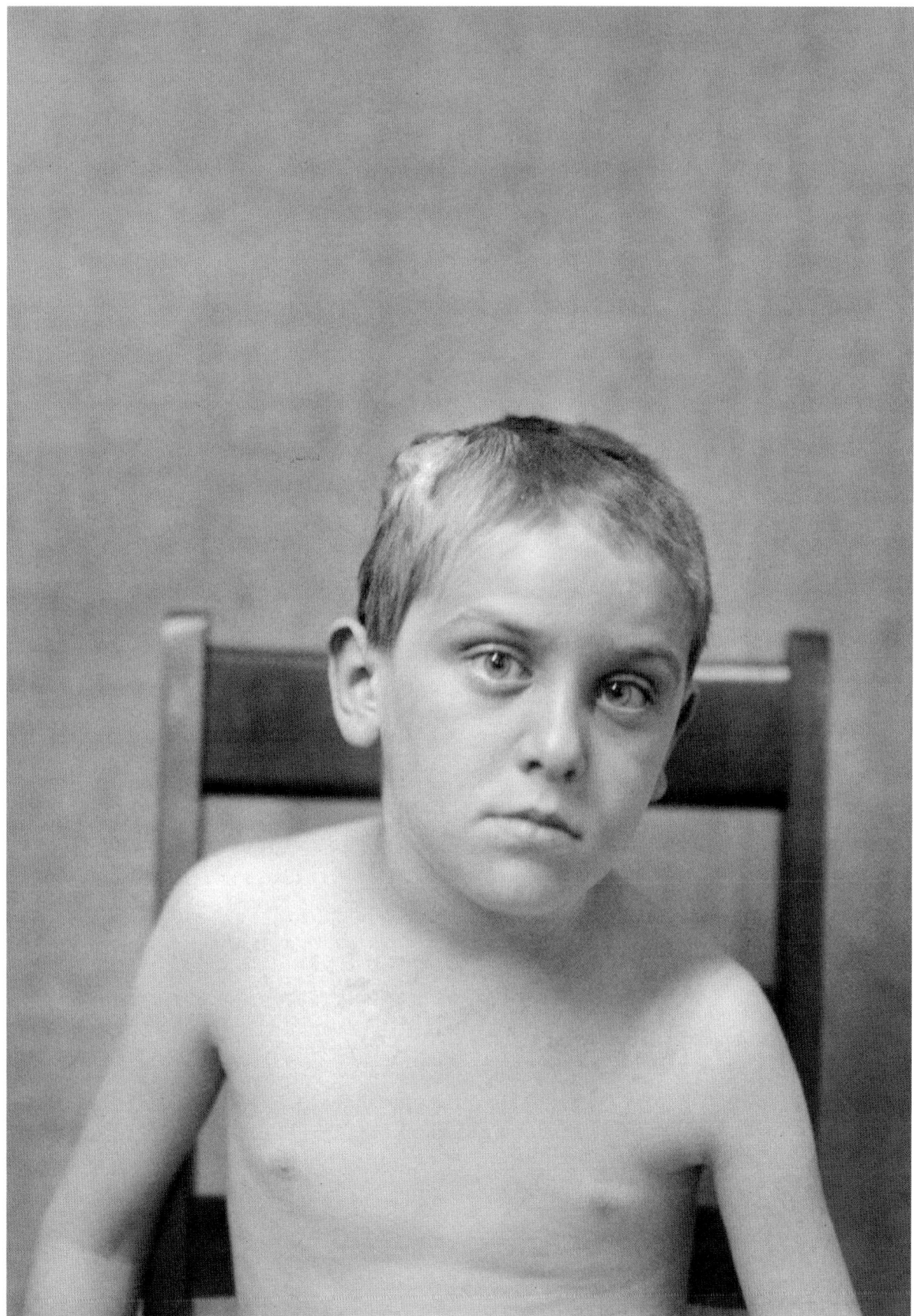

FIG. 5. TWO MONTHS POSTOPERATIVE.

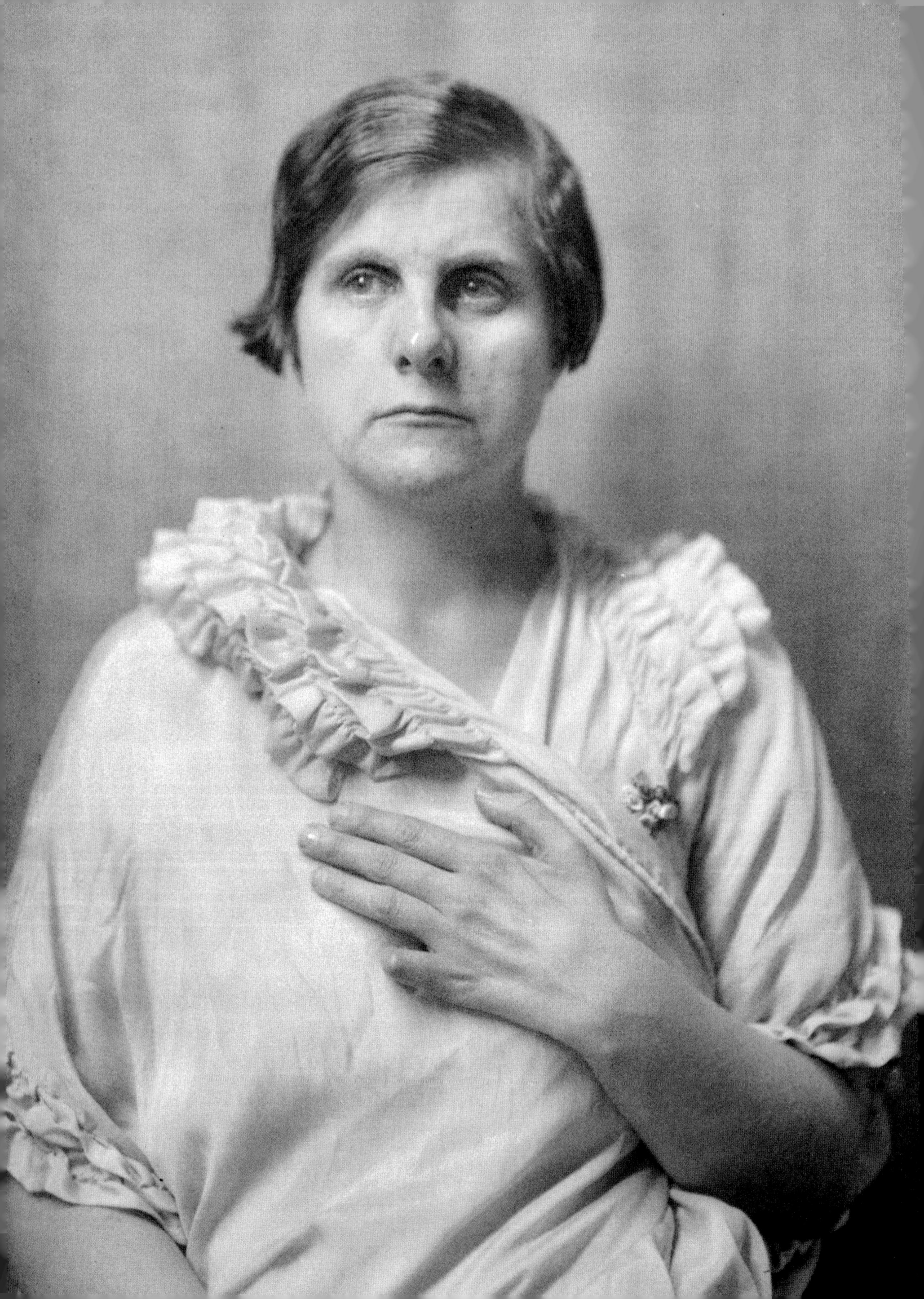

6.17 Ulnar nerve decompression

SEX: F; AGE: 30; SURG. NO. 27266

HISTORY
September 23, 1926
Dr. Cairns

A w.d. and w.n. laboratory technician of 30 re-enters the hospital complaining of weakness, atrophy and paralysis of the left hand, more particularly in the ulnar nerve distribution. In March 1925, following a hypodermic prick there was swelling and inflammation of the left forearm with numbness over the ulnar nerve distribution and motor paralysis of the muscles supplied by the ulnar nerve. It was incised about two weeks after the infection and since then she has had violent urticarial attacks. Her P.H. shows an unusual susceptibility to infection. She returns because during the past year there has been a slowly progressive loss of sensation in the other fingers of the hand and an atrophy of the ulnar muscles as well. P.E. is essentially negative except for nasty skin, hypotention, eruptions on the face, sinus arrhythmia, an early systolic whiff and the local condition. There is complete loss of sensation over the ulnar side of the palm and wrist and little finger and paralysis and contracture of the little finger. There is less sensitivity to pin prick over ...

OPERATIVE NOTE
October 2, 1926
Anesthesia – Ether – Miss Way

Neurolysis for Infection of Unknown Origin Occurring in the Depth of the Tissues of the Left Arm.

With the patient's arm in the position shown in the accompanying sketch a long incision was made finally reaching from near the external condyle 2/3rds of the distance down the arm. So soon as the scar in this situation was excised the most curious blue fascial sheaths were brought into view. It was suggested by Mr. Cairns that this might have been due to the mercurochrome which had been used. The flexor carpi ulnaris was identified and drawn outward as shown in the accompanying sketch. Finally in the midst of the scar the ulnar nerve was brought into view, though before it was cleared of its enveloping scar the nerve both distally and proximally was fully exposed. It was fortu-

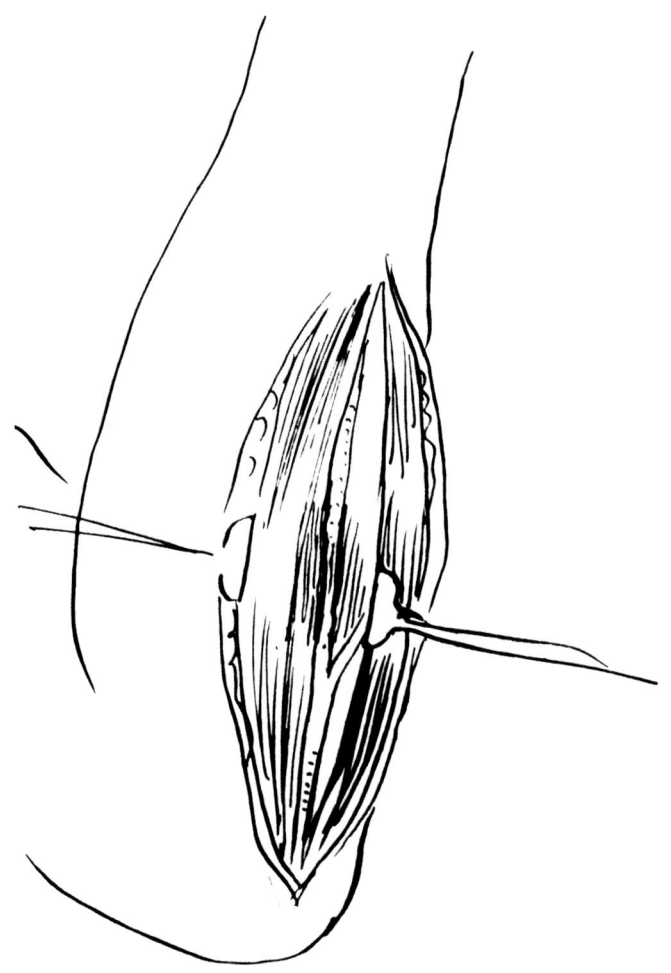

FIG. 2. SURGEON'S DRAWING.

nate that this was done; otherwise the branch to the flexor carpi ulnaris would have been divided. Whether any branches to the flexor sublimus group were divided is difficult to tell.

A fairly dense mass of scar tissue which enveloped the nerve was finally broken open and the nerve freed. The wound was then closed carefully in successive layers by fine silk sutures. No tissues.

(Dr. Cushing)

October 4, 1926
Dr. Cairns

Wound dressed by Dr. Cushing. Some overriding of the edges of the incision, nearer the upper end than the lower. At this part the wound was reopened and some fresh stitches inserted. Arm and forearm enclosed in starch casing.

October 8, 1926
Dr. Cairns

For the first time since onset of ulnar palsy there has been sensation in the ulnar side of the hand: momentary flashes of a burning, rather painful sensation in little and ring fingers. Also has pain up forearm when she passively extends the little fingers. Never had this before operation. Starch casing is very comfortable indeed. Objectively there is no change in anesthesia which is still complete over ulnar distribution of hand. In connection with the peculiar greenish color of the muscles noted at this last operation the patient states that when the infected area was opened at the first operation the surgeon noted a peculiar green color of the tissues. In subsequent treatment mercurochrome was injected locally into the tissues of the forearm.

The patient was discharged " improved."

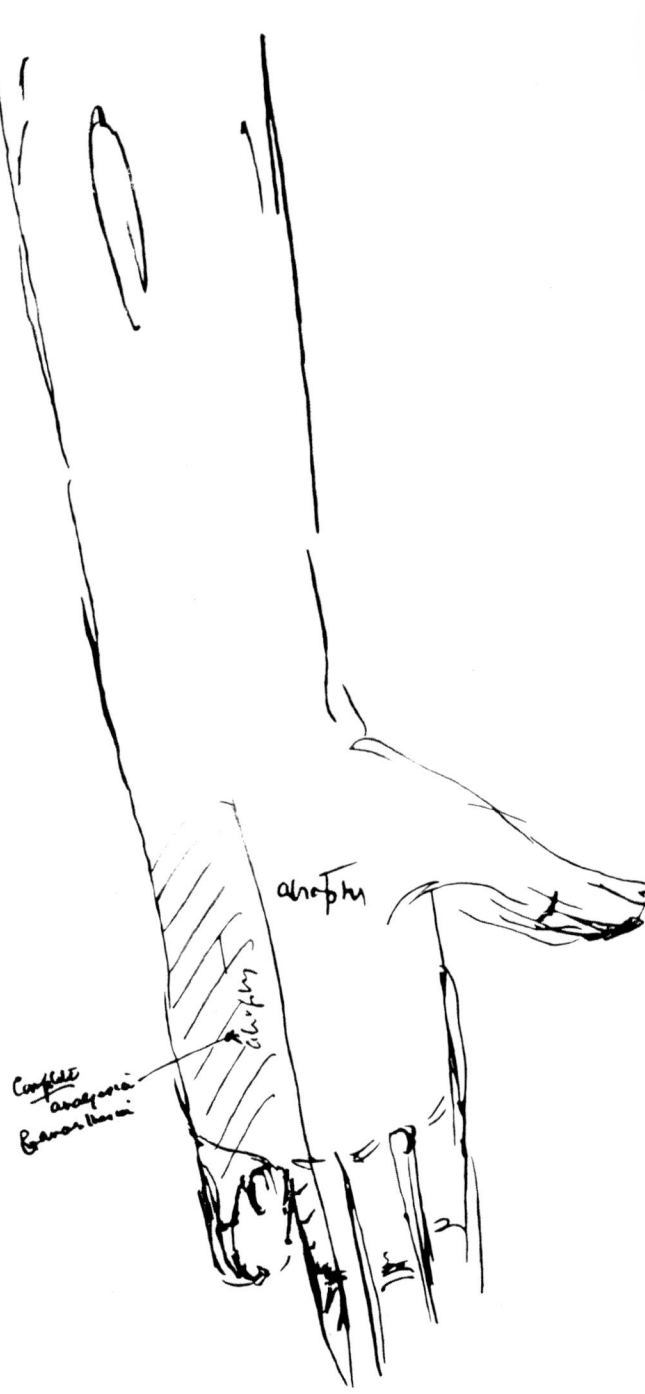

FIG. 4. PREOPERATIVE FINDINGS.

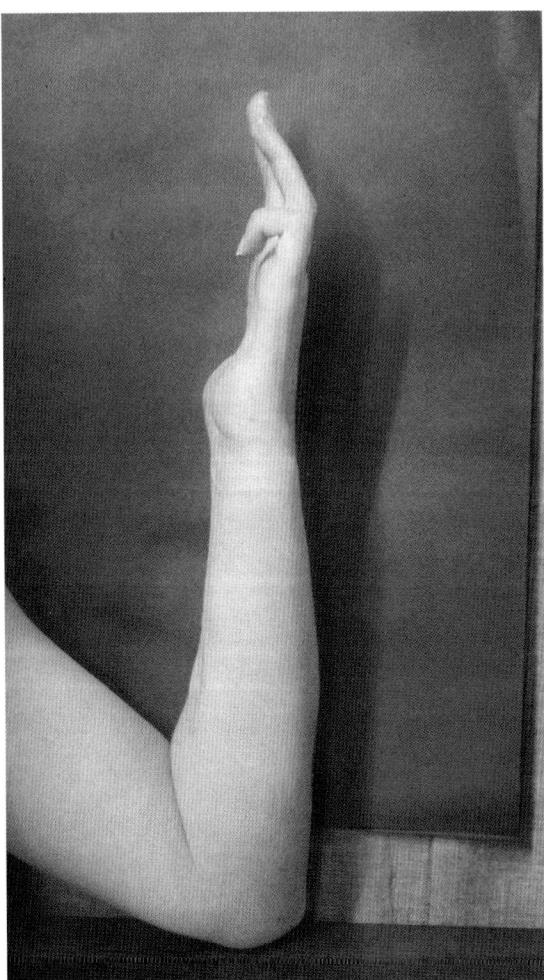

FIG. 3. PREOPERATIVE EXAM — ATROPHY AND CONTRACTURE OF THE LITTLE FINGER

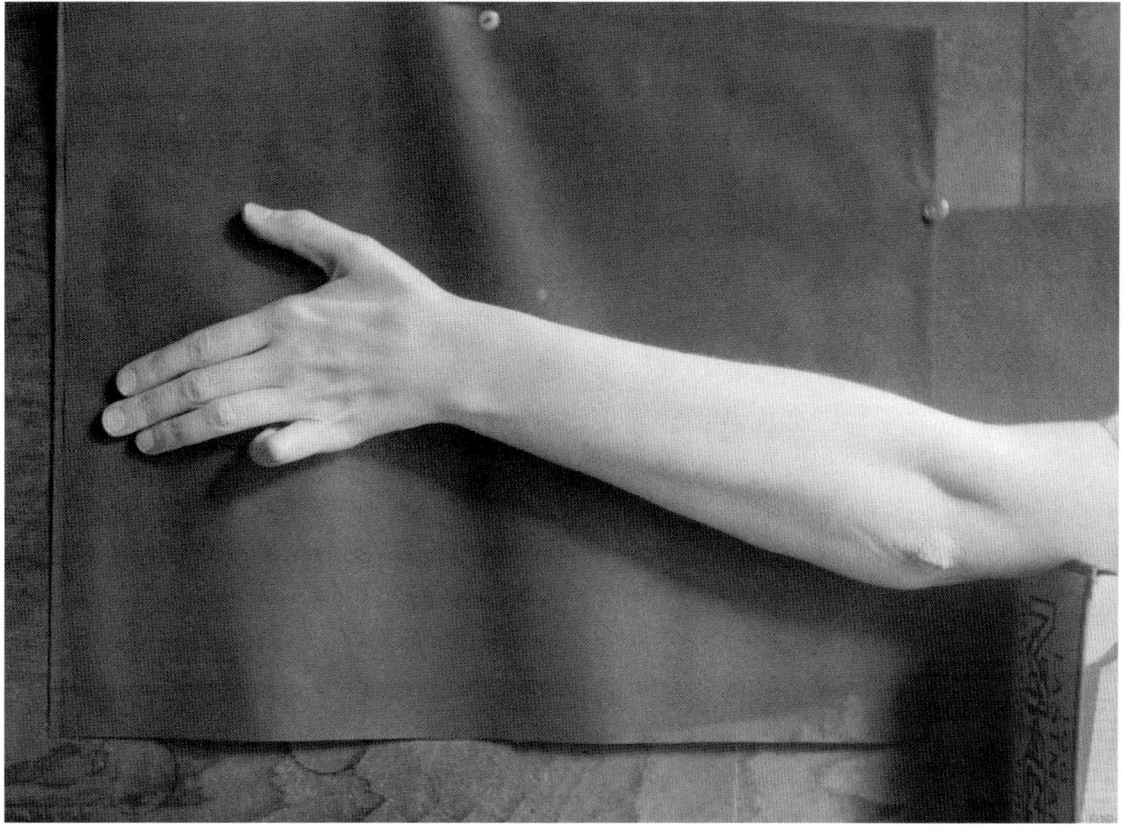

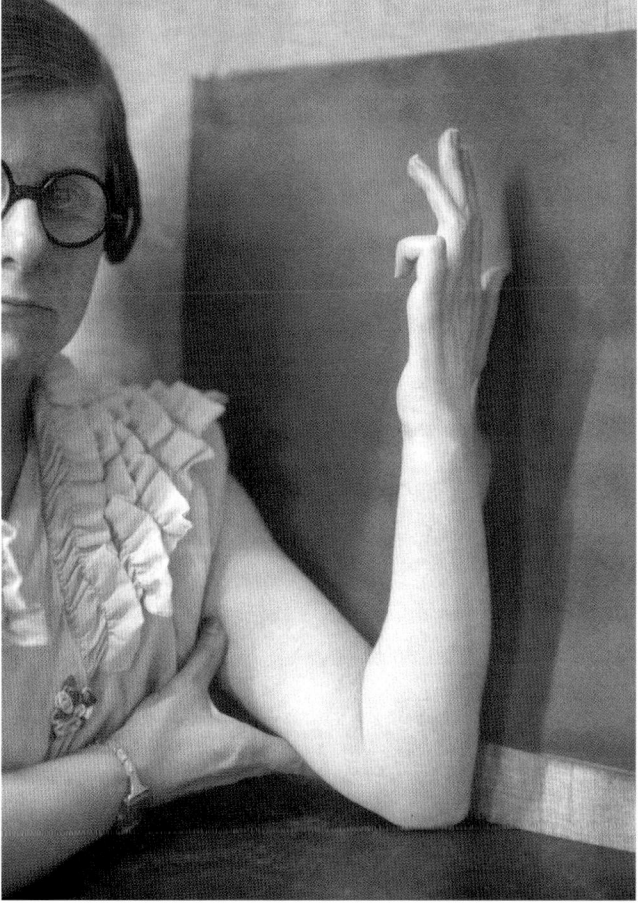

FIGS. 5 AND 6. PREOPERATIVE EXAM — ATROPHY AND CONTRACTURE OF THE LITTLE FINGER

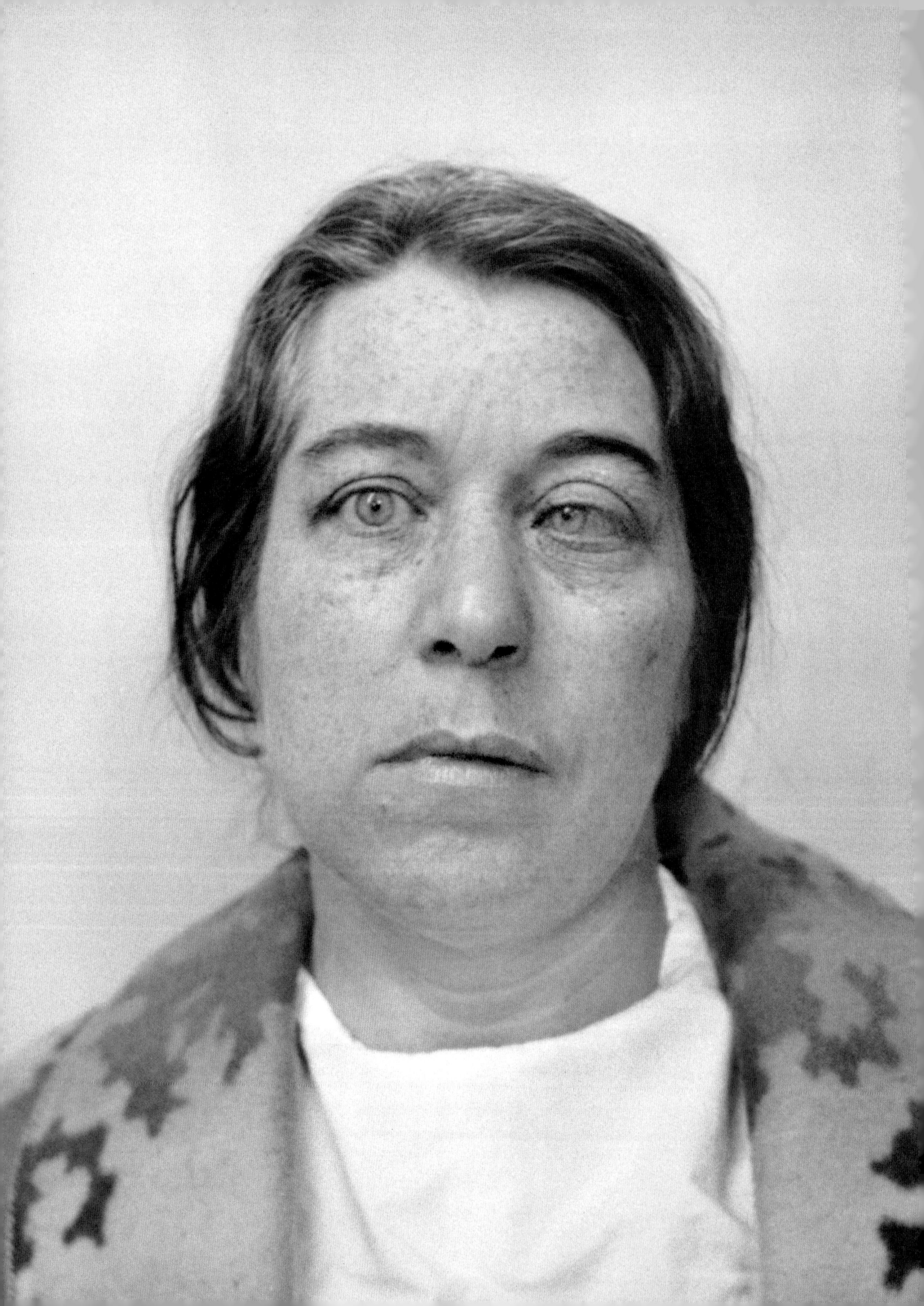

6.18 Petroclival epidermoid cholesteatoma

SEX: F; AGE: 44; SURG. NO. 32822, 35158

FIRST TWO HOSPITAL ADMISSIONS

HISTORY

In December 1926, the patient was admitted in the hospital with left facial numbness, first time noticed about the left upper lip approximately 15 months prior to this admission. This paraesthesia slowly spread to involve the left side of her face. There was diminution of hearing of the left ear. X-rays showed increased intracranial pressure, without any localizing signs. Dr. Horrax found tortuous retinal veins with absent optic cup. The laboratory findings and lumbar puncture results were non-contributory. Dr. Horrax suspected a cerebello-pontine angle tumor. The patient was discharged without treatment.

In May 1927, the patient was readmitted with the same symptoms, but slightly exaggerated. The neurological examination showed a possible partial anosmia on the left side, marked hyperaesthesia on the left side of the face, absent left corneal reflex, protrusion of the tongue to the right with a fine tremor, a lack of sensation of taste on the left side of her tongue, absent abdominal reflexes, and exaggerated deep tendon reflexes. She believed she did not receive "enough attention" in the hospital and insisted on going home and was discharged four days after entry without treatment.

After discharge, the patient did fairly well and noticed no new symptoms until three months before her third admission.

THIRD HOSPITAL ADMISSION

SUMMARY OF POSITIVE FINDINGS
December 7, 1928
Dr. Schreiber

SUBJECTIVE
1. Increasing numbness of left face, and diplopia for 4½ years.
2. Frequent dizzy spells without loss of consciousness. Three weeks ago had one with loss of consciousness.
3. Impairment of memory and cerebration.
4. Difficulty in voiding.

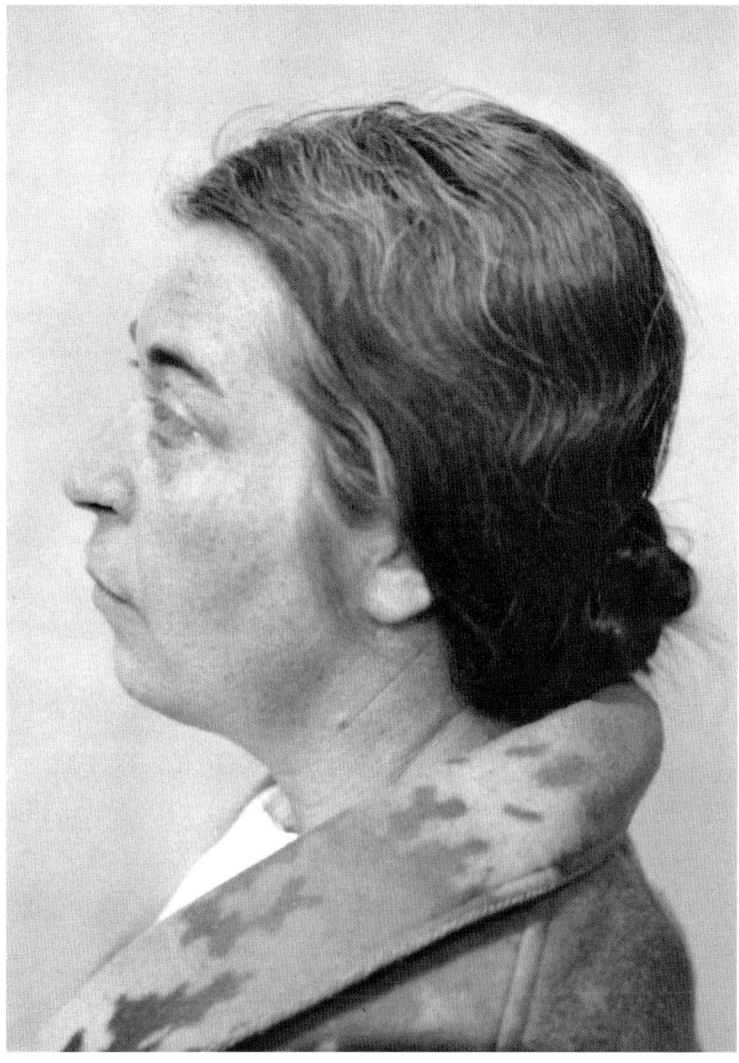

FIG. 2. PREOPERATIVE

OBJECTIVE
1. Complete impairment of left trigeminus.
2. Left external rectus palsy.
3. Reflexes: Bilateral Babinski. Absent corneal, pharyngeal, abdominal.
4. Increased right elbow jerk, and left knee kick.
5. Crusting lesion of left nares.
6. Keratitis of left eye.
7. Suggestion of aphasia.

IMPRESSION: Meningioma of left temporal fossa much in the same position as that of (the name of another patient) who was just discharged from C-2.

OPPOSITE PAGE. FIG. I. PREOPERATIVE

December 8, 1928
Dr. Schreiber

Seen in O.R. by Dr. Cushing. "Very likely temporal fossa meningioma."

SPECIAL NOTE
December 22, 1928
Dr. Cushing

This was a most interesting, encouraging, and suggestive operation in a case which offered very little more than an exploration with perhaps removal of some fragments of a meningioma. The diagnosis of a meningioma involving the Gasserian envelopes was a natural one, in view of the patient's symptomatology. The operation was relayed with Dr. Horrax who turned down the usual flap of the magnified ganglion type for operations in this region.

This case is not only interesting in itself, but illuminating to me on the ground that it shows possibly a novel way of getting at the Gasserian ganglion, absolutely free from any difficulty with bleeding, even from the meningeal artery. I think that it could be done easily enough through the ordinary ganglion opened without bone flap, though of course a bone flap would greatly facilitate the operation. Indeed, it would hardly be necessary to expose the whole ganglion as was done in this case. I feel that if the dura is put on tension down to the region of the foramen spinosum and a small puncture is then made on each side of the meningeal artery with an electric needle, while the brain is necessarily elevated, it will be possible to put a clip easily on the vessel and then to make an opening through the dura, which will allow the immediate escape of cerebrospinal fluid. Then on increasing this opening along in the direction of the third and second divisions, it would be easily possible to elevate the brain so that with the electric needle the dura can be opened over the sensory root by electrical methods and the fibers can be picked out directly from above instead of underneath the dura, as is the usual method of procedure. As a matter of fact, this is not a vastly different operation in which the dura is reflected upward, and incision is made in such a position as to directly enter the sheath of the root. However, for our method of operating, with the patient lying down, I think it would be much easier than the operation which we do. Unquestionably, it would be more awkward for those who operate with the patient sitting, one looks down upon the ganglion rather than up at it.

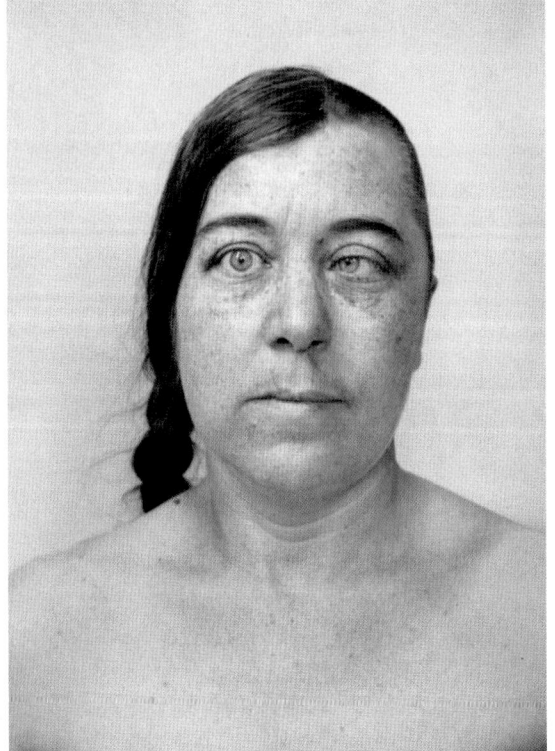
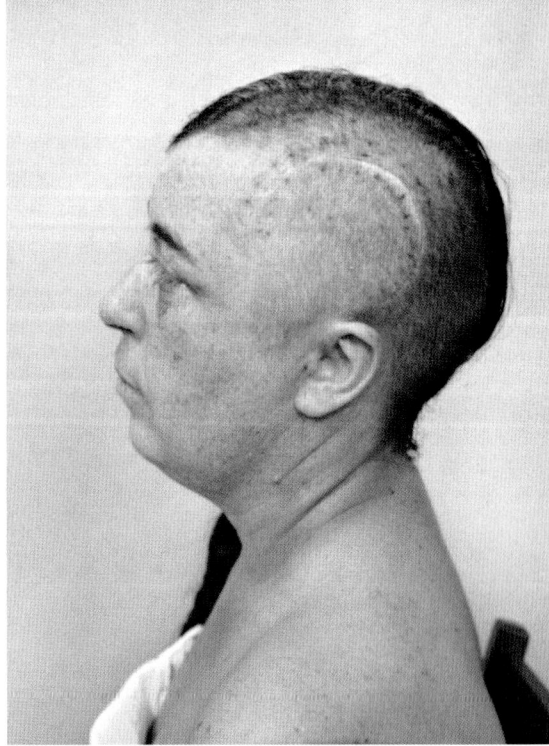

FIGS. 3–4. TWO WEEKS POSTOPERATIVE (FIRST OPERATION)

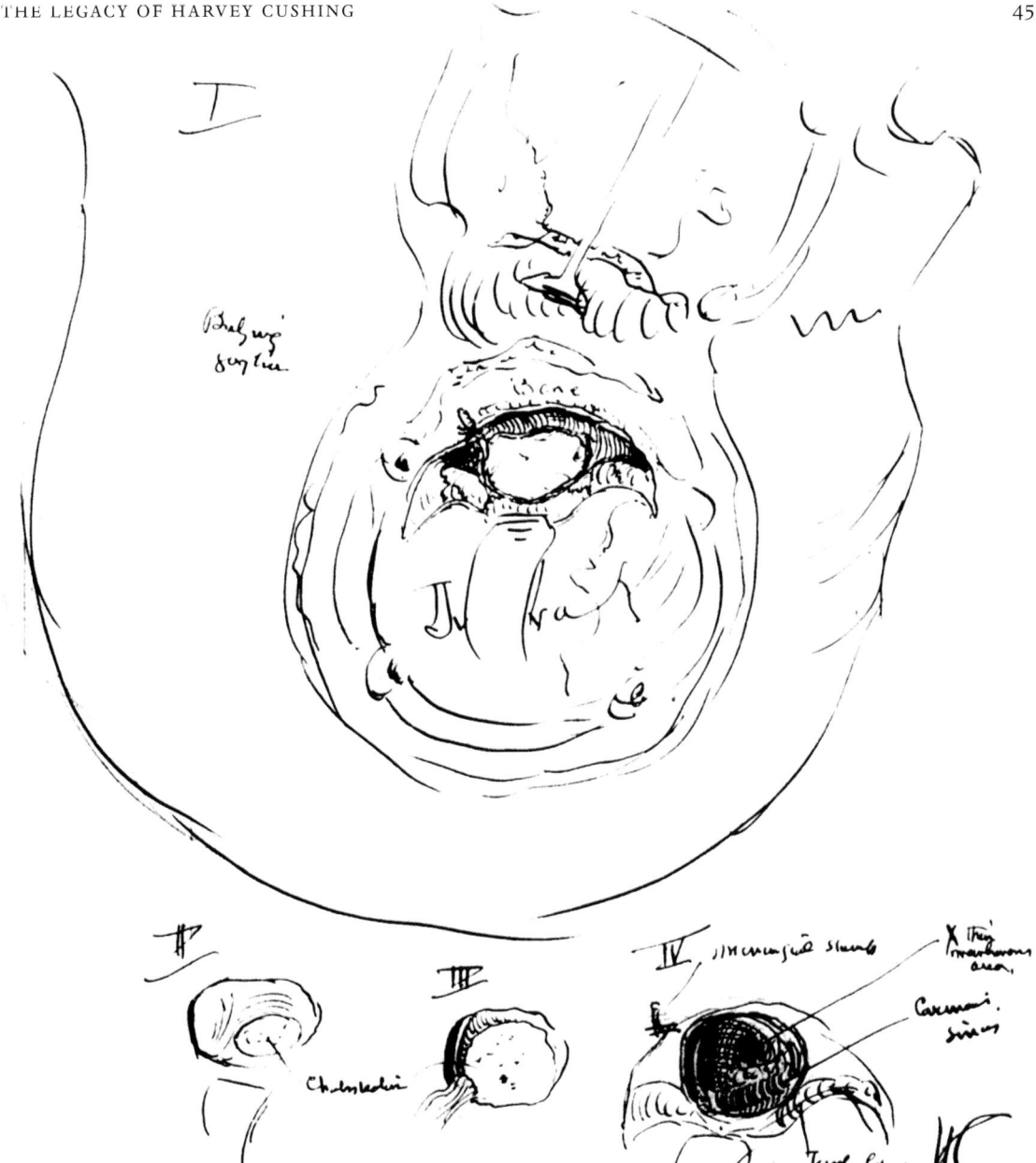

FIG. 5. OPERATIVE SKETCH (FIRST OPERATION).

OPERATIVE NOTE
December 22, 1928
Anesthesia – Novocain

Left Osteoplastic Temporal Exploration. Subtemporal Bone Defect. Negative Extradural Findings. Incision of Dura along Attachment of Gasserian Envelope. Reflection of Temporal Lobe and Dura Upward. Intradural Inspection of Gasserian Ganglion by Electrosurgical Opening of Upper Envelope. Shredded Thin Ganglion Disclosed. Ganglion Brushed Aside Exposing Subjacent Cholesteatoma about 2 cm in Diameter. Extirpation of Sac of Cholesteatoma Exposing Cavernous Sinus.

The bone flap had been turned down by Dr. Horrax without difficulty, the brain being found under considerable tension. He had made a subtemporal defect and had begun to strip the dura from the temporal fossa in the direction of the third division of the ganglion.

At this juncture I took over the procedure.

As stated, the dura was so tense that in view of the fact that the patient was not under general anaesthesia, I thought in all probability there would be an intradural tumor. I stripped the dura away from the bone well down to the attachment of the 2nd and 3rd divisions and elevated the dura enough so that had there been the margin of a meningioma in this region I certainly should have palpated it. Moreover, there was no increased vascularity which speaks against a meningioma.

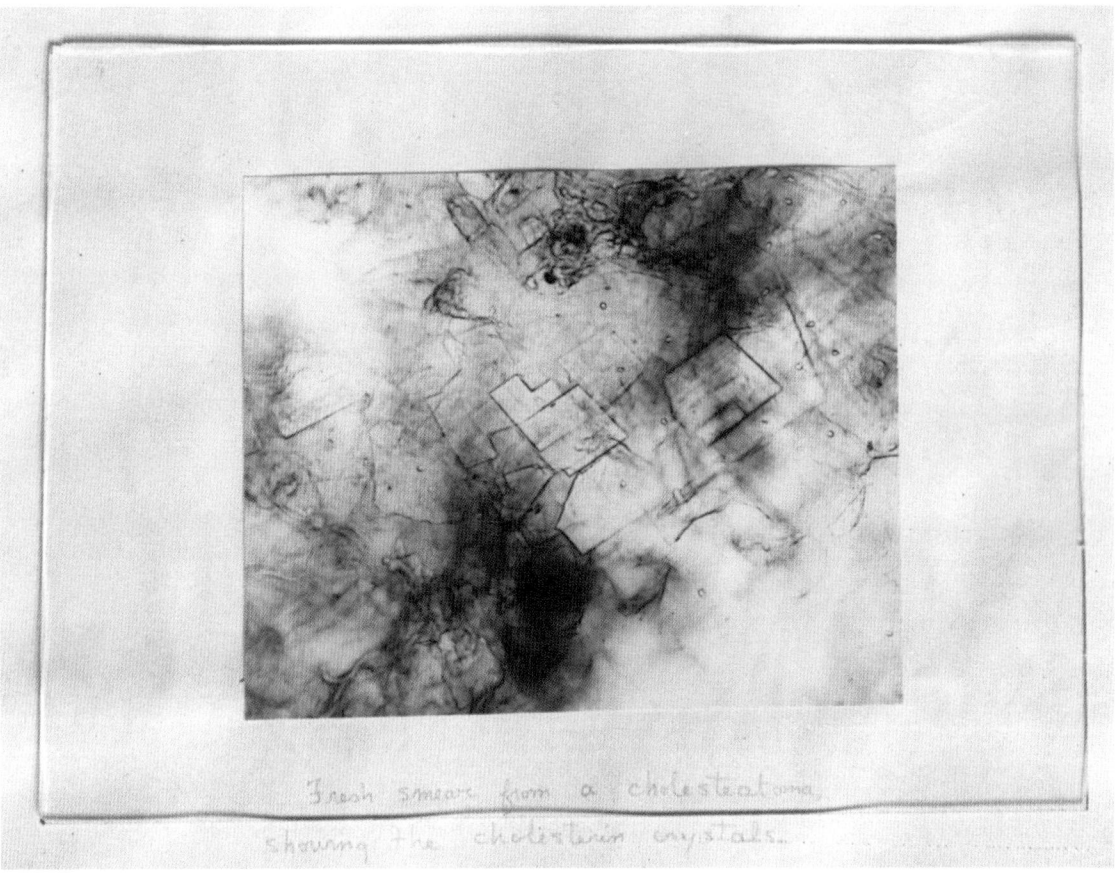

FIG. 6. HISTOLOGY SLIDE

In view of these facts, I thought I would see if I could get fluid by nicking the dura at its point of attachment just as we would in a transfrontal exploration to expose the optic nerves. I accordingly with the hook-knife, holding the brain well upward, made a short incision and an immense amount of fluid escaped, completely lowering tension. I then increased this incision in the usual fashion by putting in a pledget of cotton to hold the brain away and then incising the dura until I had an opening in the dura corresponding practically to that shown in sketch #1 (Sketch for the first operation, I). It was then possible to elevate the temporal lobe, well protected by dura, so that I could see the base of the fossa. I was surprised to find that instead of the fossa rounding out below, as I looked in toward the region of the cavernous sinus it seemed to be distinctly bulging, and though it was bulging it was soft as though it contained fluid. Never having exposed in an operation the Gasserian ganglion from this aspect, I was at a loss to know whether this was due merely to fluid or whether it was a normal condition, and I accordingly made a small incision through what I took to be the upper envelopes of the ganglion, and came down upon unmistakable nerve tissue in which I could see the fibers running in the expected direction. Tissue, however, looked edematous, and I finally enlarged the opening, brushed the dura to the side and coagulated it so that it tended to shrink up and pucker away from the field until I had the top of the ganglion exposed about as shown in Fig. #1 (Sketch for the first operation, I.)

The ganglion had a most peculiar edematous and yellowish appearance, and on gradually picking at the fibers, I found that the fibers of the first division shredded out away from the region of the cavernous sinus and there was exposed the unmistakable mass of glistening cells of the contents of a cholesteatoma, the upper wall of which I must have broken into while shredding these fibers away. This appearance is shown in sketch #2 (Sketch for the first operation, II.)

I then pulled the fibers of the first and 2nd divisions outward and cut it off at about the foramen of exit and reflected the thin and shredded ganglion upward, as shown in Fig. 3 (Sketch for the first operation, III.) This maneuver brought into view the whole upper surface of the cholesteatoma, the cellular contents of which were first scooped out for histological study and then sucked out, leaving a perfectly clean fossa. I then started to spray the wall of this fossa, hoping that I might kill off the epithelial cells of the membrane, but in so doing, the membrane began to pucker up and I found that I could pick it up and peel it out completely from the whole fossa. This small bit of tissue has been so destroyed by the spraying that it will not be worth histological study.

As a final step in the operation, the fibers of the third division were picked up, leaving the motor root intact in its bed.

Sketch #4 (Sketch for the first operation, IV) shows roughly the appearance of the conclusion of the operation, the opening possibly being a little too large. The motor root can be seen in the posterior part of the field, the cavernous sinus at the upper anterior part of the field, and at the place marked X, there was what appeared to be nothing but a thin membrane which apparently lay between the base of the skull and the tissues below without the presence of bone. I feared that this might overlie a cell in this region though it would be a peculiar place for a mastoid cell, and I consequently did not open it.

The wound was left absolutely dry and the cavity was filled with salt solution. Flap replaced and closed securely in position, the larger part of the closure being taken over by Dr. Horrax.

(Dr. Cushing)

PATHOLOGY REPORT
December 22, 1928
Dr. Eisenhardt

Examination of tissue by supravital technique shows numerous crystals, calcium deposits and debris. No epithelial cells identified.

IMPRESSION: Cholesteatoma

The patient had an uneventful postoperative course.

DISCHARGE NOTE
January 3, 1929
Dr. Schreiber

Excellent recovery. Keratitis of the left eye completely healed. Dizziness much improved. Told to wear frosted glass over left eye.

FOURTH HOSPITAL ADMISSION

SUMMARY OF POSITIVE FINDINGS
November 2, 1929
Dr. Oldberg

SUBJECTIVE

1. History of ataxia and numbness of the left side of the face 2½ yrs. duration preceding an operation performed at this hospital on Dec. 22, 1928.
2. History of low left temporal bone flap on Dec. 22, 1928, disclosing and extirpating cholesteatoma of left Gasserian ganglion.
3. Remission of many of preoperative symptoms for 6 mos. following this operation.
4. History of recurrence and exaggeration of vertigo and ataxia, with development of dysarthria and dysphagia for 3–5 mos.

OBJECTIVE

1. Low left temporal bone flap scar, well healed, with soft decompression.
2. Questionable slight bilateral chronic choked disc, with slight secondary atrophy on the right.
3. Nystagmus and left abducens paresis.
4. Right lower facial weakness of central type.
5. Bilateral moderate diminution of auditory acuity.
6. Slight dysarthria and dysphagia.
7. Ataxia, most marked in Romberg and staggering gait.

IMPRESSION: Caudal extension of cholesteatoma, originally arising in left Gasserian ganglion.

SPECIAL NOTE
November 8, 1929
Dr. Cushing

A good paper might be written on the subject of this woman's case under the title – The Pursuit of a Cholesteatoma.

If I remember the story correctly, she came in here a year or two ago with pain in the left trigeminal region associated with hypesthesia. I assumed naturally enough that she probably had a meningioma of the trigeminal sheath. At the operation, I came down upon a trigeminal nerve which was greatly thinned out and pushed upward by an

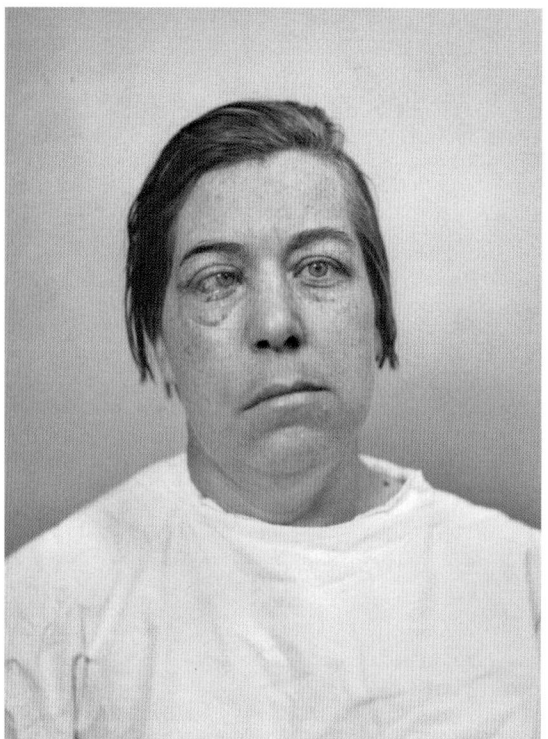
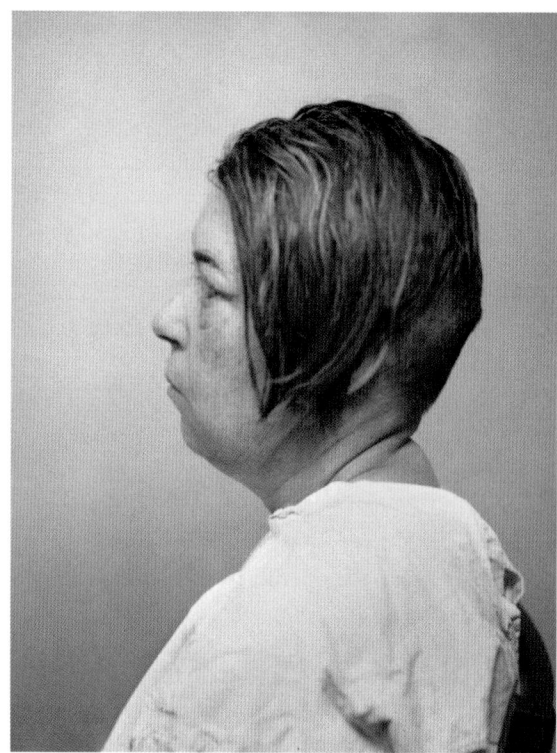

FIGS. 7–9. THREE WEEKS POSTOPERATIVE (SECOND OPERATION)

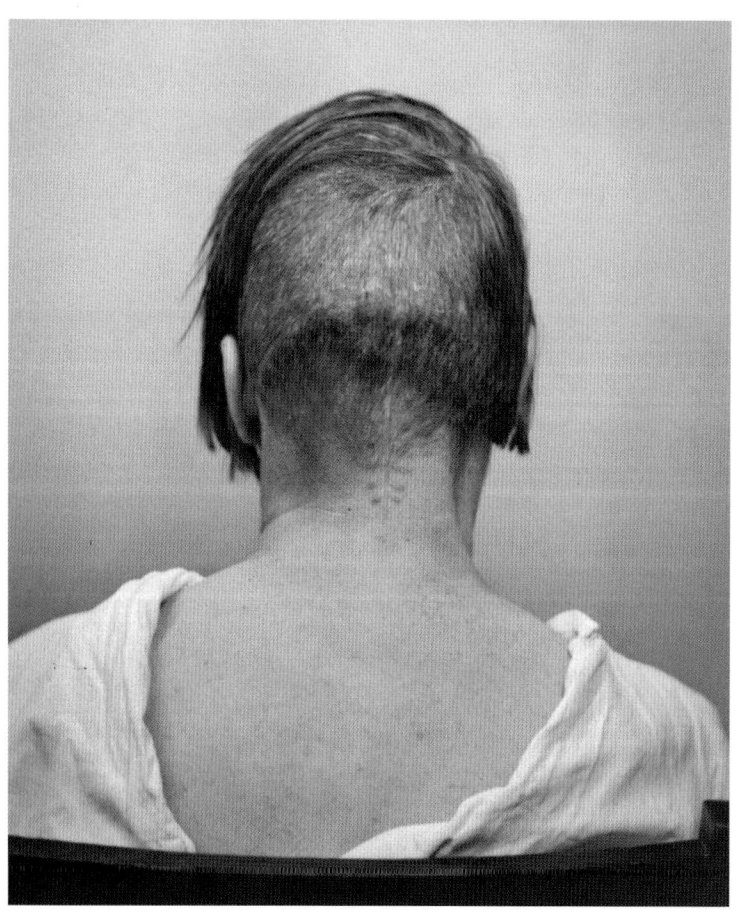

underlying cholesteatoma about as big as a marble. I cleaned this tumor out as I thought thoroughly and completely but in the process endeavored to save what I could of the trigeminal nerve. My mistake probably lay in so doing for if I had sacrificed the nerve I might have seen that tumor was passing down through the dural canal for its sensory root or perhaps better, was squeezing up from below, though I did not then consider this possibility.

She kept having trigeminal pain for a long time which mystified me and I regretted that I had not divided her sensory root.

I had lost track of the woman until I saw her a short time ago when it was perfectly evident to me that she had definite cerebellar symptoms and I consequently assumed that they must be due to the subtentorial extension of this old growth. She had no chocked disc, to be sure, and if I remember correctly, no pressure symptoms but very definite and to me unmistakable incoordination. I consequently without any great enthusiasm, suggested that I might look in behind and see if we would find some of the growth but I anticipated finding if anything a small lesion with which I could scarcely expect to deal.

The operation was relayed with Dr. Horrax.

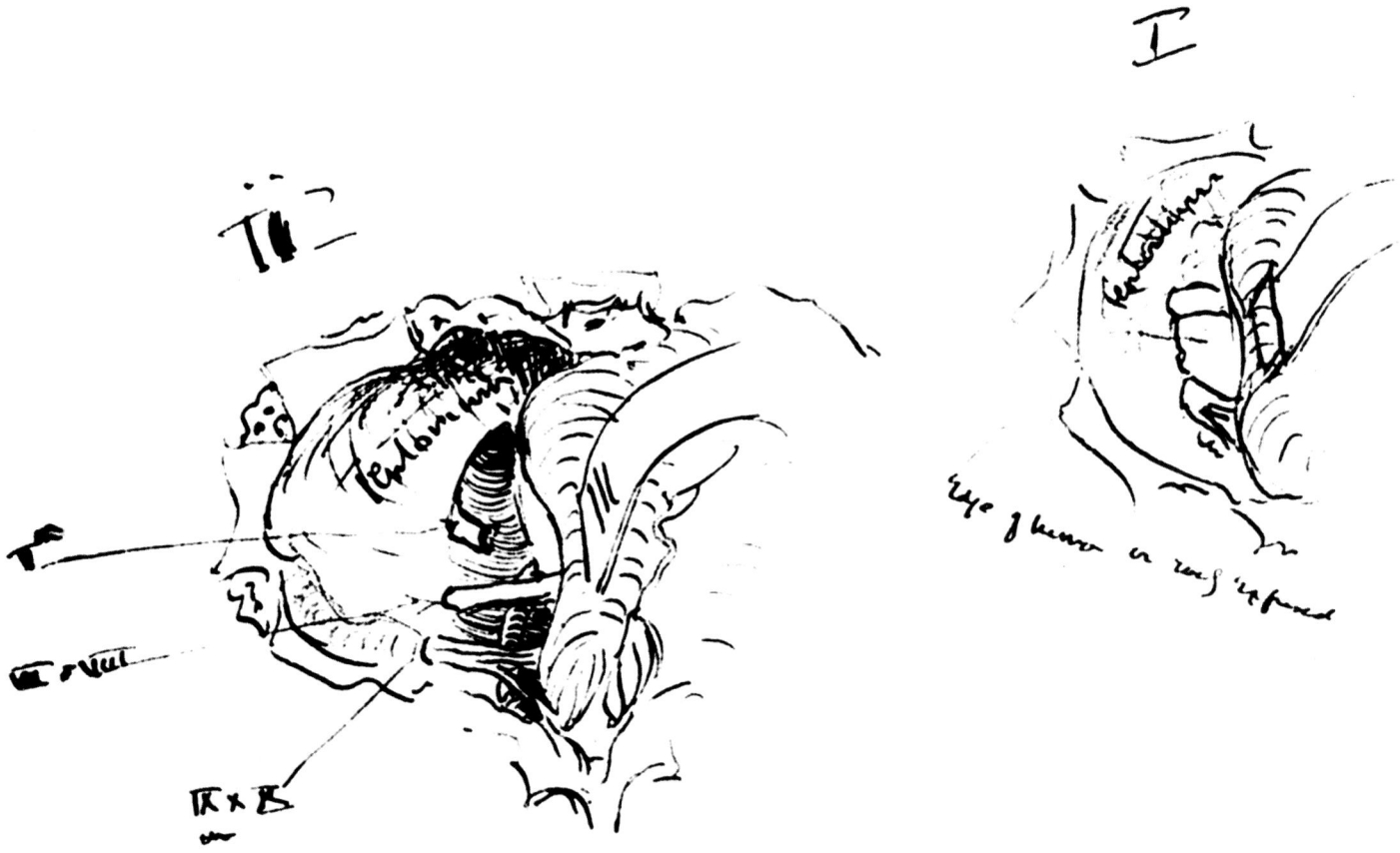

FIG. 10. OPERATIVE SKETCH (SECOND OPERATION)

OPERATIVE NOTE
November 8, 1929
Anesthesia – Novocain

Suboccipital Exploration; Disclosure of Hard Cholesteatoma Extending up Toward the Incisura and Down to the Foramen Magnum, through the Center of Which Passed the Trigeminal Nerve. Extensive Radical Removal of this Growth with the Larger Part of its Capsule. A few fragments that were adherent to the side of the pons and to the vertebral artery were left in situ.

Dr. Horrax had made a primary suboccipital exploration without opening the dura when I entered the field, the exposure having been made at my suggestion well off on the left side and without extensive exposure on the right. The dura was somewhat tense and on opening it the cerebellum was protruding so that I felt almost certainly there must be a tumor. Patient at this time began vomiting and there were occasional attacks of vomiting during the rest of the procedure. I fortunately succeeded in getting an abundance of fluid and was able to elevate the left cerebellar hemisphere and by good luck met with no anchoring veins. I retraced the cerebellum sufficiently as that I could get a view well up above the 8th nerve and there I saw a small, minute glistening point, unmistakably a cholesteatoma. I did not at this time appreciate what a large tumor we were going to find. Running across the middle of the nodule of cholesteatoma was a large anchoring vein which is unusually seen obscuring a good positive view of the trigeminal root. I clipped this vein and then divided electrically, fortunately without accident. It was then possible to brush the cerebellum in this region away from the tumor and I gradually began to clear the growth, finding it more and more widespread as it was encountered. The situation of the growth finally was exposed about as in Fig. I (Sketch for the second operation, I.) The 7th and 8th nerves were flattened up over the tumor as was also the 9th, 10th, and 11th. The major part of the growth lay headward to the 8th nerve and I finally entered the tumor and began clipping and sucking out great cholesteatomatous masses until I had a cup large enough to put in the thumb. Even so, I had not even begun to complete the enucleation. Finally I succeeded in working in between the bun-

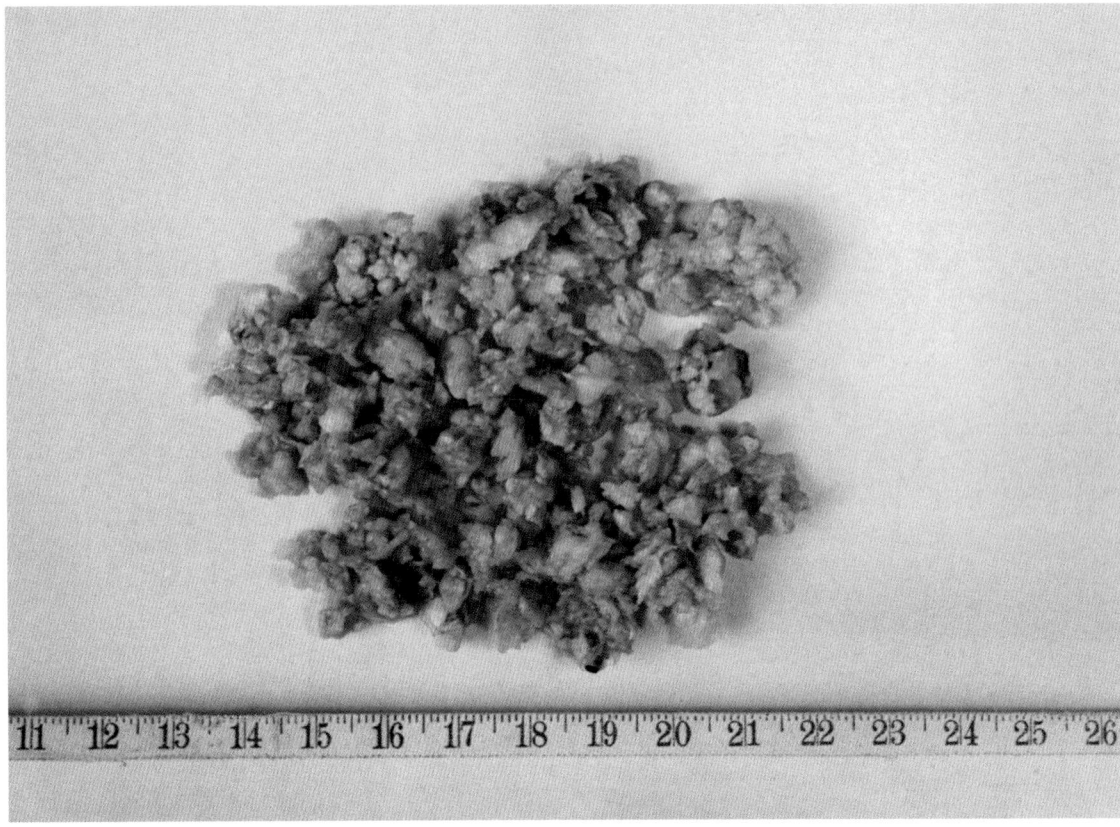

FIG. II. RESECTION SPECIMEN

dles of the 7th and 8th and the lower nerves and here again I got a large excavation. It was finally possible, by drawing out tissue with the rongeurs, gradually to begin to loosen capsule and in the course of the next two hours I succeeded in cleaning out, so far as I could tell, the entire lower capsule, meanwhile exposing the superior cerebellar peduncle to which the shell of tumor was quite definitely adherent and to get a view of the right cerebral peduncle. Some idea from this may be gained of the huge cavity. I think I may very possibly have damaged the superior cerebellar peduncle as some nerve tissue stripped away as I withdrew the capsule of the tumor from this region.

I finally was able to work in underneath the 9th, 10th, and 12th and draw out the entire lower pole of tumor, fortunately without bleeding. In this procedure, the left vertebral artery, passing up toward the basilar, was fully exposed and there were 1–2 shreds of capsule which were slightly adherent to it that I did not quite dare to remove. The 5th nerve apparently ran directly through the center of the tumor, though I did not encounter it or see it until I had begun cleaning out above the 8th nerve in the early stages of the operation. I finally divided the 5th nerve and merely left a tag of it hanging on the fossa as it entered its canal just below the incisura of the tentorium. The huge cavity was thoroughly cleared out by irrigation and the cerebellum allowed to drop back in its position. Closure was carried out by Dr. Horrax.

(Dr. Cushing)

PATHOLOGY REPORT
November 8, 1929
Dr. Eisenhardt

Examination showed numerous cholesterin crystals, the edges of which were quite distinctly outlined.

IMPRESSION: Cholesteatoma.

November 9, 1929
Dr. Oldberg

Condition excellent. Left facial somewhat more pronounced than preoperatively.

Dysphagia slightly more pronounced.

Lumbar puncture by Dr. Cushing, 33 cc of bloody fluid removed under slightly increased pressure.

November 12, 1929
Dr. Oldberg

Seen by Dr. Cushing. Cast removed.

November 26, 1929
Dr. Oldberg

Walking about ward with assistance. Her ataxia seems improved. Speaks more distinctly.

DISCHARGE NOTE
November 30, 1929
Dr. Oldberg

Patient today discharged home. Her dysarthria and dysphagia are much improved as is the ataxia. Has gained much strength and will shortly be able to perform domestic duties.

FOLLOW UP NOTE
March 11, 1930
Dr. Cushing

The patient's husband reports that she continues to have pain and needles feeling in the lower jaw and a little pain shooting up on this side. There is continued buzzing in the ear. Continues to wear a shield. The eye remains clear but there is an internal squint. She is able to walk up and down stairs alone by holding on to the rail. She sleeps soundly twelve hours a night and eats well. Still has some difficulty in swallowing. On the whole, I think her condition is as good as could be expected.

The last letter from the patient's husband was received on October 9, 1931, with the report of her death after a fall. No autopsy was done.

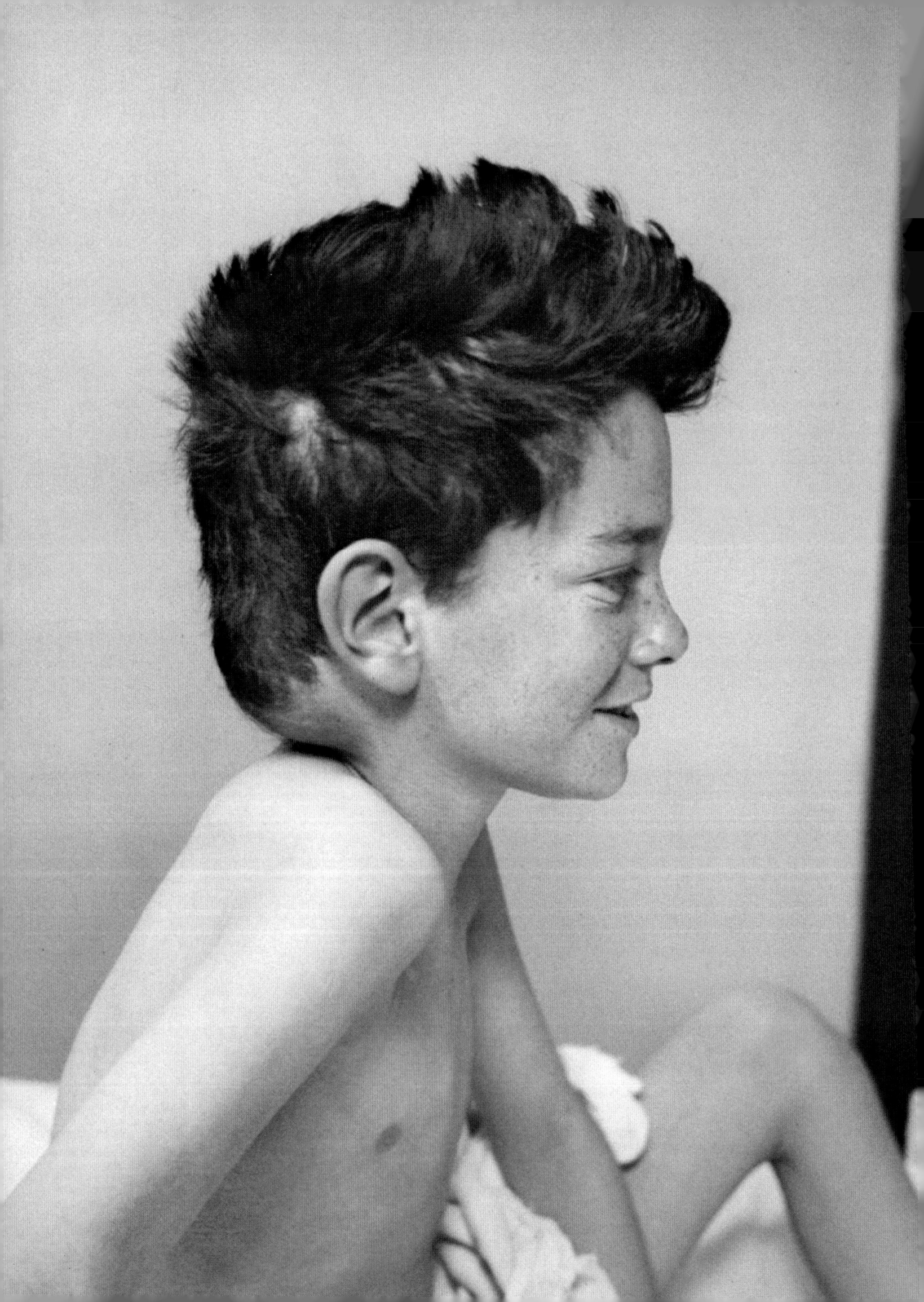

6.19 Cerebellar hemangioblastoma

SEX: M; AGE: 12; SURG. NO. 34068; 48744

HISTORY

In March 1927, this child was thought to be suffering from a cerebellar tuberculoma because of extensive calcifications noted on plain skull x-rays. In April 1927, Dr. Horrax performed a suboccipital decompression without removing any mass lesion. Two months prior to the following admission, he became restless with headaches and vomiting.

SUMMARY OF POSITIVE FINDINGS
May 23, 1929
Dr. Deery

SUBJECTIVE
1. In March 1927 a diagnosis was made of left cerebellar tumor.
2. In April 1927 Dr. Horrax did a suboccipital decompression without touching the tumor.
3. In the interval, has been cared for at the N.E. Peabody Home for Crippled Children.
4. Headaches, vomiting and restlessness in the past two months together with some increase in the size of the suboccipital hernia.

OBJECTIVE
1. A large, hydrocephalic head.
2. Rather poor general nutrition.
3. A suboccipital decompression, thru the right side of which is a soft, fluctuant hernia.
4. Fundi excessively vascular, probably a little secondary atrophy, no choking.
5. Ataxia of all four extremities more marked on the left.
6. Spasticity of the legs more marked on the right.
7. Pupils widely dilated but react promptly.

IMPRESSION: Tuberculoma of the cerebellum with severe internal hydrocephalus.

SPECIAL NOTE
June 5, 1929
Dr. Cushing

This little boy was operated upon a year or so ago by Dr. Horrax at the Children's hospital. I assume that at the time owing to some calcification that was roentgenologically visible in the cerebellum a diagnosis of tuberculoma was made, possibly under the influence of our experience with the little boy, (the name of another patient), who had a tuberculoma that has gradually been undergoing calcification. A rather low and not very complete exposure of the cerebellum was made probably under the difficulties of operating on a case of this sort in unfamiliar surroundings and with inadequate assistants. The operation was left as a decompression, a resistant tumor having been detected in the left hemisphere. The child was sent to the Peabody Home for heliotherapy, etc. There, he had been steadily going downhill, and I have encouraged the child's return under the assumption that there was a tuberculoma which we might possibly attack by electrosurgical methods inasmuch as his cerebellar symptoms have been increasing and something had to be done. The x-ray plates have shown an enormous mass of calcification filling the entire left cerebellar hemisphere and extending up so high under the tentorium that on the AP plates, it looks as though there must be

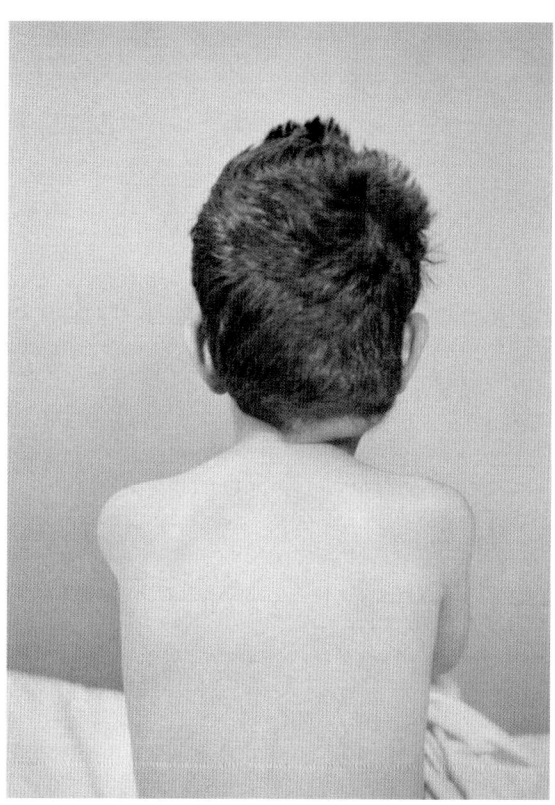

FIG. 2. PREOPERATIVE (BEFORE SECOND SURGERY)

OPPOSITE PAGE: FIG. 1. PREOPERATIVE (BEFORE SECOND SURGERY)

calcification above the tentorium. This calcification is not of the type that occurs in a healed tuberculoma but is widely scattered calcification such as we have recently, for the first time, seen in a cerebellar ependymoma. The child, moreover, has never had fever, and I felt in consequence that the lesion could hardly be tuberculous. The cerebellar symptoms were very pronounced. There has been a great deal of vomiting, and there has been marked suboccipital protrusion.

The operation was conducted wholly under local anesthesia though this at the outset did not seem possible.

OPERATIVE NOTE
June 5, 1929
Anesthesia – Novocain – Morphia

Re-opening of Suboccipital Flaps. Removal of Large Area of Previously Unremoved Bone up to Lateral Sinus. Exposure of Huge, Dense, Irregularly Surfaced Tumor at First Taken to be a Calcified Angioblastoma. Coagulation of Surface of Lesion. Partial Piecemeal Extirpation of Masses of Calcified Tissue with Muscle Replacement. Closure After Prolonged Operation.

I put this operation on for Dr. Blanco of Montevideo. The boy was put on the cerebellar table after being shaved, and as tension was considerable, I endeavored to get fluid from the ventricle by a puncture through the bulging perforation over the left occipital pole. I was unable to get fluid on 2–3 taps. I then proceeded slowly to reflect the original flaps, there being marked bleeding from the scar. I finally exposed the bone and reflected tissue up over it and was able to remove, as shown in sketch, a surprisingly large area of previously uncovered dura. The bone was extremely thin. An incision was then made in the newly uncovered dura as shown in sketch 2 (Operative Sketch II) and carried around close to the lateral sinus and across the midline. Clean bulging cerebellum was disclosed on the right, and on the left, there was nothing but a thin shell of cerebellum over the surface of the enormous tumor. The tumor was of stony hardness and had many surface irregularities. Some knobs of tissue with sessile base projected up from the surface giving it a most peculiar irregularity. The surface was covered by a tangle of large veins which bled considerably until I succeeded in coagulating them with a sparking current. The great mass of tumor as shown in sketch 3 (Operative Sketch III) was finally exposed, and I began to dig into this tissue with the electric loop. There was a surface layer of fairly soft tumor about 3–4 mm in diameter, and immediately one came down upon dense and calcareous masses. I could catch some of these masses in the loop and tear them out, but there was a good deal of bleeding, which I had to control by sparking and by coagulation. I finally succeeded in getting a fairly deep cup in the tumor as shown in sketch 4 (Operative Sketch IV), and some great masses of calcification were tilted out and torn out by the Horsely rongeurs. This whole procedure lasted a long time with as careful hemostasis as possible, but there was a rapid fall in pulse rate owing to the loss of blood, and I felt that I had gone as far as circumstances would permit. Delay on 1–2 occasions permitted the blood pressure to return once more, but on pursuing the excavation, it would fall off with great rapidity again, and I did not dare proceed. The huge tumor was quite loose, and it would rock when masses of the central concretion were grasped by the forceps. There was continued oozing from the base, and I had to implant some muscle which I had at hand, and finally the dural flaps and overlying muscle flaps were drawn together over the cavity, all tension for the time being having been relieved. The wound was closed and a small protective drain left into the cavity from between the muscle edges and led out obliquely under the scalp. The child had a precarious afternoon but on last reports was doing reasonably well.

(Dr. Cushing)

PATHOLOGY REPORT
June 5, 1929

There are great fragments of highly calcified tumor, almost certainly in view of a recent case of highly calcified ependymoma, a tumor of this same kind. The lesion had been exposed by Dr. Horrax a year ago at which time it was thought to be a tuberculoma and consequently was not verified. Although much of the tissue was treated by coagulation there are possibly ample blocks for histological study and culture. I would like to have one of the larger blocks decalcified and cut so as to show the relation of the calcification to the cellular part of the growth.

(Dr. Cushing)

DIAGNOSIS – Sclerosing, calcifying and ossifying hemangioma.

(Dr. Bennett)

SPECIAL NOTE
June 12, 1929
Dr. Cushing

This child has had a stormy convalescence, with low blood count and hemoglobin. He has just begun to pick up a little today. I did not quite dare wait any longer because I was afraid that it would be difficult to unravel the wound. I thought it would be safe to go ahead with preliminary transfusion from his father. This was carried out by Dr. Powers.

OPERATIVE NOTE
June 12, 1929
Anesthesia – Novocain

Preliminary Transfusion. Re-exposure of the Calcareous Tumor. Radical Excavation of Tumor with Partial Removal of its Wall After Coagulation. Considerable Trouble from Bleeding Shell of Tumor Plastered in Recess.

This little boy, as stated, has come along fairly well after a few days of critical condition. He was given 250 cc. of blood from his father, and studies were made of the blood just before and just after the transfusion. It seems to me that this might very possibly be an admirable way to determine bleed volume in the case of anaemia, namely by injecting or giving a quantity of blood in the bloodstream and making estimates of the percent of erythrocytes and the change in the number of erythrocytes after injection in the bloodstream. There was, as a matter of fact, in this boy's case, extremely little change in his blood count.

The child was put again face down on the cerebellar table, and after shaving the scalp and reflecting the cerebellar flap, a good exposure was obtained, as before, of the raw surface of the tumor. I proceeded to trim some of the implanted muscle away, again having considerable trouble from bleeding. We had some fairly generous muscle which was used for implantation, after tearing out some of the large secondary calcareous masses. I finally was able to get below and to the median side of the dense firmly fixed tumor, and by incision with the cutting loop, I removed a large block of the lower part of the growth. In the operative sketch, I have probably over-emphasized the amount of tumor that has been removed. Underneath the tentorium, there still remains a great mass of calcareous growth which I was tempted to attack, but the child's pressure at once had fallen off, and I thought I had better

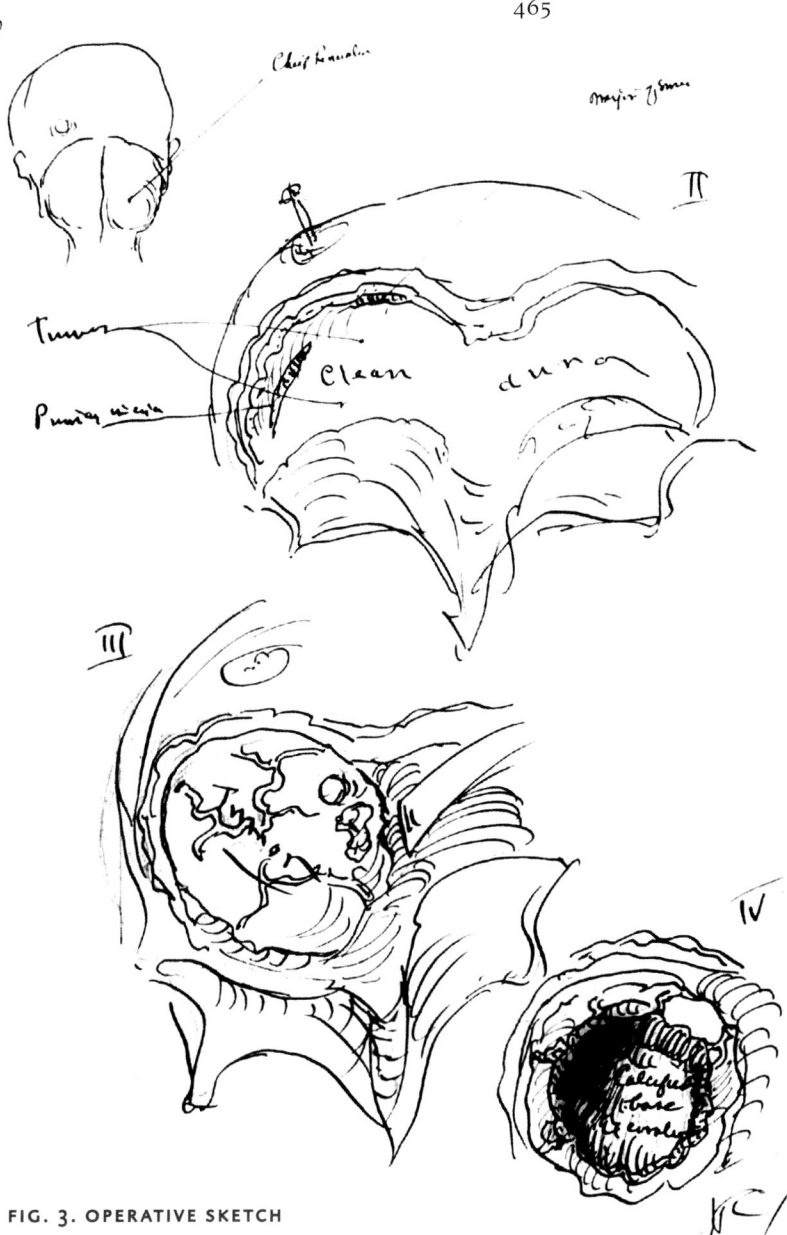

FIG. 3. OPERATIVE SKETCH

withdraw. I trust that he will be able once more to get on his feet. Whether it would be advisable to make a 3rd stage exploration after another 10 days, I am a little doubtful as there would be some apprehension of wound healing, in view of the thin flaps of muscle and thin edge of dura which were reflected at my previous operation.

The tumor seemed to be plastered in the lateral recess, and cannot quite understand why he does not have multiple paralyses from involvement of the nerves in this recess. It means, I suppose, that the tumor perhaps is less densely adherent than it appeared to be.

I got, from 2 or 3 points, quite bad bleeding and in the outer part of the field down toward the region of the mastoid emissary vessels, I had to leave a number of muscle pledgets on large spurting vessels which I,

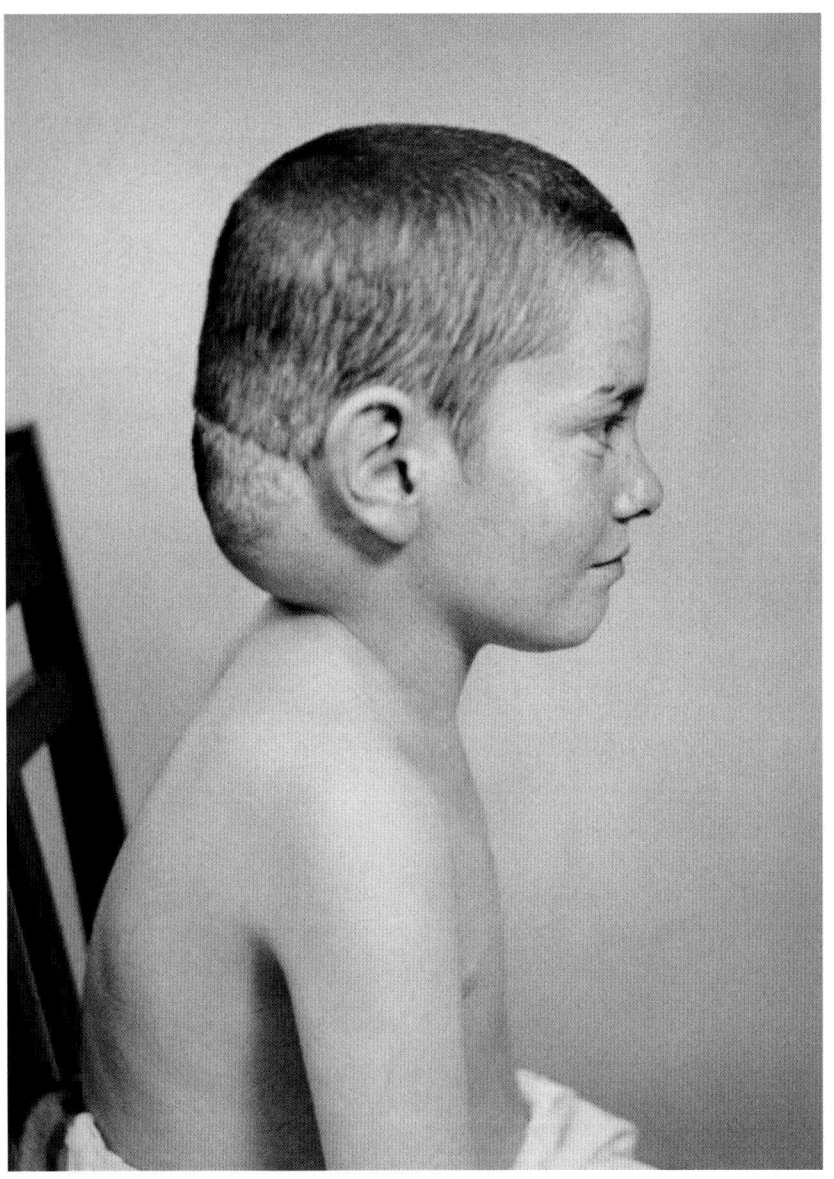

FIG. 4. THREE WEEKS POSTOPERATIVE AFTER SECOND SURGERY.

at first, crushed between Kelly clamps and then finally squeezed muscle down against it.

All through this operation, we used the cutting current on high and also freely used the coagulating current over the surface.

(Dr. Cushing)

HOSPITAL COURSE

He had a stormy hospital course, and had profound ataxia and hypotonia. His suboccipital decompression remained full and mostly tense requiring intermittent aspiration of yellow fluid. Towards the end of his hospital course, his decompression site remained full but not as tense and his ataxia improved. He was not able to walk when admitted to the hospital but was walking easily at the time of discharge.

DISCHARGE NOTE
July 3, 1929
Dr. Deery

Dr. Sosman feels that radiotherapy would not much influence this picture.

Cerebellar decompression fairly full but soft. His general nutritional state and ataxic symptoms are both much improved. He was bedridden. He now walks easily with a little support. Fundi were negative. Deep reflexes were all hyperactive but equal. He was discharged home.

FOLLOW UP VISITS

The patient underwent a series of x-ray treatments. Over the years until 1935, the patient had improved regarding his ataxia, nystagmus and general nutrition. A note in August of 1934 found him attending a trade school studying interior decorating and exam showed a "small statured aesthenic" 17 y.o. boy with a soft bulge under his right occiput and a slowly increasing hard bulge under the left occiput. He had increased general reflexes and disdiadochocinesia of his left hand. By late 1934 and early 1935 he had worsening of his cerebellar signs. More x-ray treatments were administered. He continued to deteriorate and by April 4th 1935, he was grossly ataxic, unable to walk and was admitted for cyst aspiration.

THIRD HOSPITAL ADMISSION

HISTORY

Inability to walk of 2 months duration.

SUMMARY OF POSITIVE FINDINGS
April 4, 1935
Dr. Durant

Patient exam reveals inability to walk or stand alone, markedly ataxic gait, large fluctuant bulging mass in the suboccipital region, bilateral nystagmus, optical atrophy, left; choked disc right; deficient extraocular movements; deafness; thick voice; dysphasia; underdevelopment and undernourishment; adiadochocinesis and ataxia of the tongue and extremities; markedly hyperactive tendon reflexes, more marked in the right leg; ankle clonus in the right leg, and right facial weakness.

SPECIAL NOTE
April 5, 1935
Dr. Cutler

This boy was operated on many years ago for cerebellar hemangioma; he is now in the hospital with signs of recurrence, including loud bruit over the right cerebellar lobe. He is to have X-ray therapy and then will be sent home.

DISCHARGE SUMMARY
April 17, 1935
Dr. Hyder

This patient is one of Dr. Cushing's old patients on whom in 1929 two suboccipital explorations were performed and microscopic diagnosis of hemangioblastoma, calcified, was made.

This 17-year old boy enters the hospital at the present time, complaining of inability to walk of 2 months' duration. Following discharge 2 years ago he has received a course of x-ray treatments and has been improved until Oct. 1934. Since that time the decompression has bulged markedly and inability to walk due to staggering gait has developed during the past 2 months.

P.E. shows a patient unable to walk or stand alone, markedly ataxic gait when supported, marked fluctuant bulging mass in the suboccipital region, bilateral nystagmus, optic atrophy, left, choking disc, right, dysphagia, mal-nutrition, mal-development, adiadochocinesia, generalized hyperactivity of tendon reflexes, more marked on the right, ankle clonus on the right, and right facial weakness.

HOSPITAL COURSE: While the patient was on ward he remained in bed. A definite bruit was present over the cystic suboccipital bulge. This bulge was tapped and 70 cc of clear fluid were obtained which appeared to be spinal fluid. The bulge immediately reappeared. The patient was given

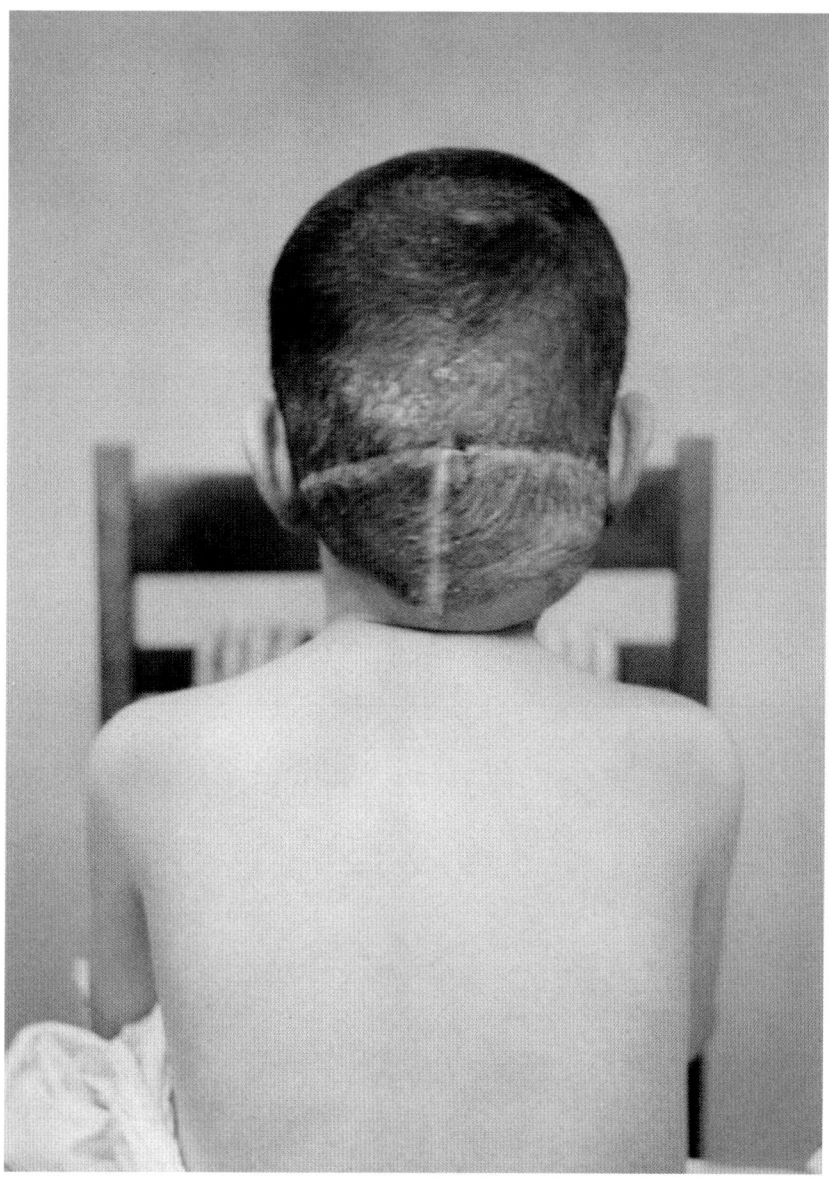

FIG. 5. THREE WEEKS POSTOPERATIVE AFTER SECOND SURGERY.

magnesium sulfate in small quantities daily. He had no vomiting except on occasions while on the ward. He was unable to walk at any time. His condition at the time of discharge was the same as at the time of entry.

DIAGNOSIS: Hemangioblastoma, calcified, recurrent, of the cerebellum.

DISPOSAL: Discharged to Tewsbury State Infirmary.

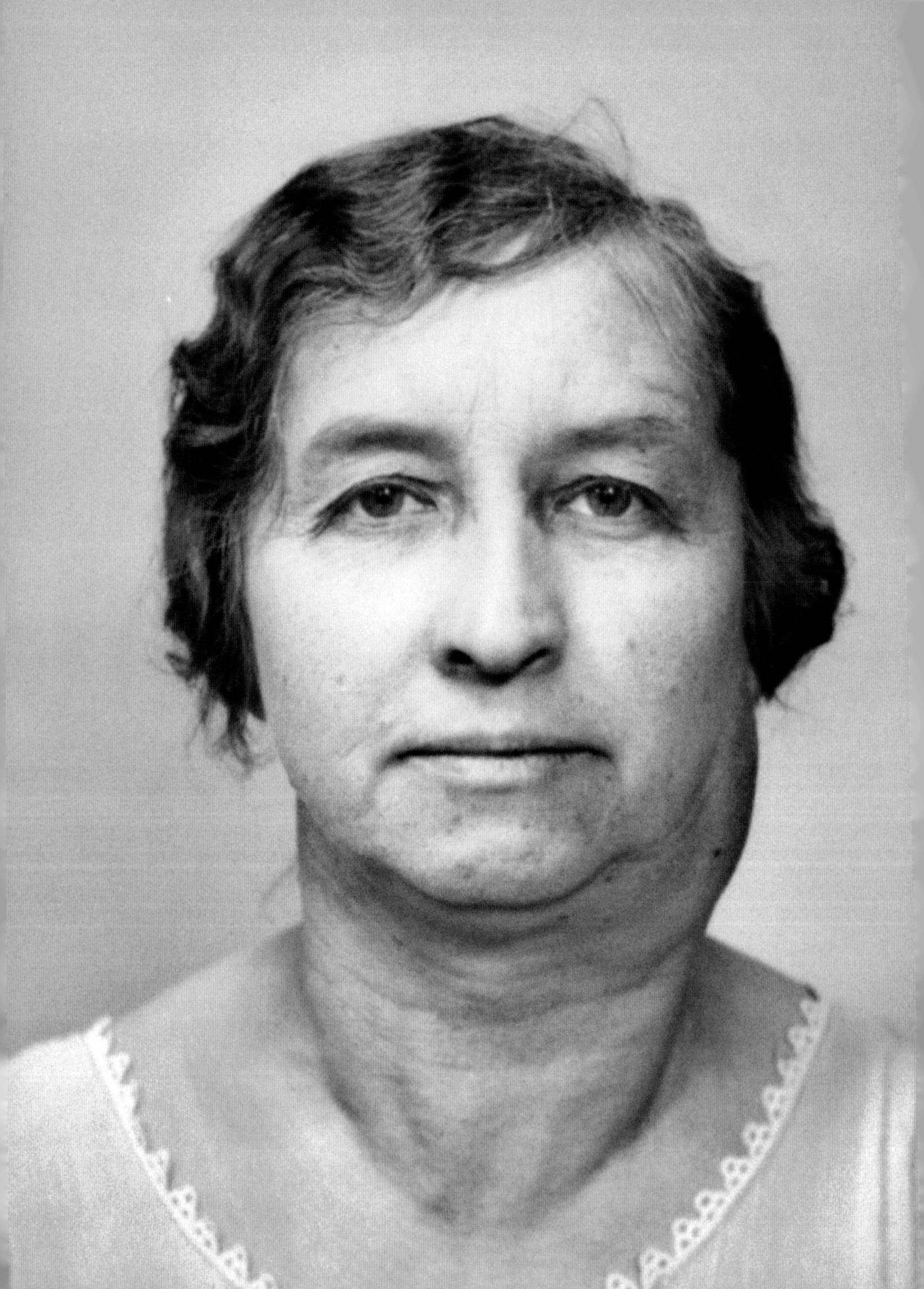

6.20 Carotid body tumor

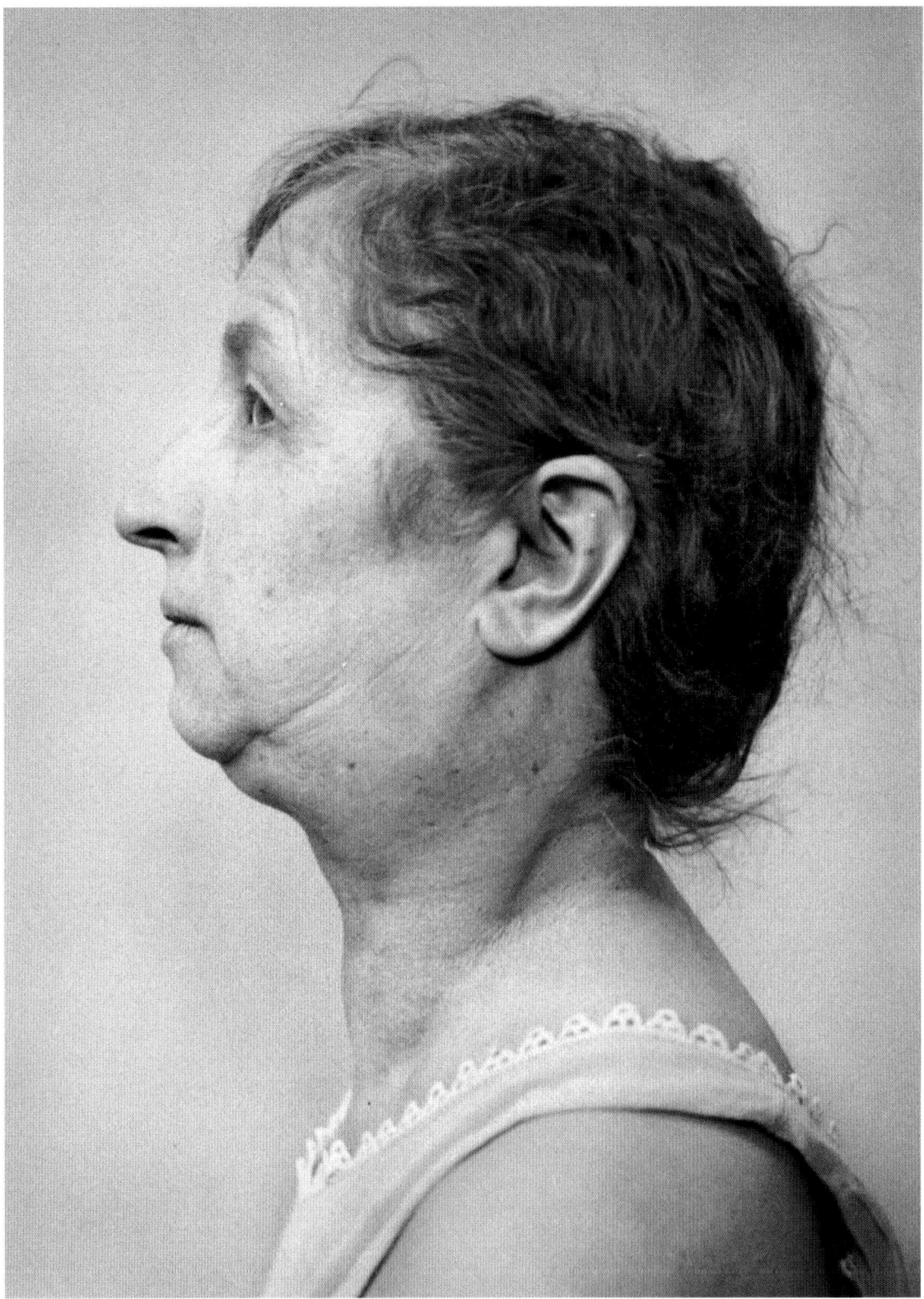

FIG. 2. PREOPERATIVE.

OPPOSITE PAGE: FIG. 1. PREOPERATIVE.

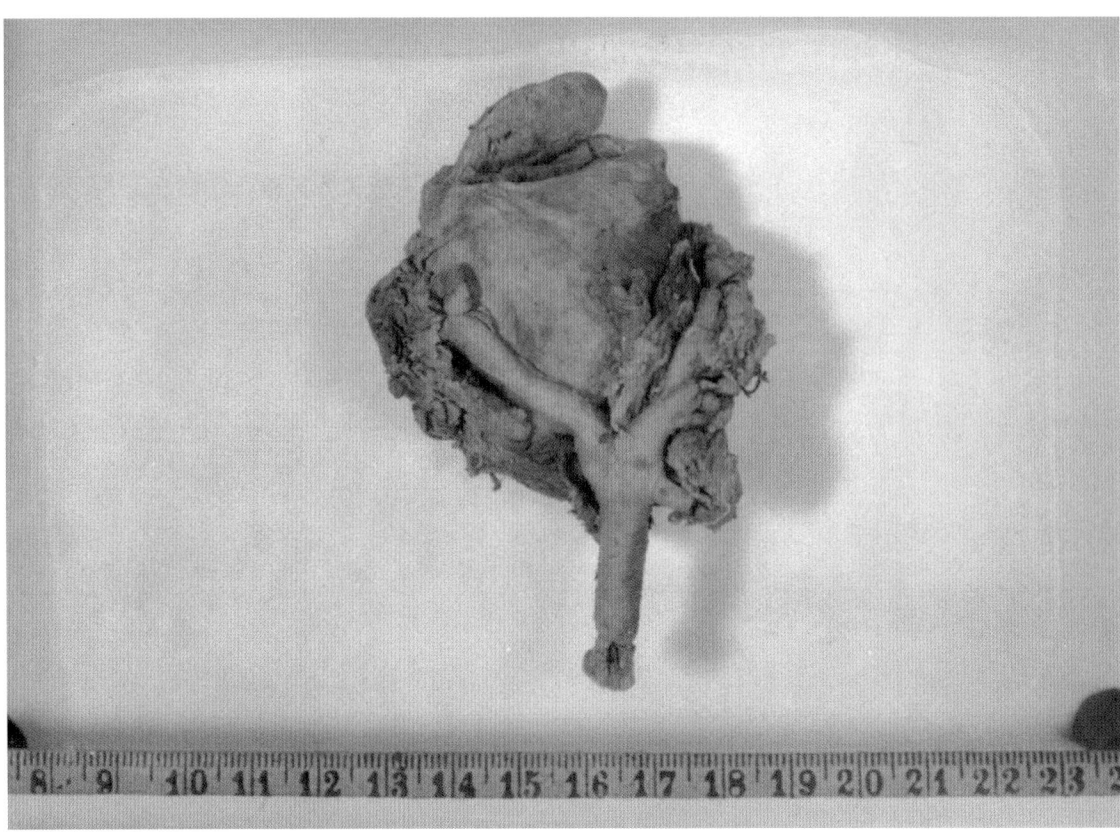

FIG. 3. RESECTED SPECIMEN.

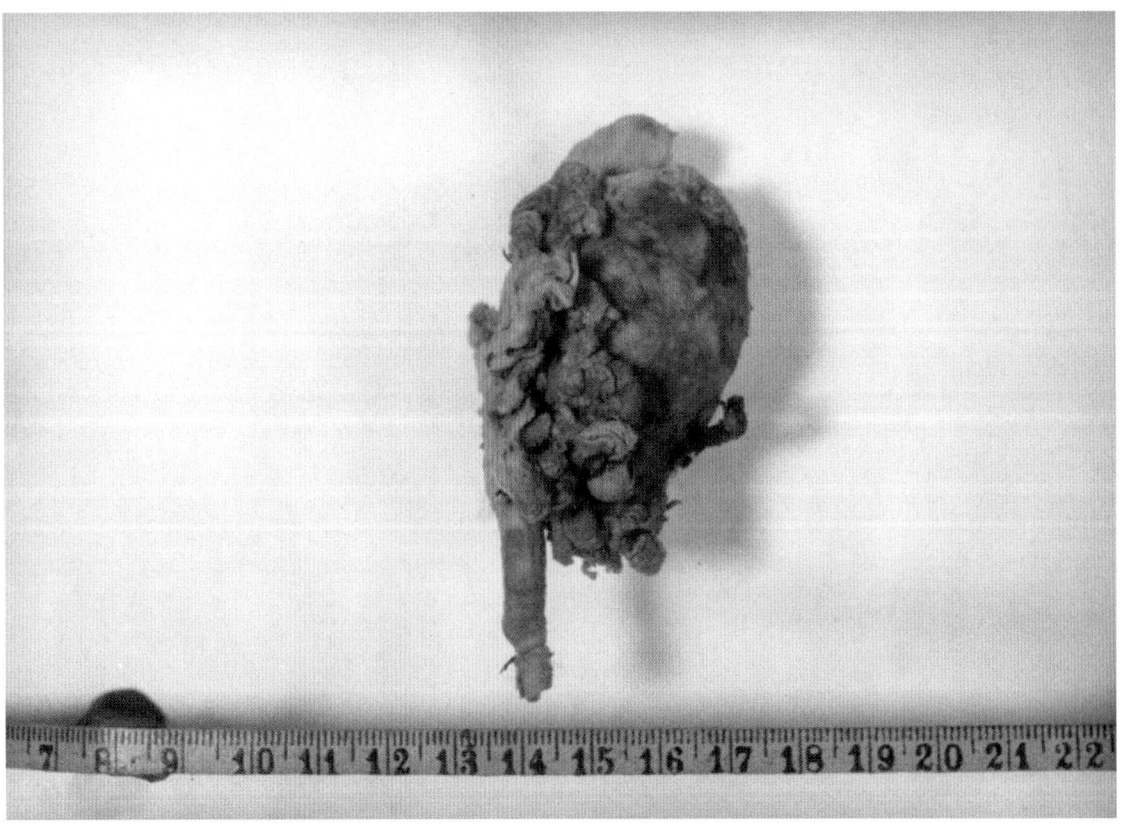

FIG. 4. RESECTED SPECIMEN.

Chapter 7

Special illustrations, additional operative sketches, teaching slides, and operating room photographs

Introduction

In the following chapter, we have summarized images which capture the spectrum in the surgical practice of Harvey Cushing.

Figures 1–8 are special elaborate illustrations which Cushing prepared for his book chapters. These illustrations depict the artistic ability of Cushing and have previously appeared in William W. Keen's *Surgery: Its Principles and Practice* published in 1908.

Additional informative operative sketches from patient records have also been included (Figures 9–48) to demonstrate Cushing's operative approach to CNS lesions. Figures 49–86 represent Cushing's lantern slides used for his lectures.

Photographs 87–111 are mainly the images of Cushing's operating room staff. These images are currently housed in the Cushing Historical Library at Yale University.

Aaron A. Cohen-Gadol, M.D., M.Sc.
Indianapolis, IN

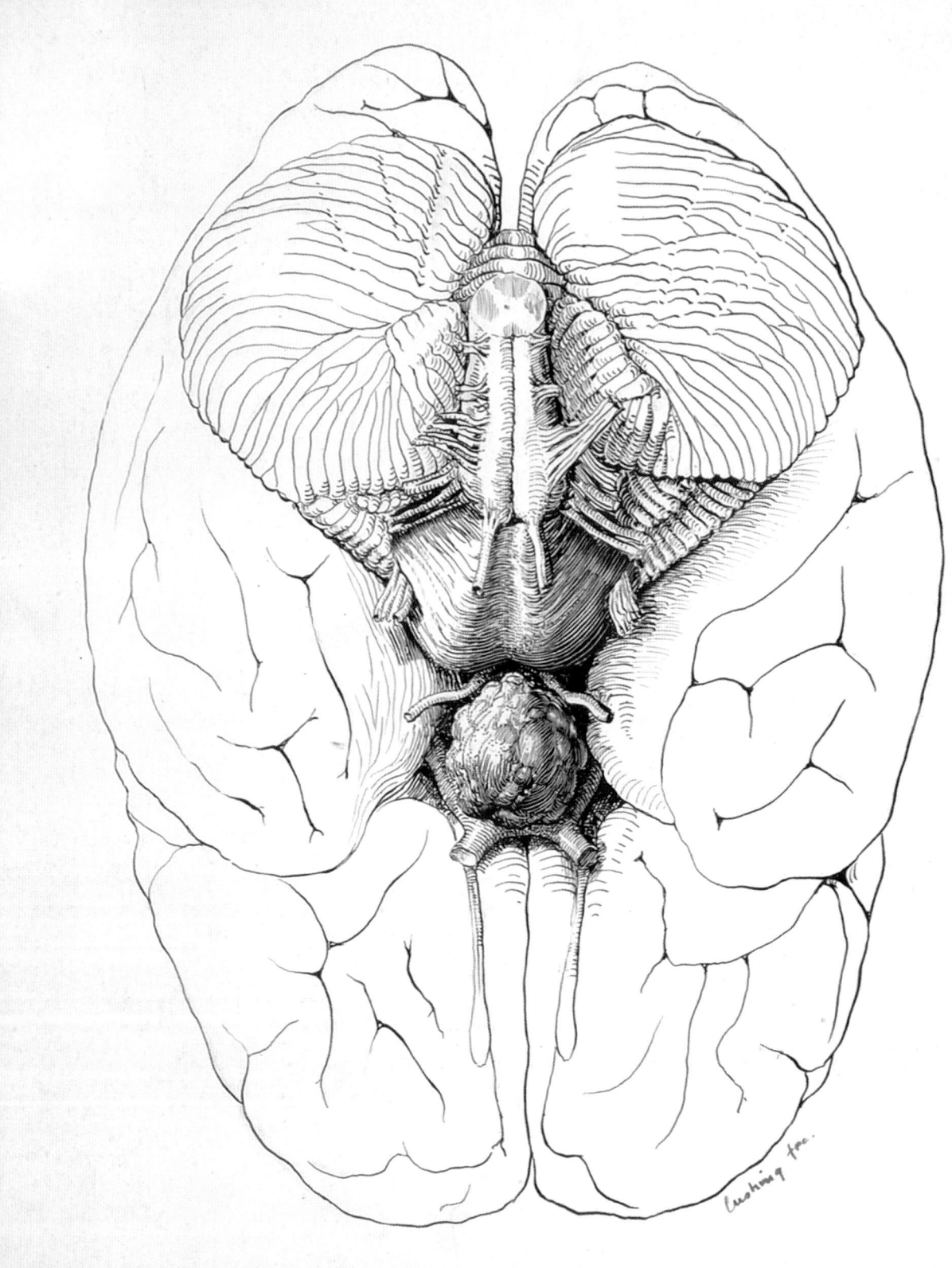

Drawing of base of Brain (Case I) and tumor, from sketch of the tissues made at the time of the autopsy.

FIG. I. SUPRASELLAR TUMOR.

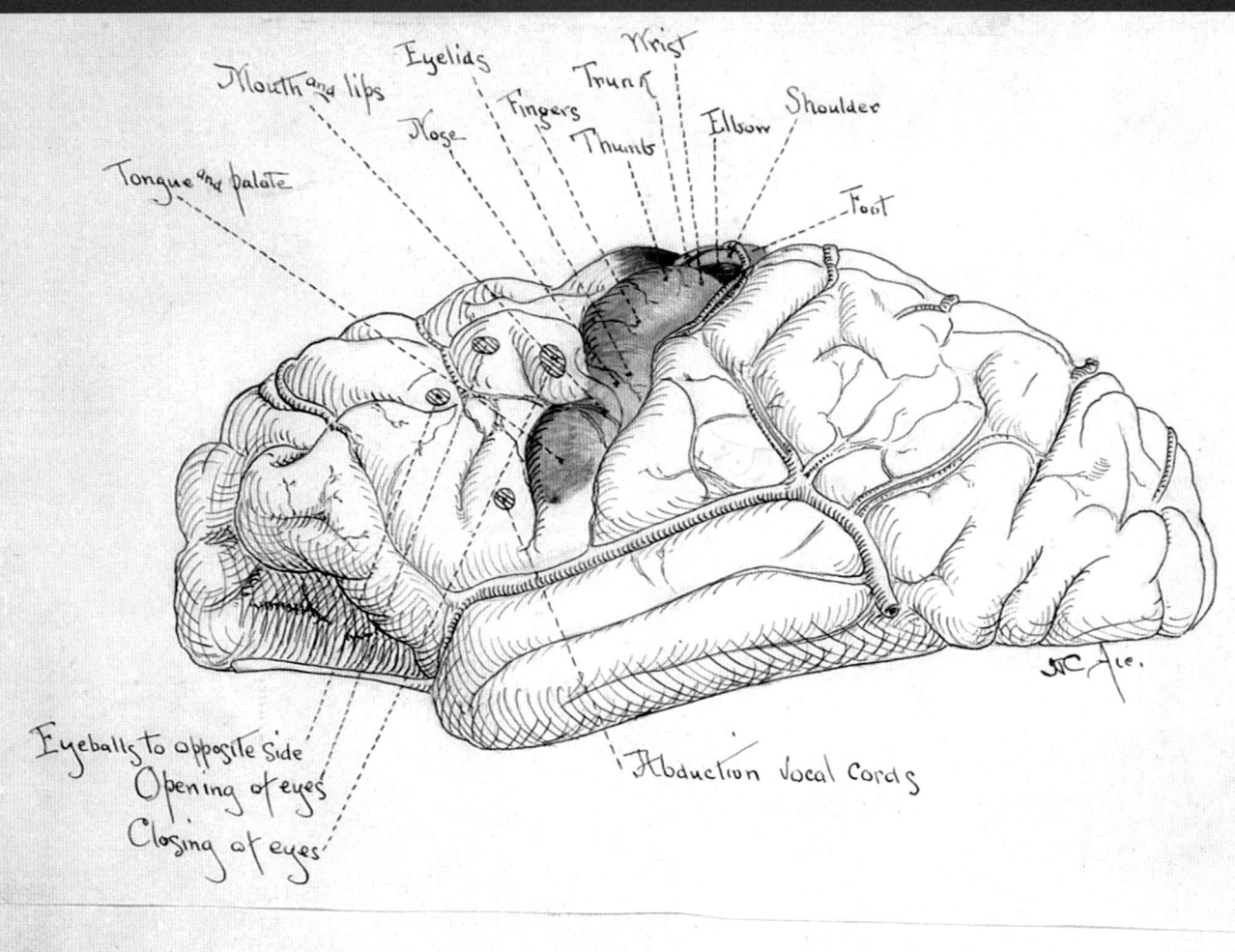
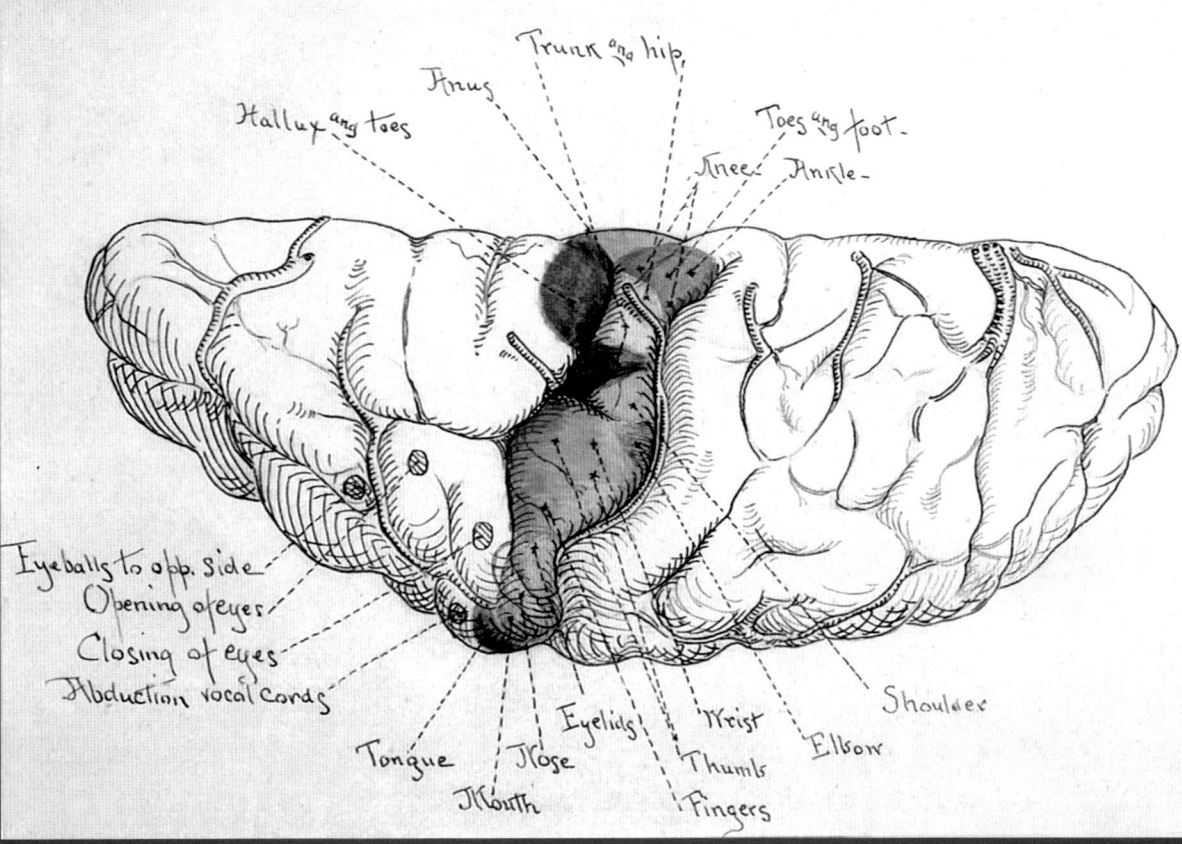

FIG. 2. ORGANIZATION OF MOTOR CORTEX.

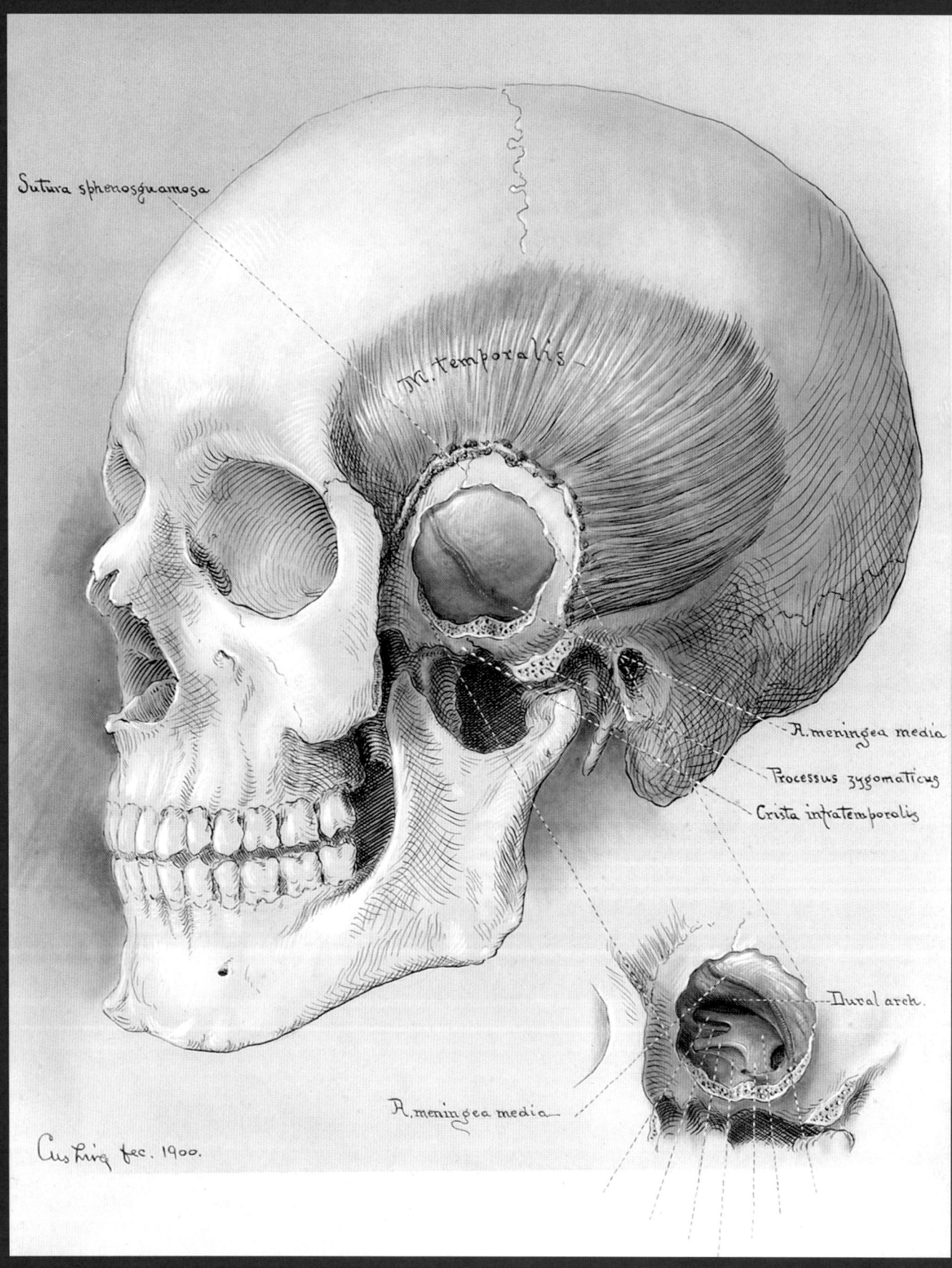

FIG. 3. APPROACH TO THE TRIGEMINAL GANGLION FOR TREATMENT OF TIGEMINAL NEURALGIA — BONY REMOVAL.

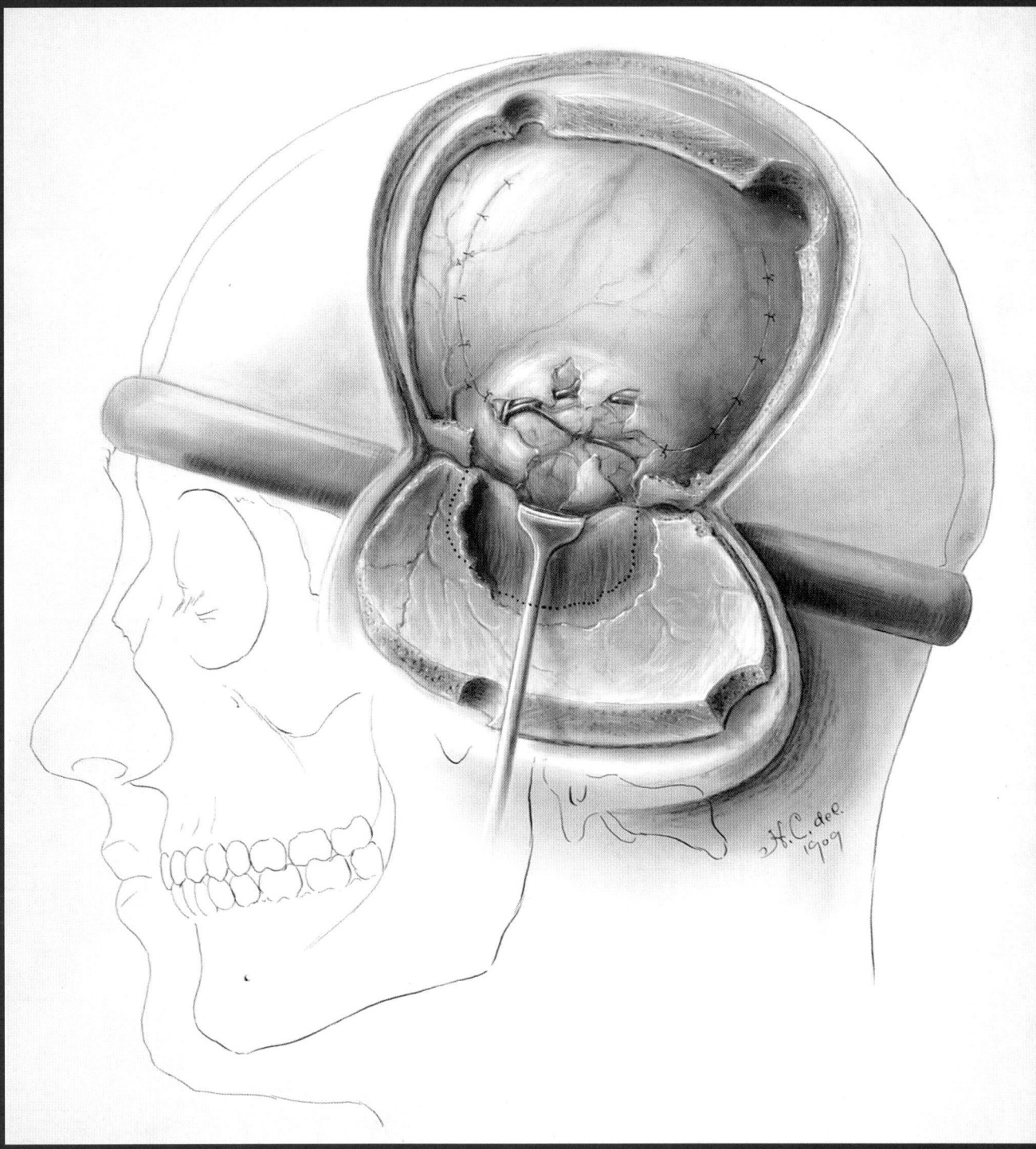

FIG. 4. DURAL CLOSURE FOR FRONTOTEMPORAL CRANIOTOMY WITH ADJUVANT SUBTEMPORAL DECOMPRESSION.

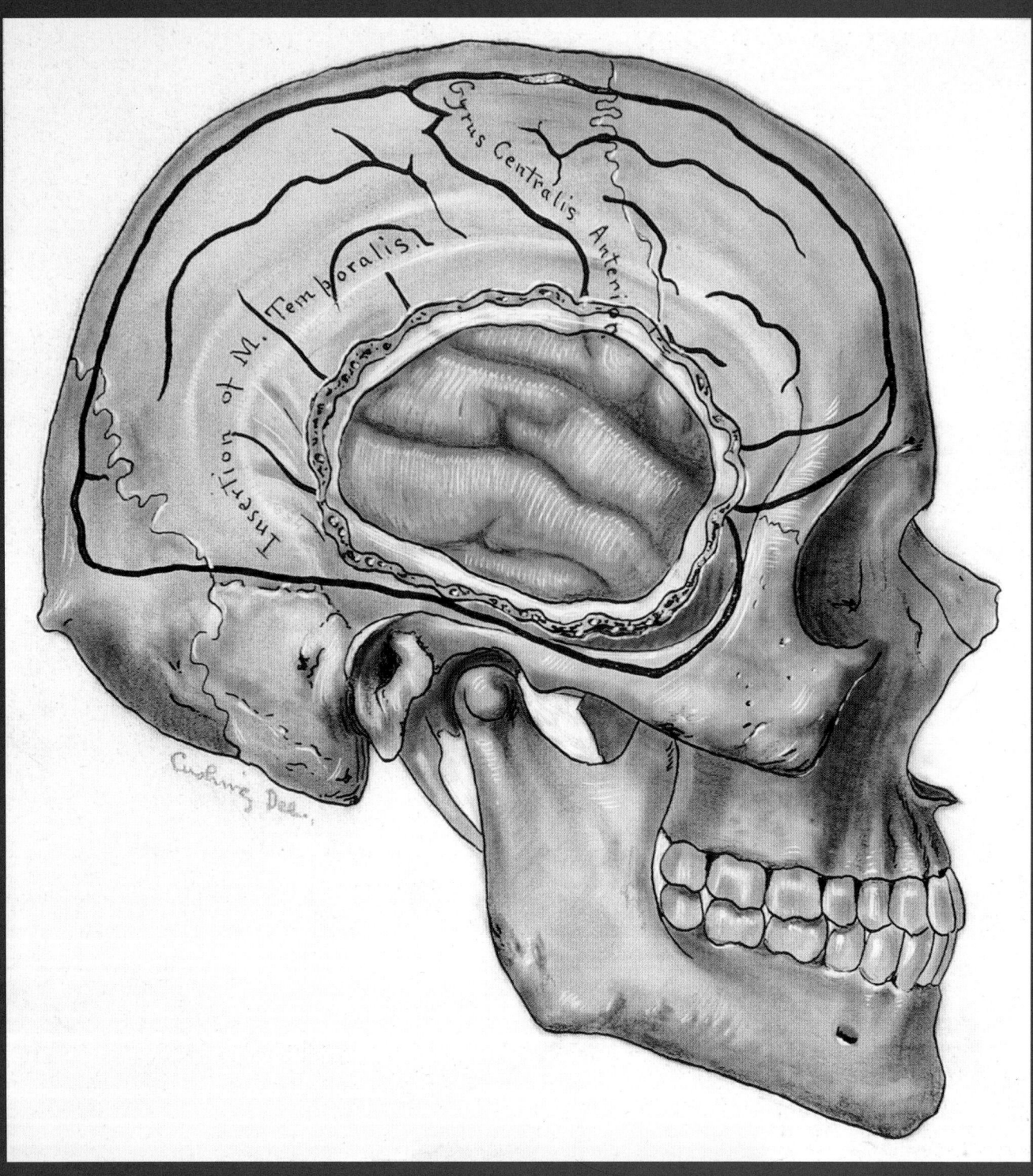

FIG. 5. SUBTEMPORAL DECOMPRESSION — THE RELATIONSHIP OF BONY EXPOSURE TO TEMPORAL GYRI.

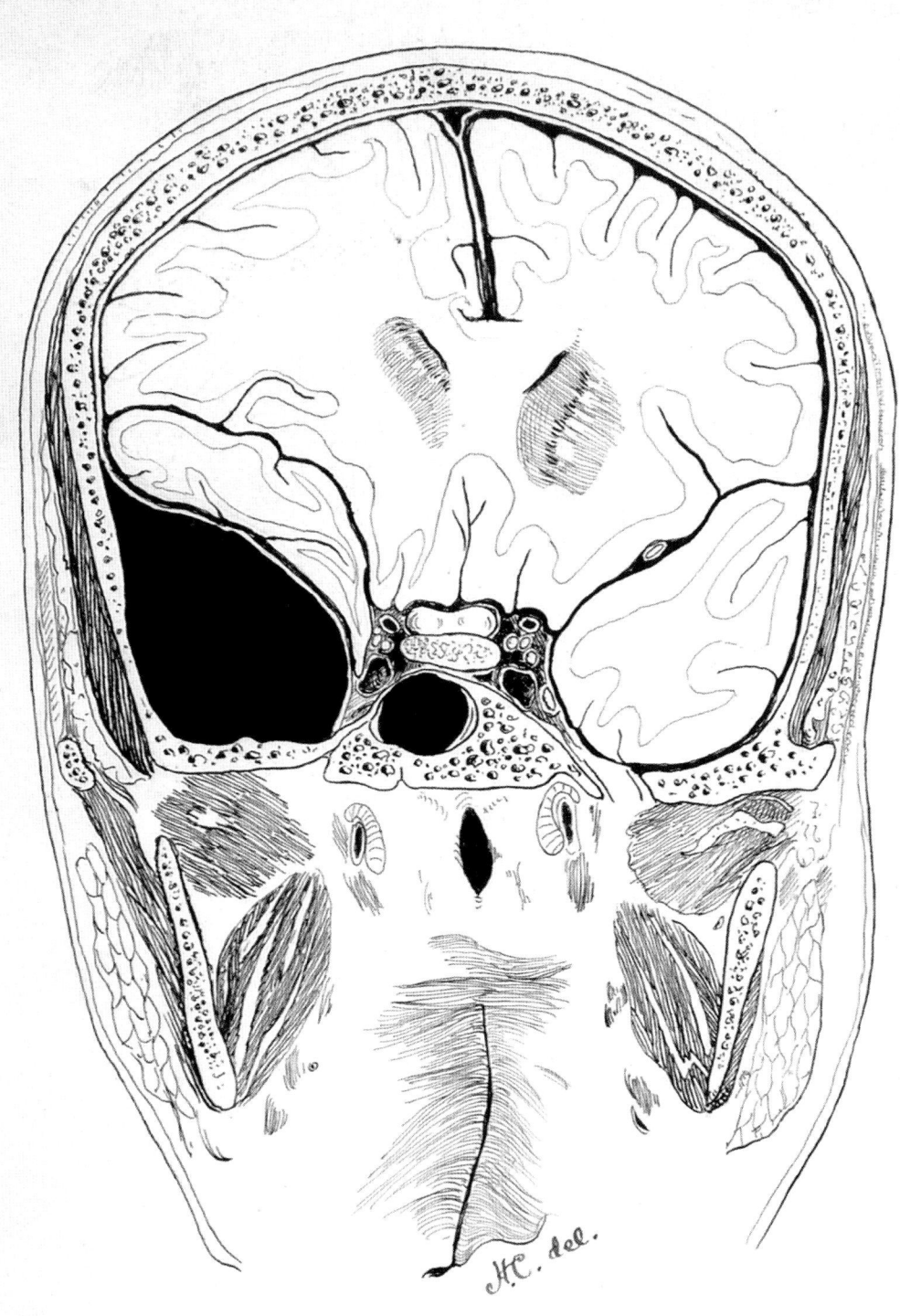

Fig 2. Coronal Section, viewed from behind, passing through the pituitary fossa. To show the situation of the extra-dural clot in Case I: also the relation of the carotid artery and cavernous sinus, anastomosed by the trauma of the fracture, and of the oculomotor nerves, injured at the same time.

FIG. 6. EPIDURAL HEMATOMA — CORONAL VIEW.

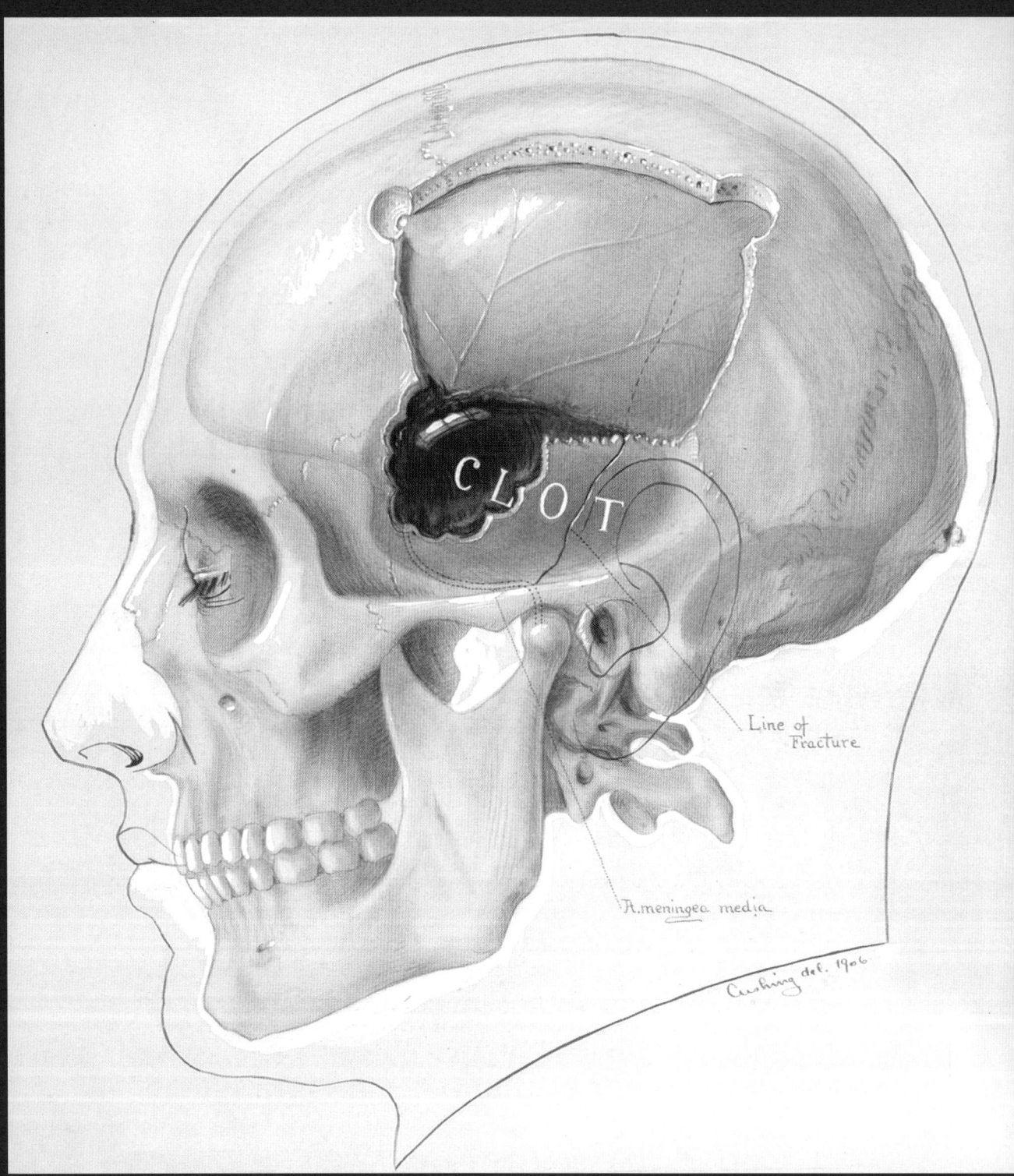

FIG. 7. EPIDURAL HEMATOMA — SAGITTAL VIEW.

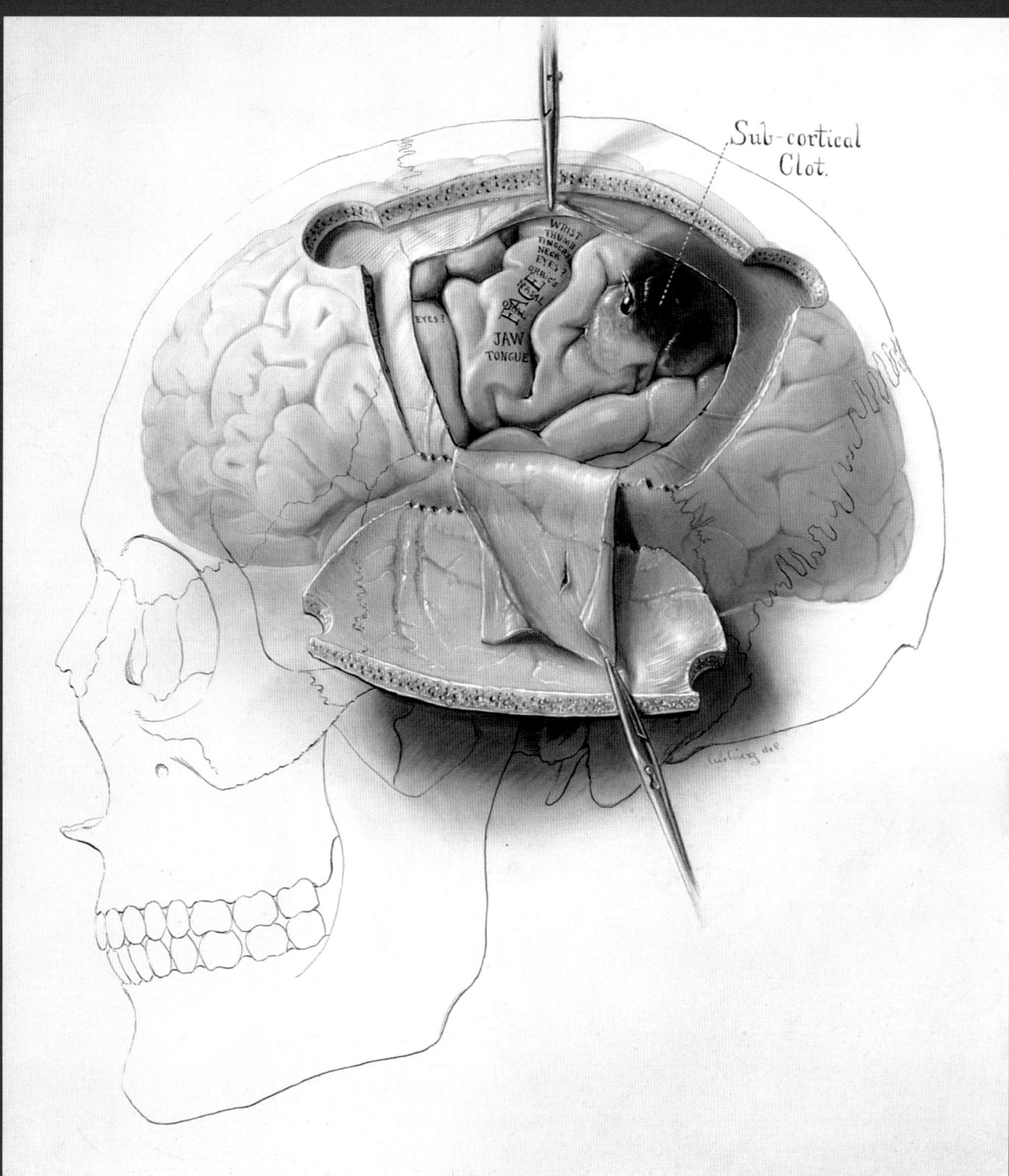

FIG. 8. SUBCORTICAL CLOT.

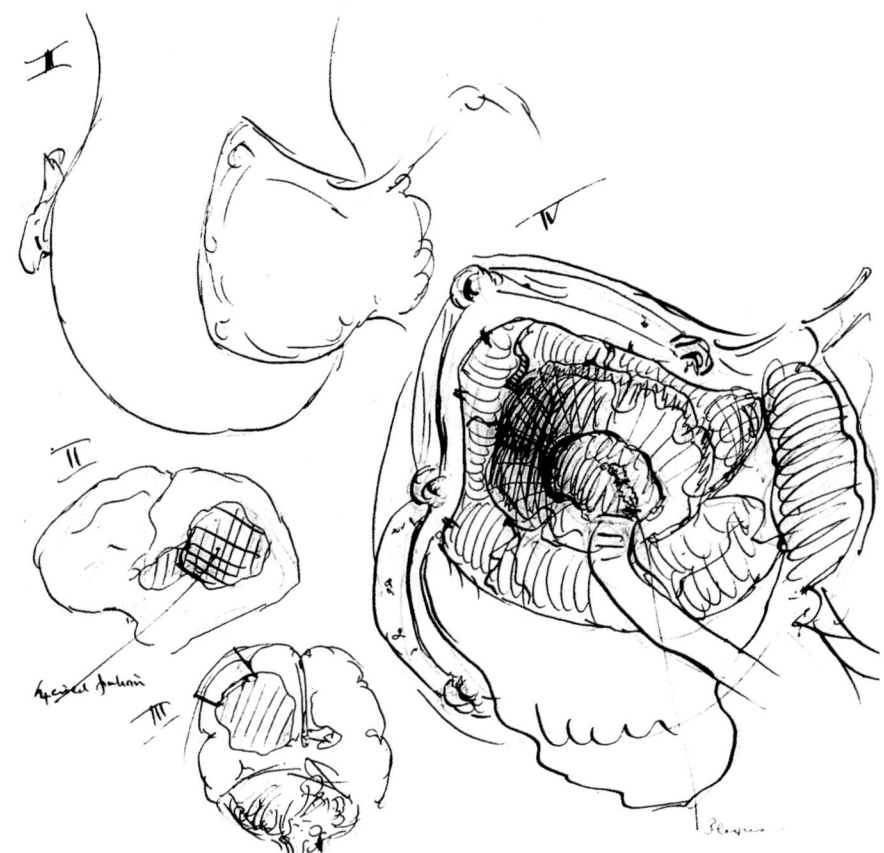

FIG. 9. LEFT OCCIPITAL GLIOMA.

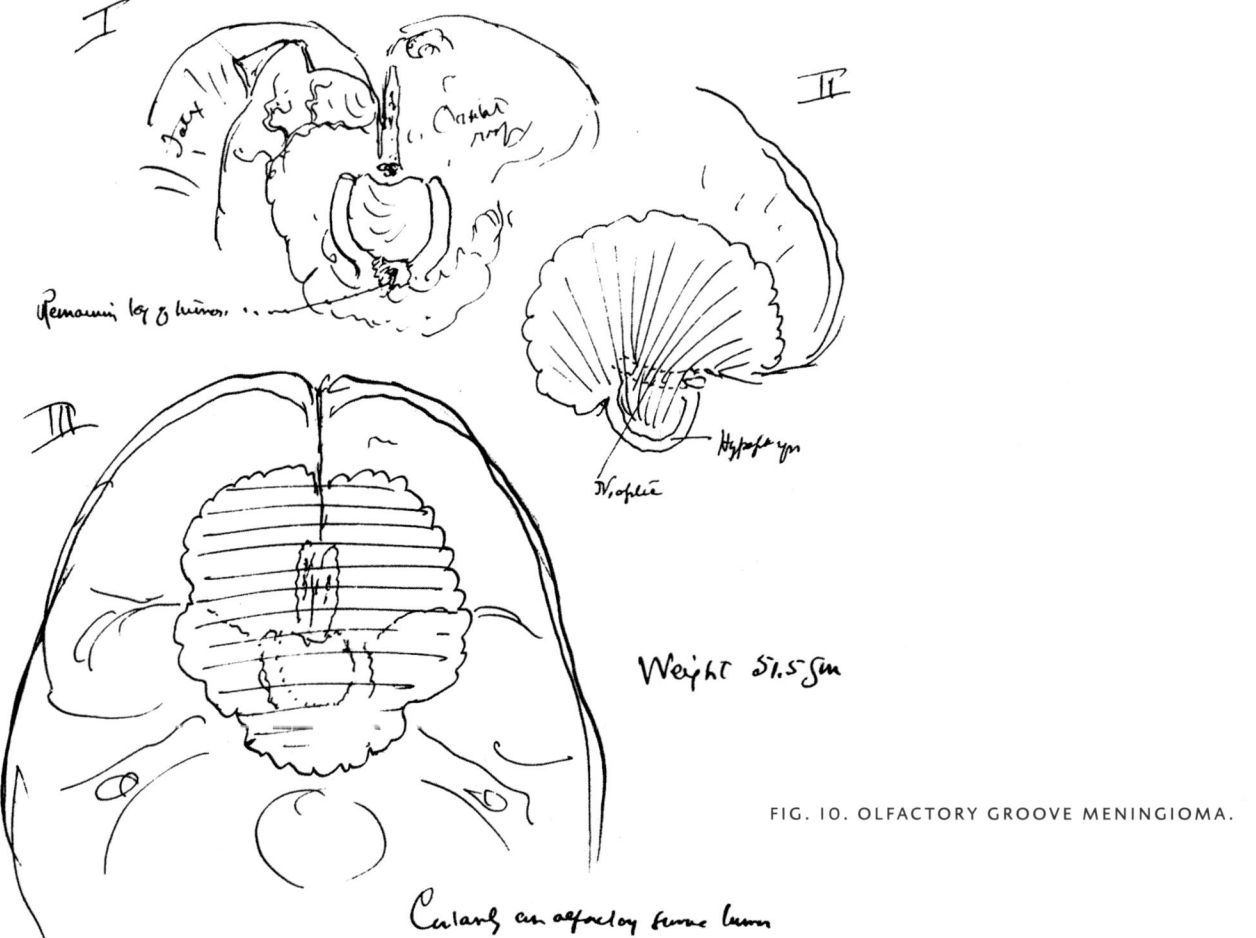

FIG. 10. OLFACTORY GROOVE MENINGIOMA.

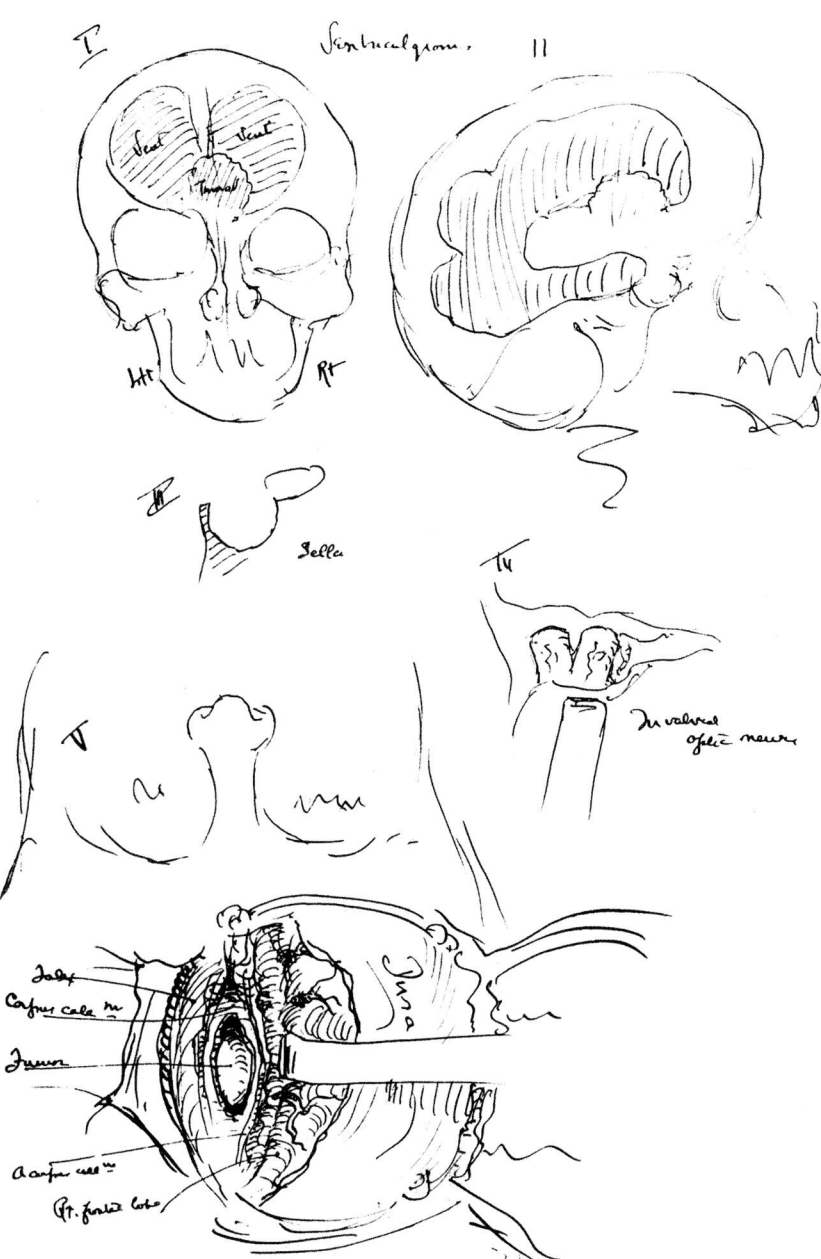

FIG. 11. GLIOMA OF THE THIRD VENTRICLE.

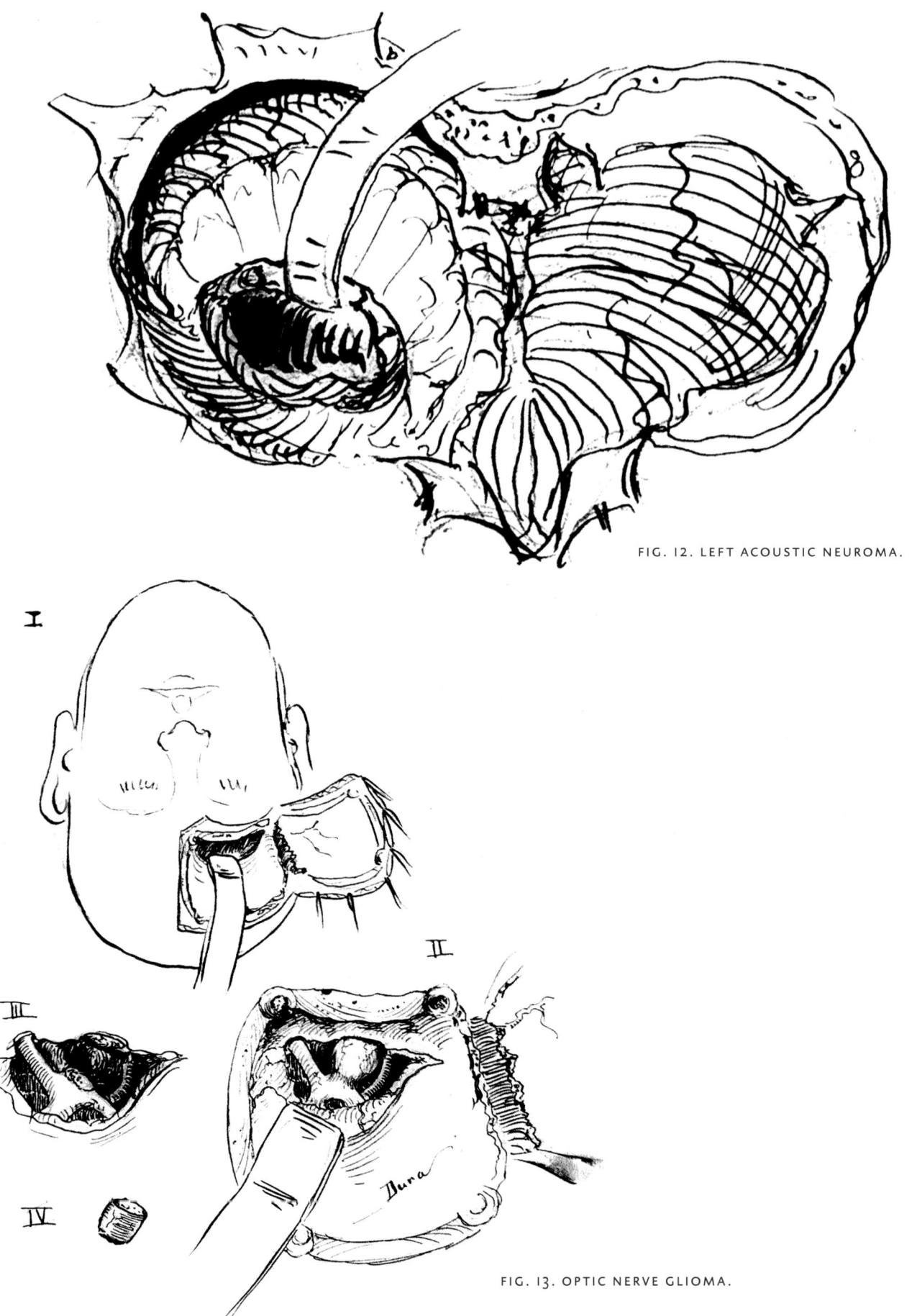

FIG. 12. LEFT ACOUSTIC NEUROMA.

FIG. 13. OPTIC NERVE GLIOMA.

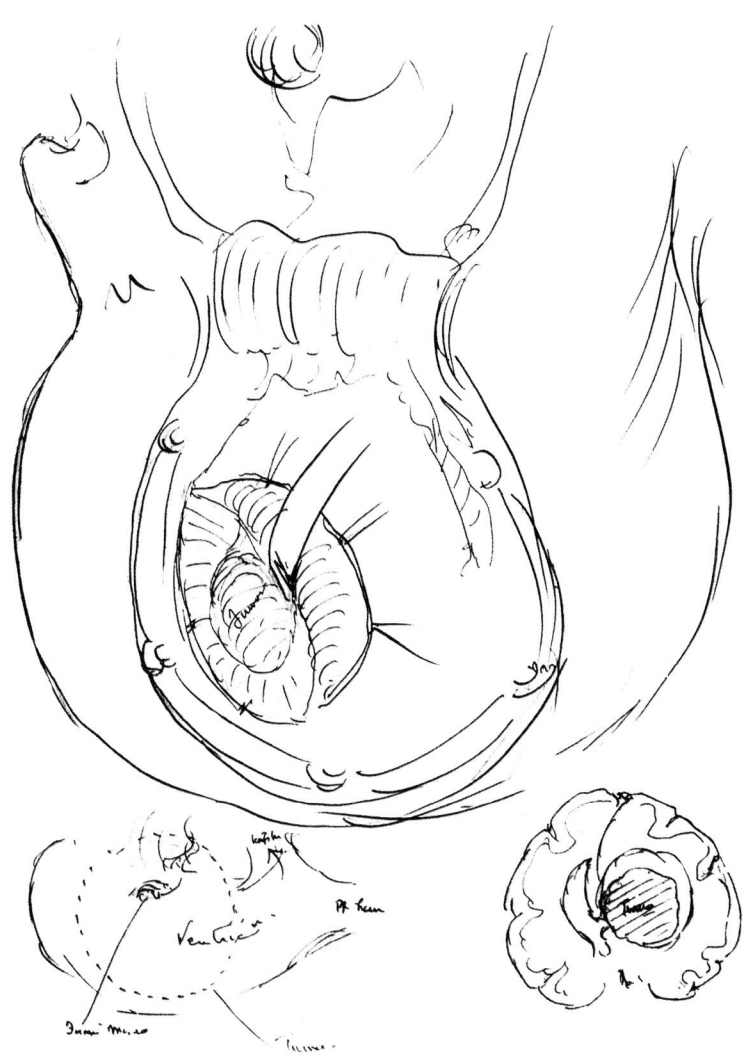

FIG. 14. RIGHT FRONTAL-INTRAVENTRICULAR GLIOMA.

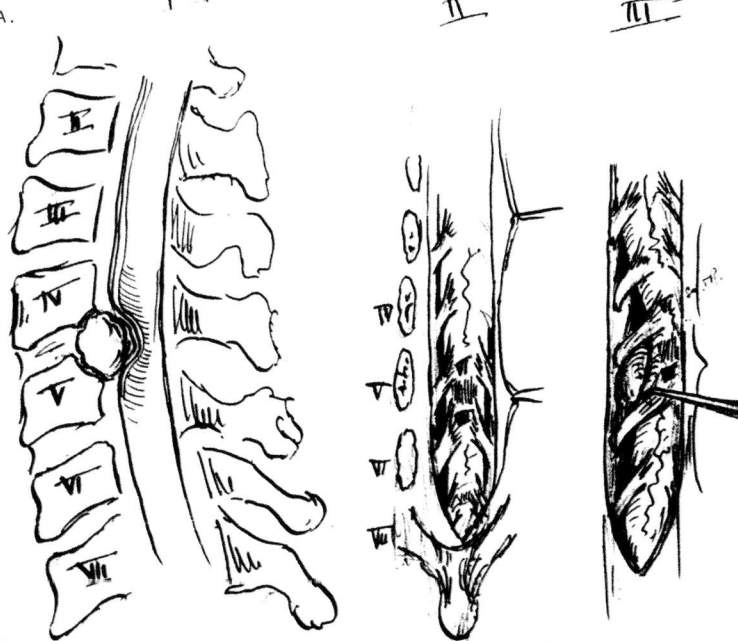

FIG. 15. CERVICAL SPINE ENCHONDROMA.

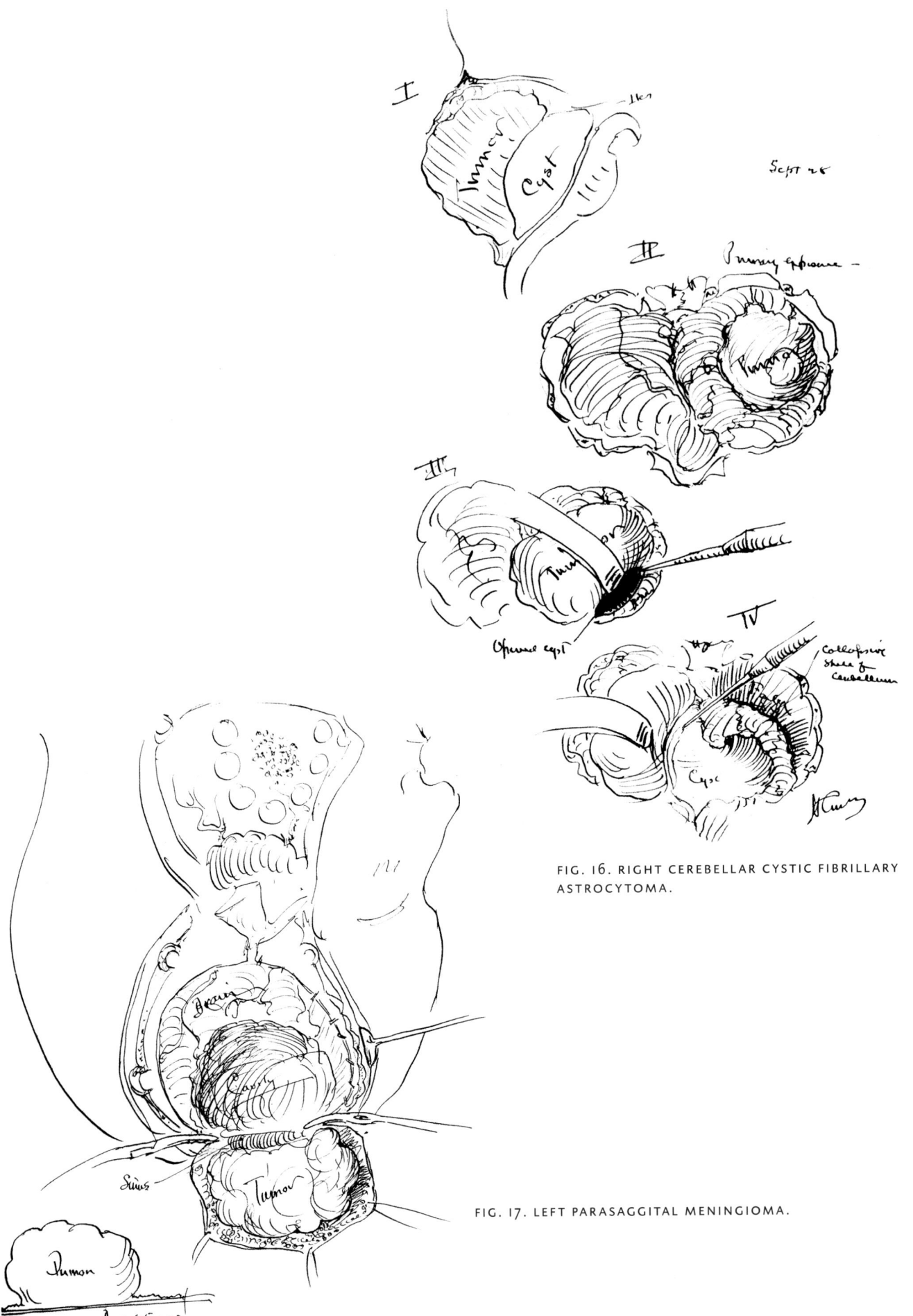

FIG. 16. RIGHT CEREBELLAR CYSTIC FIBRILLARY ASTROCYTOMA.

FIG. 17. LEFT PARASAGGITAL MENINGIOMA.

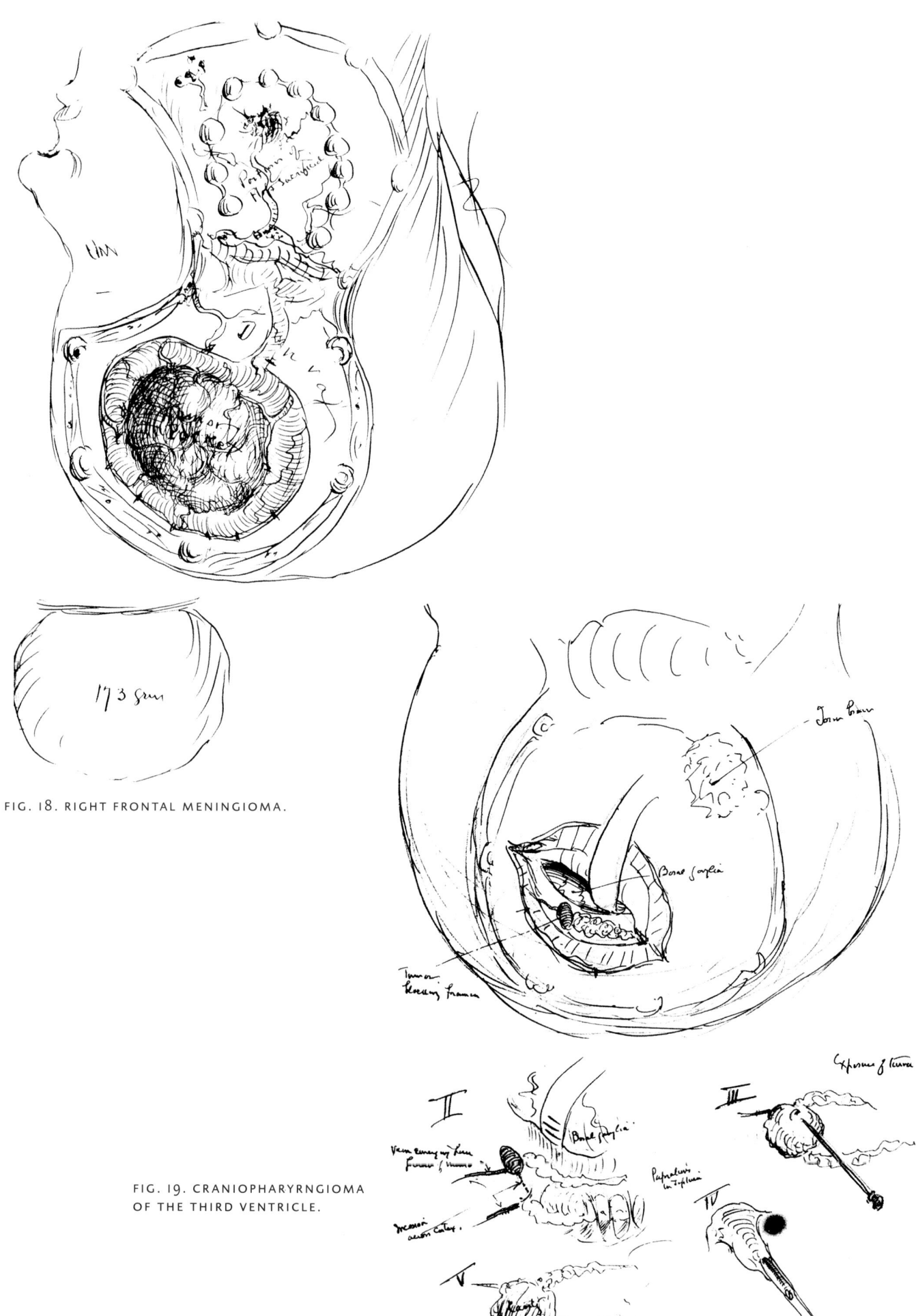

FIG. 18. RIGHT FRONTAL MENINGIOMA.

FIG. 19. CRANIOPHARYRNGIOMA OF THE THIRD VENTRICLE.

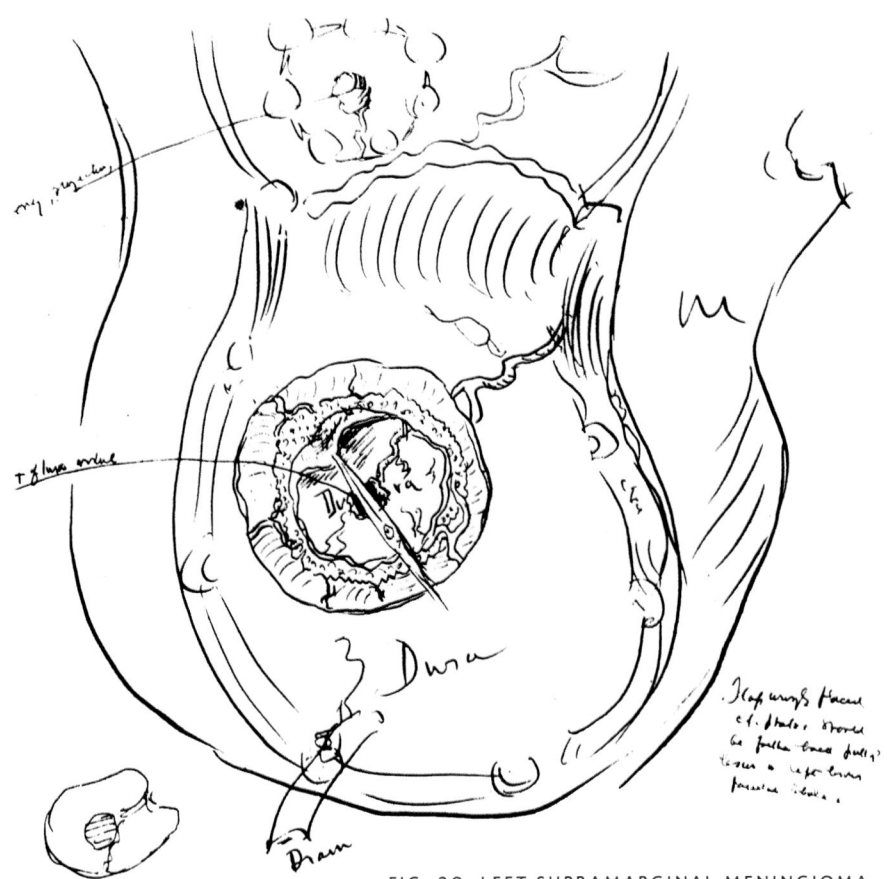

FIG. 20. LEFT SUPRAMARGINAL MENINGIOMA.

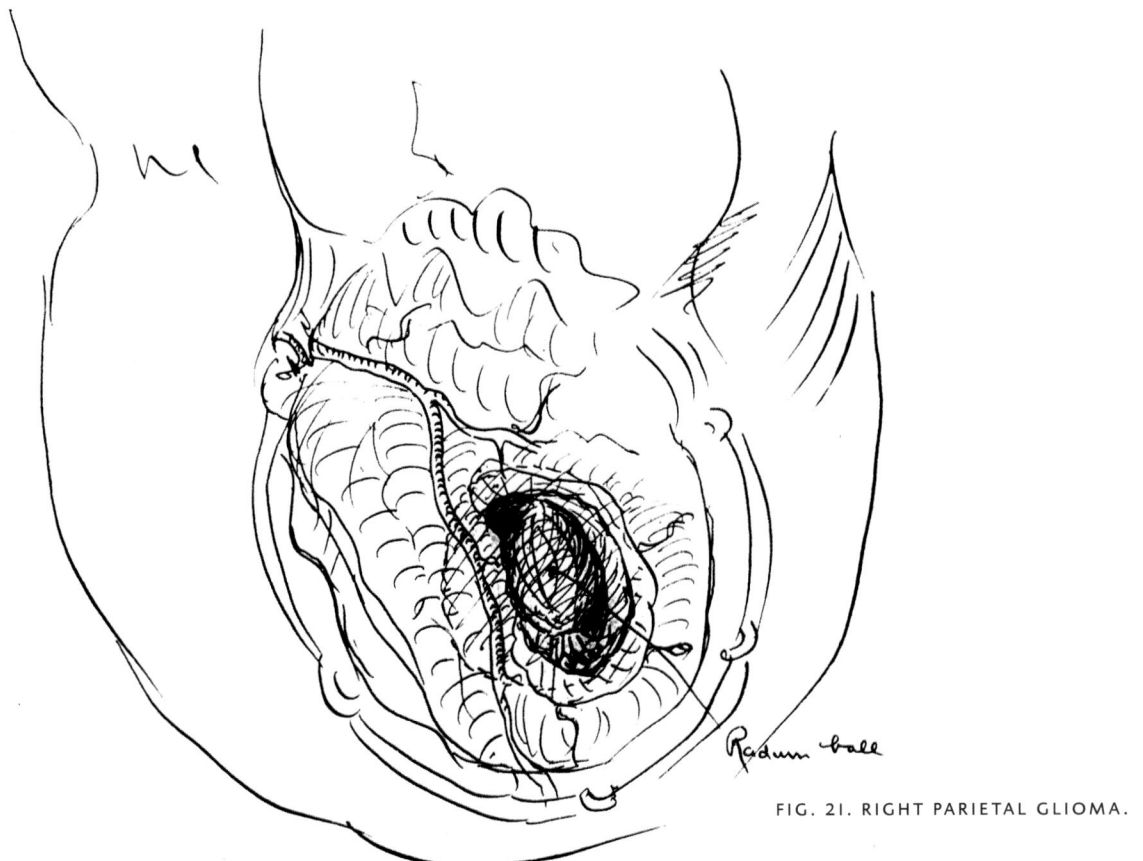

FIG. 21. RIGHT PARIETAL GLIOMA.

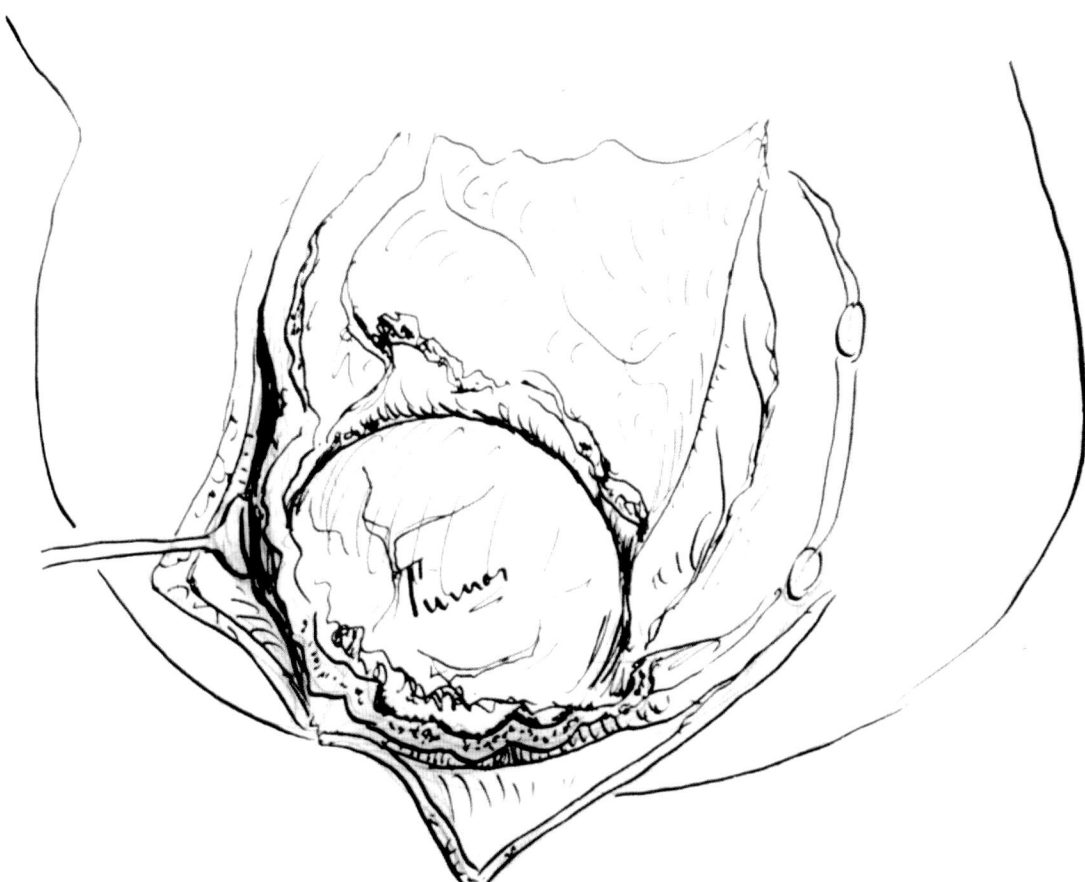

FIG. 22. RIGHT FRONTAL PARASAGITTAL MENINGIOMA.

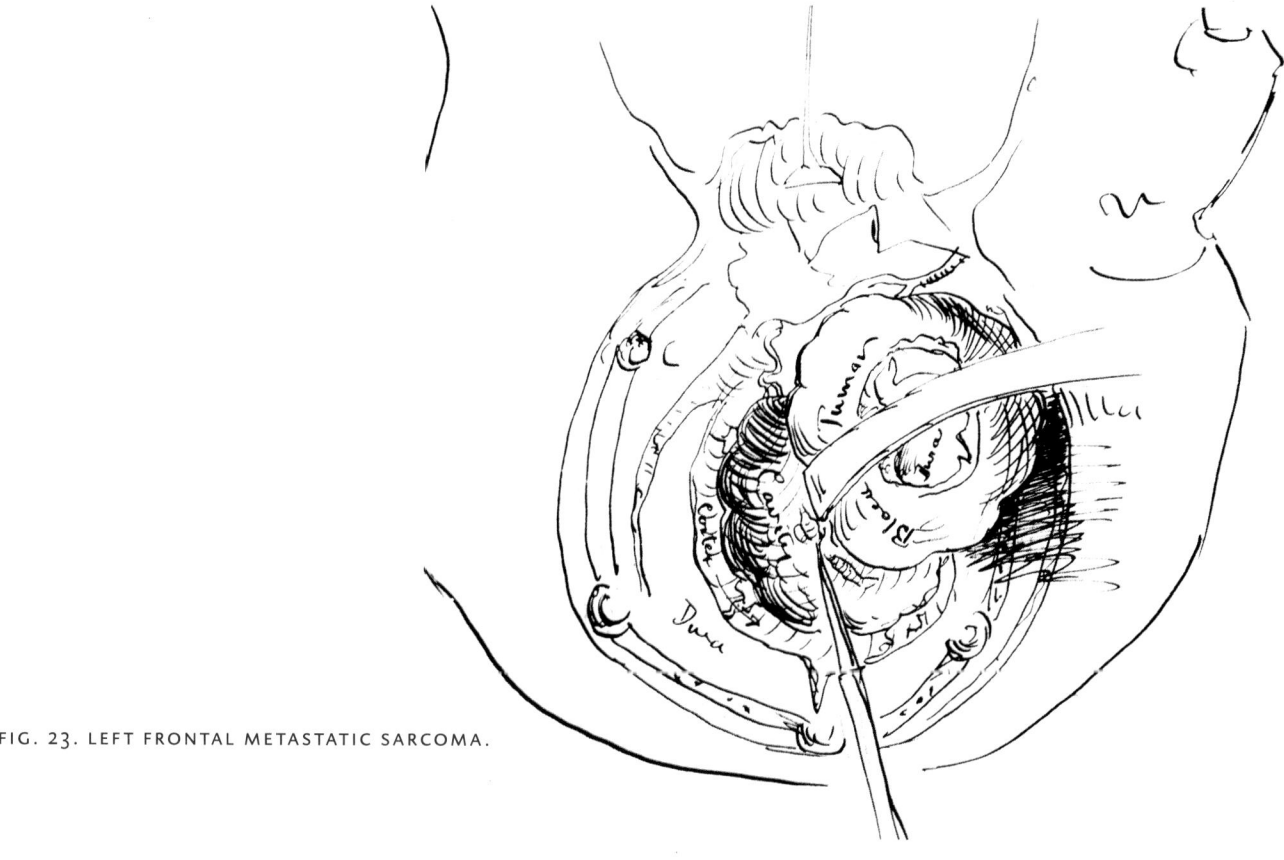

FIG. 23. LEFT FRONTAL METASTATIC SARCOMA.

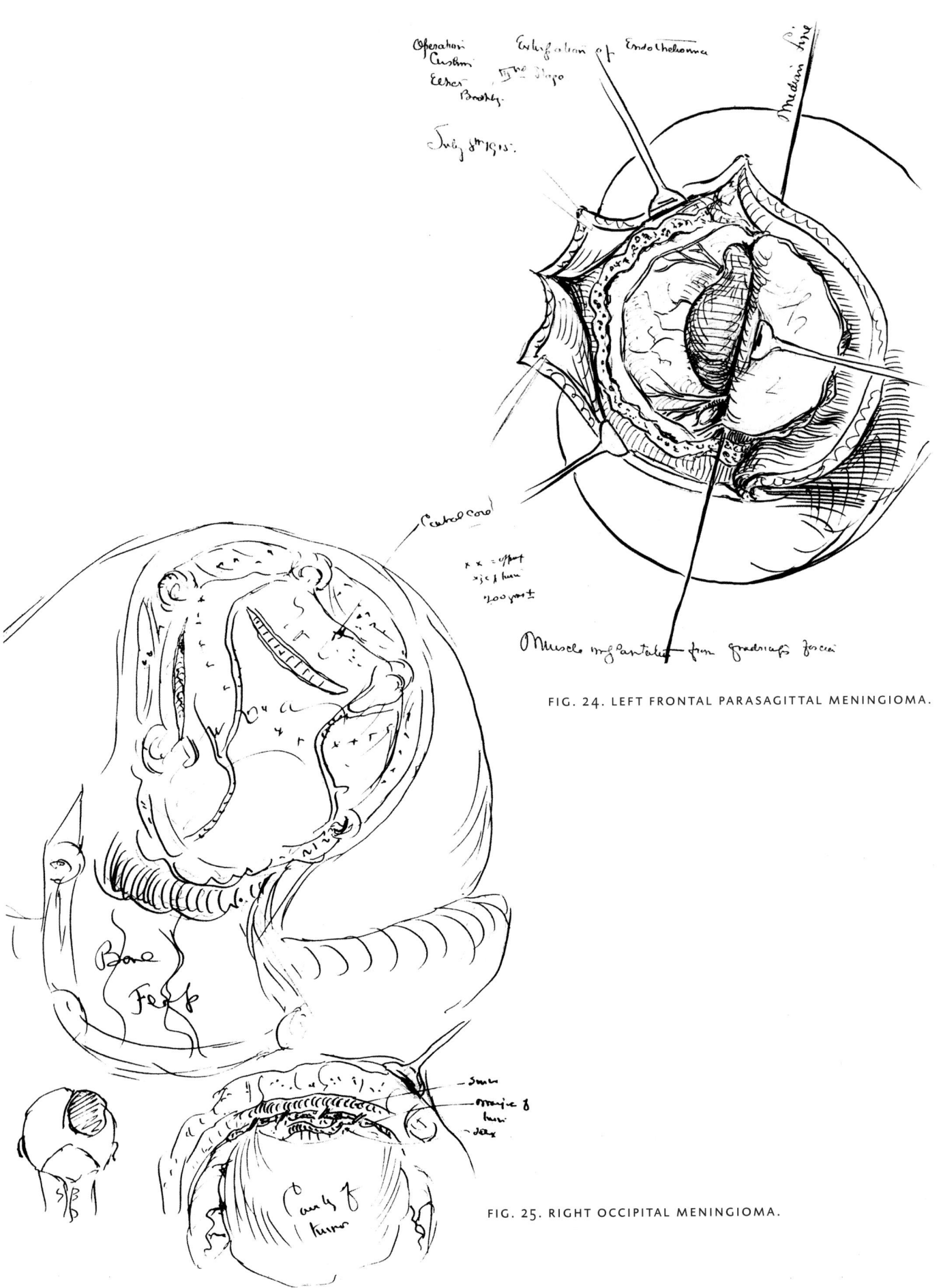

FIG. 24. LEFT FRONTAL PARASAGITTAL MENINGIOMA.

FIG. 25. RIGHT OCCIPITAL MENINGIOMA.

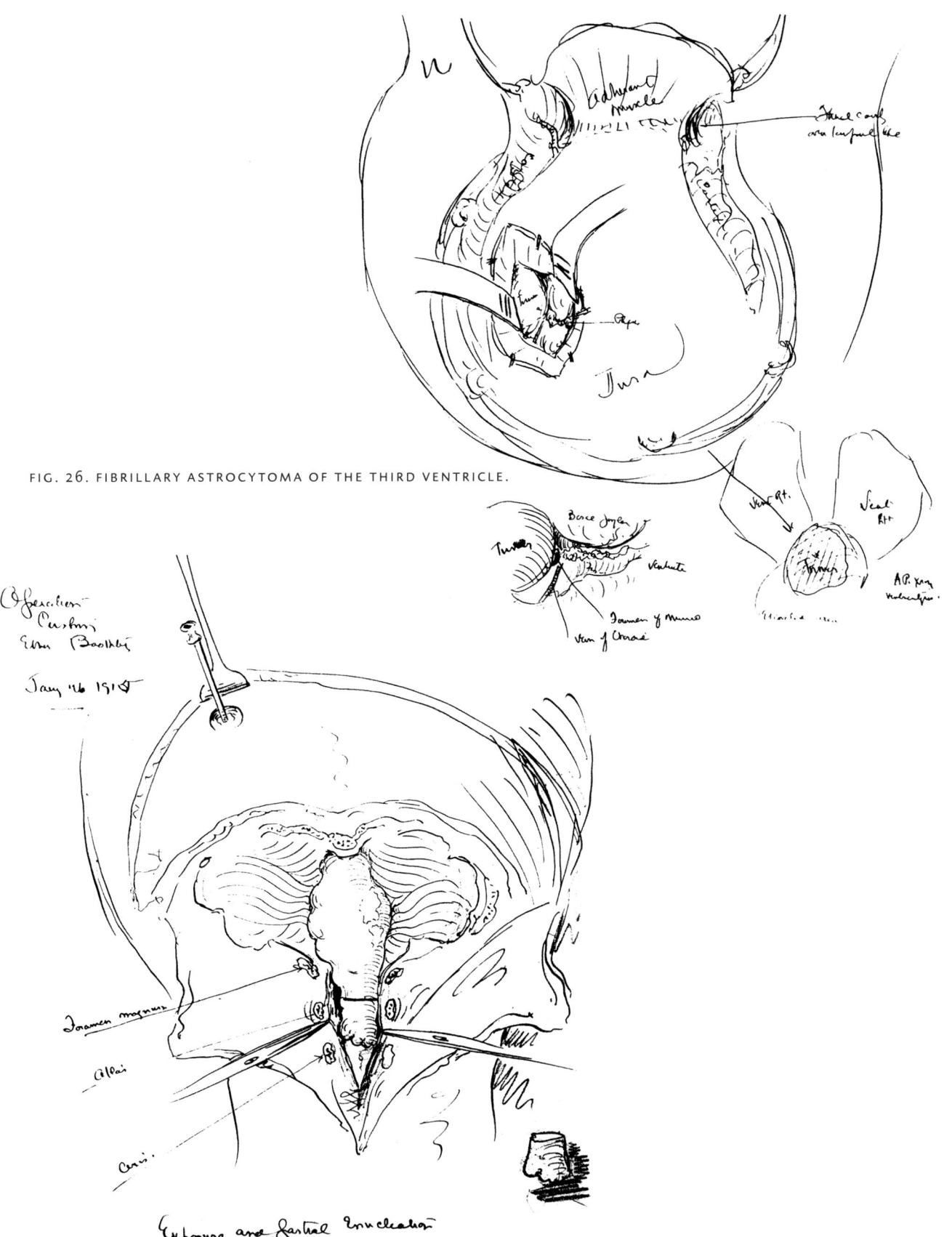

FIG. 26. FIBRILLARY ASTROCYTOMA OF THE THIRD VENTRICLE.

FIG. 27. FORAMEN MAGNUM MENINGIOMA.

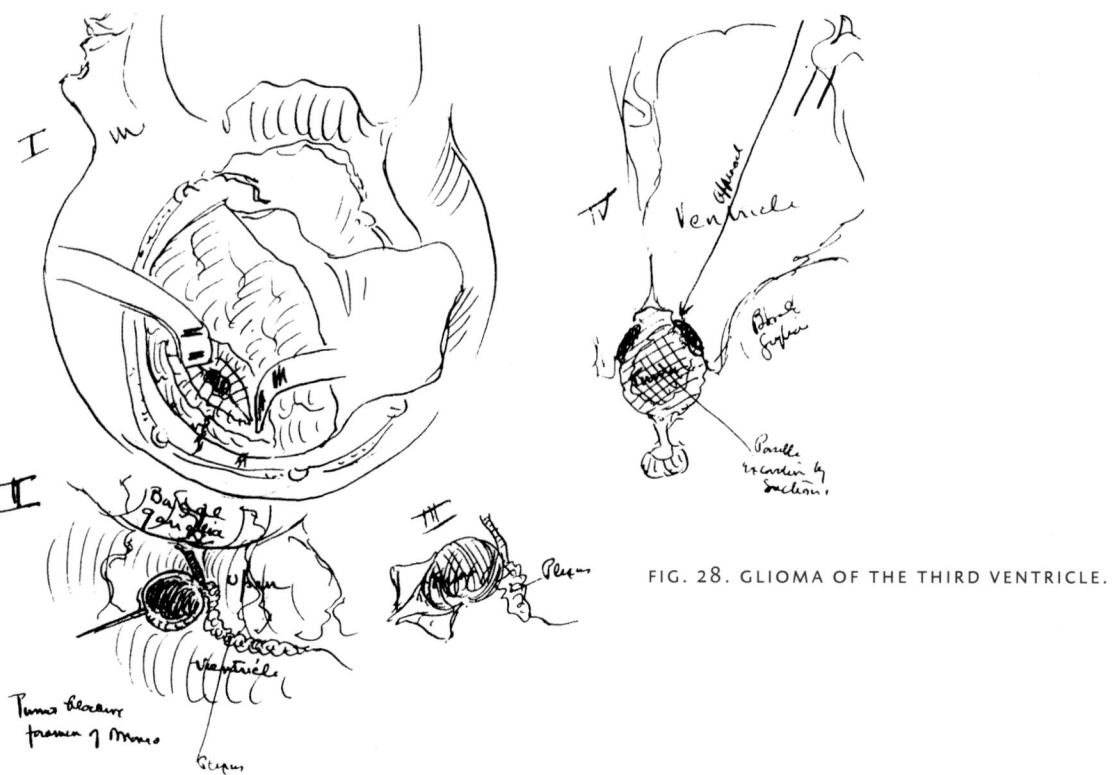

FIG. 28. GLIOMA OF THE THIRD VENTRICLE.

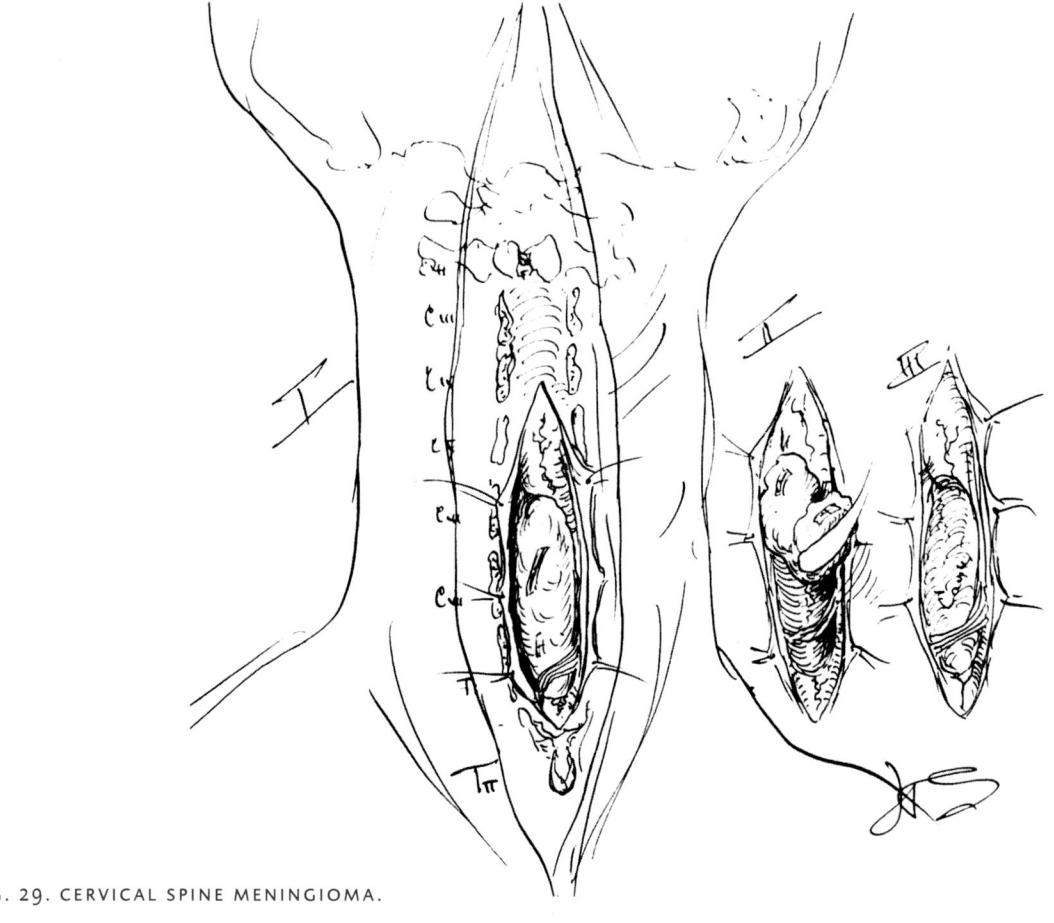

FIG. 29. CERVICAL SPINE MENINGIOMA.

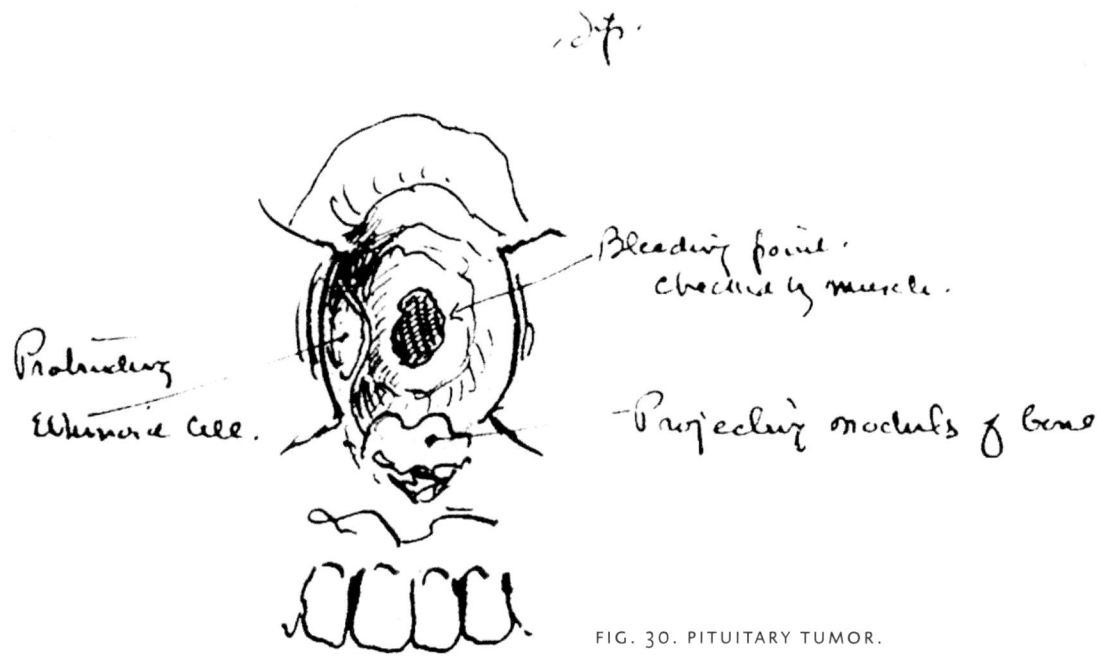

FIG. 30. PITUITARY TUMOR.

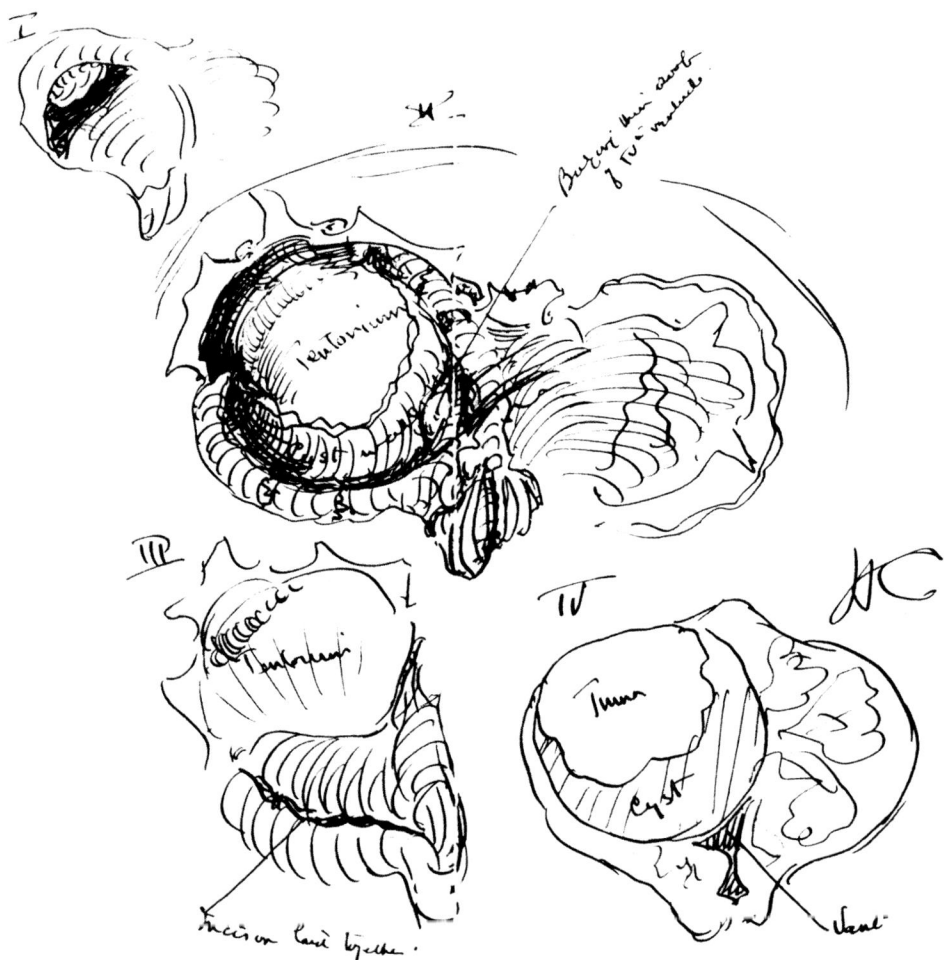

FIG. 31. LEFT CEREBELLAR MENINGIOMA.

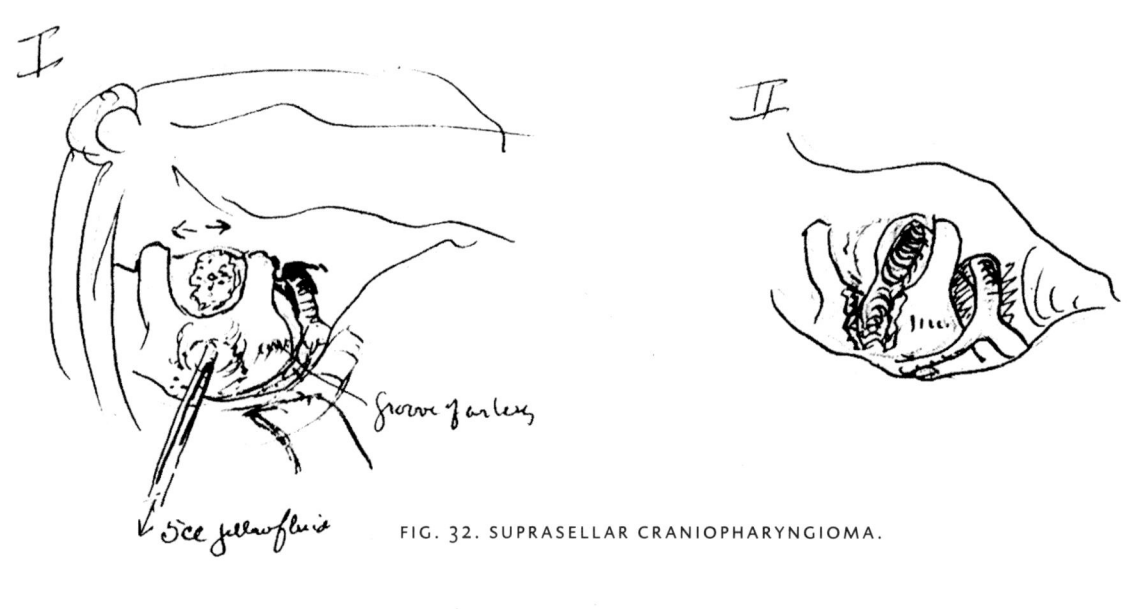

FIG. 32. SUPRASELLAR CRANIOPHARYNGIOMA.

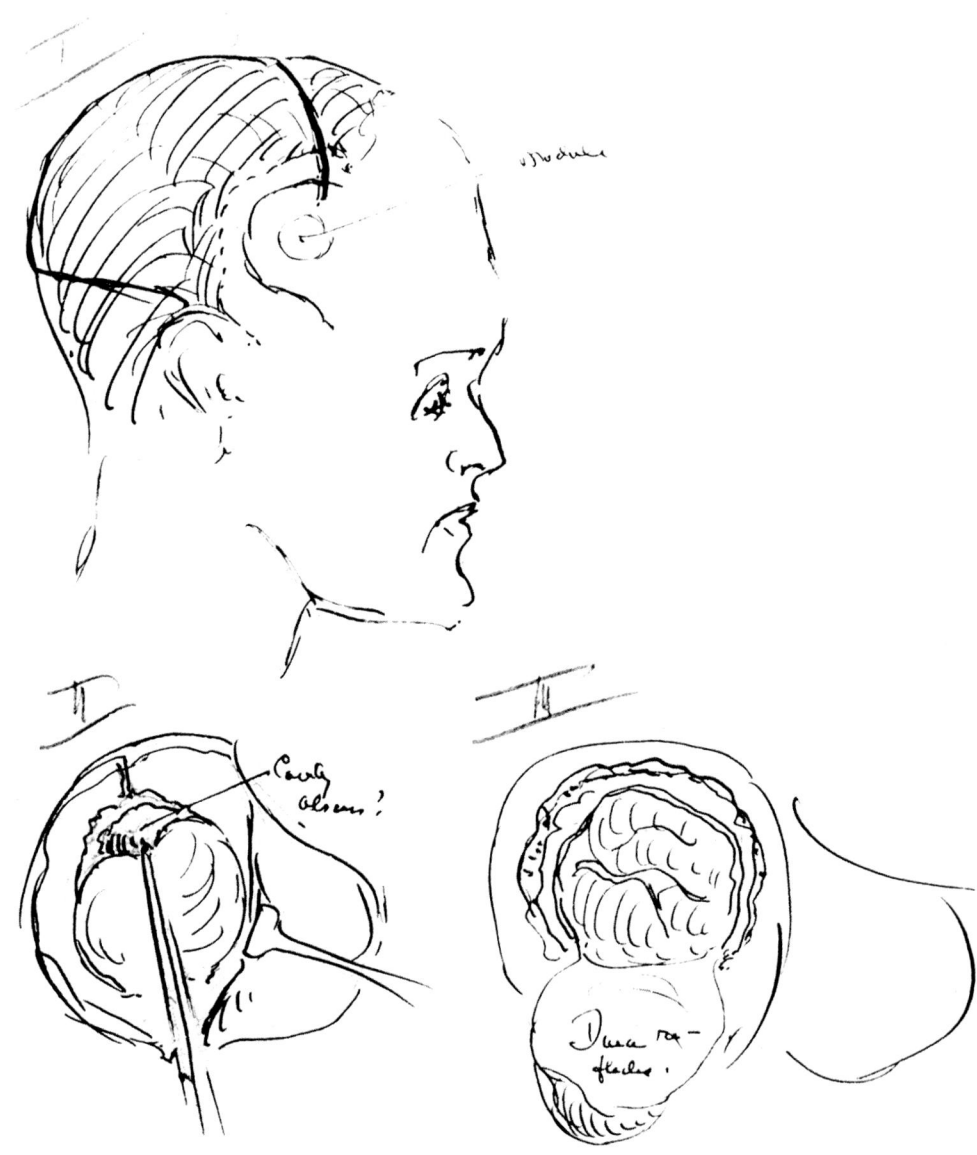

FIG. 33. RIGHT OCCIPITAL PARASAGITTAL MENINGIOMA.

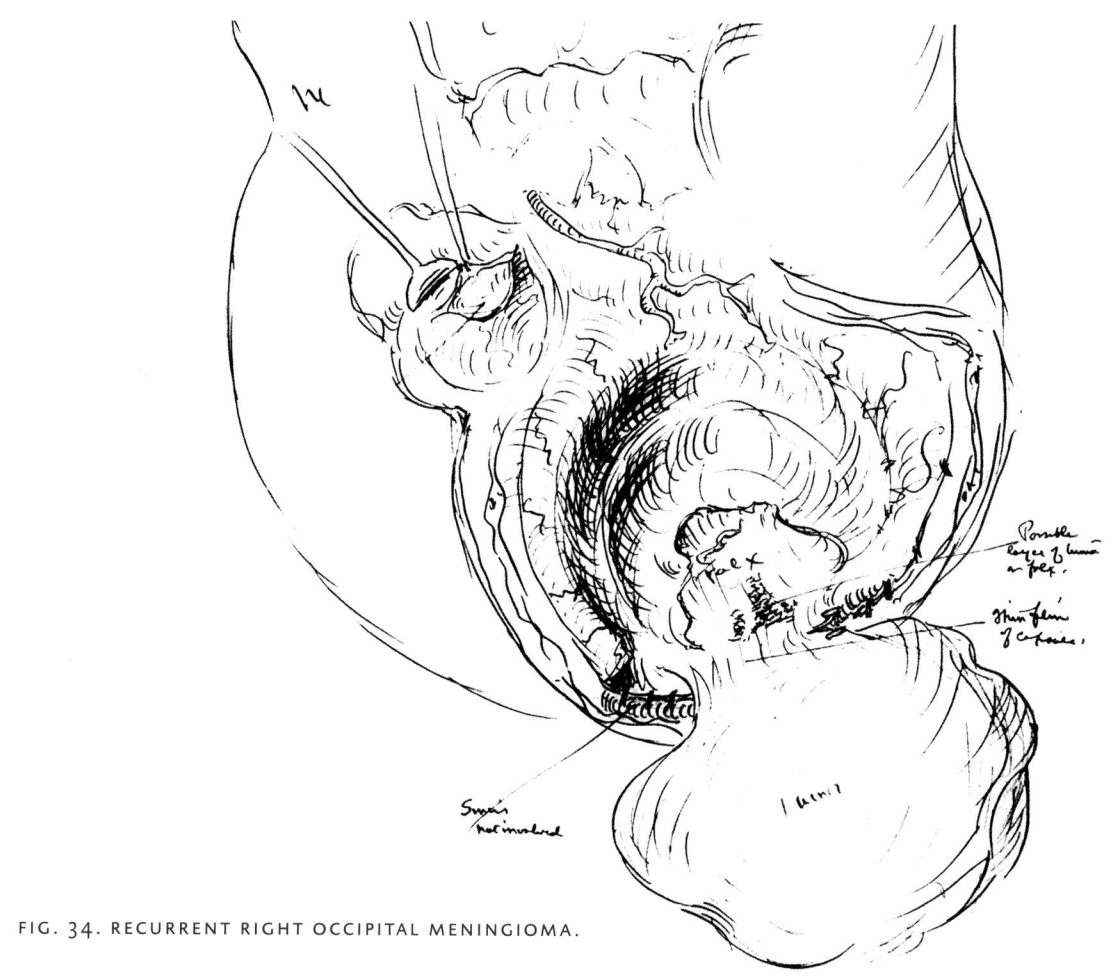

FIG. 34. RECURRENT RIGHT OCCIPITAL MENINGIOMA.

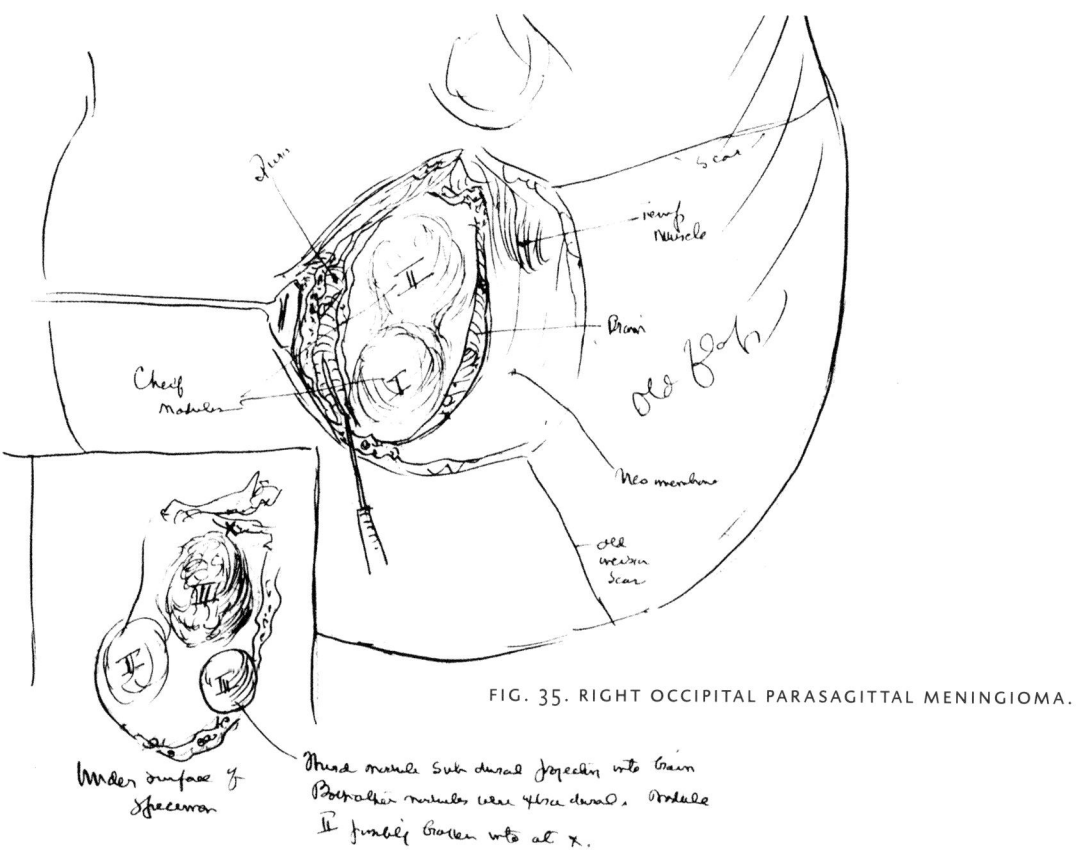

FIG. 35. RIGHT OCCIPITAL PARASAGITTAL MENINGIOMA.

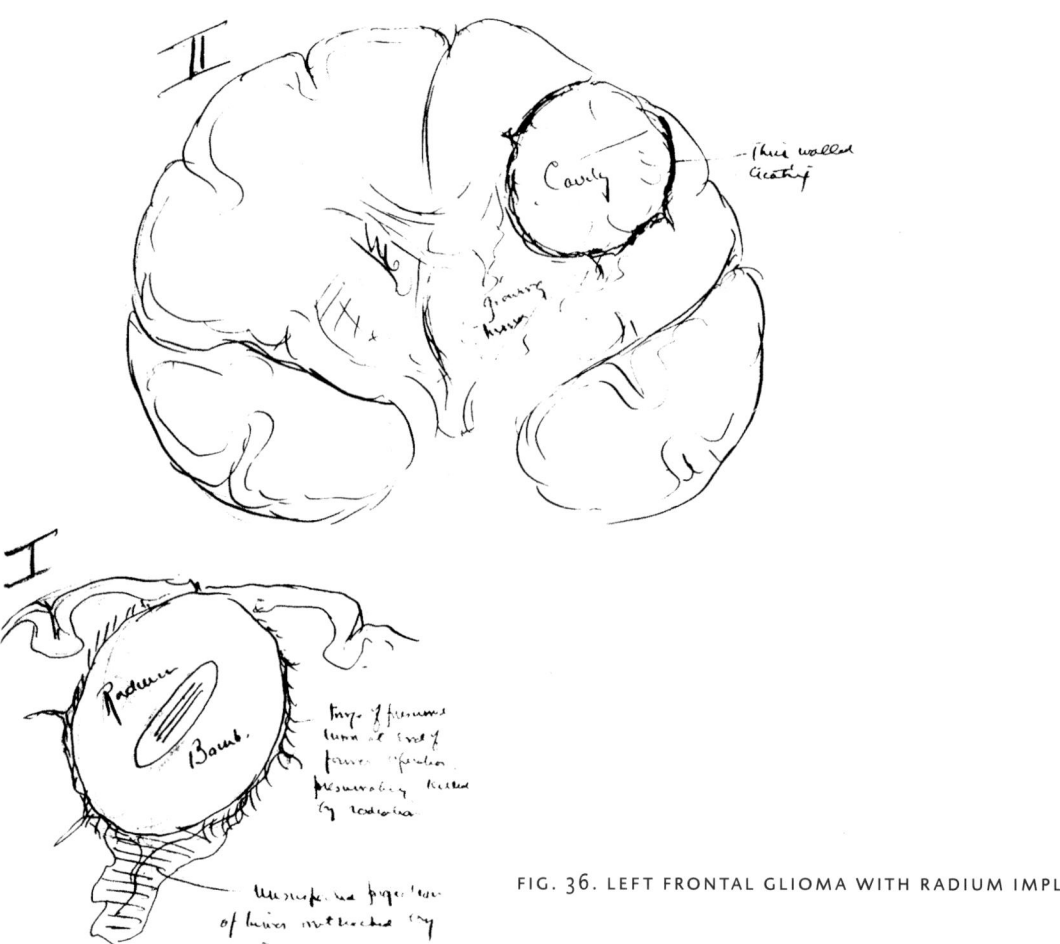

FIG. 36. LEFT FRONTAL GLIOMA WITH RADIUM IMPLANT.

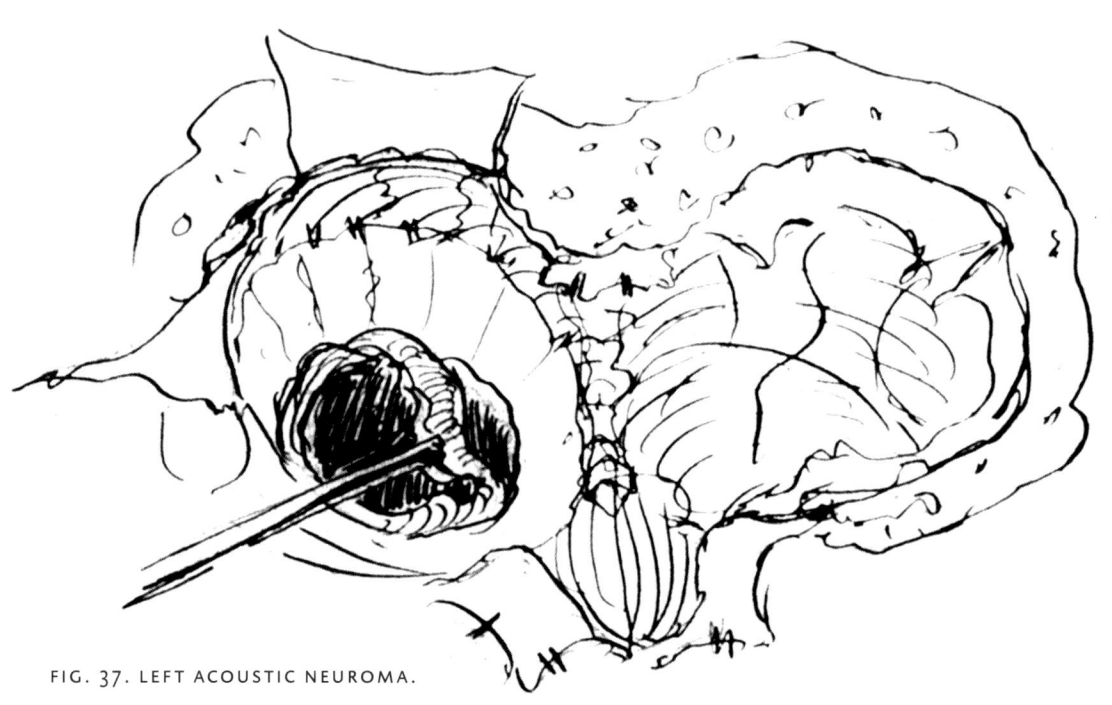

FIG. 37. LEFT ACOUSTIC NEUROMA.

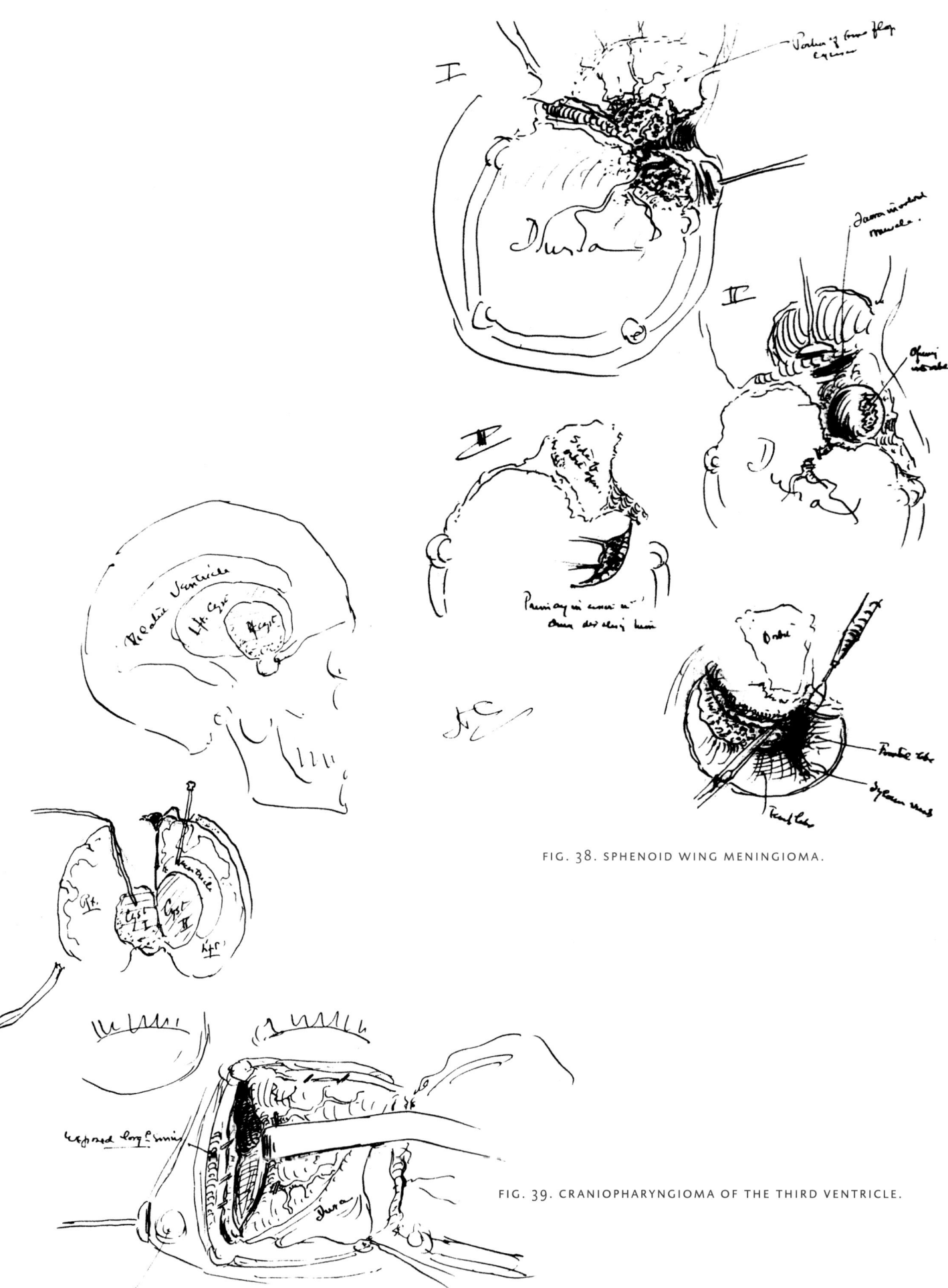

FIG. 38. SPHENOID WING MENINGIOMA.

FIG. 39. CRANIOPHARYNGIOMA OF THE THIRD VENTRICLE.

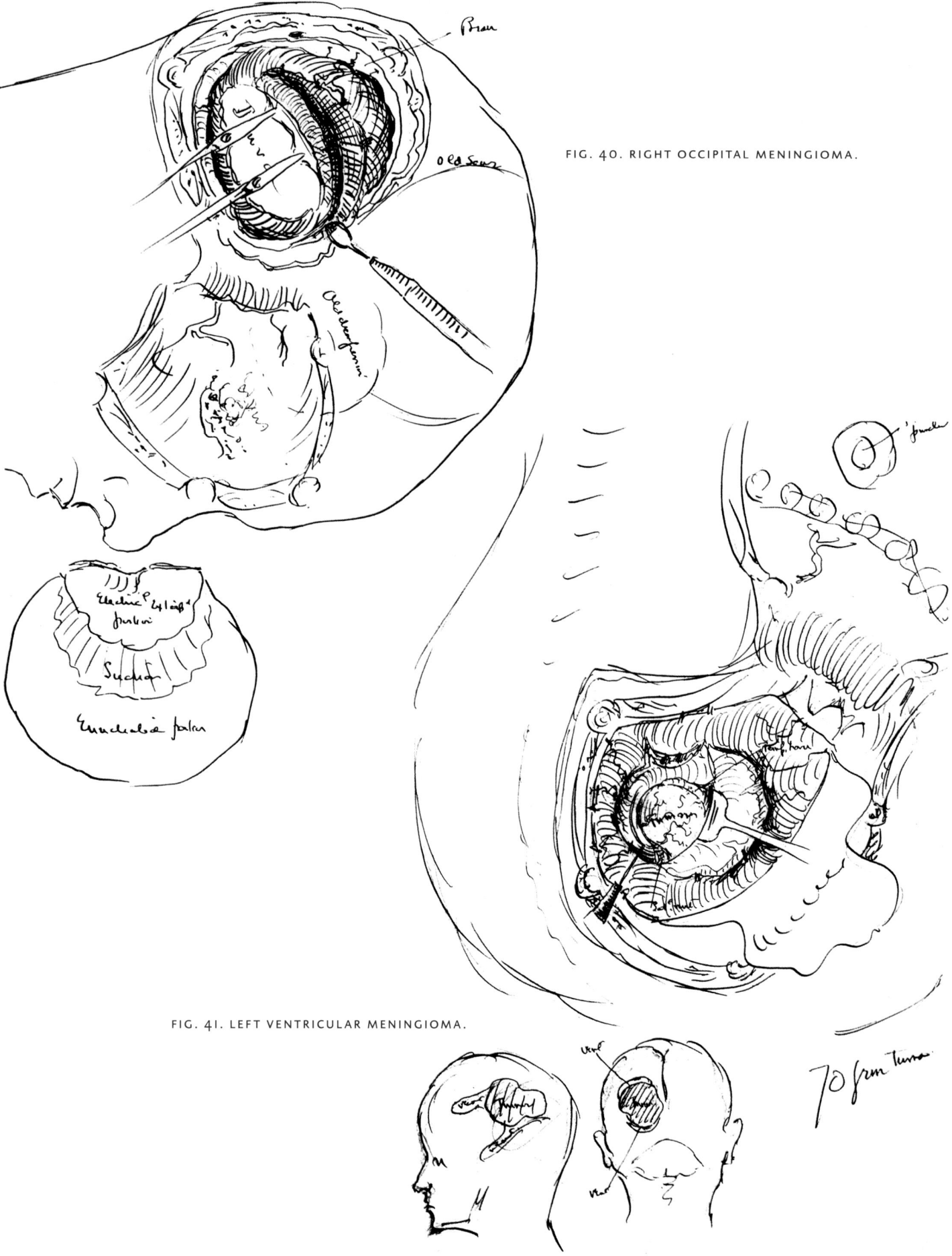

FIG. 40. RIGHT OCCIPITAL MENINGIOMA.

FIG. 41. LEFT VENTRICULAR MENINGIOMA.

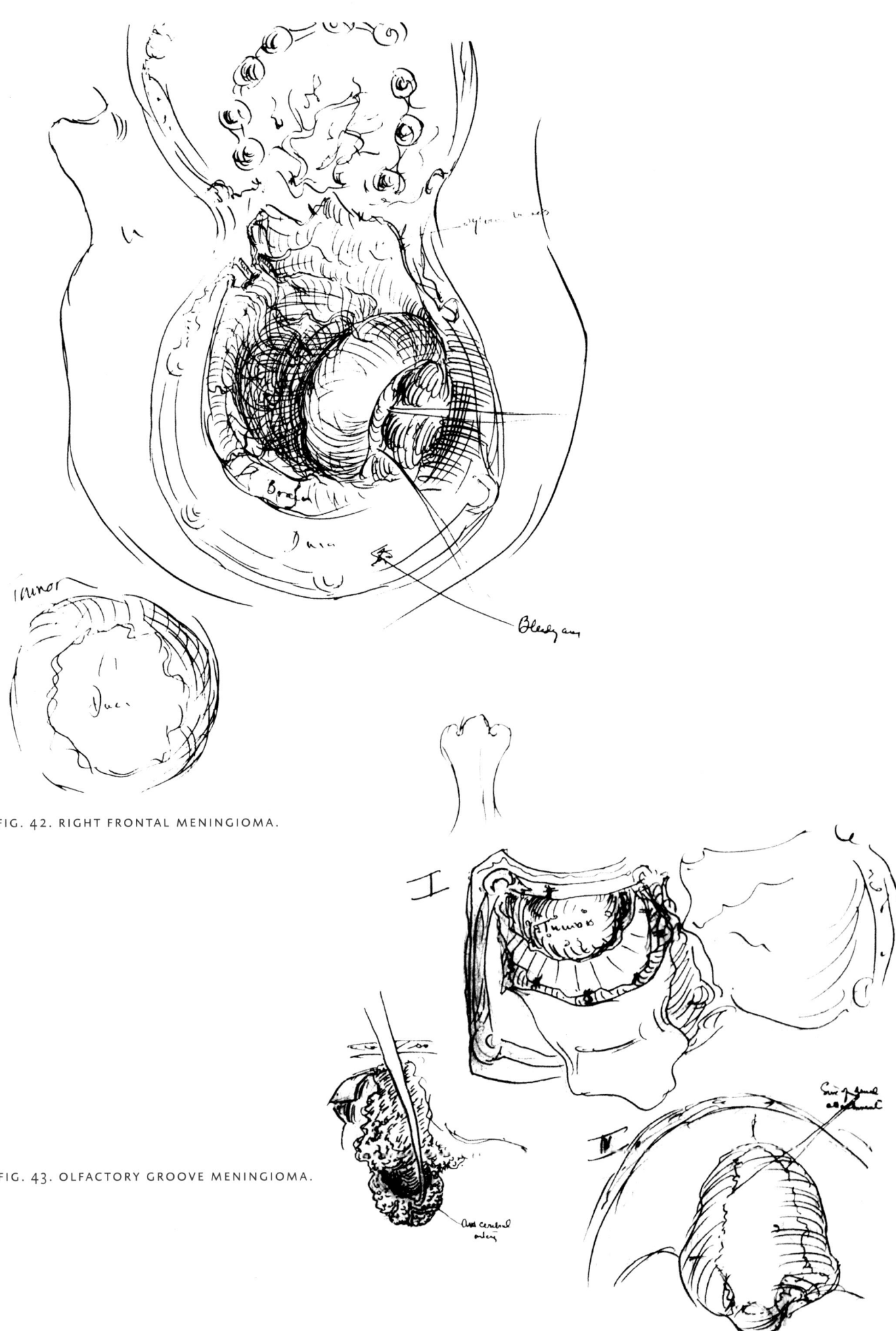

FIG. 42. RIGHT FRONTAL MENINGIOMA.

FIG. 43. OLFACTORY GROOVE MENINGIOMA.

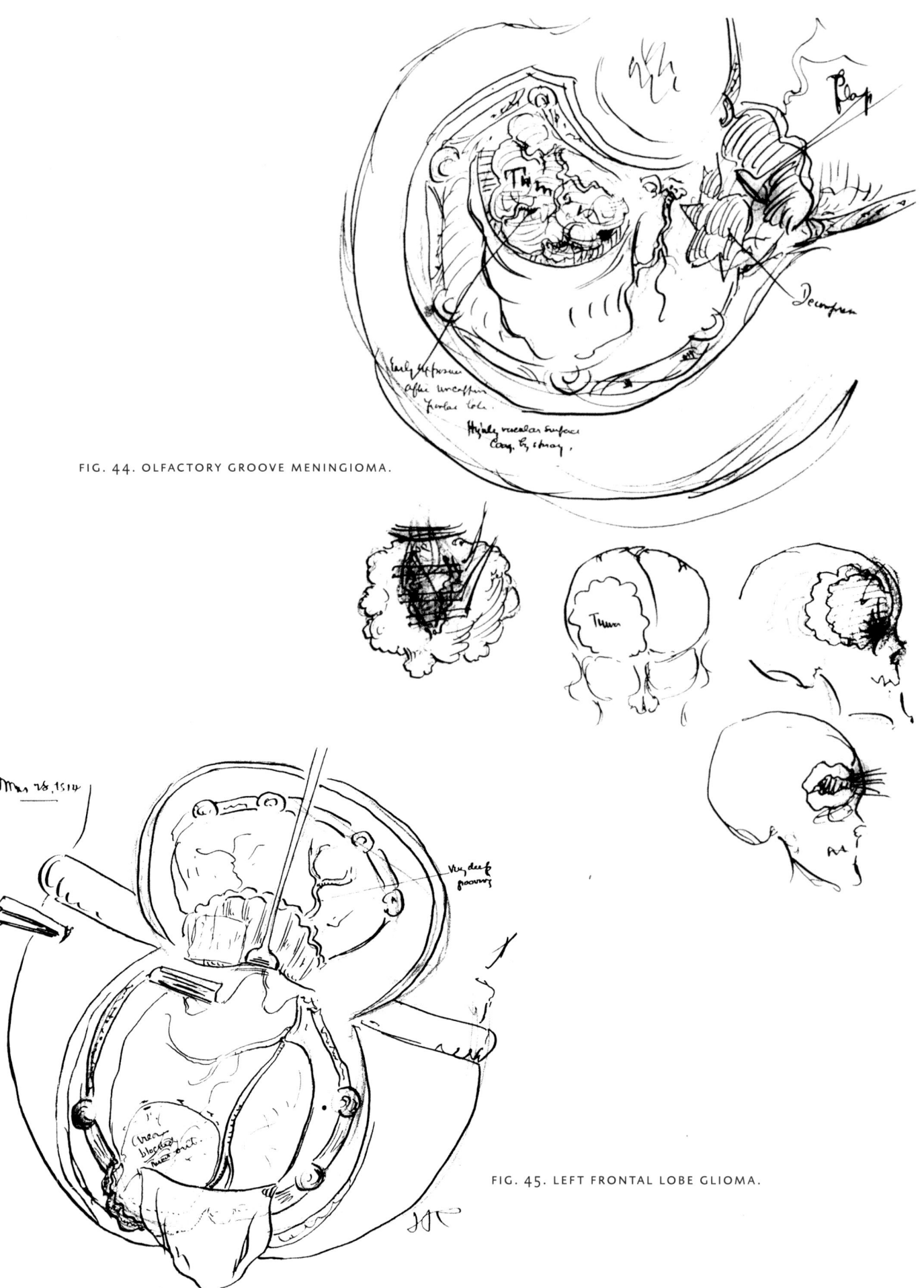

FIG. 44. OLFACTORY GROOVE MENINGIOMA.

FIG. 45. LEFT FRONTAL LOBE GLIOMA.

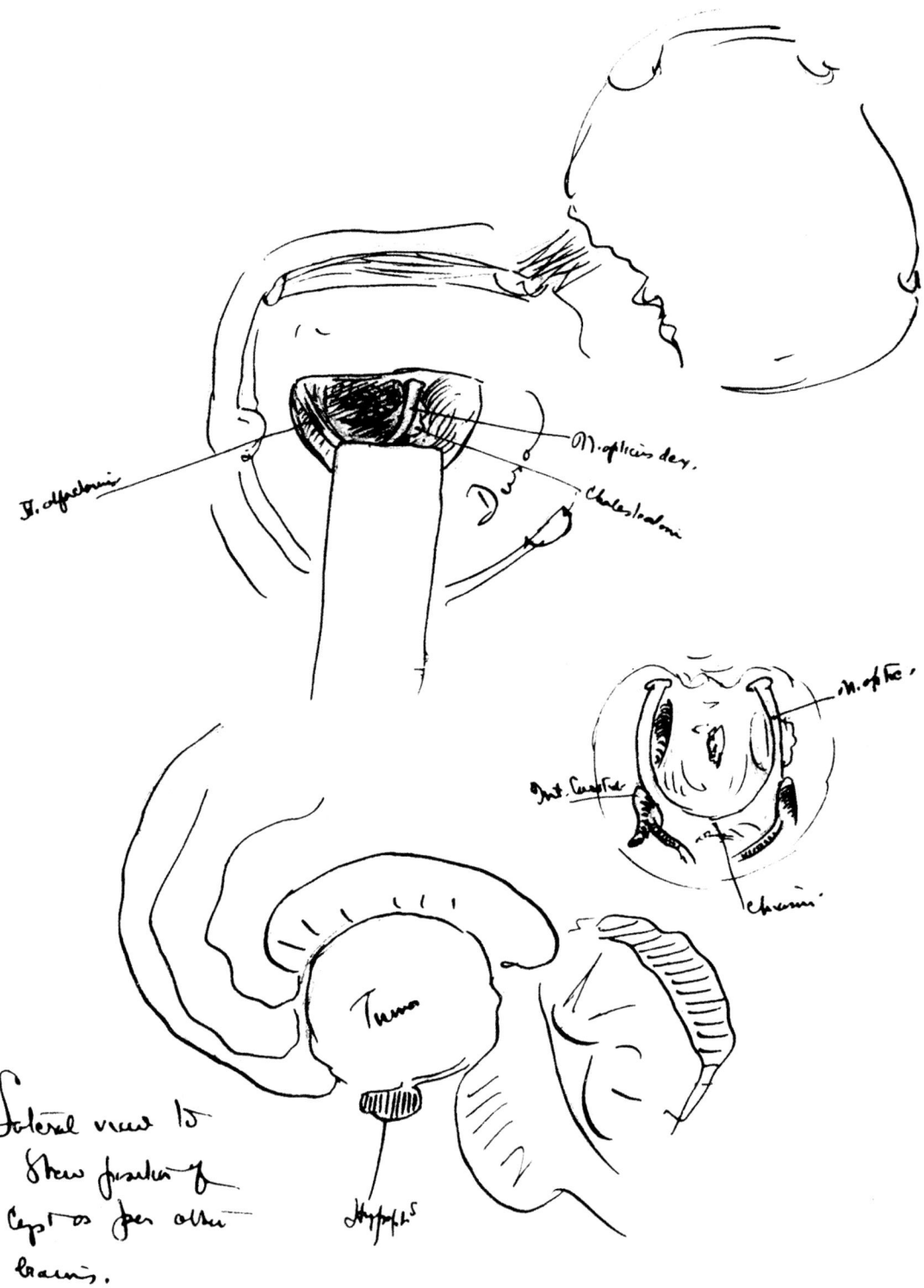

FIG. 46. SUPRASELLAR CHOLESTEATOMA.

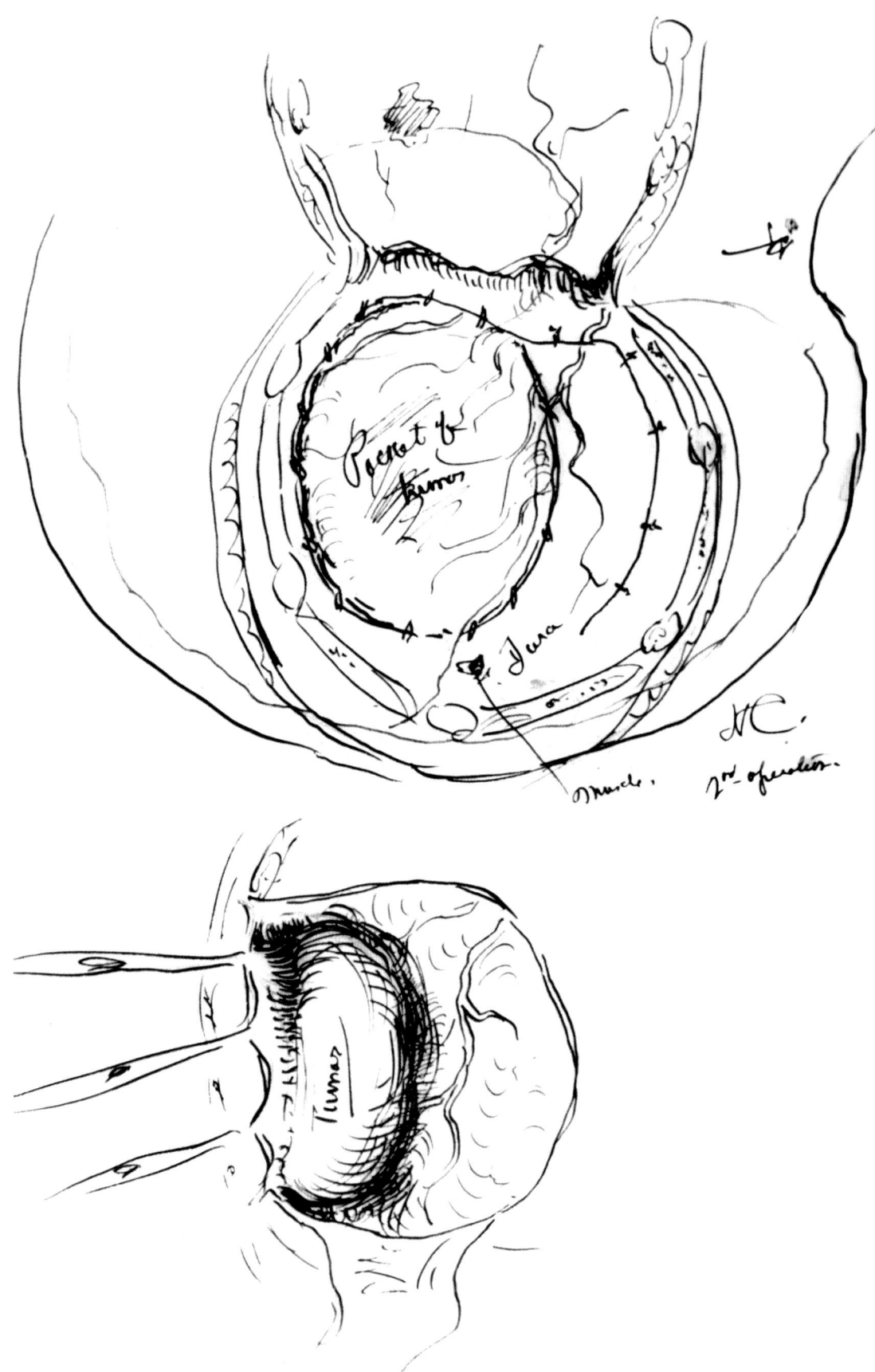

FIG. 47. RIGHT PARIETAL MENINGIOMA.

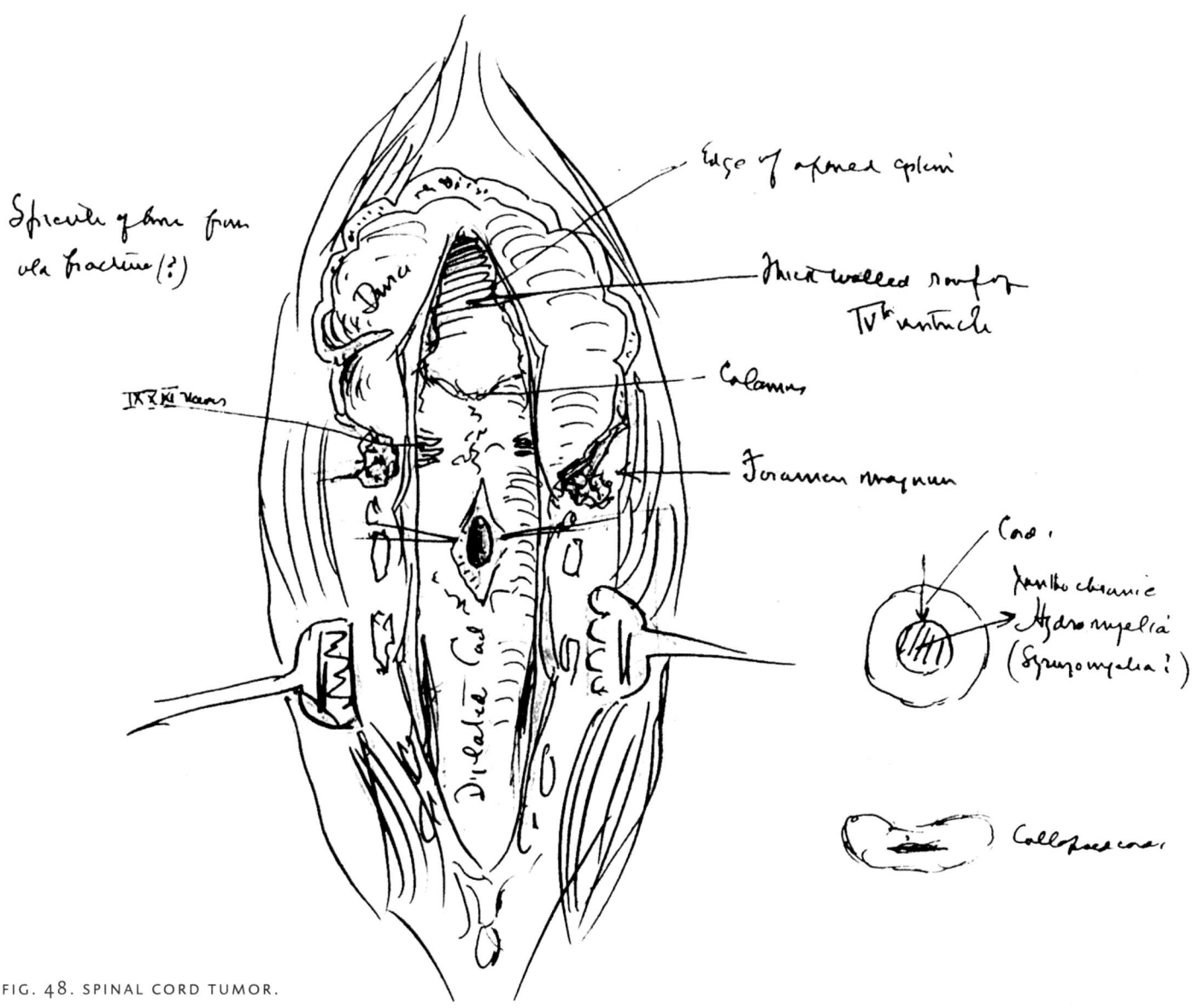

FIG. 48. SPINAL CORD TUMOR.

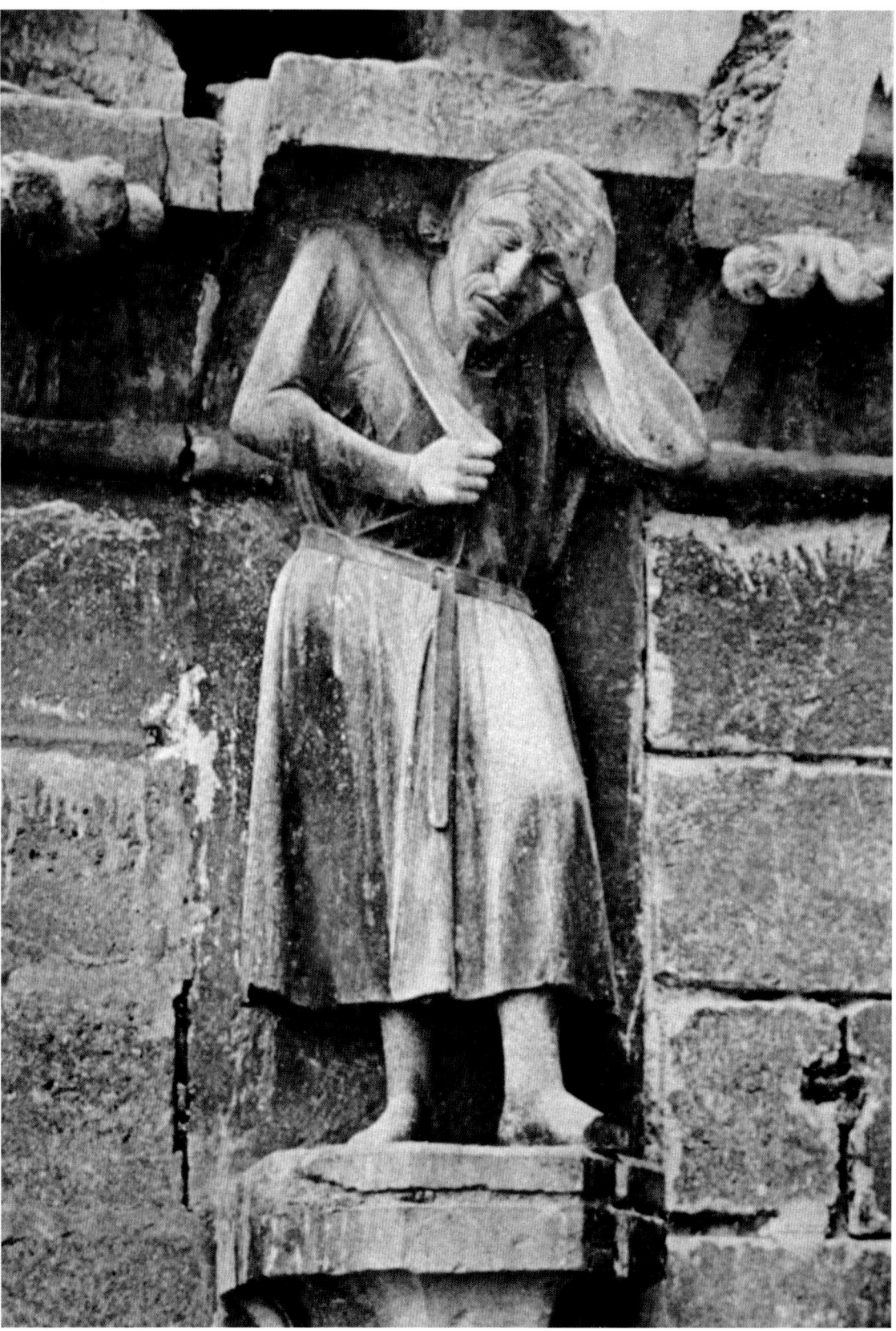

FIG. 49. A THIRTEENTH-CENTURY FIGURE ON REIMS CATHEDRAL — EXAMPLE OF ACROMEGALY.

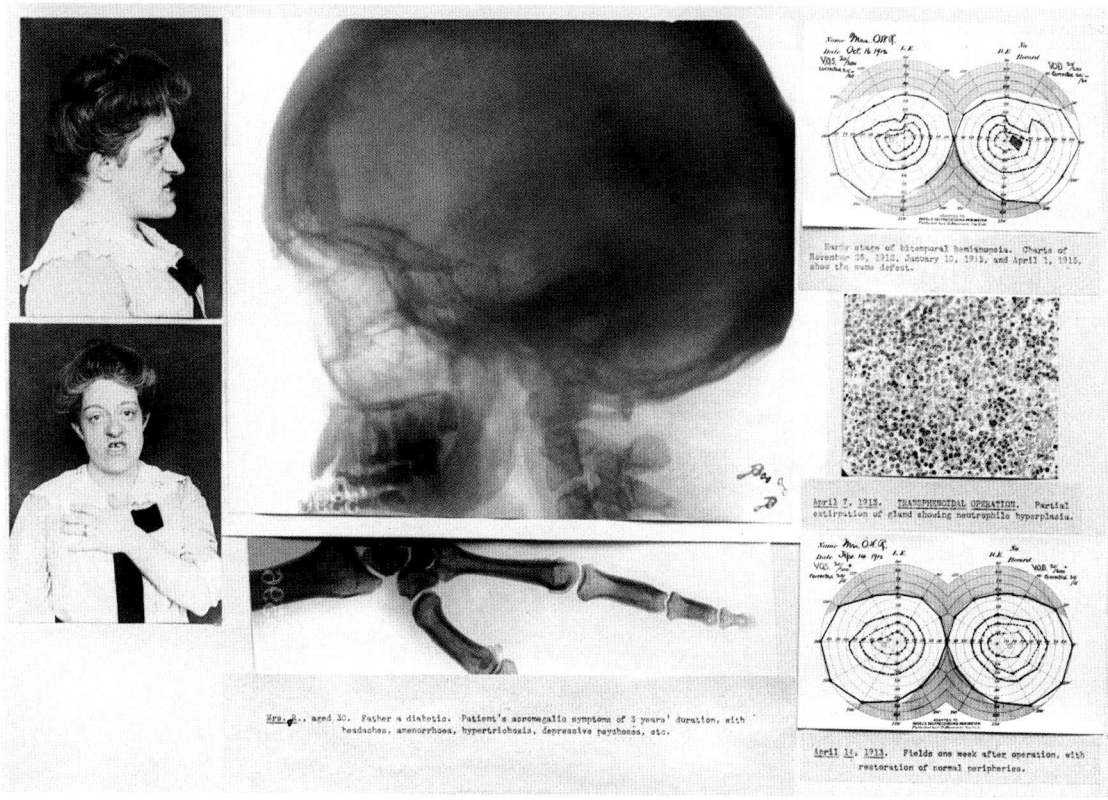

FIG. 50. ACROMEGALY.

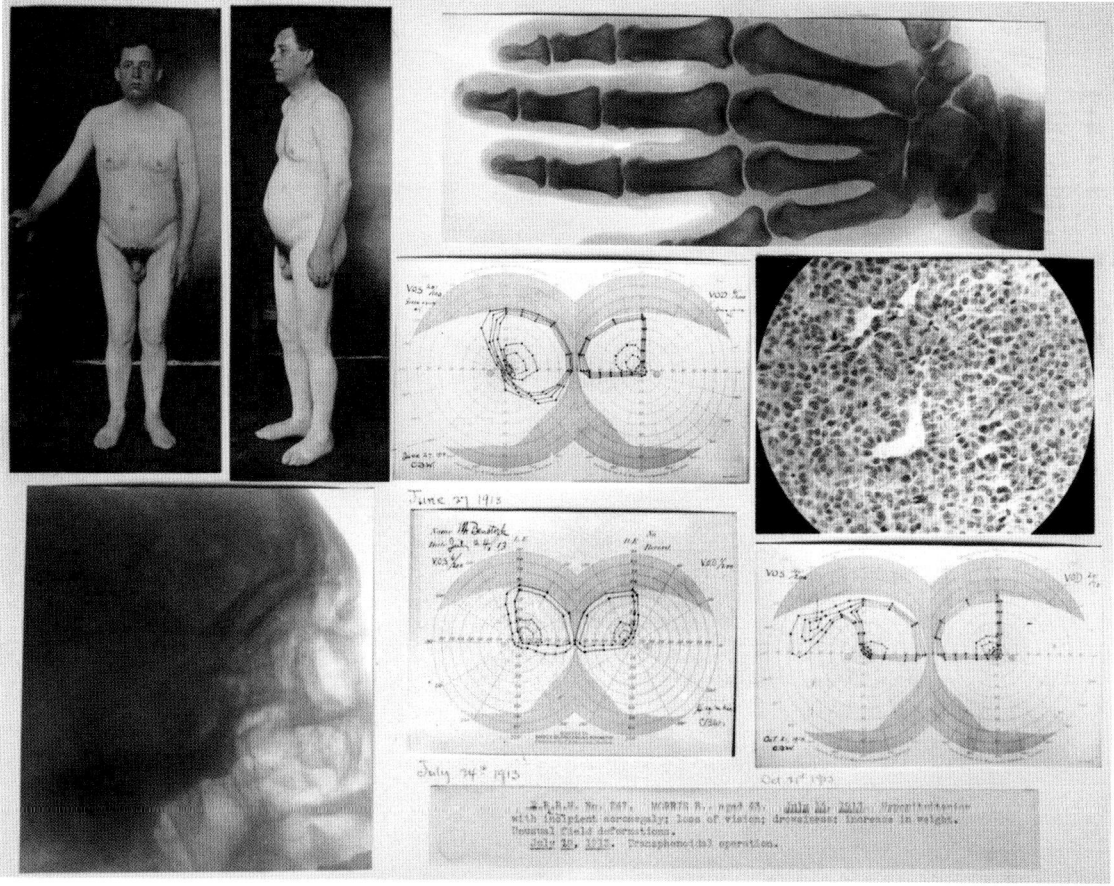

FIG. 51. ACROMEGALY ASSOCIATED WITH HYPOPITUITARISM.

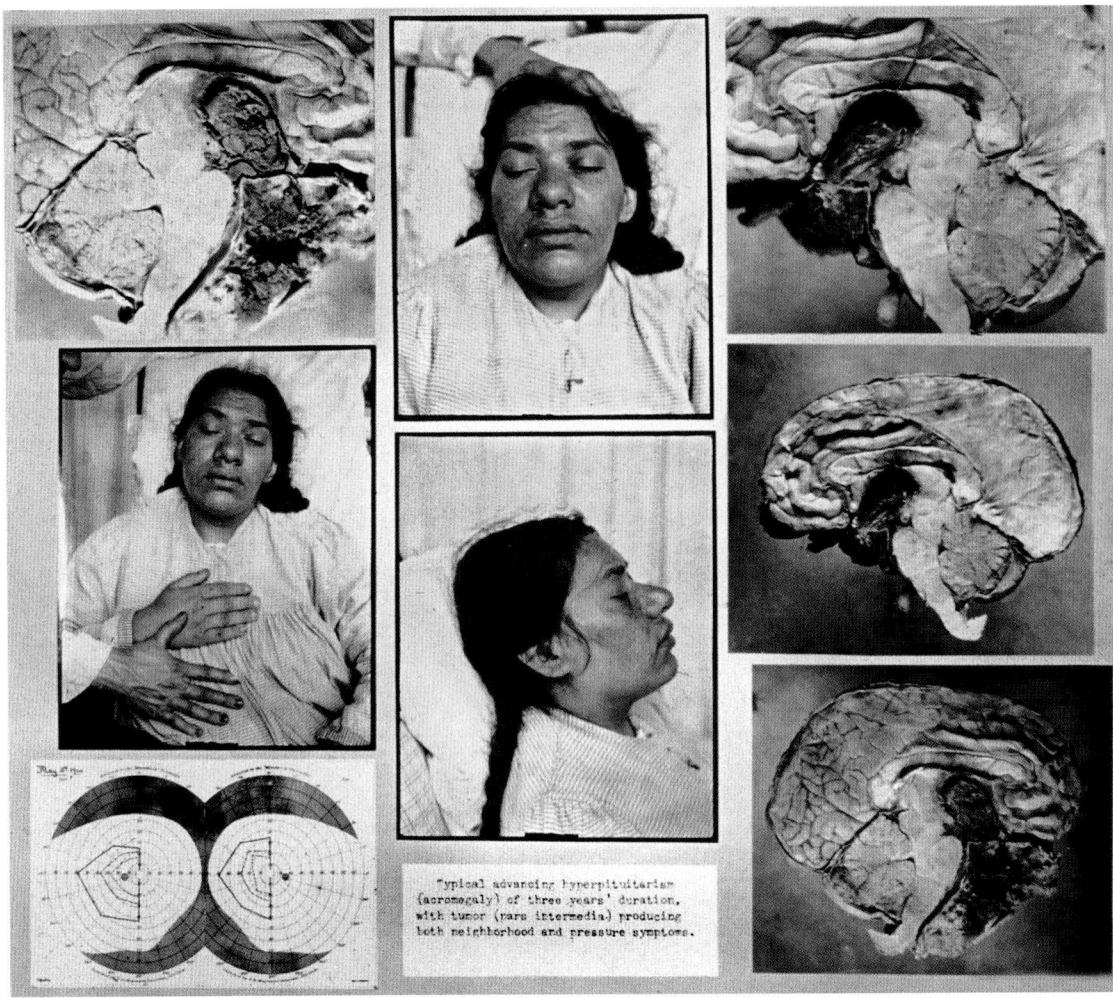

FIG. 52. ADVANCED ACROMEGALY WITH NEIGHBORHOOD PRESSURE SYMPTOMS.

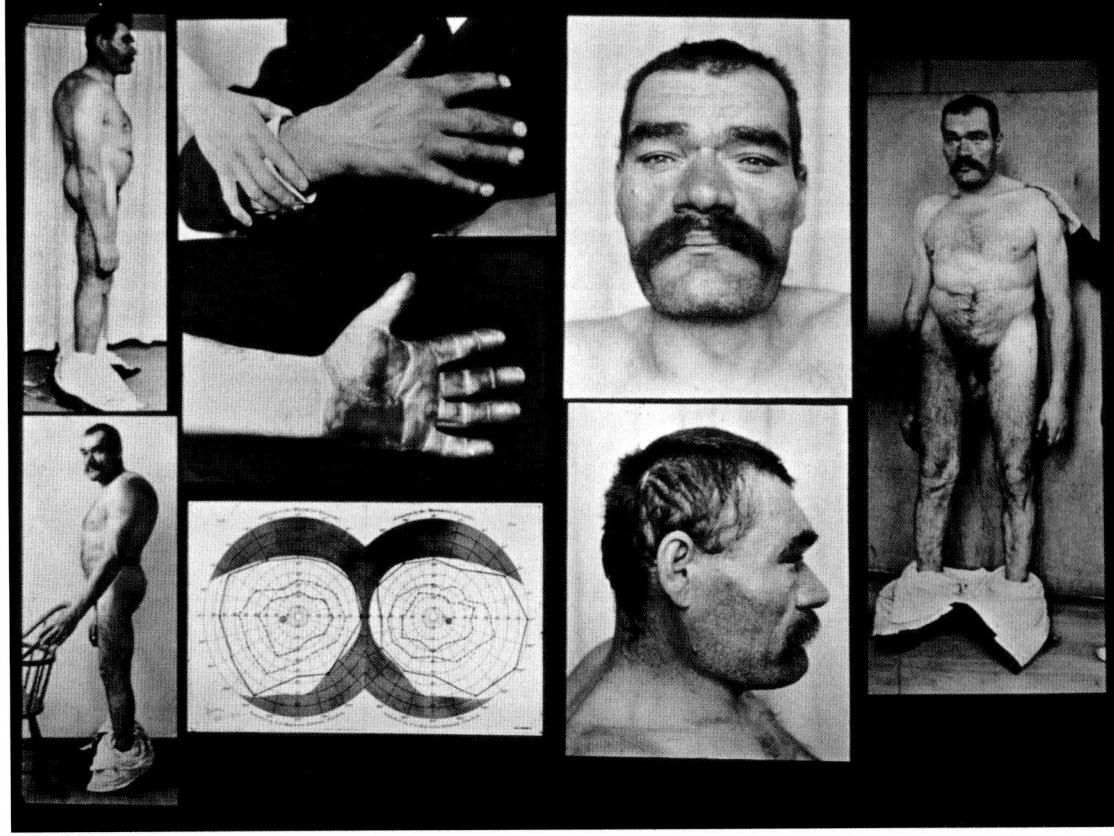

FIG. 53. ACROMEGALY.

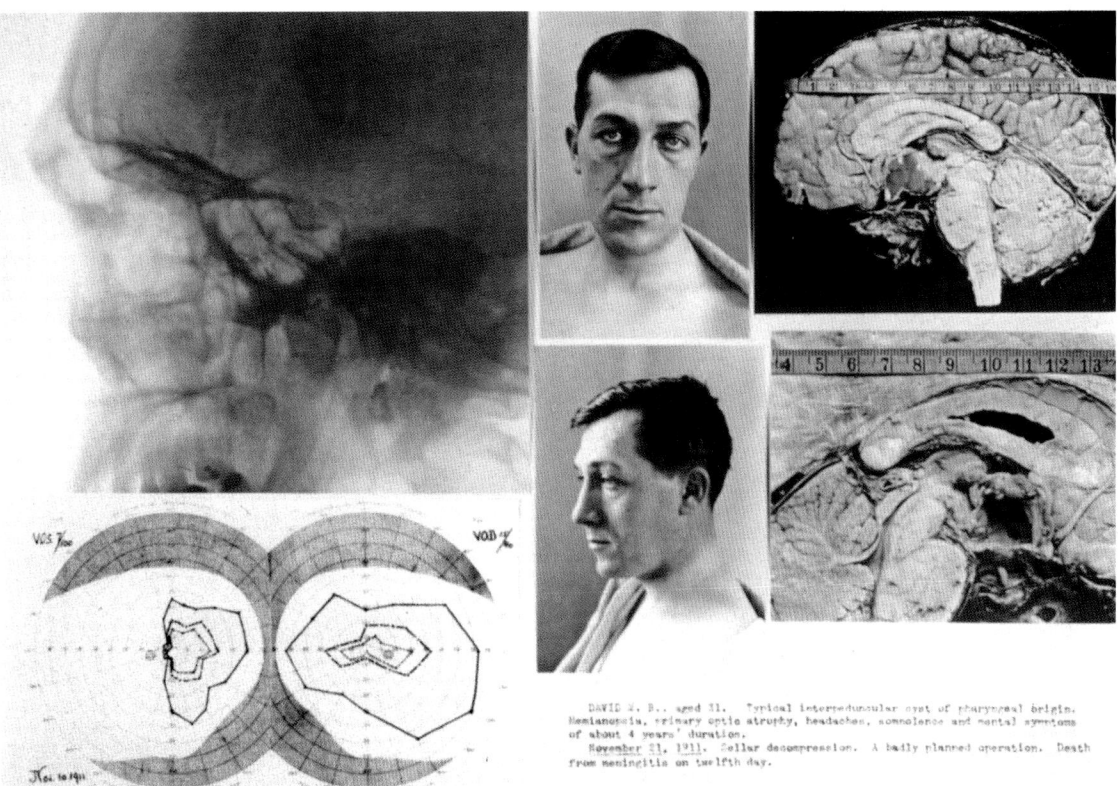

FIG. 54. CRANIOPHARYNGIOMA.

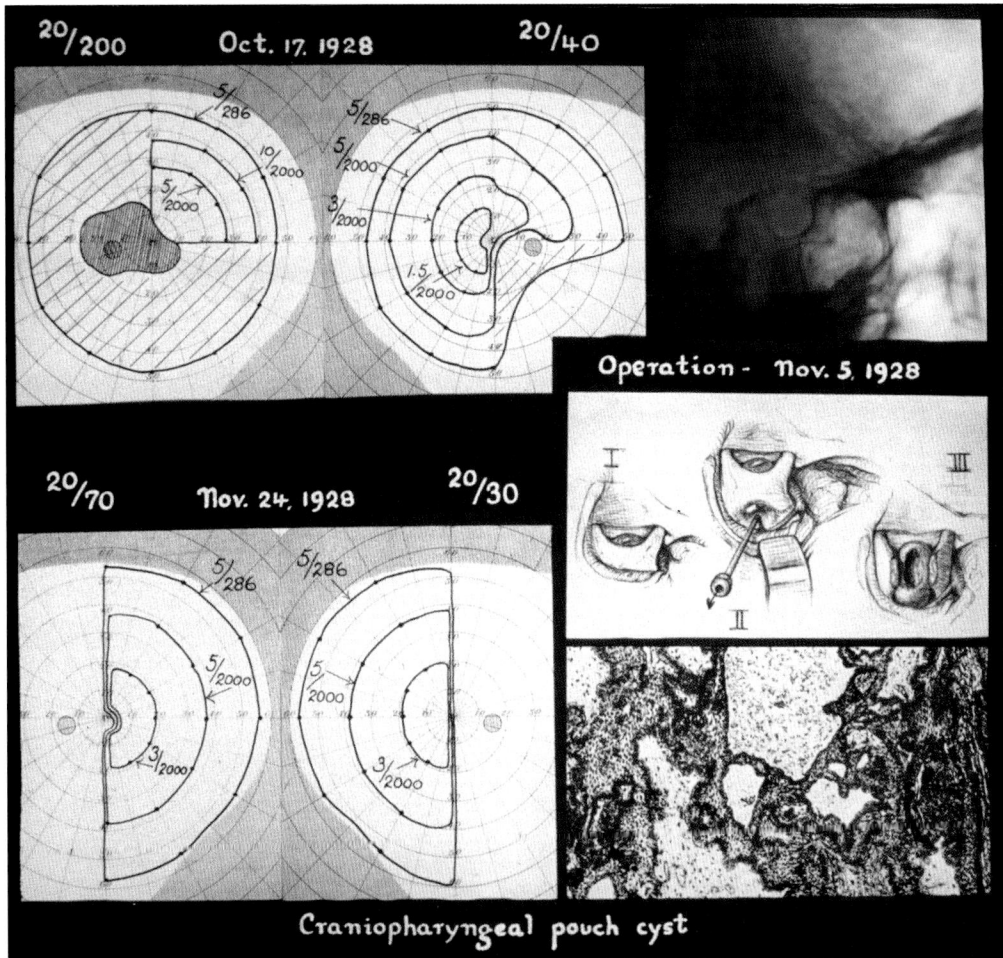

FIG. 55. CRANIOPHARYNGIOMA.

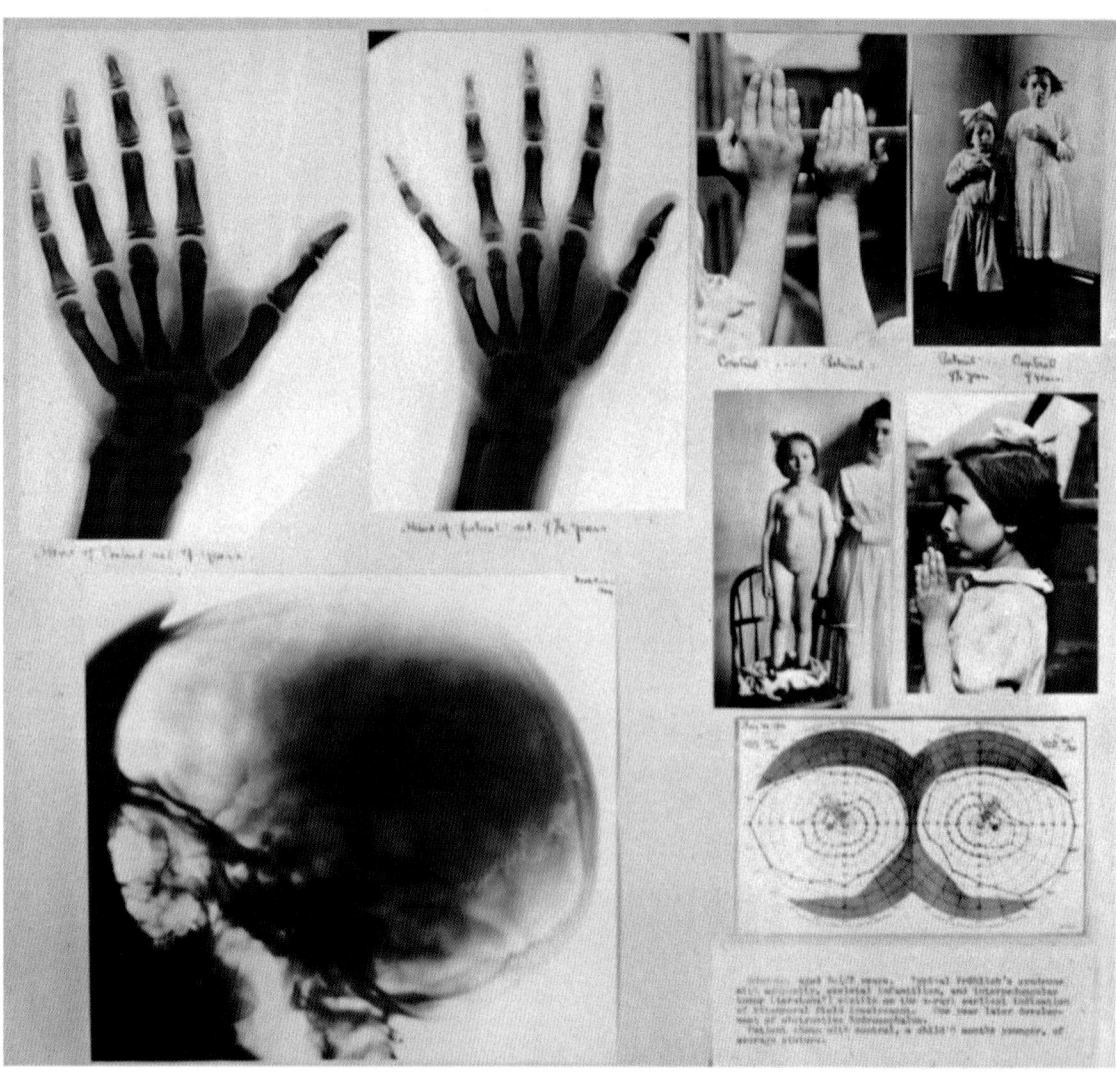

FIG. 56. CRANIOPHARYNGIOMA.

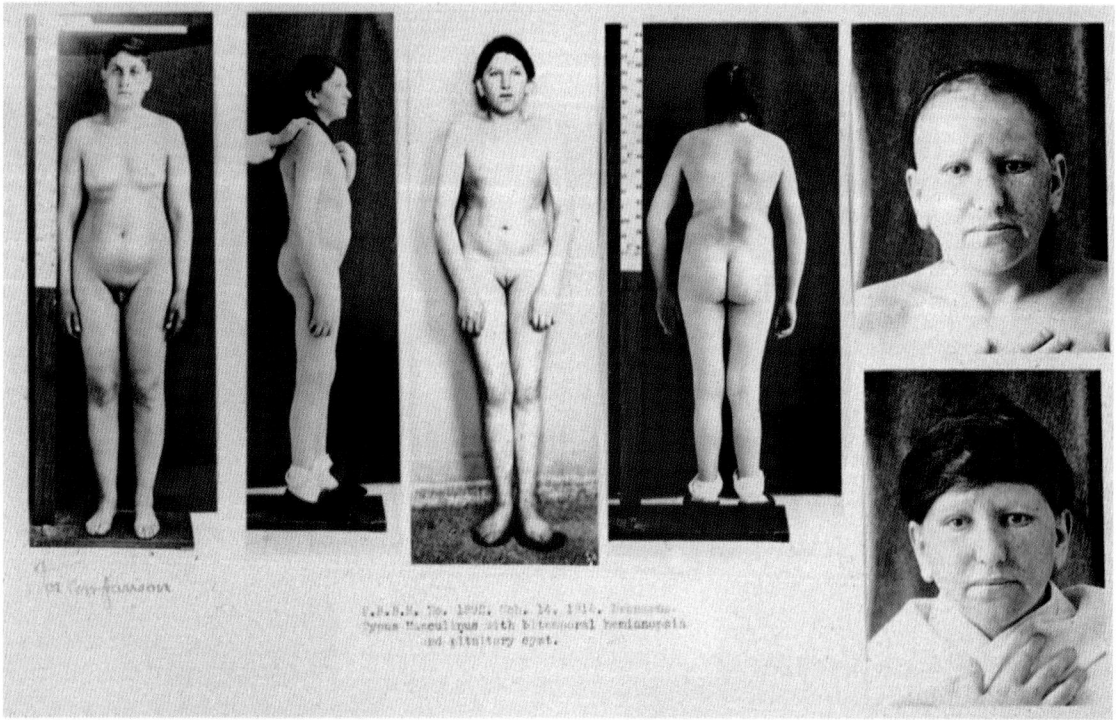

FIG. 57. CRANIOPHARYNGIOMA.

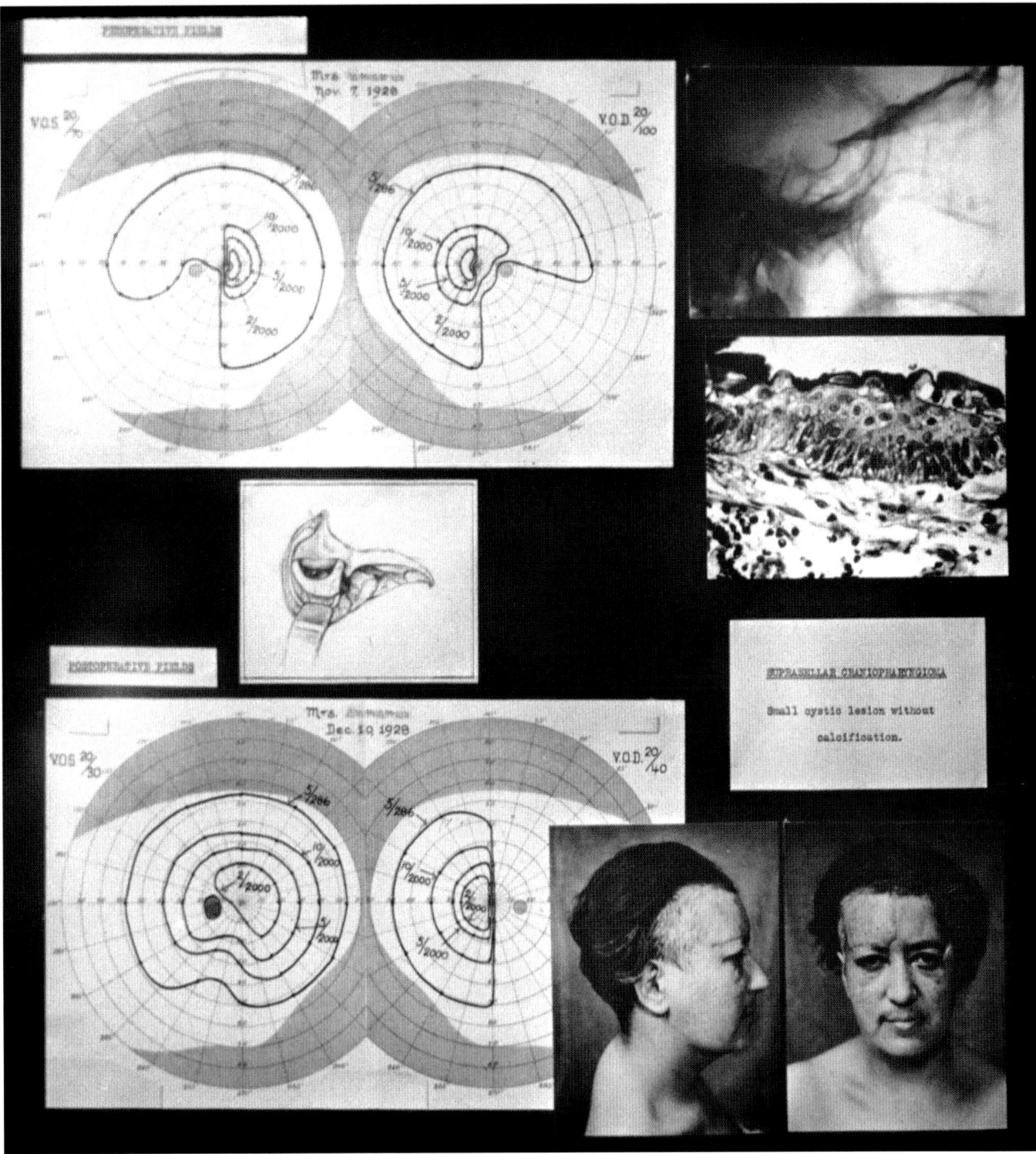

FIG. 58. CRANIOPHARYNGIOMA.

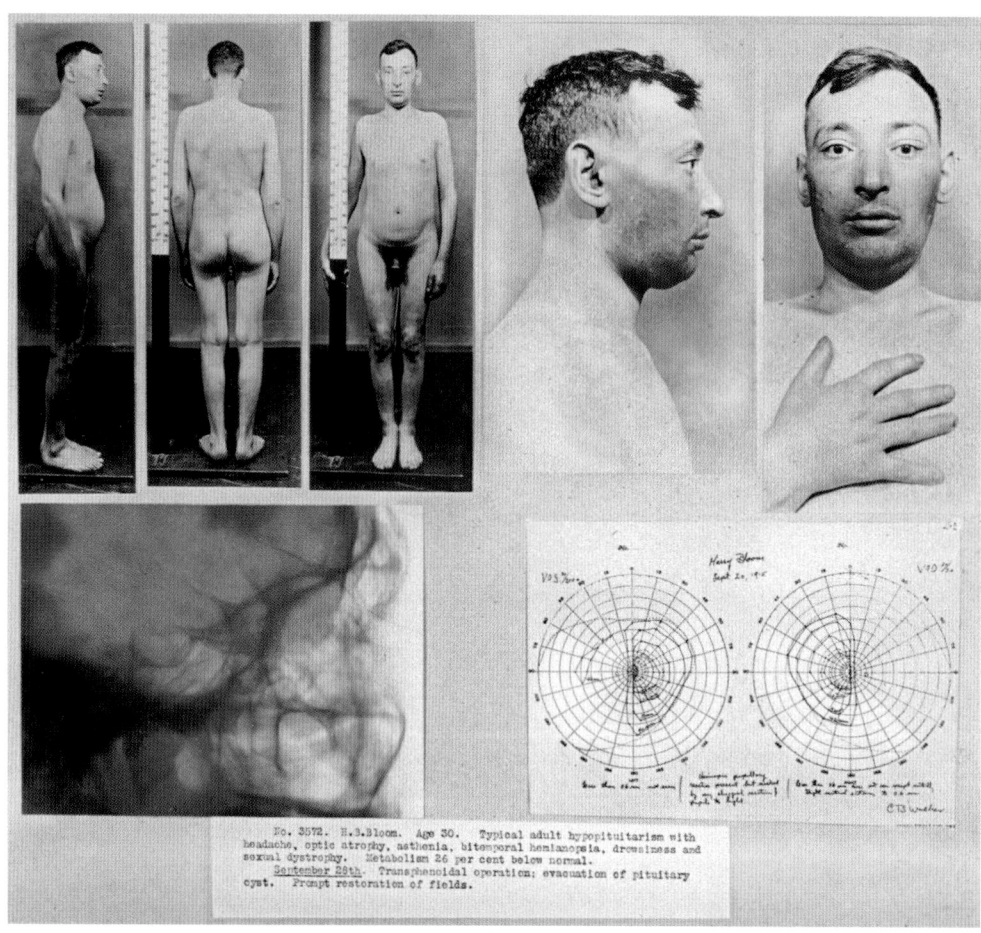

FIG. 59. CRANIOPHARYNGIOMA – HYPOPITUITARISM.

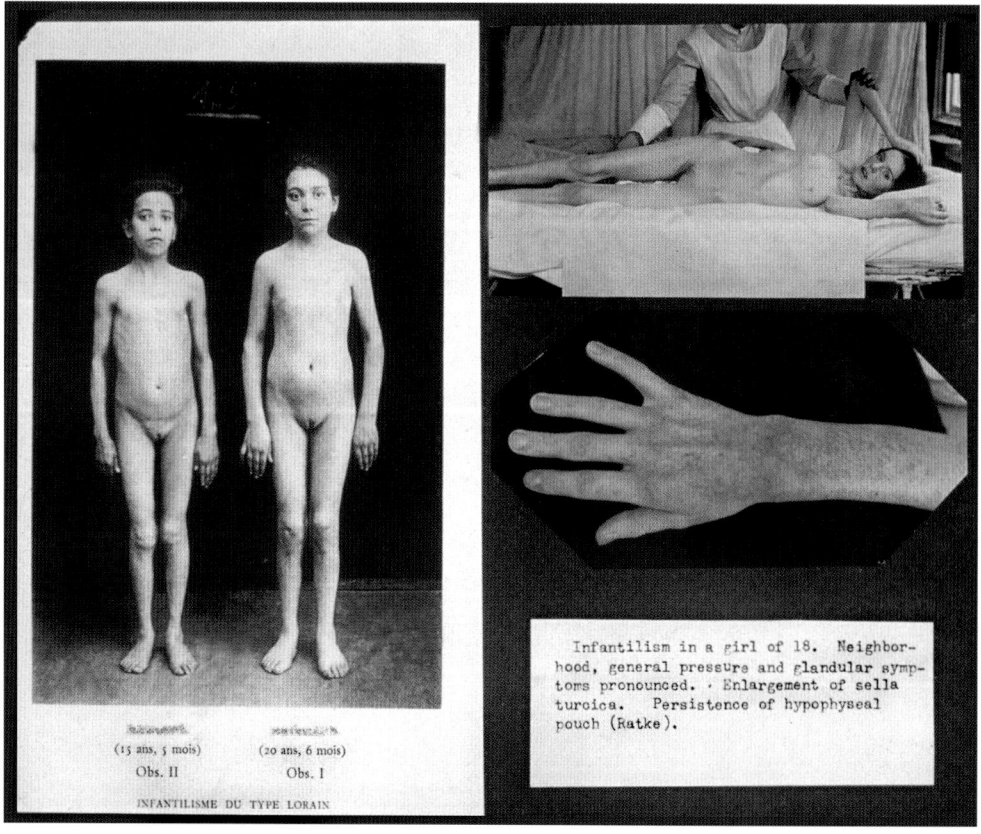

FIG. 60. CRANIOPHARYNGIOMA – HYPOPITUITARISM.

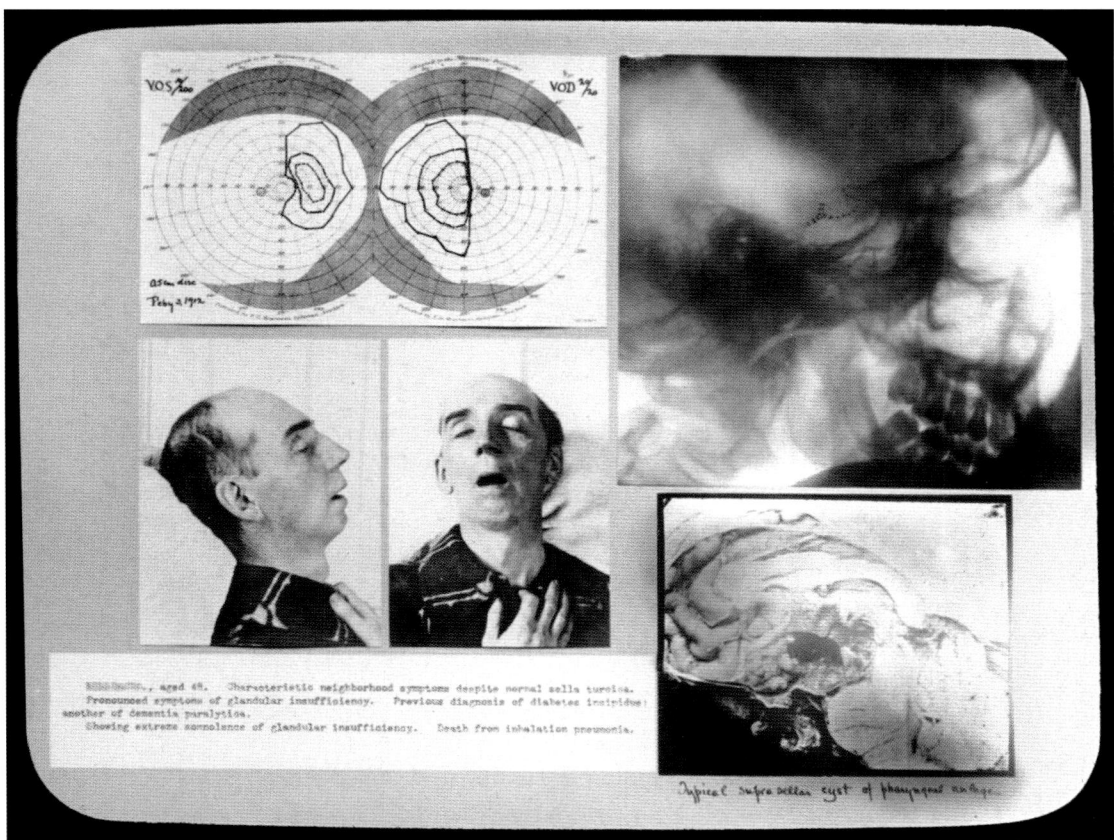

FIG. 61. CRANIOPHARYNGIOMA.

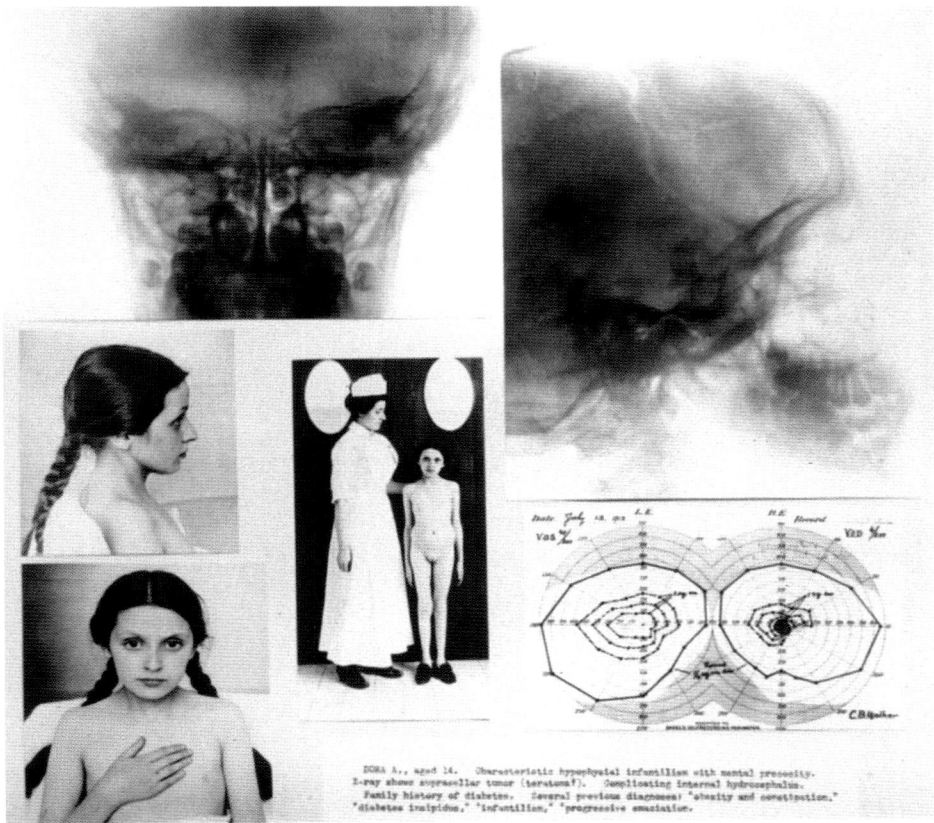

FIG. 62. CRANIOPHARYNGIOMA.

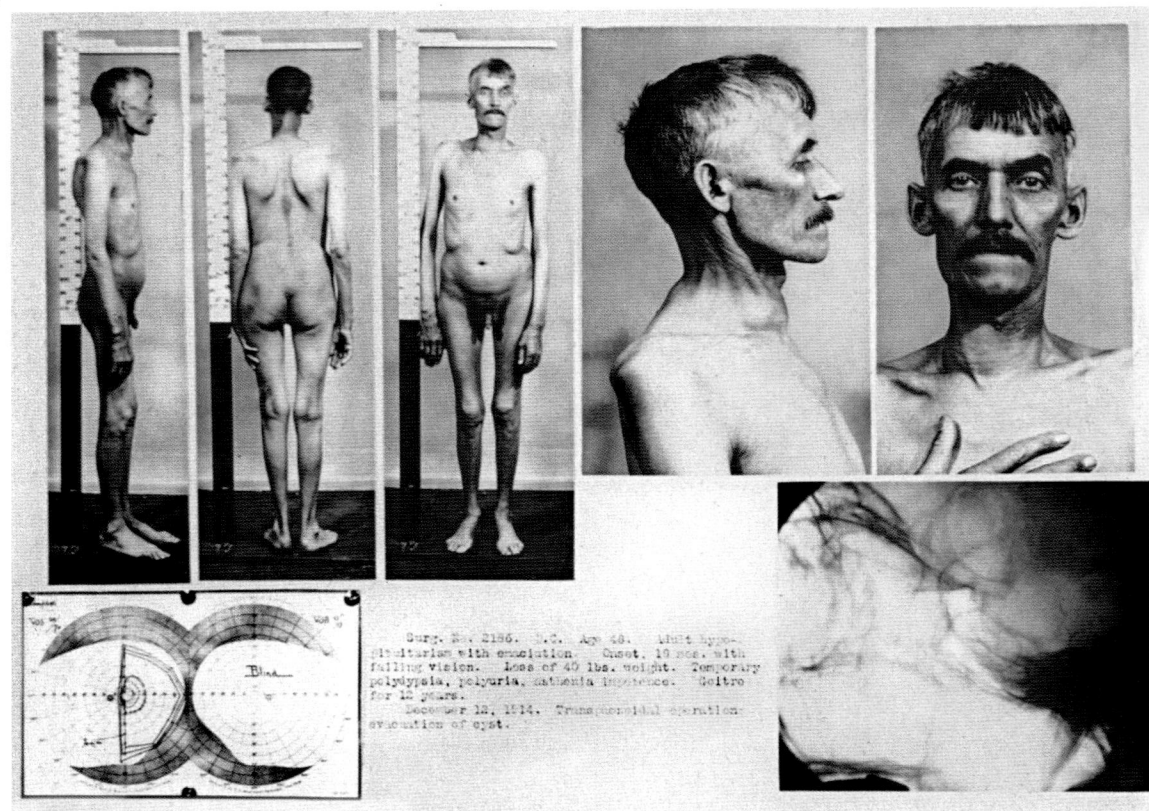

FIG. 63. SUPRASELLAR CYST ASSOCIATED WITH HYPOPITUITARISM AND EMACIATION.

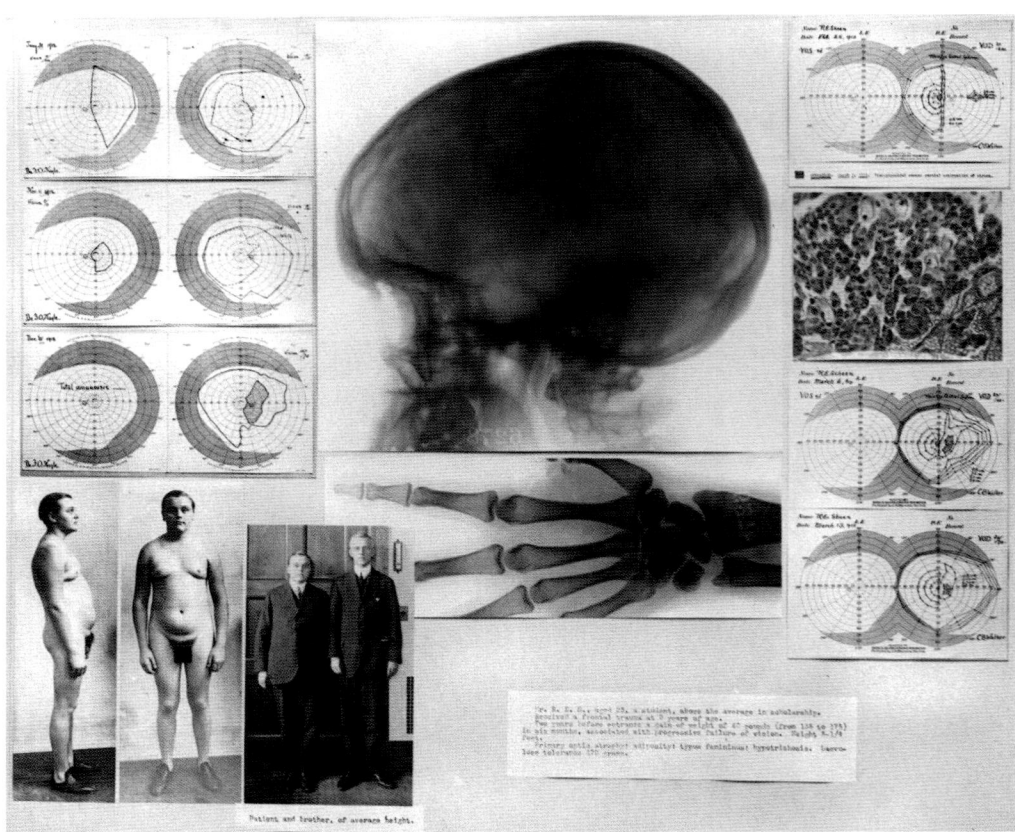

FIG. 64. HYPOPITUITARISM.

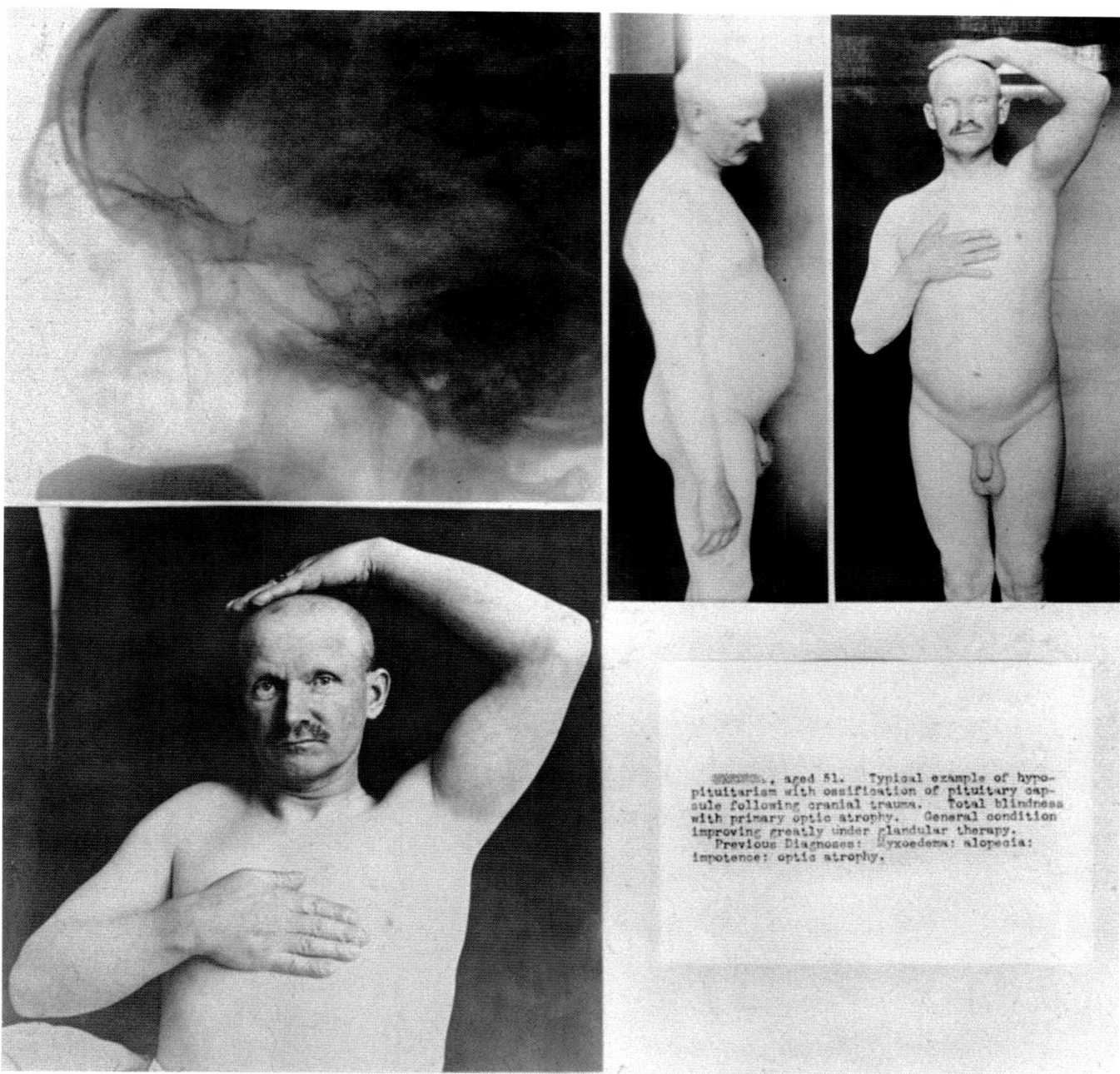

FIG. 65. HYPOPITUITARISM.

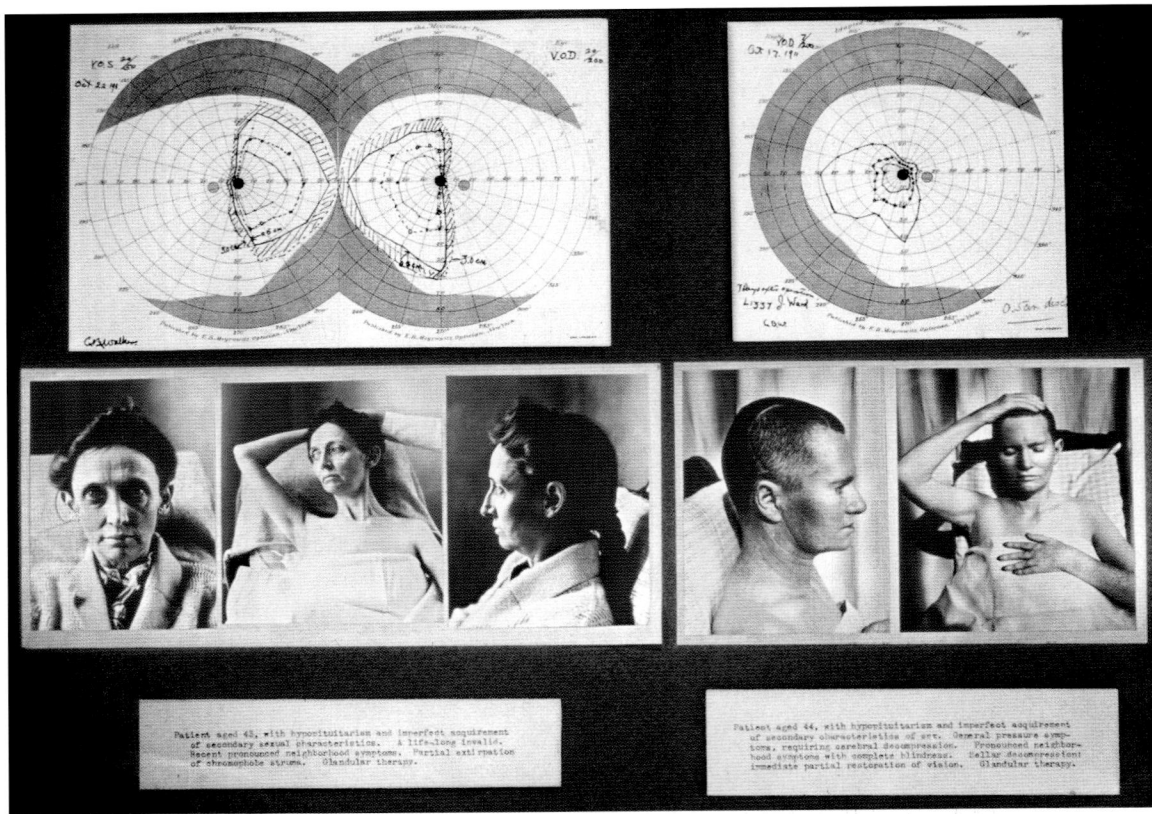

FIG. 66. HYPOPITUITARISM ASSOCIATED WITH PITUITARY ADENOMA.

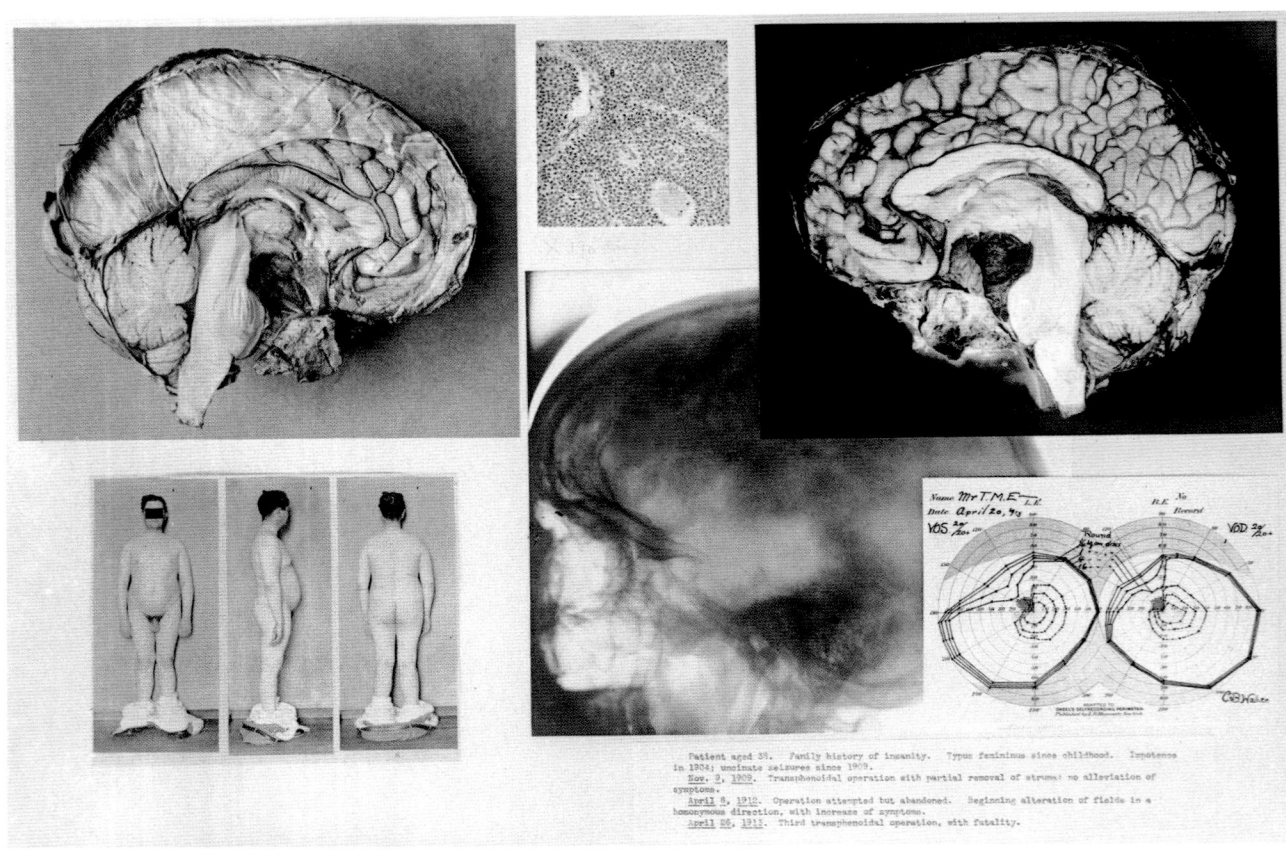

FIG. 67. MULTIPLE TRANSPHENOIDAL OPERATIONS WITH FATALITY AFTER THE LAST OPERATION.

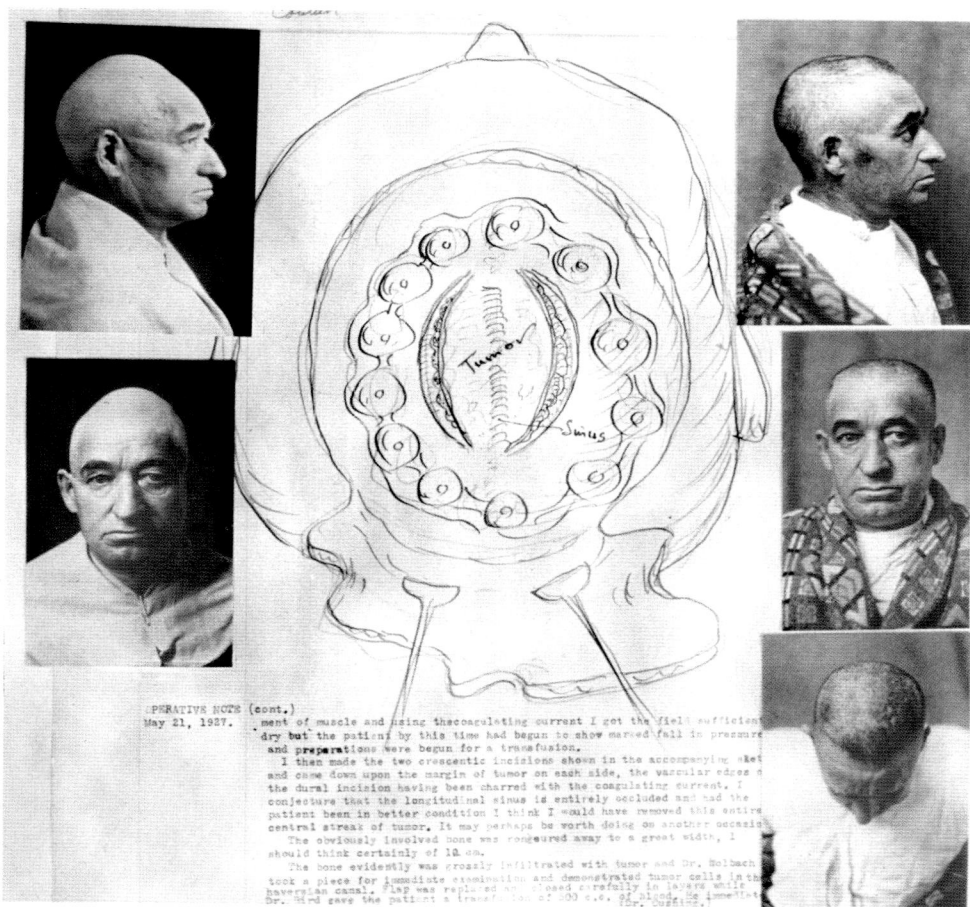

FIG. 68. PARASAGITTAL MENINGIOMA.

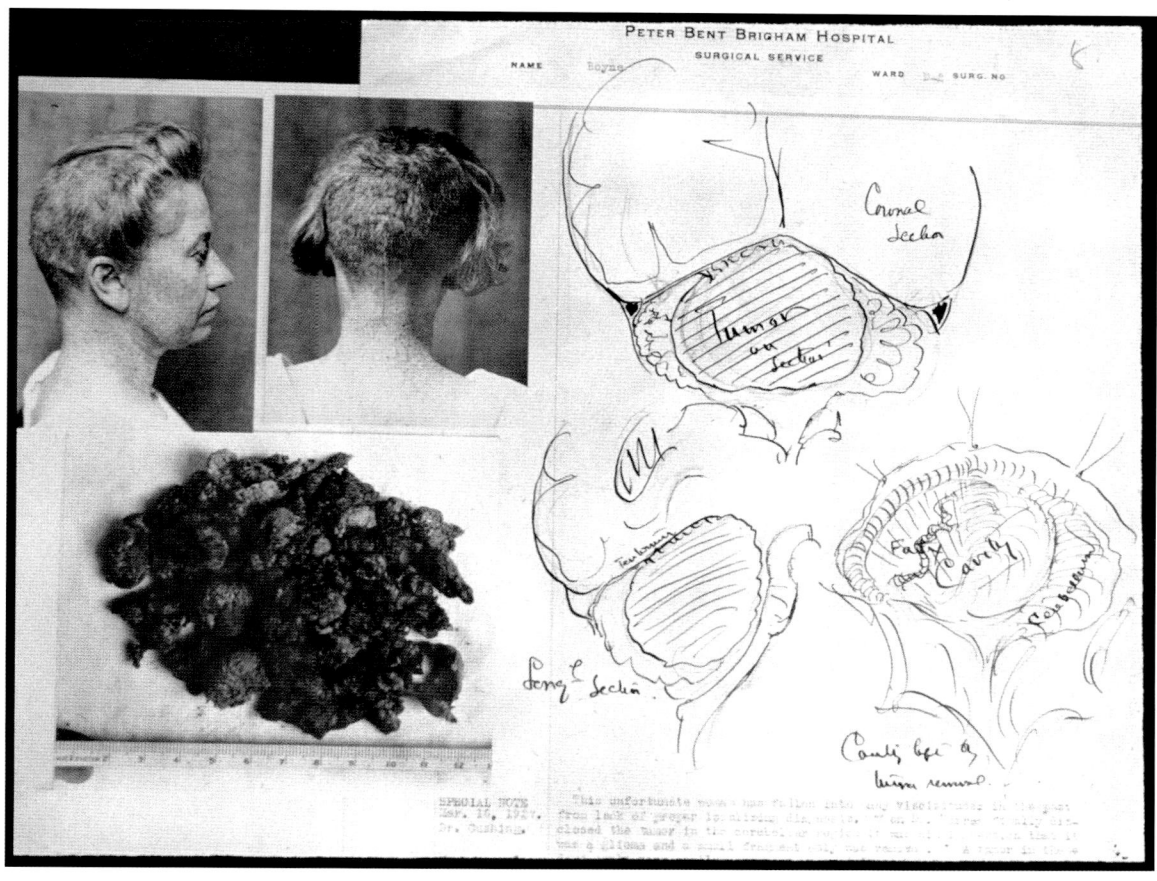

FIG. 69. CEREBELLAR MENINGIOMA.

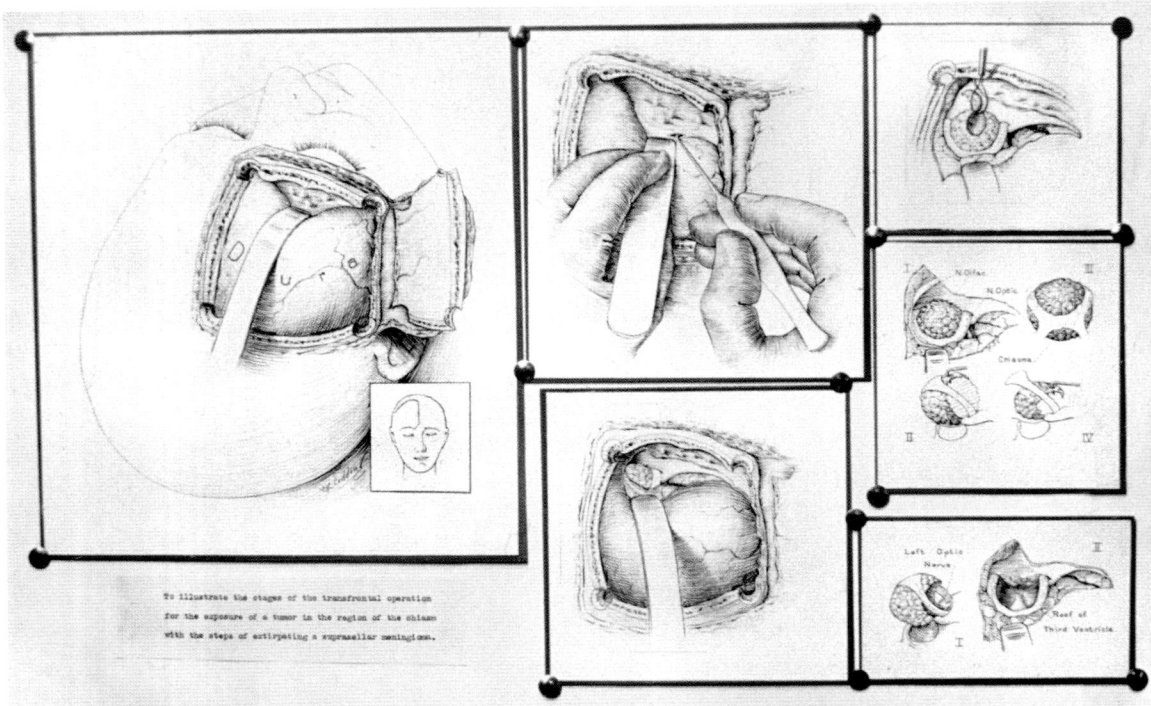

FIG. 70. STEPS INVOLVED IN EXPOSURE AND EXTIRPATION OF A SUPRASELLAR MENINGIOMA.

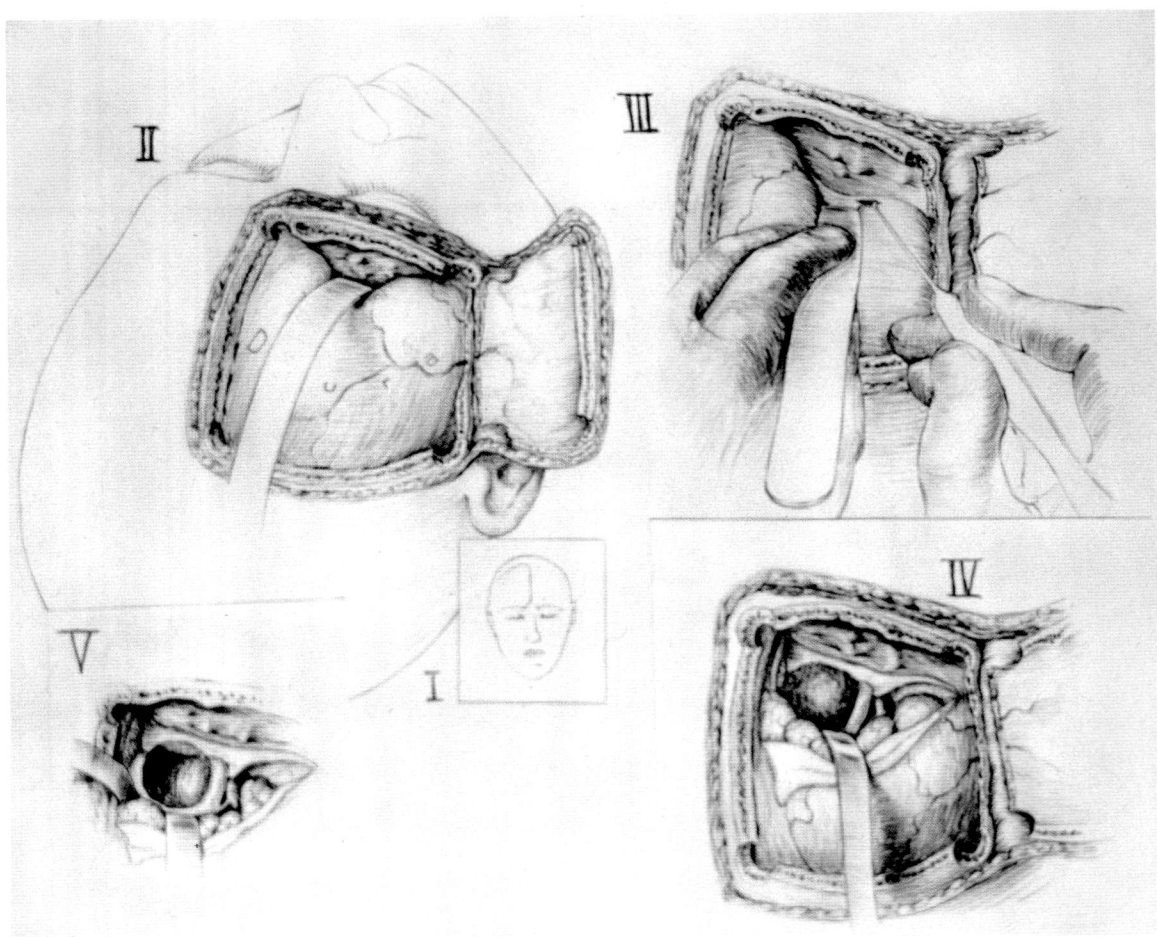

FIG. 71. TRANSFRONTAL OPERATION FOR RESECTION OF SUPRASELLAR MENINGIOMA.

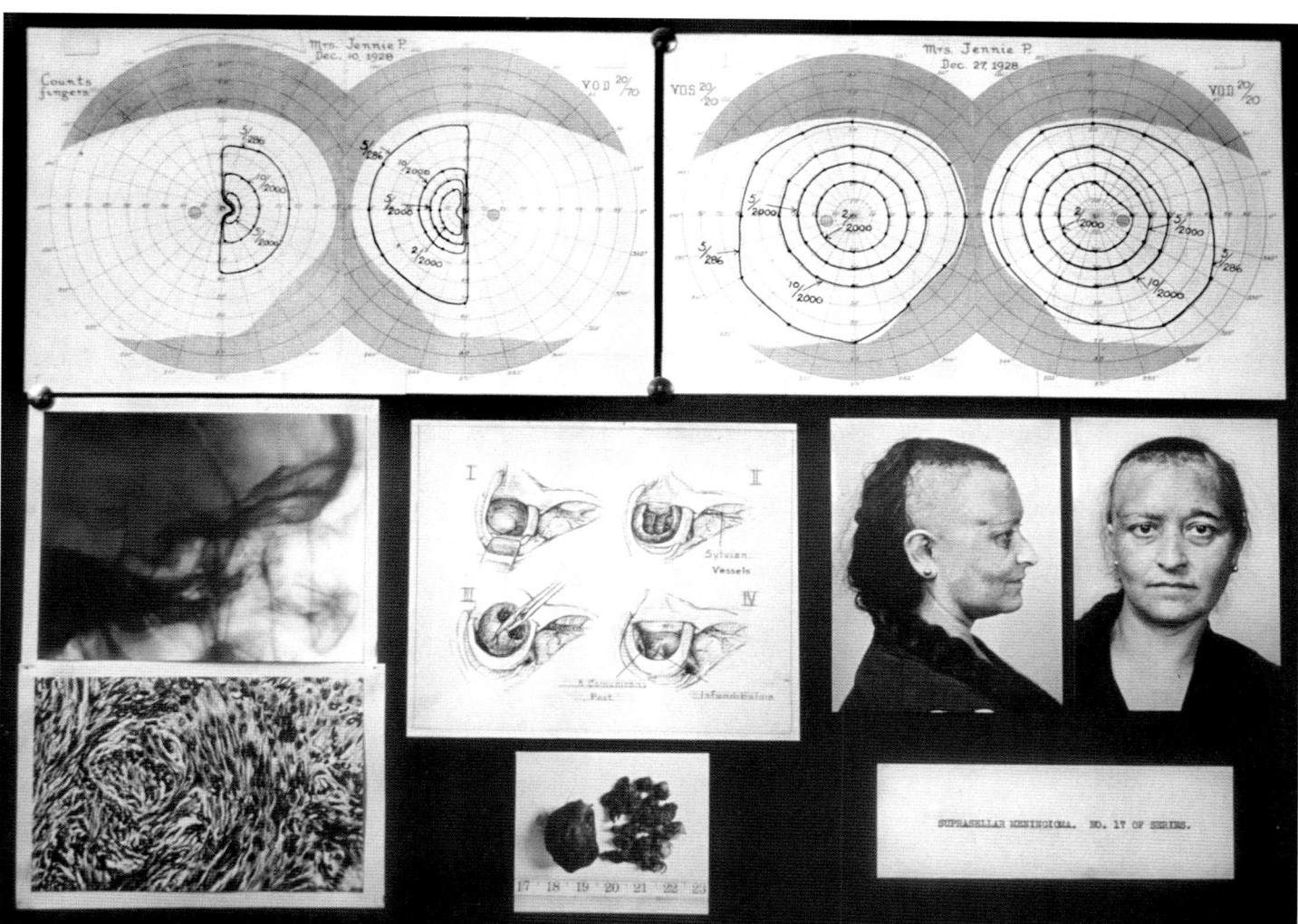

FIG. 72. SUPRASELLAR MENINGIOMA.

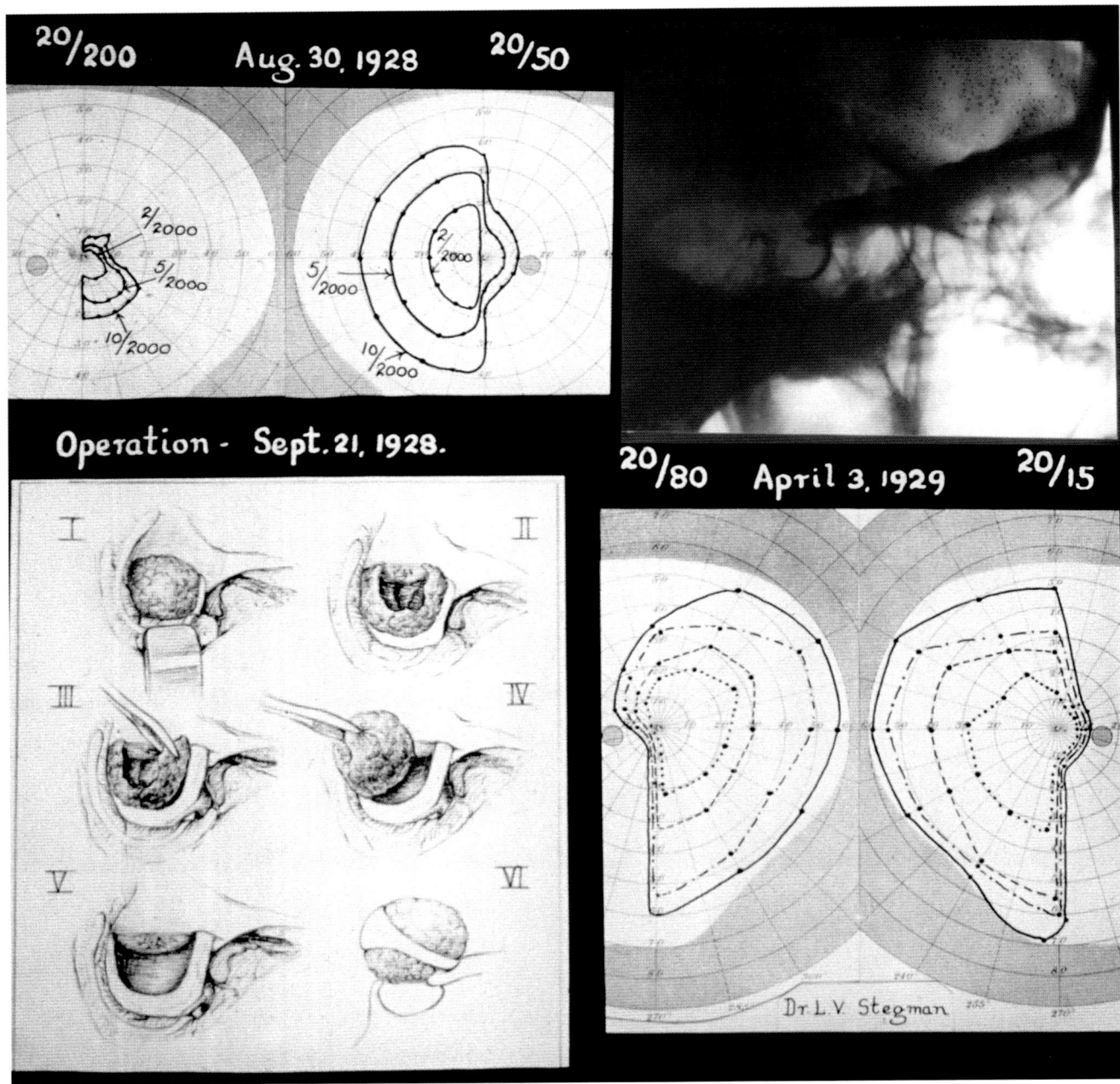

FIG. 73. SUPRASELLAR MENINGIOMA-RESTORATION OF VISUAL FIELDS AFTER SURGERY.

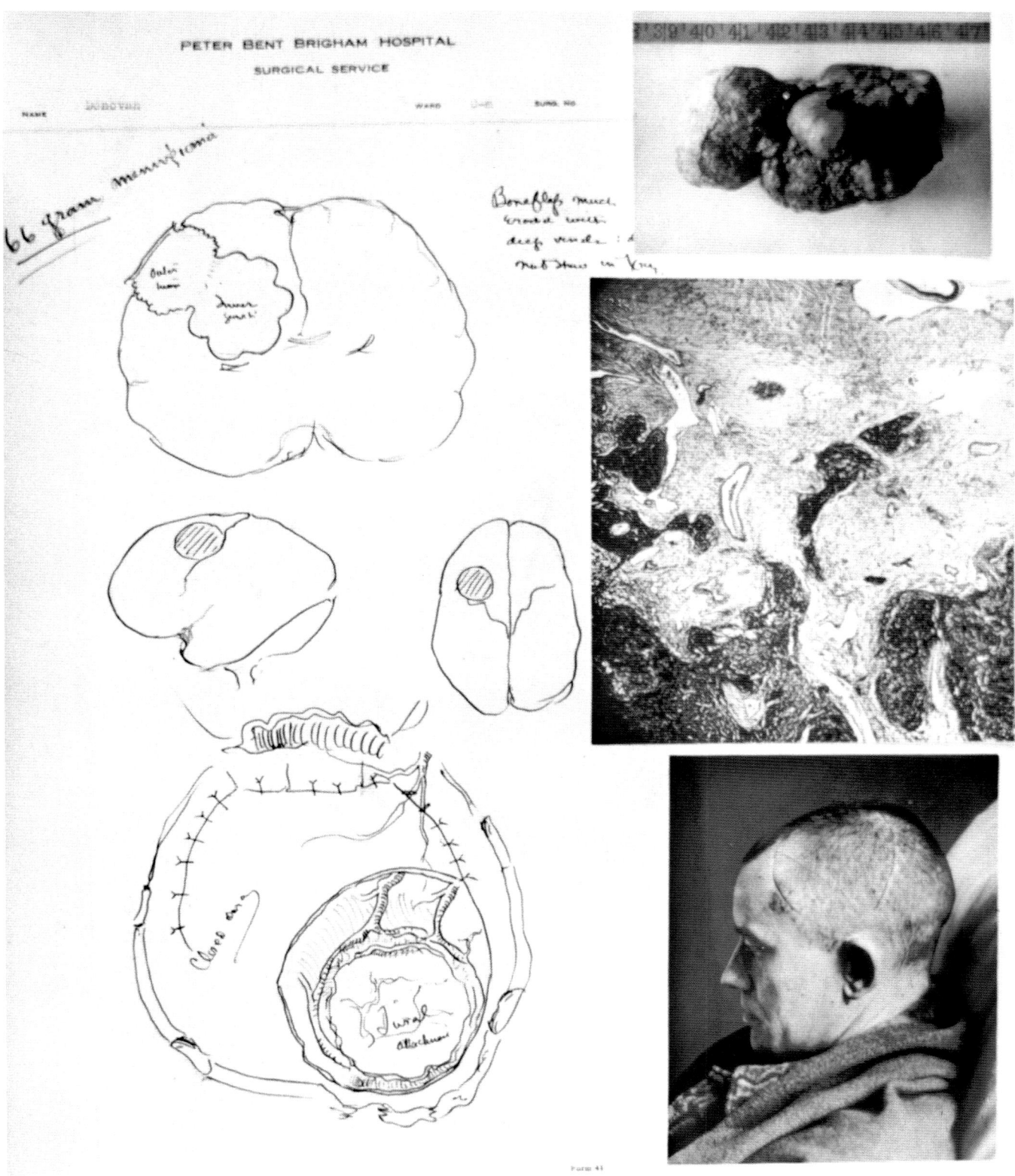

FIG. 74. LEFT FRONTAL MENINGIOMA.

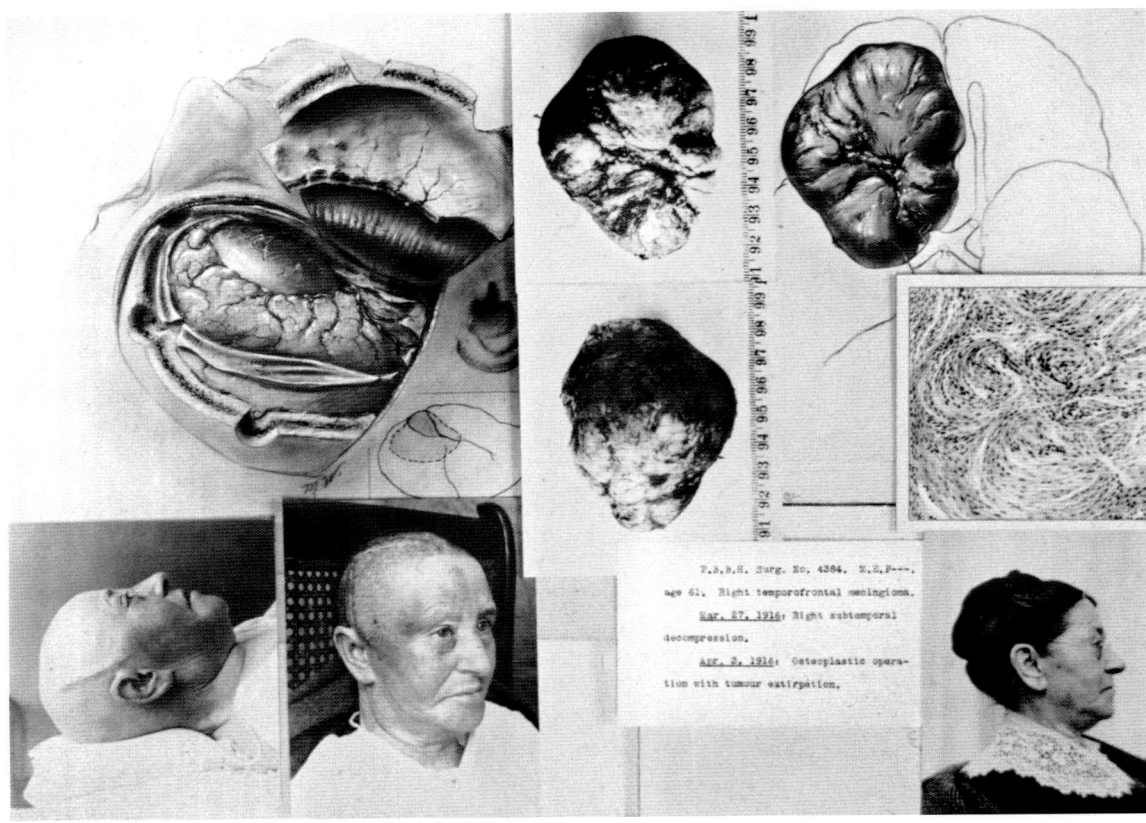

FIG. 75. RIGHT FRONTOTEMPORAL MENINGIOMA.

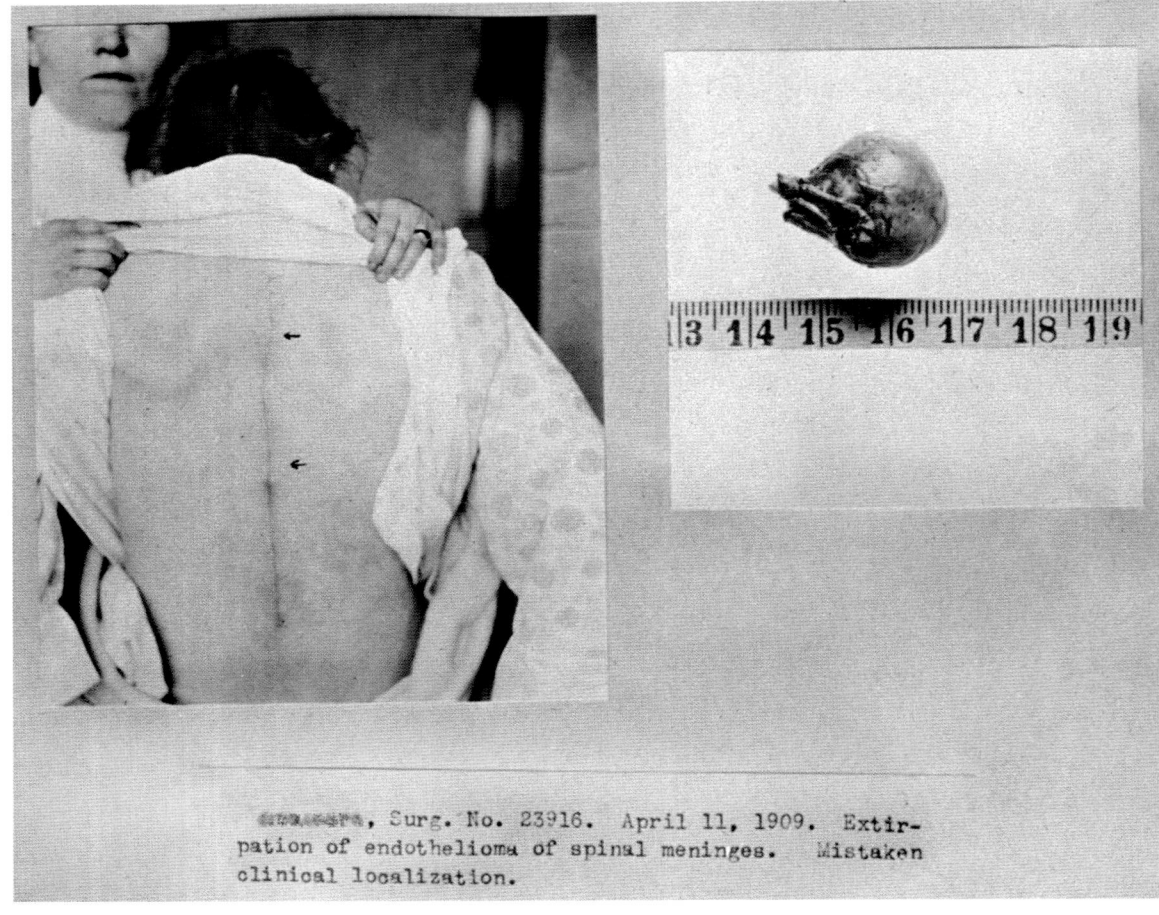

FIG. 76. SPINAL MENINGIOMA.

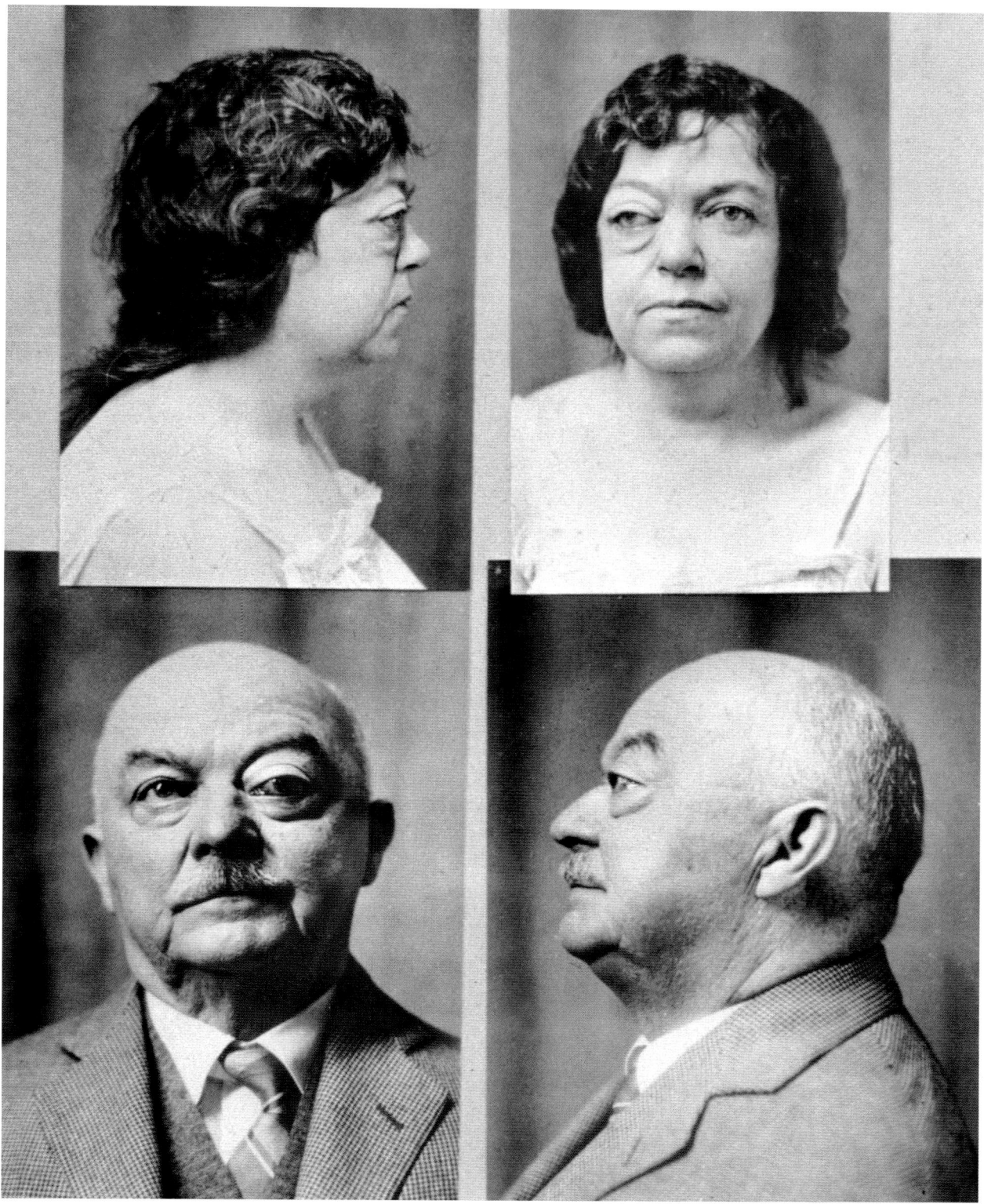

FIG. 77. HYPEROSTOSIS ASSOCIATED WITH MENINGIOMA.

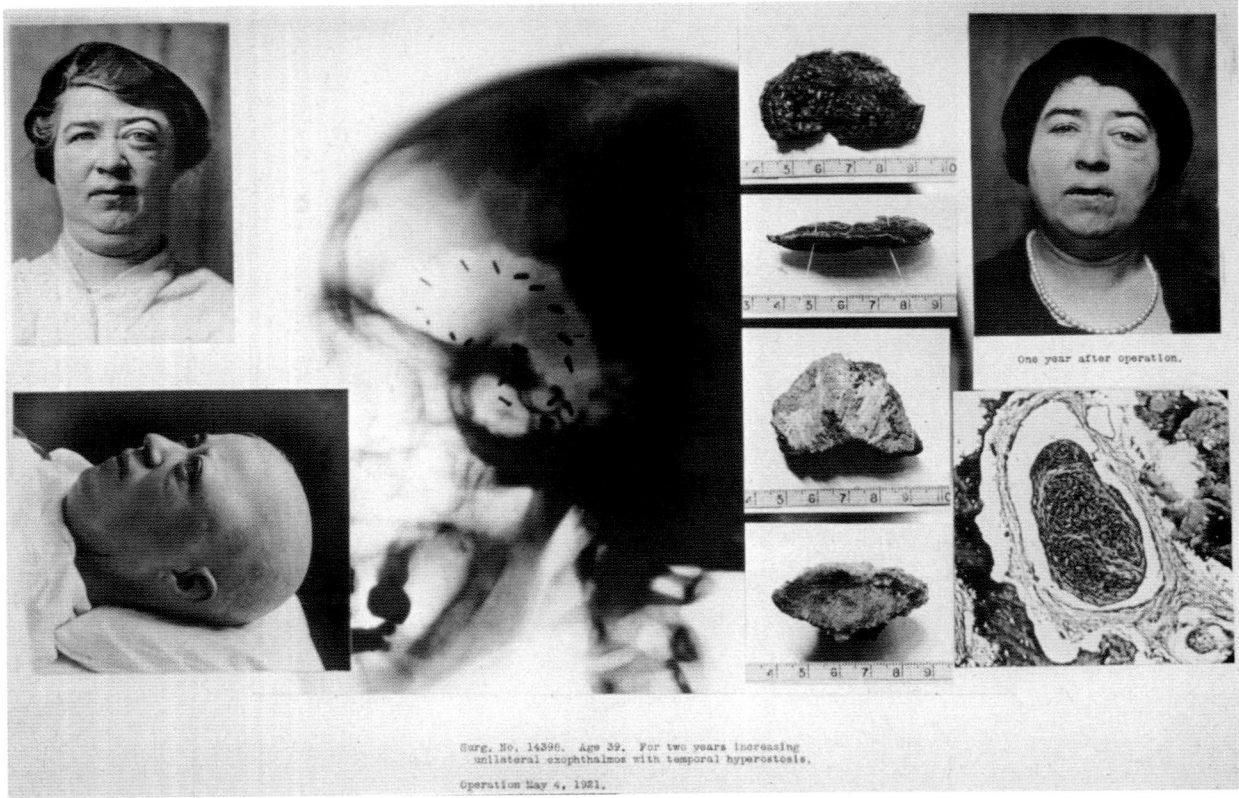

FIG. 78. LEFT SPHENOID WING MENINGIOMA.

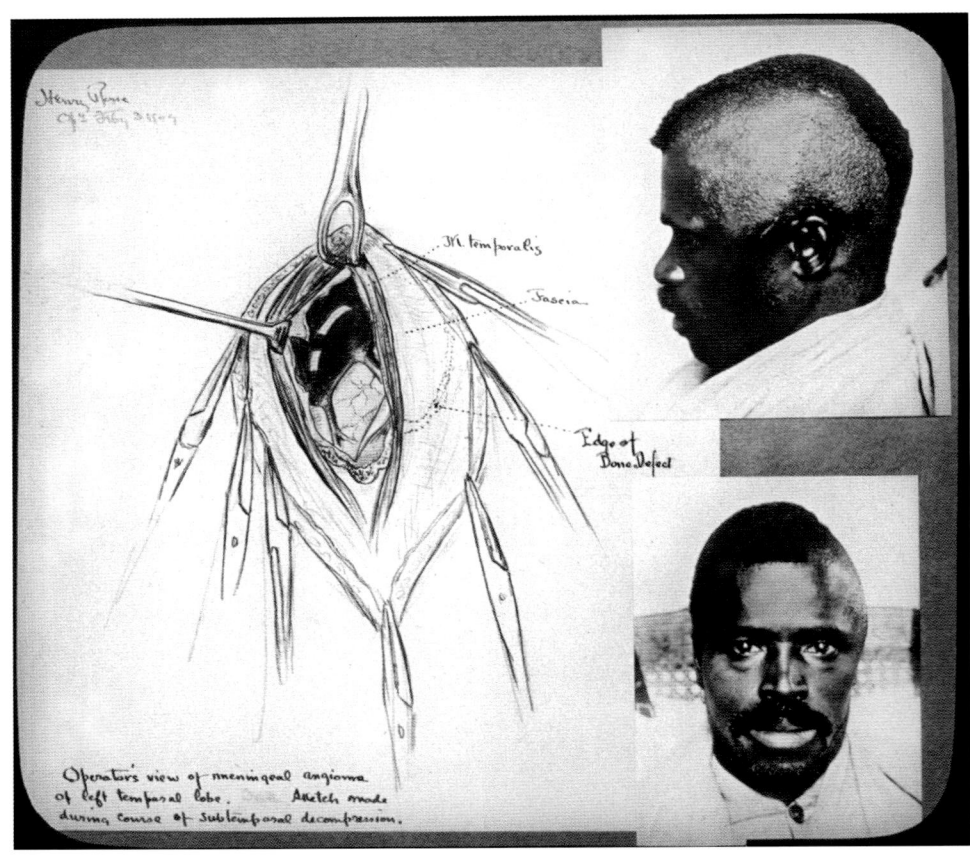

FIG. 79. LEFT TEMPORAL MENINGEAL ANGIOMA – SUBTEMPORAL DECOMPRESSION.

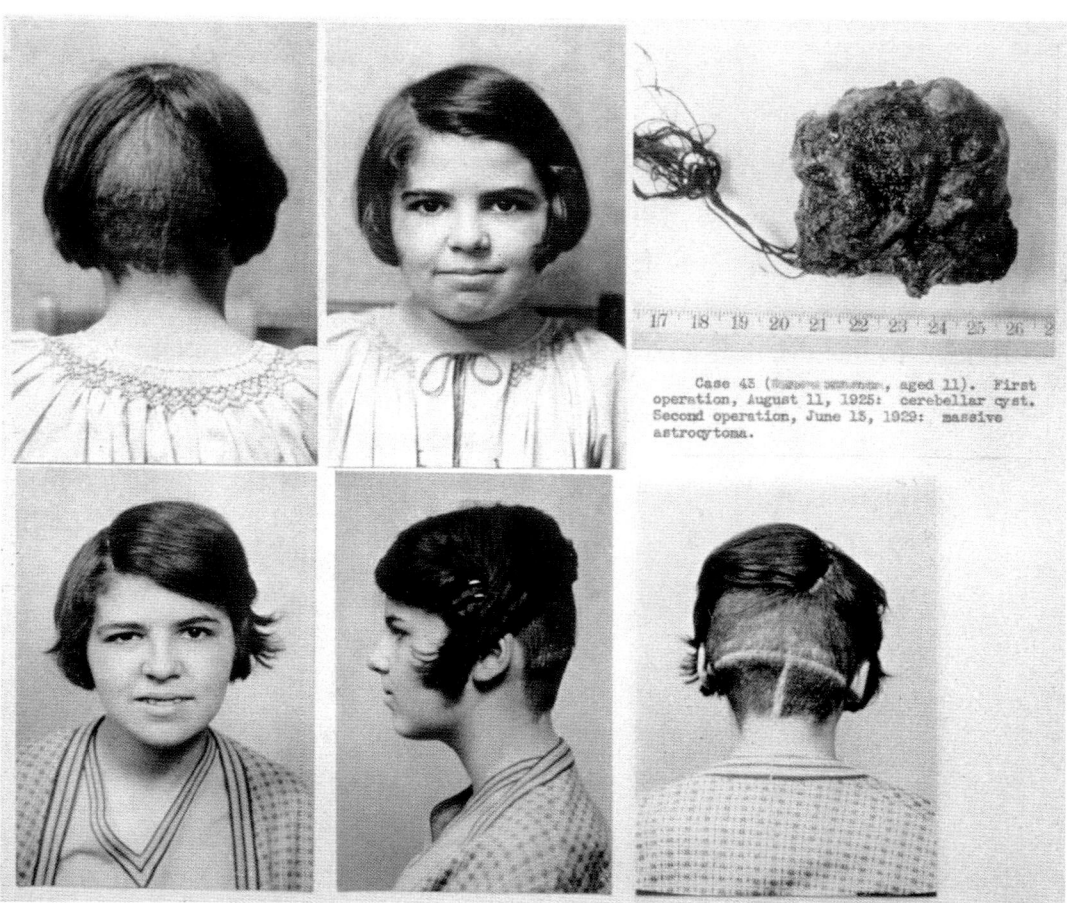

FIG. 80. CEREBELLAR ASTROCYTOMA.

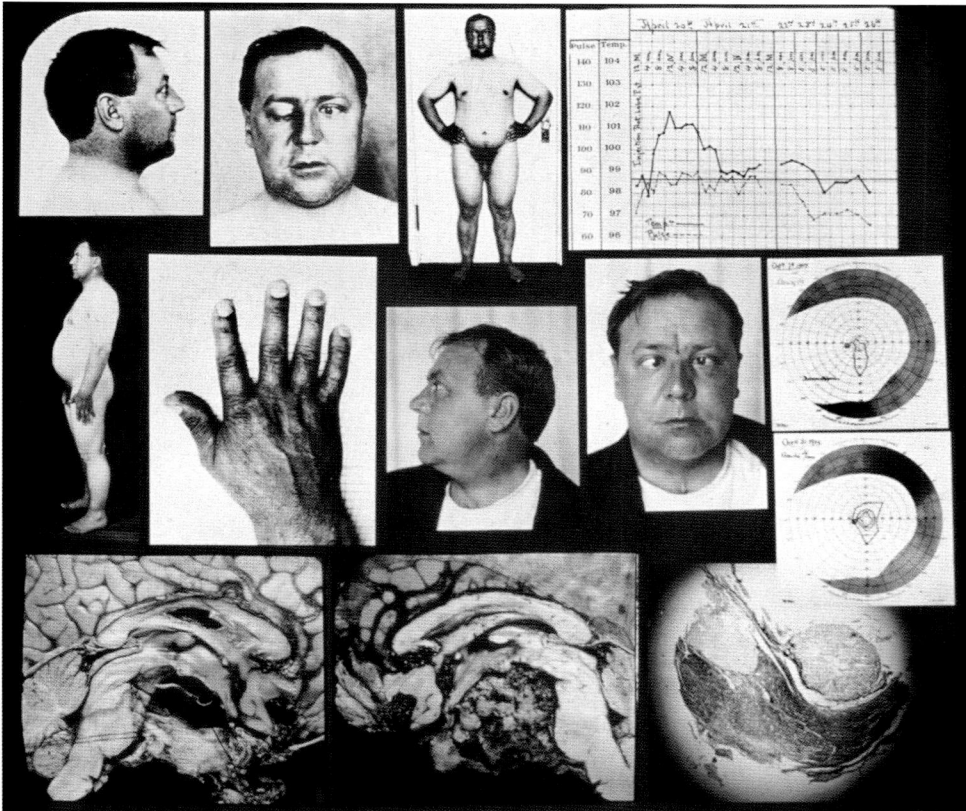

FIG. 81. PARASELLAR CHORDOMA.

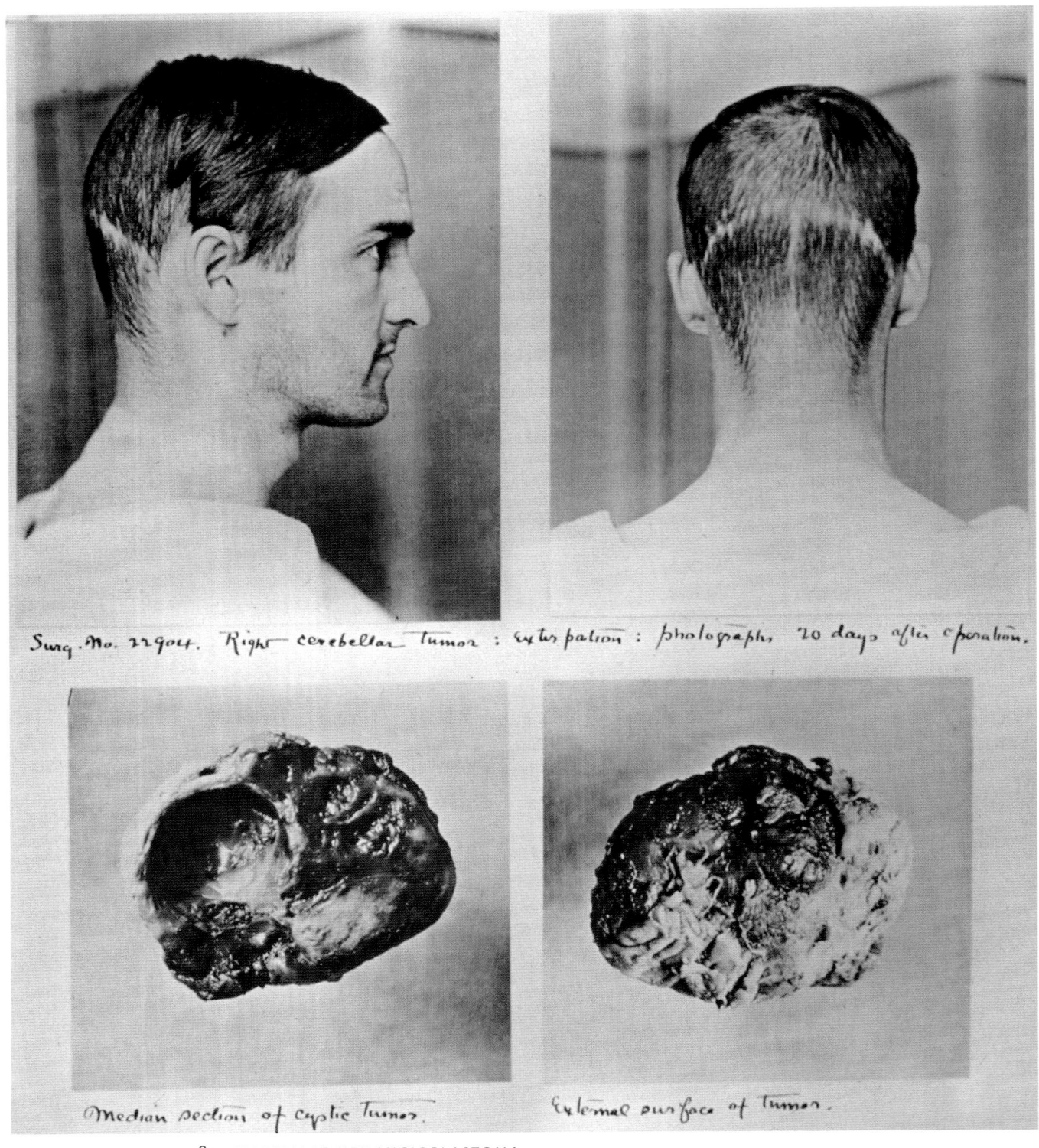

FIG. 82. CEREBELLAR HEMANGIOBLASTOMA.

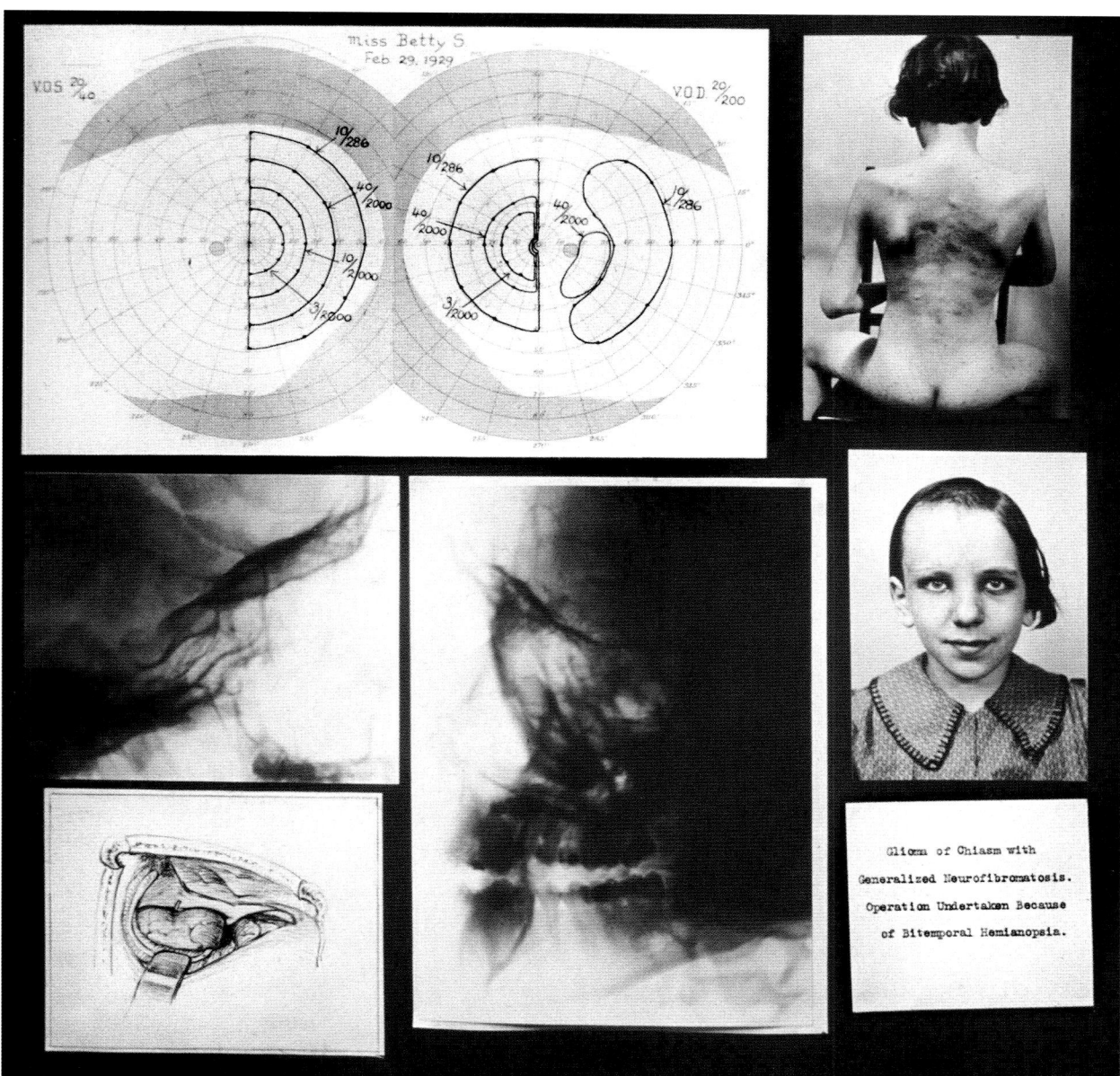

FIG. 83. OPTIC GLIOMA IN A PATIENT WITH NEUROFIBROMATOSIS.

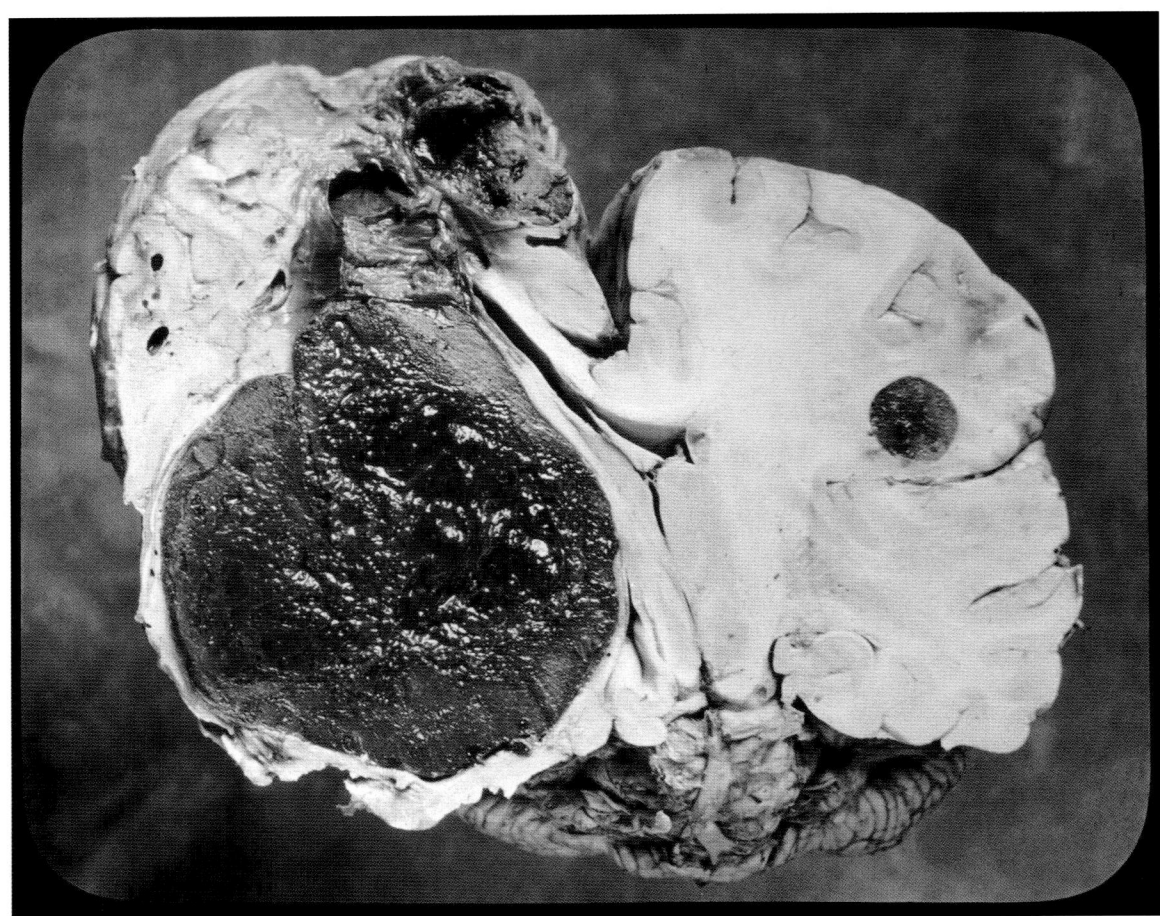

FIG. 84. METASTATIC MELANOMA-BRAIN AUTOPSY SPECIMEN.

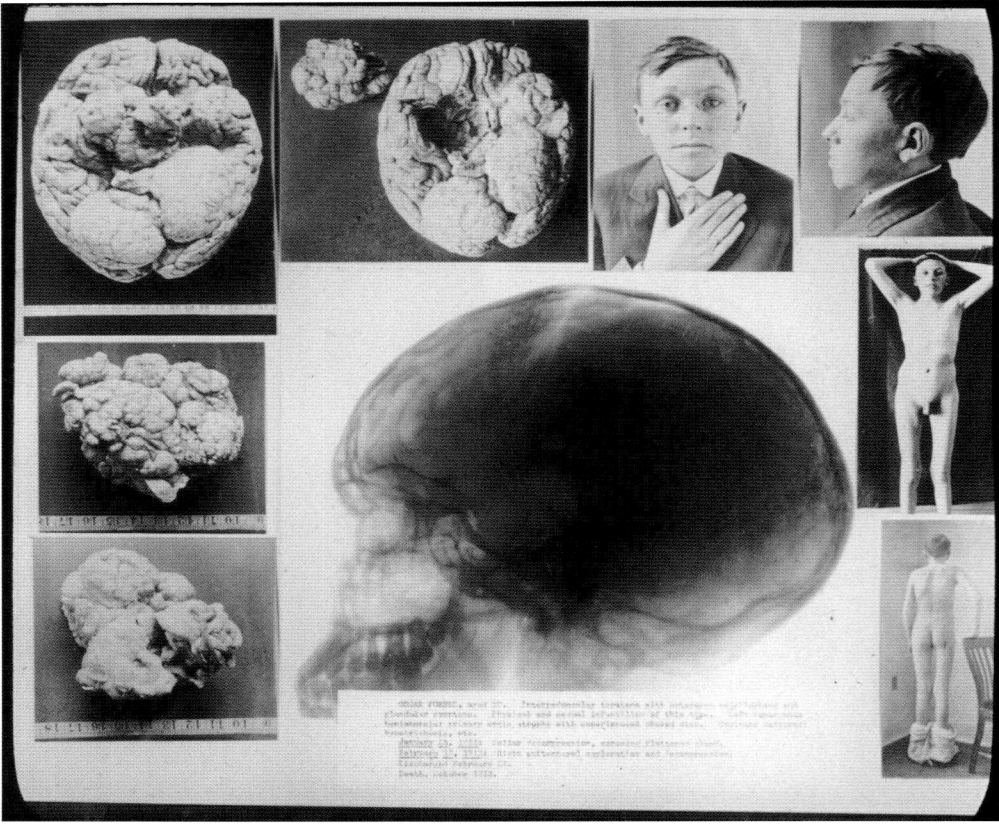

FIG. 85. TERATOMA.

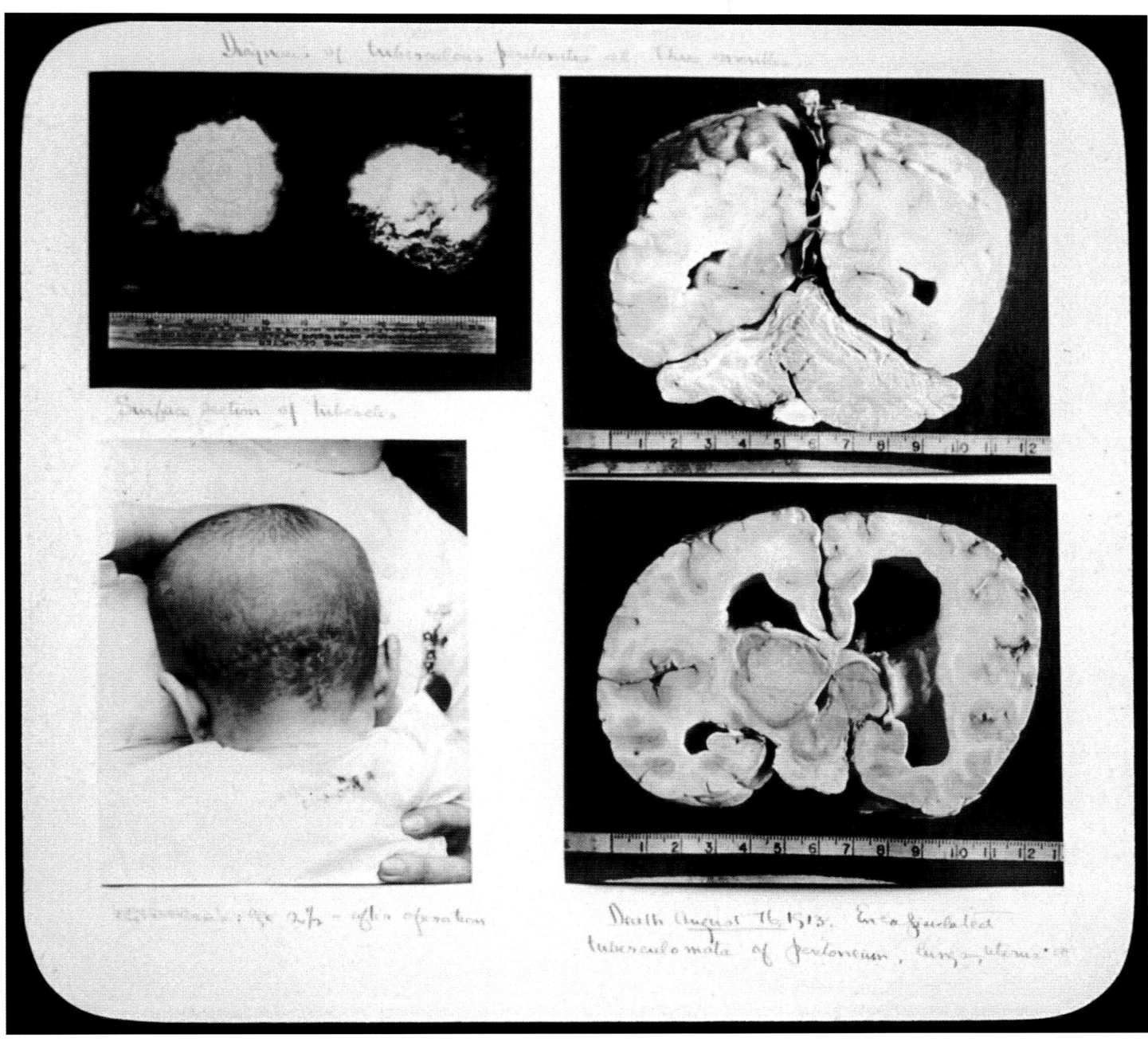

FIG. 86. DIENCEPHALIC TUBERCULOMA.

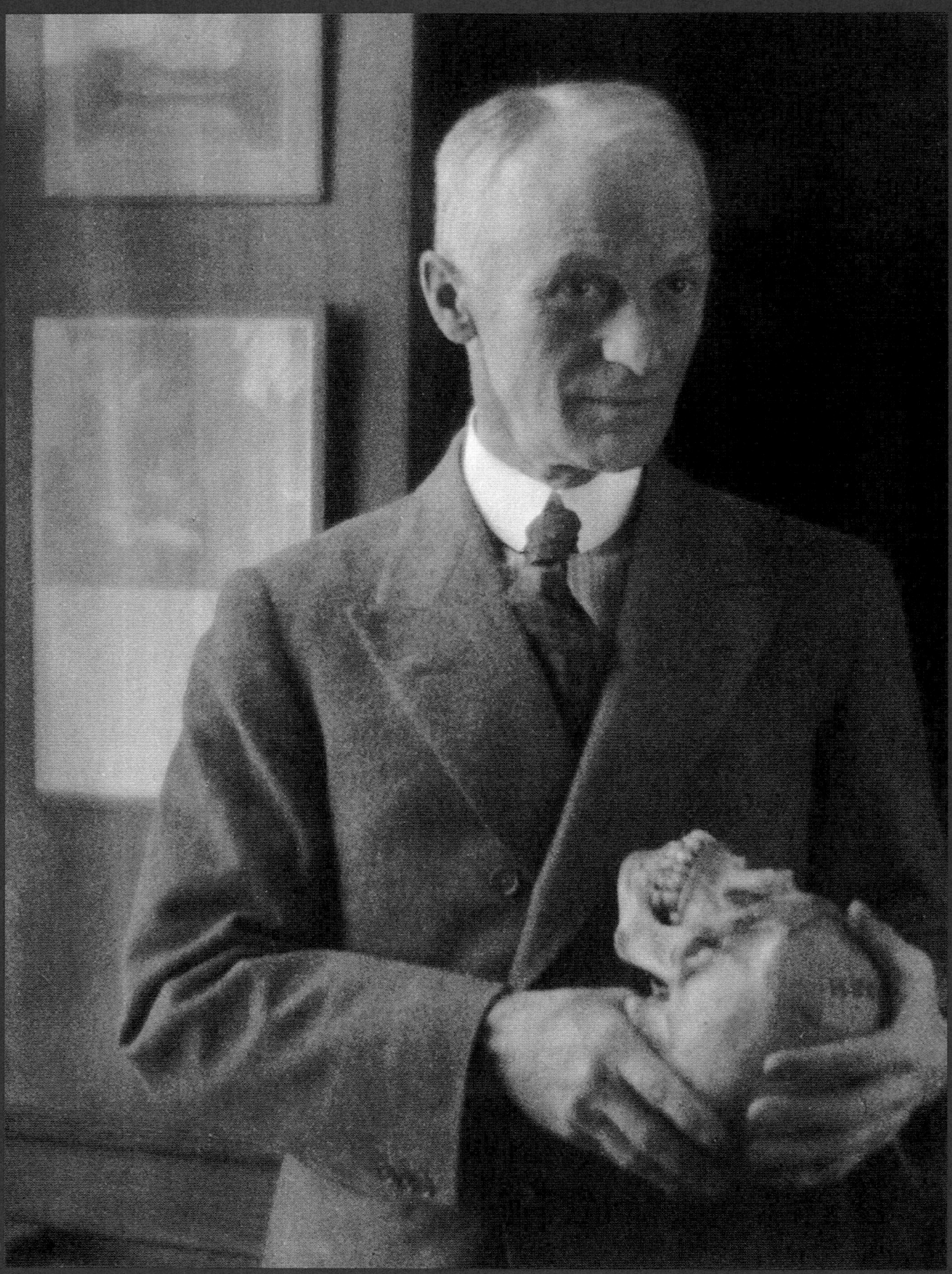

FIG. 87. DR. CUSHING POSING FOR THE CAMERA IN HIS OFFICE — DR. BOYD'S COLLECTION.

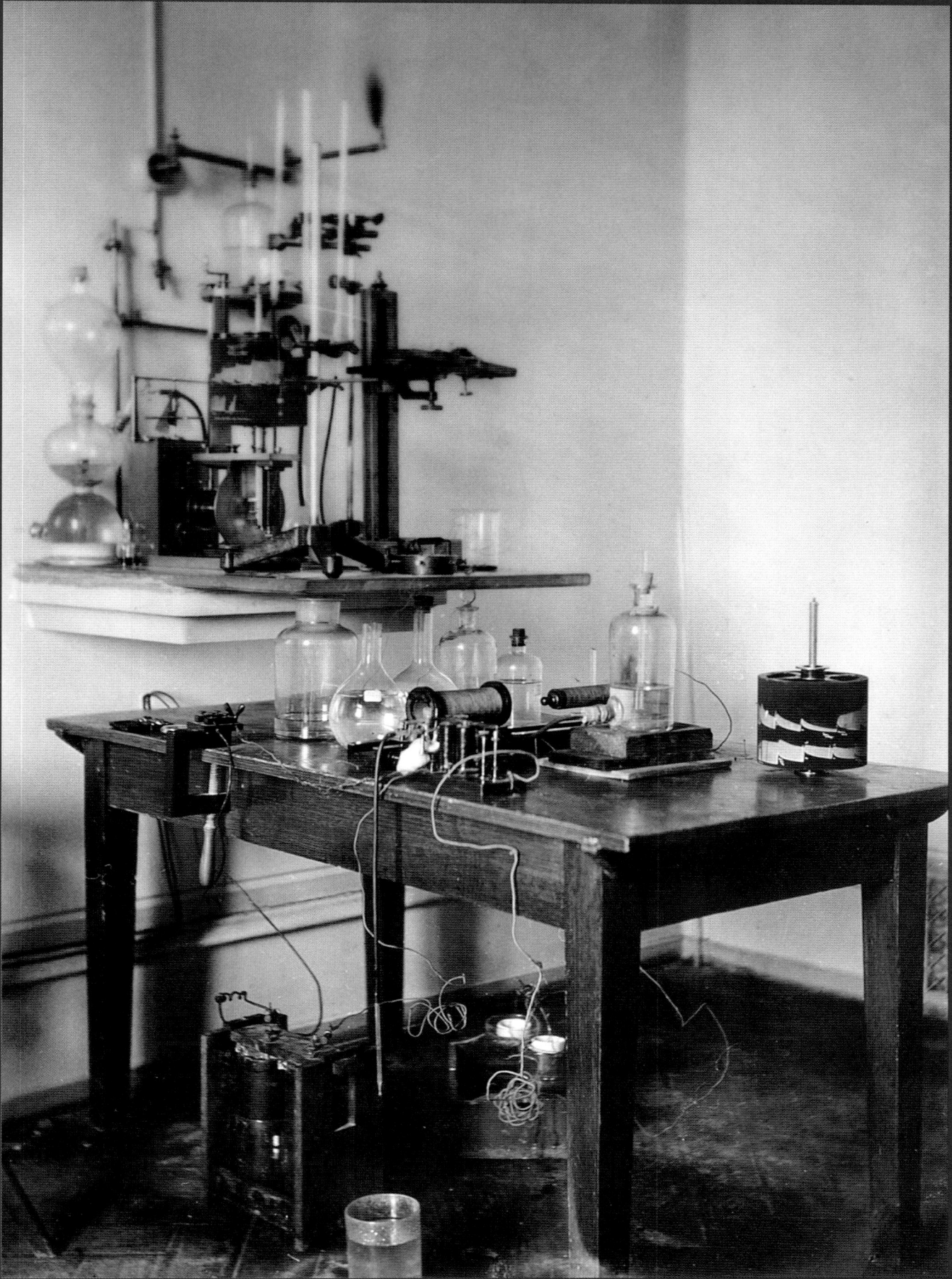

FIG. 88. HUNTERIAN LABORATORY.

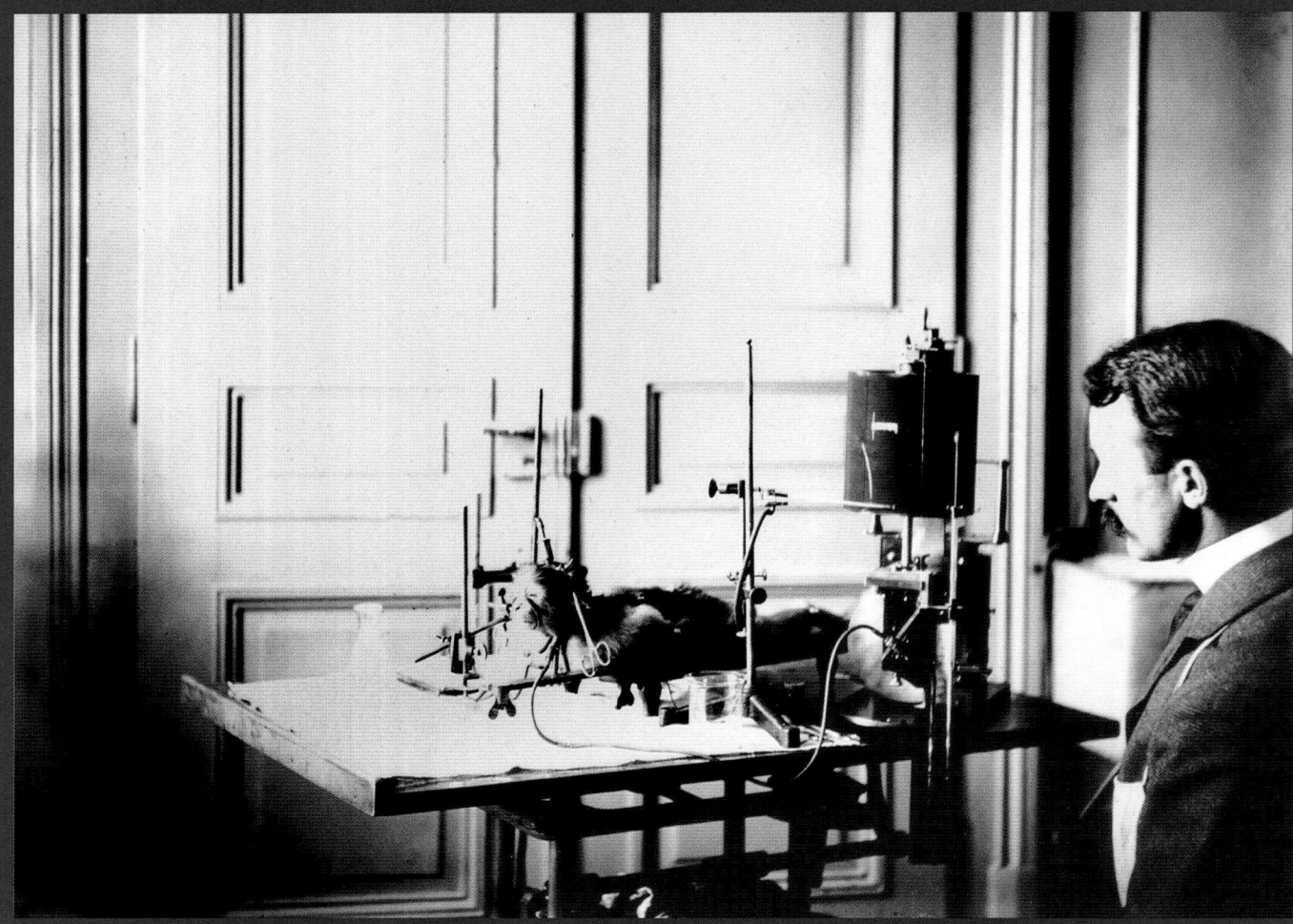
FIG. 89. HUNTERIAN LABORATORY — DR. CUSHING LOOKING OVER.

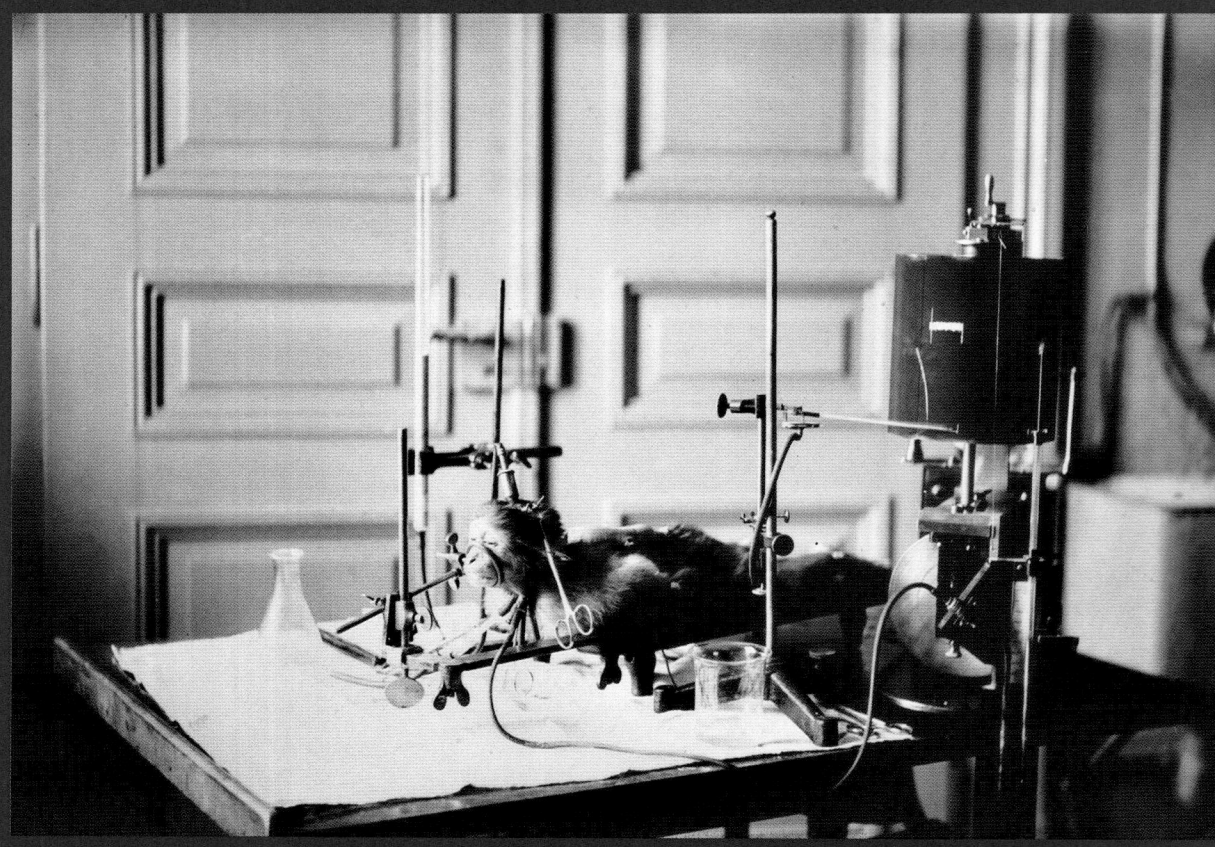
FIG. 90. HUNTERIAN LABORATORY — EXPERIMENTS ON MONKEYS.

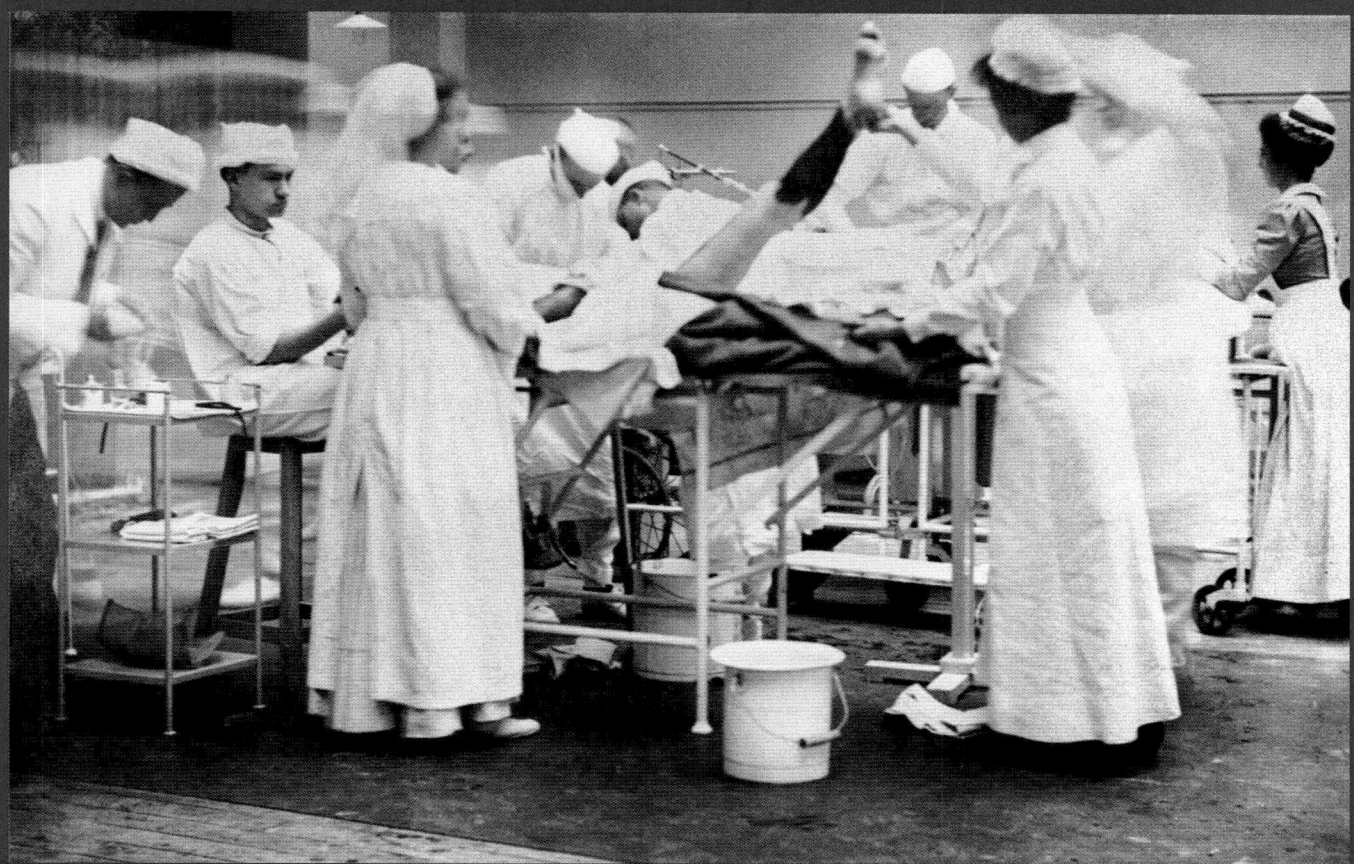

FIG. 91. DR. CUSHING'S OPERATING ROOM EARLY IN HIS CAREER.

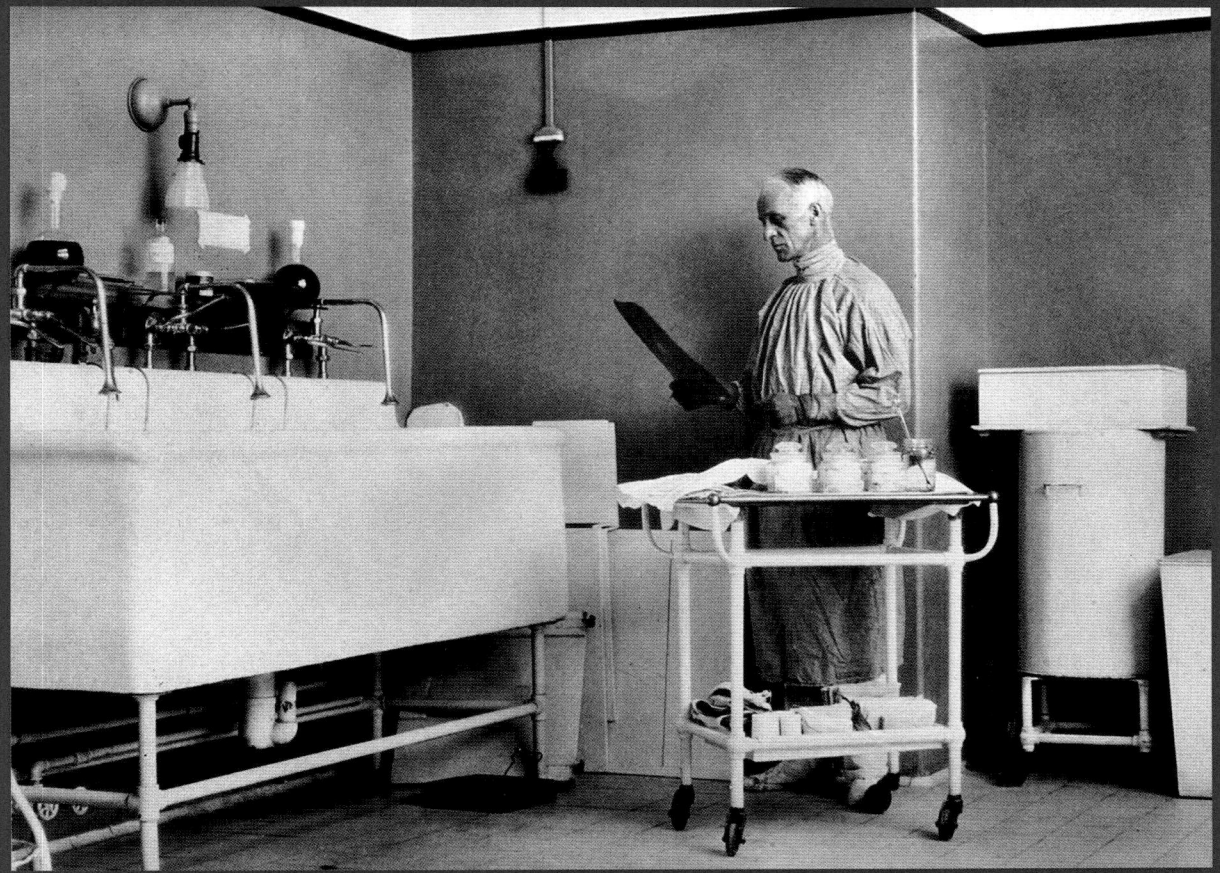

FIG. 92. DR. CUSHING LATER IN HIS CAREER.

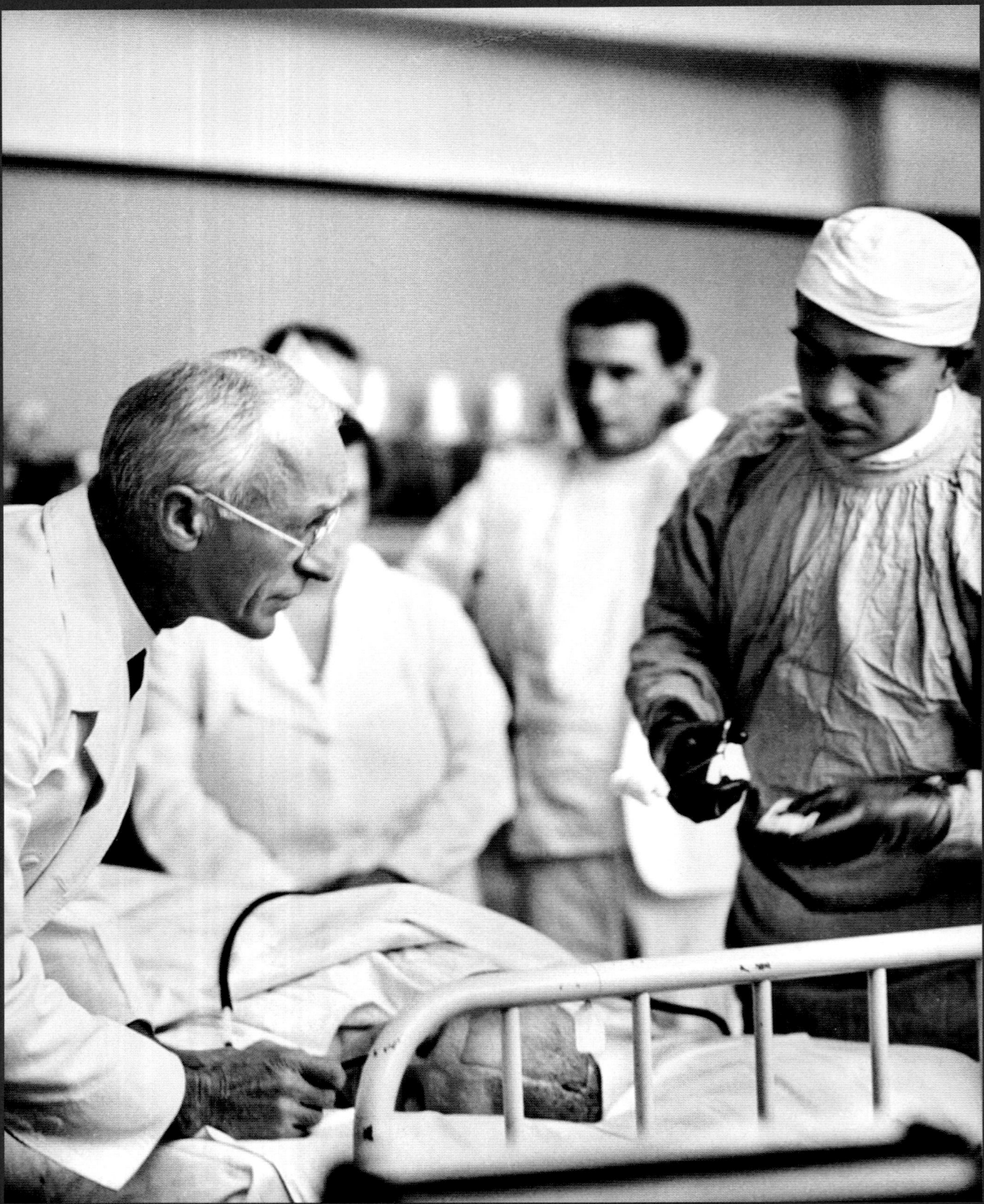
FIG. 93. DR. DECOPETT AND DR. CUSHING CONSULTING ABOUT THE PATIENT.

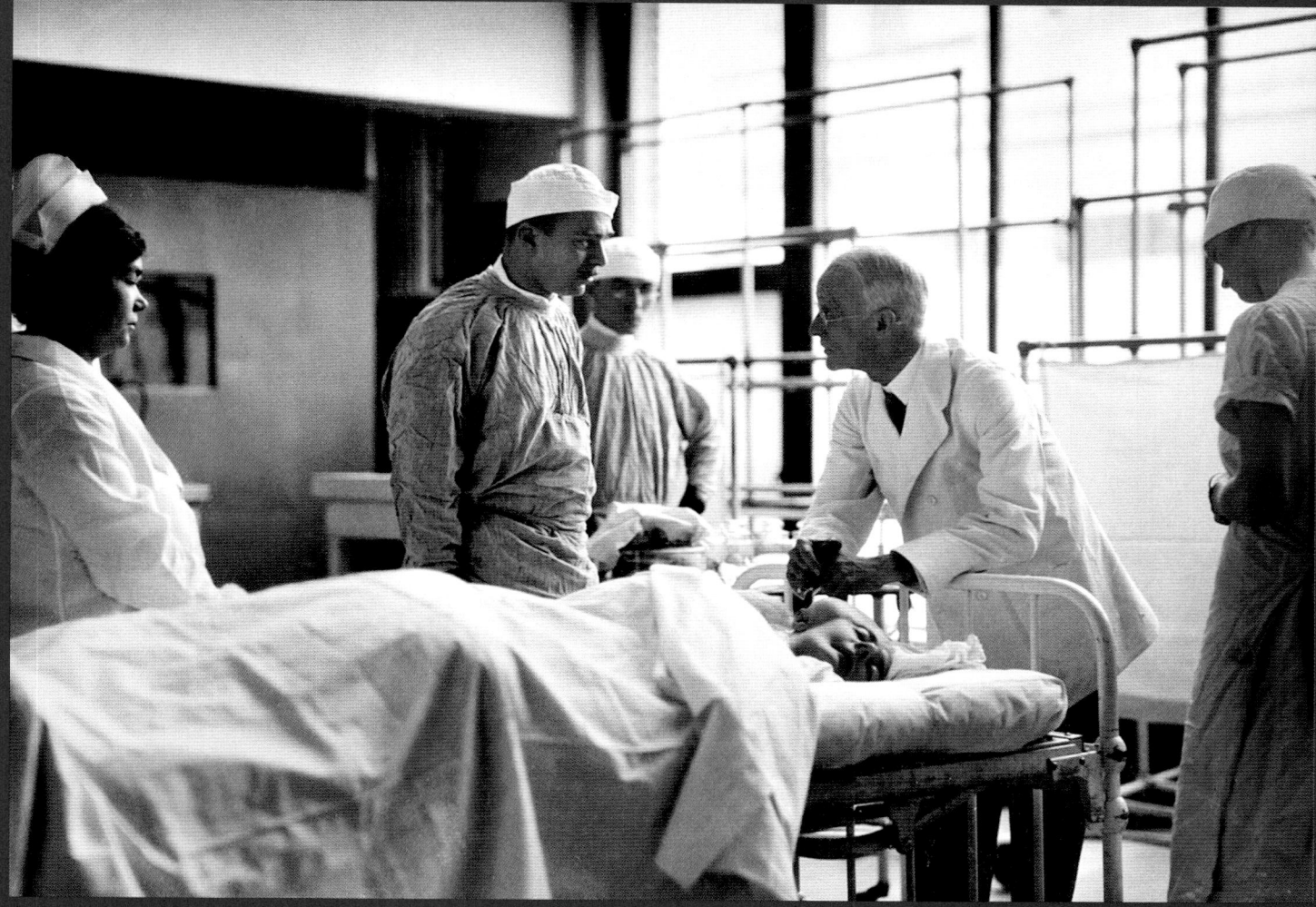
FIG. 94. DR. DECOPETT AND DR. CUSHING CONSULTING ABOUT THE PATIENT.

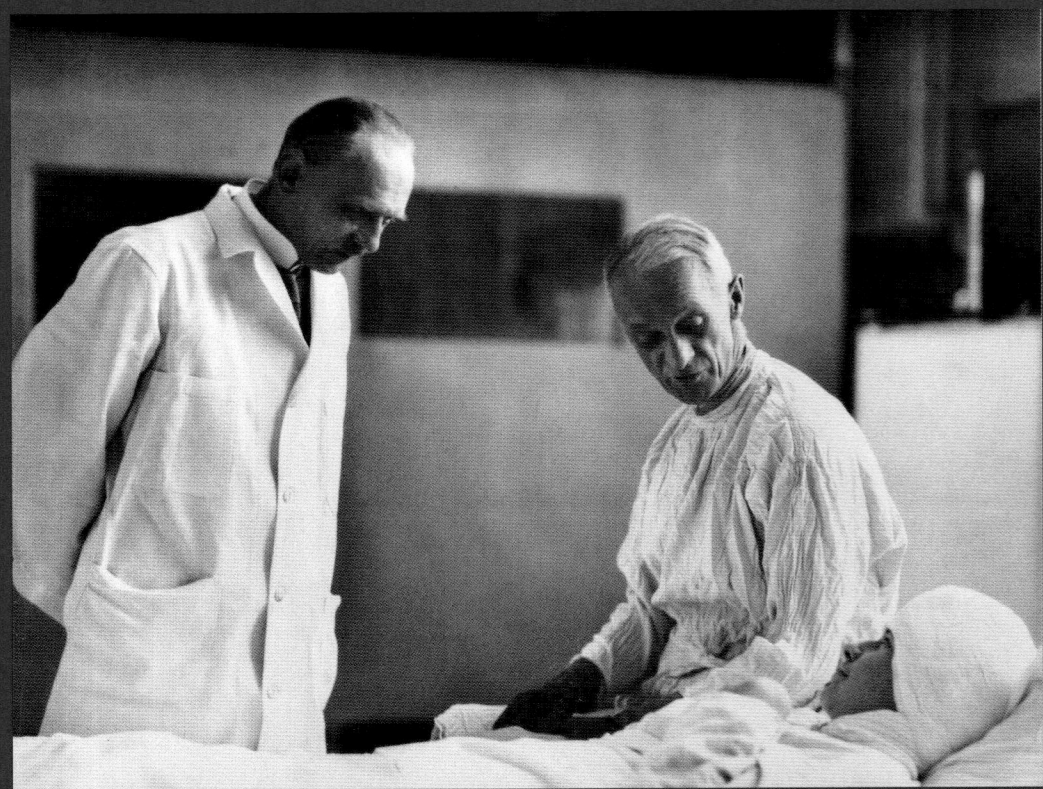
FIG. 95. DR. CUSHING AND DR. FORSTER EXAMINING A PATIENT WHO UNDERWENT A CEREBELLAR TUMOR RESECTION.

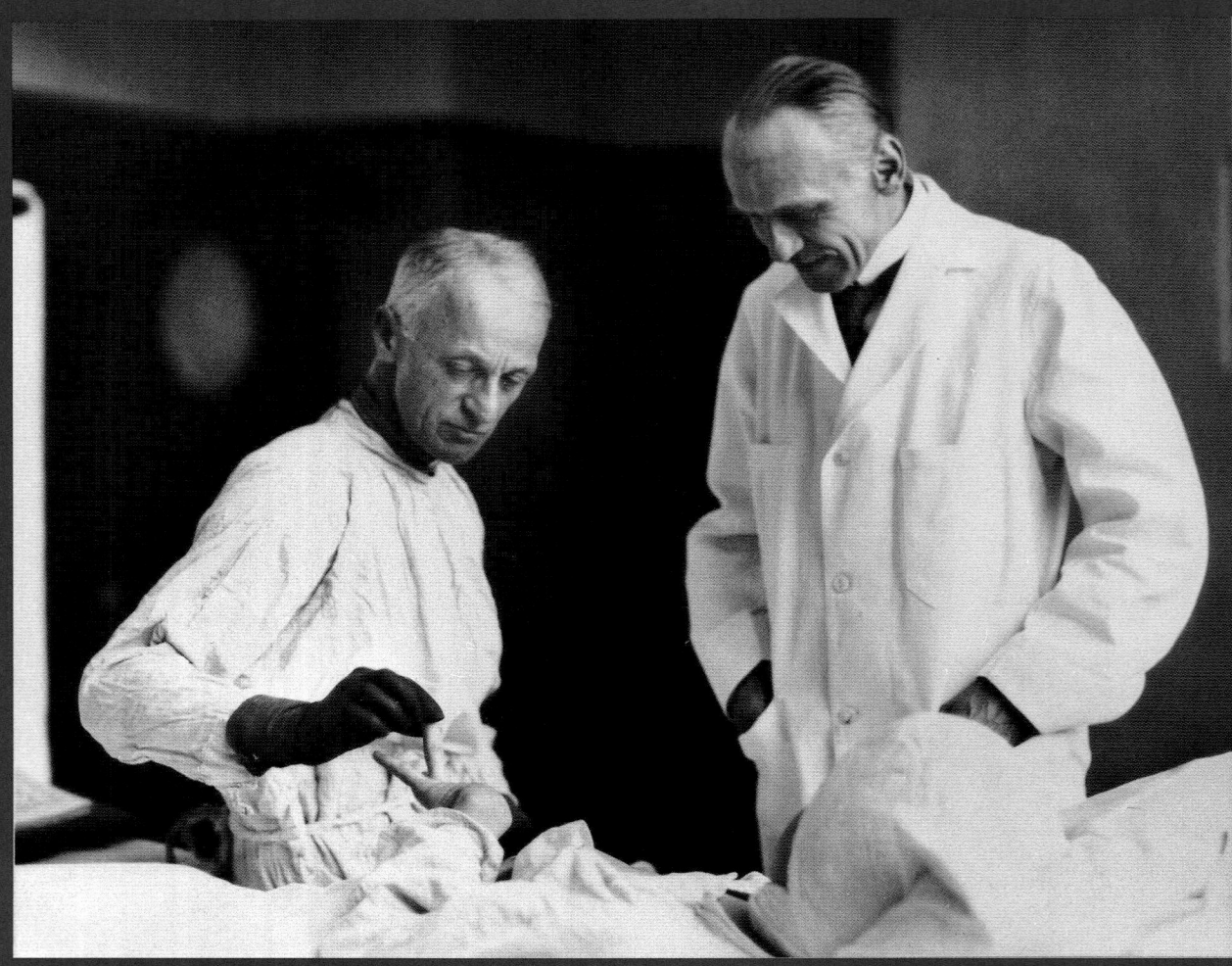
FIG. 96. DR. CUSHING AND DR. FORSTER DURING THEIR ROUNDS.

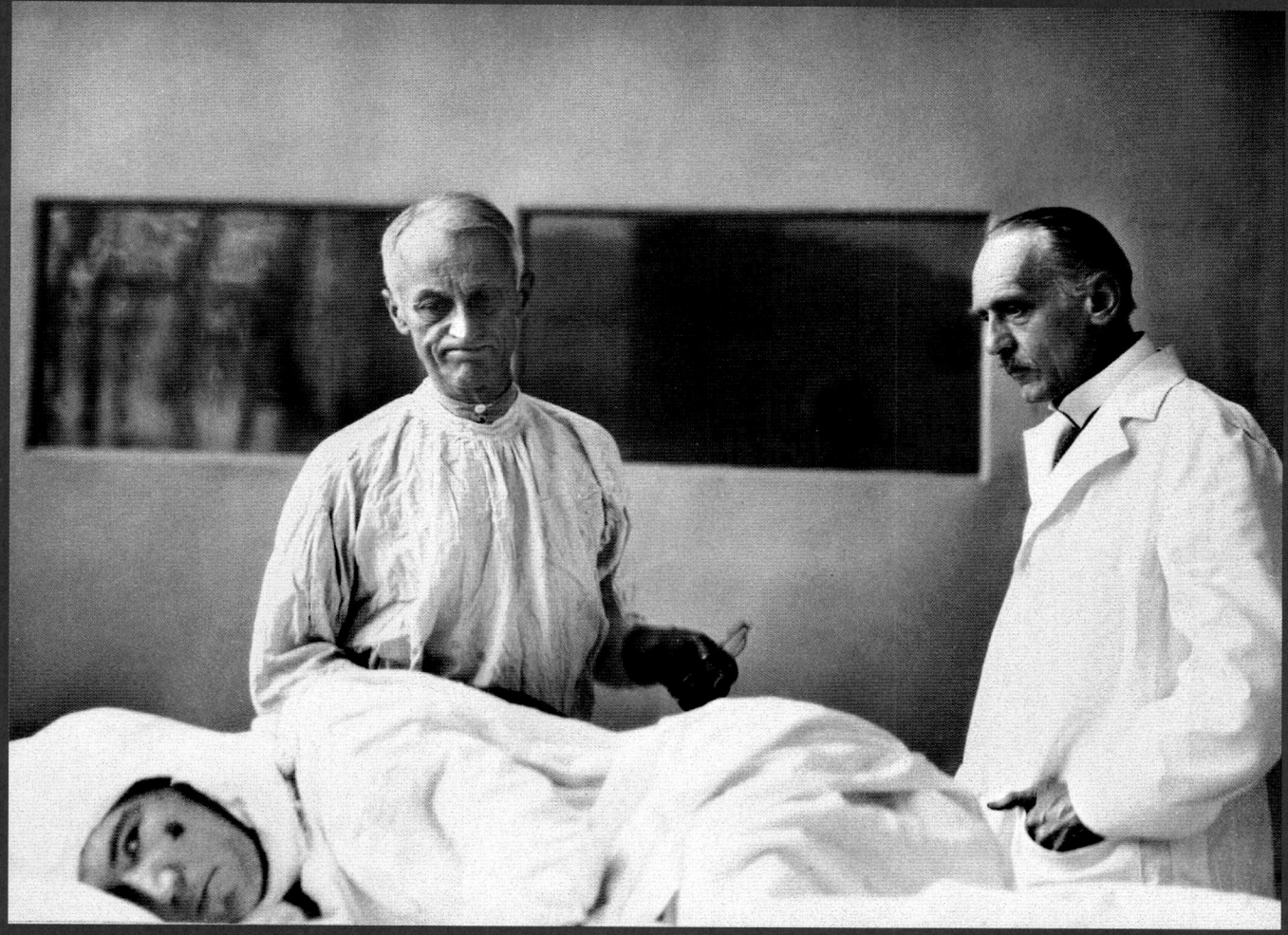
FIG. 97. DR. CUSHING AND DR. FORSTER ARE PUZZLED ABOUT THE PATIENT'S CONDITION.

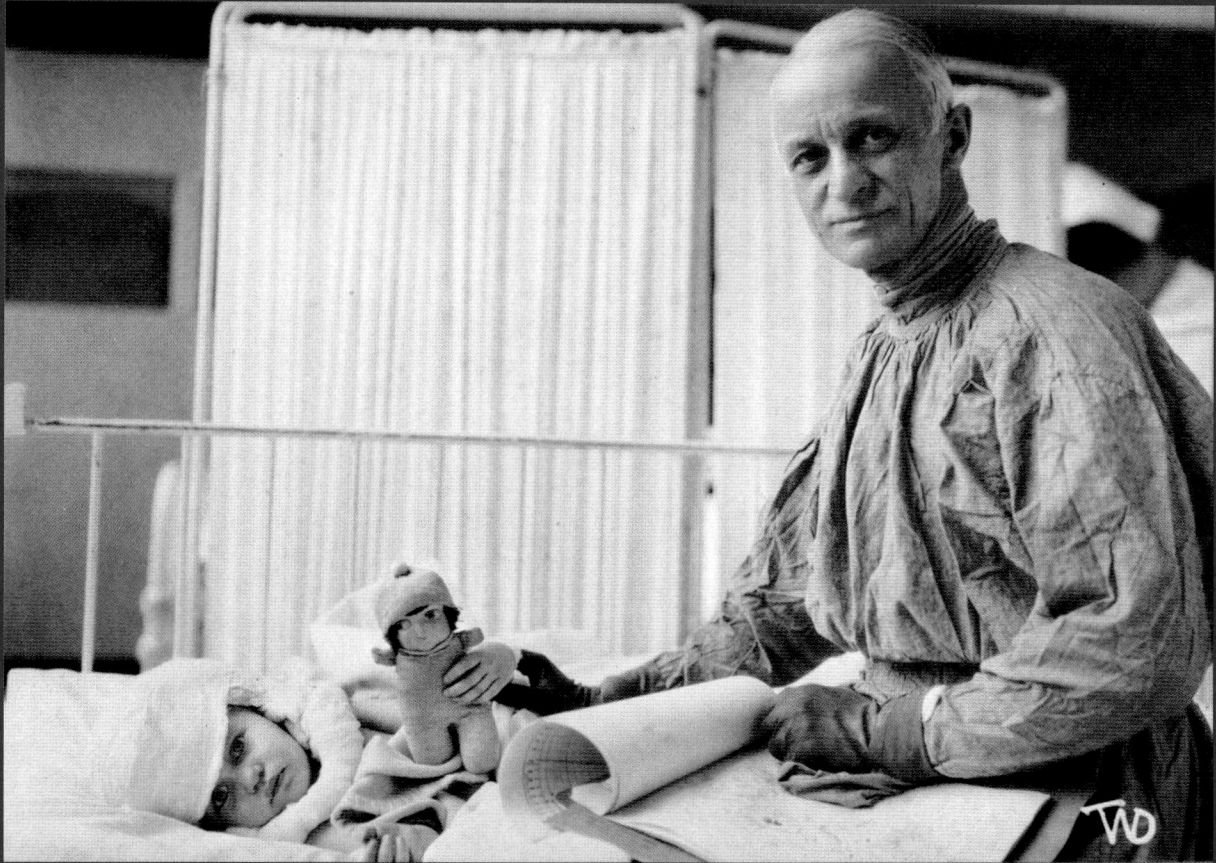
FIG. 98. DR. CUSHING VISITING A PATIENT WHO RECENTLY UNDERWENT A CEREBELLAR TUMOR OPERATION.

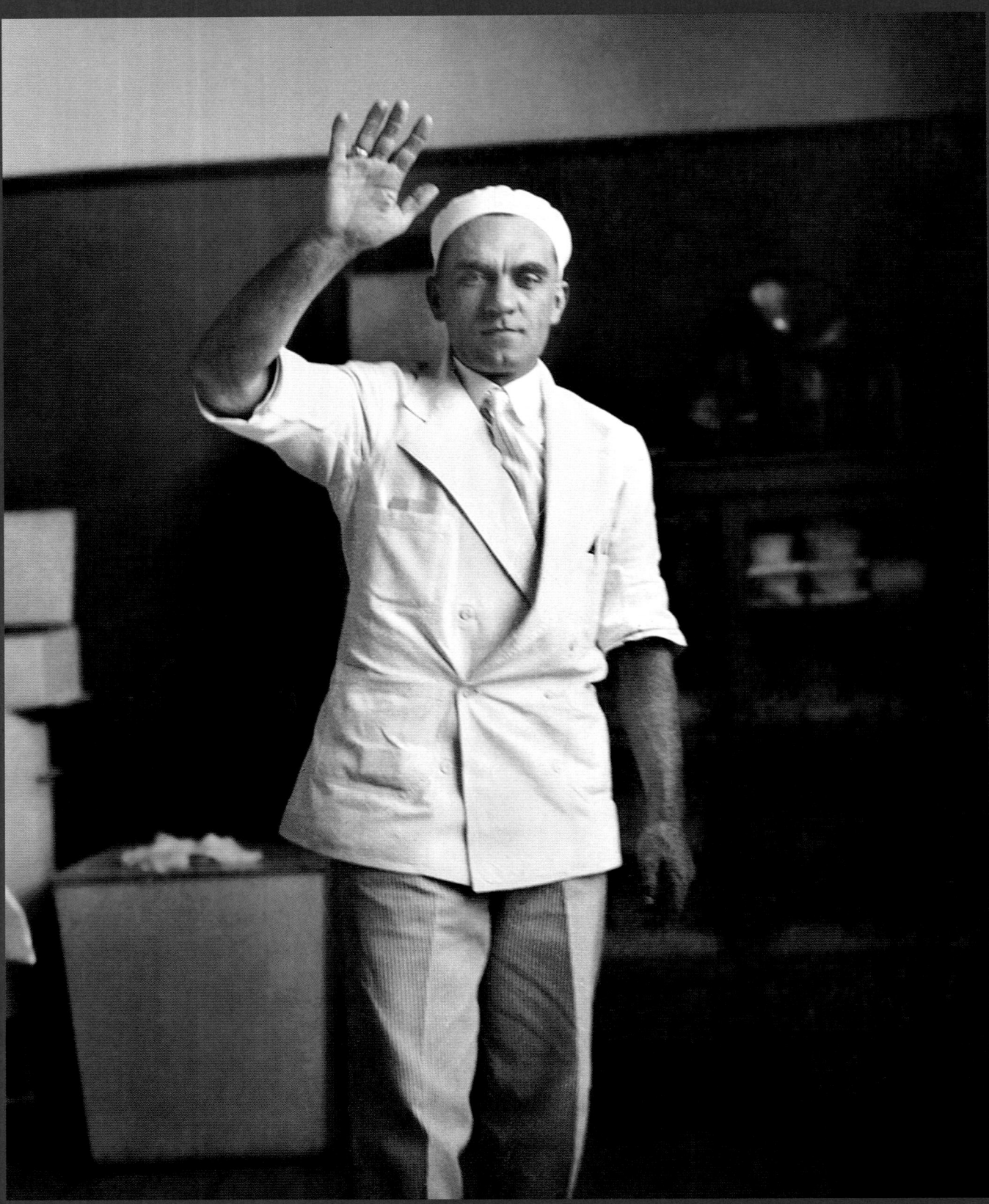
FIG. 99. ADOLPH WATZKA — DR. CUSHING'S OPERATING ROOM ORDERLY.

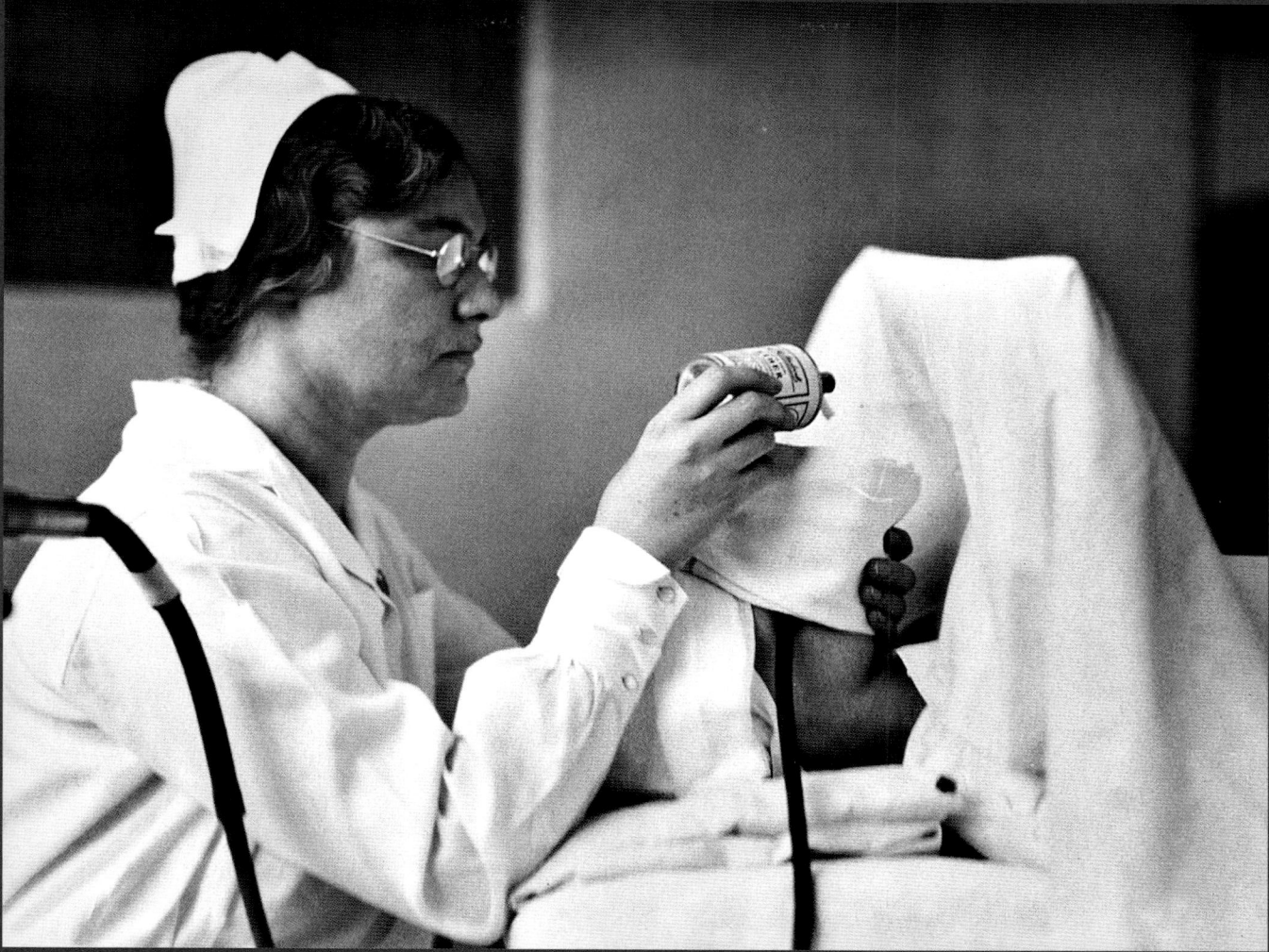
FIG. 100. MISS GERRARD — DR. CUSHING'S NURSE OF ANESTHESIA.

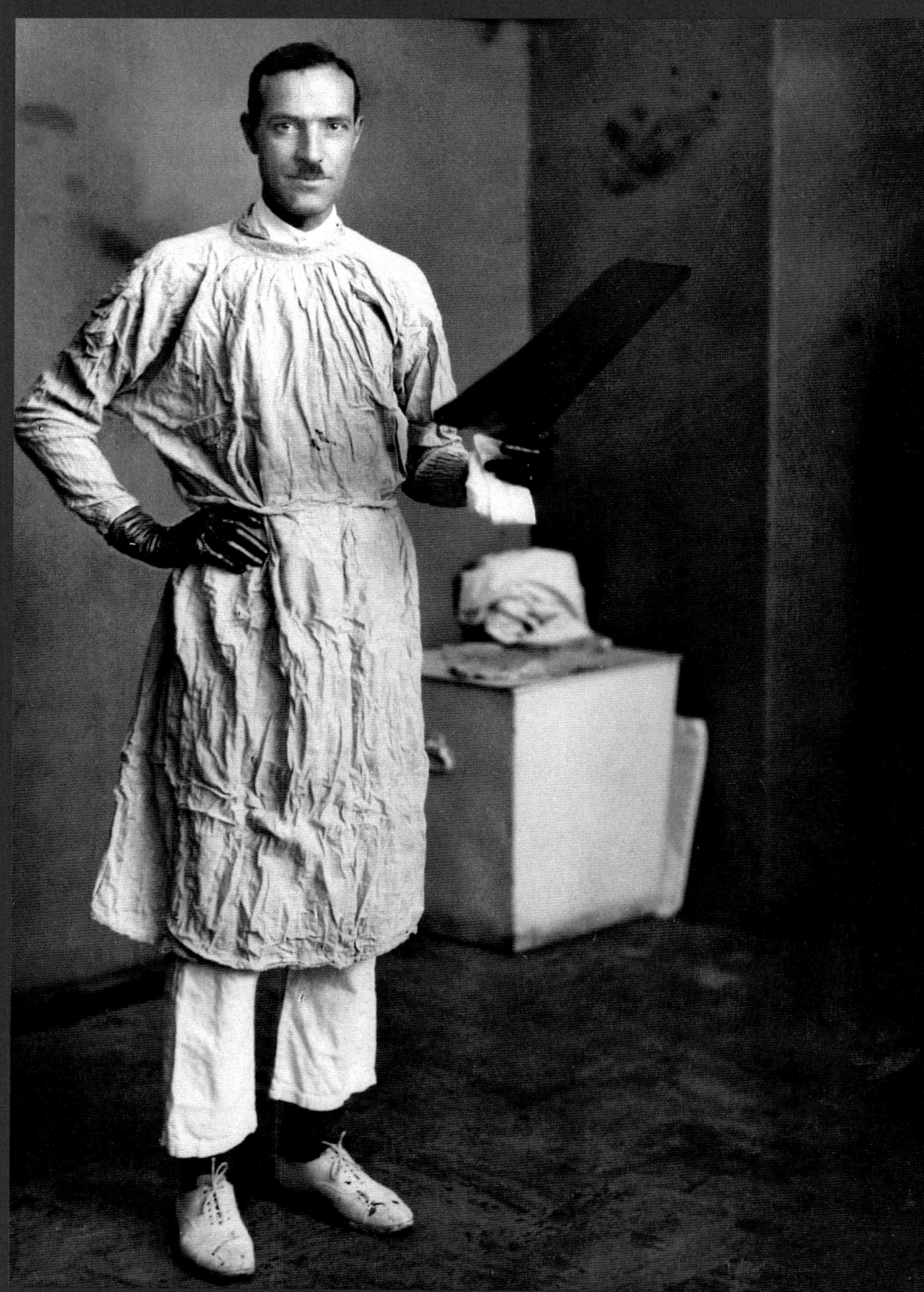

FIG. 101. DR. GILBERT HORRAX — DR. CUSHING'S LONGTIME ASSISTANT.

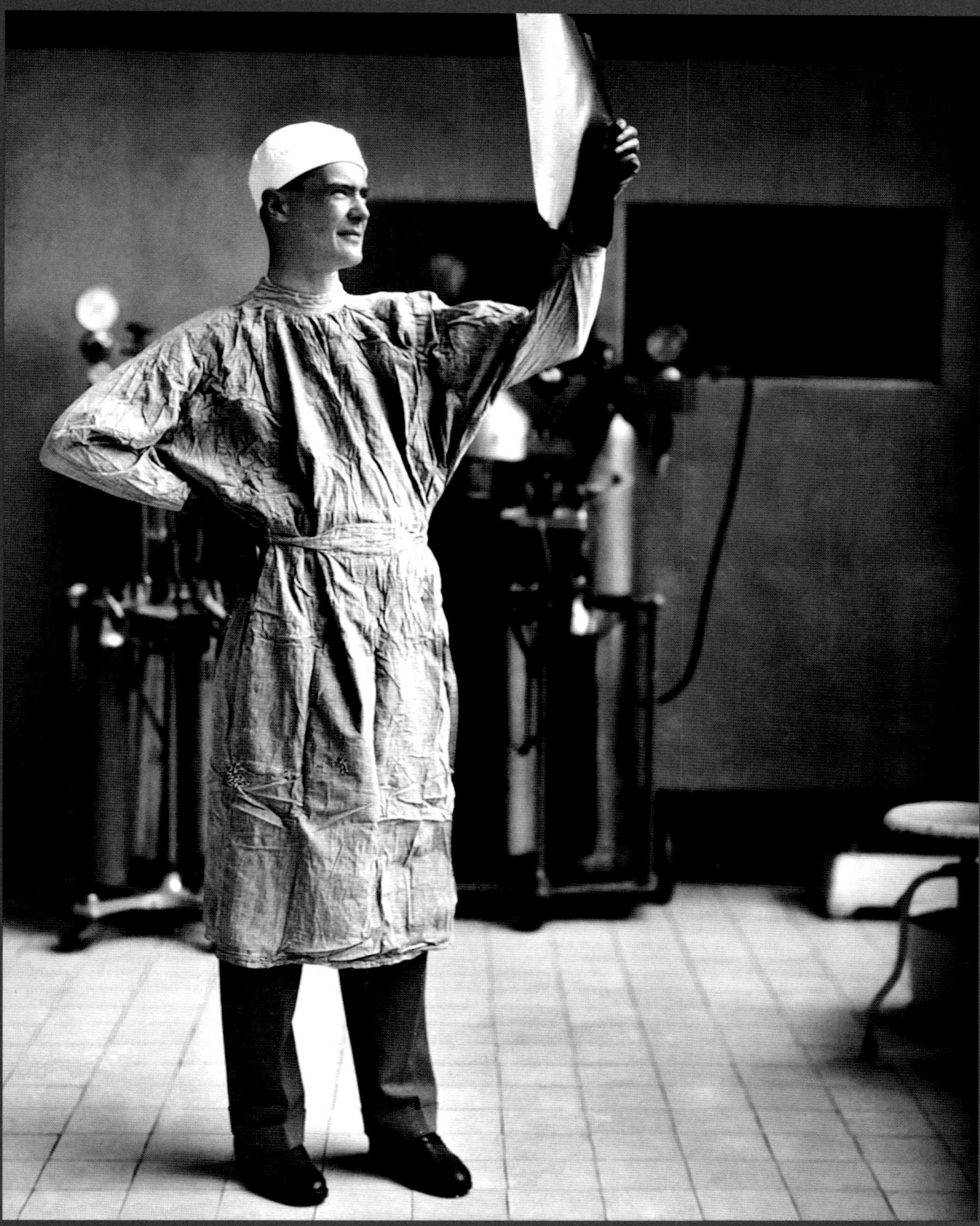

FIG. 102. DR. NORMAN DOTT — DR. CUSHING'S RESIDENT.

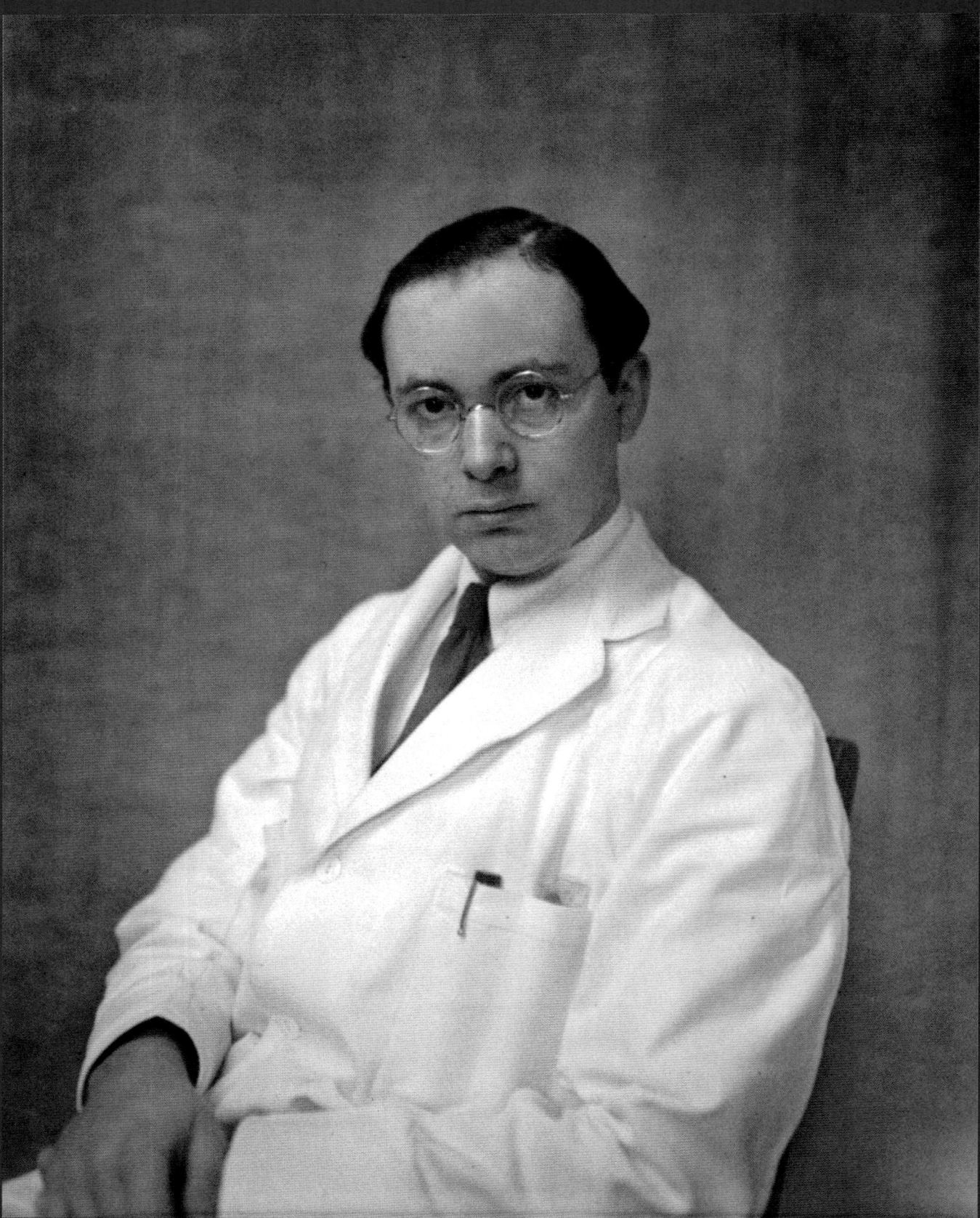

FIG. 103. DR. LEO DAVIDOFF — DR CUSHING'S RESIDENT.

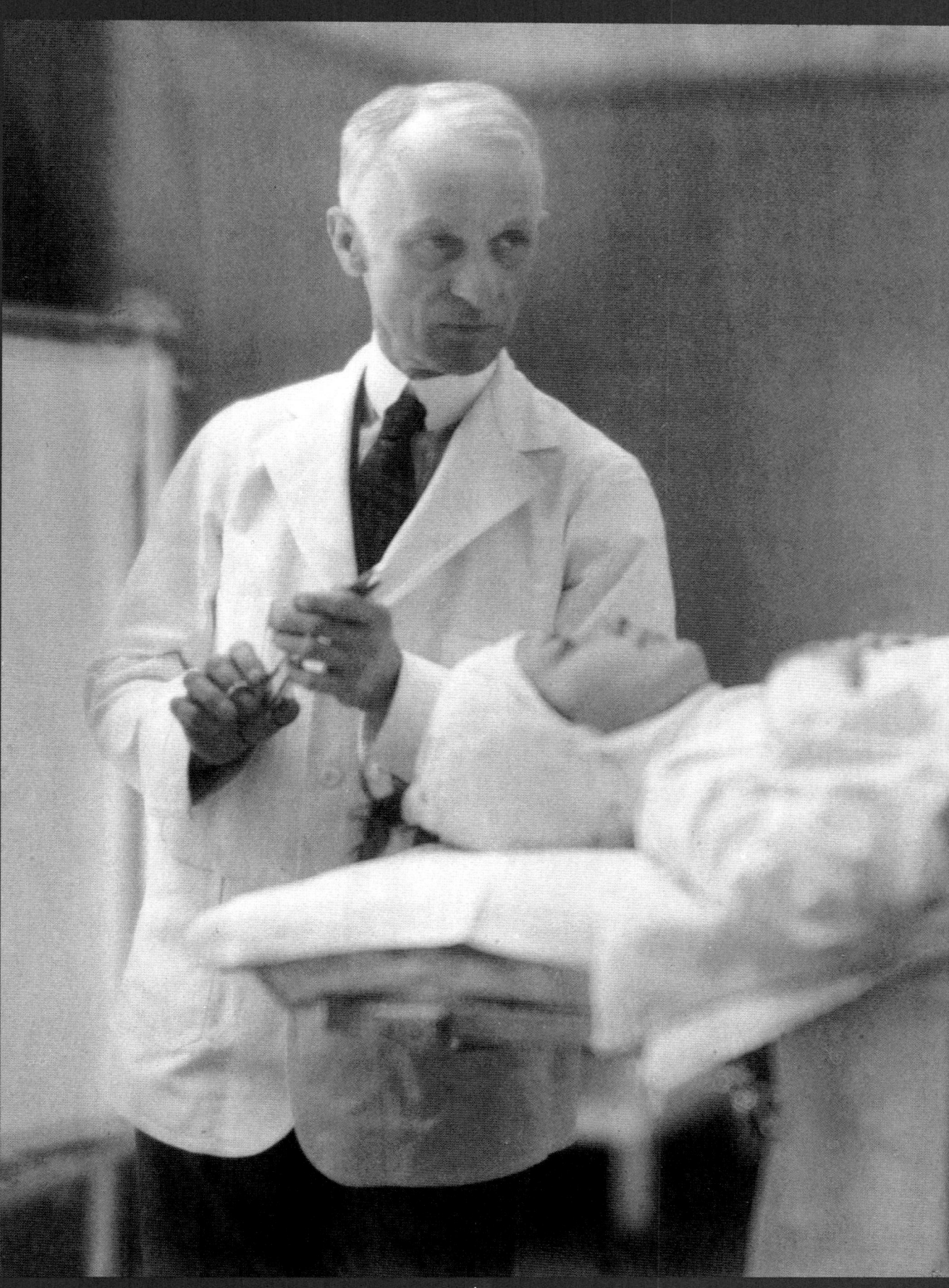
FIG. 104. DR. CUSHING FINISHING THE DRESSING — DR. BOYD'S COLLECTION.

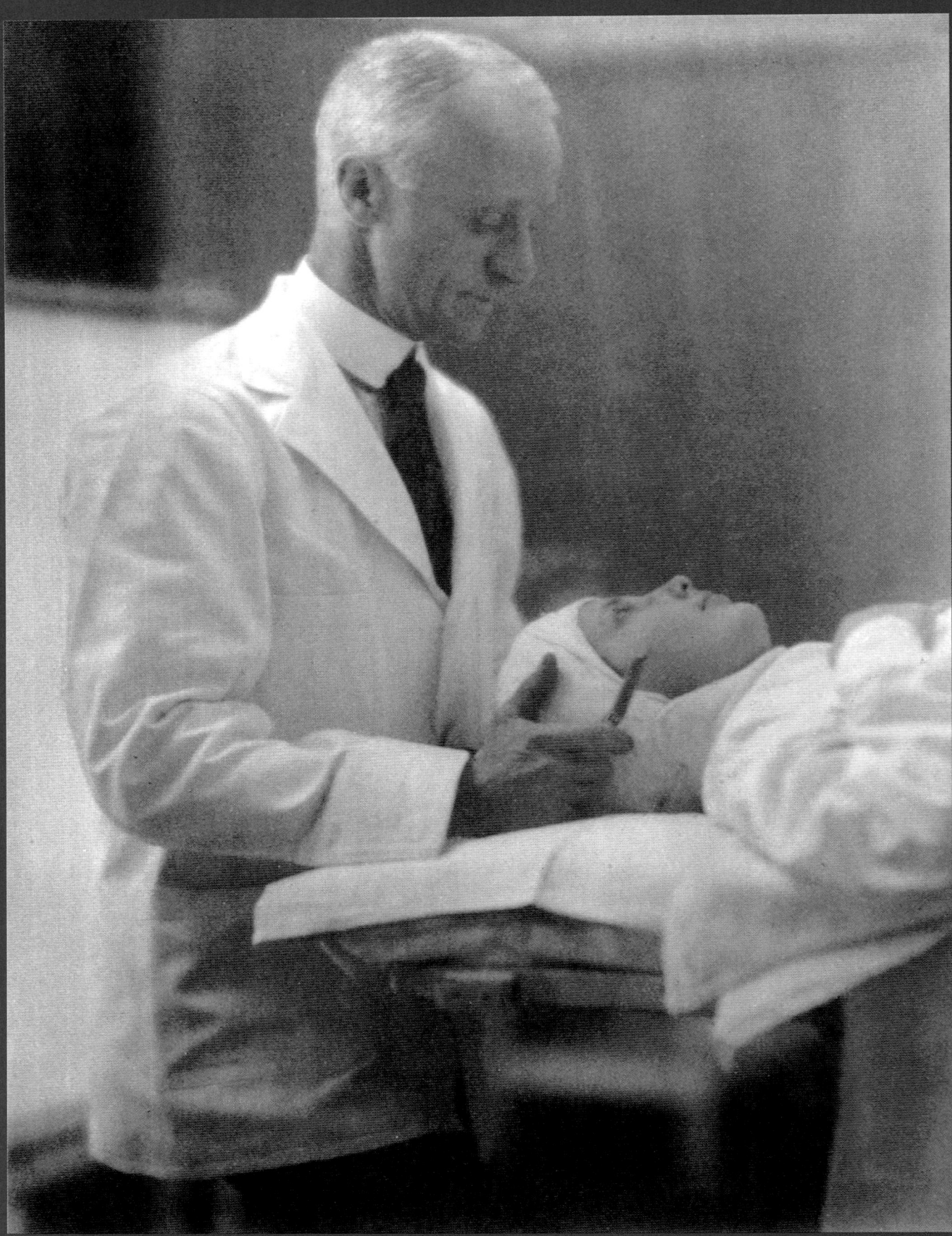

FIG. 105. DR. CUSHING FINISHING THE HEAD DRESSING — DR. BOYD'S COLLECTION.

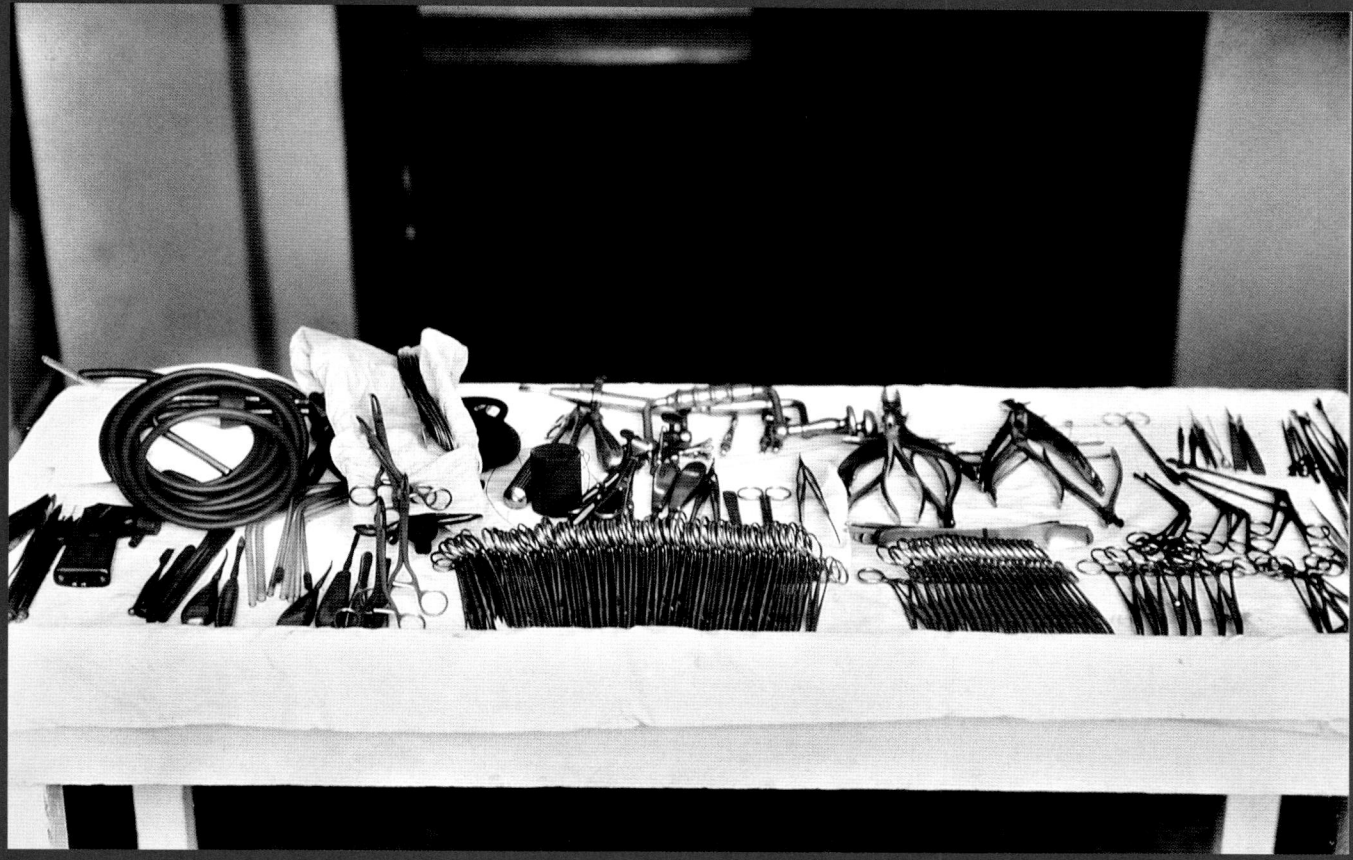

FIG. 106. OPERATING ROOM INSTRUMENT TABLE.

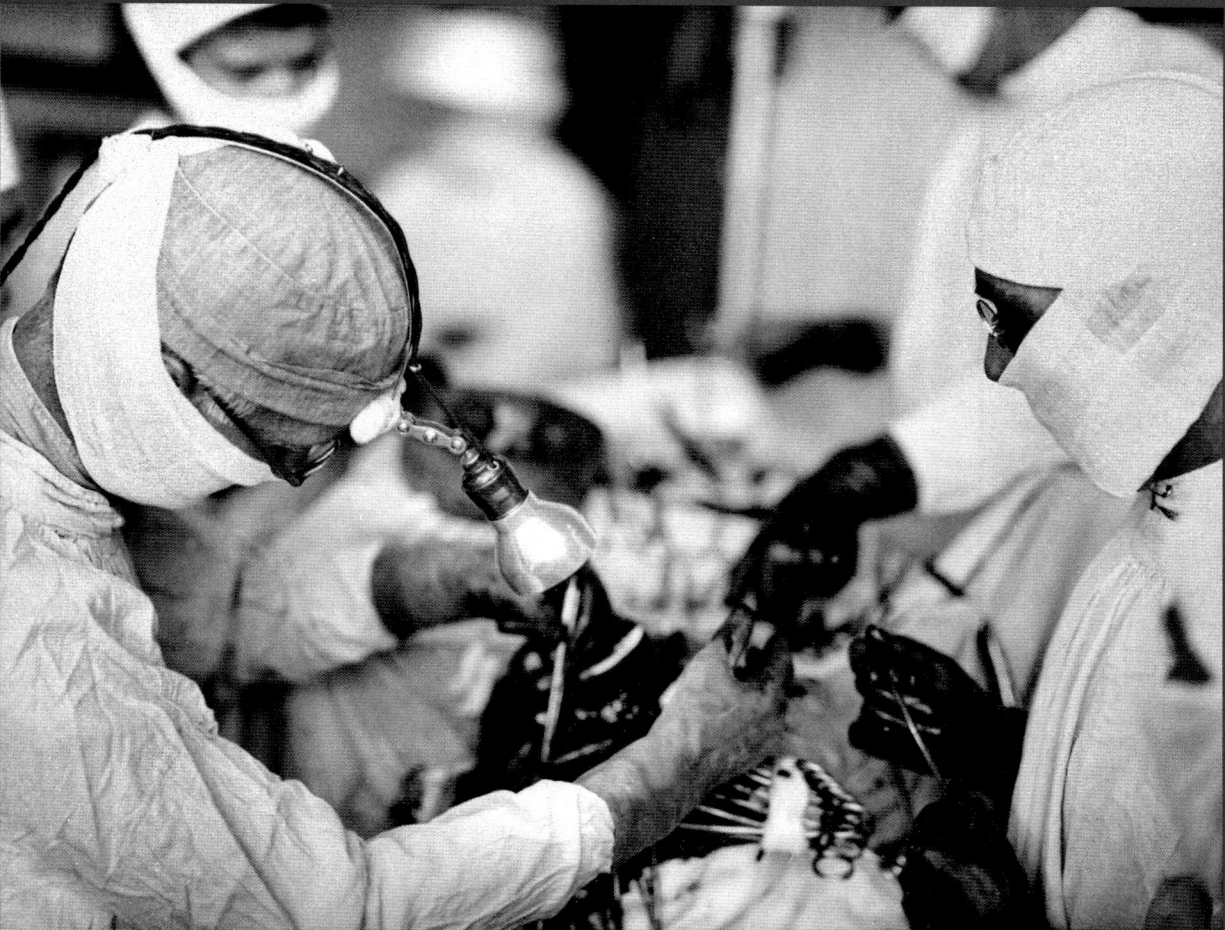

FIG. 107. DR. CUSHING IS GETTING READY TO REMOVE THE BONE FLAP.

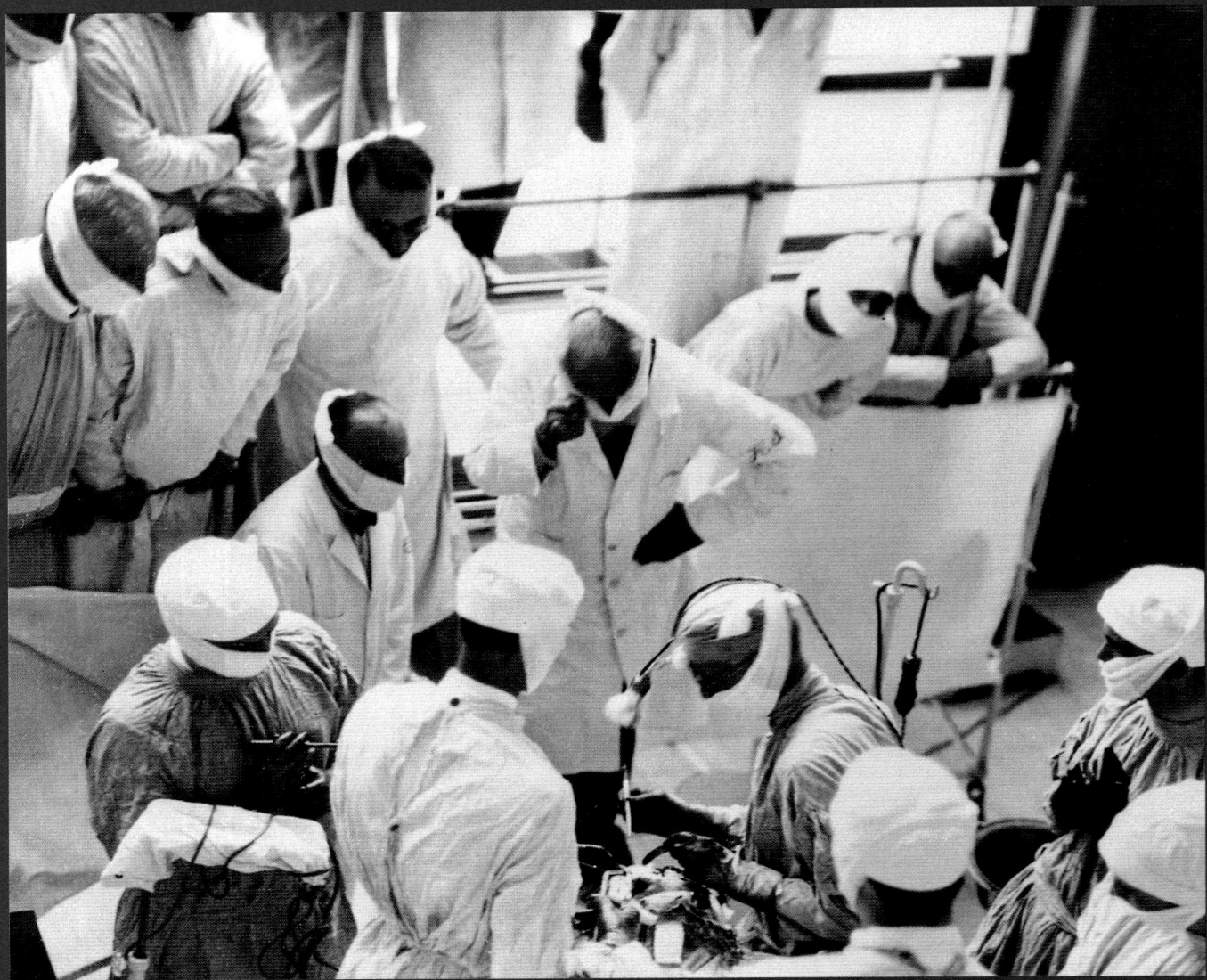
FIG. 108. DR. CUSHING OPERATING WHILE DR. PAVLOV IS LOOKING OVER.

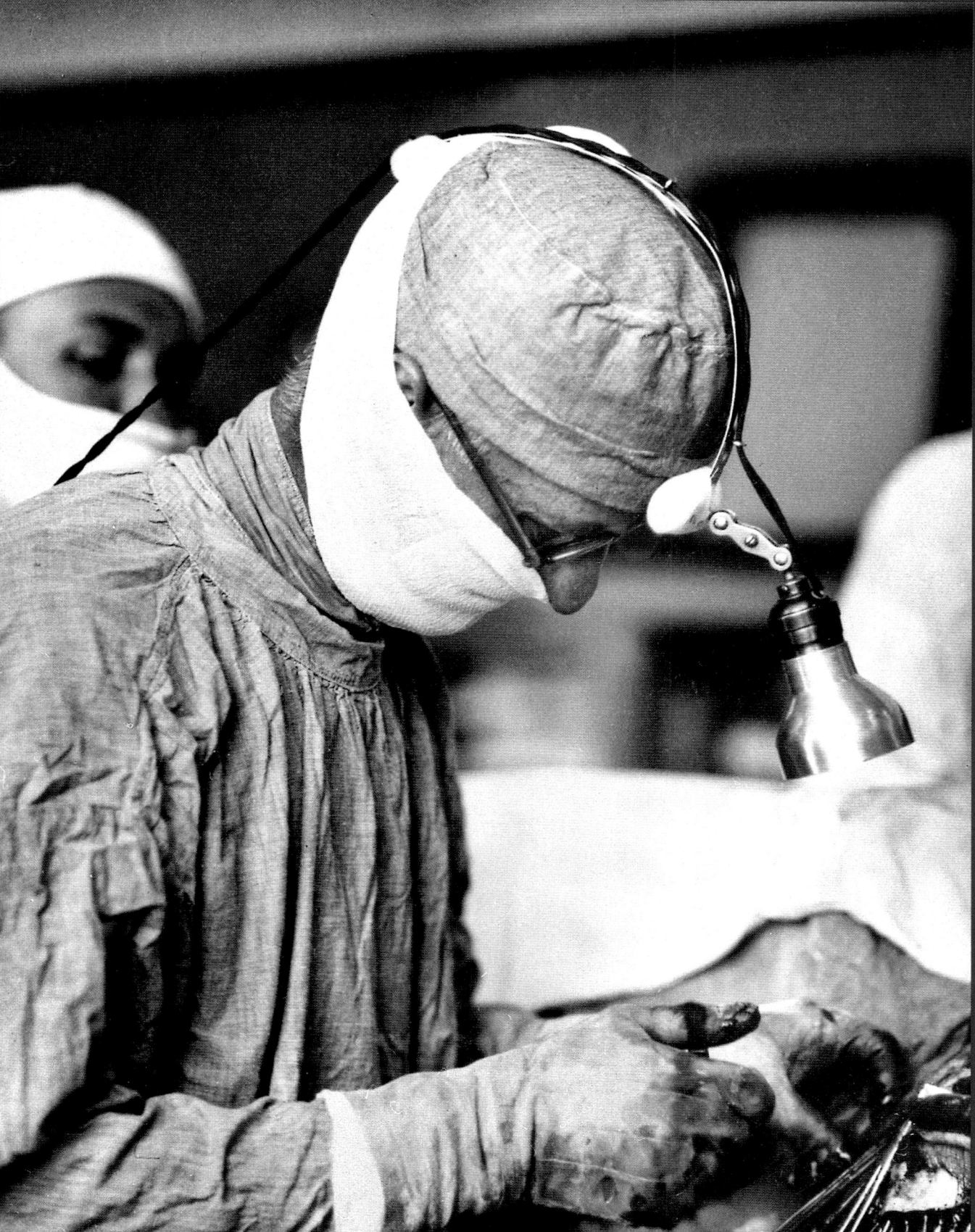

FIG. 109. DURING THE 2000TH VERIFIED BRAIN TUMOR OPERATION.

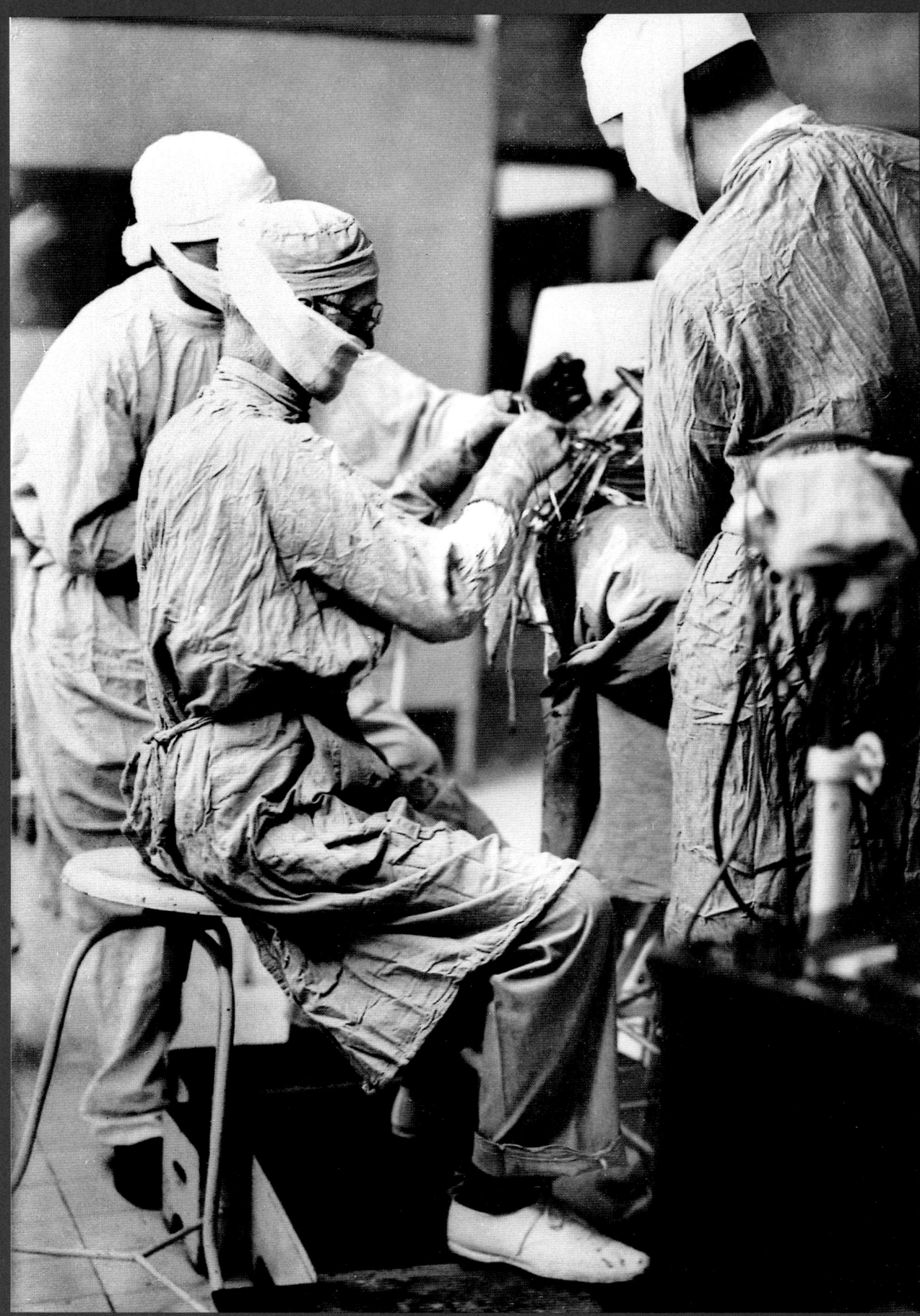

FIG. 110. CLOSING THE 2000TH VERIFIED BRAIN TUMOR OPERATION.

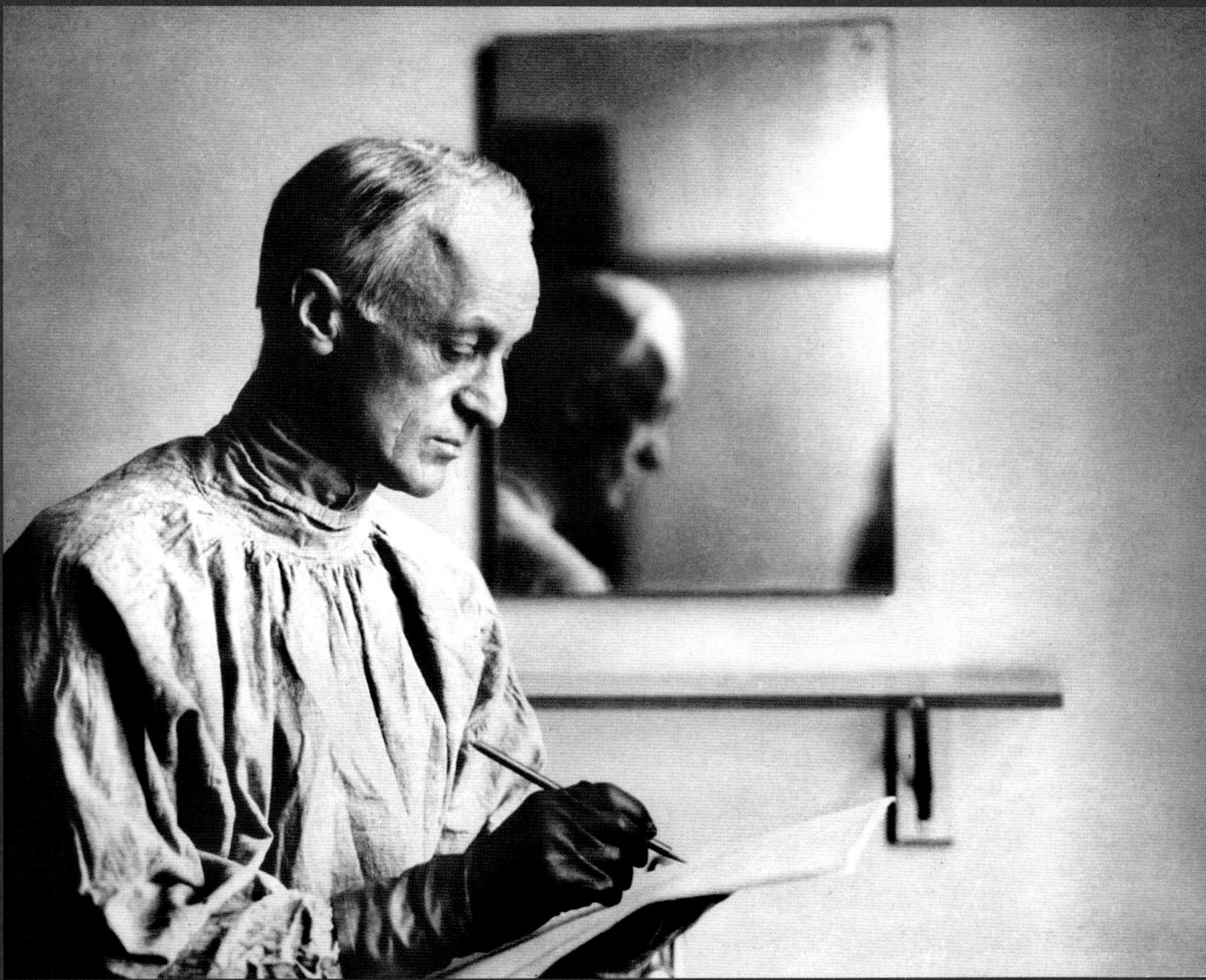
FIG. III. DR. CUSHING SKETCHING HIS OPERATIVE FINDINGS.

Index

Page numbers followed by *f* indicate entries in figures.

A

Abducent nerve (CN VI)
    pituitary adenoma and, 10
    skull base adenocarcinoma and, 126, 128
Acoustic neuroma, 394–398, 431–434
    discharge notes on, 396–398, 434
    follow-up notes on, 396–397
    gross appearance of, 433*f*
    histology of, 395–396, 396*f*, 434
    letters to Cushing on, 398, 434
    neurological exam with, 431
    objective findings with, 394, 397, 431
    operative notes on, 394–395, 432–433
    operative sketches of, 484*f*, 496*f*
    pathology report on, 395–396, 433–434
    patient histories with, 394, 431
    patient postoperative appearance, 395*f*, 432*f*
    patient preoperative appearance, 394*f*
    positive findings with, 394, 397, 431
    postoperative notes on, 434
    radiologic findings with, 394, 432
    radiotherapy for, 397
    special notes on, 394, 397, 432
    subjective findings with, 394, 397, 431
    teaching slide on, 399*f*
    ventricular puncture for, 394–395
    vision affected by, 431
Acromegaly
    Cushing's interest in, 3–4
    physician's recognition in self, 4
    pituitary adenoma and, 9–22, 87–90
    teaching slides on, 504*f*–506*f*
Adenocarcinoma, skull base, 125–129
Adenoma. *See* Pituitary adenoma
American Ophthalmological Society, 193
Anesthesia, Cushing's contributions to, 196–197
Aneurysm(s)
    anterior cerebral artery, 309–312
    bruit with, 295–296, 307–308
    congenital, of right temporal lobe, 295–296, 305–308
    Cushing on, 293–296
    first description of arterial, 293
    first ligations of, 293
    first planned intracranial operation for, 294
    incidental findings of, 293–295
    internal carotid, 300–304
    muscle grafts for, 294–295, 302, 304, 306–307, 310–312
    records on patients with, 294–295, 295*t*
    silver clips for, 294
Angiography, cerebral, 294, 296
Angioma(s), 297. *See also* Arteriovenous malformations
    arterial, 297
    arteriovenous, 297
    left hemisphere, 313–316
    venous, 297
Anterior cerebral artery aneurysm, 309–312
    discharge note on, 312
    follow-up note on, 312
    muscle graft for, 310–312
    objective findings with, 309
    operative notes on, 309–312
    operative sketches of, 309*f*, 311, 311*f*–312*f*
    patient history with, 309
    positive findings with, 309
    radiologic findings with, 309–310
    special note on, 310
    subjective findings with, 309
    ventriculogram for, 309–310
Anterior clinoid process
    craniopharyngioma and, 36
    optic chiasm glioma and, 25
    parasellar tumor and, 31
    pituitary adenoma and, 10, 16, 20
    skull base adenocarcinoma and, 125
Anterior lobe extract, for craniopharyngioma, 41–42
Antuitrin injections, for pituitary adenoma, 81–84

Arachnoid cyst, with olfactory groove meningioma, 229–230
Arterial angioma, 297
Arteriovenous malformations, 296–299
    bruit with, 297
    Cushing on, 296–299
    discharge notes on, 314
    electrosurgery for, 297, 299
    first successful removal of, 296–299, 313–314
    Gaupp on, 296
    left hemisphere, 313–316
    letters to Cushing on, 314–316
    muscle graft for, 314
    objective findings with, 313, 315
    Old Testament account of, 296
    operative notes on, 313–314, 316
    operative sketches of, 313f, 315f
    pathology report on, 316
    patient history with, 313
    positive findings with, 313, 315
    postoperative notes on, 316
    radiologic findings with, 313, 315–316
    radiotherapy for, 296–299, 314–316
    records on patients with, 297–299, 298t
    special notes on, 313, 316
    subjective findings with, 313
Astrocytoma(s)
    cerebellar
        cystic fibrillary, operative sketch of, 486f
        teaching slide on, 523f
    posterior fossa, 95
    spinal, 319
    third ventricle, fibrillary, operative sketch of, 491f
AVMS. See Arteriovenous malformations

B

Bagley, Charles, 380
Bailey, Percival
    carotid artery ligation by, 294–295, 302
    glioma classification by, 95
    home autopsy performed by, 96, 122–123
    visual field studies of, 194
Ballance, Charles, 296
Bennett and Godlee's glioma surgery, 95
Boston Children's Hospital, 35
Bovie, William T., 379
Bovie electrocautery, 194–195, 379
Brachial plexus tumor
    gross appearance of, 406f
    patient postoperative appearance, 404f–407f

Brachytherapy, 4. See also Radium implant
Bruit
    with arteriovenous malformations, 297
    with congenital aneurysm, 295–296, 307–308

C

Cairns, Hugh, 195, 197
Calcareous tissue, with pituitary adenoma, 12
Callosal puncture, for optic chiasm glioma, 25–26
Calvarium sarcoma, 135–142
    autopsy findings with, 141–142, 141f–143f
    case presentation to Neuro-Surgical Society, 138
    discharge notes on, 138
    histology of, 142
    hospital course with, 140
    objective findings with, 135
    operative notes on, 136–138
    operative sketch of, 135f
    pathology report on, 137
    patient complaint with, 140
    patient history with, 135, 138
    patient postoperative appearance, 137f–140f
    patient preoperative appearance, 134f, 136f
    pectoralis major graft for, 136–138
    positive findings with, 135
    postoperative course with, 138
    radiologic findings with, 135–136
    radiotherapy for, 138
    skeletal changes with, 135
    special note on, 137–138
    subjective findings with, 135
    vision affected by, 135
Carotid artery aneurysm, 300–304
    autopsy findings with, 302f
    discharge notes on, 302, 304
    first ligations of, 293
    follow-up notes on, 302, 304
    muscle grafts for, 302, 304
    objective findings with, 300, 303
    operative notes on, 301–304
    operative sketches of, 300f, 303f
    patient histories with, 300, 303
    positive findings with, 300, 303
    postoperative notes on, 304
    radiology findings with, 300–301, 303
    special notes on, 301, 303
    subjective findings with, 303
Carotid body tumor, 468f–470f
Caton and Paul's approach, to parasellar tumors, 3

Cauda equina fibrosarcoma, 328–331
    discharge note on, 331
    histology of, 330
    laminectomy for, 329–330
    letter to Cushing on, 331
    objective findings with, 328
    operative note on, 329–330
    operative sketch of, 328f
    pathology report on, 330
    patient history with, 328
    positive findings with, 328–329
    radiologic findings with, 329
    radiotherapy for, 331
    special note on, 329
    subjective findings with, 328
Cerebellar astrocytoma
    cystic fibrillary, operative sketch of, 486f
    teaching slide on, 523f
Cerebellar hemangioblastoma, 463–467
    discharge notes on, 466–467
    follow-up notes on, 466
    hospital course with, 466–467
    objective findings with, 463
    operative notes on, 464–466
    operative sketch of, 465f
    pathology report on, 464–465
    patient history with, 463, 466
    patient postoperative appearance, 466f–467f
    patient preoperative appearance, 462f–463f
    positive findings with, 463, 466
    special notes on, 463–465, 467
    subjective findings with, 463
    teaching slide on, 524f
Cerebellar meningioma, 204–208
    discharge notes on, 206–207
    gross appearance of, 205f
    histology of, 206, 206f
    letters to Cushing on, 207–208
    objective findings with, 204, 207
    operative notes on, 205
    operative sketches of, 204f, 493f
    pathology reports on, 206
    patient history with, 204
    patient postoperative appearance, 205f
    positive findings with, 204, 206–207
    postoperative notes on, 206
    radiologic findings with, 205
    subjective findings with, 204, 206
    teaching slide on, 207f, 515f
    vision affected by, 204, 207
Cerebellar pathology, Cushing on, 377–380

Cerebral angiography, 294, 296
Cerebral artery aneurysm, 309–312
    discharge note on, 312
    follow-up note on, 312
    muscle graft for, 310–312
    objective findings with, 309
    operative notes on, 309–312
    operative sketches of, 309f, 311, 311f–312f
    patient history with, 309
    positive findings with, 309
    radiologic findings with, 309–310
    special note on, 310
    subjective findings with, 309
    ventriculogram for, 309–310
Cervical meningocele
    patient postoperative appearance, 410f–411f
    patient preoperative appearance, 408f–411f
Cervical spine enchondroma, operative sketch of, 485f
Cervical spine meningioma, operative sketch of, 492f
Cholesteatoma
    fourth ventricle, 401–403
    petroclival epidermoid, 453–461
    suprasellar, 46–48, 501f
Chordoma, parasellar, teaching slide on, 523f
Chromophobe (chromophile) adenoma, 77–84, 88–90
Circoid angioma, 297, 313–316
A Classification of the Tumors of the Glioma Group on a Histogenetic Basis with a Correlated Study of Prognosis (Bailey and Cushing), 95
Clinoid process. *See* Anterior clinoid process; Posterior clinoid process
Codman, Emory A., 191, 197
Congenital aneurysm of right temporal lobe, 295–296, 305–308
    discharge note on, 308
    follow-up note on, 308
    muscle graft for, 306–307
    objective findings with, 305–306
    operative note on, 306–307
    operative sketch of, 305f
    patient history with, 305
    positive findings with, 305–306
    radiology findings with, 308
    special notes on, 306–307
    subjective findings with, 305
"Contributions to the clinical study of intracranial aneurysms" (Cushing and Symonds), 293
Convexity meningioma, 209–215

discharge notes on, 212, 214–215
follow-up notes on, 212, 214–215
gross appearance of, 211, 212f, 213
histology of, 211, 213–214
objective findings with, 209, 213–214
operative notes on, 209–211, 213
operative sketches of, 209f, 215f
pathology reports on, 211, 213–214
patient complaint with, 212, 214
patient history with, 209, 212
patient postoperative appearance, 208f, 210f–211f
positive findings with, 209, 213–214
postoperative notes on, 210–212, 214
radiologic findings with, 209, 213
special notes on, 213
subjective findings with, 209, 213–214
Convolutions
with craniopharyngioma, 36
with pineal region tumor, 107
Convulsions. *See* Seizures
Corphyrin injection, for craniopharyngioma, 41–42
Cranial nerve(s). *See also specific nerves*
optic chiasm glioma and, 55
pituitary adenoma and, 10
skull base adenocarcinoma and, 126–129
Craniopharyngioma, 35–43, 61–64
anterior lobe extract for, 41–42
clinic notes on, 39–40, 43
convolutions with, 36
discharge notes on, 37, 39–40, 42–43, 64
glandular symptoms of, 36
gross specimen of, 36f, 64f
histology of, 63
letters to Cushing on, 43, 64
multiple surgeries for, 35–43, 62
neighborhood symptoms of, 36
neurological symptoms of, 36
objective findings with, 40–41, 61
operative notes on, 36–38, 62
operative sketches of, 35f, 61f, 487f, 494f, 497f
pathology reports on, 37, 39, 63–64
patient complaints with, 35
patient histories with, 35, 40, 61
patient postoperative appearance, 38f, 41f, 60f–63f, 65f
patient preoperative appearance, 34f
physical findings with, 35
pituitary system analysis with, 36
polyglandular symptoms of, 36

positive findings with, 40–41, 61
postoperative course with, 39, 63–64
pressure symptoms of, 36
radiologic findings with, 35–36, 40–41, 61, 64
subjective findings with, 61
subtemporal decompression for, 35
teaching slides on, 507f–511f
transfrontal osteoplastic procedure for, 36–37, 62
ventricular puncture for, 36–39
vision affected by, 35, 37, 37f, 39f, 40, 61, 64
Craniosynostosis, 380
craniectomy flap in, 441f
craniotomy site in, 443f
patient follow-up appearance, 442f–443f
patient postoperative appearance, 419f, 441f
patient preoperative appearance, 416f–418f, 440f
resected bone fragment in, 418f
Craniotomy
exploratory
for lateral ventricle glioma, 121–122
for parasellar tumor, 29–30
frontotemporal, operative sketch of, 477f
site, in craniosynostosis, 443f
Crossbow incision, for posterior fossa lesions, 377–379
Cushing, Harvey, 528f, 530f–535f, 541f–547f. *See also specific cases*
on aneurysms, 293–296
diagnostic challenges, 294
incidental findings, 293–295
muscle pledget use, 294–295
records on patients with, 294–295, 295t
silver clip use, 294
on arteriovenous malformations, 296–299
cautious attitude, 297
classification, 297
diagnostic challenges, 297
first successful removal, 296–299, 313–314
records on patients with, 297–299, 298t
silver clip use, 297, 316
treatment armamentarium, 299
on cerebral meningiomas, 191–199
anesthesia advances, 196–197
electrosurgery techniques, 194–195
first and last operations, 191–192
hemostasis advances, 194–196
intracranial pressure control, 196
operative technique, 194–197
patients treated, 198–199
postoperative care and follow-up, 197–198, 198f

preoperative evaluation, 192–194
resection technique, 195
visual field studies, 193–194
competitive nature of, 197–198
conflict with Dandy, Walter, 96, 197
on gliomas, 95–96
aggressive approach, 95
histologic classification, 95
"Little Black Book" of, 197, 294
milestone of 2,000th surgery, 6, 545f–546f
neurovascular surgery contributions of, 293–299
operative sketches of, 474f–503f, 547f. See also Operative sketches
on parasellar tumors, 3–6
aggressive approach, 5
candid disclosure of mishaps, 5
caution and conservatism, 5
evolution of technique, 3, 5–6
fascination with disorders, 3
pediatric neurosurgery contributions of, 95
on posterior fossa pathology, 377–380
electrosurgical techniques, 377–378
lateral ventricular puncture, 377
resection of tumor mural nodule, 377–378
surgical considerations, 378–380
on spinal tumors, 319–321
admission of error, 320, 325–327
aggressive approach, 320
classification, 319–320
distrust of lipiodol myelography, 319
evolution of techniques, 319–321
gratification in procedures, 319
teaching slides of, 4, 504f–527f. See also Teaching slides
World War I service of, 4
"worst exhibition of cranial operation," 96, 186
Cushing reflex, 192
Cushing Tumor Registry, 4, 193, 197
Cutler, E. C., 280
Cysts. See specific types

D

Dandy, Walter, 96, 101, 197, 294, 296–297, 380
Danvers State Hospital, 4
Davidoff, Leo, 540f
Dermoid cyst, 35–40
Diabetes insipidus
craniopharyngioma and, 63–64
pineal region tumor and, 131–132
Diencephalic tuberculoma, teaching slide on, 527f

Dorsum sella
optic chiasm glioma and, 25
parasellar tumor and, 31
parietal neuroblastoma and, 100
pituitary adenoma and, 10, 16, 20
skull base adenocarcinoma and, 125
Dott, Norman McComish, 294, 296, 539f
Dural capsule
coagulation, with pituitary adenoma, 78–79
extirpation, with pituitary adenoma, 76–77
Dural closure, operative sketch of, 477f
Dural decompression, for pituitary adenoma, 50–53
Dwarfism, pituitary, 81–84
Dyspituitarism, 3

E

Ebers Papyrus, 293
Eisenhardt, Louise, 95–96, 197, 294
Electrosurgery
for arteriovenous malformation, 297, 299
for cerebral meningioma, 194–195
for frontal meningioma, 253–255
for occipital glioma, 186–187
for parasagittal meningioma, 275–278
for parasellar tumors, 5
for pituitary adenoma, 78–79
for posterior fossa astrocytoma, 95
for posterior fossa lesions, 377–378
for spinal tumors, 321
Elliot, John, 191–192
Elsberg, Charles A., 320
Enchondroma, cervical spine, operative sketch of, 485f
Endonasal transsphenoidal approach, to parasellar tumors, 5–6
Endothelioma. See specific tumor types
"End-results," 197–198
Ependymoma, spinal, 319, 361–369
discharge notes on, 367, 369
follow-up notes on, 367
laminectomy for, 362–367
lumbar puncture for, 362–364
neurological exam with, 361
operative notes on, 362–367
operative sketch of, 362f
patient history with, 361, 367–369
patient postoperative appearance, 363f–369f
patient preoperative appearance, 361f
positive findings with, 361
postoperative notes on, 364, 367

radiotherapy for, 369
special notes on, 361–362, 364–365, 367
subjective findings with, 361
Epidermoids
fourth ventricle, 401–403
suprasellar, 45–49
Epidural hematoma, operative sketches of, 479f–480f
Epithelial cyst of Rathke's pouch, 61–64
"Experiences with cerebellar astrocytomas: a critical review of 76 cases" (Cushing), 95, 380
External capsule, pituitary adenoma and, 17

F

Facial flushing, pituitary adenoma and, 50
Facial nerve (CN VII)
acoustic neuroma and, 431
lateral ventricle glioma and, 121
pituitary adenoma and, 10
skull base adenocarcinoma and, 128
Facial nerve rhizotomy, 380, 413–415
Femoral bowing, with pituitary adenoma, 19, 19f
Fibrillary astrocytoma
cerebellar cystic, operative sketch of, 486f
third ventricle, operative sketch of, 491f
Fibrosarcoma(s)
cauda equina, 328–331
temporal, 156–160
Fibula bowing, with optic chiasm glioma, 25
Foley, Frederick, 196
Follow-up, Cushing's emphasis on, 197–198, 198f
Foramen magnum meningioma, operative sketch of, 491f
Fourth ventricle epidermoid, 401–403
discharge note on, 403
follow-up note on, 403
histology of, 403
objective findings with, 401
operative note on, 401–402
operative sketches of, 401f–402f
pathology report on, 402–403
patient history with, 401
patient postoperative appearance, 400f, 402f–403f
positive findings with, 401
postoperative note on, 403
special note on, 403
subjective findings with, 401
Frazier, Charles, 196
Frontal bone myeloma, 179–183

autopsy findings with, 181–183, 182f–183f
discharge note on, 181
follow-up note on, 181
histology of, 183
objective findings with, 178
patient appearance, 178f–181f
patient complaint with, 178
positive findings with, 178
radiologic findings with, 178–179, 181
subjective findings with, 178
Frontal glioma
operative sketches of, 496f, 500f
radium implant for, 496f
Frontal-intraventricular glioma, right, operative sketch of, 485f
Frontal meningioma, 249–259
discharge notes on, 250–251, 256–258
electrosurgery for, 253–255
follow-up notes on, 258–259
gross appearance of, 256–257
histology of, 256
hospital course with, 256–257
objective findings with, 249–250, 252, 256–257
operative notes on, 249–250, 253–255
operative sketches of, 249f, 487f, 499f
pathology reports on, 255–257
patient history with, 249
patient postoperative appearance, 248f, 250f–252f, 257f–258f
patient preoperative appearance, 253f–256f
positive findings with, 249–252, 256–257
postoperative notes on, 254
radiologic findings with, 249–250, 252
special notes on, 252–255
subjective findings with, 249–252, 256
subtemporal decompression for, 249–250
teaching slide on, 519f
vision affected by, 249–252, 256–257
Frontal sinus
craniopharyngioma and, 36
pituitary adenoma and, 10, 20, 50, 87
Frontotemporal craniotomy, operative sketch of, 477f
Fronto-temporal medulloblastoma, left, 167–177
autopsy findings with, 175–177, 176f–177f
discharge notes on, 169, 175
follow-up notes on, 169, 175
histology of, 169, 171f
hospital course with, 169, 175
objective findings with, 167, 169–170
operative notes on, 168, 170–174
operative sketches of, 167f, 170f

osteoplastic procedure for, 168
pathology reports on, 168–169, 172
patient history with, 167, 169, 175
patient postoperative appearance, 172f–175f
patient preoperative appearance, 166f, 168f–169f
positive findings with, 167, 169–170
radiologic findings with, 167–168, 170, 174
radium implant for, 170–175, 171f
special notes on, 167–168, 170, 172
subjective findings with, 167, 169
subtemporal decompression for, 168
transcortical approach to, 170–172
ventriculogram for, 167–168
Frontotemporal meningioma, teaching slide on, 520f
Fungus cerebri, 236f, 239–241, 444f–447f

G

Galen, 293
"Galvanocautery," 194
Ganglioneuroma, spinal, 333–336
  discharge note on, 335
  follow-up note on, 336
  histology of, 335, 337f
  laminectomy for, 333–335
  objective findings with, 333
  operative note on, 333–335
  pathology debate/discussion over, 335–336
  pathology report on, 335
  patient history with, 333
  patient postoperative appearance, 332f
  physical findings with, 333, 334f
  positive findings with, 333
  radiologic findings with, 333
  subjective findings with, 333
Gasserian ganglion, alternative route to, 455–457
Glioblastoma multiforme, 185–188
Glioma(s). *See also specific types*
  Cushing and Bailey classification of, 95
  Cushing's pioneering work on, 95–96
  first reported surgery for, 95
  frontal, 496f, 500f
  frontal-intraventricular, 485f
  histology of, 95
  lateral ventricle, 113–123
  occipital, 185–188
  optic chiasm, 25–27, 55–58, 71–73
  parietal, 488f
  radiotherapy for, 95–96, 496f
  subtemporal decompression for, 95–96
  temporal, 145–149
  thalamic, 151–155
  Virchow classification of, 95
Glossopharyngeal nerve (CN IX), cerebellar meningioma and, 204, 207
Godlee, Rickman, 95, 194

H

Hallucinations
  lateral ventricle glioma and, 113
  postoperative, 12
  temporal fibrosarcoma and, 157
Halsted, William, 194
Harvey Lecture series, 3
Headache
  acoustic neuroma and, 431
  anterior cerebral artery aneurysm and, 309
  cerebellar meningioma and, 204
  convexity meningioma and, 209
  craniopharyngioma and, 35, 61
  frontal meningioma and, 249
  lateral ventricle glioma and, 113
  left fronto-temporal medulloblastoma and, 167, 169
  occipital glioma and, 185
  occipital meningioma and, 267
  olfactory groove meningioma and, 225
  parasellar tumor and, 29–30
  parietal neuroblastoma and, 99
  pineal region tumor and, 107, 131–132
  pituitary adenoma and, 9, 87
  temporal fibrosarcoma and, 156
  temporal glioma and, 147
  thalamic glioma and, 151
Hemangioblastoma, cerebellar, 463–467, 524f
Hematoma, epidural, operative sketches of, 479f–480f
Hemifacial spasm, 413–415. *See also* Trigeminal neuralgia
Herniation tapping, for parasellar tumor, 31
Hirsch, Oskar, 5–6
Hoen, Thomas, 194
Hormonal extracts
  for craniopharyngioma, 41–42
  for pineal region tumor, 161
  for pituitary adenoma, 67, 81–84
Horrax, Gilbert, 538f
Horsley, Victor, 3, 191, 194, 198, 293, 319
Horsley and Gower surgery, for spinal tumors, 319
Hunterian laboratory, 529f–530f

Hydrocephalus, 420f–421f
    with lateral ventricle glioma, 114
    with optic chiasm glioma, 25, 27
    with suprasellar epidermoid, 45
    with thalamic glioma, 152–153
Hyperostosis
    with pituitary adenoma, 10–11, 20–21
    teaching slide on, 521f
Hyperpituitarism. *See* Acromegaly
Hypopituitarism, 3
    teaching slides on, 505f, 510f, 512f–514f

I

Instruments, 543f
Internal carotid artery aneurysm, 300–304
    autopsy findings with, 302f
    discharge notes on, 302, 304
    follow-up notes on, 302, 304
    muscle grafts for, 302, 304
    objective findings with, 300, 303
    operative notes on, 301–304
    operative sketches of, 300f, 303f
    patient histories with, 300, 303
    positive findings with, 300, 303
    postoperative notes on, 304
    radiology findings with, 300–301, 303
    special notes on, 301, 303
    subjective findings with, 303
Intracranial pressure, with cerebral meningioma, 196

J

Jacksonian epilepsy, 30, 212, 243–244, 280, 289–290, 315
Jefferson, Geoffrey, 198
Johns Hopkins Hospital, 4, 101, 192–194, 297

K

Keith, Arthur, 3
Knapp Prize in Ophthalmology, 193
Krause, Fedor, 296

L

Laminectomy, 319
    for ependymoma, 362–367
    for fibrosarcoma, 329–330
    for ganglioneuroma, 333–335
    for meningioma, 322–324, 340–343, 348–349, 351–352
    for metastasis, 325–327
    for neurinoma, 372–373
    for spina bifida, 357–358
Lantern slides. *See* Teaching slides
Lateral rhinotomy approach, to parasellar tumors, 3
Lateral ventricle glioma, 113–123
    autopsy findings with, 118, 118f–119f, 122–123, 122f–123f
    discharge notes on, 114–115, 118, 122
    exploratory surgery for, 121–122
    follow-up note on, 122
    histology of, 117, 122–123
    objective findings with, 113–115, 121
    operative notes on, 114–117, 121–122
    osteoplastic procedure for, 114–116
    pathology reports on, 117, 122
    patient complaint with, 113
    patient histories with, 113, 121
    patient postoperative appearance, 112f–113f, 120f–121f
    positive findings with, 113–115, 121
    radiologic findings with, 114
    radiotherapy for, 122
    special notes on, 114–116
    subjective findings with, 113, 115, 121
    subtemporal decompression for, 114
    ventricular puncture for, 114–117
    ventriculogram for, 115–116
    vision affected by, 113, 115, 121–122
Lateral ventricular puncture
    for acoustic neuroma, 394–395
    for posterior fossa lesions, 377
Left fronto-temporal medulloblastoma, 167–177
    autopsy findings with, 175–177, 176f–177f
    discharge notes on, 169, 175
    follow-up notes on, 169, 175
    histology of, 169, 171f
    hospital course with, 169, 175
    objective findings with, 167, 169–170
    operative notes on, 168, 170–174
    operative sketches of, 167f, 170f
    osteoplastic procedure for, 168
    pathology reports on, 168–169, 172
    patient history with, 167, 169, 175
    patient postoperative appearance, 172f–175f
    patient preoperative appearance, 166f, 168f–169f
    positive findings with, 167, 169–170
    radiologic findings with, 167–168, 170, 174
    radium implant for, 170–175, 171f

special notes on, 167–168, 170, 172
  subjective findings with, 167, 169
  subtemporal decompression for, 168
  transcortical approach to, 170–172
  ventriculogram for, 167–168
Left rotational torticollis, 427–429
  objective findings with, 427
  operative notes on, 427–429
  operative sketch in, 427f
  patient histories with, 427
  patient postoperative appearance, 428f–429f, 438f–439f
  patient preoperative appearance, 426f, 436f–437f
  positive findings with, 427
  special notes on, 427
  subjective findings with, 427
Left ventricular meningioma, operative sketch of, 498f
Lipiodol myelography, Cushing's distrust of, 319
Lipoma, in spina bifida, 355–360
  discharge note on, 360
  histology of, 359
  laminectomy for, 357–358
  letter to Cushing on, 360
  neurological exam with, 356–357
  objective findings with, 355
  operative note on, 357–358
  pathology report on, 359
  patient history with, 355
  patient postoperative appearance, 358f
  patient preoperative appearance, 354f–357f
  positive findings with, 355
  postoperative notes on, 359
  radiologic findings with, 356–357
  special notes on, 355–357
  subjective findings with, 355
"Little Black Book," 197, 294
Local anesthesia, Cushing's use of, 196–197
Lumbar puncture
  for craniopharyngioma, 39
  for parasellar tumor, 31
  for posterior fossa tumors, 379
  for spinal ependymoma, 362–364

M

Magnesium sulfate enema, for posterior fossa surgery, 378–379
Magnus, Wilhelm, 297
Marie's disease. *See* Acromegaly

Mark, Leonard P., 4
Martel, Thierry de, 196
Massachusetts General Hospital, 29–30, 191–192
Mayo Clinic, 328
McKenzie, Kenneth, 193–194
Medulloblastoma(s)
  left fronto-temporal, 167–177
  radiotherapy for, 95
Melanoma, metastatic, teaching slide on, 526f
Meningioma, cerebral. *See also specific types*
  carotid artery aneurysm with, 300–304
  cerebellar, 204–208
  convexity, 209–215
  Cushing on, 191–199
  Cushing's first and last operations, 191–192
  Cushing's patients with, 198–199
  electrosurgery for, 194–195
  frontal, 249–259
  hemostasis with, 194–196
  neurological exam with, 192–193
  occipital, 267–271
  olfactory groove, 225–231
  operative technique for, 194–197
  origin of term, 194
  parasagittal, 217–223, 237–241, 260–264, 273–287
  postoperative care and follow-up with, 197–198, 198f
  preoperative evaluation of, 192–194
  sphenoid wing, 233–236
  sylvian fissure, 288–290
  visual field with, 193–194
Meningioma, spinal, 319–320, 322–324, 339–352
  Cushing's admission of mistake with, 320, 325–327
  discharge notes on, 324, 343, 349, 352
  follow-up notes on, 352
  gross appearance of, 323f, 324, 342f, 348f, 352f
  histology of, 352, 353f
  laminectomy for, 322–324, 340–343, 348–349, 351–352
  letters to Cushing on, 324, 343, 349, 352
  neurological exam with, 339, 339f, 345f, 347–348, 351
  objective findings with, 339, 347–348
  operative notes on, 322–324, 340–343, 348–349, 351–352
  operative sketches of, 322f–323f, 341f, 342–343, 347f, 492f
  pathology reports on, 324, 343, 349, 352
  patient histories with, 322, 339, 345, 351
  patient postoperative appearance, 338f, 340f, 344f, 346f, 350f–351f

positive findings with, 322, 339, 347–348
radiologic findings with, 322
special notes on, 339–340, 348–349
subjective findings with, 347
teaching slides on, 323f, 520f
Meningocele, cervical
patient postoperative appearance, 410f–411f
patient preoperative appearance, 408f–411f
Metastasis, spinal, 325–327
Metastatic melanoma, 526f
Metastatic sarcoma, operative sketch of, 489f
Mixed struma, 50–53
Moniz, Antonio Caetano de Egas, 296
Mother-of-pearl tumor, 47–48, 402
Motor cortex, operative sketch of, 475f
Mount Sinai Hospital (New York), 131–132
Muscle graft/implants
in aneurysm surgery, 294–295, 302, 304, 306–307, 310–312
in arteriovenous malformation surgery, 314
in calvarium sarcoma surgery, 136–138
in parasagittal meningioma surgery, 243–244
in spinal tumor surgery, 320
Myelography, lipiodol, Cushing's distrust of, 319
Myeloma, frontal bone, 179–183
Myelomeningocele, 379–380, 387–389
discharge note on, 388–389
follow-up note on, 389
objective findings with, 387
operative notes on, 387–388
operative sketch of, 387f
patient history with, 387
patient postoperative appearance, 388f–389f
patient preoperative appearance, 386f
positive findings with, 387
subjective findings with, 387

N

Neurinoma, spinal, 320, 371–374
discharge note on, 374
gross appearance of, 374f
laminectomy for, 372–373
letter to Cushing on, 374
neurological exam with, 371, 371f
objective findings with, 371
operative note on, 372–373
operative sketch of, 372f
pathology report on, 373–374
patient history with, 371
patient postoperative appearance, 370f, 373f
positive findings with, 371
radiologic findings with, 371
special note on, 371–372
subjective findings with, 371
Neuroblastoma, parietal, 99–105
Neurofibroma, 319
Neurological exam
with acoustic neuroma, 431
with cerebral meningioma, 192–193
with spinal tumors, 319–320
ependymoma, 361
fibrosarcoma, 328–329, 329f–331f
lipoma in spina bifida, 356–357
meningioma, 339, 339f, 345f, 347–348, 351
metastasis, 325, 326f
neurinoma, 371, 371f
with trigeminal neuralgia, 383
Neuroma, acoustic. See Acoustic neuroma
Neuro-Surgical Society, 138
Neurovascular surgery, Cushing's contributions to, 293–299
Novocaine, 196

O

Occipital glioma, 185–188
autopsy findings with, 187f, 188
craniectomy and decompression for, 185
electrosurgery for, 186–187
histology of, 186f, 188
left, operative sketch of, 482f
objective findings with, 185–186
operative notes on, 186–188
pathology report on, 188
patient appearance, 184f–185f
patient history with, 185
positive findings with, 185–186
radiologic findings with, 186
special note on, 186
transfusion required with, 187–188
ventriculogram for, 186
vision affected by, 185
"worst exhibition of cranial operation," 96, 186
Occipital meningioma, 267–271
discharge note on, 271
gross appearance of, 269–270, 269f, 270
histology of, 270, 270f
objective findings with, 267
operative note on, 268–269
operative sketches of, 267f, 490f, 494f–495f, 498f
pathology report on, 269–270

pathology reports on, 270
patient complaint with, 267
patient postoperative appearance, 271f
patient preoperative appearance, 266f–268f
positive findings with, 267
radiologic findings with, 267, 269f, 270, 270f
special note on, 268
subjective findings with, 267
vision affected by, 267
Oculomotor nerve (CN III)
lateral ventricle glioma and, 113
pituitary adenoma and, 10
skull base adenocarcinoma and, 128
trigeminal neuralgia and, 383
Oldberg, Eric, 194
Olfactory groove meningioma, 225–231
arachnoid cyst with, 229–230
discharge notes on, 229–231
gross appearance of, 225f, 227, 229, 229f, 231
histology of, 227, 231
letter to Cushing on, 231
objective findings with, 225
operative notes on, 225–228, 228f, 229–231
operative sketches of, 226f, 482f, 499f–500f
pathology reports on, 227, 229, 231
patient history with, 225
patient postoperative appearance, 224f
patient preoperative appearance, 230f–231f
positive findings with, 225
radiologic findings with, 225
special notes on, 225, 227–229
subjective findings with, 225
vision affected by, 225, 230
Olfactory nerve (CN I)
skull base adenocarcinoma and, 128
suprasellar epidermoid and, 47–48
Operating room, 531f, 543f–544f
Operative sketches, 474f–503f, 547f
acoustic neuroma, 484f, 496f
anterior cerebral artery aneurysm, 309f, 311, 311f–312f
arteriovenous malformation, 313f, 315f
calvarium sarcoma, 135f
cauda equina fibrosarcoma, 328f
cerebellar cystic fibrillary astrocytoma, 486f
cerebellar hemangioblastoma, 465f
cerebellar meningioma, 204f, 493f
cervical spine enchondroma, 485f
congenital aneurysm of right temporal lobe, 305f
convexity meningioma, 209
craniopharyngioma, 35f, 61f, 487f, 494f, 497f

dural closure, 477f
epidural hematoma, 479f–480f
foramen magnum meningioma, 491f
fourth ventricle epidermoid, 401f–402f
frontal glioma, 496f, 500f
frontal-intraventricular glioma, 485f
frontal meningioma, 249f, 487f, 499f
frontotemporal craniotomy, 477f
fronto-temporal medulloblastoma, 167f, 170f
internal carotid artery aneurysm, 300f, 303f
left rotational torticollis, 427f
left ventricular meningioma, 498f
metastatic sarcoma, 489f
motor cortex, 475f
myelomeningocele, 387f
occipital glioma, 482f
occipital meningioma, 267f, 490f, 494f–495f, 498f
olfactory groove meningioma, 226f, 228f, 482f, 499f–500f
optic chiasm glioma, 55f, 72f, 484f
parasagittal meningioma, 217f, 237f, 262f–263f, 276f, 283f, 486f, 489f–490f, 494f–495f
parietal glioma, 488f
parietal meningioma, 502f
petroclival epidermoid cholesteatoma, 455f, 459f
pituitary adenoma, 75f, 78f, 89f
pituitary tumor, 493f
sphenoid wing meningioma, 497f
spinal ependymoma, 362f
spinal meningioma, 322f–323f, 341f, 342–343, 347f, 492f
spinal metastasis, 327f
spinal neurinoma, 372f
spinal tumor, 503f
subcortical clot, 481f
subtemporal decompression, 477f–478f
supramarginal meningioma, 488f
suprasellar cholesteatoma, 501f
suprasellar epidermoid, 45f
suprasellar tumor, 474f
sylvian fissure meningioma, 288f
temporal fibrosarcoma, 156f, 159f
third ventricle fibrillary astrocytoma, 491f
third ventricle glioma, 483f, 492f
trigeminal ganglion, 476f
ulnar nerve decompression, 449f
Ophthalmology, Cushing's work in, 193–194
Optic chiasm, transfrontal approach to, 6
Optic chiasm glioma, 25–27, 55–58, 71–73
autopsy findings with, 26–27, 26f, 57–58, 59f
callosal puncture for, 25–26

cranial nerve examination with, 55
discharge notes on, 26, 57, 73
follow-up note on, 73
glandular symptoms of, 55
gross specimen of, 57f
histology of, 27, 27f, 58
neighborhood symptoms of, 55
objective findings with, 25, 55–56, 71
operative notes on, 25–26, 56–57, 72–73
operative sketches of, 55f, 72f, 484f
osteoplastic resection for, 56–57, 72
pathology report on, 27
patient complaint with, 25
patient histories with, 25, 55, 71
patient postoperative appearance, 72f–73f
patient preoperative appearance, 24f–25f, 54f, 56f, 70f–71f
pituitary symptoms of, 55
positive findings with, 25, 55–56, 71
radiologic findings with, 25, 56, 71–72
special notes on, 56, 72
subjective findings with, 25, 55, 71
teaching slide on, 525f
vision affected by, 55–56, 71
Optic nerve (CN II)
acoustic neuroma and, 431
cerebellar meningioma and, 204, 207
optic chiasm glioma and, 27, 27f, 55, 72
pituitary adenoma and, 10, 16
skull base adenocarcinoma and, 128
suprasellar epidermoid and, 47
Osler, William, 192, 319, 378
Osteoplastic procedure
for craniopharyngioma, 36–37, 62
for frontal meningioma, 253–254
for lateral ventricle glioma, 114–116
for left fronto-temporal medulloblastoma, 168
for optic chiasm glioma, 56–57, 72
for parasagittal meningioma, 218, 237–238
for petroclival epidermoid cholesteatoma, 455–457
for pituitary adenoma, 67, 76–79, 88–90
for skull base adenocarcinoma, 126
for sphenoid wing meningioma, 233
for temporal glioma, 149

P

Paget's disease, with calvarium sarcoma, 135–142
Parasagittal meningioma, 217–223, 237–241, 260–264, 273–287

Cushing's technical error on, 239–241
discharge notes on, 222–223, 241, 244–245, 261, 263, 274, 280, 286
electrosurgery for, 275–278
follow-up notes on, 222–223, 261, 280
gross appearance of, 221, 221f, 239, 245f, 261, 263, 276, 278, 278f, 284f–285f, 286
histology of, 221–222, 239, 246, 261, 263, 276, 278
large, 260–264
letters to Cushing on, 241, 244, 264
muscle graft for, 243–244
objective findings with, 217, 223, 237, 243, 260, 273, 275, 283
operative notes on, 218, 220–222, 237–241, 243–244, 260–263, 275–278, 280, 284–286
operative sketches of, 217f, 237f, 262f–263f, 276f, 283f, 486f, 489f–490f, 494f–495f
pathology reports on, 221–222, 239, 244, 246, 261, 263, 276, 278–279, 286
patient complaints with, 217, 223, 243–244
patient histories with, 237, 260, 273, 283
patient postoperative appearance, 216f, 218f–220f, 236f, 238f, 240f, 242f, 244f–245f, 277f, 286f–287f
patient preoperative appearance, 272f–274f, 282f–283f
positive findings with, 217, 223, 237, 243, 260, 273–275, 283
postoperative fungus cerebri with, 236f, 239–241
postoperative notes on, 222, 238, 263, 286
radiologic findings with, 223, 243, 245, 273, 274f–275f, 279f, 283, 284f, 286, 287f
special notes on, 218–219, 222, 243, 260–262, 275–276, 279–280, 284
subjective findings with, 217, 223, 237, 243, 273–275, 283
teaching slide on, 515f
vision affected by, 217–218, 223, 237, 273–275
Parasellar chordoma, teaching slide on, 523f
Parasellar tumors, 29–32. *See also specific types*
Cushing on, 3–6
discharge note on, 32
electrosurgery for, 5
evolution of technique for, 3, 5–6
exploratory craniotomy and decompression for, 29–30
first intracranial approach to, 3
herniation tapping for, 31
lateral rhinotomy approach to, 3
letter to Cushing on, 32

lumbar puncture for, 31
needle drainage for, 30, 31f–32f
objective findings with, 30
operative notes on, 29–31
pathology notes on, 31–32
patient history with, 29
patient preoperative appearance, 28f–32f
positive findings with, 30
postoperative course with, 32
radiologic findings with, 30–31
subjective findings with, 30
subtemporal approach to, 3
subtemporal decompression for, 3–5
transfrontal approach to, 5–6
transsphenoidal approach to, 3–6, 31
vision affected by, 6, 29–31
Parietal glioma, right, operative sketch of, 488f
Parietal meningioma, operative sketch of, 502f
Parietal neuroblastoma, 99–105
    discharge notes on, 99, 101, 103, 105
    histology of, 100–104, 104f
    letters to Cushing on, 101, 105
    objective findings with, 99–100, 103–104
    operative notes on, 99–100, 102, 104
    pathology reports on, 100–104
    patient history with, 99–103
    patient postoperative appearance, 98f–99f, 102f–103f
    positive findings with, 99–100, 103–104
    postoperative note on, 103
    radiologic findings with, 100
    subjective findings with, 99–100
    subtemporal decompression for, 99
    vision affected by, 100
Pectoralis major graft, in calvarium sarcoma surgery, 136–138
Pediatric neurosurgery, Cushing's contribution to, 95
Peripheral nerve disease, 380
Peter Bent Brigham Hospital, 30, 35, 185, 294
Petroclival epidermoid cholesteatoma, 453–461
    discharge notes on, 457, 461
    follow-up note on, 461
    gross appearance of, 460f
    histology of, 456f, 457
    objective findings with, 453, 457
    operative notes on, 455–457, 459–460
    operative sketches of, 455f, 459f
    pathology reports on, 457, 460–461
    patient history with, 453
    patient postoperative appearance, 454f, 458f
    patient preoperative appearance, 452f–453f
    positive findings with, 453, 457
    special notes on, 454, 457–458
    subjective findings with, 453, 457
Pharyngeal pouch cyst, 35–40, 56, 62
Pineal gland
    frontal bone myeloma and, 178–179
    internal carotid artery aneurysm and, 301
Pineal region tumor, 107–111, 131–133, 161–165
    autopsy findings with, 110–111, 110f–111f, 131f, 132–133, 132f, 163–165, 163f–164f
    discharge notes on, 107, 132, 162–163
    glandular symptoms of, 132
    histology of, 133, 133f, 165
    medical evaluation of, 131
    objective findings with, 107, 132, 163
    patient appearance, 106f–109f, 130f, 161f–162f
    patient complaint with, 161–162
    patient histories with, 107, 131, 161
    positive findings with, 107, 131–132, 161–163
    radiology findings with, 107, 131, 162–163
    subjective findings with, 107, 131–132, 161–163
    subtemporal decompression with, 107
    vision affected by, 107, 131–132, 162–163
Pituitary adenoma, 9–22, 50–53, 67–69, 75–90
    autopsy findings with, 12–17, 13f–16f, 20f, 22
    calcareous tissue with, 12
    chromophobe (chromophile), 77–84, 88–90
    discharge notes on, 22, 50, 53, 69, 77, 80–83
    dural capsule coagulation with, 78–79
    dural capsule extirpation with, 76–77
    dural decompression for, 50–53
    electrosurgical procedure for, 78–79
    first intracranial approach to, 3
    follow-up notes on, 77, 80, 83–84
    glandular symptoms of, 75
    gross specimen of, 79f
    histology of, 17f, 51, 68, 77, 90
    letters to Cushing on, 53, 90
    objective findings with, 9–10, 19, 50, 67, 78, 80, 87–88
    operative notes on, 11, 21–22, 50–53, 67, 76–79, 88–90
    operative sketches of, 75f, 78f, 89f
    osteoplastic procedure for, 67, 76–79, 88–90
    partial extirpation of, 67
    pathology reports on, 51, 68, 77, 79–80, 90
    patient histories with, 9, 19, 50, 67, 75, 87
    patient postoperative appearance, 66f, 68f, 76f, 82f–85f
    patient preoperative appearance, 8f–11f, 18f–21f, 50f–52f, 74f–75f, 86f–91f

polyglandular symptoms of, 75
positive findings with, 9–10, 19, 50, 67, 75, 78, 80, 87–88
postoperative course with, 80
postoperative notes on, 12, 22, 53
radiologic findings with, 10–11, 19–21, 50, 78, 79f, 81–82, 87
radiotherapy for, 19, 22
regional symptoms of, 75
right-sided decompression for, 11
skeletal changes with, 9–11, 13f–15f, 19, 19f, 67
special notes on, 67, 76, 78, 80, 88
subjective findings with, 9, 19, 67, 78, 80, 87
versus suprasellar cyst, 67
teaching slide on, 21f, 514f
transfrontal approach to, 67, 76–77, 88–90
transsphenoidal approach to, 12, 19, 21–22, 50–53
transsphenoidal decompression for, 19, 21–22
vision affected by, 9, 22, 67, 69, 75, 77–78, 80, 87–88, 90
The Pituitary Body and Its Disorders: Clinical States Produced by Disorders of the Hypophysis Cerebri (Cushing), 3–4
Pituitary struma, 50–53
Pituitary tumor. *See also specific types*
operative sketch of, 493f
Pituitrin injections, for pineal region tumor, 161
Polyclinic Hospital (New York), 45
Polydipsia
craniopharyngioma and, 40
optic chiasm glioma and, 25, 71
pineal region tumor and, 107, 132, 161
Polyphagia, with optic chiasm glioma, 25
Polyuria
craniopharyngioma and, 40, 43, 64
with optic chiasm glioma, 25
pineal region tumor and, 107, 132, 161–162
pituitary adenoma and, 67, 69
Porencephalic cyst, 391–393
discharge notes on, 392–393
follow-up note on, 393
objective findings with, 391
operative note on, 392–393
patient preoperative appearance, 390f–393f
positive findings with, 391
postoperative notes on, 393
subjective findings with, 391
ventricular puncture for, 392–393
Posterior clinoid process
internal carotid artery aneurysm and, 301
optic chiasm glioma and, 25

parasellar tumor and, 31
pituitary adenoma and, 10, 16, 20
Posterior fossa astrocytoma
Cushing's contribution to study of, 95
electrocoagulation for, 95
ventricular puncture for, 95
Posterior fossa tumors. *See also specific types*
crossbow incision for, 377–379
Cushing on, 377–380
electrosurgery for, 377–378
lateral ventricular puncture for, 377
lumbar puncture for, 379
postoperative positioning of patient, 379
resection of tumor mural nodule, 377–378
surgical considerations for, 378–380
ventriculograms for, 378
Postoperative care, Cushing's methods of, 197–198, 198f
Posturing, thalamic glioma and, 150f–153f, 153
Preoperative evaluation, Cushing's procedures and standards for, 192–194
Progeria, 422f–425f
Putnam, J. J., 191–192

R

Racemose angioma, 297
Radiotherapy
for acoustic neuroma, 397
for arteriovenous malformation, 296–299, 314–316
for calvarium sarcoma, 138
for cauda equina fibrosarcoma, 331
for glioma, 95–96, 496f
for lateral ventricle glioma, 122
for left fronto-temporal medulloblastoma, 170–175, 171f
for medulloblastoma, 95
for pituitary adenoma, 4, 19, 22
for skull base adenocarcinoma, 126–128
for spinal ependymoma, 369
for spinal tumors, 319
for temporal fibrosarcoma, 157
Radium implant
for frontal glioma, 496f
for left fronto-temporal medulloblastoma, 170–175, 171f
for pituitary adenoma, 4, 19, 22
Rathke's pouch
epithelial cyst of, 61–64
tumor of, 75–84

Rhesus monkey research, 379
Ribs, autopsy appearance of, with pituitary adenoma, 15f
Right internal carotid artery aneurysm, 300–302
    autopsy findings with, 302f
    discharge note on, 302
    follow-up note on, 302
    muscle graft for, 302
    objective findings with, 300
    operative note on, 301–302
    operative sketch of, 300f
    patient history with, 300
    positive findings with, 300
    radiology findings with, 300–301
    special note on, 301
Riva–Rocci sphygmomanometer, 196
Rotational torticollis, left, 427–429
    objective findings with, 427
    operative notes on, 427–429
    operative sketch in, 427f
    patient histories with, 427
    patient postoperative appearance, 428f–429f, 438f–439f
    patient preoperative appearance, 426f, 436f–437f
    positive findings with, 427
    special notes on, 427
    subjective findings with, 427

S

Sachs, Ernest, 196
Sarcoma(s)
    calvarium, 135–142
    metastatic, operative sketch of, 489f
    spinal, 319
Schloffler's approach, to parasellar tumors, 3
Seizures
    arteriovenous malformation and, 313, 315
    convexity meningioma and, 212
    craniopharyngioma and, 35, 43
    frontal bone myeloma and, 179
    frontal meningioma and, 257
    left fronto-temporal medulloblastoma and, 175
    optic chiasm glioma and, 71
    parasagittal meningioma and, 223, 243–244, 280
    parasellar tumor and, 30
    parietal neuroblastoma and, 99–100
    porencephalic cyst and, 391
    skull base adenocarcinoma and, 127–128
    sylvian fissure meningioma and, 289–290
    temporal fibrosarcoma and, 157
    temporal glioma and, 145, 147
    thalamic glioma and, 150f–153f, 153
Sella turcica
    craniopharyngioma and, 36, 61
    frontal bone myeloma and, 178
    internal carotid artery aneurysm and, 301
    lateral ventricle glioma and, 114
    optic chiasm glioma and, 25, 58, 72
    parasellar tumor and, 30–31
    parietal neuroblastoma and, 100
    pineal region tumor and, 131, 163
    pituitary adenoma and, 10, 20, 50, 67, 75
    skull base adenocarcinoma and, 125–126, 128
    temporal fibrosarcoma and, 158
Serpentine varices, 297
Sexuality, pituitary adenoma and, 87
Sharpe, William, 194
Silver clips
    for aneurysms, 294
    for arteriovenous malformations, 297, 316
    for cerebral meningiomas, 194, 211, 213
Skeletal changes
    with calvarium sarcoma, 135
    with optic chiasm glioma, 25
    with pituitary adenoma, 9–11, 13f–15f, 19, 19f, 50, 67
Skull, autopsy appearance of
    with calvarium sarcoma, 141, 141f–143f
    with optic chiasm glioma, 59f
    with pituitary adenoma, 13f–14f
Skull, radiology of
    with acoustic neuroma, 394
    with anterior cerebral artery aneurysm, 309–310
    with arteriovenous malformation, 315–316
    with calvarium sarcoma, 135–136
    with cerebellar meningioma, 205
    with convexity meningioma, 209, 213
    with craniopharyngioma, 35–36, 40–41, 61
    with frontal bone myeloma, 178
    with frontal meningioma, 249–250, 252
    with internal carotid artery aneurysm, 300–301, 303
    with lateral ventricle glioma, 114
    with left fronto-temporal medulloblastoma, 170, 174
    with occipital meningioma, 267, 269f–270f
    with olfactory groove meningioma, 225
    with optic chiasm glioma, 25, 56, 71–72
    with parasagittal meningioma, 223, 243, 245, 273, 274f–275f, 279f, 283, 284f, 286, 287f

with parasellar tumor, 30
with parietal neuroblastoma, 100
with pineal region tumor, 107, 131, 163
with pituitary adenoma, 10, 19–20, 50, 67, 78, 79f, 87
with skull base adenocarcinoma, 127–128
with suprasellar epidermoid, 45
with sylvian fissure meningioma, 288
with temporal fibrosarcoma, 156, 158
with thalamic glioma, 152
with trigeminal neuralgia, 415
Skull base adenocarcinoma, 125–129
    autopsy findings with, 126f–128f, 128
    cranial nerve involvement in, 126–129
    diagnoses of, 125
    discharge notes on, 127–128
    histology of, 128f
    letter to Cushing on, 127
    objective findings with, 125
    operative note on, 126
    osteoplastic resection of, 126
    patient complaint with, 125
    patient history with, 128
    patient postoperative appearance, 124f–125f
    positive findings with, 125
    radiologic findings with, 125–128
    radiotherapy for, 126–128
    special note on, 126
    subjective findings with, 125
    vision affected by, 125, 128
Society of International Surgery, Cushing surgery before, 4, 22
Sphenoid cells
    craniopharyngioma and, 36
    pituitary adenoma and, 51
Sphenoid sinus
    lateral ventricle glioma and, 114
    pituitary adenoma and, 10, 50
Sphenoid wing meningioma, 233–236
    autopsy findings with, 235, 235f
    discharge note on, 235
    gross appearance of, 234
    histology of, 234
    objective findings with, 233
    operative note on, 233
    operative sketch of, 497f
    pathology report on, 234
    patient history with, 233
    patient preoperative appearance, 232f–234f
    positive findings with, 233
    radiologic findings with, 233
    subjective findings with, 233
    teaching slide on, 522f
Spina bifida
    lipoma in, 355–360
        discharge note on, 360
        histology of, 359
        laminectomy for, 357–358
        letter to Cushing on, 360
        neurological exam with, 356–357
        objective findings with, 355
        operative note on, 357–358
        pathology report on, 359
        patient history with, 355
        patient postoperative appearance, 358f
        patient preoperative appearance, 354f–357f
        positive findings with, 355
        postoperative notes on, 359
        radiologic findings with, 356–357
        special notes on, 355–357
        subjective findings with, 355
    myelomeningocele in, 379–380, 387–389
        discharge note on, 388–389
        follow-up note on, 389
        objective findings with, 387
        operative notes on, 387–388
        operative sketch of, 387f
        patient history with, 387
        patient postoperative appearance, 388f–389f
        patient preoperative appearance, 386f
        positive findings with, 387
        subjective findings with, 387
Spinal accessory nerve rhizotomy, 380
Spinal metastasis, 325–327
    discharge note on, 327
    histology of, 327
    laminectomy for, 325–327
    letter to Cushing on, 327
    operative note on, 325–327
    operative sketch of, 327f
    pathology report on, 327
    radiological findings with, 325
Spinal tumors. *See also specific types*
    classification of, 319–320
    Cushing on, 319–321
    Cushing's admission of mistake with, 320, 325–327
    electrosurgery for, 321
    laminectomy for, 319
    localization techniques for, 319–320
    muscle grafts for, 320
    neurological exam with, 319–320

operative sketch of, 503f
radiotherapy for, 319
Spine, autopsy appearance of, with pituitary adenoma, 14f–15f
Spine, radiology of
  with calvarium sarcoma, 135
  with fibrosarcoma, 329
  with ganglioneuroma, 333
  with metastasis, 325
  with spina bifida, 356
Sternomastoid muscle graft, in aneurysm surgery, 302
Struma, pituitary, 50–53
Subcortical clot, operative sketch of, 481f
Subfrontal approach, to parasellar tumors, 5–6
Sublabial transsphenoidal approach, 4–5, 21–22
Suboccipital decompression, for posterior fossa lesions, 377
Subtemporal approach, to parasellar tumors, 3
Subtemporal decompression
  for craniopharyngioma, 35
  for frontal meningioma, 249–250
  for glioma, 95–96
  for lateral ventricle glioma, 114
  for left fronto-temporal medulloblastoma, 168
  operative sketches of, 477f–478f
  for parasellar tumors, 3–5
  with pineal region tumor, 107
  for suprasellar epidermoid, 45
  for temporal glioma, 146–147, 146f
  for thalamic glioma, 152–153
Supramarginal meningioma, operative sketch of, 488f
Suprasellar cholesteatoma, operative sketch of, 501f
Suprasellar craniopharyngioma, operative sketch of, 494f
Suprasellar cyst
  pituitary adenoma *versus*, 67
  teaching slide on, 512f
Suprasellar epidermoid, 45–49
  discharge notes on, 46, 49
  gross specimen of, 48f
  letter to Cushing on, 49
  objective findings with, 45
  operative note on, 46–48
  operative sketch of, 45f
  pathology report on, 47–48
  patient history with, 45
  patient postoperative appearance, 44f, 46f–47f
  positive findings with, 45
  radiologic findings with, 45
  special notes on, 45–46
  subjective findings with, 45
  subtemporal decompression for, 45
  transfrontal operation for, 46–48
  ventricular puncture for, 47
  vision affected by, 45–46, 48
Suprasellar extension, 6
Suprasellar meningioma, teaching slides on, 516f–518f
Suprasellar tumor, operative sketch of, 474f
Sylvian fissure meningioma, 288–290
  discharge note on, 290
  follow-up notes on, 290
  histology of, 289
  objective findings with, 288
  operative notes on, 289–290
  operative sketch of, 288f
  pathology report on, 289
  patient history with, 288
  positive findings with, 288
  postoperative note on, 290
  radiologic findings with, 288
  special notes on, 288–290
  subjective findings with, 288
  vision affected by, 288, 290
Symonds, Charles, 293

T

Teaching slides, 4, 504f–527f
  acoustic neuroma, 399f
  acromegaly, 504f–506f
  cerebellar astrocytoma, 523f
  cerebellar hemangioblastoma, 524f
  cerebellar meningioma, 207f, 515f
  craniopharyngioma, 507f–511f
  diencephalic tuberculoma, 527f
  frontal meningioma, 519f
  frontotemporal meningioma, 520f
  hyperostosis, 521f
  hypopituitarism, 505f, 510f, 512f–514f
  metastatic melanoma, 526f
  optic glioma, 525f
  parasagittal meningioma, 515f
  parasellar chordoma, 523f
  pituitary adenoma, 21f, 514f
  sphenoid wing meningioma, 522f
  spinal meningioma, 323f, 520f
  suprasellar cyst, 512f
  suprasellar meningioma, 516f–518f
  temporal fibrosarcoma, 159f
  temporal meningeal angioma, 522f

teratoma, 526f
transsphenoidal operation, 514f
Telangiectases, 297
Temporal fibrosarcoma, 156–160
    discharge notes on, 157, 160
    follow-up note on, 160
    hospital course with, 157
    letter to Cushing on, 160
    objective findings with, 156–158
    operative notes on, 158–160
    operative sketch of, 156f, 159f
    pathology report on, 159–160
    patient history with, 156–157
    patient preoperative appearance, 157f, 159f
    positive findings with, 156–158
    radiologic findings with, 156, 158
    radiotherapy for, 157
    special notes on, 156, 158, 160
    subjective findings with, 156–157
    teaching slide on, 159f
    visual effects of, 156–158
Temporal glioma, 145–149
    discharge notes on, 147, 149
    letters to Cushing on, 149
    objective findings with, 145, 147–148
    operative notes on, 146–147, 149
    osteoplastic procedure for, 149
    patient history with, 145, 147
    patient postoperative appearance, 144f–148f
    positive findings with, 145, 147–148
    radiology findings with, 145
    special notes on, 146, 148–149
    subjective findings with, 145, 147
    subtemporal decompression for, 146–147, 146f
    ventriculogram for, 146
    vision affected by, 145, 147
Temporal lobe, congenital aneurysm of, 295–296, 305–308
    discharge note on, 308
    follow-up note on, 308
    muscle graft for, 306–307
    objective findings with, 305–306
    operative note on, 306–307
    operative sketch of, 305f
    patient history with, 305
    positive findings with, 305–306
    radiology findings with, 308
    special notes on, 306–307
    subjective findings with, 305
Temporal meningeal angioma, teaching slide on, 522f

Teratoma, teaching slide on, 526f
Thalamic glioma, 151–155
    autopsy findings with, 153–154, 153f–154f
    exploratory surgery for, 152–153
    operative notes on, 152–153
    patient history with, 151
    patient postoperative appearance, 150f–153f
    positive findings with, 151–152
    posturing or convulsing with, 150f–153f, 153
    radiologic findings with, 151–152
    subjective findings with, 151
    subtemporal decompression for, 152–153
    ventriculogram for, 153–154
    vision affected by, 151
Thalamus, pituitary adenoma and, 17
Third ventricle, pituitary adenoma and, 17
Third ventricle astrocytoma, fibrillary, operative sketch of, 491f
Third ventricle craniopharyngioma, operative sketches of, 487f, 497f
Third ventricle glioma, operative sketches of, 483f, 492f
Thomas, Henry, 192
Tibial bowing
    with optic chiasm glioma, 25
    with pituitary adenoma, 19, 19f
Tinnitus
    acoustic neuroma and, 431
    calvarium sarcoma and, 135
    cerebellar meningioma and, 204
    frontal meningioma and, 251
    parietal neuroblastoma and, 99–100
Tooth, H. H., 191
Torticollis, left rotational, 427–429
    objective findings with, 427
    operative notes on, 427–429
    operative sketch in, 427f
    patient histories with, 427
    patient postoperative appearance, 428f–429f, 438f–439f
    patient preoperative appearance, 426f, 436f–437f
    positive findings with, 427
    special notes on, 427
    subjective findings with, 427
Transcortical approach, to left fronto-temporal medulloblastoma, 170–172
Transfrontal approach
    to craniopharyngioma, 36–37, 62
    to parasellar tumors, 5–6
    to pituitary adenoma, 67, 76–77, 88–90
    to suprasellar epidermoid, 46–48

Transsphenoidal approach
    endonasal, 5–6
    to parasellar tumors, 3–6, 31
    to pituitary adenoma, 12, 19, 21–22
    sublabial, 4–5, 21–22
    teaching slide on, 514f
Transsphenoidal decompression, for pituitary adenoma, 19, 21–22
Transvermian approach, to posterior fossa, 95, 377
Trigeminal nerve (CN V)
    acoustic neuroma and, 431
    cerebellar meningioma and, 204
    discharge note on, 415
    follow-up note on, 415
    skull base adenocarcinoma and, 127–128
Trigeminal neuralgia, 379, 383–384, 413–415
    discharge notes on, 384
    letter to Cushing on, 384
    neurological exam in, 383
    objective findings with, 383, 413
    operative notes on, 384, 413–415
    operative sketches in, 383f, 476f
    patient histories with, 383, 413
    patient preoperative appearance, 382f, 412f
    positive findings with, 383, 413
    postoperative notes on, 384, 413–414
    radiologic findings with, 415
    special note on, 414
    subjective findings with, 383, 413
Trochlear nerve (CN IV), skull base adenocarcinoma and, 128
Tuberculoma, diencephalic, teaching slide on, 527f
Tumors. *See specific types*
Tumors Arising from the Blood-Vessels of the Brain: Angiomatous Malformations and Hemangioblastomas (Cushing), 296

U

Ulnar nerve decompression, 449–451
    operative note on, 449–450
    operative sketch of, 449f
    patient history in, 449
    preoperative findings for, 448f, 450f–451f

V

Vagus nerve (CN X), cerebellar meningioma and, 204, 207
Varices, 297
Vasopressin, for polyuria, 43
Venous angioma, 297
Ventricular puncture
    for acoustic neuroma, 394–395
    for craniopharyngioma, 36–39
    for lateral ventricle glioma, 114–117
    for optic chiasm glioma, 25–26
    for porencephalic cyst, 392–393
    for posterior fossa astrocytoma, 95
    for posterior fossa lesions, 377
    for suprasellar epidermoid, 47
Ventriculogram
    for anterior cerebral artery aneurysm, 309–310
    for congenital temporal lobe aneurysm, 306
    Cushing's reluctance to use, 96, 378
    for lateral ventricle glioma, 115–116
    for left fronto-temporal medulloblastoma, 167–168
    for occipital glioma, 186
    for posterior fossa tumor, 378
    for temporal glioma, 146
    for thalamic glioma, 153–154
Vestibulocochlear nerve (CN VIII)
    acoustic neuroma and, 431
    cerebellar meningioma and, 204, 207
    skull base adenocarcinoma and, 128
Virchow classification, of gliomas, 95
Vision
    acoustic neuroma and, 431
    calvarium sarcoma and, 135
    cerebellar meningioma and, 204, 207
    cerebral aneurysm and, 300, 303, 305–306, 308
    craniopharyngioma and, 35, 37, 37f, 39f, 40, 61, 64
    frontal meningioma and, 249–252, 256–257
    lateral ventricle glioma and, 113, 115, 121–122
    occipital glioma and, 185
    occipital meningioma and, 267
    olfactory groove meningioma and, 225, 230
    optic chiasm glioma and, 55–56, 71
    parasagittal meningioma and, 217–218, 223, 237, 273–275
    parasellar tumors and, 6, 29–31
    parietal neuroblastoma and, 100
    pineal region tumor and, 107, 131–132, 162–163
    pituitary adenoma and, 9, 22, 67, 69, 75, 77–78, 80, 87–88, 90
    skull base adenocarcinoma and, 125, 128
    suprasellar epidermoid and, 45–46, 48
    sylvian fissure meningioma and, 288, 290
    temporal fibrosarcoma and, 156–158
    temporal glioma and, 145, 147
    thalamic glioma and, 151

Visual fields, Cushing's work on, 193–194
Visual hallucinations
    lateral ventricle glioma and, 113
    postoperative, 12
    temporal fibrosarcoma and, 157

W

Watzka, Adolph, 409*f*, 536*f*
Weed, Lewis, 196
Wood, Leonard, 198

X

Xenograft research, 379